Clinical Periodontology and Implant Dentistry

Clinical Periodontology and Implant Dentistry

4th edition

Jan Lindhe

Thorkild Karring • Niklaus P. Lang

Editors

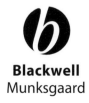

Blackwell
Munksgaard

© 2003 by Blackwell Munksgaard, a Blackwell
Publishing company (Fourth edition) ©1983 by
Munksgaard (First edition), © 1989 by Munksgaard
(Second edition), © 1997 by Munksgaard (Third edition)

Editorial Offices:
Blackwell Publishing Ltd, 9600 Garsington Road,
    Oxford OX4 2DQ, UK
    Tel: +44 (0) 1865 776868
Blackwell Publishing Professional, 2121 State Avenue,
    Ames, Iowa 50014-8300, USA
    Tel: +1 515 292 0140
Blackwell Publishing Asia Pty Ltd, 550 Swanston Street,
    Carlton, Victoria 3053, Australia
    Tel: +61 (0)3 8359 1011

First edition published 1983 by Munksgaard
Second edition published 1989
Third edition published 1997
Fourth edition published by Blackwell Munksgaard, a
Blackwell Publishing Company
Reprinted 2003, 2005, 2006

Library of Congress Cataloging-in-Publication Data

Clinical periodontology and implant dentistry /
Jan Lindhe, Thorkild Karring, Niklaus P. Lang,
editors. – 4th ed.
        p. ; cm.
    Includes bibliographical references and index.
    ISBN 1-4051-0236-5
    1. Periodontics. 2. Periodontal disease. 3. Dental
implants. I. Lindhe, Jan. II. Karring, Thorkild. III. Lang,
Niklaus Peter.
(DNLM: 1. Periodontal Diseases. 2. Dental
Implantation. 3. Dental Implants. WU 240 C6415 2003)
RK361.C54 2003
617.6′32 – dc21
                                    2003044334

ISBN-10: 1-4051-0236-5
ISBN-13: 978-14051-0236-0

A catalogue record for this title is available from the
British Library

Set in 9.5/12 pt Palatino
by Tegneren Jens ApS, Vejle, Denmark
Printed and bound in Denmark
by Narayana Press, Odder, Denmark

The publisher's policy is to use permanent paper from
mills that operate a sustainable forestry policy, and
which has been manufactured from pulp processed
using acid-free and elementary chlorine-free practices.
Furthermore, the publisher ensures that the text
paper and cover board used have met acceptable
invironmental accreditation standards.

For further information on Blackwell Munksgaard, visit
our website: www.dentistry.blackwellmunksgaard.com

Contents

Basic Concepts

Clinical Concepts

Implant Concepts

Foreword

It often happens that a textbook is obsolete by the time it is published. Furthermore, a book written by several authors is frequently lacking in both style and methodology.

This textbook, *Clinical Periodontology and Implant Dentistry*, is therefore an unusual and stimulating surprise to the reader. The many chapters included are all written by authors who apparently share an epistemological approach that guides the logic of research and scientific discovery. Each chapter tells the story of how different problems related to etiology, pathogenesis, treatment and prevention of different lesions in the periodontal tissues led to the formulation of hypotheses or theories that were subsequently subjected to testing.

We know that the formulation of a novel hypothesis requires fantasy and creativity and that experiments (testing) can be planned and meaningful observations can be made after an intelligent hypothesis is formulated. The authors of this book seem convinced, for logical reasons, that observations and experiments are always best performed after the formulation of hypotheses, and that "science will never grow by merely multiplying data and observations". Experiments are performed to examine if the theories proposed were correct, close to the truth or false.

The history of periodontology – as of any scientific domain – is also and above all the history of its errors. Indeed, the errors form the walls of our base of knowledge and allow us to appreciate the closeness to the truth, once unraveled.

The reading of *Clinical Periodontology and Implant Dentistry* invites student and specialist to take a fascinating intellectual journey that in the end allows her or him to understand how knowledge in various fields of this discipline of medicine was progressed and how it should be used in the practice of dentistry. Those reading this book will not only learn what to do or not to do in diagnosing, treating and preventing periodontal pathologies, but they will never cease to undertake its activity of rational criticism and critical control, being continuously reminded of Einstein's words that "all our knowledge remains fallible".

Giorgio Vogel
Professor
Department of Medicine, Surgery and Dentistry
University of Milan
Italy

Preface

Preparations for the 4th edition of *Clinical Periodontology and Implant Dentistry* started in 2001 when all senior authors of the various chapters of the current text were identified and invited to join the team of contributors. The authors were selected because of their reputations as leading researchers, clinicians or teachers in Periodontology, Prosthetic Dentistry, Implant Dentistry and associated domains. Their task was simple but demanding; within your field of expertise, find all relevant information, digest the knowledge and present to the reader a "state of the art" text that can be appreciated by (i) the student of dentistry and dental hygiene, (ii) the graduate student of Periodontology and related domains and (iii) the practicing dentist; the general practitioner and the specialist in Periodontology and/or Implant Dentistry.

I am proud to present the outcome of this collective effort as it appears in this 4th edition of *Clinical Periodontology and Implant Dentistry.*

As was the case in the 3rd edition, this textbook consists of three separate parts; *Basic Concepts, Clinical Concepts* and *Implant Concepts;* that together illustrate most, if not all, important aspects of contemporary Periodontology. Several chapters from the 3rd edition of this book have been thoroughly revised, some have required only modest amendment, while several chapters in each separate part are entirely new. The amendments and additions illustrate that Periodontology is continuously undergoing change and that the authors of the textbook are at the forefront of this conversion.

Classification of Periodontal Diseases

Denis F. Kinane and Jan Lindhe

In 1999 the American Academy of Periodontology staged an International Workshop, the sole purpose of which was to reach a consensus on the classification of periodontal disease and conditions. The most notable changes are in the terminology of the various disease categories which reflect a better understanding of the disease presentations and their differences but also in the acceptance that adult and early-onset forms of periodontitis can occur at any age. Thus we have: adult periodontitis becoming chronic periodontitis; early-onset forms of periodontitis becoming aggressive forms of periodontitis; systemic disease forms of periodontitis; and necrotizing forms of periodontitis.

ADULT PERIODONTITIS - CHRONIC PERIODONTITIS

The International Workshop recommended that the term "adult periodontitis" be discarded since this form of periodontal disease can occur over a wide range of ages and can be found in both the primary and secondary dentition (Consensus Report 1999). The term "chronic periodontitis" was chosen as it was considered less restrictive than the age-dependent designation of "adult periodontitis". It was agreed that chronic periodontitis could be designated as localized or generalized depending on whether less than or more than 30% of sites within the mouth were affected.

EARLY-ONSET FORMS OF PERIODONTITIS - AGGRESSIVE PERIODONTITIS

The International Workshop recommended that the term "early-onset periodontitis" be discarded since this form of disease can occur at various ages and can persist in older adults. Thus aggressive periodontitis can be considered either localized or generalized. Thus the term "localized aggressive periodontitis" replaces the older term "localized juvenile periodontitis" or "localized early-onset periodontitis". The new term "generalized aggressive periodontitis" replaces "generalized juvenile periodontitis" or "generalized early-onset periodontitis". The classification term "prepubertal periodontitis" has been discarded and these forms of periodontitis are described as localized or generalized aggressive periodontitis occurring prepubertally.

SYSTEMIC DISEASE FORMS OF PERIODONTITIS

The International Workshop agreed that certain systemic conditions (such as smoking, diabetes, etc.) can modify periodontitis (chronic or aggressive) and that certain systemic conditions can cause destruction of the periodontium (which may or may not be histopathologically periodontitis), for example neutropenias or leukaemias.

NECROTIZING FORMS OF PERIODONTITIS – NECROTIZING FORMS OF PERIODONTAL DISEASES

It was accepted by the International Workshop that "necrotizing ulcerative gingivitis" (NUG) and "necrotizing ulcerative periodontitis" (NUP) be collectively referred to as "necrotizing periodontal diseases". It was agreed that NUG and NUP were likely to be different stages of the same infection and may not be separate disease categories. Both of these diseases are associated with diminished systemic resistance to bacterial infection of periodontal tissues. A crucial difference between NUG and NUP is whether the disease is limited to the gingiva or also involves the attachment apparatus.

REFERENCE

Consensus Report on Chronic Periodontitis (1999). *Annals of Periodontology*, **4**, p. 38.

Contributors

MARTIN ADDY
Division of Restorative Dentistry
Department of Oral and Dental Science
Bristol Dental Hospital and School
UK

TOMAS ALBREKTSSON
Department of Biomaterials
Facultaty of Medicine
The Sahlgrenska Academy at Göteborg University
Sweden

MAURÍCIO ARAÚJO
Department of Odontology
State University of Maringá
Maringá
Brazil

ROLF ATTSTRÖM
Department of Periodontology
Centre for Oral Health Sciences
Malmö University
Sweden

URS BELSER
Department of Prosthetic Dentistry
School of Dental Medicine
University of Geneva
Switzerland

GUNNAR BERGENHOLTZ
Department of Endodontology and Oral Diagnosis
Faculty of Odontology
The Sahlgrenska Academy at Göteborg University
Sweden

TORD BERGLUNDH
Department of Periodontology
Faculty of Odontology
The Sahlgrenska Academy at Göteborg University
Sweden

JEAN-PIERRE BERNARD
Department of Stomatology and Oral Surgery
School of Dental Medicine
University of Geneva
Switzerland

URS BRÄGGER
Department of Periodontology and Fixed
Prosthodontics
School of Dental Medicine
University of Berne
Switzerland

DANIEL BUSER
Department of Oral Surgery and Stomatology
School of Dental Medicine
University of Berne
Switzerland

GIANFRANCO CARNEVALE
Via Ridolfino Venuti 38
Rome
Italy

NOEL CLAFFEY
Dublin Dental School and Hospital
Trinity College
Dublin
Republic of Ireland

PIERPAOLO CORTELLINI
Via C. Botta 16
Florence
Italy

JOSÉ ECHEVERRÍA
Department of Periodontics
School of Dentistry
University of Barcelona
Spain

INGVAR ERICSSON
Department of Prosthetic Dentistry
Faculty of Odontology
Malmö University
Sweden

HANS-GÖRAN GRÖNDAHL
Department of Oral and Maxillofacial Radiology
Faculty of Odontology
The Sahlgrenska Academy at Göteborg University
Sweden

Anne Haffajee
Department of Periodontology
The Forsyth Institute
Boston, MA
USA

Christoph H.F. Hämmerle
Clinic for Fixed and Removable Prosthodontics
Centre for Dental and Oral Medicine and
Cranio-Maxillofacial Surgery
University of Zürich
Switzerland

Gunnar Hasselgren
Division of Endodontics
School of Dental and Oral Surgery
Columbia University
New York, NY
USA

Lars Heijl
Department of Periodontology
Faculty of Odontology
The Sahlgrenska Academy at Göteborg University
Sweden

David Herrera
Facultad de Odontología
Ciudad Universitaria, Madrid
Spain

Palle Holmstrup
Faculty of Health Sciences
School of Dentistry, Department of Periodontology
University of Copenhagen
Denmark

Thorkild Karring
Department of Periodontology
Royal Dental College
Faculty of Health Sciences
University of Aarhus
Denmark

Denis F. Kinane
Department of Periodontics, Endodontics and
Dental Hygiene
School of Dentistry
University of Louisville
Kentucky, KY
USA

Niklaus P. Lang
Department of Periodontology and Fixed
Prosthodontics
School of Dental Medicine
University of Berne
Switzerland

Ulf Lekholm
Department of Oral Maxillofacial Surgery
Faculty of Odontology
The Sahlgrenska Academy at Göteborg University
Sweden

Jan Lindhe
Department of Periodontology
Faculty of Odontology
The Sahlgrenska Academy at Göteborg University
Sweden

Bruno G. Loos
Department of Periodontology
ACTA, Amsterdam
The Netherlands

Lisa Mayfield
Department of Periodontics and Fixed
Prosthodontics
School of Dental Medicine
University of Berne
Switzerland

Andrea Mombelli
Department of Periodontology and Oral
Pathophysiology
University of Geneva
Switzerland

Sture Nyman
Deceased

Richard Palmer
Department of Periodontology
Guy's, King's and St Thomas' Dental Institute
King's College London
UK

Panos N. Papapanou
Division of Periodontics
School of Dental and Oral Surgery
Columbia University
New York, NY
USA

David W. Paquette
Department of Periodontology
School of Dentistry
University of North Carolina
Chapel Hill
North Carolina, NC
USA

Roberto Pontoriero
Galleria Passarella 2
Milan
Italy

GIOVAN PAULO PINI PRATO
Department of Odontology
University of Florence
Italy

MARC QUIRYNEN
School of Dentistry, Oral Pathology and
Maxillofacial Surgery
Faculty of Medicine
Catholic University of Leuven
Belgium

JESPER REIBEL
Department of Oral Pathology and Oral Medicine
School of Dentistry
University of Copenhagen
Denmark

HARALD RYLANDER
Department of Periodontology
Faculty of Odontology
The Sahlgrenska Academy at Göteborg University
Sweden

GIOVANNI SALVI
Department of Periodontology and Fixed
Prosthodontics
School of Dental Medicine
University of Berne
Switzerland

MARIANO SANZ
Facultad de Odontontología
Ciudad Universitaria, Madrid
Spain

MASSIMO SIMION
Department of Periodontology and Implant
Rehabilitation
School of Dental Medicine
University of Milan
Italy

SIGMUND SOCRANSKY
Department of Periodontology
The Forsyth Institute
Boston, MA
USA

MENA SOORY
Department of Periodontology
Guy's, King's and St. Thomas' Dental Institute
King's College London
UK

MAURIZIO S. TONETTI
Department of Periodontology
Eastman Dental Institute
University College, University of London
UK

UBELE VAN DER VELDEN
Department of Periodontology
ACTA, Amsterdam
The Netherlands

DANIEL VAN STEENBERGHE
School of Dentistry, Oral Pathology and
Maxillofacial Surgery
Faculty of Medicine
Catholic University of Leuven
Belgium

ARIE J. VAN WINKELHOFF
Department of Oral Microbiology
ACTA
Amsterdam
The Netherlands

GIORGIO VOGEL
Department of Medicine, Surgery and Dentistry
University of Milan
Italy

HEINER WEHRBEIN
Poliklinik für Kieferorthopaedie
Augustusplatz 2
Mainz
Germany

ANN WENNERBERG
Department of Biomaterials
Department of Prosthetic Dentistry/Dental Material
Science
Facultuty of Medicine
The Sahlgrenska Academy at Göteborg University
Sweden

JAN L. WENNSTRÖM
Department of Periodontology
Faculty of Odontology
The Sahlgrenska Academy at Göteborg University
Sweden

JYTTE WESTERGAARD
Panum Instituttet
School of Dentistry
University of Copenhagen
Denmark

RAY C. WILLIAMS
Department of Periodontology
School of Dentistry
University of North Carolina
Chapel Hill
North Carolina, NC
USA

BJÖRN ZACHRISSON
Stortingsgatan 10
Oslo
Norway

BASIC CONCEPTS

CHAPTER 1

Anatomy of the Periodontium

JAN LINDHE, THORKILD KARRING AND MAURÍCIO ARAÚJO

INTRODUCTION

This chapter includes a brief description of the characteristics of the normal periodontium. It is assumed that the reader has prior knowledge of oral embryology and histology. The periodontium (pert = around, odontos = tooth) comprises the following tissues (Fig. 1-1): (1) the *gingiva* (G), (2) the *periodontal ligament* (PL), (3) the *root cementum* (RC), and (4) the *alveolar bone* (AP). The alveolar bone consists of two components, the *alveolar bone proper* (ABP) and the alveolar process. The alveolar bone proper, also called "bundle bone" is continuous with the alveolar process and forms the thin bone plate that lines the alveolus of the tooth.

The main function of the periodontium is to attach the tooth to the bone tissue of the jaws and to maintain the integrity of the surface of the masticatory mucosa of the oral cavity. The periodontium, also called "the attachment apparatus" or "the supporting tissues of the teeth", constitutes a developmental, biologic, and functional unit which undergoes certain changes with age and is, in addition, subjected to morphologic changes related to functional alterations and alterations in the oral environment.

The development of the periodontal tissues occurs during the development and formation of teeth. This process starts early in the embryonic phase when cells from the neural crest (from the neural tube of the embryo) migrate into the first branchial arch. In this position the neural crest cells form a band of *ectomesenchyme* beneath the epithelium of the stomatodeum (the primitive oral cavity). After the uncommitted neural crest cells have reached their location in the jaw space, the epithelium of the stomatodeum releases

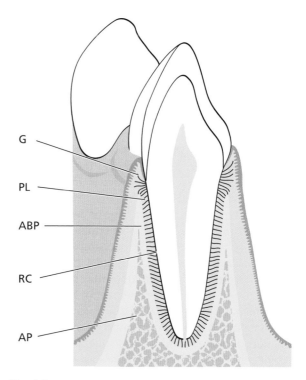

Fig. 1-1.

factors which initiate epithelial-ectomesenchymal interactions. Once these interactions have occurred, the ectomesenchyme takes the dominating role in the further development. Following the formation of the *dental lamina*, a series of processes are initiated (bud stage, cap stage, bell stage with root development) which result in the formation of a tooth and its surrounding periodontal tissues, including the alveolar bone proper. During the cap stage, condensation of ectomesenchymal cells appears in relation to the den-

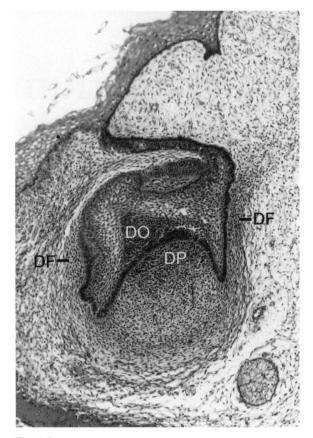

Fig. 1-2.

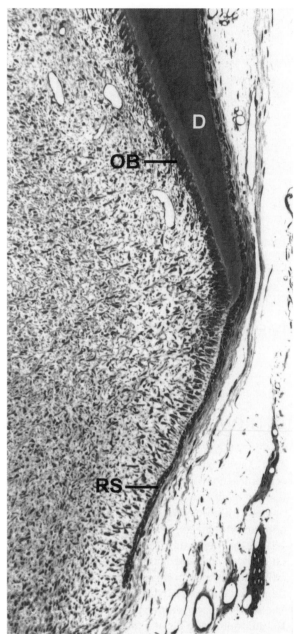

Fig. 1-3.

tal epithelium (the dental organ (DO)), forming the *dental papilla* (DP) that gives rise to the dentin and the pulp, and the *dental follicle* (DF) that gives rise to the periodontal supporting tissues (Fig. 1-2). The decisive role played by the ectomesenchyme in this process is further established by the fact that the tissue of the dental papilla apparently also determines the shape and form of the tooth.

If a tooth germ in the bell stage of development is dissected and transplanted to an ectopic site (e.g. the connective tissue or the anterior chamber of the eye), the tooth formation process continues. The crown and the root are formed, and the supporting structures, i.e. cementum, periodontal ligament and a thin lamina of alveolar bone proper, also develop. Such experiments document that all information necessary for the formation of a tooth and its attachment apparatus is obviously residing within the tissues of the dental organ and the surrounding ectomesenchyme. The dental organ is the formative organ of enamel, the dental papilla is the formative organ of the dentin-pulp complex, and the dental follicle is the formative organ of the attachment apparatus (the cementum, the periodontal ligament and the alveolar bone proper).

The development of the root and the periodontal supporting tissues follows that of the crown. Epithelial cells of the external and internal dental epithelium (the dental organ) proliferate in apical direction forming a double layer of cells named *Hertwig's epithelial root sheath* (RS). The odontoblasts (OB) forming the dentin of the root differentiate from ectomesenchy-

mal cells in the dental papilla under inductive influence of the inner epithelial cells (Fig. 1-3). The dentin (D) continues to form in apical direction producing the framework of the root. During formation of the root, the periodontal supporting tissues including acellular cementum develop. Some of the events in the cementogenesis are still unclear, but the following concept is gradually emerging.

At the start of dentin formation, the inner cells of Hertwig's epithelial root sheath synthesize and secrete enamel-related proteins, probably belonging to the amelogenin family. At the end of this period, the epithelial root sheath becomes fenestrated and through these fenestrations ectomesenchymal cells from the dental follicle penetrate and contact the root surface. The ectomesenchymal cells in contact with the enamel-related proteins differentiate into cementoblasts and start to form cementoid. This cementoid

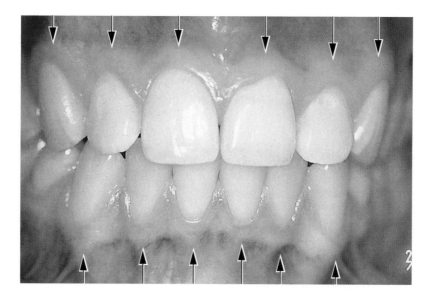

Fig. 1-4.

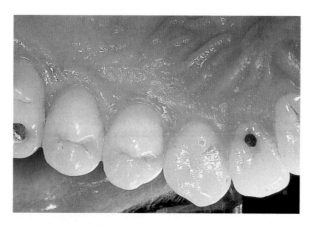

Fig. 1-5.

represents the organic matrix of the cementum and consists of a ground substance and collagen fibers, which intermingle with collagen fibers in the not yet fully mineralized outer layer of the dentin. It is assumed that the cementum becomes firmly attached to the dentin through these fiber interactions. The formation of the cellular cementum, which covers the apical third of the dental roots, differs from that of acellular cementum in that some of the cementoblasts become embedded in the cementum.

The remaining parts of the periodontium are formed by ectomesenchymal cells from the dental follicle lateral to the cementum. Some of them differentiate into periodontal fibroblasts and form the fibers of the periodontal ligament while others become osteoblasts producing the alveolar bone proper in which the periodontal fibers are anchored. In other words, the primary alveolar wall is also an ectomesenchymal product. It is likely, but still not conclusively documented, that ectomesenchymal cells remain in the mature periodontium and take part in the turnover of this tissue.

GINGIVA

Macroscopic anatomy

The oral mucosa (mucous membrane) is continuous with the skin of the lips and the mucosa of the soft palate and pharynx. The oral mucosa consists of (1) the *masticatory mucosa*, which includes the gingiva and the covering of the hard palate, (2) the *specialized mucosa*, which covers the dorsum of the tongue, and (3) the remaining part, called the *lining mucosa*.

Fig. 1-4. The gingiva is that part of the masticatory mucosa which covers the alveolar process and surrounds the cervical portion of the teeth. It consists of an epithelial layer and an underlying connective tissue layer called the *lamina propria*. The gingiva obtains its final shape and texture in conjunction with eruption of the teeth.

In the coronal direction the coral pink gingiva terminates in the *free gingival margin,* which has a scalloped outline. In the apical direction the gingiva is continuous with the loose, darker red *alveolar mucosa* (lining mucosa) from which the gingiva is separated by a, usually, easily recognizable borderline called

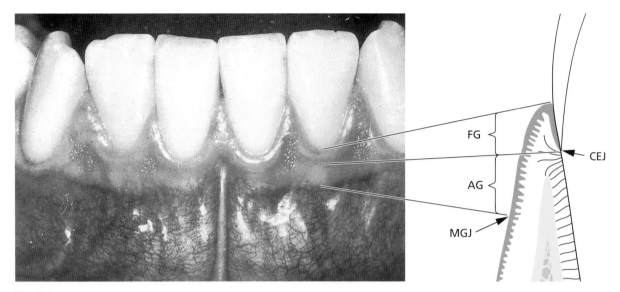

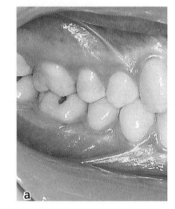

Fig. 1-6.

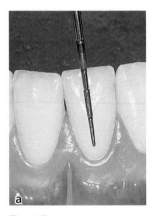
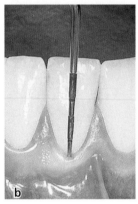

Fig. 1-7.

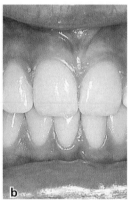

Fig. 1-8.

either the *mucogingival junction* (arrows) or the *mucogingival line*.

Fig. 1-5. There is no mucogingival line present in the palate since the hard palate and the maxillary alveolar process are covered by the same type of masticatory mucosa.

Fig. 1-6. Two parts of the gingiva can be differentiated:

1. the *free gingiva* (FG)
2. the *attached gingiva* (AG)

The free gingiva is coral pink, has a dull surface and firm consistency. It comprises the gingival tissue at the vestibular and lingual/palatal aspects of the teeth, and the *interdental gingiva* or the *interdental papillae*. On the vestibular and lingual side of the teeth, the free gingiva extends from the gingival margin in apical direction to the *free gingival groove* which is positioned at a level corresponding to the level of the *cemento-enamel junction* (CEJ). The attached gingiva is in apical direction demarcated by the mucogingival junction (MGJ).

Fig. 1-7. The free gingival margin is often rounded in such a way that a small invagination or sulcus is formed between the tooth and the gingiva (Fig. 1-7a).

When a periodontal probe is inserted into this invagination and, further apically, towards the cemento-enamel junction, the gingival tissue is separated from the tooth, and a "*gingival pocket*" or "*gingival crevice*" is artificially opened. Thus, in normal or clinically healthy gingiva there is in fact no "gingival pocket" or "gingival crevice" present but the gingiva is in close contact with the enamel surface. In the illustration to the right (Fig. 1-7b), a periodontal probe has been inserted in the tooth/gingiva interface and a "gingival crevice" artificially opened approximately to the level of the cemento-enamel junction.

After completed tooth eruption, the free gingival margin is located on the enamel surface approximately 1.5 to 2 mm coronal to the cemento-enamel junction.

Fig. 1-8. The shape of the interdental gingiva (the interdental papilla) is determined by the contact relationships between the teeth, the width of the approximal tooth surfaces, and the course of the cemento-

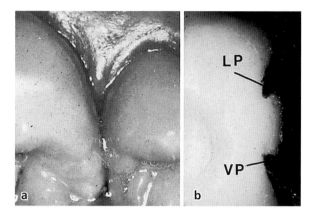

Fig. 1-9.

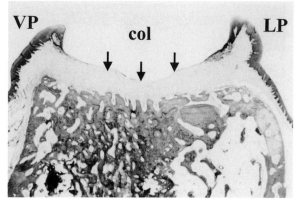

Fig. 1-9c.

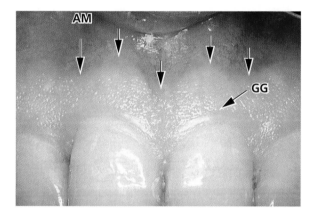

Fig. 1-10.

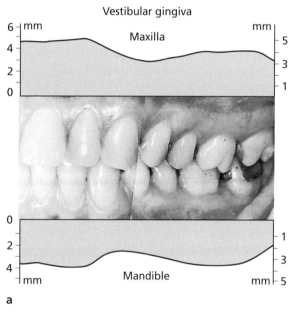

a

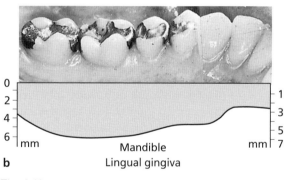

b

Fig. 1-11.

enamel junction. In anterior regions of the dentition, the interdental papilla is of pyramidal form (Fig. 1-8b) while in the molar regions, the papillae are more flattened in buccolingual direction (Fig. 1-8a). Due to the presence of interdental papillae, the free gingival margin follows a more or less accentuated, scalloped course through the dentition.

Fig. 1-9. In the premolar/molar regions of the dentition, the teeth have approximal contact surfaces (Fig. 1-9a) rather than contact points. Since the interdental papilla has a shape in conformity with the outline of the interdental contact surfaces, a concavity – *a col* – is established in the premolar and molar regions, as demonstrated in Fig. 1-9b, where the distal tooth has been removed. Thus, the interdental papillae in these areas often have one vestibular (VP) and one lingual/palatal portion (LP) separated by the col region. The col region, as demonstrated in the histological section (Fig. 1-9c), is covered by a thin non-keratinized epithelium (arrows). This epithelium has many features in common with the junctional epithelium (see Fig. 1-34).

Fig. 1-10. The attached gingiva is, in coronal direction, demarcated by the free gingival groove (GG) or, when such a groove is not present, by a horizontal plane placed at the level of the cemento-enamel junction. In clinical examinations it was observed that a free gingival groove is only present in about 30-40% of adults.

The free gingival groove is often most pronounced on the vestibular aspect of the teeth, occurring most frequently in the incisor and premolar regions of the mandible, and least frequently in the mandibular molar and maxillary premolar regions.

The attached gingiva extends in the apical direction to the mucogingival junction (arrows), where it becomes continuous with the alveolar (lining) mucosa (AM). It is of firm texture, coral pink in color, and often shows small depressions on the surface. The depressions, named "stippling", give the appearance

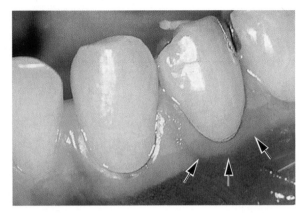

Fig. 1-12.

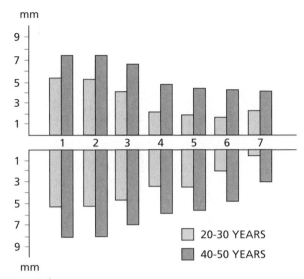

Fig. 1-13.

of orange peel. It is firmly attached to the underlying alveolar bone and cementum by connective tissue fibers, and is, therefore, comparatively immobile in relation to the underlying tissue. The darker red alveolar mucosa (AM) located apical to the mucogingival junction, on the other hand, is loosely bound to the underlying bone. Therefore, in contrast to the attached gingiva, the alveolar mucosa is mobile in relation to the underlying tissue.

Fig. 1-11 describes how the width of the gingiva varies in different parts of the mouth. In the maxilla (Fig. 1-11a) the vestibular gingiva is generally widest in the area of the incisors and most narrow adjacent to the premolars. In the mandible (Fig. 1-11b) the gingiva on the lingual aspect is particularly narrow in the area of the incisors and wide in the molar region. The range of variation is 1-9 mm.

Fig. 1-12 illustrates an area in the mandibular premolar region where the gingiva is extremely narrow. The arrows indicate the location of the mucogingival junction. The mucosa has been stained with an iodine solution in order to distinguish more accurately between the gingiva and the alveolar mucosa.

Fig. 1-13 depicts the result of a study in which the width of the attached gingiva was assessed and related to the age of the patients examined. It was found that the gingiva in 40 to 50-year-olds was significantly wider than that in 20 to 30-year-olds. This observation indicates that the width of the gingiva tends to increase with age. Since the mucogingival junction remains stable throughout life in relation to the lower border of the mandible, the increasing width of the gingiva may suggest that the teeth, as a result of occlusal wear, slowly erupt throughout life.

Microscopic anatomy

Oral epithelium

Fig. 1-14a presents a schematic drawing of a histologic section (see Fig. 1-14b) describing the composition of

the gingiva and the contact area between the gingiva and the enamel (E).

Fig. 1-14b. The free gingiva comprises all epithelial and connective tissue structures (CT) located coronal to a horizontal line placed at the level of the cemento-enamel junction (CEJ). The epithelium covering the free gingiva may be differentiated as follows:

- *oral epithelium* (OE), which faces the oral cavity
- *oral sulcular epithelium* (OSE), which faces the tooth without being in contact with the tooth surface
- *junctional epithelium* (JE), which provides the contact between the gingiva and the tooth.

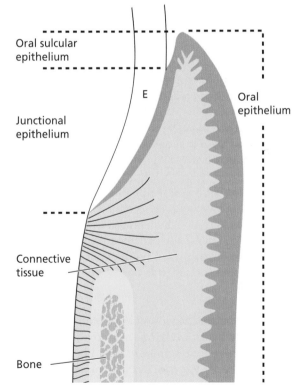

Fig. 1-14a.

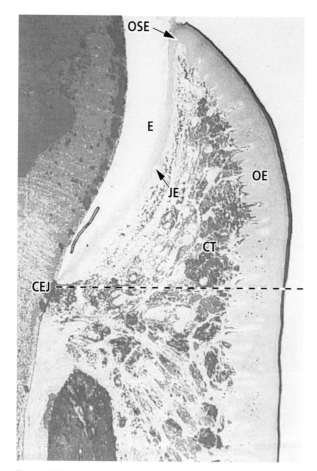

Fig. 1-14b.

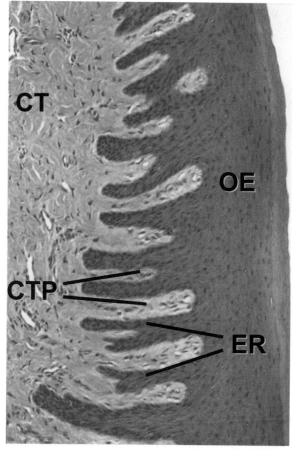

Fig. 1-14c.

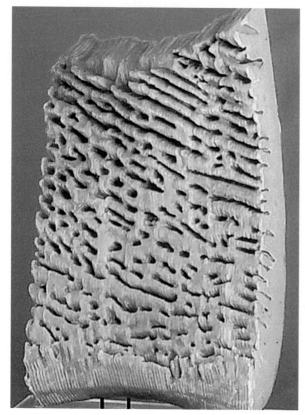

Fig. 1-15.

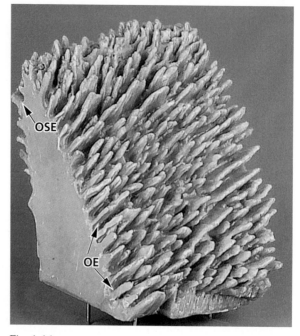

Fig. 1-16.

Fig. 1-14c. The boundary between the oral epithelium (OE) and the underlying connective tissue (CT) has a wavy course. The connective tissue portions which project into the epithelium are called *connective tissue papillae* (CTP) and are separated from each other by

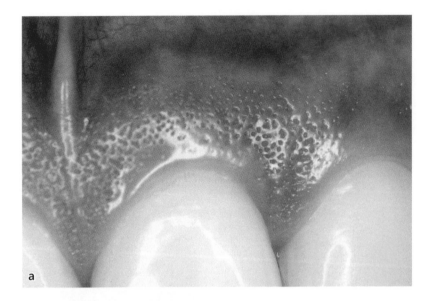

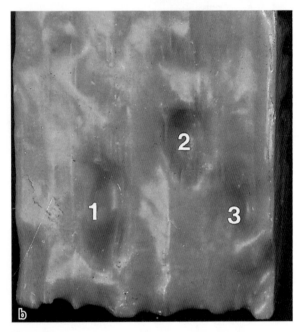

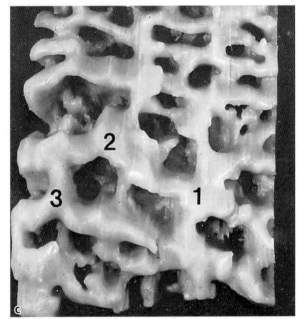

Fig. 1-17.

epithelial ridges – so-called *rete pegs* (ER). In normal, non-inflamed gingiva, rete pegs and connective tissue papillae are lacking at the boundary between the junctional epithelium and its underlying connective tissue (Fig. 1-14b). Thus, a characteristic morphologic feature of the oral epithelium and the oral sulcular epithelium is the presence of rete pegs, while these structures are lacking in the junctional epithelium.

Fig. 1-15 presents a model, constructed on the basis of magnified serial histologic sections, showing the subsurface of the oral epithelium of the gingiva after the connective tissue has been removed. The subsurface of the oral epithelium (i.e. the surface of the epithelium facing the connective tissue) exhibits several depressions corresponding to the connective tissue papillae (in Fig. 1-16) which project into the epithelium. It can be seen that the epithelial projections, which in histologic sections separate the connective tissue papil-

lae, constitute a continuous system of epithelial ridges.

Fig. 1-16 presents a model of the connective tissue, corresponding to the model of the epithelium shown in Fig. 1-15. The epithelium has been removed, thereby making the vestibular aspect of the gingival connective tissue visible. Notice the connective tissue papillae which project into the space that was occupied by the oral epithelium (OE) in Fig. 1-15 and by the oral sulcular epithelium (OSE) on the back of the model.

Fig. 1-17a. In 40% of adults the attached gingiva shows a stippling on the surface. The photograph shows a case where this stippling is conspicuous (see also Fig. 1-10).

Fig. 1-17b presents a magnified model of the outer

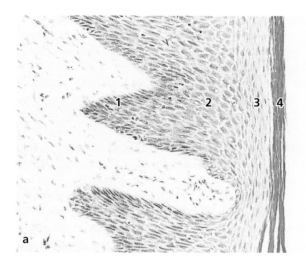
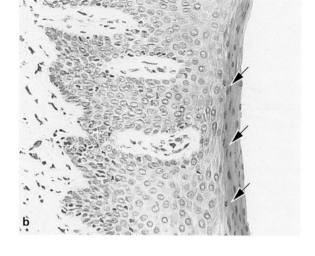

Fig. 1-18.

surface of the oral epithelium of the attached gingiva. The surface exhibits the minute depressions (1-3) which, when present, give the gingiva its characteristic stippled appearance.

Fig. 1-17c shows a photograph of the subsurface (i.e. the surface of the epithelium facing the connective tissue) of the same model as that shown in Fig. 1-17b. The subsurface of the epithelium is characterized by the presence of epithelial ridges which merge at various locations (1-3). The depressions (1-3) seen on the outer surface of the epithelium (shown in Fig. 1-17b) correspond with the fusion sites (1-3) between epithelial ridges. Thus, the depressions on the surface of the gingiva occur in the areas of fusion between various epithelial ridges.

Fig. 1-18a. A portion of the oral epithelium covering the free gingiva is illustrated in this photomicrograph. The oral epithelium is a *keratinized, stratified, squamous epithelium* which, on the basis of the degree to which the keratin-producing cells are differentiated, can be divided into the following cell layers:

1. *basal layer* (stratum basale or stratum germinativum)
2. *prickle cell layer* (stratum spinosum)
3. *granular cell layer* (stratum granulosum)
4. *keratinized cell layer* (stratum corneum)

It should be observed that in this section, cell nuclei are lacking in the outer cell layers. Such an epithelium is denoted *orthokeratinized*. Often, however, the cells of the stratum corneum of the epithelium of human gingiva contain remnants of the nuclei (arrows) as seen in Fig. 1-18b. In such a case, the epithelium is denoted *parakeratinized*.

Fig. 1-19. In addition to the keratin-producing cells which comprise about 90% of the total cell population, the oral epithelium contains the following types of cell:

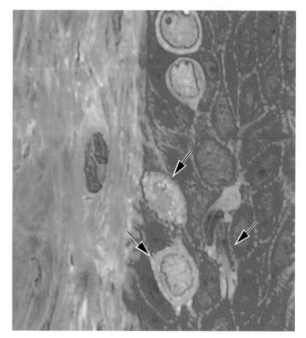

Fig. 1-19.

1. *melanocytes*
2. *Langerhans cells*
3. *Merkel's cells*
4. *inflammatory cells*

These cell types are often stellate and have cytoplasmic extensions of various size and appearance. They are also called "clear cells" since in histologic sections, the zone around their nuclei appears lighter than that in the surrounding keratin-producing cells.

The photomicrograph shows "clear cells" (arrows) located in or near the stratum basale of the oral epithelium. Except the Merkel's cells, these "clear cells", which are not producing keratin, lack desmosomal attachment to adjacent cells. The melanocytes are pigment-synthesizing cells and are responsible for the melanin pigmentation occasionally seen on the gingiva. However, both lightly and darkly pigmented individuals present melanocytes in the epithelium.

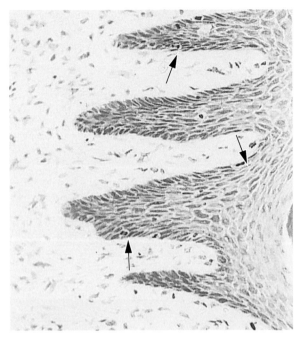

Fig. 1-20.

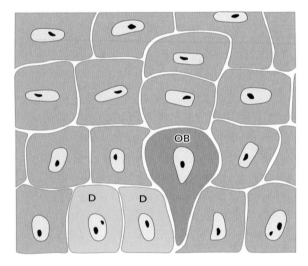

Fig. 1-21.

The Langerhans cells are believed to play a role in the defense mechanism of the oral mucosa. It has been suggested that the Langerhans cells react with antigens which are in the process of penetrating the epithelium. An early immunologic response is thereby initiated, inhibiting or preventing further antigen penetration of the tissue. The Merkel's cells have been suggested to have a sensory function.

Fig. 1-20. The cells in the basal layer are either cylindric or cuboid, and are in contact with the *basement membrane* that separates the epithelium and the connective tissue. The basal cells possess the ability to divide, i.e. undergo mitotic cell division. The cells marked with arrows in the photomicrograph are in the process of

dividing. It is in the basal layer that the epithelium is renewed. Therefore, this layer is also termed *stratum germinativum*, and can be considered the *progenitor cell compartment* of the epithelium.

Fig. 1-21. When two daughter cells (D) have been formed by cell division, an adjacent "older" basal cell (OB) is pushed into the spinous cell layer and starts, as a *keratinocyte*, to traverse the epithelium. It takes approximately 1 month for a keratinocyte to reach the outer epithelial surface, where it becomes shed from the stratum corneum. Within a given time, the number of cells which divide in the basal layer equals the number of cells which become shed from the surface. Thus, under normal conditions there is complete equilibrium between cell renewal and cell loss so that the epithelium maintains a constant thickness. As the basal cell migrates through the epithelium, it becomes flattened with its long axis parallel to the epithelial surface.

Fig. 1-22. The basal cells are found immediately adjacent to the connective tissue and are separated from this tissue by the basement membrane, probably produced by the basal cells. Under the light microscope this membrane appears as a structureless zone approximately 1 to 2 μm wide (arrows) which reacts positively to a PAS stain (periodic acid-Schiff stain). This positive reaction demonstrates that the basement membrane contains carbohydrate (glycoproteins). The epithelial cells are surrounded by an extracellular substance which also contains protein-polysaccharide complexes. At the ultrastructural level, the basement membrane has a complex composition.

Fig. 1-23 is an electronmicrograph (magnification × 70 000) of an area including part of a basal cell, the basement membrane and part of the adjacent connective tissue. The basal cell (BC) occupies the upper portion of the picture. Immediately beneath the basal cell an approximately 400 Å wide electron lucent zone can be seen which is called *lamina lucida* (LL). Beneath the lamina lucida an electron dense zone of approximately the same thickness can be observed. This zone is called *lamina densa* (LD). From the lamina densa so-called *anchoring fibers* (AF) project in a fan-shaped fashion into the connective tissue. The anchoring fibers are approximately 1 μm in length and terminate freely in the connective tissue. The basement membrane, which appeared as an entity under the light microscope, thus, in the electronmicrograph, appears to comprise one lamina lucida and one lamina densa with adjacent connective tissue fibers (anchoring fibers). The cell membrane of the epithelial cells facing the lamina lucida harbors a number of electron-dense, thicker zones appearing at various intervals along the cell membrane. These structures are called *hemidesmosomes* (HD). The cytoplasmic *tonofilaments* (CT) in

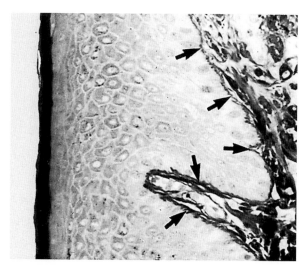

Fig. 1-22.

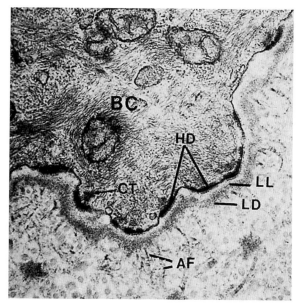

Fig. 1-23.

the cell converge towards such hemidesmosomes. The hemidesmosomes are involved in the attachment of the epithelium to the underlying basement membrane.

Fig. 1-24 illustrates an area of stratum spinosum in the gingival oral epithelium. Stratum spinosum consists of 10-20 layers of relatively large, polyhedral cells, equipped with short cytoplasmic processes resembling spines. The cytoplasmic processes (arrows) occur at regular intervals and give the cells a prickly appearance. Together with intercellular protein-carbohydrate complexes, cohesion between the cells is provided by numerous "desmosomes" (pairs of hemidesmosomes) which are located between the cytoplasmic processes of adjacent cells.

Fig. 1-25 shows an area of stratum spinosum in an electronmicrograph. The dark-stained structures between the individual epithelial cells represent the *desmosomes* (arrows). A desmosome may be considered to be two hemidesmosomes facing one another. The presence of a large number of desmosomes indicates that the cohesion between the epithelial cells is solid. The light cell (LC) in the center of the illustration harbors no hemidesmosomes and is, therefore, not a keratinocyte but rather a "clear cell" (see also Fig. 1-19).

Fig. 1-26 is a schematic drawing describing the composition of a desmosome. A desmosome can be con-

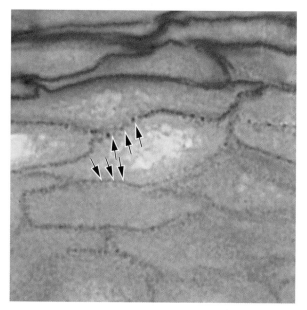

Fig. 1-24.

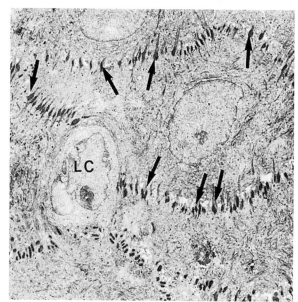

Fig. 1-25.

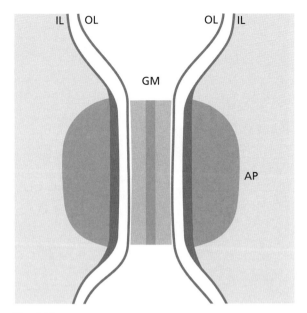

Fig. 1-26.

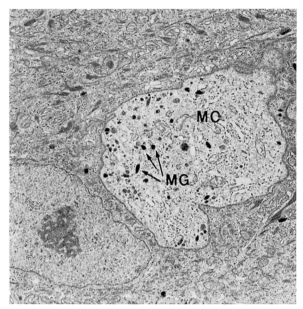

Fig. 1-27.

sidered to consist of two adjoining hemidesmosomes separated by a zone containing electron-dense granulated material (GM). Thus, a desmosome comprises the following structural components: (1) the *outer leaflets* (OL) of the cell membrane of two adjoining cells, (2) the thick *inner leaflets* (IL) of the cell membranes and (3) the *attachment plaques* (AP), which represent granular and fibrillar material in the cytoplasm.

Fig. 1-27. As mentioned previously, the oral epithelium also contains melanocytes, which are responsible for the production of the pigment melanin. Melanocytes are present in individuals with marked pigmentation of the oral mucosa (Indians and Negroes) as well as in individuals where no clinical signs of pigmentation can be seen. In this electronmicrograph a melanocyte (MC) is present in the lower portion of the stratum spinosum. In contrast to the keratinocytes, this cell contains melanin granules (MG) and has no tonofilaments or hemidesmosomes. Note the large amount of tonofilaments in the cytoplasm of the adjacent keratinocytes.

Fig. 1-28. When traversing the epithelium from the basal layer to the epithelial surface, the keratinocytes undergo continuous differentiation and specialization. The many changes which occur during this process are indicated in this diagram of a keratinized stratified squamous epithelium. From the basal layer (stratum basale) to the granular layer (stratum granulosum) both the number of tonofilaments (F) in the cytoplasm and the number of desmosomes (D) increase. In contrast, the number of organelles such as mitochondria (M), lamellae of rough endoplasmic reticulum (E) and Golgi complexes (G) decrease in the keratinocytes on their way from the basal layer towards the surface. In the stratum granulosum, electron dense *keratohyalin bodies* (K) and clusters of glycogen containing granules start to occur. Such gran-

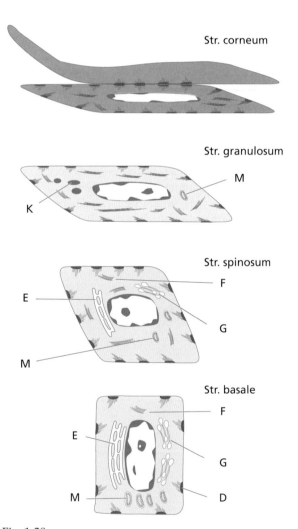

Fig. 1-28.

ules are believed to be related to the synthesis of keratin.

Fig. 1-29 is a photomicrograph of the stratum granulosum and stratum corneum. Keratohyalin granules (arrows) are seen in the stratum granulosum. There is an abrupt transition of the cells from the stratum granulosum to the stratum corneum. This is indicative of a very sudden keratinization of the cytoplasm of the keratinocyte and its conversion into a horny squame. The cytoplasm of the cells in the stratum corneum (SC) is filled with keratin and the entire apparatus for protein synthesis and energy production, i.e. the nucleus, the mitochondria, the endoplasmic reticulum and the Golgi complex, is lost. In a parakeratinized epithelium, however, the cells of the stratum corneum contain remnants of nuclei. Keratinization is considered a process of differentiation rather than degeneration. It is a process of protein synthesis which requires energy and is dependent on functional cells, i.e. cells containing a nucleus and a normal set of organelles.

Summary
The keratinocyte undergoes continuous differentiation on its way from the basal layer to the surface of the epithelium. Thus, once the keratinocyte has left the basement membrane it can no longer divide but maintains a capacity for production of protein (tonofilaments and keratohyalin granules). In the granular layer, the keratinocyte is deprived of its energy- and protein-producing apparatus (probably by enzymatic breakdown) and is abruptly converted into a keratin-filled cell which via the stratum corneum is shed from the epithelial surface.

Fig. 1-30 illustrates a portion of the epithelium of the alveolar (lining) mucosa. In contrast to the epithelium of the gingiva, the lining mucosa has no stratum corneum. Notice that cells containing nuclei can be identified in all layers, from the basal layer to the surface of the epithelium.

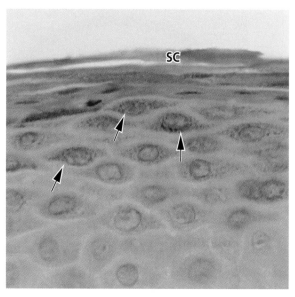

Fig. 1-29.

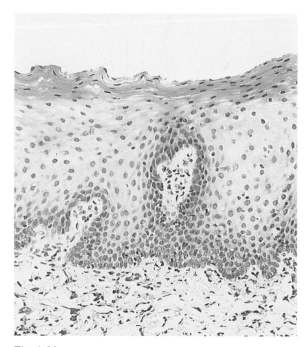

Fig. 1-30.

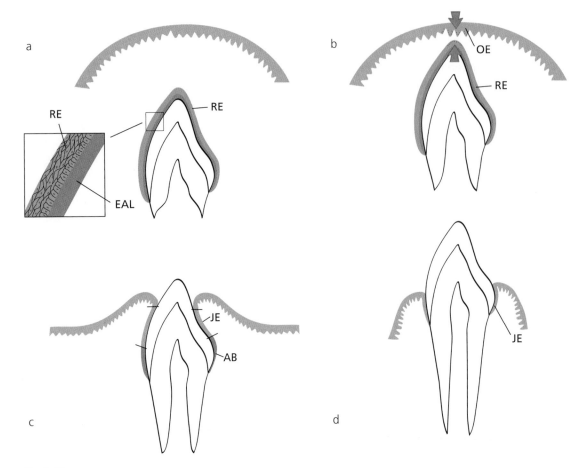

Fig. 1-31.

Dento-gingival epithelium

The tissue components of the dento-gingival region achieve their final structural characteristics in conjunction with the eruption of the teeth. This is illustrated in Fig. 1-31a-d.

Fig. 1-31a. When the enamel of the tooth is fully developed, the enamel-producing cells (ameloblasts) become reduced in height, produce a basal lamina and form, together with cells from the outer enamel epithelium, the so-called reduced dental epithelium (RE). The basal lamina (epithelial attachment lamina: EAL) lies in direct contact with the enamel. The contact between this lamina and the epithelial cells is maintained by hemidesmosomes. The reduced enamel epithelium surrounds the crown of the tooth from the moment the enamel is properly mineralized until the tooth starts to erupt.

Fig. 1-31b. As the erupting tooth approaches the oral epithelium, the cells of the outer layer of the reduced dental epithelium (RE), as well as the cells of the basal layer of the oral epithelium (OE), show increased mitotic activity (arrows) and start to migrate into the underlying connective tissue. The migrating epithelium produces an epithelial mass between the oral epithelium and the reduced dental epithelium so that the tooth can erupt without bleeding. The former ameloblasts do not divide.

Fig. 1-31c. When the tooth has penetrated into the oral cavity, large portions immediately apical to the incisal area of the enamel are covered by a junctional epithelium (JE) containing only a few layers of cells. The cervical region of the enamel, however, is still covered by ameloblasts (AB) and outer cells of the reduced dental epithelium.

Fig. 1-31d. During the later phases of tooth eruption, all cells of the reduced enamel epithelium are replaced

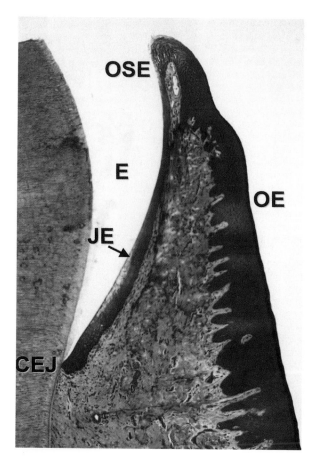

Fig. 1-32.

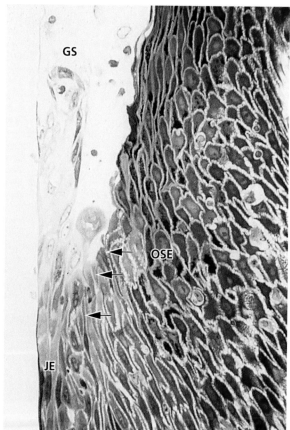

Fig. 1-33.

by a junctional epithelium. This epithelium is continuous with the oral epithelium and provides the attachment between the tooth and the gingiva. If the free gingiva is excised after the tooth has fully erupted, a new junctional epithelium, indistinguishable from that found following tooth eruption, will develop during healing. The fact that this new junctional epithelium has developed from the oral epithelium indicates that the cells of the oral epithelium possess the ability to differentiate into cells of junctional epithelium.

Fig. 1-32 is a histologic section cut through the border area between the tooth and the gingiva, i.e. the *dento-gingival region*. The enamel (E) is to the left. Towards the right follow the *junctional epithelium* (JE), the *oral sulcular epithelium* (OSE) and the *oral epithelium* (OE). The oral sulcular epithelium covers the shallow groove, the gingival sulcus located between the enamel and the top of the free gingiva. The junctional epithelium differs morphologically from the oral sulcular epithelium and oral epithelium, while the two

latter are structurally very similar. Although individual variation may occur, the junctional epithelium is usually widest in its coronal portion (about 15-20 cell layers), but becomes thinner (3-4 cells) towards the cemento-enamel junction (CEJ). The borderline between the junctional epithelium and the underlying connective tissue does not present epithelial rete pegs except when inflamed.

Fig. 1-33. The junctional epithelium has a free surface at the bottom of the *gingival sulcus* (GS). Like the oral sulcular epithelium and the oral epithelium, the junctional epithelium is continuously renewed through cell division in the basal layer. The cells migrate to the base of the gingival sulcus from where they are shed. The border between the junctional epithelium (JE) and the oral sulcular epithelium (OSE) is indicated by arrows. The cells of the oral sulcular epithelium are cuboidal and the surface of this epithelium is keratinized.

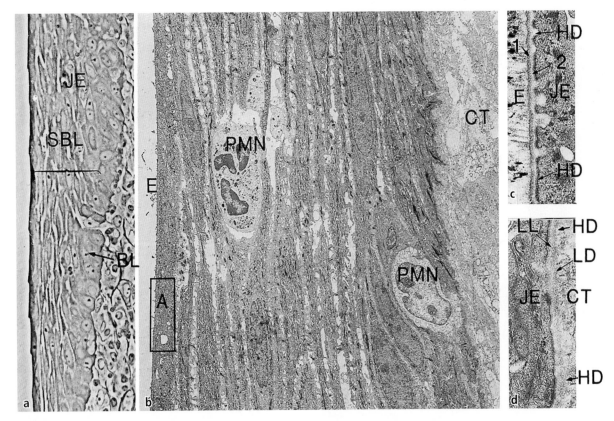

Fig. 1-34.

Fig. 1-34 illustrates different characteristics of the junctional epithelium. As can be seen in Fig. 1-34a, the cells of the junctional epithelium (JE) are arranged into one basal layer (BL) and several suprabasal layers (SBL). Fig. 1-34b demonstrates that the basal cells as well as the suprabasal cells are flattened with their long axis parallel to the tooth surface. (CT = connective tissue, E = enamel space.)

There are distinct differences between the oral sulcular epithelium, the oral epithelium and the junctional epithelium:

1. The size of the cells in the junctional epithelium is, relative to the tissue volume, larger than in the oral epithelium.
2. The intercellular space in the junctional epithelium is, relative to the tissue volume, comparatively wider than in the oral epithelium.
3. The number of desmosomes is smaller in the junctional epithelium than in the oral epithelium.

Note the comparatively wide intercellular spaces between the oblong cells of the junctional epithelium, and the presence of two neutrophilic granulocytes (PMN) which are traversing the epithelium.

The framed area (A) is shown in a higher magnification in Fig. 1-34c, from which it can be seen that the basal cells of the junctional epithelium are not in direct contact with the enamel (E). Between the enamel and the epithelium (JE) one electron-dense zone (1) and one electron-lucent zone (2) can be seen. The electron-lucent zone is in contact with the cells of the junctional

epithelium (JE). These two zones have a structure very similar to that of the lamina densa (LD) and lamina lucida (LL) in the basement membrane area (i.e. the epithelium (JE)-connective tissue (CT) interface) described in Fig. 1-23. Furthermore, as seen in Fig. 1-34d, the cell membrane of the junctional epithelial cells harbors hemidesmosomes (HD) towards the enamel as it does towards the connective tissue. Thus, the interface between the enamel and the junctional epithelium is similar to the interface between the epithelium and the connective tissue.

Fig. 1-35 is a schematic drawing of the most apically positioned cell in the junctional epithelium. The enamel (E) is depicted to the left in the drawing. It can be seen that the electron-dense zone (1) between the junctional epithelium and the enamel can be considered a continuation of the lamina densa (LD) in the basement membrane of the connective tissue side. Similarly, the electron-lucent zone (2) can be considered a continuation of the lamina lucida (LL). It should be noted, however, that at variance with the epithelium-connective tissue interface, there are no anchoring fibers (AF) attached to the lamina densa-like structure (1) adjacent to the enamel. On the other hand, like the basal cells adjacent to the basement membrane (at the connective tissue interface), the cells of the junctional epithelium facing the lamina lucida-like structure (2) harbor hemidesmosomes. Thus, the interface between the junctional epithelium and the enamel is structurally very similar to the epithelium-connective tissue interface, which means that the junctional epi-

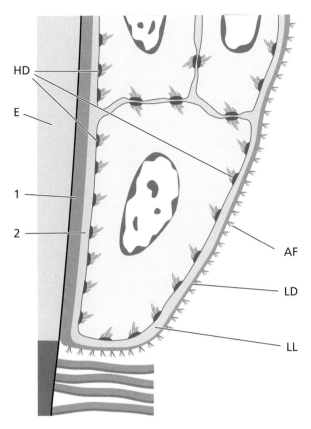

Fig. 1-35.

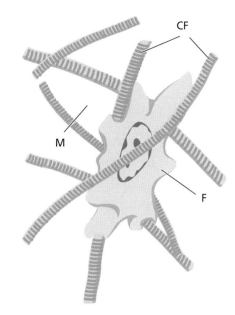

Fig. 1-36.

thelium is not only in contact with the enamel but is actually physically attached to the tooth via hemidesmosomes.

Lamina propria
The predominant tissue component of the gingiva is the connective tissue (lamina propria). The major components of the connective tissue are *collagen fibers* (around 60% of connective tissue volume), *fibroblasts* (around 5%), *vessels and nerves* (around 35%) which are embedded in an amorphous ground substance (matrix).

Fig. 1-36. The drawing illustrates a fibroblast (F) residing in a network of connective tissue fibers (CF). The intervening space is filled with matrix (M) which constitutes the "environment" for the cell.

Cells
The different types of cell present in the connective tissue are: (1) *fibroblasts*, (2) *mast cells*, (3) *macrophages* and (4) *inflammatory cells*.

Fig. 1-37. The *fibroblast* is the most predominant connective tissue cell (65% of the total cell population). The fibroblast is engaged in the production of various types of fibers found in the connective tissue, but is also instrumental in the synthesis of the connective tissue matrix. The fibroblast is a spindle-shaped or stellate cell with an oval-shaped nucleus containing one or more nucleoli. A part of a fibroblast is shown in electron microscopic magnification. The cytoplasm

contains a well-developed granular endoplasmic reticulum (E) with ribosomes. The Golgi complex (G) is usually of considerable size and the mitochondria (M) are large and numerous. Furthermore, the cytoplasm contains many fine tonofilaments (F). Adjacent to the cell membrane, all along the periphery of the cell, a large number of vesicles (V) can be found.

Fig. 1-38. The *mast cell* is responsible for the production of certain components of the matrix. This cell also produces vasoactive substances, which can affect the function of the microvascular system and control the flow of blood through the tissue. A mast cell is presented in electron microscopic magnification. The cytoplasm is characterized by the presence of a large number of vesicles (V) of varying size. These vesicles contain biologically active substances such as proteolytic enzymes, histamine and heparin. The Golgi

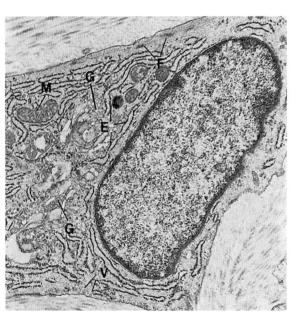

Fig. 1-37.

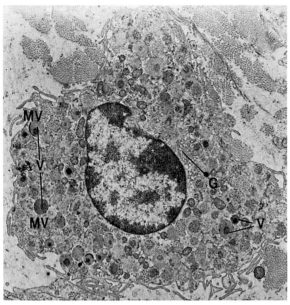

Fig. 1-38.

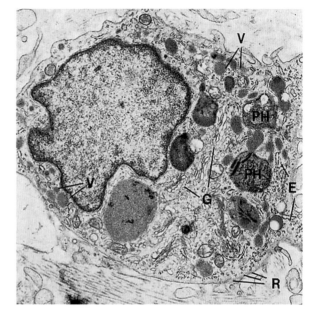

Fig. 1-39.

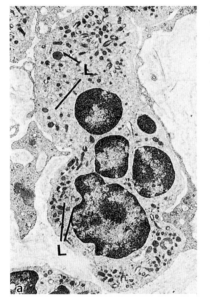

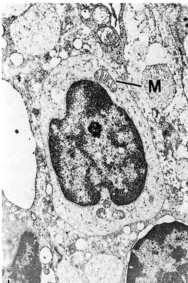

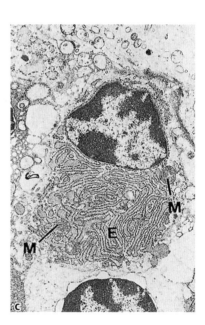

Fig. 1-40.

complex (G) is well developed, while granular endoplasmic reticulum structures are scarce. A large number of small cytoplasmic projections, i.e. microvilli (MV), can be seen along the periphery of the cell.

Fig. 1-39. The *macrophage* has a number of different phagocytic and synthetic functions in the tissue. A macrophage is shown in electron microscopic magnification. The nucleus is characterized by numerous invaginations of varying size. A zone of electron-dense chromatin condensations can be seen along the periphery of the nucleus. The Golgi complex (G) is

well developed and numerous vesicles (V) of varying size are present in the cytoplasm. Granular endoplasmic reticulum (E) is scarce, but a certain number of free ribosomes (R) are evenly distributed in the cytoplasm. Remnants of phagocytosed material are often found in lysosomal vesicles: phagosomes (PH). In the periphery of the cell, a large number of microvilli of varying size can be seen. Macrophages are particularly numerous in inflamed tissue. They are derived from circulating blood monocytes which migrate into the tissue.

Fig. 1-40. Besides fibroblasts, mast cells and macro-

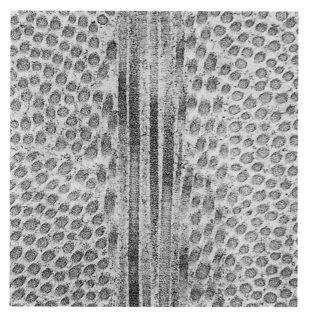

Fig. 1-41.

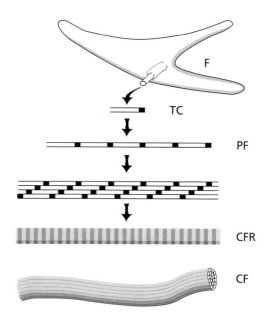

Fig. 1-42.

phages, the connective tissue also harbors *inflammatory cells* of various types, for example neutrophilic granulocytes, lymphocytes and plasma cells.

The *neutrophilic granulocytes*, also called *polymorphonuclear leukocytes*, have a characteristic appearance (Fig. 1-40a). The nucleus is lobulate and numerous lysosomes (L), containing lysosomal enzymes, are found in the cytoplasm.

The *lymphocytes* (Fig. 1-40b) are characterized by an oval to spherical nucleus containing localized areas of electron-dense chromatin. The narrow border of cytoplasm surrounding the nucleus contains numerous free ribosomes, a few mitochondria (M) and, in localized areas, endoplasmic reticulum with fixed ribosomes. Lysosomes are also present in the cytoplasm.

The *plasma cells* (Fig. 1-40c) contain an eccentrically located spherical nucleus with radially deployed electron-dense chromatin. Endoplasmic reticulum (E) with numerous ribosomes is found randomly distributed in the cytoplasm. In addition, the cytoplasm contains numerous mitochondria (M) and a well-developed Golgi complex.

Fibers

The connective tissue fibers are produced by the fibroblasts and can be divided into: (1) *collagen fibers*, (2) *reticulin fibers*, (3) *oxytalan fibers* and (4) *elastic fibers*.

Fig. 1-41. The *collagen fibers* predominate in the gingival connective tissue and constitute the most essential components of the periodontium. The electronmicrograph shows cross- and longitudinal sections of collagen fibers. The collagen fibers have a characteristic cross-banding with a periodicity of 700 Å between the individual dark bands.

Fig. 1-42 illustrates some important features of the synthesis and the composition of collagen fibers produced by fibroblasts (F). The smallest unit, the collagen molecule, is often referred to as *tropocollagen*. A tropocollagen molecule (TC) which is seen in the upper portion of the drawing is approximately 3000 Å long and has a diameter of 15 Å. It consists of three polypeptide chains intertwined to form a helix. Each chain contains about 1000 amino acids. One third of these are glycine and about 20% proline and hydroxyproline, the latter being found practically only in collagen. Tropocollagen synthesis takes place inside the fibroblast from which the tropocollagen molecule is secreted into the extracellular space. Thus, the polymerization of tropocollagen molecules to collagen fibers takes place in the extracellular compartment. First, tropocollagen molecules are aggregated longitudinally to *protofibrils* (PF), which are subsequently laterally aggregated parallel to *collagen fibrils* (CFR), with an overlapping of the tropocollagen molecules by about 25% of their length. Due to the fact that special refraction conditions develop after staining at the sites where the tropocollagen molecules adjoin, a cross-banding with a periodicity of approximately 700 Å occurs under light microscopy. The *collagen fibers* (CF) are bundles of collagen fibrils, aligned in such a way that the fibers also exhibit a cross-banding with a periodicity of 700 Å. In the tissue, the fibers are usually arranged in bundles. As the collagen fibers mature, covalent crosslinks are formed between the tropocollagen molecules, resulting in an age-related reduction in collagen solubility.

Cementoblasts and *osteoblasts* are cells which also possess the ability to produce collagen.

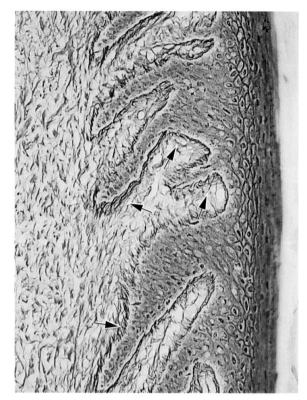

Fig. 1-43.

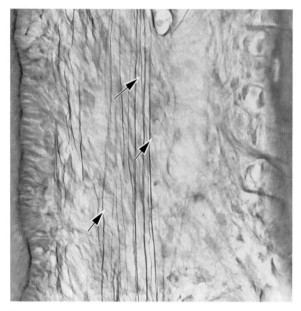

Fig. 1-44.

Fig. 1-43. Reticulin fibers – as seen in this photomicrograph – exhibit argyrophilic staining properties and are numerous in the tissue adjacent to the basement membrane (arrows). However, reticulin fibers also occur in large numbers in the loose connective tissue surrounding the blood vessels. Thus, reticulin fibers are present at the epithelium-connective tissue and the endothelium-connective tissue interfaces.

Fig 1-44. Oxytalan fibers are scarce in the gingiva but numerous in the periodontal ligament. They are composed of long thin fibrils with a diameter of approximately 150 Å. These connective tissue fibers can be demonstrated light microscopically only after previous oxidation with peracetic acid. The photomicrograph illustrates oxytalan fibers (arrows) in the periodontal ligament, where they have a course mainly parallel to the long axis of the tooth. The function of these fibers is as yet unknown. The cementum is seen to the left and the alveolar bone to the right.

Fig. 1-45. Elastic fibers in the connective tissue of the gingiva and periodontal ligament are only present in association with blood vessels. However, as seen in this photomicrograph, the lamina propria and submucosa of the alveolar (lining) mucosa contain numerous elastic fibers (arrows). The gingiva (G) seen coronal to the mucogingival junction (MGJ) contains no elastic fibers except in association with the blood vessels.

Fig. 1-46. Although many of the collagen fibers in the gingiva and the periodontal ligament are irregularly or randomly distributed, most tend to be arranged in groups of bundles with a distinct orientation. According to their insertion and course in the tissue, the oriented bundles in the gingiva can be divided into the following groups:

1. *Circular fibers* (CF) are fiber bundles which run their course in the free gingiva and encircle the tooth in a cuff- or ring-like fashion.
2. *Dentogingival fibers* (DGF) are embedded in the cementum of the supra-alveolar portion of the root and project from the cementum in a fan-like configuration out into the free gingival tissue of the facial, lingual and interproximal surfaces.
3. *Dentoperiosteal fibers* (DPF) are embedded in the same portion of the cementum as the dentogingival fibers, but run their course apically over the vestibular and lingual bone crest and terminate in the tissue of the attached gingiva. In the border area between the free and attached gingiva, the epithelium often lacks support by underlying oriented collagen fiber bundles. In this area the free gingival groove (GG) is often present.
4. *Transseptal fibers* (TF), seen on the drawing to the right, extend between the supra-alveolar cementum of approximating teeth. The transseptal fibers run straight across the interdental septum and are embedded in the cementum of adjacent teeth.

Fig. 1-47 illustrates in a histologic section the orientation of the transseptal fiber bundles (arrows) in the supra-alveolar portion of the interdental area. It should be observed that, besides connecting the cementum (C) of adjacent teeth, the transseptal fibers

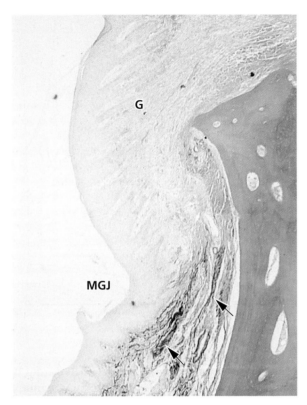

Fig. 1-45.

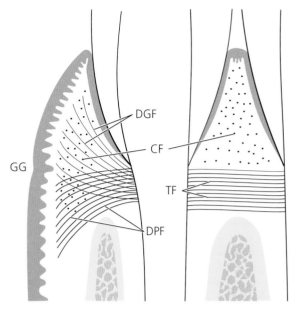

Fig. 1-46.

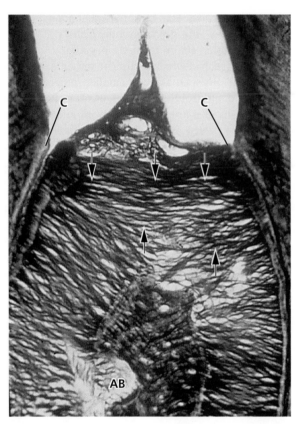

Fig. 1-47.

also connect the supra-alveolar cementum (C) with the crest of the alveolar bone (AB). The four groups of collagen fiber bundles presented in Fig. 1-46 reinforce the gingiva and provide the resilience and tone which is necessary for maintaining its architectural form and the integrity of the dento-gingival attachment.

Matrix
The *matrix* of the connective tissue is produced mainly by the fibroblasts, although some constituents are produced by mast cells, and other components are derived from the blood. The matrix is the medium in which the connective tissue cells are embedded and it is essential for the maintenance of the normal function of the connective tissue. Thus, the transportation of water, electrolytes, nutrients, metabolites, etc., to and from the individual connective tissue cells occurs within the matrix. The main constituents of the connective tissue matrix are protein carbohydrate macromolecules. These complexes are normally divided into *proteoglycans* and *glycoproteins*. The proteoglycans contain *glycosaminoglycans* as the carbohydrate units (hyaluronan sulfate, heparan sulfate, etc.), which, via covalent bonds, are attached to one or more protein chains. The carbohydrate component is always predominant in the proteoglycans. The glycosaminoglycan called hyaluronan or "hyaluronic acid" is probably not bound to protein. The glycoproteins (fibronectin, osteonectin, etc.) also contain polysaccha-

rides, but these macromolecules are different from glycosaminoglycans. The protein component is predominating in glycoproteins. In the macromolecules, mono- or oligosaccharides are, via covalent bonds, connected with one or more protein chains.

Fig. 1-48. Normal function of the connective tissue depends on the presence of proteoglycans and gly-

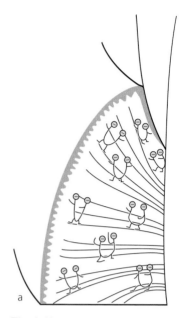
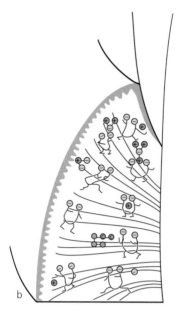
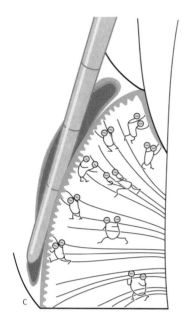

Fig. 1-48.

cosaminoglycans. The carbohydrate moiety of the proteoglycans, the glycosaminoglycans ( ), are large, flexible, chain formed, negatively charged molecules, each of which occupies a rather large space (Fig. 1-48a). In such a space, smaller molecules, e.g. water and electrolytes, can be incorporated while larger molecules are prevented from entering (Fig. 1-48b). The proteoglycans thereby regulate diffusion and fluid flow through the matrix and are important determinants for the fluid content of the tissue and the maintenance of the osmotic pressure. In other words, the proteoglycans act as a molecule filter and, in addition, play an important role in the regulation of cell migration (movements) in the tissue. Due to their structure and hydration, the macromolecules exert resistance towards deformation, thereby serving as regulators of the consistency of the connective tissue (Fig. 1-48c). If the gingiva is suppressed, the macromolecules become deformed. When the pressure is eliminated, the macromolecules regain their original form. Thus, the macromolecules are important for the resilience of the gingiva.

Epithelial mesenchymal interaction

There are many examples of the fact that during the embryonic development of various organs, a mutual inductive influence occurs between the epithelium and the connective tissue. The development of the teeth is a characteristic example of such phenomena. The connective tissue is, on the one hand, a determining factor for normal development of the tooth bud while, on the other, the enamel epithelia exert a definite influence on the development of the mesenchymal components of the teeth.

It has been suggested that tissue differentiation in the adult organism can be influenced by environmental factors. The skin and mucous membranes, for instance, often display increased keratinization and hyperplasia of the epithelium in areas which are exposed to mechanical stimulation. Thus, the tissues seem to adapt to environmental stimuli. The presence of keratinized epithelium on the masticatory mucosa has been considered to represent an adaptation to mechanical irritation released by mastication. However, research has demonstrated that the characteristic

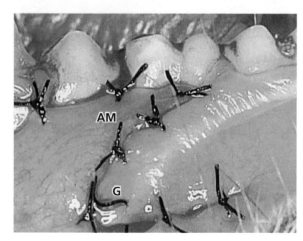

Fig. 1-49.

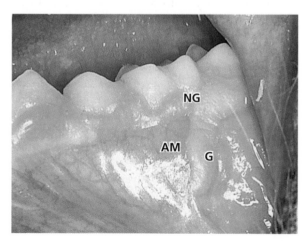

Fig. 1-50.

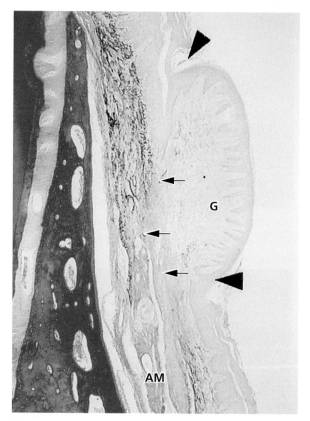

Fig. 1-51.

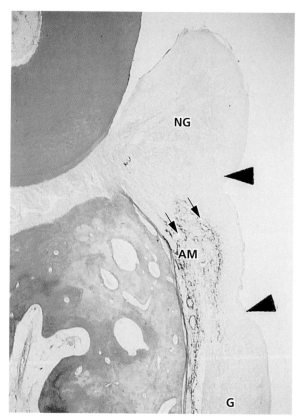

Fig. 1-52.

features of the epithelium in such areas are genetically determined. Some pertinent observations are reported in the following:

Fig. 1-49 shows an area in a monkey where the gingiva (G) and the alveolar mucosa (AM) have been transposed by a surgical procedure. The alveolar mucosa is placed in close contact with the teeth while the gingiva is positioned in the area of the alveolar mucosa.

Fig. 1-50 shows the same area, as seen in Fig. 1-49, 4 months later. Despite the fact that the transplanted gingiva (G) is mobile in relation to the underlying bone, like the alveolar mucosa, it has retained its characteristic, morphologic features of a masticatory mucosa. However, a narrow zone of new keratinized gingiva (NG) has regenerated between the transplanted alveolar mucosa (AM) and the teeth.

Fig. 1-51 presents a histologic section cut through the transplanted gingiva seen in Fig. 1-50. Since elastic fibers are lacking in the gingival connective tissue (G), but are numerous (small arrows) in the connective tissue of the alveolar mucosa (AM), the transplanted gingival tissue can readily be identified. The epithelium covering the transplanted gingival tissue exhibits a distinct keratin layer (between large arrows) on the surface, and also the configuration of the epithelium-connective tissue interface (i.e. rete pegs and connective tissue papillae) is similar to that of normal non-transplanted gingiva. Thus, the heterotopically located gingival tissue has maintained its original

specificity. This observation demonstrates that the characteristics of the gingiva are genetically determined rather than being the result of functional adaptation to environmental stimuli.

Fig. 1-52 shows a histologic section cut through the coronal portion of the area of transplantation (shown in Fig. 1-50). The transplanted gingival tissue (G) shown in Fig. 1-51 can be seen in the lower portion of the photomicrograph. The alveolar mucosa transplant (AM) is seen between the large arrows in the middle of the illustration. After surgery, the alveolar mucosa transplant was positioned in close contact with the teeth as seen in Fig. 1-49. After healing, a narrow zone of keratinized gingiva (NG) developed coronal to the alveolar mucosa transplant (see Fig. 1-50). This new zone of gingiva (NG), which can be seen in the upper portion of the histologic section, is covered by keratinized epithelium and the connective tissue contains no purple-stained elastic fibers. In addition, it is important to notice that the junction between keratinized and non-keratinized epithelium (large arrows) corresponds exactly to the junction between "elastic" and "inelastic" connective tissue (small arrows). The connective tissue of the new gingiva has regenerated from the connective tissue of the supra-alveolar and periodontal ligament compartments and has separated the alveolar mucosal transplant (AM) from the tooth (see Fig. 1-53). However, it is most likely that the epithelium which covers the new gingiva has migrated from the adjacent epithelium of the alveolar mucosa.

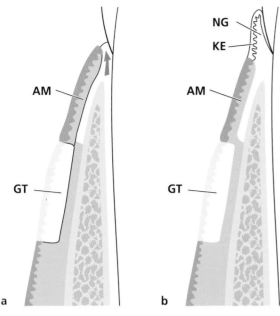

Fig. 1-53.

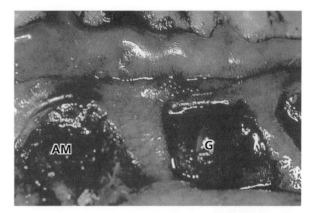

Fig. 1-54.

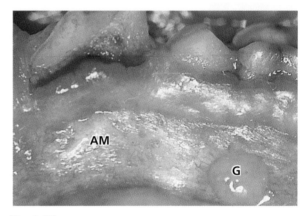

Fig. 1-55.

Fig. 1-53 presents a schematic drawing of the development of the new, narrow zone of keratinized gingiva (NG) seen in Figs. 1-50 and 1-52.

Fig. 1-53a. Granulation tissue has proliferated coronally along the root surface (arrow) and has separated the alveolar mucosa transplant (AM) from its original contact with the tooth surface.

Fig. 1-53b. Epithelial cells have migrated from the alveolar mucosal transplant (AM) onto the newly formed gingival connective tissue (NG). Thus, the newly formed gingiva has become covered with a keratinized epithelium (KE) which has originated from the non-keratinized epithelium of the alveolar mucosa (AM). This implies that the newly formed gingival connective tissue (NG) possesses the ability to induce changes in the differentiation of the epithelium originating from the alveolar mucosa. This epithelium, which is normally non-keratinized, apparently differentiates to keratinized epithelium because of stimuli arising from the newly formed gingival connective tissue (NG). (GT: gingival transplant.)

Fig. 1-54 illustrates a portion of gingival connective tissue (G) and alveolar mucosal connective tissue (AM) which, after transplantation, has healed into wound areas in the alveolar mucosa. Epithelialization of these transplants can only occur through migration of epithelial cells from the surrounding alveolar mucosa.

Fig. 1-55 shows the transplanted gingival connective tissue (G) after re-epithelialization. This tissue portion has attained an appearance similar to that of the normal gingiva, indicating that this connective tissue is now covered by keratinized epithelium. The trans-

planted connective tissue from the alveolar mucosa (AM) is covered by non-keratinized epithelium, and has the same appearance as the surrounding alveolar mucosa.

Fig. 1-56 presents two histologic sections through the area of the transplanted gingival connective tissue. The section shown in Fig. 1-56a is stained for elastic fibers (arrows). The tissue in the middle without elastic fibers is the transplanted gingival connective tissue (G). Fig. 1-56b shows an adjacent section stained with hematoxylin and eosin. By comparing Figs. 1-56a and 1-56b it can be seen that:

1. the transplanted gingival connective tissue is covered by keratinized epithelium (between arrowheads)
2. the epithelium-connective tissue interface has the same wavy course (i.e. rete pegs and connective tissue papillae) as seen in normal gingiva.

The photomicrographs seen in Figs. 1-56c and 1-56d illustrate, at a higher magnification, the border area between the alveolar mucosa (AM) and the transplanted gingival connective tissue (G). Note the distinct relationship between keratinized epithelium (arrow) and "inelastic" connective tissue (arrowheads), and between non-keratinized epithelium and "elas-

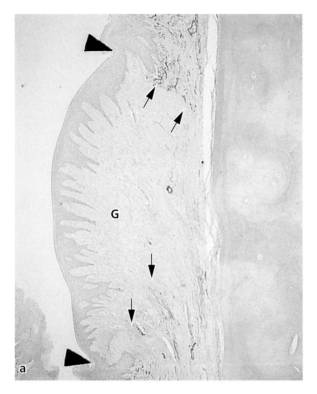

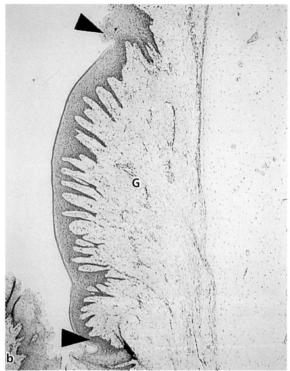

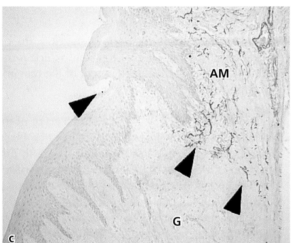

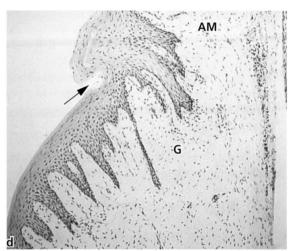

Fig. 1-56.

tic" connective tissue. The establishment of such a close relationship during healing implies that the transplanted gingival connective tissue possesses the ability to alter the differentiation of epithelial cells as previously suggested (Fig. 1-53). From being non-keratinizing cells, the cells of the epithelium of the alveolar mucosa have evidently become keratinizing cells. This means that the specificity of the gingival epithelium is determined by genetic factors inherent in the connective tissue.

PERIODONTAL LIGAMENT

The periodontal ligament is the soft, richly vascular and cellular connective tissue which surrounds the roots of the teeth and joins the root cementum with the

socket wall. In the coronal direction, the periodontal ligament is continuous with the lamina propria of the gingiva and is demarcated from the gingiva by the collagen fiber bundles which connect the alveolar bone crest with the root (the alveolar crest fibers).

Fig. 1-57 is a radiograph of a mandibular premolar-molar region. In radiographs, two types of alveolar bone can be distinguished:

1. The part of the alveolar bone which covers the alveolus, called "lamina dura" (arrows).
2. The portion of the alveolar process which, in the radiograph, has the appearance of a meshwork. This is called the "spongy bone".

The periodontal ligament is situated in the space between the roots (R) of the teeth and the lamina dura or

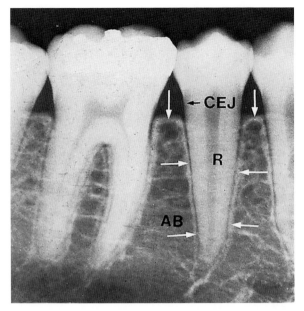

Fig. 1-57.

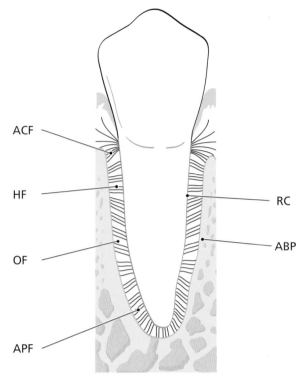

Fig. 1-58.

the alveolar bone proper (arrows). The alveolar bone (AB) surrounds the tooth to a level approximately 1 mm apical to the cemento-enamel junction (CEJ). The coronal border of the bone is called the *alveolar crest* (arrows).

The periodontal ligament space has the shape of an hourglass and is narrowest at the mid-root level. The width of the periodontal ligament is approximately 0.25 mm (range 0.2-0.4 mm). The presence of a periodontal ligament permits forces, elicited during masticatory function and other tooth contacts, to be distributed to and resorbed by the alveolar process via the alveolar bone proper. The periodontal ligament is also essential for the mobility of the teeth. Tooth mobility is to a large extent determined by the width, height and quality of the periodontal ligament (see Chapters 18 and 30).

Fig. 1-58 illustrates in a schematic drawing how the periodontal ligament is situated between the alveolar bone proper (ABP) and the root cementum (RC). The tooth is joined to the bone by bundles of collagen fibers which can be divided into the following main groups according to their arrangement:

1. *alveolar crest fibers* (ACF)
2. *horizontal fibers* (HF)
3. *oblique fibers* (OF)
4. *apical fibers* (APF)

Fig. 1-59. The periodontal ligament and the root cementum develop from the loose connective tissue (the follicle) which surrounds the tooth bud. The sche-

matic drawing depicts the various stages in the organization of the periodontal ligament which forms concomitantly with the development of the root and the eruption of the tooth.

Fig. 1-59a. The tooth bud is formed in a crypt of the bone. The collagen fibers produced by the fibroblasts in the loose connective tissue around the tooth bud are, during the process of their maturation, embedded into the newly formed cementum immediately apical to the cemento-enamel junction (CEJ). These fiber bundles oriented towards the coronal portion of the bone crypt will later form the dentogingival fiber group, the dentoperiosteal fiber group and the transseptal fiber group which belong to the oriented fibers of the gingiva (see Fig. 1-46).

Fig. 1-59b. The true periodontal ligament fibers, the *principal fibers*, develop in conjunction with the eruption of the tooth. First, fibers can be identified entering the most marginal portion of the alveolar bone.

Fig. 1-59c. Later, more apically positioned bundles of oriented collagen fibers are seen.

Fig. 1-59d. The orientation of the collagen fiber bundles alters continuously during the phase of tooth eruption. First, when the tooth has reached contact in

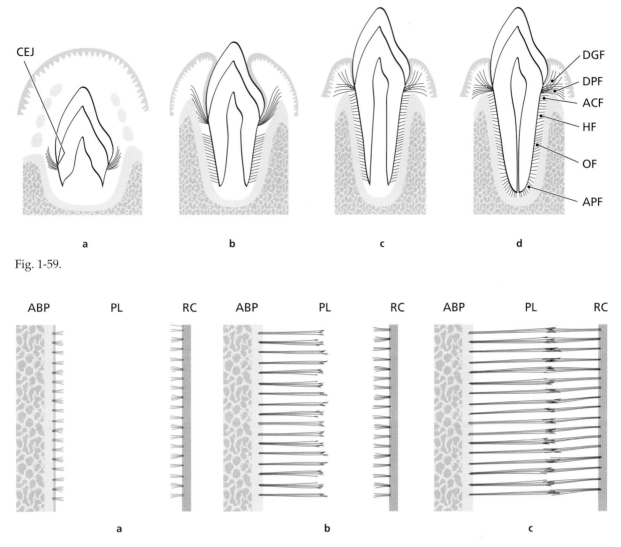

Fig. 1-59.

Fig. 1-60.

occlusion and is functioning properly, the fibers of the periodontal ligament associate into groups of well-oriented dentoalveolar collagen fibers demonstrated in Fig. 1-58. These collagen structures undergo constant remodeling (i.e. resorption of old fibers and formation of new ones).

Fig. 1-60. This schematic drawing illustrates the development of the principal fibers of the periodontal ligament. The alveolar bone proper (ABP) is seen to the left, the periodontal ligament (PL) is depicted in the center and the root cementum (RC) is seen to the right.

Fig. 1-60a. First, small, fine, brush-like fibrils are detected arising from the root cementum and projecting into the PL space. The surface of the bone is, at this stage, covered by osteoblasts. From the surface of the bone only a small number of radiating, thin collagen fibrils can be seen.

Fig. 1-60b. Later on, the number and thickness of fibers entering the bone increase. These fibers radiate towards the loose connective tissue in the mid-portion of the periodontal ligament area (PL), which contains more or less randomly oriented collagen fibrils. The fibers originating from the cementum are still short while those entering the bone gradually become longer. The terminal portions of these fibers carry finger-like projections.

Fig. 1-60c. The fibers originating from the cementum subsequently increase in length and thickness and fuse in the periodontal ligament space with the fibers originating from the alveolar bone. When the tooth, following eruption, reaches contact in occlusion and starts to function, the principal fibers become organized in bundles and run continuously from the bone to the cementum.

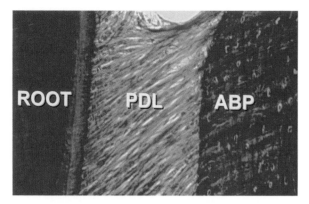

Fig. 1-61a.

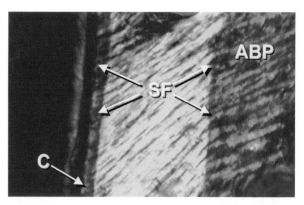

Fig. 1-61b.

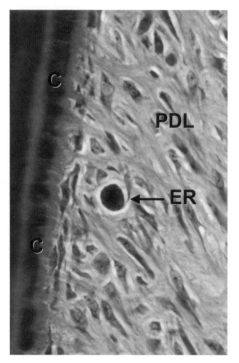

Fig. 1-62a.

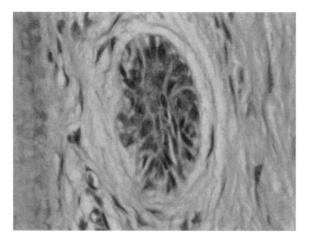

Fig. 1-62b.

Fig. 1-61a illustrates how the principal fibers of the periodontal ligament (PDL) run continuously from the root cementum to the alveolar bone proper (ABP). The principal fibers embedded in the cementum

(Sharpey's fibers) have a smaller diameter but are more numerous than those embedded in the alveolar bone proper (Sharpey's fibers).

Fig. 1-61b presents a polarized version of Fig. 1-61a. In this illustration the Sharpey's fibers (SF) can be seen penetrating not only the cementum (C) but also the entire width of the alveolar bone proper (ABP). The periodontal ligament also contains a few elastic fibers associated with the blood vessels. Oxytalan fibers (see Fig. 1-44) are also present in the periodontal ligament. They have a mainly apico-occlusal orientation and are located in the ligament closer to the tooth than to the alveolar bone. Very often they insert into the cementum. Their function has not been determined.

The cells of the periodontal ligament are: *fibroblasts, osteoblasts, cementoblasts, osteoclasts,* as well as *epithelial cells* and *nerve fibers*. The fibroblasts are aligned along the principal fibers, while cementoblasts line the surface of the cementum, and the osteoblasts line the bone surface.

Fig. 1-62a shows the presence of clusters of epithelial cells (ER) in the periodontal ligament (PDL). These cells, called the *epithelial cell rests of Mallassez*, represent remnants of the Hertwig's epithelial root sheath. The epithelial cell rests are situated in the periodontal ligament at a distance of 15-75 μm from the cementum (C) on the root surface. A group of such epithelial cell rests is seen in a higher magnification in Fig. 1-62b.

Fig. 1-63. Electron microscopically it can be seen that the epithelial cell rests are surrounded by a basement membrane (BM) and that the cell membranes of the epithelial cells exhibit the presence of desmosomes (D) as well as hemidesmosomes (HD). The epithelial cells contain only few mitochondria and have a poorly developed endoplasmic reticulum. This means that they are vital, but resting, cells with minute metabolism.

Fig. 1-64 is a photomicrograph of a periodontal ligament removed from an extracted tooth. This specimen prepared tangential to the root surface shows that the epithelial cell rests of Mallassez, which in ordinary

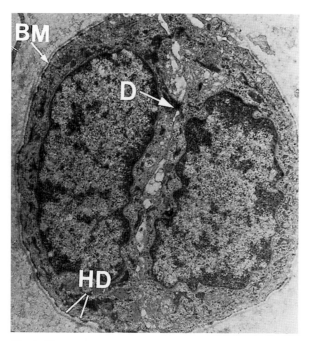

Fig. 1-63.

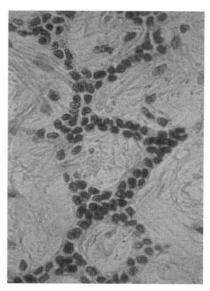

Fig. 1-64.

histologic sections appear as isolated groups of epithelial cells, in fact form a continuous network of epithelial cells surrounding the root. Their function is at present unknown.

ROOT CEMENTUM

The cementum is a specialized mineralized tissue covering the root surfaces and, occasionally, small portions of the crown of the teeth. It has many features in common with bone tissue. However, the cementum contains no blood or lymph vessels, has no innervation, does not undergo physiologic resorption or remodeling, but is characterized by continuing deposition throughout life. Like other mineralized tissues, it contains collagen fibers embedded in an organic matrix. Its mineral content, which is mainly hydroxyapatite, is about 65% by weight; a little more than that of bone (i.e. 60%). Cementum serves different functions. It attaches the periodontal ligament fibers to the root and contributes to the process of repair after damage to the root surface.

Different forms of cementum have been described:

1. *Acellular, extrinsic fiber cementum* (AEFC) is found in the coronal and middle portions of the root and contains mainly bundles of Sharpey's fibers. This type of cementum is an important part of the attachment apparatus and connects the tooth with the alveolar bone proper.
2. *Cellular, mixed stratified cementum* (CMSC) occurs in the apical third of the roots and in the furcations. It contains both extrinsic and intrinsic fibers as well as cementocytes.
3. *Cellular, intrinsic fiber cementum* (CIFC) is found mainly in resorption lacunae and it contains intrinsic fibers and cementocytes.

Fig. 1-65a shows a portion of a root with adjacent periodontal ligament (PDL). A thin layer of acellular, extrinsic fiber cementum (AEFC) with densely packed extrinsic fibers covers the peripheral dentin. Cementoblasts and fibroblasts can be observed adjacent to the cementum.

Fig. 1-65b represents a scanning electron micrograph of AEFC. Note that the extrinsic fibers attach to the dentin (left) and are continous with the collagen fiber bundles (CB) of the periodontal ligament (PDL). The

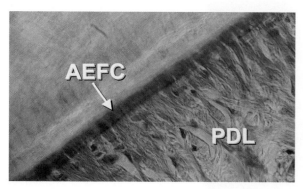

Fig. 1-65a.

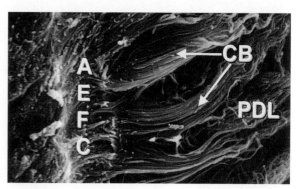

Fig. 1-65b.

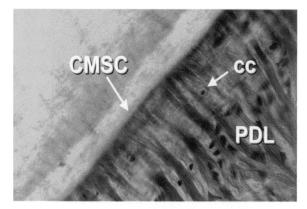

Fig. 1-66.

AEFC is formed concomitantly with the formation of the root dentin. At a certain stage during tooth formation, the epithelial sheath of Hertwig, which lines the newly formed predentin, is fragmented. Cells from the dental follicle then penetrate the epithelial sheath of Hertwig and occupy the area next to the predentin. In this position, the ectomesenchymal cells from the dental follicle differentiate into cementoblasts and begin to produce collagen fibers at right angles to the surface. The first cementum is deposited on the highly mineralized superficial layer of the mantle dentin called the "hyaline layer" which contains enamel matrix proteins and the initial collagen fibers of the cementum. Subsequently, cementoblasts drift away from the surface resulting in increased thickness of the cementum and incorporation of principal fibers.

Fig. 1-66 demonstrates the structure of cellular, mixed stratified cementum (CMSC) which, in contrast to AEFC, contains cells and intrinsic fibers. The CMSC is laid down throughout the functional period of the

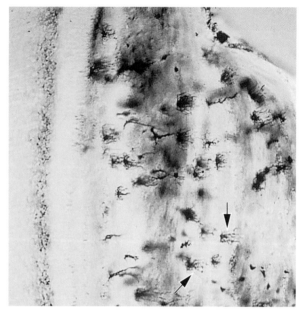

Fig. 1-67.

tooth. The various types of cementum are produced by cementoblasts or periodontal ligament (PDL) cells lining the cementum surface. Some of these cells become incorporated into the cementoid, which subsequently mineralizes to form cementum. The cells which are incorporated in the cementum are called *cementocytes* (CC).

Fig. 1-67 illustrates how cementocytes (black cells) reside in lacunae in CMSC or CIFC. They communicate with each other through a network of cytoplasmic processes (arrows) running in canaliculi in the cementum. The cementocytes also, through cytoplasmic processes, communicate with the cementoblasts on

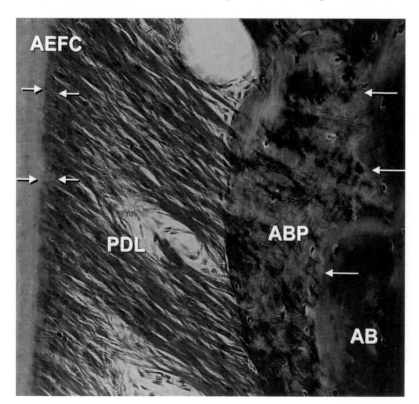

Fig. 1-68a.

the surface. The presence of cementocytes allows transportation of nutrients through the cementum, and contributes to the maintenance of the vitality of this mineralized tissue.

Fig. 1-68a is a photomicrograph of a section through the periodontal ligament (PDL) in an area where the root is covered with acellular, extrinsic fiber cementum (AEFC). The portions of the principal fibers of the periodontal ligament which are embedded in the root cementum (arrows) and in the alveolar bone proper (ABP) are called *Sharpey's fibers*. The arrows to the right indicate the border between ABP and the alveolar bone (AB). In AEFC the Sharpey's fibers have a smaller diameter and are more densely packed than their counterparts in the alveolar bone. During the continuous formation of AEFC, portions of the periodontal ligament fibers (principal fibers) adjacent to the root become embedded in the mineralized tissue. Thus, the Sharpey's fibers in the cementum are a direct continuation of the principal fibers in the periodontal ligament and the supra-alveolar connective tissue.

Fig. 1-68b. The Sharpey's fibers constitute the *extrinsic fiber system* (E) of the cementum and are produced by fibroblasts in the periodontal ligament. The *intrinsic fiber system* (I) is produced by cementoblasts and is composed of fibers oriented more or less parallel to the long axis of the root.

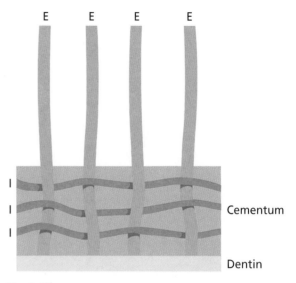

Fig. 1-68b.

Fig. 1-69 shows extrinsic fibers penetrating acellular, extrinsic fiber cementum (AEFC). The characteristic crossbanding of the collagen fibers is masked in the cementum because apatite crystals have become deposited in the fiber bundles during the process of mineralization.

Fig. 1-70. In contrast to the bone, the cementum (C) does not exhibit alternating periods of resorption and apposition, but increases in thickness throughout life by deposition of successive new layers. During this

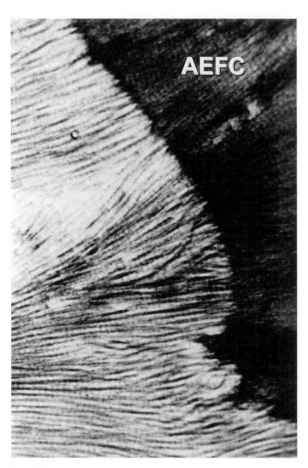

Fig. 1-69.

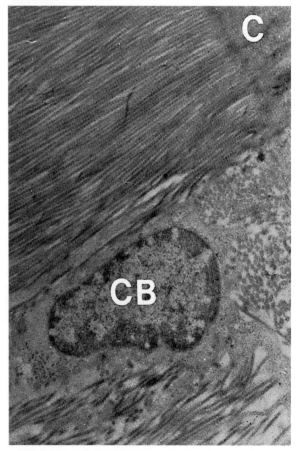

Fig. 1-70.

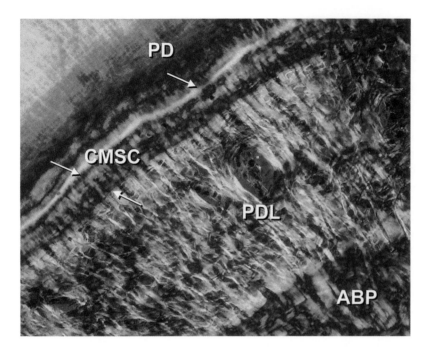

Fig. 1-71.

process of gradual apposition, the particular portion of the principal fibers which resides immediately adjacent to the root surface becomes mineralized. Mineralization occurs by the deposition of hydroxyapatite crystals, first within the collagen fibers, later upon the fiber surface and finally in the interfibrillar matrix. The electronphotomicrograph shows a cementoblast (CB) located near the surface of the cementum (C) and between two inserting principal fiber bundles. Generally, the AEFC is more mineralized than CMSC and CIFC. Sometimes only the periphery of the Sharpey's fibers of the CMSC is mineralized, leaving an unmineralized core within the fiber.

Fig. 1-71 is a photomicrograph of the periodontal ligament (PDL) which resides between the cementum (CMSC) and the alveolar bone proper (ABP). The CMSC is densely packed with collagen fibers oriented parallel to the root surface (intrinsic fibers) and Sharpey's fibers (extrinsic fibers), oriented more or less perpendicularly to the cementum-dentine junction (predentin (PD)). The various types of cementum increase in thickness by gradual apposition throughout life. The cementum becomes considerably wider in the apical portion of the root than in the cervical portion, where the thickness is only 20-50 μm. In the apical root portion the cementum is often 150-250 μm wide. The cementum often contains incremental lines indicating alternating periods of formation. The CMSC is formed after the termination of tooth eruption, and after a response to functional demands.

ALVEOLAR BONE

The alveolar process is defined as the parts of the maxilla and the mandible that form and support the sockets of the teeth. The alveolar process develops in conjunction with the development and eruption of the teeth. The alveolar process consists of bone which is formed both by cells from the dental follicle (alveolar bone proper) and cells which are independent of tooth development. Together with the root cementum and the periodontal membrane, the alveolar bone constitutes the attachment apparatus of the teeth, the main function of which is to distribute and resorb forces generated by, for example, mastication and other tooth contacts.

Fig. 1-72 illustrates a cross-section through the alveolar process (pars alveolaris) of the maxilla at the midroot level of the teeth. Note that the bone which covers the root surfaces is considerably thicker at the palatal than at the buccal aspect of the jaw. The walls of the sockets are lined by *cortical bone* (arrows), and the area between the sockets and between the compact jaw bone walls is occupied by *cancellous bone*. The cancellous bone occupies most of the interdental septa but only a relatively small portion of the buccal and palatal bone plates. The cancellous bone contains *bone trabeculae*, the architecture and size of which are partly genetically determined and partly the result of the forces to which the teeth are exposed during function. Note how the bone on the buccal and palatal aspects of the alveolar process varies in thickness from one region to another. The bone plate is thick at the palatal aspect and on the buccal aspect of the molars but thin in the buccal anterior region.

Fig. 1-73 shows cross-sections through the mandibular alveolar process at levels corresponding to the coronal (Fig. 1-73a) and apical (Fig. 1-73b) thirds of the roots. The bone lining the wall of the sockets (alveolar bone proper) is often continuous with the compact or cortical bone at the lingual (L) and buccal (B) aspects of the

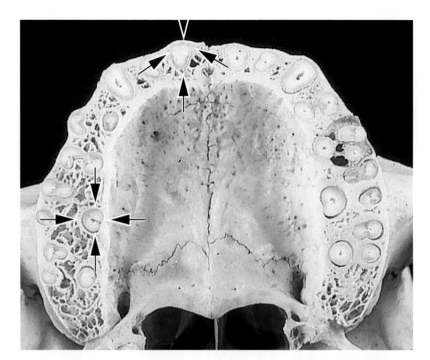

Fig. 1-72.

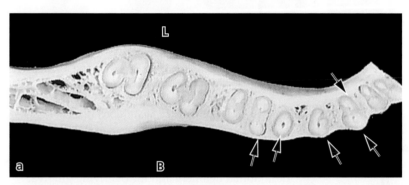

Fig. 1-73.

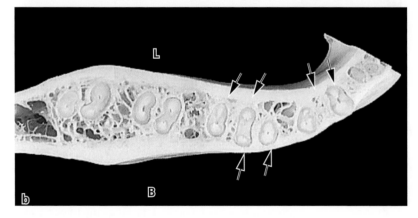

alveolar process (arrows). Note how the bone on the buccal and lingual aspects of the alveolar process varies in thickness from one region to another. In the incisor and premolar regions, the bone plate at the buccal aspects of the teeth is considerably thinner than

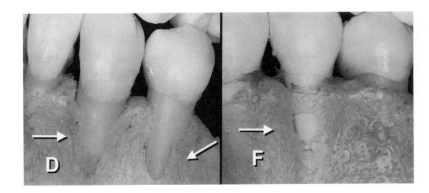

Fig. 1-74.

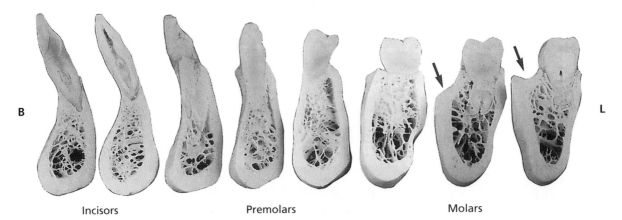

Incisors   Premolars   Molars

Fig. 1-75.

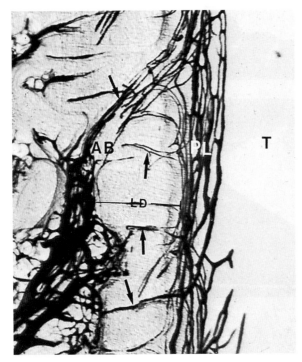

Fig. 1-76.

at the lingual aspect. In the molar region, the bone is thicker at the buccal than at the lingual surfaces.

Fig. 1-74. At the buccal aspect of the jaws, the bone coverage is sometimes missing at the coronal portion of the roots, forming a so-called *dehiscence* (D). If some bone is present in the most coronal portion of such an area the defect is called a *fenestration* (F). These defects often occur where a tooth is displaced out of the arch and are more frequent over anterior than posterior teeth. The root in such defects is covered only by periodontal ligament and the overlying gingiva.

Fig. 1-75 presents vertical sections through various regions of the mandibular dentition. The bone wall at the buccal (B) and lingual (L) aspects of the teeth varies considerably in thickness, e.g. from the premolar to the molar region. Note, for instance, how the presence of the oblique line (*linea obliqua*) results in a shelf-like bone process (arrows) at the buccal aspect of the second and third molars.

Fig. 1-76 shows a section through the periodontal ligament (PL), tooth (T), and the alveolar bone (AB). The blood vessels in the periodontal ligament and the alveolar bone appear black because the blood system was perfused with ink. The compact bone (alveolar bone proper) which lines the tooth socket, and in a radiograph (Fig. 1-57) appears as "lamina dura" (LD), is perforated by numerous *Volkmann's canals* (arrows) through which blood vessels, lymphatics, and nerve fibers pass from the alveolar bone (AB) to the periodontal ligament (PL). This layer of bone into which the principal fibers are inserted (Sharpey's fibers) is sometimes called "bundle bone". From a functional and structural point of view, this "bundle bone" has many features in common with the cementum layer on the root surfaces.

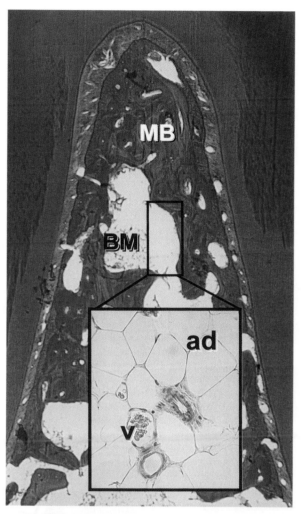

Fig. 1-77.

Fig. 1-77. The alveolar process starts to form early in fetal life, with mineral deposition at small foci in the mesenchymal matrix surrounding the tooth buds. These small mineralized areas increase in size, fuse, and become resorbed and remodeled until a continuous mass of bone has formed around the fully erupted teeth. The mineral content of bone, which is mainly hydroxyapatite, is about 60% on a weight basis. The photomicrograph illustrates the bone tissue within the furcation area of a mandibular molar. The bone tissue can be divided into two compartments: mineralized bone (MB) and bone marrow (BM). The mineralized bone is made up of lamellae – lamellar bone – while the bone marrow contains adipocytes (ad), vascular structures (v), and undifferentiated mesenchymal cells (see insertion).

Fig. 1-78. The mineralized, lamellar bone includes two types of bone tissue: the bone of the alveolar process (AB) and the alveolar bone proper (ABP), which covers the alveolus. The ABP or the bundle bone has a varying width and is indicated with white arrows. The alveolar bone (AB) is a tissue of mesenchymal origin and it is not considered as part of the genuine attachment apparatus. The alveolar bone proper (ABP), on the other hand, together with the periodontal ligament (PDL) and the cementum (C) is responsible for the attachment between the tooth and the skeleton. AB and ABP may, as a result of altered functional demands, undergo adaptive changes.

Fig. 1-79 describes a portion of lamellar bone. The lamellar bone at this site contains *osteons* (white cir-

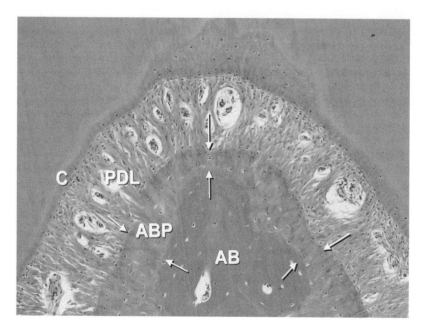

Fig. 1-78.

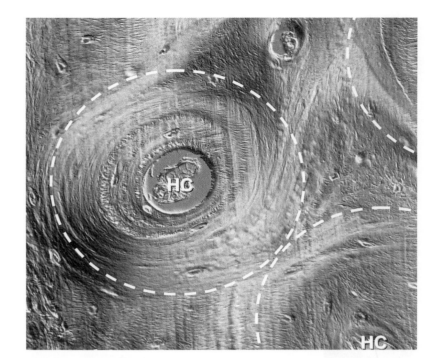

Fig. 1-79.

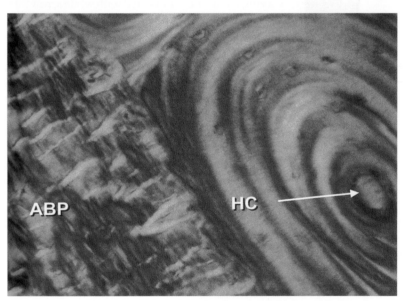

Fig. 1-80a.

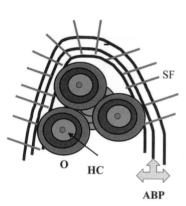

Fig. 1-80b.

cles) each of which harbors a blood vessel located in a Haversian canal (HC). The blood vessel is surrounded by concentric, mineralized lamellae to form the osteon. The space between the different osteons is filled with so-called interstitial lamellae. The osteons in the lamellar bone are not only structural units but also metabolic units. Thus, the nutrition of the bone is secured by the blood vessels in the Haversian canals and connecting vessels in the Volkmann canals.

Fig. 1-80. The histologic section (Fig. 1-80a) shows the borderline between the alveolar bone proper (ABP) and lamellar bone with an osteon. Note the presence of the Haversian canal (HC) in the center of the osteon.

The alveolar bone proper (ABP) includes circumferential lamella and contains Sharpey's fibers which extend into the periodontal ligament. The schematic drawing (Fig. 1-80b) is illustrating three active osteons (brown) with a blood vessel (red) in the Haversian canal (HC). Interstitial lamella (green) is located between the osteons (O) and represents an old and partly remodelled osteon. The alveolar bone proper (ABP) is presented by the dark lines into which the Sharpey's fibers (SF) insert.

Fig. 1-81 illustrates an osteon with osteocytes (OC) residing in osteocyte lacunae in the lamellar bone. The osteocytes connect via canaliculi (can) which contain

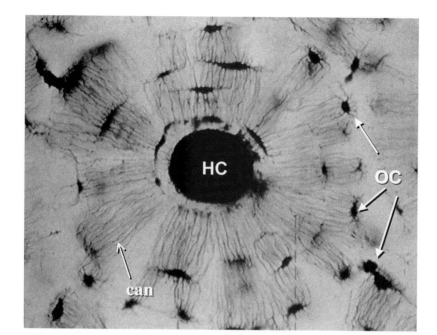

Fig. 1-81.

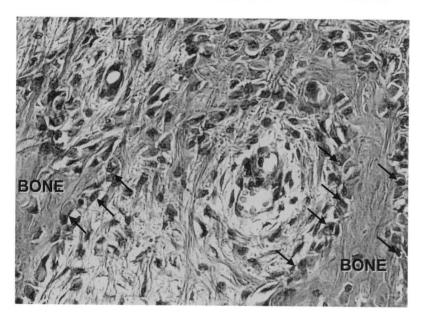

Fig. 1-82.

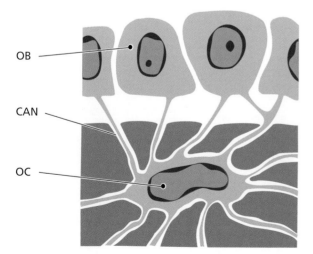

Fig. 1-83.

cytoplasmatic projections of the osteocytes. A Haversian canal (HC) is seen in the middle of the osteon.

Fig. 1-82 illustrates an area of the alveolar bone in which bone formation occurs. The osteoblasts (arrows), the bone-forming cells, are producing bone matrix (osteoid) consisting of collagen fibers, glycoproteins and proteoglycans. The bone matrix or the osteoid undergoes mineralization by the deposition of minerals such as calcium and phosphate, which are subsequently transformed into hydroxyapatite.

Fig. 1-83. The drawing illustrates how osteocytes, present in the mineralized bone, communicate with osteoblasts on the bone surface through canaliculi.

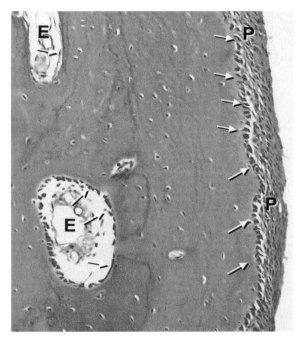

Fig. 1-84.

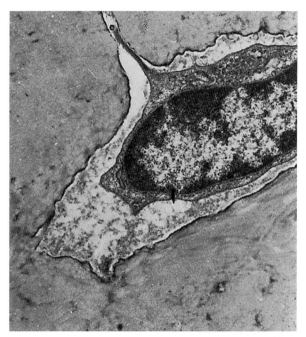

Fig. 1-85.

Fig. 1-84. All active bone forming sites harbor osteoblasts. The outer surface of the bone is lined by a layer of such osteoblasts which, in turn, are organized in a periosteum (P) that contains densely packed collagen fibers. On the "inner surface" of the bone, i.e. in the bone marrow space, there is an endosteum (E), which presents similar features as the periosteum.

Fig. 1-85 illustrates an osteocyte residing in a lacuna in the bone. It can be seen that cytoplasmic processes radiate in different directions.

Fig. 1-86 illustrates osteocytes (OC) and how their long and delicate cytoplasmic processes communicate through the canaliculi (CAN) in the bone. The resulting canalicular-lacunar system is essential for cell metabolism by allowing diffusion of nutrients and waste products. The surface between the osteocytes with their cytoplasmic processes on the one side, and the mineralized matrix on the other, is very large. It has

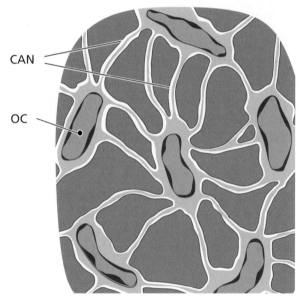

Fig. 1-86.

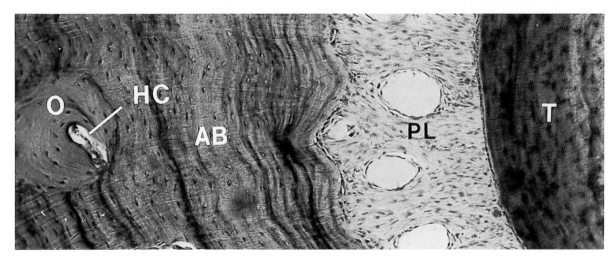

Fig. 1-87.

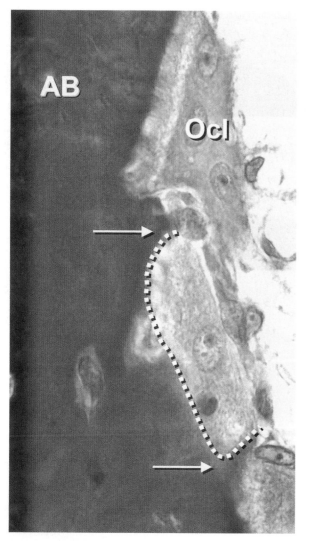

Fig. 1-88.

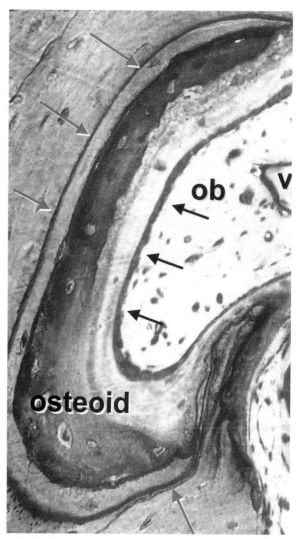

Fig. 1-89.

been calculated that the interface between cells and matrix in a cube of bone, $10 \times 10 \times 10$ cm, amounts to approximately 250 m^2. This enormous surface of exchange serves as a regulator, e.g. for the serum calcium and the serum phosphate levels via hormonal control mechanisms.

Fig. 1-87. The alveolar bone is constantly renewed in response to functional demands. The teeth erupt and migrate in a mesial direction throughout life to compensate for attrition. Such movement of the teeth implies remodelling of the alveolar bone. During the process of remodelling, the bone trabeculae are continuously resorbed and reformed and the cortical bone mass is dissolved and replaced by new bone. During breakdown of the cortical bone, resorption canals are formed by proliferating blood vessels. Such canals, which in their center contain a blood vessel, are subsequently refilled with new bone by the formation of lamellae arranged in concentric layers around the blood vessel. A new Haversian system (O) is seen in the photomicrograph of a horizontal section through the alveolar bone (AB), periodontal ligament (PL) and tooth (T).

Fig. 1-88. The resorption of bone is always associated with *osteoclasts* (Ocl). These cells are giant cells specialized in the breakdown of mineralized matrix (bone, dentin, cementum) and are probably developed from blood monocytes. The resorption occurs by the release of acid substances (lactic acid, etc.) which forms an acidic environment in which the mineral salts of the bone tissue become dissolved. Remaining organic substances are eliminated by enzymes and osteoclastic phagocytosis. Actively resorbing osteoclasts adhere to the bone surface and produce lacunar pits called *Howship's lacunae* (dotted line). They are mobile and capable of migrating over the bone surface. The photomicrograph demonstrates osteoclastic activity at the surface of alveolar bone (AB).

Fig. 1-89 illustrates a so-called bone multicellular unit (BMU), which is present in bone tissue undergoing active remodeling. The reversal line, indicated by red arrows, demonstrates to which level bone resorption has occurred. From the reversal line new bone has started to form and has the character of osteoid. Note the presence of osteoblasts (ob) and vascular structures (v). The osteoclasts resorb organic as well as inorganic substances.

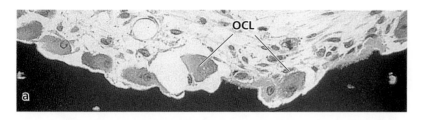

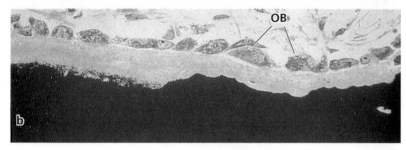

Fig. 1-90.

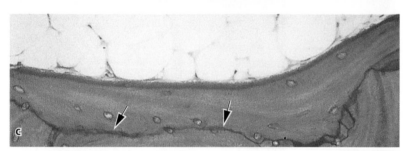

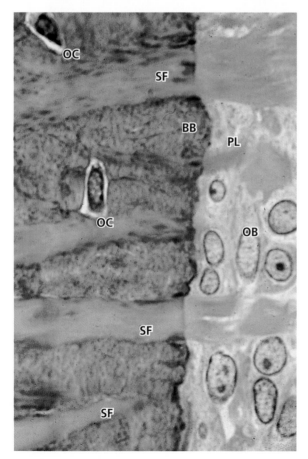

Fig. 1-91.

Fig. 1-90. Both the cortical and cancellous alveolar bone are constantly undergoing remodeling (i.e. re-sorption followed by formation) in response to tooth drifting and changes in functional forces acting on the teeth. Remodeling of the trabecular bone starts with resorption of the bone surface by osteoclasts (OCL) as seen in Fig. 1-90a. After a short period, osteoblasts (OB) start depositing new bone (Fig. 1-90b) and finally a new bone multicellular unit is formed, clearly deli-neated by a reversal line (arrows) as seen in Fig. 1-90c.

Fig. 1-91. Collagen fibers of the periodontal ligament (PL) are inserting in the mineralized bone which lines the wall of the tooth socket. This bone, which as previously described is called alveolar bone proper or bundle bone (BB), has a high turnover rate. The por-tions of the collagen fibers which are inserted inside the bundle bone are called Sharpey's fibers (SF). These fibers are mineralized at their periphery, but often have a non-mineralized central core. The collagen fiber bundles inserting in the bundle bone generally have a larger diameter and are less numerous than the corresponding fiber bundles in the cementum on the opposite side of the periodontal ligament. Individual bundles of fibers can be followed all the way from the alveolar bone to the cementum. However, despite being in the same bundle of fibers, the collagen adja-cent to the bone is always less mature than that adja-cent to the cementum. The collagen on the tooth side has a low turnover rate. Thus, while the collagen adjacent to the bone is renewed relatively rapidly, the collagen adjacent to the root surface is renewed slowly or not at all. Note the occurrence of osteoblasts (OB) and osteocytes (OC).

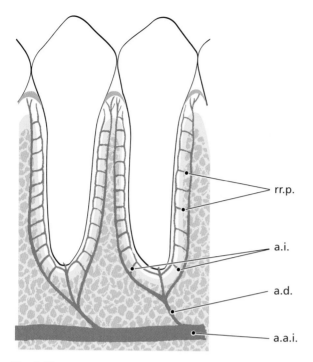

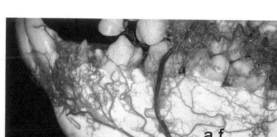

Fig. 1-92.

Fig. 1-93.

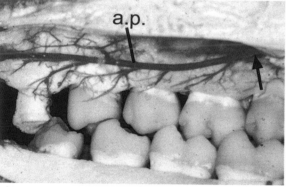

Fig. 1-94.

Fig. 1-95.

Blood supply of the periodontium

Fig. 1-92. The schematic drawing depicts the blood supply to the teeth and the periodontal tissues. The *dental artery* (a.d.), which is a branch of the *superior* or *inferior* alveolar artery (a.a.i.), dismisses the *intraseptal artery* (a.i.) before it enters the tooth socket. The terminal branches of the *intraseptal artery* (*rami perforantes*, rr.p.) penetrate the alveolar bone proper in canals at all levels of the socket (see Fig. 1-76). They anastomose in the periodontal ligament space, together with blood vessels originating from the apical portion of the periodontal ligament and with other terminal branches, from the intraseptal artery (a.i.). Before the dental artery (a.d.) enters the root canal it puts out branches which supply the apical portion of the periodontal ligament.

Fig. 1-93. The gingiva receives its blood supply mainly

through *supraperiosteal* blood vessels which are terminal branches of the *sublingual artery* (a.s.), the *mental artery* (a.m.), the *buccal artery* (a.b.), the *facial artery* (a.f.), the *greater palatine artery* (a.p.), the *infra orbital artery* (a.i.) and the *posterior superior dental artery* (a.ap.).

Fig. 1-94 depicts the course of the greater palatine artery (a.p.) in a specimen of a monkey which at sacrifice was perfused with plastic. Subsequently, the soft tissue was dissolved. The greater palatine artery (a.p.), which is a terminal branch of the *ascending palatine artery* (from the *maxillary*, "internal maxillary", artery), runs through the *greater palatine canal* (arrow) to the palate. As this artery runs in a frontal direction it puts out branches which supply the gingiva and the masticatory mucosa of the palate.

Fig. 1-95. The various arteries are often considered to supply certain well-defined regions of the dentition. In reality, however, there are numerous anastomoses

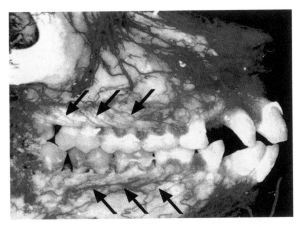

Fig. 1-96.

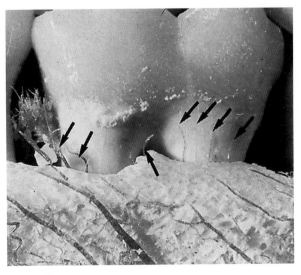

Fig. 1-97.

present between the different arteries. Thus, the *entire system of blood vessels*, rather than individual groups of vessels, should be regarded as the unit supplying the soft and hard tissue of the maxilla and the mandible, e.g. in this figure there is an anastomosis (arrow) between the *facial artery* (a.f.) and the blood vessels of the mandible.

Fig. 1-96 illustrates a vestibular segment of the maxilla and mandible from a monkey which at sacrifice was perfused with plastic. Notice that the vestibular gingiva is supplied with blood mainly through *supraperiosteal* blood vessels (arrows).

Fig. 1-97. As can be seen, blood vessels (arrows) origi-

nating from vessels in the periodontal ligament are passing the alveolar bone crest and contribute to the blood supply of the free gingiva.

Fig. 1-98 shows a specimen from a monkey which at the time of sacrifice was perfused with ink. Subsequently, the specimen was treated to make the tissue transparent (cleared specimen). To the right, the supraperiosteal blood vessels (sv) can be seen. During their course towards the free gingiva they put forth numerous branches to the *subepithelial plexus* (sp) located immediately beneath the oral epithelium of the

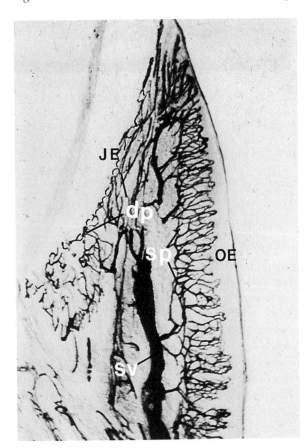

Fig. 1-98.

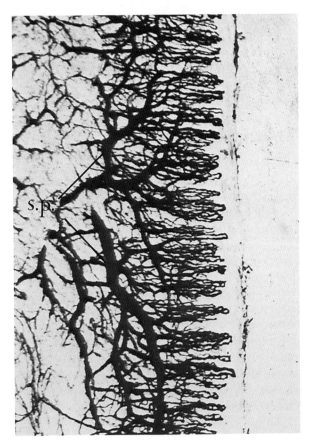

Fig. 1-99.

free and attached gingiva. This subepithelial plexus in turn yields thin *capillary loops* to each of the connective tissue papillae projecting into the oral epithelium (OE). The number of such capillary loops is constant over a very long time and is not altered by application of epinephrine or histamine to the gingival margin. This implies that the blood vessels of the lateral portions of the gingiva, even under normal circumstances, are fully utilized and that the blood flow to the free gingiva is regulated entirely by velocity alterations. In the free gingiva, the supraperiosteal blood vessels (sv) anastomose with blood vessels from the periodontal ligament and the bone. Beneath the junctional epithelium (JE) seen to the left, is a plexus of blood vessels termed the *dentogingival plexus* (dp). The blood vessels in this plexus have a thickness of approximately 40 μm, which means that they are mainly venules. In healthy gingiva, no capillary loops occur in the dentogingival plexus.

Fig. 1-99. This specimen illustrates how the subepithelial plexus (sp), beneath the oral epithelium of the free and attached gingiva, yields thin capillary loops to each connective tissue papilla. These capillary loops have a diameter of approximately 7 μm, which means they are the size of true capillaries.

Fig. 1-100 illustrates the dentogingival plexus in a section cut parallel to the subsurface of the junctional epithelium. As can be seen, the dentogingival plexus consists of a fine-meshed network of blood vessels. In the upper portion of the picture, capillary loops can be detected belonging to the subepithelial plexus beneath the oral sulcular epithelium.

Fig. 1-101 is a schematic drawing of the blood supply to the free gingiva. As stated above, the main blood supply of the free gingiva derives from the *supraperiosteal* blood vessels (SV) which, in the gingiva, anastomose with blood vessels from the *alveolar bone* (ab) and *periodontal ligament* (pl). To the right in the drawing, the oral epithelium (OE) is depicted with its underlying subepithelial plexus of vessels (sp). To the left beneath the junctional epithelium (JE), the dentogingival plexus (dp) can be seen, which, under normal conditions, comprises a fine-meshed network without capillary loops.

Fig. 1-102 shows a section prepared through a tooth (T) with its periodontium. Blood vessels (perforating

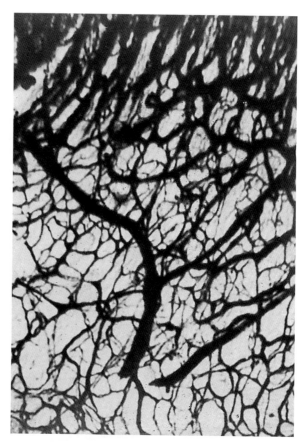

Fig. 1-100.

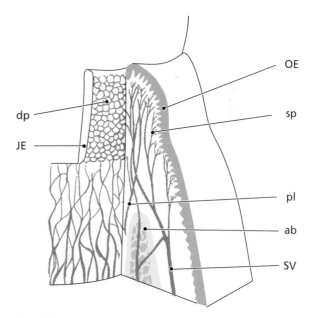

Fig. 1-101.

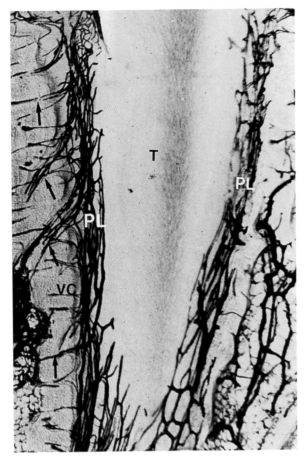

Fig. 1-102.

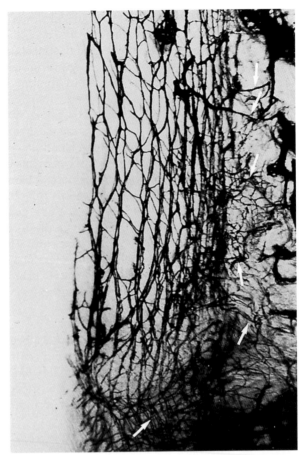

Fig. 1-103.

rami; arrows) arising from the intraseptal artery in the alveolar bone run through canals (Volkmann's canals) in the socket wall (VC) into the periodontal ligament (PL), where they anastomose.

Fig. 1-103 shows blood vessels in the periodontal ligament in a section cut parallel to the root surface. After entering the periodontal ligament, the blood vessels (perforating rami; arrows) anastomose and form a polyhedral network which surrounds the root like a stocking. The majority of the blood vessels in the periodontal ligament are found close to the alveolar bone. In the coronal portion of the periodontal ligament, blood vessels run in coronal direction, passing the alveolar bone crest, into the free gingiva (see Fig. 1-97).

Fig. 1-104 is a schematic drawing of the blood supply of the periodontium. The blood vessels in the periodontal ligament form a polyhedral network surrounding the root. Note that the free gingiva receives its blood supply from (1) supraperiosteal blood vessels, (2) the blood vessels of the periodontal ligament and (3) the blood vessels of the alveolar bone.

Fig. 1-105 illustrates schematically the so-called *extravascular* circulation through which nutrients and other substances are carried to the individual cells and metabolic waste products are removed from the tissue. In the arterial (A) end of the capillary, to the left in the drawing, a hydraulic pressure of approximately 35 mm Hg is maintained as a result of the pumping function of the heart. Since the hydraulic pressure is higher than the osmotic pressure (OP) in the tissue (which is approximately 30 mm Hg), a transportation of substances will occur from the blood vessels to the extravascular space (ES). In the venous (V) end of the capillary system, to the right in the drawing, the hydraulic pressure has decreased to approximately 25 mm Hg (i.e. 5 mm lower than the osmotic pressure in the tissue). This allows a transportation of substances from the extravascular space to the blood vessels. Thus, the difference between the hydraulic pressure and the osmotic pressure (OP) results in a transportation of substances from the blood vessels to the extravascular space in the arterial part of the capillary while, in the venous part, a transportation of substances occurs from the extravascular space to the blood vessels. Hereby an extravascular circulation is established (small arrows).

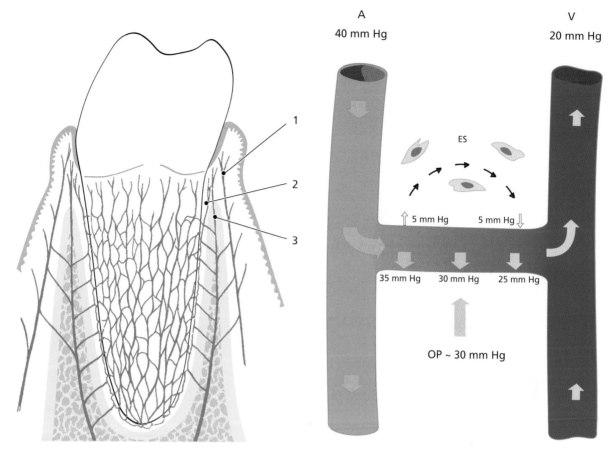

Fig. 1-104.

Fig. 1-105.

LYMPHATIC SYSTEM OF THE PERIODONTIUM

Fig. 1-106. The smallest lymph vessels, the *lymph capillaries*, form an extensive network in the connective tissue. The wall of the lymph capillary consists of a single layer of endothelial cells. For this reason such capillaries are difficult to identify in an ordinary histologic section. The lymph is absorbed from the tissue fluid through the thin walls into the lymph capillaries. From the capillaries, the lymph passes into larger lymph vessels which are often in the vicinity of corresponding blood vessels. Before the lymph enters the blood stream it passes through one or more *lymph nodes* in which the lymph becomes filtered and supplied with lymphocytes. The lymph vessels are like veins provided with valves. The lymph from the periodontal tissues is drained to the lymph nodes of the head and the neck. The labial and lingual gingiva of the mandibular incisor region is drained to the *submental lymph nodes* (sme). The palatal gingiva of the maxilla is drained to the *deep cervical lymph nodes* (cp). The buccal gingiva of the maxilla and the buccal and lingual gingiva in the mandibular premolar-molar region are drained to *submandibular lymph nodes* (sma). Except for the third molars and mandibular incisors, all teeth with their adjacent periodontal tissues are drained to the submandibular lymph nodes (sma).

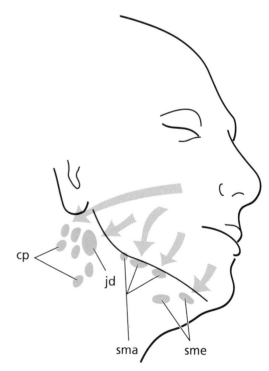

Fig. 1-106.

The third molars are drained to the *jugulodigastric lymph node* (jd) and the mandibular incisors to the *submental lymph nodes* (sme).

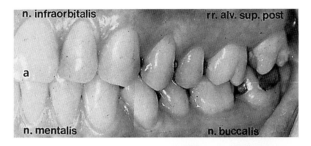

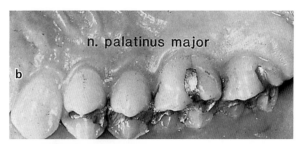

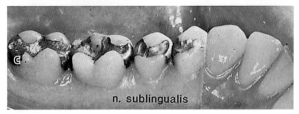

Fig. 1-107.

NERVES OF THE PERIODONTIUM

Like other tissues in the body, the periodontium contains receptors which record pain, touch and pressure (*nociceptors* and *mechanoreceptors*). In addition to the different types of sensory receptors, nerve components are found innervating the blood vessels of the periodontium. Nerves recording pain, touch, and pressure have their trophic center in the *semilunar ganglion* and are brought to the periodontium via the *trigeminal nerve* and its end branches. Owing to the presence of receptors in the periodontal ligament, small forces applied on the teeth may be identified. For example, the presence of a very thin (10-30 μm) metal foil (strip) placed between the teeth during occlusion can readily be identified. It is also well known that a movement which brings the teeth of the mandible in contact with the occlusal surfaces of the maxillary teeth is arrested reflexively and altered into an opening movement if a hard object is detected in the chew. Thus, the receptors in the periodontal ligament, together with the proprioceptors in muscles and tendons, play an essential role in the regulation of chewing movements and chewing forces.

Fig. 1-107 shows the various regions of the gingiva which are innervated by end branches of the trigeminal nerve. The gingiva on the labial aspect of maxillary incisors, canines and premolars is innervated by *superior labial branches* from the *infraorbital nerve*, n. infraorbitalis (Fig. 1-107a). The buccal gingiva in the maxillary molar region is innervated by branches from the *posterior superior dental nerve*, rr. alv. sup. post (Fig. 1-107a). The palatal gingiva is innervated by the *greater palatal nerve*, n. palatinus major (Fig. 1-107b), except for the area of the incisors, which is innervated by the *long sphenopalatine nerve*, n. pterygopalatini. The lingual gingiva in the mandible is innervated by the *sublingual nerve*, n. sublingualis (Fig. 1-107c), which is an end branch of the *lingual nerve*. The gingiva at the

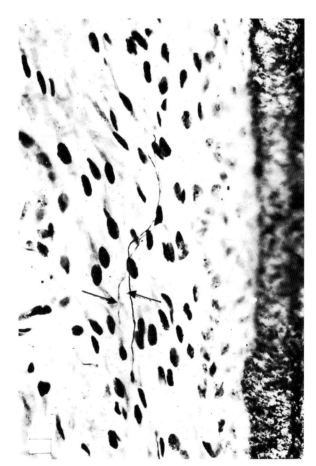

Fig. 1-108.

labial aspect of mandibular incisors and canines is innervated by the *mental nerve*, n. mentalis, and the gingiva at the buccal aspect of the molars by the *buccal nerve*, n. buccalis (Fig. 1-107a). The innervation areas of these two nerves frequently overlap in the premolar region. The teeth in the mandible including their periodontal ligament are innervated by the *inferior alveolar nerve*, n. alveolaris inf., while the teeth in the maxilla are innervated by the *superior alveolar plexus*, n. alveolares sup.

Fig. 1-108. The small nerves of the periodontium follow almost the same course as the blood vessels. The nerves to the gingiva run in the tissue superficial to the periosteum and put out several branches to the oral epithelium on their way towards the free gingiva. The nerves enter the periodontal ligament through the perforations (Volkmann's canals) in the socket wall (see Fig. 1-102). In the periodontal ligament, the nerves join larger bundles which take a course parallel to the long axis of the tooth. The photomicrograph illustrates small nerves (arrows) which have emerged from larger bundles of ascending nerves in order to supply certain parts of the periodontal ligament tissue. Various types of neural terminations such as free nerve endings and Ruffini's corpuscles have been identified in the periodontal ligament.

REFERENCES

Ainamo, J. & Talari, A. (1976). The increase with age of the width of attached gingiva. *Journal of Periodontal Research* **11**, 182-188.

Anderson, D.T., Hannam, A.G. & Matthews, G. (1970). Sensory mechanisms in mammalian teeth and their supporting structures. *Physiological Review* **50**, 171-195.

Bartold, P.M. (1995). Turnover in periodontal connective tissue: dynamic homeostasis of cells, collagen and ground substances. *Oral Diseases* **1**, 238-253.

Beertsen, W., McCulloch, C.A.G. & Sodek, J. (1997). The periodontal ligament: a unique, multifunctional connective tissue. *Periodontology 2000* **13**, 20-40.

Bosshardt, D.D. & Schroeder, H.E. (1991). Establishment of acellular extrinsic fiber cementum on human teeth. A light- and electron-microscopic study. *Cell Tissue Research* **263**, 325-336.

Bosshardt, D.D. & Selvig, K.A. (1997). Dental cementum: the dynamic tissue covering of the root. *Periodontology 2000* **13**, 41-75.

Carranza, E.A., Itoiz, M.E., Cabrini, R.L. & Dotto, C.A. (1966). A study of periodontal vascularization in different laboratory animals. *Journal of Periodontal Research* **1**, 120-128.

Egelberg, J. (1966). The blood vessels of the dentogingival junction. *Journal of Periodontal Research* **1**, 163-179.

Fullmer, H.M., Sheetz, J.H. & Narkates, A.J. (1974). Oxytalan connective tissue fibers. A review. *Journal of Oral Pathology* **3**, 291-316.

Hammarström, L. (1997). Enamel matrix, cementum development and regeneration. *Journal of Clinical Periodontology* **24**, 658-677.

Karring, T. (1973). Mitotic activity in the oral epithelium. *Journal of Periodontal Research, Suppl.* **13**, 1-47.

Karring, T., Lang, N.R. & Löe, H. (1974). The role of gingival connective tissue in determining epithelial differentiation. *Journal of Periodontal Research* **10**, 1-11.

Karring, T. & Löe, H. (1970). The three-dimensional concept of the epithelium-connective tissue boundary of gingiva. *Acta Odontologica Scandinavia* **28**, 917-933.

Karring, T., Ostergaard, E. & Löe, H. (1971). Conservation of tissue specificity after heterotopic transplantation of gingiva and alveolar mucosa. *Journal of Periodontal Research* **6**, 282-293.

Kvam, E. (1973). Topography of principal fibers. *Scandinavian Journal of Dental Research* **81**, 553-557.

Lambrichts, I., Creemers, J. & van Steenberghe, D. (1992). Morphology of neural endings in the human periodontal ligament: an electron microscopic study. *Journal of Periodontal Research* **27**, 191-196.

Listgarten, M.A. (1966). Electron microscopic study of the gingivo-dental junction of man. *American Journal of Anatomy* **119**, 147-178.

Listgarten, M.A. (1972). Normal development, structure, physiology and repair of gingival epithelium. *Oral Science Review* **1**, 3-67.

Lozdan, J. & Squier, C.A. (1969). The histology of the mucogingival junction. *Journal of Periodontal Research* **4**, 83-93.

Melcher, A.H. (1976). Biological processes in resorption, deposition and regeneration of bone. In: Stahl, S.S., ed. *Periodontal Surgery, Biologic Basis and Technique.* Springfield: C.C. Thomas, pp. 99-120.

Page, R.C., Ammons, W.F., Schectman, L.R. & Dillingham, L.A. (1974). Collagen fiber bundles of the normal marginal gingiva in the marmoset. *Archives of Oral Biology* **19**, 1039-1043.

Palmer, R.M. & Lubbock, M.J. (1995). The soft connective tissue of the gingiva and periodontal ligament: are they unique? *Oral Diseases* **1**, 230-237.

Saffar, J.L., Lasfargues, J.J. & Cherruah, M. (1997). Alveolar bone and the alveolar process: the socket that is never stable. *Periodontology 2000* **13**, 76-90.

Schenk, R.K. (1994). Bone regeneration: Biologic basis. In: Buser, D., Dahlin, C. & Schenk, R. K., eds. *Guided Bone Regeneration in Implant Dentistry.* Berlin: Quintessence Publishing Co.

Schroeder, H.E. (1986). The periodontium. In: Schroeder, H. E., ed. *Handbook of Microscopic Anatomy.* Berlin: Springer, pp. 47-64.

Schroeder, H.E. & Listgarten, M.A. (1971). *Fine Structure of the Developing Epithelial Attachment of Human Teeth,* 2nd edn. Basel: Karger, p. 146.

Schroeder, H.E. & Listgarten, M.A. (1997). The gingival tissues: the architecture of periodontal protection. *Periodontology 2000* **13**, 91-120.

Schroeder, H.E. & Münzel-Pedrazzoli, S. (1973). Correlated morphometric and biochemical analysis of gingival tissue. Morphometric model, tissue sampling and test of stereologic procedure. *Journal of Microscopy* **99**, 301-329.

Schroeder, H.E. & Theilade, J. (1966). Electron microscopy of normal human gingival epithelium. *Journal of Periodontal Research* **1**, 95-119.

Selvig, K.A. (1965). The fine structure of human cementum. *Acta Odontologica Scandinavica* **23**, 423-441.

Valderhaug, J.R. & Nylen, M.U. (1966). Function of epithelial rests as suggested by their ultrastructure. *Journal of Periodontal Research* **1**, 67-78.

Acknowledgement

We thank the following for contributing to the illustrations in Chapter 1:

M. Listgarten, R.K. Schenk, H.E. Schroeder, K.A. Selvig and K. Josephsen.

Chapter 2

Epidemiology of Periodontal Diseases

Panos N. Papapanou and Jan Lindhe

The term epidemiology is of Hellenic origin; it consists of the preposition "epi", which means "among" or "against" and the noun "demos" which means "people". As denoted by its etymology, epidemiology is defined as "the study of the distribution of disease or a physiological condition in human populations and of the factors that influence this distribution" (Lilienfeld 1978). A more inclusive description by Frost (1941) emphasizes that "epidemiology is essentially an inductive science, concerned not merely with describing the distribution of disease, but equally or more with fitting it into a consistent philosophy". Thus, the information obtained from an epidemiologic investigation should extend beyond a mere description of the distribution of the disease in different populations (*descriptive* epidemiology): it should be further utilized to (1) elucidate the etiology of a specific disease by combining epidemiologic data with information from other disciplines such as genetics, biochemistry, microbiology, sociology, etc. (*etiologic* epidemiology); (2) evaluate the consistency of epidemiologic data with hypotheses developed clinically or experimentally (*analytical* epidemiology); and (3) provide the basis for developing and evaluating preventive procedures and public health practices (*experimental/interventive* epidemiology).

Based on the above, epidemiological research in periodontics must (1) fulfill the task of providing data on the *prevalence* of periodontal diseases in different populations, i.e. the frequency of their occurrence, as well as on the *severity* of such conditions, i.e. the level of occurring pathologic changes; (2) elucidate aspects related to the *etiology* and the *determinants of development* of these diseases (*causative* and *risk* factors); and (3) provide documentation concerning the effectiveness of preventive and therapeutic measures aimed against these diseases on a population basis.

METHODOLOGICAL ISSUES

Examination methods – index systems

Examination of the periodontal status of a given individual includes clinical assessments of inflammation in the periodontal tissues, registration of probing depths and clinical attachment levels and radiographic assessments of remaining alveolar bone. A variety of index systems for the scoring of these parameters has been developed over the years. A number of such systems was designed exclusively for examination of patients in a dental practice set-up, while others were to be utilized in epidemiological research.

The design of the index systems and the definition of the various scores inevitably reflected the knowledge on the etiology and pathogenesis of periodontal disease of the time they were introduced, as well as concepts related to the current therapeutic approaches and strategies. This section will not provide a complete list of all available scoring systems, but rather give a brief description of a limited number of indices that are either currently used or are likely to be encountered in the recent literature. For description of earlier scoring systems and a historical perspective of their development, the reader is referred to Ainamo (1989).

Assessment of inflammation of the periodontal tissues

Presence of inflammation in the marginal portion of the gingiva is usually recorded by means of probing assessments, according to the principles of the Gingival Index outlined in the publication by Löe (1967). According to this system, entire absence of visual signs of inflammation in the gingival unit is scored as 0, while a slight change in color and texture is scored as 1. Visual inflammation and bleeding tendency from the gingival margin right after a periodontal probe is briefly run along the gingival margin is scored as 2, while overt inflammation with tendency for spontaneous bleeding is scored as 3. A parallel index for scoring plaque deposits (Plaque Index) in a scale from 0 to 3 (Silness & Löe 1964) was introduced, according to which absence of plaque deposits is scored as 0, plaque disclosed after running the periodontal probe along the gingival margin as 1, visible plaque as 2 and abundant plaque as 3. Simplified variants of both the Gingival and the Plaque Index (Ainamo & Bay 1975) have been extensively used, assessing presence/absence of inflammation or plaque respectively in a binomial fashion (*dichotomous scoring*). In such systems, bleeding from the gingival margin and visible plaque score "1", while absence of bleeding and no visible plaque score "0".

Bleeding after probing to the base of the probeable pocket (Gingival Sulcus Bleeding Index) has been a common way of assessing presence of subgingival inflammation (Mühlemann & Son 1971). In this dichotomous registration, "1" is scored in case bleeding emerges within 15 seconds after probing. Presence/absence of bleeding on probing to the base of the pocket tends to increasingly substitute the use of the Gingival Index in epidemiological studies.

Assessment of loss of periodontal tissue support

One of the early indices providing indirect information on the loss of periodontal tissue support was the Periodontal Index (PI) developed in the 1950s by Russell (1956), and until the 1980s it was the most widely used index in epidemiological studies of periodontal disease. Its criteria are applied to each tooth and the scoring is as follows: a tooth with healthy periodontium scores (0), a tooth with gingivitis around only part of the tooth circumference (1), a tooth with gingivitis encircling the tooth (2), pocket formation (6) and loss of function due to excessive tooth mobility (8). Due to the nature of the criteria used, the PI is a reversible scoring system, i.e. a tooth or an individual can, after treatment, have the score lowered or reduced to 0.

In contrast to the PI system, the Periodontal Disease Index (PDI), developed by Ramfjord (1959), is a system designed to assess *destructive* disease, measures *loss of attachment* instead of *pocket depth* and is, therefore, an irreversible index. The scores, ranging from 0-6, denote periodontal health or gingivitis (scores 0-3) and various levels of attachment loss (scores 4-6).

In contemporary epidemiological studies, loss of periodontal tissue support is assessed by measurements of pocket depth and attachment level. Probing pocket depth (PPD) is defined as the distance from the gingival margin to the location of the tip of a periodontal probe inserted in the pocket with moderate probing force. Likewise, probing attachment level (PAL) or clinical attachment level (CAL) is defined as the distance from the cemento-enamel junction (CEJ) to the location of the inserted probe tip. Probing assessments may be carried out at different locations of the tooth circumference (buccal, lingual, mesial or distal sites). The number of probing assessments per tooth has varied in epidemiological studies from two to six, while the examination may either include all present teeth (*full-mouth*) or a subset of *index* teeth (*partial-mouth* examination).

Carlos et al. (1986) proposed an index system which records loss of periodontal tissue support. The index was denoted the Extent and Severity Index (ESI) and consists of two components (*bivariate* index): (1) the *Extent*, describing the proportion of tooth sites of a subject examined showing signs of destructive periodontitis, and (2) the *Severity*, describing the amount of attachment loss at the diseased sites, expressed as a mean value. An attachment loss threshold of ≥ 1 mm was set as the criterion for a tooth site to qualify as affected by the disease. Although arbitrary, the introduction of a threshold value serves a dual purpose: (1) it readily distinguishes the fraction of the dentition affected by disease at levels exceeding the error inherent in the clinical measurement of attachment loss, and (2) it prevents unaffected tooth sites from contributing to the individual subject's mean attachment loss value. In order to limit the assessments to be performed, a partial examination comprising the mid-buccal and mesio-buccal aspects of the upper right and lower left quadrants was recommended. It has to be emphasized that the system was designed to assess the cumulative effect of destructive periodontal disease rather than the presence of the disease itself. The bivariate nature of the index facilitates a rather detailed description of attachment loss patterns: for example an ESI of (90, 2.5) suggests a generalized but rather mild form of destructive disease, in which 90% of the tooth sites are affected by an average attachment loss of 2.5 mm. In contrast, an ESI of (20, 7.0) describes a severe, localized form of disease. Validation of various partial extent and severity scoring systems against the full-mouth estimates has been also performed (Papapanou et al. 1993).

Radiographic assessment of alveolar bone loss
The potential and limitations of intraoral radiography to describe loss of supporting periodontal tissues were reviewed by Lang & Hill (1977) and Benn (1990). Radiographs have been commonly employed in cross-sectional epidemiologic studies to evaluate the result of periodontal disease on the supporting tissues rather than the presence of the disease itself. Radiographic assessments have been particularly common as screening methods for detecting subjects suffering from juvenile periodontitis as well as a means for monitoring periodontal disease progression in longitudinal studies. Assessments of bone loss in intraoral radiographs are usually performed by evaluating a multitude of qualitative and quantitative features of the visualized interproximal bone, e.g. (1) presence of an intact lamina dura, (2) the width of the periodontal ligament space, (3) the morphology of the bone crest ("even" or "angular" appearance), and (4) the distance between the cemento-enamel junction (CEJ) and the most coronal level at which the periodontal ligament space is considered to retain a normal width. The threshold for bone loss, i.e. the CEJ-bone crest distance considered to indicate that bone loss has occurred, varies between 1 and 3 mm in different studies. Radiographic data are usually presented as (1) mean bone loss scores per subject (or group of subjects), and (2) number or percentage of tooth surfaces per subject (or group of subjects) exhibiting bone loss exceeding certain thresholds. In early studies, bone loss was frequently recorded using "ruler" devices, describing the amount of lost or remaining bone as a percentage of the length of the root or the tooth (Lavstedt et al. 1975; Schei et al. 1959).

Assessment of periodontal treatment needs
An index system aimed at assessing the need for periodontal treatment in large population groups was developed, at the initiative of the World Health Organisation (WHO), by Ainamo et al. (1982). The principles of the Community Periodontal Index for Treatment Needs (CPITN) can be summarized as follows:

1. The dentition is divided into six *sextants* (one anterior and two posterior tooth regions in each dental arch). The treatment need in a sextant is recorded when two or more teeth – not intended for extraction – are present. If only one tooth remains in the sextant, the tooth is included in the adjoining sextant.
2. Probing assessments are performed either around all teeth in a sextant or around certain index teeth (the latter approach has been recommended for epidemiologic surveys). However, only the most

severe measure in the sextant is chosen to represent the sextant.
3. The periodontal conditions are scored as follows:
   - *Code 1* is given to a sextant with no pockets, calculus or overhangs of fillings but in which bleeding occurs after gentle probing in one or several gingival units.
   - *Code 2* is assigned to a sextant if there are no pockets exceeding 3 mm, but in which dental calculus and plaque retaining factors are seen or recognized subgingivally.
   - *Code 3* is given to a sextant that harbors 4-5 mm deep pockets.
   - *Code 4* is given to a sextant that harbors pockets 6 mm deep or deeper.
4. The treatment needs are scores based on the most severe code in the dentition as TN 0, in case of gingival health, TN 1 indicating need for improved oral hygiene if Code 1 has been recorded, TN 2 indicating need for scaling, removal of overhangs and improved oral hygiene (Codes 2+3) and TN 3 indicating complex treatment (Code 4).

Although not designed for epidemiological purposes, this index system has been extensively used worldwide and particularly in developing countries. A substantial amount of data generated by its use has been accumulated in the WHO Global Oral Data Bank (Miyazaki et al. 1992, Pilot & Miyazaki 1994).

Critical evaluation

A fundamental prerequisite for any epidemiological study is an accurate definition of the disease under investigation. Unfortunately, no uniform criteria have been established in periodontal research for this purpose. Epidemiological studies have employed a wide array of symptoms including gingivitis, probing depth, clinical attachment level and radiographically assessed alveolar bone loss in an inconsistent manner. Considerable variation characterizes the threshold values employed for defining periodontal pockets as "deep" or "pathological", or the clinical attachment level and alveolar bone scores required for assuming that "true" loss of periodontal tissue support has, in fact, occurred. In addition, the number of "affected" tooth surfaces required for assigning an individual subject as a "case", i.e. as suffering from periodontal disease, has varied. These inconsistencies in the definitions inevitably affect the figures describing the distribution of the disease (Papapanou 1996). A review of the literature charged with the task to compare disease prevalence or incidence in different populations or at different time periods must first be confronted with the interpretation of the figures reported and literally "decode" the published data in order to identify the state of periodontal health or disease that these figures reflect. These problems have been addressed in the literature and two specific aspects have attracted special attention, namely (1) the ability of partial recording methodologies to reflect the full mouth conditions, and (2) the use of the CPITN system in epidemiological studies of periodontal disease.

There is little doubt that an optimal examination of the periodontal conditions should include circumferential probing assessments around all teeth. Nevertheless, the majority of epidemiological studies have, for practical reasons, employed partial recording methodologies. The rationale for the use of partial examinations has been the assumption that (1) the time required for the performance of a partial survey – and consequently its cost – is significantly decreased, and (2) the amount of information lost is kept to a minimum, provided that the examined segments adequately reflect the periodontal condition of the entire dentition. However, attempts to accurately quantify the amount of information lost through the different partial recording systems made by several investigators (Diamanti-Kipioti et al. 1993, Eaton et al. 2001, Hunt 1987, Hunt & Fann 1991, Kingman et al. 1988, Stoltenberg et al. 1993a) have revealed that the discrepancy between the findings obtained by means of partial and full-mouth surveys may be substantial. These studies have typically employed full-mouth data for a series of periodontal parameters and compared them with the values obtained by assessments performed at a subset of teeth or tooth surfaces. Their results suggest that:

1. high correlations between full-mouth and half-mouth attachment loss scores should be expected in adult populations, due to the apparent symmetry of periodontal conditions around the midline;
2. the performance of a partial recording system is directly dependent on the actual prevalence of periodontal disease in the population in question and, consequently, on the age of the subjects examined; the less frequent the disease in the population and the lower the number of sites that are affected in each individual mouth, the more difficult it becomes for the partial examination to detect the periodontal lesions;
3. a full-mouth examination provides the best means of accurately assessing the prevalence and severity of periodontal disease in a population.

The use of the CPITN system in epidemiological studies of periodontal disease was critically evaluated in a number of publications (Baelum et al. 1993a,b, 1995, Benigeri et al. 2000, Butterworth & Sheiham 1991, Grytten & Mubarak 1989, Holmgren & Corbet 1990, Schürch et al. 1990). At the time the system was designed, the conversion of periodontal health to disease was thought to include a continuum of conditions, ranging from an inflammation-free state developing through gingivitis (bleeding), calculus deposition, shallow and deep pocket formation to progressive, destructive disease. The treatment concepts were based on the assumption that probing depths determined the choice between non-surgical and more complicated, surgical periodontal therapy. It should also be remembered that this particular index was clearly intended for screening large population groups in order to determine treatment needs and to facilitate preventive and therapeutic strategies and not for describing prevalence and severity of periodontal disease.

In view of the revised, contemporary views on the pathogenesis and treatment of the periodontal diseases, studies have questioned the suitability of the CPITN for such purposes. For example, Baelum et al. (1993b) examined the validity of the hierarchical principle of the CPITN by using data originating from a cross-sectional study of a random sample of 1121 Kenyans aged 15 to 65 years. According to the CPITN, a tooth with calculus is assumed to be positive also for bleeding on probing and a tooth with moderately deep or deep pockets is assumed to be positive for both calculus and bleeding. The data showed, however, that calculus as the most severe finding overestimated the occurrence of bleeding by up to 18%, while pocketing overestimated the occurrence of calculus by up to 54% and of bleeding by up to 13%. In a companion paper based on the same subject sample (Baelum et al. 1993a), results from a full-mouth examination were compared with those generated by the use of the 10 index teeth recommended by the WHO for surveys of adults. It was revealed that the partial recording underestimated the prevalence of pockets (moderate or deep) in virtually all groups. The proportion of persons with ≥ 6 mm pockets that would have been overlooked if only the index teeth had been examined was 55% in the 25 to 29 year age group, 39% (40 to 44 years) and 23% (50 to 54 years). It was concluded that the partial CPITN methodology seriously underestimates the more severe periodontal conditions both in terms of prevalence and severity, since it fails to detect a substantial proportion of subjects with periodontal pockets. Finally, in another report from this rural Kenyan sample (Baelum et al. 1995), the authors examined the relationship between CPITN findings and the prevalence and severity of clinical attachment loss (CAL). They reported that, in ages over 40 years, over 90% of the persons with a CPITN score of 2 had attachment loss of ≥ 4 mm and that, in ages over 50 years, more than half of such subjects had attachment loss of ≥ 6 mm. While less than 20% of the 15 to 29 year olds with a CPITN score of 3 had CAL of ≥ 6 mm, 10% of the sextants with a CPITN score of 0 in subjects over 35 years had CAL of ≥ 4 mm. It was thus demonstrated that the CPITN scores do not consistently correlate with attachment loss scores, but tend to overestimate prevalence and severity among younger subjects while they underestimate such parameters in elderly populations.

Another publication (Butterworth & Sheiham 1991) addressed the suitability of CPITN to record changes in the periodontal conditions. The authors examined attendants of a general dental practice before and after therapy and reported that, despite a substantial improvement in the state of health of the periodontal tissues, assessed through gingivitis, calculus and pocketing scores, the CPITN scores were only marginally improved. The latter observation clearly illustrates the unsuitability of the CPITN system to reflect distinct differences in periodontal conditions and its inappropriateness as a method for assessing treatment needs.

Prevalence of periodontal diseases

Introduction

As discussed in detail in Chapter 9, a workshop that took place in 1999 was charged with the specific task of revising the classification of periodontal diseases (Workshop on the Classification of Periodontal Diseases 1999). The resulting new classification encompasses eight main categories:

I. Gingival diseases
II. Chronic periodontitis
III. Aggressive periodontitis
IV. Periodontitis as a manifestation of systemic diseases
V. Necrotizing periodontal diseases
VI. Abscesses of the periodontium
VII. Periodontitis associated with endodontic lesions
VIII. Developmental or acquired deformities and conditions.

Obviously, a review of the existing literature on the prevalence of periodontal diseases in various populations is doomed to encounter the new nomenclature infrequently. For example, no epidemiological studies of aggressive periodontitis in adult subjects are available yet. Similarly, studies distinguishing between plaque-induced and non-plaque-induced gingival diseases, or between chronic periodontitis in young subjects and adults, are not available. Thus, this chapter must inevitably rely on the use of evidence generated by the use of old terminology, but attempts to utilize the new terms whenever feasible. Primarily, the following text is focused on the epidemiology of conditions currently classified as either chronic or aggressive periodontitis. Although these diagnoses no longer rely on the subject's age as a primary determinant, the following text and tables utilize age as a secondary descriptor to facilitate accurate data extraction from the original studies.

Periodontitis in adults

In an epidemiologic survey performed during the 1950s in India, Marshall-Day et al. (1955) used assessments of alveolar bone height to distinguish between gingivitis and destructive periodontal disease in a sample involving 1187 dentate subjects. The authors reported (1) a decrease in the percentage of subjects with "gingival disease without any bone involvement" with increasing age concomitant with an increase in the percentage of subjects with "chronic, destructive periodontal disease", and (2) a 100% occurrence of destructive periodontitis after the age of 40 years. Findings from other epidemiologic studies from the same period verified a high prevalence of destructive periodontal disease in the adult population in general and a clear increase in disease prevalence with age. In the 1960s Scherp (1964) reviewed the available literature on the epidemiology of periodontal disease and concluded that (1) periodontal disease appears to be a major, global public health problem affecting the majority of the adult population after the age of 35-40 years, (2) the disease starts as gingivitis in young age which, if left untreated, leads to progressive destructive periodontitis, and (3) more than 90% of the variance of the periodontal disease severity in the population can be explained by age and oral hygiene. These notions, based on the currently established concepts on the pathogenesis of periodontal disease, dominated the periodontal literature for a time period extending into the late 1970s.

Studies performed during the 1980s provided a more thorough description of the site-specific features of periodontal disease and the high variation in periodontal conditions between and within different populations. Contrary to what was customary until then, the prevalence issue was no longer addressed through a mere assignment of individuals to a "periodontitis-affected" or a "disease-free" group, based on presence or absence of attachment or alveolar bone loss. Instead, studies began to unravel details concerning the *extent* at which the dentition was affected by destructive disease (i.e. the percentage of tooth sites involved), and the *severity* of the defects (expressed through the amount of lost tissue support). The traditional description of pocket depth and attachment loss scores through subject mean values was soon complemented by frequency distributions, revealing percentages of tooth sites exhibiting probing depth or attachment level of varying severity. Such an additional analysis appeared necessary after it had been realized that mean values offer a crude description of periodontal conditions and fail to reflect the variability in the severity of periodontal disease within and between individuals. In an article presenting different methods of evaluating periodontal disease data in epidemiological research, Okamoto et al. (1988) proposed the use of *percentile plots* in the graphic illustration of attachment loss data. As exemplified by Fig. 2-1, such plots make it possible to illustrate simultaneously both the proportion of subjects exhibiting attachment loss of different levels and the severity of the loss within the subjects. Similar plots may be

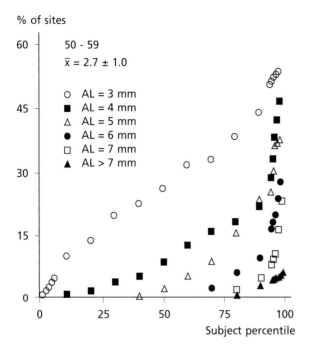

Fig. 2-1. Attachment loss in a group of Japanese subjects 50-59 years of age. The mean value of attachment level and the standard deviation are shown in the top of the figure. The x-axis represents the subject percentile and the y-axis represents the percentage of sites in the subjects showing attachment loss of 3, 4, 5, 6, 7 and > 7 mm (represented by 8). Subjects with no or only minor signs of attachment loss are reported to the left and subjects with increasing amounts of periodontal destruction are reported to the right of the graph. For example, the median subject (50th percentile), exhibited 5 mm attachment loss at 2%, 4 mm loss at 8%, and 3 mm attachment loss at 25% of its sites. From Okamoto et al. (1988), reproduced with permission.

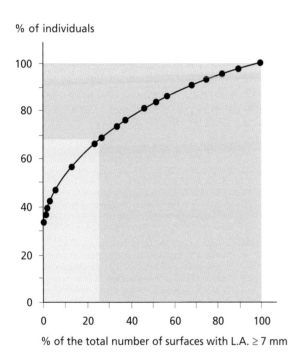

Fig. 2-2. Cumulative distribution of individuals aged ≥ 50 years according to the cumulated proportion of surfaces with L.A. ≥ 7 mm. All individuals are arranged according to increasing number of surfaces with L.A. ≥ 7 mm present in each individual. Thus, individuals with few such surfaces are represented by the dots in the left side of the diagram and those with many such surfaces by dots in the right side. It is seen that 31% (100% – 69%) of the individuals account for 75% (100% – 25%) of the total number of surfaces with L.A. ≥ 7 mm present (shaded area). From Baelum et al. (1986), reproduced with permission.

produced for other parameters such as gingivitis, probing depths and gingival recession and may provide a comprehensive description of both the prevalence and the severity of periodontal disease in a given sample.

Pioneering research by a Danish research group, made significant contributions to our current understanding of epidemiological issues in periodontal research. Baelum et al. (1986) described cross-sectional findings on dental plaque, calculus, gingivitis, loss of attachment, periodontal pockets and tooth loss in a sample of adult Tanzanians aged 30-69 years. Despite the fact that subjects examined exhibited large amounts of plaque and calculus, pockets deeper than 3 mm and attachment loss of ≥ 6 mm occurred at less than 10% of the tooth surfaces. None of the subjects examined was edentulous and very few had experienced any major loss of teeth. Of particular interest was the analysis of the distribution of sites within subjects (Fig. 2-2). This analysis revealed that 75% of the tooth sites with attachment loss of ≥ 7 mm were found in 31% of the subjects, indicating that a subfraction of the sample was responsible for the major part of the observed periodontal breakdown. In other words, advanced periodontal disease was not evenly distributed in the population and not readily correlated to supragingival plaque levels; instead, the majority of the subjects examined exhibited negligible periodontal problems while a limited group was affected by advanced disease.

Table 2-1. Cross-sectional studies of periodontitis in adults

Authors/Country	Sample/Methodology	Findings
Löe et al. (1978) Norway/Sri Lanka	Two samples, one comprising 565 Norwegian students and academicians and the other 480 Sri Lankan tea laborers, in ages 16-30+ yrs; assessments of plaque, gingivitis, calculus, probing depth (PD) and attachment loss (AL) at the mesial and facial aspects of all teeth	Norwegian group: excellent oral hygiene, negligible amounts of plaque and gingivitis, virtually no deep pockets and minimal attachment loss; mean AL at the age of 30 < 1 mm; Sri Lankan group: poor oral hygiene, abundant plaque and calculus, attachment loss present at the age of 16, increasing with age; mean AL at the age of 30 ≈ 3 mm, a substantial number of teeth with AL of > 10 mm
Baelum et al. (1988a) Kenya	A stratified random sample of 1131 subjects, 15-65 yrs; full-mouth assessments of tooth mobility, plaque, calculus, bleeding on probing (BoP), PD and AL	Plaque in 75-95% and calculus in 10-85% of all surfaces; PD ≥ 4 mm in < 20% of the sites; AL of ≥ 1 mm in 10-85% of the sites; the % of sites/subject with PD or AL of of ≥ 4 mm or of ≥ 7 mm conspicuously skewed
Yoneyama et al. (1988) Japan	A random sample of 319 subjects, 20-79 yrs old; full-mouth probing assessments of PD, AL and gingival recession	0.2% of the sites in subjects 30-39 yrs and 1.2% of the sites in subjects 70-79 yrs had a PD of > 6 mm; AL > 5 mm affected 1% of the sites in the youngest group and 12.4% of the sites in the oldest group; skewed distribution of advanced AL; advanced disease more prevalent and widespread in older ages
Brown et al. (1990) USA	A sample of 15 132 subjects, stratified by geographic region, representing 100 million employed adults aged 18-64 yrs; probing assessments at mesial and buccal sites in one upper and one lower quadrant; mesial assessments performed from the buccal aspect of the teeth; assessments of gingivitis, PD, AL and gingival recession	44% of all subjects had gingivitis at an average of 2.7 sites/subject and at < 6% of all sites assessed; pockets 4-6 mm were observed in 13.4% of the subjects at an average of 0.6 sites/person and at 1.3% of all sites assessed; corresponding figures for pockets ≥ 7 mm were 0.6%, 0.01 and 0.03%; AL ≥ 3 mm was prevalent in 44% of the subjects (increasing with age from 16% to 80%) affecting an average of 3.4 sites/subject; corresponding figures for AL ≥ 5 mm were 13% (2-35%) and 0.7 sites/subject
Salonen et al. (1991) Sweden	A random sample of 732 subjects, 20-80+ yrs, representing 0.8% of the population of a southern geographic region; full-mouth radiographic examination; alveolar bone level expressed as a percentage of the root length (B/R ratio); B/R of ≥ 80% represents intact periodontal bone support	Age group of 20-29 yrs: 38% of the subjects had no sites with B/R < 80% and 8% of the subjects had ≥ 5 sites below this threshold; corresponding figures for the age group 50-59 yrs were 5% and 75%; after the age of 40, women displayed more favorable B/R ratios than men
Hugoson et al. (1998) Sweden	Three random samples of 600, 597 and 584 subjects in ages 20-70 yrs, examined in 1973, 1983 and 1993, respectively; full-mouth clinical and radiographic examination; based on clinical and radiographic findings, the subjects were classified according to severity of periodontal disease in five groups, where group 1 included subjects with close to faultless periodontal tissues and group 5 subjects with severe disease	Edentulousness decreased over the 20-year period from 11% to 8% to 5%; % distribution of the subjects in the five groups in 1973, 1983 and 1993 respectively, was as follows: G1: 8%/23%/22%, G2: 41%/22%/38%, G3: 47%/41%/27%, G4: 2%/11%/10%, G5: 1%/2%/3%; the increase in the prevalence of subjects with severe disease was apparently due to increase of dentate subjects in older ages
Albandar et al. (1999) USA	A nationally representative, multistage probability sample comprising 9689 subjects, 30-90 years old (NHANES III study); probing assessments at mesial and buccal sites in one upper and one lower quadrant; mesial assessments performed from the buccal aspect of the teeth; assessments of gingivitis, PD, and location of the gingival margin in relation to the CEJ	Pockets ≥ 5 mm were found in 8.9% of all subjects (7.6% in non-Hispanic whites, 18.4% in non-Hispanic blacks, and 14.4% in Mexican Americans); AL ≥ 5mm occurred in 19.9% of all subjects (19.9% in non-Hispanic whites, 27.9% in non-Hispanic blacks, and 28.34% in Mexican Americans)

PD: probing depth; AL: attachment level; CEJ: cemento-enamel junction

In a study of similar design performed in Kenya, the same investigators (Baelum et al. 1988a) analyzed data from 1131 subjects aged 15-65 years and confirmed their earlier observations. Poor oral hygiene in the sample was reflected by high plaque, calculus and gingivitis scores. However, pockets ≥ 4 mm deep were found in less than 20% of the surfaces and the proportion of sites per individual with deep pockets and advanced loss of attachment revealed a pronounced skewed distribution. The authors suggested that "destructive periodontal disease should not be perceived as an inevitable consequence of gingivitis which ultimately leads to considerable tooth loss" and called for a more specific characterization of the features of peri-odontal breakdown in those individuals who seem particularly susceptible.

Several epidemiological studies have been published in the last twenty years, verifying the above principles. In these studies, periodontal disease has been assessed by means of clinical examination of the periodontal tissues (Albandar et al. 1999, Albandar & Kingman 1999, Anagnou Vareltzides et al. 1996, Bagramian et al. 1993, Beck et al. 1990, Brown et al. 1989, 1990, Douglass et al. 1993, Gilbert et al. 1992, Horning et al. 1990, Hunt et al. 1990, Kiyak et al. 1993, Locker & Leake 1993a, Löe et al. 1992, Matthesen et al. 1990, McFall et al. 1989, Oliver et al. 1998, Querna et al. 1994, Slade et al. 1993, Söder et al. 1994, Stuck et al. 1989,

Weyant et al. 1993); radiographic assessments of alveolar bone loss (Diamanti-Kipioti et al. 1995, Jenkins & Kinane 1989, Papapanou et al. 1988, Salonen et al. 1991, Wouters et al. 1989); or a combination of clinical and radiographic means (Hugoson et al. 1992, Hugoson et al. 1998, Papapanou et al. 1990).

Table 2-1 summarizes the design and main findings from a number of cross-sectional studies in adults from geographically divergent areas that involve samples of a relatively large size. Most of the studies focus on assessments of prevalence of "advanced periodontitis", the definition of which is, however, far from identical among the studies, rendering comparisons difficult. Nevertheless, it appears that severe forms of periodontitis affect a minority of the subjects in the industrialized countries, at proportions probably not exceeding 10% of the population. The percentage of such subjects increases considerably with age and appears to reach its peak at the age of 50 to 60 years. The increased tooth loss occurring after this age appears to account for the subsequent decline in prevalence.

It is worth pointing out that, among the studies reviewed in Table 2-1, the study employing circumferential probing assessments around all teeth (Horning et al. 1990) reported the highest prevalence of advanced disease, suggesting that the impact of the methodology used may have been decisive. The interesting issue of disparities in the severity of periodontitis was brought up by Baelum et al. (1996). The authors recalculated their own data from a Kenyan (Baelum et al. 1988a) and a Chinese (Baelum et al. 1988b) adult population to conform with the methods of examination and data presentation utilized in each of six other surveys (from Japan, Yoneyama et al. 1988; Norway, Löe et al. 1978; New Mexico, Ismail et al. 1987; Sri Lanka, Löe et al. 1978; and two South Pacific islands, Cutress et al. 1982). Among the samples included in this analysis, only the Sri Lankan and the South Pacific subjects appeared to suffer a severe periodontal tissue breakdown, while the distribution of advanced disease was strikingly similar in six out of the eight samples, despite marked differences in oral hygiene conditions. Hence the data failed to corroborate the traditional generalization that the prevalence and severity of periodontitis is markedly increased in African and Asian populations. On the other hand, data from the Third National Health and Nutrition Study (NHANES III; Albandar et al. (1999)), which examined a large nationally representative, stratified, multistage probability sample in the USA, clearly showed that the prevalence of deep pockets and advanced attachment loss was more pronounced in non-Hispanic blacks and Hispanics than in non-Hispanic white subjects. This observation was consistent even when several alternative thresholds defining advanced disease were employd. Thus, current evidence suggests that the prevalence of severe periodontitis is not uniformly distributed among various races, ethnicities, or socio-economic groups (Hobdell, 2001).

Table 2-2 summarizes a number of prevalence studies of periodontal disease in elderly subjects. In five studies (Beck et al. 1990; Gilbert & Heft 1992; Hunt et al. 1990; Locker & Leake 1993a; Weyant et al. 1993) data on attachment loss have been used to calculate extent and severity index scores (ESI), which appear to be relatively consistent between the surveys. It is evident that attachment loss of moderate magnitude was frequent and widespread in these subject samples; however, severe disease was again found to affect relatively limited proportions of the samples and generally only a few teeth per subject.

The limitations of the findings from studies using the CPITN system were discussed above. However, a substantial part of the available information from the developing countries has been collected by the use of this index. An article providing a summary of almost 100 CPITN surveys from more than 50 countries performed over the period 1981-89 for the age group of 35 to 44 years was published by Miyazaki et al. (1991b). These studies indicate a huge variation in the percentage of subjects with one or several deep (≥ 6 mm) pockets both between and within different geographic areas. Hence, the percentage of subjects with such pockets ranged between 1% and 74% in Africa (data from 17 surveys), 8% and 22% in North and South America (4 surveys), 2% and 36% in the Eastern Mediterranean (6 surveys), 2% and 40% in Europe (38 surveys), 2% and 64% in South-East Asia, and between 1% and 22% in the Western Pacific area (17 surveys). The average number of sextants per subject with ≥ 6 mm deep pockets also varied considerably and ranged between 0 and 2.1 in Africa, 0.1 and 0.4 in America, 0.1 and 0.6 in the East Mediterranean, 0.1 and 0.8 in Europe, 0.1 and 2.1 in South-East Asia and 0 and 0.4 in the Western Pacific area. However, it is difficult to assess the extent to which these values reflect true differences in the periodontal conditions between the samples and not the methodological limitations of the CPITN system.

Periodontitis in children and adolescents

The form of periodontal disease that affects the *primary* dentition, the condition formerly called *prepubertal periodontitis,* has been reported to appear in both a generalized and a localized form (Page et al. 1983). Information about this disease was mainly provided by clinical case reports and no data related to the prevalence and the distribution of the disease in the general population are available. However, a few studies involving samples of children have provided limited data on the frequency with which deciduous teeth may be affected by loss of periodontal tissue support. The criteria used in these studies are by no means uniform, hence the prevalence data vary significantly. In an early study, Jamison (1963) examined by the use of the Periodontal Disease Index the "prevalence of destructive periodontal disease" (indicated

Table 2-2. Cross-sectional studies of periodontitis in elderly subjects

Authors/Country	Sample/Methodology	Findings
Baelum et al. (1988b) China	544 persons, aged 60+, from two urban and one rural area of Beijing area; assessments of plaque, calculus, gingivitis, loss of attachment, pocket depth and tooth mobility	0-29% edentulous; mean no. of teeth 6.9-23.9, depending on age and sex; ≈ 50% of all surfaces with plaque and calculus; 50% of all sites with AL of ≥ 4 mm, < 15% with PD ≥ 4 mm; conspicuously skewed % of sites/person with AL of ≥ 7 mm and PD ≥ 4 mm
Locker & Leake (1993a) Canada	907 subjects, in ages 50-75+ yrs, living independently in four communities; probing assessments at mesiobuccal and mid-buccal aspects of all teeth; mid-palatal and mesio-palatal probing assessments in upper molars; 23% of the subjects edentulous; calculation of extent and severity index (ESI) with AL threshold set at ≥ 2 mm; "Severe disease": > 4 sites with AL ≥ 5 mm and PD ≥ 4 mm at ≥ 1 of those sites	59% of the subjects with PD of ≥ 4 mm, 16% with ≥ 6 mm and 3% with ≥ 8 mm; 86% of the subjects with PAL of ≥ 4 mm, 42% with ≥ 6 mm and 16% with ≥ 8 mm; 20% of the subjects with a mean PAL of ≥ 4 mm; severe disease in 22% of the subjects; mean ESI: 77, 2.44
Beck et al. (1990) USA	690 community dwelling adults, age 65+; probing assessments at mesio- and mid-buccal surfaces, all teeth; "Advanced disease": ≥ 4 sites with AL of ≥ 5 mm and ≥ 1 of these sites with PD of ≥ 4 mm	Mean ESI in blacks: 78, 4; in whites: (65, 3.1); advanced disease in 46% of the blacks and 16% of the whites
Gilbert & Heft (1992) USA	671 dentate subjects, 65-97 yrs old, attending senior activity centers; probing assessments at mesial and buccal surfaces of one upper and one lower quadrant; questionnaire data; calculation of ESI	An average of 17.0 teeth/subject; 50.7% of the subjects with most severe mesial pocket of 4-6 mm and 3.4% with pockets ≥ 7 mm; 61.6% with most severe AL of 4.6 mm and 24.2% with AL of ≥ 7 mm; ESI increased with age: 84.8, 3.6 (65-69 yrs); 88.7, 3.8 (75-79 yrs); 91.2, 3.9 (85+ yrs)
Douglass et al. (1993) USA	1151 community-dwelling elders, age 70+ yrs; probing assessments at ≥ 3 sites/tooth, all teeth; 57% of the sample female, predominantly white (95%); 37.6% edentulous; mean no. of teeth present between 21.5 and 17.9, depending on age	85% of the subjects with BOP; 66% with 4-6 mm deep pockets affecting an average of 5.3 teeth/subject; 21% with pockets of > 6 mm affecting an average of 2.2 teeth; 39% with AL of 4-6 mm at 6.7 sites/subject and 56% AL of > 6 mm at 2.7 teeth/subject
Kiyak et al. (1993) USA	1063 residents in 31 nursing homes, 72-98 yrs old; visual inspection of the oral cavity; periodontal status assessed indirectly through registration of intraoral swelling or suppuration, sore or bleeding gums, increased tooth mobility, and poor oral hygiene	42% of the subjects with remaining natural teeth; 43% of those with sore or bleeding gums, 18% with significant tooth mobility, 6% with intraoral swelling or suppuration and 72% with poor oral hygiene
Weyant et al. (1993) USA	650 long-term residents of nursing home care units, mean age 72 yrs; probing assessments at mesial and buccal surfaces, all teeth; demographic, oral and general health data recorded; sample predominantly male and white; calculation of ESI scores	42% of the sample edentulous; 60% of the subjects with PD of > 3 mm at an average of 5.8 sites/person; 3.7% with PD of ≥ 6 mm at < 1 site/person; overall mean mesial ESI: 74, 2.91
Bourgeois et al. (1999) France	603 non-institutionalized elderly, 65-74 yrs old; stratified sample with respect to gender, place of residence and socio-economic group; periodontal conditions assessed by means of the CPITN	16.3% of the sample edentulous; 31.5% of the subjects had pockets ≥ 4 mm; 2.3% had pockets ≥ 6 mm
Pajukoski et al. (1999) Finland	181 hospitalized patients (mean age 81.9 yrs) and 254 home-living patients (mean age 76.9 yrs); periodontal conditions assessed by means of the CPITN	66.3% of the hospitalized and 42.1% of the non-hospitalized subjects were edentulous; 26% of both the hospitalized and the non-hospitalized subjects had pockets ≥ 6 mm

PD: probing depth; AL: attachment level; CEJ: cemento-enamel junction; ESI: Extent and Severity Index; CPITN: Community Periodontal Index of Treatment Needs

by PDI scores > 3) in a sample of 159 children in Michigan, USA and reported figures of 27% for 5-7 year old children, 25% for 8-10 year olds and 21% for 11-14 year olds. Shlossman et al. (1986) used an attachment level value of ≥ 2 mm as a cut-off point and reported in a sample of Pima Indians a prevalence of 7.7% in 5-9 year olds and 6.1% in 10-14 year olds. Sweeney et al. (1987) examined radiographs obtained from 2264 children 5-11 years old, who were referred to a university clinic for routine dental treatment, and reported that a distinct radiographic bone loss was evident at one or more primary molars in 19 children

(0.8%), 16 of whom were black, 2 Caucasian and 1 Asian.

In contrast, relatively uniform criteria have been used in epidemiological studies of *aggressive periodontitis* in young subjects, the condition formerly termed *juvenile periodontitis* (JP), and particularly the *localized* form, formerly termed *localized juvenile periodontitis* (LJP). Typically, a two-stage approach has been adopted in these surveys: first, bite-wing radiographs were used to screen for bone lesions adjacent to molars and incisors and then a clinical examination was performed to verify the diagnosis. As illustrated by the

Table 2-3. Cross-sectional studies of localized and generalized aggressive periodontitis (LAP and GAP) in adolescents and young adults

Authors/Country	Sample/Methodology	Findings
Saxén (1980) Finland	A random sample of 8096 16 year olds; radiographic and clinical criteria (bone loss adjacent to first molars without any obvious iatrogenic factors and presence of pathological pockets)	Prevalence of LAP 0.1% (8 subjects, 5 of whom were females)
Kronauer et al. (1986) Switzerland	A representative sample of 7604 16 year olds; two step examination (radiographic detection of bone lesion on bite-wing radiographs, clinical verification of presence of pathological pockets)	Prevalence of LAP of 0.1%; 1:1 sex ratio
Saxby (1987) UK	A sample of 7266 schoolchildren; initial screening by probing assessments around incisors and first molars; LAP cases diagnosed definitively by full-mouth clinical and radiographic examination	Overall prevalence of LAP of 0.1%, 1:1 sex ratio; however, prevalence varied in different ethnic groups (0.02% in Caucasians, 0.2% in Asians and 0.8% in Afro-Caribbeans)
Neely (1992) USA	1038 schoolchildren 10-12 years old, volunteers in a dentifrice trial; three-stage examination including radiographic and clinical assessments; bite-wing radiographs screened for possible cases; bone loss measurements of the CEJ-bone crest distance of ≥ 2 mm used to identify probable cases; LAP diagnosed clinically as PD of ≥ 3 mm at ≥ 1 first permanent molars in absence of local irritants	117 possible and 103 probable cases identified in step 1 and 2, respectively; out of 99 probable cases contacted, 43 were examined clinically; two cases of LAP could be confirmed in stage 3, yielding a prevalence rate of 0.46%
Cogen et al. (1992) USA	4757 children, age < 15 yrs, from the pool of a children's hospital; retrospective radiographic examination of two sets of bite-wings; LAP diagnosed in case of arc-shaped alveolar bone loss in molars and/or incisors	Whites: LAP prevalence 0.3%, female: male ratio 4:1; blacks: LAP prevalence 1.5%, female: male ratio $\approx$ 1:1; among black LAP cases with available radiographs from earlier examinations, 85.7% showed evidence of bone loss in the mixed dentition and 71.4% in the deciduous dentition
Albandar (1989) Denmark, Norway, Iraq	Denmark: 561 7th grade schoolchildren; Norway: 241 14 year olds; Iraq: 516 7th grade children; two bite-wings/subject; "Incipient lesions" considered present if the CEJ-alveolar crest distance > 2 mm and/or "vertical" pattern of bone loss	6% of the Iraqi, 3.6% of the Danish, and 1.7% of the Norwegian schoolchildren had ≥ 1 proximal surfaces of the first molars with vertical bone loss
Cappelli et al. (1994) USA	470 students, 13-17 yrs old; two-stage examination; probing assessments at the proximal surfaces of all teeth; subjects with loss of attachment examined with respect to subgingival A.a. and systemic antibodies; 94% of the examined of Hispanic ethnicity; 47% male; early-onset disease defined as ≥ 1 pockets with PD ≥ 5 mm	25.7% of the subjects suffered from periodontitis; 16.2% had multiple sites with PD ≥ 5 mm; 1.7% diagnosed as LAP; 85% of all subjects with periodontitis showed elevated antibodies against A.a. serotype b; subjects with detectable A.a. were 4.5 times more likely to suffer from EOP than being healthy or having gingivitis
Löe & Brown (1991) USA	National Survey of US children, multistage probability sampling representing 45 million schoolchildren; 40 694 subjects, 14-17 yrs old examined; probing assessments at mesial and buccal sites, all teeth; LAP: ≥ 1 first molar and ≥ 1 incisor or second molar and ≤ 2 cuspids or premolars with ≥ 3 mm AL; GAP: if LAP criteria not met and ≥ 4 teeth (of which ≥ 2 were second molars, cuspids or premolars) with ≥ 3 mm attachment loss (AL); Incidental loss of attachment (ILA): if neither LAP nor GAP criteria met but ≥ 1 teeth with ≥ 3 mm AL; bivariate and multivariate analysis	Population estimates: LAP 0.53%; GAP 0.13%; ILA 1.61%; altogether 2.27% representing almost 300 000 adolescents; blacks at much higher risk for all forms of early-onset disease than whites; males more likely (4.3:1) to have GAP than females, after adjusting for other variables; black males 2.9 times as likely to have LAP than black females; white females more likely to have LAP than white males by the same odds
Bhat (1991) USA	A sample of 11 111 schoolchildren, 14-17 yrs old; probing assessments at mesial and buccal surfaces of all teeth; multistage cluster sampling stratified by age, sex, seven geographic regions, and rural or urban residence; not stratified by race or ethnicity	22% of children with ≥ 1 site with AL of ≥ 2 mm, 0.72% of ≥ 4 mm and 0.04% of ≥ 6 mm; supra- and subgingival calculus in 34% and 23% of the children, respectively
van der Velden et al. (1989) The Netherlands	4565 subjects 14-17 yrs old examined; randomization among high school students; probing assessments at the mesio- and distofacial surfaces of first molars and incisors; one bacterial sample from the dorsum of the tongue and one subgingival plaque sample from the site with maximal attachment loss obtained from 103 out of the 230 subjects with AL and cultured for identification of A. actinomycetemcomitans	Overall, AL occurred in 5% of the sample and was more frequent in males; 16 subjects (0.3%) had ≥ 1 site with AL of 5-8 mm; female:male ratio in this group 1.3:1; A. actinomycetemcomitans was identified in 17% of the sampled subjects with AL

Table 2-3 (*contd*)

Authors/Country	Sample/Methodology	Findings
Lopez et al. (1991) Chile	2500 schoolchildren in Santiago (1318 male, 1182 female), 15-19 yrs of age; clinical and radiographic assessments; three-stage screening: (1) clinical assessments of probing depth at incisors and molars, (2) children with ≥ 2 teeth with PD of ≥ 5.5 mm subjected to a limited radiographic examination, and (3) children with alveolar bone loss of ≥ 2 mm invited for a full-mouth clinical and radiographic examination	After screening, 27 subjects had a tentative diagnosis of LJP out of which 8 were confirmed (7 female, 1 male); overall prevalence of LJP 0.32%, 95% confidence limits between 0.22% and 0.42%; LJP significantly more frequent in the low socio-economic group
Ben Yehouda et al. (1991) Israel	1160 male Israeli army recruits, in ages 18-19 yrs; panoramic radiography; juvenile periodontitis diagnosed on the basis of bone loss involving ≥ 30% of the root length adjacent to first molars or incisors	10 recruits (0.86%, 95% confidence interval 0.84%-0.88%) had a bone loss pattern consistent with localized juvenile periodontitis
Joss et al. (1992) Switzerland	757 male army recruits, 19-20 yrs old; half-mouth examination, probing assessments at four sites/tooth; bite-wing radiographs of the right mouth half; representative sample of the young male Swiss population, with respect to ethnic background, profession and socio-economic status	Only one subject suffered from LJP (0.13%); 0.4% of the recruits showed PD of ≥ 5 mm and 1% of the subjects showed AL of ≥ 4 mm
Melvin et al. (1991) USA	5013 military recruits, 17-26 yrs old; panoramic radiography followed by full-mouth clinical examination; diagnosis of JP if bone loss and attachment loss was greater at first molars and/or incisors than at other teeth	Overall prevalence of JP 0.76%, female:male ratio 1.1:1; prevalence in blacks 2.1%, female:male ratio 0.52:1; prevalence in whites 0.09%, female:male ratio 4.3:1
Tinoco et al. (1997) Brazil	7843 schoolchildren, 12-19 yrs old; two-stage screening: (1) clinical assessment of PD at first molars, (2) children with ≥ 1 tooth with PF ≥ 5 mm examined futher; LAP diagnosed if a person with no systemic disease presented with > 2 mm at ≥ 1 sites with radiographic evidence of bone loss and ≥ 1 infrabony defects at molars/incisors	119 subjects identified at initial screening; 25 confirmed cases of LAP; overall prevalence 0.3%; ethnic origins and gender ratios not reported

Terms used in the original publications:"localized juvenile periodontitis" instead of "localized aggressive periodontitis", and "generalized juvenile periodontitis" instead of "generalized aggressive periodontitis".
PD: probing depth; AL: attachment level; CEJ: cemento-enamel junction

data in Table 2-3, the prevalence of localized aggressive periodontitis (LAP) varies in geographically and/or racially different populations. In Caucasians, the disease appears to affect females more frequently than males and the prevalence is low (≈ 0.1%). In other races, and in particular in black subjects, the disease is more prevalent (probably at levels over 1%) and the sex ratio appears to be reversed, since males are affected more frequently than females.

The progression pattern of periodontitis in adolescents was studied in an interesting longitudinal study by Brown et al. (1996), which in fact is the follow-up of the study by Löe & Brown (1991) presented in Table 2-3. In a nationally representative sample comprising 14 013 adolescents in the USA, the authors studied the pattern of progression of the disease entity formerly termed *early-onset periodontitis*, i.e. the kind of periodontitis that occurs in individuals of young age. Subjects were diagnosed at baseline as free from periodontitis, or suffering from localized aggressive periodontitis (LAP), generalized aggressive periodontitis (GAP), or incidental attachment loss (IAL). Of the individuals diagnosed with localized aggressive periodontitis at baseline, 62% continued to display localized periodontitis lesions 6 years later, but 35% developed a generalized disease pattern. Among the group initially diagnosed as suffering from IAL, 28% developed localized or generalized aggressive periodontitis, while 30% were reclassified in the no attachment

loss group. Molars and incisors were the teeth most often affected in all three affected groups. Thus, the study indicated that these three forms of periodontitis may progress in a similar fashion, and that certain cases of localized, aggressive disease may develop into generalized aggressive periodontitis.

The possibility that *localized aggressive periodontitis* and *prepubertal periodontitis* are associated conditions, i.e. that the former is a development of the latter, has also attracted attention. Sjödin et al. (1989) examined retrospectively radiographs of the primary dentition of 17 subjects with LAP and reported that 16 of the subjects showed a CEJ-bone crest distance of ≥ 3 mm in at least one tooth site of their deciduous dentition. The same research group (Sjödin & Mattson 1992) examined the CEJ-bone crest distance in radiographs from 128 periodontally healthy children in ages 7-9 years, in order to define a threshold value which, if exceeded, would with high probability entail periodontal pathology around the deciduous teeth. Having set this threshold value to 2 mm, Sjödin et al. (1993) examined radiographs of the deciduous dentition retrospectively from 118 patients with aggressive periodontitis and 168 age- and sex-matched periodontally healthy controls. The patients were divided into two groups, one comprising subjects with only one affected site (45 subjects) and another (73 subjects) including subjects with 2 to 15 sites with bone loss in their permanent dentition. It was found that 52% of the subjects in the latter group, 20% of the subjects in the former group and only 5% of the controls exhibited at least one site with bone loss in their primary dentition. The authors concluded that, at least in some young subjects with aggressive periodontitis, the onset of the disease may be manifested in the primary dentition. Similar results were reported by Cogen et al. (1992), from a study in the US. Among systemically healthy young black people with aggressive periodontitis and with radiographs available of the primary dentition, 71% showed alveolar bone loss adjacent to one or several primary teeth.

Epidemiological studies of periodontal conditions in adolescents have also been carried out by means of the CPITN system. Miyazaki et al. (1991a) presented an overview of 103 CPITN surveys of subjects aged 15-19 years from over 60 countries. The most frequent finding in these groups was the presence of calculus which was much more prevalent in subjects from non-industrialized than industrialized countries. Probing pocket depths of 4-5 mm were present in about two thirds of the populations examined. However, deep pockets ($\geq$ 6 mm) were relatively infrequent: score 4 quadrants were reported to occur in only 10 of the examined populations (in 4 out of 9 examined American samples, 1 out of 16 African, 1 out of 10 East Mediterranean, 2 out of 35 European, 2 out of 15 South-East Asian and in none out of 18 Western Pacific samples).

For an extensive recent review of the epidemiology of periodontal diseases in children and adolescents the reader is referred to the publication by Jenkins & Papapanou (2001).

Periodontitis and tooth loss

Tooth loss may be the ultimate consequence of destructive periodontal disease. Teeth lost due to the sequelae of the disease are obviously not amenable to registration in epidemiological surveys and may, hence, lead to an underestimation of the prevalence and the severity of the disease. The well-established concept of *selection bias* in epidemiology (indicating that the comparatively healthier subjects will present for an examination while the more diseased will refuse participation) is in this context applicable on the individual tooth level (since the severely affected teeth may have already been extracted/lost). Aspects related to tooth loss on a population basis have been addressed in numerous publications. Important questions that were analyzed included (1) the relative contribution of periodontitis as a reason underlying tooth extractions in subjects retaining a natural dentition (Bailit et al. 1987, Brown et al. 1989, Cahen et al. 1985, Corbet & Davies 1991, Heft & Gilbert 1991, Klock & Haugejorden 1991, McCaul et al. 2001, Reich & Hiller 1993, Stephens et al. 1991), (2) its role in cases of full-mouth extractions, the so called *total tooth clearance* (Eklund & Burt 1994, Takala et al. 1994), and (3)

risk factors for tooth loss (Burt et al. 1990, Drake et al. 1995, Hunt et al. 1995, Krall et al. 1994, Phipps et al. 1991).

Typically, surveys addressing the first topic have utilized questionnaire data obtained from general practitioners instructed to document the reasons for which teeth were extracted over a certain time period. The results indicate that the reason underlying the vast majority of extractions in ages up to 40 to 45 years is dental caries. However, in older age cohorts, periodontal disease becomes about equally responsible for tooth loss. Overall, periodontitis is thought to account for 30-35% of all tooth extractions while caries and its sequelae account for up to 50%. In addition, caries appears to be the principal reason for extractions in cases of total tooth clearance. Finally, identified risk factors for tooth loss include smoking, perceived poor dental health, socio-behavioral traits, and periodontitis scores.

Obviously, it is hardly feasible to "translate" tooth loss data into prevalence figures of periodontal disease. An evaluation, however, of the problem conferred to populations – and in particular older age cohorts – due to the disease should weight in information provided by tooth loss data, otherwise underestimation of the occurrence and the consequences of the disease seems inevitable.

RISK FACTORS FOR PERIODONTITIS

Introduction and definitions

There is an abundance of both empirical evidence and substantial theoretical justification for accepting the widespread belief that many diseases have more than one cause, i.e. that they are of *multifactorial etiology* (Kleinbaum et al. 1982). Consequently, in any particular instance when a *causal relationship* is investigated, the specificity of the relation between exposure to an etiological agent and effect, i.e. the *necessity* or the *sufficiency* of the condition, may be challenged. In the case of most infectious diseases for example, it is known that the presence of the microbial agent – which we define as the necessary condition – is not always accompanied by signs or symptoms characteristic of that disorder. Thus, the agent itself is not sufficient to cause any pathological occurrence; rather, the disease development may be dependent on several other factors, including nutritional deficiencies, toxic exposures, emotional stress and the complex impact of social influences. In non-infectious diseases (except for genetic abnormalities), there is usually no factor known to be present in every single case of the disease. For example, smoking is not necessary for the development of lung cancer, and no degree of coro-

	Exposed	Non-exposed	
Cases	155	25	180
Disease-free	40	80	120
	195	105	300

Fig. 2-3. Contingency table describing the distribution of a group of 300 subjects according to exposure to a particular factor and disease status.

nary atherosclerosis is a necessary condition for myocardial infarction.

The *causal inference*, i.e. the procedure of drawing conclusions related to the cause(s) of a disease, is a particularly complicated issue in epidemiological research. In the 1970s, Hill (1971) formalized the criteria that have to be fulfilled in order to accept a causal relation. These included:

1. *Strength of the association.* The stronger the association is between the potential (*putative*) risk factor and disease presence, the more likely it is that the anticipated causal relation is valid.
2. *Dose-response effect.* An observation that the frequency of the disease increases with the dose or level of exposure to a certain factor supports a causal interpretation.
3. *Temporal consistency.* It is important to establish that the exposure to the anticipated causative factor occurred prior to the onset of the disease. This may be difficult in case of diseases with long latent periods or factors that change over time.
4. *Consistency of the findings.* If several studies investigating a given relationship generate similar results, the causal interpretation is strengthened.
5. *Biological plausibility.* It is advantageous if the anticipated relationship makes sense in the context of current biological knowledge. However, it must be realized that the less that is known about the etiology of a given disease, the more difficult it becomes to satisfy this particular criterion.
6. *Specificity of the association.* If the factor under investigation is found to be associated with only one disease, or if the disease is found to be associated with only one factor among a multitude of factors tested, the causal relation is strengthened. However, this criterion can by no means be used to reject a causal relation, since many factors have multiple effects and most diseases have multiple causes.

It is important to realize that the criteria described above are meant as guidelines when a causal inference is established. None of them, however, is either necessary or sufficient for a causal interpretation. Strict adherence to any of them without concomitant consideration of the other may result in incorrect conclusions.

A distinction has to be drawn between a *causal* factor, assessed as above, and a *risk* factor. In a broad sense, the term risk factor may indicate an aspect of personal behavior or lifestyle, an environmental exposure, or an inborn or inherited characteristic which, on the basis of epidemiologic evidence, is known to be associated with disease-related conditions. Such an attribute or exposure may be associated with an increased probability of occurrence of a particular disease without necessarily being a causal factor. A risk factor may be modified by intervention, thereby reducing the likelihood that the particular disease will occur.

The principles of the *risk assessment process* were discussed by Beck (1994) and should consist of the following four steps:

1. The *identification* of one or several individual factors that appear to be associated with the disease.
2. In the case of multiple factors, a *multivariate risk assessment model* must be developed that discloses which combination of factors does most effectively discriminate between health and disease.
3. The *assessment* step, in which new populations are screened for this particular combination of factors, with a subsequent comparison of the level of the disease assessed with the one predicted by the model.
4. The *targeting* step, in which exposure to the identified factors is modified by prevention or intervention and the effectiveness of this particular regimen is evaluated.

Thus, according to this flow chart, *potential* or *putative risk factors* (often also referred to as *risk indicators*) are first identified and thereafter tested until their significance as *true risk factors* is proven.

Finally, distinction must be made between *prognostic* factors (or *disease predictors*), i.e. characteristics related to the progression of *pre-existing* disease and *true risk factors*; i.e. exposures related to the *onset* of the disease. For example, it is established in longitudinal studies of periodontal disease (Papapanou et al. 1989) that the amount of alveolar bone loss or the number of teeth present at baseline may be used to predict further progression of the disease. These variables are, in fact, alternative measures of the disease itself and express the level of susceptibility of a given subject to periodontal diseases. Although they may be excellent predictors for further disease progression, they can clearly not be considered as risk factors.

There are several ways to study the relation between exposure to a certain factor and the development of a particular disease, as required under point 1. One of these is described in Fig. 2-3 which illustrates a hypothetical situation where exposure to the potential risk factor Z is studied among 180 subjects found to suffer from the disease D ("cases") and 120 disease-free individuals ("controls"). It was observed that 155 out of the 180 diseased subjects had been exposed to factor Z, as was also the case for 40 non-diseased subjects. The association between exposure and disease may in this example be expressed by the *odds ratio* (OR), which is the ratio of exposure among the cases to exposure among the controls. For the data in Fig. 2-3, the odds ratio is calculated as

$$(155/25){:}(40/80) = (155 \times 80){:}(40 \times 25) = 12.4$$

This indicates that the cases were 12.4 times more likely to have been exposed to factor Z than the controls.

In a study of the association between exposure to a risk factor and the occurrence of disease, *confounding* can occur when an additional factor, associated with the disease, exists and is unevenly distributed among the groups under investigation. For instance, in a study between radon exposure and lung cancer, smoking may act as a confounder if the smoking habits of the subjects exposed to radon are different from those of the subjects not exposed.

There are various ways to assess simultaneously the effect of a number of putative risk factors identified in step 1 and generate the multivariate model required for step 2. For example, the association between exposure and disease may for reasons of simplicity have the form of the following linear equation:

$$y = a + b_1x_1 + b_2x_2 + b_3x_3 + \ldots b_nx_n$$

where y represents occurrence or severity of the disease, a is the intercept (a constant value), $x_1, x_2, \ldots x_n$ describe the different exposures (putative risk factors), and $b_1, b_2, \ldots b_n$ are *estimates* defining the relative importance of each individual exposure as determinant of disease, after taking all other factors into account. Such an approach may identify factors with statistically and biologically significant effect and may eliminate the effect of confounders.

In the third step (assessment step), a new population sample that is independent of the one used in the construction of the multivariate model is screened for occurrence of disease and presence of the relevant factors included in the multivariate model. Subsequently, the predictions of disease are compared with the observed disease, and the *external validity* of the model (i.e. the "behavior" or "fitness" of the model in the new population) is evaluated. Alternatively, exposure to the relevant factors is assessed among the subjects of the new sample, and disease *incidence*, i.e. the number of new cases of disease, is determined over a time period after a longitudinal follow-up of the subjects.

A number of significant issues may be elucidated during the targeting step. Hence, aspects of causality or risk are verified if disease occurrence is suppressed when exposure is impeded. Importantly, an evaluation of the particular preventive/therapeutic strategy from a "cost-benefit" point of view is facilitated.

In the case of periodontitis, it should be realized that none of the putative risk factors has been subjected to the scrutiny of all four steps. In fact, risk assessment studies in dental research in general have been confined to the first two steps. In other words, while numerous cross-sectional studies identifying potential factors are available, a relatively limited number of longitudinal studies has involved a multivariate approach for identifying true risk factors while simultaneously controlling for the effect of possible confounders. In the following text, the issue of risk factors is addressed according to the principles described above. Results from cross-sectional studies are considered to provide evidence for putative risk factors which may be further enhanced if corroborated by longitudinal studies involving multivariate techniques.

Studies of putative risk factors for periodontitis

Multiple factors

In a relatively large number of cross-sectional studies, multiple risk markers/putative risk factors for periodontal disease have been examined (Beck et al. 1990, Grossi et al. 1994, 1995, Horning et al. 1992, Ismail & Szpunar 1990, Källestål & Matsson 1990, Locker & Leake 1993b, Mumghamba et al. 1995, Oliver et al. 1991, Tervonen et al. 1991, Wheeler et al. 1994). A selection of such studies and an outline of their design and main findings is presented in Table 2-4. A common feature of these studies is the use of a multivariate approach when seeking associations between factors and outcome variables (i.e. the extent and severity of periodontal disease). Increased odds ratios for severe disease have been documented for certain "background" factors such as male sex and black or Filipino origin; older age; low socio-economic or educational status; certain systemic conditions such as diabetes; smoking; and occurrence of certain bacteria such as

Table 2-4. Putative risk factors for periodontitis in cross-sectional studies

Authors/Country	Sample/Methodology	Findings
Ismail & Szpunar (1990) USA	Two random samples of dentate Mexican-Americans, 12-74 yrs old; 395 with low and 1894 high acculturation status; probing assessments at mesial sites, all teeth (Russell's periodontal index); data from HHANES survey; acculturation index (AI) in a scale from 1 to 5; the two groups comprised the lower 8.6% of the sample with AI of 1 and upper 46.8% with an AI score of 3.1-4.9	Logistic regression revealed that subjects with low AI had significantly more gingivitis and periodontal pocketing than subjects with high AI, even after accounting for the effects of age, sex, debris and calculus index scores, income and education
Beck et al. (1990) USA	690 community dwelling adults, age 65+; probing assessments at mesio- and mid-buccal surfaces, all teeth; logistic regression for advanced AL and deep pocketing; "advanced disease": ≥ 4 sites with AL of ≥ 5 mm and ≥ 1 of these sites with PD of ≥ 4 mm	Blacks: 78% of their sites with attachment loss, mean AL on these sites 4 mm; whites: 65%, 3.1 mm; odds ratios in blacks: tobacco use 2.9; P. gingivalis > 2% 2.4; P. intermedia > 2% 1.9; last dental visit > 3 yrs 2.3; bleeding gums 3.9; in whites: tobacco use 6.2; presence of P. gingivalis (+) 2.4; no dental visits for > 3 years plus BANA (+) 16.8
Tervonen et al. (1991) Finland	895 subjects in ages 25, 35, 50 and 65 yrs; CPITN; interview and questionnaire; logistic regression to evaluate the associations between periodontal pocketing (PD ≥ 4 mm) and dietary and oral hygiene habits, social factors, appreciation of natural teeth, use and availability of dental services	Periodontal pocketing was correctly classified in 65% of the cases and was significantly associated with social variables and behavioral factors; adjusted odds ratios for periodontal pocketing: age 1.7 to 4.3, male sex 2.0
Oliver et al. (1991) USA	15 132 employed adults, 18-64 yrs; partial recording; probing assessments at mesial and buccal sites in one upper and one lower quadrant; pair-wise associations between the prevalence and extent of PD with race, education, income, dental insurance and dental visits	Periodontal disease was more prevalent and extensive in subjects who were black, had lower education, and had not seen a dentist for the past three years or more
Horning et al. (1992) USA	1783 subjects, 13-84 yrs old, presenting for examination in a military dental clinic; full-mouth, circumferential probing assessments; logistic regression in a predictive model for periodontal disease by use of a number of putative risk indicators	Age over 30 yrs, Filipino background, male sex and current smoker status were significant predictors with adjusted odds ratios 5.0, 1.7, 1.8 and 1.8, respectively
Locker & Leake (1993b) Canada	907 subjects, age 50+ yrs, in two metropolitan and two non-metropolitan communities; probing assessments at mesio-buccal and buccal sites, recession at four sites/tooth, all teeth; in upper molars, palatal probing assessments as well; stepwise linear regression and logistic regression analysis to seek associations between certain socio-demographic, general health, psychosocial, oral health variables, and three indicators of periodontal disease experience (mean AL, % of sites with AL ≥ 2 mm, and "severe" disease)	34% of the subjects had attachment loss of ≥ 2 mm in > 80% of their sites; in the multivariate analysis, age, education, current smoking status and number of teeth had the most consistent independent effects; odds ratios for severe disease: age over 75 yrs 3.9, low educational level 2, current smoking 2.9
Grossi et al. (1994) USA	Random sample of 1426 subjects, age 25-74 yrs, in a metropolitan community; full-mouth probing assessments; multivariate analysis of risk indicators for attachment loss; associations to the right remain valid after controlling for gender, socio-economic status, education, and oral hygiene levels	Significant odds ratios for severe attachment loss (model including exclusively systemic diseases): allergy 0.6, anaemia 0.7, diabetes 2.0, age 1.9 to 9.1; significant odds ratios in a model including potential risk indicators: Capnocytophaga spp. 0.6, anaemia 0.6, high education 0.6, male sex 1.4, P. gingivalis 1.6, age 1.7 to 9.0, smoking 2.0 to 4.7, diabetes 2.3, B. forsythus 2.4
Grossi et al. (1995) USA	Same sample as in Grossi et al. (1994); 1361 subjects, age 25-74 yrs; assessments of interproximal bone loss from full-mouth radiographs; the degree of association between bone loss and explanatory variables was analyzed by stepwise logistic regression	Odds ratios for severe bone loss: kidney disease 0.55, high education 0.7, allergy 0.8, male sex 1.3, smoking 1.5 to 7.3, P. gingivalis 1.73, race 2.4, B. forsythus 2.52, age 2.6 to 24.1

PD: probing depth; AL: attachment level; CEJ: cemento-enamel junction; CPITN: Community Periodontal Index of Treatment Needs; BANA: N-benzoyl-DL-arginine-2-naphthylamide; a substrate hydrolyzed in the presence of *Treponema denticola*, *Porphyromonas gingivalis* and *Bacteroides forsythus*

Porphyromonas gingivalis, *Bacteroides forsythus* and *Prevotella intermedia* in the subgingival plaque. Another interesting observation is that different factors may be of importance in distinct population groups; hence, race (Beck et al. 1990) or age (Grossi et al. 1994) appears to influence the interaction between certain factors and disease expression.

Tobacco smoking

The biological plausibility of an association between tobacco smoking and periodontitis was founded on the potential effects of several tobacco-related substances, notably nicotine, carbon monoxide and hydrogen cyanide. It is increasingly clear that smoking may affect the vasculature, the humoral immune sys-

Table 2-5. Studies focused on the role of tobacco smoking as a risk factor for periodontitis

Authors/Country	Sample/Methodology	Findings
Bergström (1989) Sweden	Patients referred for periodontal therapy (155 subjects, 30, 40 and 50 yrs old); a random sample of the Stockholm population served as controls; full-mouth probing assessments; sites with PD ≥ 4 mm considered diseased; recording of plaque and gingivitis scores	56% of the patients and 34% of the controls were smokers (odds ratio 2.5); significantly higher frequency of periodontally involved teeth in smokers; no notable difference between smokers and non-smokers with respect to plaque and gingivitis
Haber & Kent (1992) USA	196 patients with periodontal disease in a periodontal practice and 209 patients from five general practices; probing assessments at six sites/tooth and full-mouth radiographs; questionnaire on smoking habits; patients with negative history of periodontal therapy from the general practices included as controls; comparison of (1) the prevalence of smoking among the two patient groups, and (2) periodontal disease severity among current and never smokers	Overall smoking history in the periodontal practice 75%; in the general practice 54%; summary odds ratio for positive smoking history in perio versus general practice patients was 2.6; in the perio group, frequency of current smoking increased with increasing severity of periodontal disease
Locker (1992) Canada	907 adults, ≥ 50 yrs old, living independently in four Ontario communities; partial, probing assessments; half of the participants reported a positive history of smoking and 20% were current smokers	Current smokers had fewer teeth, were more likely to have lost all their natural teeth and had higher extent and severity of periodontal disease than those who had never smoked
Haber et al. (1993) USA	132 diabetics and 95 non-diabetics, 19-40 yrs old; probing assessments at six sites/tooth, all teeth; questionnaire on smoking habits; calculation of the population attributable risk percent (PAR%), as an estimate of the excess prevalence of periodontitis in the study population that is associated with smoking	The prevalence of periodontitis was markedly higher among smokers than non-smokers within both the diabetic and non-diabetic groups; PAR% among non-diabetics was 51% in ages 19-30 yrs and 32% in ages 31-40 yrs
Stoltenberg et al. (1993b) USA	Out of 615 medically healthy adults, 28-73 yrs old, attending a health maintenance organization, selection of 63 smokers and 126 non-smokers of similar age, sex, plaque and calculus scores; probing assessments at the proximal surfaces of premolars and molars in a randomly selected posterior sextant; detection of P. gingivalis, P. intermedia, A. actinomycetemcomitans, E. corrodens and F. nucleatum by a semi-quantitative fluorescence immunoassay, in one buccal and one lingual sample per tooth examined; logistic regression to determine if any of the bacteria or smoking were indicators of mean posterior probing depth of ≥ 3.5 mm	Odds ratio for a smoker having a mean PD of ≥ 3.5 mm was 5.3 (95% CI 2.0 to 13.8); no statistically significant difference between smokers and non-smokers with respect to prevalence of the bacteria examined; the logistic model revealed that a mean PD of ≥ 3.5 mm was significantly associated with the presence of A.a., P.i., E.c. and smoking; smoking was a stronger indicator than any of the bacteria examined
Jette et al. (1993) USA	1156 community dwellers, age 70+ yrs; probing assessments at four sites/tooth, all teeth; evaluation if lifelong tobacco use is a modifiable risk factor for poor dental health; multiple regression analysis	18.1% of men and 7.9% of women were tobacco users (overall 12.3%; including 1% smokeless tobacco users); years of exposure to tobacco products was a statistically significant factor for tooth loss, coronal root caries and periodontal disease, regardless of other social and behavioral factors; periodontal disease (no. of affected teeth) was predicted by longer duration of tobacco use, male sex and more infrequent practice of oral hygiene
Martinez Canut et al. (1995) Spain	889 periodontitis patients, in ages 21-76 yrs; probing assessments at six sites/tooth, all teeth; analysis of variance to examine the role of smoking on the severity of periodontitis	Smoking was statistically related to increased severity of periodontitis in multivariate analysis; a dose-response effect was demonstrated, with subjects smoking > 20 cigarettes/day showing significantly higher attachment loss
Axelsson et al. (1998) Sweden	A random sample of 1093 subjects, in ages 35, 50, 65 and 75 yrs; prevalence of smoking in the four age groups was 35%, 35%, 24% and 12%, respectively; recordings included AL, CPITN scores, DMF surfaces, plaque and stimulated salivary secretion rate (SSSR)	In the oldest age group, 41% of the smokers and 35% of the non-smokers were edentulous; in every age group, mean attachment loss was statistically significantly increased in smokers by 0.37, 0.88, 0.85 and 1.33 mm, respectively; smokers had higher CPITN and DMF scores, increased SSSR, but similar plaque levels
Tomar & Asma (2000) USA	12 329 subjects, in age ≥ 18 yrs, participants in the NHANES III study; probing assessments at mesial and buccal sites in one upper and one lower quadrant; mesial assessments performed from the buccal aspect of the teeth; assessments of gingivitis, PD, and location of the gingival margin in relation to the CEJ; "periodontitis" was defined as ≥ 1 site with AL ≥ 4 mm and PD ≥ 4 mm	27.9% of the participants were current smokers and 9.2% met the definition for periodontitis; current smokers were four times as likely to suffer from periodontitis than never smokers, after adjustments for age, gender, race/ethnicity, education and income:poverty ratio; among current smokers, there was a dose-response relationship between cigarettes/day and periodontitis; 41.9% of periodontitis cases were attributable to current smoking and 10.9% to former smoking

PD: probing depth; AL: attachment level; CEJ: cemento-enamel junction; CPITN: Community Periodontal Index of Treatment Needs; DMF: decayed, missing, filled

Odds ratio

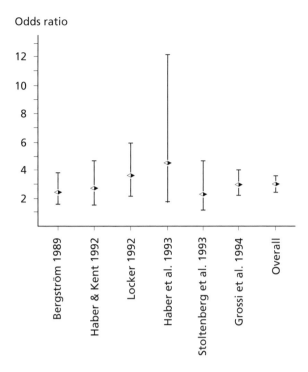

Fig. 2-4. Meta-analysis of smoking as a risk factor for periodontal disease. The studies included are: Bergström (1989), Haber & Kent (1992), Locker (1992), Haber et al. (1993), Stoltenberg et al. (1993b) and Grossi et al. (1994). Bars indicate the 95% confidence limits for the depicted odds ratios.

tem, the cellular immune and inflammatory systems, and exercise effects through the cytokine and adhesion molecule network (for recent reviews see Gelskey 1999, Kinane & Chestnutt 2000, Palmer et al. 1999). A substantial number of studies, a selection of which is summarized in Table 2-5, established the association of smoking with impaired periodontal conditions (Axelsson et al. 1998, Bergström 1989, Goultschin et al. 1990, Haber & Kent 1992, Haber et al. 1993, Jette et al. 1993, Locker 1992, Martinez Canut et al. 1995, Ragnarsson et al. 1992, Stoltenberg et al. 1993b, Tomar & Asma 2000, Wouters et al. 1993).

It is important to emphasize that the multivariate techniques employed in several studies reveal that the inferior periodontal status of smokers cannot be attributed to poorer plaque control or more severe gingivitis (Bergström 1989). Earlier reports suggested a rather similar composition of the subgingival microflora in smokers and non-smokers (Stoltenberg et al. 1993b); however, recent studies demonstrated that shallow sites in smokers are colonized at higher levels by periodontal pathogens, such as *B. forsythus, Treponema denticola,* and *P. gingivalis,* and that these differences were obscured in deep, diseased pockets. In an attempt to quantitate the effects of smoking on the periodontal conditions, Haber et al. (1993) suggested that the excess prevalence of periodontal disease in the population attributed solely to smoking is by far greater than the one owed to other systemic predispositions, such as diabetes mellitus. Data derived from the NHANES III study (Tomar & Asma 2000) suggested that as many as 42% of periodontitis cases in the USA can be attributed to current smoking, and another 11% to former smoking. Interestingly, smoking cessation was shown to be beneficial to the periodontal tissues. In a longitudinal study (Bolin et al. 1993), 349 subjects with ≥ 20 remaining teeth were

examined on two occasions 10 years apart (1970 and 1980). Progression of periodontal disease was assessed on radiographs at all approximal tooth surfaces and was revealed to be almost twice as rapid in smokers than in non-smokers. It was also observed that subjects who quit smoking at some time point within the observation period had a significantly retarded progression of bone loss than the one occurring in smokers. Similar observations were made by Krall et al. (1997) who reported that, over a mean follow-up period of 6 years, subjects who continued to smoke had a 2.4-fold (men) to 3.5-fold risk of tooth loss when compared to non-smokers. Finally, in a 10-year follow-up study, Bergström et al. (2000) observed an increase of periodontally diseased sites concomitant with loss of periodontal bone height in current smokers, as compared to non-smokers whose periodontal health condition remained unaltered throughout the period of investigation. The periodontal health condition in former smokers was similarly stable to that of non-smokers, underscoring the beneficial effects of smoking cessation.

Fig. 2-4 describes a *meta-analysis* of data from studies studying the association between smoking and periodontal conditions. In essence, meta-analysis is a statistical method which combines results from different studies of similar design, in order to gain an overall increased *power,* i.e. an enhanced potential to reveal biological associations which, in fact, exist but are difficult to detect (Chalmers 1993, Oakes 1993, Proskin & Volpe 1994). This analysis incorporated data from six studies, including a total of 2361 subjects, with known smoking habits and periodontal status (Bergström & Eliasson 1989, Grossi et al. 1994, Haber & Kent 1992, Haber et al. 1993, Locker 1992; Stoltenberg et al. 1993b). It can be observed that smoking entailed an overall increased, statistically and biologi-

Table 2-6. Studies focused on the role of diabetes mellitus as a risk factor for periodontitis

Authors/Country	Sample/Methodology	Findings
Hugoson et al. (1989) Sweden	82 subjects with long and 72 with short duration IDDM; 77 non-diabetics (age 20-70 yrs); full-mouth, probing assessments at four sites/tooth; radiographs of lower molar-premolar regions; subjects assigned into five groups according to increasing severity of periodontal disease; no multifactorial analysis	No notable difference in plaque, calculus and no. of teeth between diabetics and non-diabetics; long duration diabetics were more frequently classified in groups 4 and 5 and had significantly more tooth surfaces with PD of ≥ 6 mm than non-diabetics; significantly more extensive ABL in long duration diabetics 40-49 yrs old
Shlossman et al. (1990) USA	3219 Pima Indians, ≥ 5 yrs; prevalence of NIDDM 23% (20% in men, 25% in women); probing assessments at six sites/tooth, at six index teeth; alveolar bone loss from panoramic radiographs; 2878 subjects with available radiographic data, probing assessments or both; comparison between diabetics and non-diabetics with respect to AL and ABL	Median attachment loss and alveolar bone loss higher in diabetics for all age groups and in both sexes
Emrich et al. (1991) USA	Sample and methodology same as above (Shlossman et al. 1990); 1342 Pima Indians, 15 yrs and older, with natural teeth; 19% (254) with diabetes and 12% (158) with impaired glucose tolerance; linear logistic models to predict prevalence and severity of periodontal disease; prevalence: ≥ 1 sites with AL of ≥ 5 mm or ABL $\geq 25\%$ of the root length; severity: square root of average AL or ABL	Diabetes, age and calculus were significant risk markers for periodontitis; odds ratios for a diabetic to have periodontal disease were 2.8 (clinically assessed) and 3.4 (radiographically)
de Pommereau et al. (1992) France	85 adolescents with IDDM in ages 12-18 yrs and 38 healthy age-matched controls; probing assessments at six sites/tooth, all teeth; bite-wing radiographs at molars and sites with AL > 2 mm; patients divided according to disease duration (more or less than 6 yrs); sexual maturation according to Tanner's classification; metabolic control expressed through glycosylated hemoglobin (HbA1c); non-parametric pair-wise analysis	None of the subjects had sites with AL ≥ 3 mm or radiographic signs of periodontitis; despite similar plaque scores, diabetic children had significantly more gingival inflammation; no significant relation between gingival condition and age, Tanner's index, HbA1c level or disease duration
Oliver & Tervonen (1993) USA	114 diabetic patients, 20-64 yrs old (60% with IDDM and 40% with NIDDM); half mouth, probing assessments at four sites/tooth; data from the 1985-86 National Survey served as controls	Tooth loss was similar among diabetics and US employed adults; 60% of the diabetics and 16% of the controls had ≥ 1 site with PD ≥ 4 mm; attachment level data were comparable in both groups
Thorstensson & Hugoson (1993) Sweden	83 IDDM patients and 99 age and sex-matched non-diabetics (age 40-70 yrs); full-mouth, probing assessments at four sites/tooth; radiographs of lower molar-premolar regions; subjects assigned into five groups according to increasing severity of periodontal disease; univariate analysis	Diabetics 40-49 yrs old (mean disease duration 25.6 yrs) had more periodontal pockets ≥ 6 mm and more extensive alveolar bone loss than non-diabetics, but this was not the case for subjects aged 50-59 or 60-69 yrs (mean disease duration 20.5 and 18.6 years, respectively). Disease duration appeared to be a significant determinant of periodontitis development
Pinson et al. (1995) USA	26 IDDM children, 7-18 yrs old and 24 controls, 20 of whom were siblings of the diabetic patients; full-mouth, probing assessments at six sites/tooth; metabolic control assessed through glycosylated hemoglobin (GHb); analysis of co-variance	Overall, no statistically significant differences between cases and controls; no association between GHb and clinical variables; after correcting for plaque, diabetics showed more severe gingival inflammation in specific tooth regions
Taylor et al. (1998) USA	2-year longitudinal study of 24 subjects with NIDDM and 362 subjects without diabetes, aged 15-57 yrs; degree of bone loss on panoramic radiographs was assessed on a scale of 0-4	A regression model having progression of bone loss as the dependent variable revealed a cumulative odds ratio for NIDDM of 4.23 (95% C.I. 1.80-9.92)

PD: probing depth; AL: attachment level; CEJ: cemento-enamel junction
IDDM and NIDDM insulin-dependent and non-insulin dependent diabetes mellitus, respectively; both terms have been abolished and replaced by type 1 and type 2 diabetes

cally significant risk for severe disease (estimated overall odds-ratio of 2.82; 95% confidence limits 2.36 to 3.39).

Diabetes mellitus
Diabetes as a risk factor for periodontitis has been addressed and debated for several years (Genco & Löe 1993), but a number of biological mechanisms have been recently identified by which the disease may contribute to impaired periodontal conditions (for re-

view see Lalla et al. (2000)). Table 2-6 summarizes some epidemiological evidence based on a number of case-control and cohort studies that examine the periodontal status of patients with diabetes (de Pommereau et al. 1992, Emrich et al. 1991, Hugoson et al. 1989, Oliver & Tervonen 1993, Pinson et al. 1995, Shlossman et al. 1990, Thorstensson & Hugoson 1993). Two of these studies (de Pommereau et al. 1992, Pinson et al. 1995) deal with diabetes in children and adolescents and, apart from a more pronounced gingivitis in patients with insulin dependent diabetes mellitus (IDDM), fail to detect notable differences in the periodontal conditions between the diabetics and the healthy subjects. All remaining studies but one (Oliver & Tervonen 1993) demonstrate more severe periodontal conditions in adult patients with diabetes. Of special interest appears to be the study by Emrich et al. (1991) who employed a multivariate analysis in a large subject sample with high prevalence of type II diabetes. These investigators showed that diabetics were three times more likely to suffer attachment and alveolar bone loss than non-diabetics. The studies in Table 2-6 further indicate that diabetes of long duration, early onset and poor metabolic control confers an increased risk for periodontitis.

Evidence from longitudinal studies corroborating the role of diabetes mellitus as a risk factor for periodontitis is also available. A 2-year follow-up study of patients with diabetes and healthy controls by Taylor et al. (1998) demonstrated that diabetes conferred an odds ratio of 4.2 for progression of bone loss over the observation period. Studies have further related the progression of periodontitis to the level of metabolic control (Seppälä et al. 1993, Tervonen & Oliver 1993). In the study by Seppälä et al. (1993), IDDM patients with long diabetes duration were followed for a period of 2 to 3 years. It was demonstrated that patients with good metabolic control exhibited less longitudinal attachment loss and bone loss than poorly controlled patients, despite similar levels of plaque control. In a retrospective study of patients with long-term records of metabolic control, Tervonen & Oliver (1993) showed that calculus and long-term control of diabetes were significant predictors of probing depth of ≥ 4 mm in a multiple regression model.

HIV infection

A number of cross-sectional studies in the 1990s addressed the issue of prevalence of periodontal disease in HIV seropositive subjects (Friedman et al. 1991, Klein et al. 1991, Lamster et al. 1994, Masouredis et al. 1992, Swango et al. 1991). Contrary to early reports demonstrating very severe periodontal conditions in HIV positive subjects, these studies failed to document any notable difference in prevalence and severity of periodontal disease in such subjects when compared to HIV negative controls. A possible explanation may be the fact that the majority of the more recent studies involved random samples of HIV positive subjects and not AIDS patients presenting for examination after manifestation of oral symptoms. It is possible, therefore, that the earlier studies suffer from a certain degree of selection bias.

Two companion publications reporting from a short-term longitudinal study (Cross & Smith 1995, Smith et al. 1995) involved a group of 29 HIV seropositive subjects who were examined at baseline and 3 months. No notably high prevalence or incidence of attachment loss was recorded and their subgingival microflora resembled that obtained from non-

systemically affected subjects, while it was not correlated to their CD4+ and CD8+ lymphocyte counts. However, a 20-month follow-up study of 114 homosexual/bisexual men by Barr et al. (1992) revealed a clear relationship between incidence of attachment loss and immunosuppression, expressed through T4 cell counts. The authors suggested that seropositivity in combination with older age confers an increased risk for attachment loss. Similar observations were drawn by Lamster et al. (1997) who concluded that periodontitis in the presence of HIV infection is dependent upon the immunologic competency of the host as well as the local inflammatory response to both typical and atypical subgingival microbiota. Finally, a cross-sectional study of 326 HIV-infected adults (McKaig et al. 1998) revealed an overall high prevalence of periodontitis, with 62% of the subjects having probing depths of ≥ 5 mm and 66% having attachment loss > 5 mm. Interestingly, after adjustments for CD4+ counts, persons taking HIV-antiretroviral medication were five times less likely to suffer from periodontitis as those not taking such medication, which further demonstrates the importance of the host's immunologic competency in this context.

Other factors

Factors that are increasingly investigated in recent studies include osteopenia/osteoporosis, especially in conjunction with hormone replacement therapy in postmenopausal women (Reinhardt et al. 1999, Ronderos et al. 2000, Tezal et al. 2000), as well as psychosocial stress and coping behaviors (Genco et al. 1999).

Longitudinal studies and conclusions

Table 2-7 presents the design and results of a number of studies involving longitudinal assessments of clinical attachment level or alveolar bone loss and multivariate techniques to identify factors associated with the progression of periodontitis. It is apparent that several features vary considerably between the studies; e.g. the time periods for which the subjects were followed, the size of the samples, the number of sites studied (full-mouth or partial recordings). Examined together, however, the studies allow the following conclusions:

1. It is important to distinguish between risk factors and disease predictors. The use of the latter will undoubtedly increase the coefficient of determination of the multivariate models, (i.e. the proportion of the variance explained by means of the models) but may mask the significance of true etiologic factors. As shown by Ismail et al. (1990a), factors identified by the bivariate analysis which, in addition, bear a biologically plausible etiologic potential (such as dental plaque) do not retain their significance in a multivariate model when predictors such as tooth mobility are also included. As dem-

Table 2-7. Risk factors/predictors in longitudinal clinical and radiographic studies

Authors/Country	Sample/Methodology	Findings
Ismail et al. (1990) USA	526 subjects examined in 1959, 5-50 yrs old, 167 re-examined in 1987; 28-year follow-up; probing assessments at four sites/tooth, all teeth; incidence of attachment loss expressed as: (1) mean LAL, (2) % of sites and subjects with LAL ≥ 2 mm, (3) ≥ 3 mm and (4) ≥ 4 mm; markers of LAL in (5) bivariate analysis and (6) logistic regression	(1) 13% of the subjects, mean LAL ≥ 2 mm (2) 33% of sites, 97% of the subjects (3) 15% of the sites, 88% of the subjects (4) 5% of the sites, 57% of the subjects (5) age, smoking, high tooth mobility/plaque/gingivitis/calculus at baseline, lower education, irregular dental attendance (6) age, smoking, tooth mobility; significant odds ratios for LAL: gender 2.2, education 3.0, dental visits 3.1, smoking 6.3, age 3.9 to 5.4
Haffajee et al. (1991a) Japan	271 randomly selected subjects, 20-59+ yrs old; 1-year follow-up; probing assessments at six sites/tooth, all teeth; chi-square analysis, log linear regression, discriminant analysis; progression threshold: ≥ 3 mm of LAL	27% of the subjects had ≥ 1 site with ≥ 3 mm LAL; older subjects at greater risk than younger; the greater the % of sites with visible plaque or BoP, the greater the risk for LAL; log-linear analysis suggested that the association between BoP, age or plaque with LAL may be explained by their association with baseline AL
Haffajee et al. (1991b) USA	38 subjects, 14-71 yrs old, with prior evidence of attachment loss; 2 month follow-up; probing assessments at six sites/tooth, all teeth; 28 subgingival samples per subject at baseline, DNA-probe analysis with respect to 14 bacterial species; progression threshold: ≥ 3 mm of LAL; the mean % of the total cultivable microbiota was averaged across active and inactive sites; odds ratios computed at different thresholds for each species	Significant odds ratios for new disease: *P. gingivalis* 5.6, *C. rectus* 3.8, *V. parvula* 0.16 and *C. ochracea* 0.08; discriminant analysis using the significantly related species was useful in predicting subjects at risk for new attachment loss
Halazonetis et al. (1989) USA	23 patients with pocket depths monitored for 5 to 12 months prior to therapy; probing assessments at six sites/tooth, all teeth; based on amount and distribution of prior attachment loss the subjects were divided into three groups: minor periodontitis, predominantly molar periodontitis and generalized periodontitis	Subjects with minor periodontitis and predominantly molar periodontitis exhibited LAL more frequently in molar sites, proximal sites and sites with baseline AL ≥ 4 mm; in subjects with generalized periodontitis, LAL was related to tooth surface and baseline AL but not to tooth type
Papapanou et al. (1989) Sweden	201 subjects in ages 25-70 yrs at baseline; 10-year follow-up; randomization among subjects referred for a full-mouth radiographic examination; assessments of alveolar bone loss (ABL) at the approximal surfaces of all teeth; incidence of longitudinal bone loss (LBL); multiple regression using parameters known at baseline to predict bone level status at the second examination	3% of the subjects became edentulous; 7% showed a mean LBL of ≥ 3 mm; 16% of the sites lost ≥ 2 mm of bone support; 15% of the subjects accounted for 50% of all sites with LBL of ≥ 6 mm; 70-year olds showed a statistically significantly higher rate of bone loss when compared to all other groups; remaining teeth and bone loss at baseline were the best predictors of end status
Albandar (1990) Norway	142 subjects, 18-67 yrs old at baseline; 6-year follow-up; randomization among the employees of an industrial plant in Oslo; 6 periapical radiographs per subject; assessments of ABL; radiographs available from baseline, 2 and 6 yrs; contingency tables to analyze disease progression according to tooth type, age and presence of bone loss at baseline; analysis of variance to study the rate of LBL according to the classification variables	Similar degree of LBL in all four age groups; LBL varied according to tooth type and was more pronounced at sites with bone loss at baseline; 90% of the sites were stable over the entire observation period, 3% were active during the first period, 6% over the second period, and 1% during both periods
Papapanou & Wennström (1991) Sweden	Sample and methodology as in Papapanou et al. (1989); classification of the bone loss pattern at baseline as angular or even; angular defects scored in a scale from 1-3 with increasing depth; multiple regression to predict LBL over the 10-year period; diagnostic test for progression based on presence of an angular bony defect at baseline	Sites with an angular bone loss pattern showed more LBL than sites with even bone loss, after adjusting for the subject's and the site's initial amount of bone loss; while 13% of the sites with an even pattern lost bone, this percentage increased to 22%, 46%, and 68% for sites with angular defects of degree 1, 2 and 3, respectively; presence of an angular bony defect at baseline identified LBL with 8% sensitivity, 94% specificity, 28% positive and 77% negative predictability
Beck & Koch (1994) USA	263 blacks, 229 whites, age 65+ yrs; 18-month follow-up; probing assessments at mesio-buccal and buccal sites, all teeth; progression threshold: ≥ 3 mm of LAL; risk factors for LAL manifested through increasing pocket depths were compared to those that conferred progression via increased gingival recession; logistic regression	Subjects with LAL manifested through deepening pockets had different characteristics than those whose LAL was primarily expressed as increased gingival recession; thus, different etiologies may be involved in the two processes
Brown et al. (1994) USA	The same sample as in Beck & Koch (1994); 18-month follow-up; probing assessments at mesio-buccal and buccal sites, all teeth; progression threshold: ≥ 3 mm of LAL; incidence of LAL and risk/predictive factors were studied by logistic regression	50% of the subjects harbored ≥ 1 "loser" site (third of the blacks, quarter of the whites); 24% of the blacks and 16% of the whites harbored ≥ 3 "loser" sites. Risk factors: blacks: *P. gingivalis, P. intermedia*, no flossing, worsening memory, no dental visits for the past 3 years; Whites: *P. gingivalis*, medical care within the last 6 months, depression, regular smoking; advanced disease at baseline was a good predictor of attachment loss

Table 2-7 (contd)

Authors/Country	Sample/Methodology	Findings
Elter et al. (1999) USA	Five sequential examinations of 697 blacks and whites, age 65+ yrs, over a 7-year period; multivariate regression models to examine factors of importance for LAL	For both whites and blacks, factors significantly associated with LAL were *P. gingivalis* amounting to > 2% of the total microbial count, no dental care, smoking and high BANA scores
Bergström et al. (2000) Sweden	A 10-year prospective follow-up of a cohort of 101 professional musicians (16 subjects who smoked at baseline and throughout the follow-up period, 28 former smokers who had quit smoking prior to baseline, 40 never smokers, and 17 subjects who changed smoking habits over the follow-up period); clinical and radiographic examination of periodontal status available at baseline and follow-up	Smoking was significantly associated with both clinical and radiographic periodontal deterioration after controlling for age and baseline severity of periodontitis; periodontal status remained stable in non-smokers and former smokers during the 10-year period

PD: probing depth; AL: attachment level; CEJ: cemento-enamel junction; LAL: longitudinal attachment loss; LBL: longitudinal bone loss
BANA: N-benzoyl-DL-arginine-2-naphthylamide; a substrate hydrolyzed in the presence of *Treponema denticola*, *Porphyromonas gingivalis* and *Bacteroides forsythus*

onstrated by Haffajee et al. (1991a), age, plaque or bleeding are related to both the baseline disease levels as well as to the incidence of the disease. Inclusion of a factor in a model may, thus, eliminate a co-varying, biologically significant other factor.

2. The same risk factors do not necessarily have to be verified in every single study in order to be accepted as such, since the interaction between environmental and subject-related factors (alternatively referred to as "susceptibility" to the disease) does not have to be constant in geographically or racially different populations.

3. Factors identified as "disease markers" in cross-sectional studies do also emerge as such in the longitudinal studies. Hence, smoking appears to be a true risk factor. Results obtained by studies employing improved microbiological methods indicate that certain subgingival species are risk/etiological factors. According to the Consensus Report of the latest World Workshop in Periodontics (1996), there is sufficient evidence to incriminate three bacterial species (*P. gingivalis*, *B. forsythus* and *Actinobacillus actinomycetemcomitans*) as *causative factors* for periodontitis. The exact role of age is more difficult to assess; it is unclear if aging *per se* is a risk factor, or if its effect is due to the prolonged exposure of older subjects to true etiological factors. Angular bony defects appear to be risk markers for progressing disease (Papapanou & Wennström 1991, Papapanou & Tonetti 2000).

4. Assessment of incident periodontitis is directly associated with the progression threshold employed on both the tooth site level (mm of additional attachment loss or bone loss required to characterize a site as "progressing" or "active") and on the subject level (number of "active" sites). It appears that a majority of subjects harbor sites which progress over time. However, it is a small subfraction of subjects that suffer substantial longitudinal attachment loss at multiple sites.

Finally, an interesting issue was brought up in a report by Beck et al. (1995). In a longitudinal study, the authors compared characteristics of patients experiencing attachment loss at previously non-diseased sites with those of patients suffering progression of already established disease. While low income and medication with drugs associated with soft tissue reactions were features in common for both groups of patients, new lesions were more frequent in patients who used smokeless tobacco and had a history of oral pain. Risk for progression of established disease was higher in cigarette smokers, subjects with high levels of subgingival *Porphyromonas gingivalis* and individuals with worsening financial problems. These data suggest that periodontitis may be like other diseases for which the factors associated with the initiation of the disease may be different from the ones involved in its progression. If this observation is verified in other studies, such a distinction may have implications for future assessment strategies and may improve the accuracy of the risk/prediction models.

PERIODONTAL INFECTIONS AND RISK FOR SYSTEMIC DISEASE

During the past few years, a whole new area of periodontal research has emerged, commonly referred to as "periodontal medicine". Following some initial reports linking periodontal infections to cardiovascular disease, researchers are increasingly dwelling on the exploration of additional epidemiological and experimental evidence as well as possible underlying pathogenic mechanisms. The biological plausibility of these associations and the epidemiological evidence available today are briefly summarized in the following text.

Atherosclerosis – cardiovascular/cerebrovascular disease

A wealth of data originating from diverse areas of investigation has implicated chronic, low-level inflammation as an important factor in atherosclerotic cardiovascular disease (CVD) (Ross 1999). Supporting studies stemming from a variety of disciplines such as cell biology, epidemiology, clinical trials and experimental animal research have consistently revealed that atherosclerotic lesions involve an inflammatory component. The cellular interactions in atherogenesis are fundamentally similar to those in chronic inflammatory-fibroproliferative diseases, and atherosclerotic lesions represent a series of highly specific cellular and molecular responses that can best be described, in aggregate, as an inflammatory disease (Ross, 1993, 1999).

It is well established that the periodontal diseases represent mixed infections of the periodontal tissues caused by primarily anaerobic, Gram-negative bacteria (Haffajee & Socransky 1994). As discussed above, the prevalence of these infections may be substantial in certain populations. The deepening of the periodontal sulcus occurring during the course of these infections is concurrent with a marked bacterial proliferation, resulting in bacterial cell levels reaching 10^9 or 10^{10} bacteria within a single pathological periodontal pocket. The ulcerated epithelial lining of the periodontal pocket provides a gate through which lipopolysaccharide (LPS) and other antigenic structures of bacterial origin challenge the immune system and elicit a local and systemic host response (Ebersole & Taubman 1994). Importantly, a number of pathogenic species involved in the periodontal infections display tissue invasion properties (Meyer et al. 1991, Sandros et al. 1994). Frequent transient bacteremias occurring as a result of daily activities such as tooth brushing or chewing (Silver et al. 1977) may confer a significant systemic bacterial challenge to the host.

Emerging evidence indicates that periodontal infections do, in fact, have systemic consequences. Periodontitis patients display higher white blood cell counts (Kweider et al., 1993, Loos et al. 2000) and C-reactive protein (Ebersole et al. 1997, Loos et al. 2000, Slade et al. 2000) levels (CRP) than periodontally healthy controls. Wu et al. (2000) examined the relation between periodontal health status and cardiovascular risk factors, including serum total and high density lipoprotein cholesterol, CRP, and plasma fibrinogen. Based on an analysis of a total of 10 146 subjects from NHANES III with available cholesterol and CRP and 4461 with available fibrinogen, poor periodontal status was significantly associated with increased CRP and fibrinogen levels. Slade et al. (2000) explored the same database and reported (1) that people with extensive periodontal disease had an increase of approximately one-third in mean CRP and a doubling in prevalence of elevated CRP compared with periodontally healthy people, and (2) similarly raised CRP levels in edentulous subjects. In line with the observation that chronic infection may contribute to a pro-coagulant state, Torgano et al. (1999) and Mattila et al. (1989) demonstrated elevated von Willebrand factor antigen, a measure of endothelial cell damage, in individuals with multiple dental infections. Circulating levels of several cytokines (IL-1beta, IL-2, IL-6 and IL-8), induced by several infections (Endo et al. 1992, Humar et al. 1999, Otto et al. 1999) but locally in the periodontal tissues also by periodontitis (Salvi et al. 1998), have been identified as biomarkers of ischemic atherosclerotic disease (Biasucci et al. 1999, Kanda et al. 1996). Interestingly, these pro-inflammatory cytokines have also been detected within atheromatous lesions (Barath et al. 1990a,b, Galea et al. 1996).

The presence of oral bacteria in atheromatic plaque lesions has been examined. Chiu (1999) investigated the relation between the presence of multiple infectious agents in human carotid endarterectomy specimens and pathoanatomic features of the corresponding carotid plaques, and reported positive immunostainings for *P. gingivalis* and *Streptococcus sanguis* in several carotid plaque specimens. The bacteria were immunolocalized in plaque shoulders and lymphohistiocytic infiltrate, associated with ulcer and thrombus formation, and adjacent to areas of strong labeling for apoptotic bodies. A similar study using the polymerase chain reaction (Haraszthy et al. 2000) reported that 30% of the carotid endarderectomy specimens examined were positive for *B. forsythus*, 26% for *P. gingivalis*, 18% for *A. actinomycetemcomitans*, and 14% for *P. intermedia*.

Importantly, periodontal disease has been also associated with clinical events. DeStefano et al. (1993) used a prospective cohort of 9760 subjects and found a nearly two-fold higher risk of coronary heart disease for individuals with periodontal disease. In a case-control study, Syrjanen et al. (1989) compared the level of dental disease in 40 patients who had suffered a cerebrovascular accident with 40 randomly selected community controls, matched for gender and age, and reported that severe chronic dental infection was associated with cerebral infarction in males under 50 years of age. Beck et al. (1996) used data from a cohort of 1147 subjects who were medically healthy at baseline, of whom 207 developed CHD over an average follow-up of 18 years. Radiographic evidence of alveolar bone loss was used to stratify the subjects according to minimal and severe periodontitis. The results, presented as incidence odds ratios adjusted for age and race, showed a significant association between severe bone loss and total CHD, fatal CHD, and stroke. In another case-control study (Grau et al. 1997), multiple logistic regression adjusted for age, social status and a number of established vascular risk factors revealed that poor dental status was independently associated with cerebrovascular ischemia (odds ratio of 2.6; 95% CI 1.18 to 5.7). Beck et al. (2001) have provided the first evidence that periodontitis may be linked to subclinical atherosclerosis. The authors analyzed cross-sectional data on 6017 persons, participants in the Atherosclerosis Risk in Communities Study, and demonstrated that severe periodontitis conferred increased odds for higher carotid artery intima-media wall thickness (OR 2.09, 95% CI 1.73-2.53 for IMT of ≥ 1 mm).

Taken together, the studies above strongly suggest

a biologically plausible association between periodontal infections and the pathogenesis of cardiovascular disease. Studies do exist, however, which have failed to document such an association and point to a possibility of a more complex, conditional relationship. For example, Hujoel et al. (2000) analyzed data from the first NHANES follow-up study, and reported that periodontitis was associated with a non-significant increased risk for a coronary heart disease event (hazard ratio, 1.14; 95% CI 0.96-1.36). One of the shortcomings of this study, however, was the way periodontal disease was measured, namely by means of a crude index system that did not employ probing assessments. Another report (Mattila et al. 2000) described in detail assessments of dental pathology found in various CHD categories, including elderly patients. Although presence of dental pathology was in this study more frequent among CHD patients than controls, the differences were not statistically significant. This absence of effect was contrary to earlier results from the same group of investigators (Mattila 1993, Mattila et al. 1993) and could not be explained by potential confounding factors. Instead, it was suggested that the higher age of the participants in this study was the most likely reason for the discrepancy.

Preterm birth

Preterm infants are born prior to completion of 37 weeks of gestation. Based on weight at birth, preterm infants can be further classified as very low birth weight (< 1500 g) or moderately low birth weight (between 1500 g and 2500 g). An estimated 11% of pregnancies end in preterm birth (Goldenberg & Rouse 1998), and this rate appears to increase despite significant advances in obstetrical medicine and improvements in prenatal care utilization. The contribution of PTB to infant mortality and morbidity is substantial and includes a number of acute and chronic disorders such as respiratory distress syndrome, cerebral palsy, pathologic heart conditions, epilepsy, blindness and severe learning problems (McCormick 1985).

Genito-urinary tract infections, such as bacterial vaginosis, and inflammatory mediators resulting from such infections have been established to play a role in the pathogenesis of PTB. However, women with preterm labor do not invariably present with positive amniotic fluid cultures (Romero et al. 1988), leading to the hypothesis that PTB may be indirectly mediated through *distant* infections resulting in translocation of bacteria, bacterial vesicles and lipopolysaccharide (LPS) in the systemic circulation. The possibility that periodontal infections may constitute such maternal infections that may adversely influence birth outcome was raised for the first time in the late 1980s (McGregor et al. 1988). Transient bacteremias occur commonly in subjects with inflamed gingiva (Ness & Perkins 1980) and may conceivably

reach the placental tissues, providing the inflammatory impetus for labor induction (Offenbacher et al. 1998). An interesting observation in this context was provided in a publication by Hill (1998), who reported that amniotic fluid cultures from women with vaginosis rarely contained bacteria common to the vaginal tract but frequently harbored fusobacteria which are common constituents of the periodontal microbiota. Thus, these authors proposed that oral bacteria may reach amniotic fluids and influence maternal fetal tissues via a hematogenous spread resulting in a chorioamniotic challenge.

So far, there is only limited evidence available in the literature suggesting a positive association between periodontal infections and preterm birth. In a case-control study, Offenbacher et al. (1996) examined 124 mothers, of whom 93 ("cases") gave birth to children with birth weight of less than 2500 g, prior to 37 weeks of gestation. "Controls" were 46 mothers who delivered at term infants of normal birth weight. Assessments included a broad range of known obstetric risk factors, such as tobacco use, drug use, alcohol consumption, level of prenatal care, parity, genitourinary infections and nutrition. The data showed a small, albeit statistically significant, difference in attachment loss between cases and controls (3.1 v. 2.8 mm). Multivariate logistic regression models, controlling for other risk factors and covariates, demonstrated that periodontitis, defined in this publication as ≥ 60% of all sites with attachment loss of ≥ 3 mm, conferred adjusted odds ratios of 7.9 for preterm, low birth weight babies.

A second study by Mitchell-Lewis et al. (2001) examined the relationship between periodontal infections and preterm low birth weight (PLBW) in a cohort of young, minority, pregnant and postpartum women; and the effect of periodontal interventions on pregnancy outcome. A total of 213 women were examined clinically for dental plaque, calculus, bleeding on probing and probing depth. Birth outcome data were available for 164 women, including one group (n = 74) subjected to oral prophylaxis during pregnancy, and a second group (n = 90) who received no prenatal periodontal treatment. In this cohort of women with high incidence of PLBW (16.5%), the data showed that no differences in clinical periodontal status were observed between PLBW cases and women with normal birth outcome. However, PLBW mothers had statistically significantly higher levels of *B. forsythus* and *C. rectus*, and consistently elevated counts for a number of species examined. Interestingly, PLBW occurred in 18.9% of the women who did not receive periodontal intervention, and in 13.5% (10 cases) of those who received such therapy, reflecting a substantial incidence reduction of approximately 30%. However, these results, albeit consistent with the hypothesis that periodontal infections confer risk for preterm birth, should be interpreted with caution due to the small sample size in this study.

In a large prospective study, Jeffcoat et al. (2001)

assessed the periodontal conditions of 1313 pregnant women at 21 to 24 weeks' gestation and followed them until delivery. The authors reported that for women with generalized periodontitis, defined as ≥ 90% of all sites with attachment loss of 3 mm or more, adjusted odds ratios were 4.45 for delivery prior to 37 weeks' gestational age, 5.28 for delivery before 35 weeks' gestational age, and 7.07 for delivery before 32 weeks' gestational age. Finally, a recent study by Dasanayake et al. (2001) reported data on IgG serum antibody levels in 17 women who delivered preterm and 63 women who delivered at term. Cases were found to display statistically significantly higher titers against *P. gingivalis* and *B. forsythus*.

Apparently, the available data are inadequate in establishing any firm conclusion on the issue. A particularly important piece of evidence that needs to be unequivocally established is the effect of periodontal interventions on the incidence of preterm birth in a randomized clinical trial. Fulfillment of the targeting step of the risk assessment process by means of an interventional strategy may not be realistic in the study of the role of periodontal infections in the pathogenesis of atheromatic vascular disease, since (1) these processes may take several years to develop, and (2) the appropriate timing of the interventions may be difficult to determine. In the study of preterm birth, however, the short duration of gestation renders such a study design clearly feasible.

Diabetes mellitus

The role of diabetes as a risk factor for periodontitis has been discussed above; however, limited data seem to suggest that an inverse relationship may also be present. In line with the concept that infections may contribute to impaired metabolic control of diabetes (Lang 1992, Ling et al. 1994, Rayfield et al. 1982), studies of both type 1 (Thorstensson et al. 1996) and type 2 (Taylor et al. 1996) diabetic subjects have indicated that periodontal infections may also be detrimental in this context. The former study involved 39 diabetic subjects with severe periodontitis and the same number of diabetic subjects with gingivitis or mild periodontitis. Both groups had a median duration of diabetes of 25 years. Over a median follow-up period of 6 years, significantly higher prevalence of proteinuria and cardiovascular complications was observed in the severe periodontitis group. A 2-year follow-up study of 90 subjects with type 2 diabetes with good to moderate metabolic control revealed that severe periodontitis at baseline was associated with increased risk for poor glycemic control.

A limited number of studies have examined the effect of treatment of periodontitis on diabetic metabolic control, as reflected by levels of glycated hemoglobin A1c (HbA1c) or plasma glucose. Interestingly, all studies that solely included mechanical periodontal therapy (Aldridge et al. 1995, Christgau et al. 1998,

Grossi et al. 1997, Seppälä et al. 1993, Smith et al. 1996) except one (Stewart et al. 2001), reveal no effect on diabetes metabolic control, regardless of periodontal disease severity, baseline level of metabolic control, or type and duration of diabetes. In contrast, studies including antibiotics as an adjunct to mechanical therapy (Grossi et al. 1997, Miller et al. 1992, Williams & Mahan 1960) reported a limited, short-term improvement in metabolic control. Additional and larger randomized clinical trials are required to clearly establish and quantify such potential effects.

CONCLUDING REMARKS

One of the issues still debated is whether the worldwide prevalence of periodontal disease is increasing or decreasing. Unfortunately, no simple answer can be given for a number of reasons. First, no universal answer is possible, since the prevalence of periodontal disease appears to vary with race and geographic region. Second, the quality of the data available from the developing and the developed countries is clearly not comparable. While a number of well-conducted epidemiological surveys that provide detailed information has been carried out in certain western countries, the majority of the studies in the third world have used the CPITN system, which produced data of inadequate detail and questionable value. Moreover, wherever high quality studies do exist, no earlier studies of comparable quality are usually available from the same populations. Therefore, a definitive evaluation of a possible increase or decrease in the prevalence of periodontal diseases is not feasible. What is well documented, however, is that the rate of edentulousness has decreased over the past 20 years and that people today tend to retain higher numbers of natural teeth than their natives several generations back. This fact *per se* entails that, if anything, the figures of prevalence of periodontal disease should be expected to increase rather than decrease, as long as the disease is measured by means of cumulative clinical attachment loss (Douglass & Fox 1993). Such an increase, however, may not necessarily result in increased need for periodontal therapy (Oliver et al. 1989). Future research is expected to further elucidate these issues, provided that an adequate and consistent epidemiological methodology is utilized.

The need for description of prevalence and incidence of periodontal diseases in every conceivable population has been questioned (Baelum & Papapanou 1996), although such information may be of value for local oral health planners. The principal task of future epidemiological research should, therefore, be the identification of risk factors for disease development. Although a number of risk factors has already been established and a wide array of disease markers recognized, the impact of the intervention with such factors on the state of periodontal health has yet to be documented. To assess the magnitude of the clinical benefit achieved by such modulation, detailed examinations of the periodontal tissues must be adopted in prospective, long-term epidemiological surveys.

Somewhat provocatively, it has been stated that modern science has a tendency to rediscover issues brought up a long time back and (then) rejected. One cannot help bringing the "focal infection" theory into mind, when encountering the emerging plethora of publications dealing with the role of periodontal infections as a risk factor for other pathological conditions. At this stage, albeit the proposed associations appear biologically plausible, we cannot draw any

definitive conclusions on whether these associations are in fact causal, and if so, on the magnitude of their biological effects. Nevertheless, these studies underscore that the oral cavity is an integral part of the human body, and that systemic health must encompass oral – and periodontal – health as well. Last but certainly not least, these studies have provided a unique opportunity for us oral health researchers to expand our investigative sphere, interact fruitfully with our colleagues in medicine, and acquire more knowledge. Irrespective of the definitive conclusions of these research efforts, their byproducts may prove to be just as important as the elucidation of the research task *per se*.

References

Ainamo, J. (1989). Epidemiology of Periodontal Disease. In: Lindhe, J., ed. *Textbook of Clinical Periodontology*, 2nd edn. Copenhagen: Munksgaard, pp. 70-91.

Ainamo, J., Barmes, D., Beagrie, G., Cutress, T., Martin, J. & Sardo-Infirri, J. (1982). Development of the World Health Organization (WHO) community periodontal index of treatment needs (CPITN). *International Dental Journal* **32**, 281-291.

Ainamo, J. & Bay, I. (1975). Problems and proposals for recording gingivitis and plaque. *International Dental Journal* **25**, 229-235.

Albandar, J.M. (1989). Prevalence of incipient radiographic periodontal lesions in relation to ethnic background and dental care provisions in young adults. *Journal of Clinical Periodontology* **16**, 625-629.

Albandar, J.M. (1990). A 6-year study on the pattern of periodontal disease progression. *Journal of Clinical Periodontology* **17**, 467-471.

Albandar, J.M., Brunelle, J.A. & Kingman, A. (1999). Destructive periodontal disease in adults 30 years of age and older in the United States, 1988-1994. *Journal of Periodontology* **70**, 13-29.

Albandar, J.M. & Kingman, A. (1999). Gingival recession, gingival bleeding, and dental calculus in adults 30 years of age and older in the United States, 1988-1994. *Journal of Periodontology* **70**, 30-43.

Aldridge, J.P., Lester, V., Watts, T.L., Collins, A., Viberti, G. & Wilson, R.F. (1995). Single-blind studies of the effects of improved periodontal health on metabolic control in type 1 diabetes mellitus. *Journal of Clinical Periodontology* **22**, 271-275.

Anagnou Vareltzides, A., Diamanti-Kipioti, A., Afentoulidis, N., Moraitaki Tsami, A., Lindhe, J., Mitsis, F. & Papapanou, P.N. (1996). A clinical survey of periodontal conditions in Greece. *Journal of Clinical Periodontology* **23**, 758-763.

Axelsson, P., Paulander, J. & Lindhe, J. (1998). Relationship between smoking and dental status in 35-, 50-, 65-, and 75-year-old individuals. *Journal of Clinical Periodontology* **25**, 297-305.

Baelum, V., Chen, X., Manji, F., Luan, W-M. & Fejerskov, O. (1996). Profiles of destructive periodontal disease in different populations. *Journal of Periodontology Research* **31**, 16-26.

Baelum, V., Fejerskov, O. & Karring, T. (1986). Oral hygiene, gingivitis and periodontal breakdown in adult Tanzanians. *Journal of Periodontal Research* **21**, 221-232.

Baelum, V., Fejerskov, O. & Manji, F. (1988a). Periodontal diseases in adult Kenyans. *Journal of Clinical Periodontology* **15**, 445-452.

Baelum, V., Fejerskov, O., Manji, F. & Wanzala, P. (1993a). Influence of CPITN partial recordings on estimates of prevalence and severity of various periodontal conditions in adults. *Community Dentistry and Oral Epidemiology* **21**, 354-359.

Baelum, V., Luan, W-M., Fejerskov, O. & Xia, C. (1988b). Tooth

mortality and periodontal conditions in 60 to 80-year-old Chinese. *Scandinavian Journal of Dental Research* **96**, 99-107.

Baelum, V., Manji, F., Fejerskov, O. & Wanzala, P. (1993b). Validity of CPITN's assumptions of hierarchical occurrence of periodontal conditions in a Kenyan population aged 15-65 years. *Community Dentistry and Oral Epidemiology* **21**, 347-353.

Baelum, V., Manji, F., Wanzala, P. & Fejerskov, O. (1995). Relationship between CPITN and periodontal attachment loss findings in an adult population. *Journal of Clinical Periodontology* **22**, 146-152.

Baelum, V. & Papapanou, P.N. (1996). CPITN and the epidemiology of periodontal disease. *Community Dentistry and Oral Epidemiology* **24**, 367-368.

Bagramian, R.A., Farghaly, M.M., Lopatin, D., Sowers, M., Syed, S.A. & Pomerville, J.L. (1993). Periodontal disease in an Amish population. *Journal of Clinical Periodontology* **20**, 269-272.

Bailit, H.L., Braun, R., Maryniuk, G.A. & Camp, P. (1987). Is periodontal disease the primary cause of tooth extraction in adults? *Journal of the American Dental Association* **114**, 40-45.

Barath, P., Fishbein, M.C., Cao, J., Berenson, J., Helfant, R.H. & Forrester, J.S. (1990a). Detection and localization of tumor necrosis factor in human atheroma. *American Journal of Cardiology* **65**, 297-302.

Barath, P., Fishbein, M.C., Cao, J., Berenson, J., Helfant, R.H. & Forrester, J.S. (1990b). Tumor necrosis factor gene expression in human vascular intimal smooth muscle cells detected by in situ hybridization. *American Journal of Pathology* **137**, 503-509.

Barr, C., Lopez, M.R. & Rua Dobles, A. (1992). Periodontal changes by HIV serostatus in a cohort of homosexual and bisexual men. *Journal of Clinical Periodontology* **19**, 794-801.

Beck, J., Garcia, R., Heiss, G., Vokonas, P. & Offenbacher, S. (1996). Periodontal disease and cardiovascular disease. *Journal of Periodontology* **67**, 1123-1137.

Beck, J.D. (1994). Methods of assessing risk for periodontitis and developing multifactorial models. *Journal of Periodontology* **65**, 468-478.

Beck, J.D., Elter, J.R., Heiss, G., Couper, D., Mauriello, S.M. & Offenbacher, S. (2001). Relationship of periodontal disease to carotid artery intima-media wall thickness: the atherosclerosis risk in communities (ARIC) study. *Arteriosclerosis, Thrombosis Vascular Biology* **21**, 1816-1822.

Beck, J.D. & Koch, G.G. (1994). Characteristics of older adults experiencing periodontal attachment loss as gingival recession or probing depth. *Journal of Periodontal Research* **29**, 290-298.

Beck, J.D., Koch, G.G. & Offenbacher, S. (1995). Incidence of attachment loss over 3 years in older adults – new and progressing lesions. *Community Dentistry and Oral Epidemiology* **23**, 291-296.

Beck, J.D., Koch, G.G., Rozier, R.G. & Tudor, G.E. (1990). Prevalence and risk indicators for periodontal attachment loss in a population of older community-dwelling blacks and whites. *Journal of Periodontology* **61**, 521-528.

Ben Yehouda, A., Shifer, A., Katz, J., Kusner, W., Machtei, E. & Shmerling, M. (1991). Prevalence of juvenile periodontitis in Israeli military recruits as determined by panoramic radiographs. *Community Dentistry and Oral Epidemiology* **19**, 359-360.

Benigeri, M., Brodeur, J.M., Payette, M., Charbonneau, A. & Ismail, A.I. (2000). Community periodontal index of treatment needs and prevalence of periodontal conditions. *Journal of Clinical Periodontology* **27**, 308-312.

Benn, D.K. (1990). A review of the reliability of radiographic measurements in estimating alveolar bone changes. *Journal of Clinical Periodontology* **17**, 14-21.

Bergström, J. (1989). Cigarette smoking as risk factor in chronic periodontal disease. *Community Dentistry and Oral Epidemiology* **17**, 245-247.

Bergström, J. & Eliasson, S. (1989). Prevalence of chronic periodontal disease using probing depth as a diagnostic test. *Journal of Clinical Periodontology* **16**, 588-592.

Bergström, J., Eliasson, S. & Dock, J. (2000). A 10-year prospective study of tobacco smoking and periodontal health. *Journal of Periodontology* **71**, 1338-1347.

Bhat, M. (1991). Periodontal health of 14 to 17-year-old US schoolchildren. *Journal of Public Health Dentistry* **51**, 5-11.

Biasucci, L.M., Liuzzo, G., Fantuzzi, G., Caligiuri, G., Rebuzzi, A.G., Ginnetti, F., Dinarello, C.A. & Maseri, A. (1999). Increasing levels of interleukin (IL)-1Ra and IL-6 during the first 2 days of hospitalization in unstable angina are associated with increased risk of in-hospital coronary events. *Circulation* **99**, 2079-2084.

Bolin, A., Eklund, G., Frithiof, L. & Lavstedt, S. (1993). The effect of changed smoking habits on marginal alveolar bone loss. A longitudinal study. *Swedish Dental Journal* **17**, 211-216.

Bourgeois, D.M., Doury, J. & Hescot, P. (1999). Periodontal conditions in 65-74 year old adults in France, 1995. *International Dental Journal* **49**, 182-186.

Brown, L.F., Beck, J.D. & Rozier, R.G. (1994). Incidence of attachment loss in community-dwelling older adults. *Journal of Periodontology* **65**, 316-323.

Brown, L.J., Albandar, J.M., Brunelle, J.A. & Löe, H. (1996). Early-onset periodontitis: progression of attachment loss during 6 years. *Journal of Periodontology* **67**, 968-975.

Brown, L.J., Oliver, R.C. & Löe, H. (1989). Periodontal diseases in the US in 1981: Prevalence, severity, extent, and role in tooth mortality. *Journal of Periodontology* **60**, 363-370.

Brown, L.J., Oliver, R.C. & Löe, H. (1990). Evaluating periodontal status of US employed adults. *Journal of the American Dental Association* **121**, 226-232.

Burt, B.A., Ismail, A.I., Morrison, E.C. & Beltran, E.D. (1990). Risk factors for tooth loss over a 28-year period. *Journal of Dental Research* **69**, 1126-1130.

Butterworth, M. & Sheiham, A. (1991). Changes in the Community Periodontal Index of Treatment Needs (CPITN) after periodontal treatment in a general dental practice. *British Dental Journal* **171**, 363-366.

Cahen, P.M., Frank, R.M. & Turlot, J.C. (1985). A survey of the reasons for dental extractions in France. *Journal of Dental Research* **64**, 1087-1093.

Cappelli, D.P., Ebersole, J.L. & Kornman, K.S. (1994). Early-onset periodontitis in Hispanic-American adolescents associated with *A. actinomycetemcomitans*. *Community Dentistry and Oral Epidemiology* **22**, 116-121.

Carlos, J.P., Wolfe, M.D. & Kingman, A. (1986). The extent and severity index: A simple method for use in epidemiologic studies of periodontal disease. *Journal of Clinical Periodontology* **13**, 500-505.

Chalmers, T.C. (1993). Meta-analytic stimulus for changes in clinical trials. *Statistical Methods in Medical Research* **2**, 161-172.

Chiu, B. (1999). Multiple infections in carotid atherosclerotic plaques. *American Heart Journal* **138**, S534-536.

Christgau, M., Palitzsch, K-D., Schmalz, G., Kreiner, U. & Frenzel, S. (1998). Healing response to non-surgical periodontal therapy in patients with diabetes mellitus: clinical, microbiological, and immunological results. *Journal of Clinical Periodontology* **25**, 112-124.

Cogen, R.B., Wright, J.T. & Tate, A.L. (1992). Destructive periodontal disease in healthy children. *Journal of Periodontology* **63**, 761-765.

Consensus report. World Workshop in Periodontics (1996). Periodontal diseases: pathogenesis and microbial factors. *Annals of Periodontology* **1**, 926-932.

Corbet, E.F. & Davies, W.I. (1991). Reasons given for tooth extraction in Hong Kong. *Community Dental Health* **8**, 121-130.

Cross, D.L. & Smith, G.L.F. (1995). Comparison of periodontal disease in HIV seropositive subjects and controls (II). Microbiology, immunology and prediction of disease progression. *Journal of Clinical Periodontology* **22**, 569-577.

Cutress, T.W., Powell, R.N. & Ball, M.E. (1982). Differing profiles of periodontal disease in two similar South Pacific island populations. *Community Dentistry and Oral Epidemiology* **10**, 193-203.

Dasanayake, A.P., Boyd, D., Madianos, P.N., Offenbacher, S. & Hills, E. (2001). The association between Porphyromonas gingivalis-specific maternal serum IgG and low birth weight. *Journal of Periodontology* **72**, 1491-1497.

de Pommereau, V., Dargent-Paré, C., Robert, J.J. & Brion, M. (1992). Periodontal status in insulin-dependent diabetic adolescents. *Journal of Clinical Periodontology* **19**, 628-632.

DeStefano, F., Anda, R.F., Kahn, H.S., Williamson, D.F. & Russell, C.M. (1993). Dental disease and risk of coronary heart disease and mortality. *British Medical Journal* **306**, 688-691.

Diamanti-Kipioti, A., Afentoulidis, N., Moraitaki-Tsami, A., Lindhe, J., Mitsis, F. & Papapanou, P.N. (1995). A radiographic survey of periodontal conditions in Greece. *Journal of Clinical Periodontology* **22**, 385-390.

Diamanti-Kipioti, A., Papapanou, P.N., Moraitaki Tsami, A., Lindhe, J. & Mitsis, F. (1993). Comparative estimation of periodontal conditions by means of different index systems. *Journal of Clinical Periodontology* **20**, 656-661.

Douglass, C.W. & Fox, C.H. (1993). Cross-sectional studies in periodontal disease: current status and implications for dental practice. *Advances in Dental Research* **7**, 25-31.

Douglass, C.W., Jette, A.M., Fox, C.H., Tennstedt, S.L., Joshi, A., Feldman, H.A., McGuire, S.M. & McKinlay, J.B. (1993). Oral health status of the elderly in New England. *Journal of Gerontology* **48**, 0022-1422.

Drake, C.W., Hunt, R.J. & Koch, G.G. (1995). Three-year tooth loss among black and white older adults in North Carolina. *Journal of Dental Research* **74**, 675-680.

Eaton, K.A., Duffy, S., Griffiths, G.S., Gilthorpe, M.S. & Johnson, N.W. (2001). The influence of partial and full-mouth recordings on estimates of prevalence and extent of lifetime cumulative attachment loss: a study in a population of young male military recruits. *Journal of Periodontology* **72**, 140-145.

Ebersole, J.L., Machen, R.L., Steffen, M.J. & Willmann, D.E. (1997). Systemic acute-phase reactants, C-reactive protein and haptoglobin, in adult periodontitis. *Clinical Experimental Immunology* **107**, 347-352.

Ebersole, J.L. & Taubman, M.A. (1994). The protective nature of host responses in periodontal diseases. *Periodontology 2000* **5**, 112-141.

Eklund, S.A. & Burt, B.A. (1994). Risk factors for total tooth loss in the United States; longitudinal analysis of national data. *Journal of Public Health Dentistry* **54**, 5-14.

Elter, J.R., Beck, J.D., Slade, G.D. & Offenbacher, S. (1999). Etiologic models for incident periodontal attachment loss in older adults. *Journal of Clinical Periodontology* **26**, 113-123.

Emrich, L.J., Shlossman, M. & Genco, R.J. (1991). Periodontal disease in non-insulin-dependent diabetes mellitus. *Journal of Periodontology* **62**, 123-131.

Endo, S., Inada, K., Inoue, Y., Kuwata, Y., Suzuki, M., Yamashita, H., Hoshi, S. & Yoshida, M. (1992). Two types of septic shock classified by the plasma levels of cytokines and endotoxin. *Circulation and Shock* **38**, 264-274.

Friedman, R.B., Gunsolley, J., Gentry, A., Dinius, A., Kaplowitz, L. & Settle, J. (1991). Periodontal status of HIV-seropositive and AIDS patients. *Journal of Periodontology* **62**, 623-627.

Frost, W.H. (1941). Epidemiology. In: Maxcy, K.E., ed. *Papers of Wade Hampton Frost, M.D.* New York: The Commonwealth Fund, pp. 493-542.

Galea, J., Armstrong, J., Gadsdon, P., Holden, H., Francis, S.E. & Holt, C.M. (1996). Interleukin-1 beta in coronary arteries of patients with ischemic heart disease. *Arteriosclerosis Thrombosis Vascular Biology* **16**, 1000-1006.

Gelskey, S.C. (1999). Cigarette smoking and periodontitis: methodology to assess the strength of evidence in support of a causal association. *Community Dentistry and Oral Epidemiology* **27**, 16-24.

Genco, R.J., Ho, A. W., Grossi, S.G., Dunford, R.G. & Tedesco, L.A. (1999). Relationship of stress, distress and inadequate coping behaviors to periodontal disease. *Journal of Periodontology* **70**, 711-723.

Genco, R.J. & Löe, H. (1993). The role of systemic conditions and disorders in periodontal disease. *Periodontology 2000* **2**, 98-116.

Gilbert, G.H. & Heft, M.W. (1992). Periodontal status of older Floridians attending senior activity centers. *Journal of Clinical Periodontology* **19**, 249-255.

Goldenberg, R.L. & Rouse, D.J. (1998). Prevention of premature birth. *New England Journal of Medicine* **339**, 313-320.

Goultschin, J., Cohen, H.D., Donchin, M., Brayer, L. & Soskolne, W.A. (1990). Association of smoking with periodontal treatment needs. *Journal of Periodontology* **61**, 364-367.

Grau, A.J., Buggle, F., Ziegler, C., Schwarz, W., Meuser, J., Tasman, A.J., Buhler, A., Benesch, C., Becher, H. & Hacke, W. (1997). Association between acute cerebrovascular ischemia and chronic and recurrent infection. *Stroke* **28**, 1724-1729.

Grossi, S.G., Genco, R.J., Machtei, E.E., Ho, A.W., Koch, G., Dunford, R., Zambon, J.J. & Hausmann, E. (1995). Assessment of risk for periodontal disease. II. Risk indicators for alveolar bone loss. *Journal of Periodontology* **66**, 23-29.

Grossi, S.G., Skrepcinski, F.B., DeCaro, T., Robertson, D.C., Ho, A.W., Dunford, R.G. & Genco, R.J. (1997). Treatment of periodontal disease in diabetics reduces glycated hemoglobin. *Journal of Periodontology* **68**, 713-719.

Grossi, S.G., Zambon, J.J., Ho, A.W., Koch, G., Dunford, R.G., Machtei, E.E., Norderyd, O.M. & Genco, R.J. (1994). Assessment of risk for periodontal disease. I. Risk indicators for attachment loss. *Journal of Periodontology* **65**, 260-267.

Grytten, J. & Mubarak, A. (1989). CPITN (Community Periodontal Index of Treatment Needs) – what is its use and what does it mean? *Nor Tannlaegeforen Tid* **99**, 338-343.

Haber, J. & Kent, R.L. (1992). Cigarette smoking in a periodontal practice. *Journal of Periodontology* **63**, 100-106.

Haber, J., Wattles, J., Crowley, M., Mandell, R., Joshipura, K. & Kent, R.L. (1993). Evidence for cigarette smoking as a major risk factor for periodontitis. *Journal of Periodontology* **64**, 16-23.

Haffajee, A.D. & Socransky, S.S. (1994). Microbial etiological agents of destructive periodontal diseases. *Periodontology 2000* **5**, 78-111.

Haffajee, A.D., Socransky, S.S., Lindhe, J., Kent, R.L., Okamoto, H. & Yoneyama, T. (1991a). Clinical risk indicators for periodontal attachment loss. *Journal of Clinical Periodontology* **18**, 117-125.

Haffajee, A.D., Socransky, S.S., Smith, C. & Dibart, S. (1991b). Relation of baseline microbial parameters to future periodontal attachment loss. *Journal of Clinical Periodontology* **18**, 744-750.

Halazonetis, T.D., Haffajee, A.D. & Socransky, S.S. (1989). Relationship of clinical parameters to attachment loss in subsets of subjects with destructive periodontal diseases. *Journal of Clinical Periodontology* **16**, 563-568.

Haraszthy, V.I., Zambon, J.J., Trevisan, M., Zeid, M. & Genco, R.J. (2000). Identification of periodontal pathogens in atheromatous plaques. *Journal of Periodontology* **71**, 1554-1560.

Heft, M.W. & Gilbert, G.H. (1991). Tooth loss and caries prevalence in older Floridians attending senior activity centers. *Community Dentistry and Oral Epidemiology* **19**, 228-232.

Hill, A.B. (1971). *Principles of Medical Statistics*, 9th edn. New York: Oxford University Press.

Hill, G.B. (1998). Preterm birth: associations with genital and possibly oral microflora. *Annals of Periodontology* **3**, 222-232.

Hobdell, M.H. (2001). Economic globalization and oral health. *Oral Diseases*, **7**, 137-143.

Holmgren, C.J. & Corbet, E.F. (1990). Relationship between periodontal parameters and CPITN scores. *Community Dentistry and Oral Epidemiology* **18**, 322-323.

Horning, G.M., Hatch, C.L. & Cohen, M.E. (1992). Risk indicators for periodontitis in a military treatment population. *Journal of Periodontology* **63**, 297-302.

Horning, G.M., Hatch, C.L. & Lutskus, J. (1990). The prevalence of periodontitis in a military treatment population. *Journal of the American Dental Association* **121**, 616-622.

Hugoson, A., Laurell, L. & Lundgren, D. (1992). Frequency distribution of individuals aged 20-70 years according to severity of periodontal disease experience in 1973 and 1983. *Journal of Clinical Periodontology* **19**, 227-232.

Hugoson, A., Norderyd, O., Slotte, C. & Thorstensson, H. (1998). Distribution of periodontal disease in a Swedish adult population 1973, 1983 and 1993. *Journal of Clinical Periodontology* **25**, 542-548.

Hugoson, A., Thorstensson, H., Falk, H. & Kuylenstierna, J. (1989). Periodontal conditions in insulin-dependent diabetics. *Journal of Clinical Periodontology* **16**, 215-223.

Hujoel, P.P., Drangsholt, M., Spiekerman, C. & DeRouen, T.A. (2000). Periodontal disease and coronary heart disease risk. *JAMA* **284**, 1406-1410.

Humar, A., St Louis, P., Mazzulli, T., McGeer, A., Lipton, J., Messner, H. & MacDonald, K.S. (1999). Elevated serum cytokines are associated with cytomegalovirus infection and disease in bone marrow transplant recipients. *Journal of Infectious Diseases* **179**, 484-488.

Hunt, R.J. (1987). The efficiency of half-mouth examinations in estimating the prevalence of periodontal disease. *Journal of Dental Research* 1044-1048.

Hunt, R.J., Drake, C.W. & Beck, J.D. (1995). Eighteen-month incidence of tooth loss among older adults in North Carolina. *American Journal of Public Health* **85**, 561-563.

Hunt, R.J. & Fann, S.J. (1991). Effect of examining half the teeth in a partial periodontal recording of older adults. *Journal of Dental Research* **70**, 1380-1385.

Hunt, R.J., Levy, S.M. & Beck, J.D. (1990). The prevalence of periodontal attachment loss in an Iowa population aged 70 and older. *Journal of Public Health Dentistry* **50**, 251-256.

Ismail, A.I., Eklund, S.A., Striffler, D.F. & Szpunar, S.M. (1987). The prevalence of advanced loss of periodontal attachment in two New Mexico populations. *Journal of Periodontal Research* **22**, 119-124.

Ismail, A.I., Morrison, E.C., Burt, B.A., Caffesse, R.G. & Kavanagh, M.T. (1990). Natural history of periodontal disease in adults: Findings from the Tecumseh Periodontal Disease Study, 1959-87. *Journal of Dental Research* **69**, 430-435.

Ismail, A.I. & Szpunar, S.M. (1990). Oral health status of Mexican-Americans with low and high acculturation status: findings from southwestern HHANES, 1982-84. *Journal of Public Health Dentistry* **50**, 24-31.

Jamison, H.C. (1963). Prevalence of periodontal disease in the deciduous teeth. *Journal of American Dental Association* **66**, 208-215.

Jeffcoat, M.K., Geurs, N.C., Reddy, M.S., Cliver, S.P., Goldenberg, R.L. & Hauth, J.C. (2001). Periodontal infection and preterm birth: results of a prospective study. *Journal of American Dental Association* **132**, 875-880.

Jenkins, W.M. & Kinane, D.F. (1989). The "high risk" group in periodontitis. *British Dental Journal* **167**, 168-171.

Jenkins, W.M.M. & Papapanou, P.N. (2001). Epidemiology of periodontal diseases in children and adolescents. *Periodontology 2000* **26**, 16-32.

Jette, A.M., Feldman, H.A. & Tennstedt, S.L. (1993). Tobacco use: A modifiable risk factor for dental disease among the elderly. *American Journal of Public Health* **83**, 1271-1276.

Joss, A., Weber, H.P., Gerber, C., Siegrist, B., Curilovic, Z., Saxer, U.P. & Lang, N.P. (1992). Periodontal conditions in Swiss Army recruits. *Schweizer Monatsschrift für Zahnmedizin* **102**, 541-548.

Källestål, C. & Matsson, L. (1990). Periodontal conditions in a group of Swedish adolescents. (II). Analysis of data. *Journal of Clinical Periodontology* **17**, 609-612.

Kanda, T., Hirao, Y., Oshima, S., Yuasa, K., Taniguchi, K., Nagai, R. & Kobayashi, I. (1996). Interleukin-8 as a sensitive marker of unstable coronary artery disease. *American Journal of Cardiology* **77**, 304-307.

Kinane, D.F. & Chestnutt, I.G. (2000). Smoking and periodontal disease. *Critical Review of Oral Biology and Medicine*, **11**, 356-365.

Kingman, A., Morrison, E., Löe, H. & Smith, J. (1988). Systematic errors in estimating prevalence and severity of periodontal disease. *Journal of Periodontology* **59**, 707-713.

Kiyak, H.A., Grayston, M.N. & Crinean, C.L. (1993). Oral health problems and needs of nursing home residents. *Community Dentistry and Oral Epidemiology* **21**, 49-52.

Klein, R.S., Quart, A.M. & Small, C.B. (1991). Periodontal disease in heterosexuals with acquired immunodeficiency syndrome. *Journal of Periodontology* **62**, 535-540.

Kleinbaum, D.G., Kupper, L.L. & Morgenstern, H. (1982). *Epidemiologic Research. Principles and quantitative methods*, 1st edn. New York: Van Nostrand Reinhold.

Klock, K.S. & Haugejorden, O. (1991). Primary reasons for extraction of permanent teeth in Norway: changes from 1968 to 1988. *Community Dentistry and Oral Epidemiology* **19**, 336-341.

Krall, E.A., Dawson-Hughes, B., Garvey, A.J. & Garcia, R.I. (1997). Smoking, smoking cessation, and tooth loss. *Journal of Dental Research* **76**, 1653-1659.

Krall, E.A., Dawson-Hughes, B., Papas, A. & Garcia, R.I. (1994). Tooth loss and skeletal bone density in healthy postmenopausal women. *Osteoporosis International* **4**, 104-109.

Kronauer, E., Borsa, G. & Lang, N.P. (1986). Prevalence of incipient juvenile periodontitis at age 16 years in Switzerland. *Journal of Clinical Periodontology* **13**, 103-108.

Kweider, M., Lowe, G.D., Murray, G.D., Kinane, D.F. & McGowan, D.A. (1993). Dental disease, fibrinogen and white cell count; links with myocardial infarction? *Scottish Medical Journal* **38**, 73-74.

Lalla, E., Lamster, I.B., Drury, S., Fu, C. & Schmidt, A.M. (2000). Hyperglycemia, glycoxidation and receptor for advanced glycation endproducts: potential mechanisms underlying diabetic complications, including diabetes-associated periodontitis. *Periodontology 2000* **23**, 50-62.

Lamster, I.B., Begg, M.D., Mitchell-Lewis, D., Fine, J.B., Grbic, J.T., Todak, G.G., el Sadr, W., Gorman, J.M., Zambon, J.J. & Phelan, J.A. (1994). Oral manifestations of HIV infection in homosexual men and intravenous drug users. Study design and relationship of epidemiologic, clinical, and immunologic parameters to oral lesions. *Oral Surgery, Oral Medicine, Oral Pathology* **78**, 163-174.

Lamster, I.B., Grbic, J.T., Bucklan, R.S., Mitchell-Lewis, D., Reynolds, H.S. & Zambon, J.J. (1997). Epidemiology and diagnosis of HIV-associated periodontal diseases. *Oral Diseases* **3** (Suppl. 1) S141-148.

Lang, C.H. (1992). Sepsis-induced insulin resistance in rats is mediated by a beta-adrenergic mechanism. *American Journal of Physiology* **263**, E703-711.

Lang, N.P. & Hill, R.G. (1977). Radiographs in periodontics. *Journal of Clinical Periodontology* **4**, 16-28.

Lavstedt, S., Eklund, G. & Henrikson, C-O. (1975). Partial recording in conjunction with roentgenologic assessment of proximal marginal bone loss. *Acta Odontologica Scandinavica* **33**, 90-113.

Lilienfeld, D.E. (1978). Definitions of epidemiology. *American Journal of Epidemiology* **107**, 87-90.

Ling, P.R., Bistrian, B.R., Mendez, B. & Istfan, N.W. (1994). Effects of systemic infusions of endotoxin, tumor necrosis factor, and interleukin-1 on glucose metabolism in the rat: relationship to endogenous glucose production and peripheral tissue glucose uptake. *Metabolism* **43**, 279-284.

Locker, D. (1992). Smoking and oral health in older adults. *Canadian Journal of Public Health* **83**, 429-432.

Locker, D. & Leake, J.L. (1993a). Periodontal attachment loss in independently living older adults in Ontario, Canada. *Journal of Public Health Dentistry* **53**, 6-11.

Locker, D. & Leake, J.L. (1993b). Risk indicators and risk markers for periodontal disease experience in older adults living independently in Ontario, Canada. *Journal of Dental Research* **72**, 9-17.

Löe, H. (1967). The Gingival Index, the Plaque Index and the Retention Index system. *Journal of Periodontology* **38**, 610-616.

Löe, H., Ånerud, Å. & Boysen, H. (1992). The natural history of periodontal disease in man: prevalence, severity, and extent of gingival recession. *Journal of Periodontology* **63**, 489-495.

Löe, H., Ånerud, Å., Boysen, H. & Smith, M. (1978). The natural history of periodontal disease in man. Study design and baseline data. *Journal of Periodontal Research* **13**, 550-562.

Löe, H. & Brown, L.J. (1991). Early onset periodontitis in the United States of America. *Journal of Periodontology* **62**, 608-616.

Loos, B.G., Craandijk, J., Hoek, F.J., Wertheim-van Dillen, P.M. & van der Velden, U. (2000). Elevation of systemic markers related to cardiovascular diseases in the peripheral blood of periodontitis patients. *Journal of Periodontology* **71**, 1528-1534.

Lopez, N.J., Rios, V., Pareja, M.A. & Fernandez, O. (1991). Prevalence of juvenile periodontitis in Chile. *Journal of Clinical Periodontology* **18**, 529-533.

Marshall-Day, C.D., Stephens, R.G. & Quigley, L.F. Jr. (1955). Periodontal disease: prevalence and incidence. *Journal of Periodontology* **26**, 185-203.

Martinez Canut, P., Lorca, A. & Magan, R. (1995). Smoking and periodontal disease severity. *Journal of Clinical Periodontology* **22**, 743-749.

Masouredis, C.M., Katz, M.H., Greenspan, D., Herrera, C., Hollander, H., Greenspan, J.S. & Winkler, J.R. (1992). Prevalence of HIV-associated periodontitis and gingivitis in HIV-infected patients attending an AIDS clinic. *Journal of Acquired Immune Deficiency Syndrome* **5**, 479-483.

Matthesen, M., Baelum, V., Aarslev, I. & Fejerskov, O. (1990). Dental health of children and adults in Guinea-Bissau, West Africa, in 1986. *Community Dental Health* **7**, 123-133.

Mattila, K., Rasi, V., Nieminen, M., Valtonen, V., Kesaniemi, A., Syrjala, S., Jungell, P. & Huttunen, J.K. (1989). von Willebrand factor antigen and dental infections. *Thrombosis Research* **56**, 325-329.

Mattila, K.J. (1993). Dental infections as a risk factor for acute myocardial infarction. *European Heart Journal* **14**, 51-53.

Mattila, K.J., Asikainen, S., Wolf, J., Jousimies-Somer, H., Valtonen, V. & Nieminen, M. (2000). Age, dental infections, and coronary heart disease. *Journal of Dental Research* **79**, 756-760.

Mattila, K.J., Valle, M.S., Nieminen, M.S., Valtonen, V.V. & Hietaniemi, K.L. (1993). Dental infections and coronary atherosclerosis. *Atherosclerosis* **103**, 205-211.

McCaul, L.K., Jenkins, W.M. & Kay, E.J. (2001). The reasons for the extraction of various tooth types in Scotland: a 15-year follow-up. *Journal of Dentistry* **29**, 401-407.

McCormick, M.C. (1985). The contribution of low birth weight to infant mortality and childhood morbidity. *New England Journal of Medicine* **312**, 82-90.

McFall, W.T.J., Bader, J.D., Rozier, R.G., Ramsey, D., Graves, R.,

Sams, D. & Sloame, B. (1989). Clinical periodontal status of regularly attending patients in general dental practices. *Journal of Periodontology* **60**, 145-150.

McGregor, J.A., French, J.I., Lawellin, D. & Todd, J.K. (1988). Preterm birth and infection: pathogenic possibilities. *American Journal of Reproductive Immunology* **16**, 123-132.

McKaig, R.G., Thomas, J.C., Patton, L.L., Strauss, R.P., Slade, G.D. & Beck, J.D. (1998). Prevalence of HIV-associated periodontitis and chronic periodontitis in a southeastern US study group. *Journal of Public Health Dentistry* **58**, 294-300.

Melvin, W.L., Sandifer, J.B. & Gray, J.L. (1991). The prevalence and sex ratio of juvenile periodontitis in a young racially mixed population. *Journal of Periodontology* **62**, 330-334.

Meyer, D.H., Sreenivasan, P.K. & Fives-Taylor, P.M. (1991). Evidence for invasion of a human oral cell line by *Actinobacillus actinomycetemcomitans*. *Infection and Immunity* **59**, 2719-2726.

Miller, L.S., Manwell, M.A., Newbold, D., Reding, M.E., Rasheed, A., Blodgett, J. & Kornman, K.S. (1992). The relationship between reduction in periodontal inflammation and diabetes control: a report of nine cases. *Journal of Periodontology* **63**, 843-848.

Mitchell-Lewis, D., Engebretson, S.P., Chen, J., Lamster, I.B. & Papapanou, P.N. (2001). Periodontal infections and pre-term birth: Early findings from a cohort of young minority women in New York. *European Journal of Oral Sciences* **109**, 34-39.

Miyazaki, H., Pilot, T. & Leclercq, M-H. (1992). *Periodontal profiles. An overview of CPITN data in the WHO Global Oral Data Bank for the age group 15-19 years, 35-44 years and 65-75 years*. World Health Organization.

Miyazaki, H., Pilot, T., Leclercq, M.H. & Barmes, D.E. (1991a). Profiles of periodontal conditions in adolescents measured by CPITN. *International Dental Journal* **41**, 67-73.

Miyazaki, H., Pilot, T., Leclercq, M.H. & Barmes, D.E. (1991b). Profiles of periodontal conditions in adults measured by CPITN. *International Dental Journal* **41**, 74-80.

Mühlemann, H.R. & Son, S. (1971). Gingival sulcus bleeding – a leading symptom in initial gingivitis. *Helvetica Odontologica Acta* **15**, 107-113.

Mumghamba, E.G.S., Markkanen, H.A. & Honkala, E. (1995). Risk factors for periodontal diseases in Ilala, Tanzania. *Journal of Clinical Periodontology* **22**, 347-354.

Neely, A.L. (1992). Prevalence of juvenile periodontitis in a circumpubertal population. *Journal of Clinical Periodontology* **19**, 367-372.

Ness, P.M. & Perkins, H.A. (1980). Transient bacteremia after dental procedures and other minor manipulations. *Transfusion* **20**, 82-85.

Oakes, M. (1993). The logic and role of meta-analysis in clinical research. *Statistical Methods in Medical Research* **2**, 147-160.

Offenbacher, S., Jared, H.L., O'Reilly, P.G., Wells, S.R., Salvi, G.E., Lawrence, H.P., Socransky, S.S. & Beck, J.D. (1998). Potential pathogenic mechanisms of periodontitis associated pregnancy complications. *Annals of Periodontology* **3**, 233-250.

Offenbacher, S., Katz, V., Fertik, G., Collins, J., Boyd, D., Maynor, G., McKaig, R. & Beck, J. (1996). Periodontal infection as a possible risk factor for preterm low birth weight. *Journal of Periodontology* **67**, 1103-1113.

Okamoto, H., Yoneyama, T., Lindhe, J., Haffajee, A. & Socransky, S. (1988). Methods of evaluating periodontal disease data in epidemiological research. *Journal of Clinical Periodontology* **15**, 430-439.

Oliver, R.C., Brown, L.J. & Löe, H. (1989). An estimate of periodontal treatment needs in the US based on epidemiologic data. *Journal of Periodontology* **60**, 371-380.

Oliver, R.C., Brown, L.J. & Löe, H. (1991). Variations in the prevalence and extent of periodontitis. *Journal of American Dental Association* **122**, 43-48.

Oliver, R.C., Brown, L.J. & Loe, H. (1998). Periodontal diseases in the United States population. *Journal of Periodontology* **69**, 269-278.

Oliver, R.C. & Tervonen, T. (1993). Periodontitis and tooth loss:

comparing diabetics with the general population. *Journal of American Dental Association* **124**, 71-76.

Otto, G., Braconier, J., Andreasson, A. & Svanborg, C. (1999). Interleukin-6 and disease severity in patients with bacteremic and nonbacteremic febrile urinary tract infection. *Journal of Infectious Diseases* **179**, 172-179.

Page, R.C., Bowen, T., Altman, L., Vandesteen, E., Ochs, H., Mackenzie, P., Osterberg, S., Engel, L.D. & Williams, B.L. (1983). Prepubertal periodontitis. I. Definition of a clinical disease entity. *Journal of Periodontology* **54**, 257-271.

Pajukoski, H., Meurman, J.H., Snellman-Grohn, S. & Sulkava, R. (1999). Oral health in hospitalized and nonhospitalized community-dwelling elderly patients. *Oral Surgery, Oral Medicine, Oral Pathology, Oral Radiology and Endodontology* **88**, 437-443.

Palmer, R.M., Scott, D.A., Meekin, T.N., Poston, R.N., Odell, E.W. & Wilson, R.F. (1999). Potential mechanisms of susceptibility to periodontitis in tobacco smokers. *Journal of Periodontal Research* **34**, 363-369.

Papapanou, P.N. (1996). Periodontal diseases: epidemiology. *Annals of Periodontology* **1**, 1-36.

Papapanou, P.N. & Tonetti, M.S. (2000). Epidemiology of osseous periodontal lesions. *Periodontology 2000* **22**, 8-21.

Papapanou, P.N. & Wennström, J.L. (1991). The angular bony defect as indicator of further alveolar bone loss. *Journal of Clinical Periodontology* **18**, 317-322.

Papapanou, P.N., Wennström, J.L. & Gröndahl, K. (1988). Periodontal status in relation to age and tooth type. A cross-sectional radiographic study. *Journal of Clinical Periodontology* **15**, 469-478.

Papapanou, P.N., Wennström, J.L. & Gröndahl, K. (1989). A 10-year retrospective study of periodontal disease progression. *Journal of Clinical Periodontology* **16**, 403-411.

Papapanou, P.N., Wennström, J.L. & Johnsson, T. (1993). Extent and severity of periodontal destruction based on partial clinical assessments. *Community Dentistry and Oral Epidemiology* **21**, 181-184.

Papapanou, P.N., Wennström, J.L., Sellén, A., Hirooka, H., Gröndahl, K. & Johnsson, T. (1990). Periodontal treatment needs assessed by the use of clinical and radiographic criteria. *Community Dentistry and Oral Epidemiology* **18**, 113-119.

Phipps, K.R., Reifel, N. & Bothwell, E. (1991). The oral health status, treatment needs, and dental utilization patterns of Native American elders. *Journal of Public Health Dentistry* **51**, 228-233.

Pilot, T. & Miyazaki, H. (1994). Global results: 15 years of CPITN epidemiology. *International Dental Journal* **44**, 553-560.

Pinson, M., Hoffman, W.H., Garnick, J.J. & Litaker, M.S. (1995). Periodontal disease and type I diabetes mellitus in children and adolescents. *Journal of Clinical Periodontology* **22**, 118-123.

Proskin, H.M. & Volpe, A.R. (1994). Meta-analysis in dental research: A paradigm for performance and interpretation. *Journal of Clinical Dentistry* **5**, 19-26.

Querna, J.C., Rossmann, J.A. & Kerns, D.G. (1994). Prevalence of periodontal disease in an active duty military population as indicated by an experimental periodontal index. *Military Medicine* **159**, 233-236.

Ragnarsson, E., Eliasson, S.T. & Olafsson, S.H. (1992). Tobacco smoking, a factor in tooth loss in Reykjavik, Iceland. *Scandinavian Journal of Dental Research* **100**, 322-326.

Ramfjord, S.P. (1959). Indices for prevalence and incidence of periodontal disease. *Journal of Periodontology* **30**, 51-59.

Rayfield, E.J., Ault, M.J., Keusch, G.T., Brothers, M.J., Nechemias, C. & Smith, H. (1982). Infection and diabetes: the case for glucose control. *American Journal of Medicine* **72**, 439-450.

Reich, E. & Hiller, K.A. (1993). Reasons for tooth extraction in the western states of Germany. *Community Dentistry and Oral Epidemiology* **21**, 379-383.

Reinhardt, R.A., Payne, J.B., Maze, C.A., Patil, K.D., Gallagher, S.J. & Mattson, J.S. (1999). Influence of estrogen and osteopenia/osteoporosis on clinical periodontitis in postmenopausal women. *Journal of Periodontology* **70**, 823-828.

Romero, R., Quintero, R., Oyarzun, E., Wu, Y.K., Sabo, V., Mazor,

M. & Hobbins, J.C. (1988). Intraamniotic infection and the onset of labor in preterm premature rupture of the membranes. *American Journal of Obstetrics and Gynecology* **159**, 661-666.

Ronderos, M., Jacobs, D.R., Himes, J.H. & Pihlstrom, B.L. (2000). Associations of periodontal disease with femoral bone mineral density and estrogen replacement therapy: cross-sectional evaluation of US adults from NHANES III. *Journal of Clinical Periodontology* **27**, 778-786.

Ross, R. (1993). The pathogenesis of atherosclerosis: a perspective for the 1990s. *Nature* **362**, 801-809.

Ross, R. (1999). Atherosclerosis – an inflammatory disease. *New England Journal of Medicine* **340**, 115-126.

Russell, A.L. (1956). A system for classification and scoring for prevalence surveys of periodontal disease. *Journal of Dental Research* **35**, 350-359.

Salonen, L.W., Frithiof, L., Wouters, F.R. & Helldén, L.B. (1991). Marginal alveolar bone height in an adult Swedish population. A radiographic cross-sectional epidemiologic study. *Journal of Clinical Periodontology* **18**, 223-232.

Salvi, G.E., Brown, C.E., Fujihashi, K., Kiyono, H., Smith, F.W., Beck, J.D. & Offenbacher, S. (1998). Inflammatory mediators of the terminal dentition in adult and early onset periodontitis. *Journal of Periodontal Research* **33**, 212-225.

Sandros, J., Papapanou, P.N., Nannmark, U. & Dahlén, G. (1994). Porphyromonas gingivalis invades human pocket epithelium in vitro. *Journal of Periodontal Research* **29**, 62-69.

Saxby, M.S. (1987). Juvenile periodontitis: an epidemiological study in the West Midlands of the United Kingdom. *Journal of Clinical Periodontology* **14**, 594-598.

Saxén, L. (1980). Prevalence of juvenile periodontitis in Finland. *Journal of Clinical Periodontology* **7**, 177-186.

Schei, O., Waerhaug, J., Lövdal, A. & Arno, A. (1959). Alveolar bone loss related to oral hygiene and age. *Journal of Periodontology* **30**, 7-16.

Scherp, H.W. (1964). Current concepts in periodontal disease research: Epidemiological contributions. *Journal of American Dental Association* **68**, 667-675.

Schürch, E., Jr., Minder, C.E., Lang, N.P. & Geering, A.H. (1990). Comparison of clinical periodontal parameters with the Community Periodontal Index for Treatment Needs (CPITN) data. *Schweizer Monatsschrift für Zahnmedizin* **100**, 408-411.

Seppälä, B., Seppälä, M. & Ainamo, J. (1993). A longitudinal study on insulin-dependent diabetes mellitus and periodontal disease. *Journal of Clinical Periodontology* **20**, 161-165.

Shlossman, M., Knowler, W.C., Pettitt, D.J. & Genco, R.J. (1990). Type 2 diabetes mellitus and periodontal disease. *Journal of American Dental Association* **121**, 532-536.

Shlossman, M., Pettitt, D., Arevalo, A. & Genco, R.J. (1986). Periodontal disease in children and young adults on the Gila River Indian Reservation. *Journal of Dental Research* **65**, special issue, abstract no. 1127.

Silness, J. & Löe, H. (1964). Periodontal disease in pregnancy. II Correlation between oral hygiene and periodontal condition. *Acta Odontologica Scandinavica* **22**, 112-135.

Silver, J.G., Martin, A.W. & McBride, B.C. (1977). Experimental transient bacteraemias in human subjects with varying degrees of plaque accumulation and gingival inflammation. *Journal of Clinical Periodontology* **4**, 92-99.

Sjödin, B., Crossner, C.G., Unell, L. & Ostlund, P. (1989). A retrospective radiographic study of alveolar bone loss in the primary dentition in patients with localized juvenile periodontitis. *Journal of Clinical Periodontology* **16**, 124-127.

Sjödin, B. & Matsson, L. (1992). Marginal bone level in the normal primary dentition. *Journal of Clinical Periodontology* **19**, 672-678.

Sjödin, B., Matsson, L., Unell, L. & Egelberg, J. (1993). Marginal bone loss in the primary dentition of patients with juvenile periodontitis. *Journal of Clinical Periodontology* **20**, 32-36.

Slade, G.D., Offenbacher, S., Beck, J.D., Heiss, G. & Pankow, J.S. (2000). Acute-phase inflammatory response to periodontal disease in the US population. *Journal of Dental Research* **79**, 49-57.

Slade, G.D., Spencer, A.J., Gorkic, E. & Andrews, G. (1993). Oral health status and treatment needs of non-institutionalized persons aged 60+ in Adelaide, South Australia. *Australian Dental Journal* **38**, 373-380.

Smith, G.L.F., Cross, D.L. & Wray, D. (1995). Comparison of periodontal disease in HIV seropositive subjects and controls (I). Clinical features. *Journal of Clinical Periodontology* **22**, 558-568.

Smith, G.T., Greenbaum, C.J., Johnson, B.D. & Persson, G.R. (1996). Short-term responses to periodontal therapy in insulin-dependent diabetic patients. *Journal of Periodontology* **67**, 794-802.

Söder, P.O., Jin, L.J., Söder, B. & Wikner, S. (1994). Periodontal status in an urban adult population in Sweden. *Community Dentistry and Oral Epidemiology* **22**, 106-111.

Stephens, R.G., Kogon, S.L. & Jarvis, A.M. (1991). A study of the reasons for tooth extraction in a Canadian population sample. *Journal of Canadian Dental Association* **57**, 501-504 (erratum published in **57**, 611).

Stewart, J.E., Wager, K.A., Friedlander, A.H. & Zadeh, H.H. (2001). The effect of periodontal treatment on glycemic control in patients with type 2 diabetes mellitus. *Journal of Clinical Periodontology* **28**, 306-310.

Stoltenberg, J.L., Osborn, J.B., Pihlstrom, B.L., Hardie, N.A., Aeppli, D.M., Huso, B.A., Bakdash, M.B. & Fischer, G.E. (1993a). Prevalence of periodontal disease in a health maintenance organization and comparisons to the national survey of oral health. *Journal of Periodontolgy* **64**, 853-858.

Stoltenberg, J.L., Osborn, J.B., Pihlstrom, B.L., Herzberg, M.C., Aeppli, D.M., Wolff, L.F. & Fischer, G.E. (1993b). Association between cigarette smoking, bacterial pathogens, and periodontal status. *Journal of Periodontology* **64**, 1225-1230.

Stuck, A.E., Chappuis, C., Flury, H. & Lang, N.P. (1989). Dental treatment needs in an elderly population referred to a geriatric hospital in Switzerland. *Community Dentistry and Oral Epidemiology* **17**, 267-272.

Swango, P.A., Kleinman, D.V. & Konzelman, J.L. (1991). HIV and periodontal health. A study of military personnel with HIV. *Journal of American Dental Association* **122**, 49-54.

Sweeney, E.A., Alcoforado, G.A.P., Nyman, S. & Slots, J. (1987). Prevalence and microbiology of localized prepubertal periodontitis. *Oral Microbiology and Immunology* **2**, 65-70.

Syrjanen, J., Peltola, J., Valtonen, V., Iivanainen, M., Kaste, M. & Huttunen, J.K. (1989). Dental infections in association with cerebral infarction in young and middle-aged men. *Journal of Internal Medicine* **225**, 179-184.

Takala, L., Utriainen, P. & Alanen, P. (1994). Incidence of edentulousness, reasons for full clearance, and health status of teeth before extractions in rural Finland. *Community Dentistry and Oral Epidemiology* **22**, 254-257.

Taylor, G.W., Burt, B.A., Becker, M.P., Genco, R.J., Shlossman, M., Knowler, W.C. & Pettitt, D.J. (1996). Severe periodontitis and risk for poor glycemic control in patients with non-insulin-dependent diabetes mellitus. *Journal of Periodontology* **67**, 1085-1093.

Taylor, G.W., Burt, B.A., Becker, M.P., Genco, R.J., Shlossman, M., Knowler, W.C. & Pettitt, D.J. (1998). Non-insulin dependent diabetes mellitus and alveolar bone loss progression over 2 years. *Journal of Periodontology* **69**, 76-83.

Tervonen, T., Knuuttila, M. & Nieminen, P. (1991). Risk factors associated with abundant dental caries and periodontal pocketing. *Community Dentistry and Oral Epidemiology* **19**, 82-87.

Tervonen, T. & Oliver, R.C. (1993). Long-term control of diabetes mellitus and periodontitis. *Journal of Clinical Periodontology* **20**, 431-435.

Tezal, M., Wactawski-Wende, J., Grossi, S.G., Ho, A.W., Dunford, R. & Genco, R.J. (2000). The relationship between bone mineral density and periodontitis in postmenopausal women. *Journal of Periodontology* **71**, 1492-1498.

Thorstensson, H. & Hugoson, A. (1993). Periodontal disease

experience in adult long-duration insulin-dependent diabetics. *Journal of Clinical Periodontology* **20**, 352-358.

Thorstensson, H., Kuylenstierna, J. & Hugoson, A. (1996). Medical status and complications in relation to periodontal disease experience in insulin-dependent diabetics. *Journal of Clinical Periodontology* **23**, 194-202.

Tinoco, E.M., Beldi, M.I., Loureiro, C.A., Lana, M., Campedelli, F., Tinoco, N.M., Gjermo, P. & Preus, H.R. (1997). Localized juvenile periodontitis and *Actinobacillus actinomycetemcomitans* in a Brazilian population. *European Journal of Oral Science* **105**, 9-14.

Tomar, S.L. & Asma, S. (2000). Smoking-attributable periodontitis in the United States: findings from NHANES III. National Health and Nutrition Examination Survey. *Journal of Periodontology* **71**, 743-751.

Torgano, G., Cosentini, R., Mandelli, C., Perondi, R., Blasi, F., Bertinieri, G., Tien, T.V., Ceriani, G., Tarsia, P., Arosio, C. & Ranzi, M.L. (1999). Treatment of Helicobacter pylori and Chlamydia pneumoniae infections decreases fibrinogen plasma level in patients with ischemic heart disease. *Circulation* **99**, 1555-1559.

van der Velden, U., Abbas, F., Van Steenbergen, T.J., De Zoete, O.J., Hesse, M., De Ruyter, C., De Laat, V.H. & De Graaff, J. (1989). Prevalence of periodontal breakdown in adolescents and presence of *Actinobacillus actinomycetemcomitans* in subjects with attachment loss. *Journal of Periodontology* **60**, 604-610.

Weyant, R.J., Jones, J.A., Hobbins, M., Niessen, L.C., Adelson, R. & Rhyne, R.R. (1993). Oral health status of a long-term-care, veteran population. *Community Dentistry and Oral Epidemiology* **21**, 227-233.

Wheeler, T.T., McArthur, W.P., Magnusson, I., Marks, R.G., Smith, J., Sarrett, D.C., Bender, B.S. & Clark, W.B. (1994). Modeling the relationship between clinical, microbiologic, and immunologic parameters and alveolar bone levels in an elderly population. *Journal of Periodontology* **65**, 68-78.

Williams, R. & Mahan, C. (1960). Periodontal disease and diabetes in young adults. *JAMA*, **172**, 776-778.

Workshop on the Classification of Periodontal Diseases (1999). *Annals of Periodontology* **4**, 1-112.

Wouters, F.R., Salonen, L.E., Helldén, L.B. & Frithiof, L. (1989). Prevalence of interproximal periodontal intrabony defects in an adult population in Sweden. A radiographic study. *Journal of Clinical Periodontology* **16**, 144-149.

Wouters, F.R., Salonen, L.W., Frithiof, L. & Helldén, L.B. (1993). Significance of some variables on interproximal alveolar bone height based on cross-sectional epidemiologic data. *Journal of Clinical Periodontology* **20**, 199-206.

Wu, T., Trevisan, M., Genco, R.J., Falkner, K.L., Dorn, J.P. & Sempos, C.T. (2000). Examination of the relation between periodontal health status and cardiovascular risk factors: serum total and high density lipoprotein cholesterol, C-reactive protein, and plasma fibrinogen. *American Journal of Epidemiology* **151**, 273-282.

Yoneyama, T., Okamoto, H., Lindhe, J., Socransky, S.S. & Haffajee, A.D. (1988). Probing depth, attachment loss and gingival recession. Findings from a clinical examination in Ushiku, Japan. *Journal of Clinical Periodontology* **15**, 581-591.

CHAPTER 3

Dental Plaque and Calculus

NIKLAUS P. LANG, ANDREA MOMBELLI AND ROLF ATTSTRÖM

Microbial considerations

General introduction to plaque formation

Dental plaque as a biofilm

Structure of dental plaque
  Supragingival plaque
  Subgingival plaque
  Peri-implant plaque

Dental calculus
  Clinical appearance, distribution and clinical diagnosis
  Attachment to tooth surfaces and implants
  Mineralization, composition and structure
  Clinical implications

MICROBIAL CONSIDERATIONS

Throughout life, all the interface surfaces of the body are exposed to colonization by a wide range of microorganisms. In general, the establishing microbiota live in harmony with the host. Constant renewal of the surfaces by shedding prevents the accumulation of large masses of microorganisms. In the mouth, however, teeth provide hard, non-shedding surfaces for the development of extensive bacterial deposits. The accumulation and metabolism of bacteria on hard oral surfaces is considered the primary cause of dental caries, gingivitis, periodontitis, peri-implant infec-

tions and stomatitis. Massive deposits are regularly associated with localized disease of the subjacent hard or soft tissues. In 1 mm^3 of dental plaque weighing approximately 1 mg, more than 10^8 bacteria are present. Although over 300 species have been isolated and characterized in these deposits, it is still not possible to identify all the species present. In the context of the oral cavity, the bacterial deposits have been termed *dental plaque* or *bacterial plaque*. Classical experiments have demonstrated that accumulation of bacteria on teeth reproducibly induces an inflammatory response in associated gingival tissues (Fig. 3-1a,b). Removal of plaque leads to the disappearance of the clinical signs of this inflammation (Löe et al.

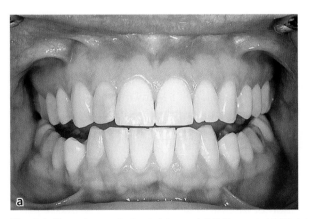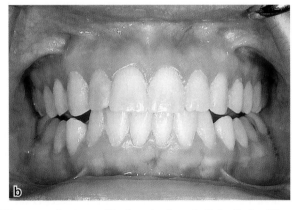

Fig. 3-1. Experimental gingivitis model (Löe et al. 1965) (a) Human volunteer with clean teeth and clinically healthy gingival tissues at the start of the period of experimental plaque accumulation. (b) Same human volunteer after 21 days of abolished oral hygiene practices leading to plaque deposits covering almost all tooth surfaces and consequently developing a generalized marginal gingival inflammation.

1965, Theilade et al. 1966). Similar cause and effect relationships have been demonstrated for plaque and peri-implant mucositis (Pontoriero et al. 1994).

Germ-free animals provide an experimental model which has demonstrated that the absence of bacteria is associated with optimal dental and gingival health. Clinical studies have convincingly demonstrated that regular daily removal of dental plaque in most patients prevents further dental disease. Dental professionals and patients, therefore, consider regular mechanical removal of all bacterial deposits from non-shedding oral surfaces the primary means to prevent disease.

At first, a direct relationship was often assumed to exist between the total number of accumulated bacteria and the amplitude of the pathogenic effect; biologically relevant differences in the composition of plaque usually were not considered. This bacterial mass, termed *plaque*, was shown to produce a variety of irritants, such as acids, endotoxins and antigens, which, over time, invariably dissolved teeth and destroyed the supporting tissues. Consequently, the need to discriminate among bacterial deposits from different patients or at healthy or diseased sites was not yet recognized in detail. Individuals with extensive periodontal disease were either suspected of having a weak resistance to bacterial plaque as a whole or were blamed for inadequate home care. Such a view of dental plaque as a biomass is referred to as the *non-specific plaque hypothesis* (Theilade 1986).

The propensity of inflamed sites to undergo permanent tissue destruction was recognized later to be more specific in nature, because not all gingivitis lesions seemed invariably to progress to periodontitis. Most periodontal sites in most subjects do not always show clinical signs of active tissue destruction with loss of connective tissue fiber attachment to the root surface, even though they may constantly be colonized by varying numbers and species of bacteria. Possible pathogens have been suggested among the organisms regularly found at elevated levels in periodontal lesions in relation to those observed under clinically healthy conditions. Longitudinal studies have indicated an increased risk for periodontal breakdown in sites colonized by some potentially pathogenic organisms. Treatment outcomes were better if these organisms could no longer be detected at follow-up examinations (see Chapter 4). If periodontal disease is indeed due to a limited number of bacterial species, the continuous and maximal suppression of plaque as a whole may not be the only possibility to prevent or treat periodontitis. Hence, specific elimination or reduction of presumptive pathogenic bacteria from plaque may become a valid alternative. Treatment may only be necessary in those patients diagnosed as having the specific infection and may be terminated once the pathogenic agents are eliminated. Such a view of periodontitis being caused by specific

pathogens is referred to as the *specific plaque hypothesis* (Loesche 1979).

The term *infection* refers to the presence and multiplication of a microorganism in body tissues. The uniqueness of bacterial plaque-associated dental diseases as infections relates to the lack of massive bacterial invasion of tissues. Infections caused by the normal microbiota are sometimes called endogenous infections. Endogenous infections result when indigenous microbes thrust from their normal habitats into unusual anatomic regions. *Staphylococcus epidermidis*, for instance, is a non-pathogenic, commensal saprophyte on the skin. If this organism reaches the surface of a vascular prosthesis or an orthopedic implant, a serious infection may emerge. Infections caused by endogenous microbes are called *opportunistic infections* if they occur at the usual habitat of the microorganisms. Such infections may be the result of changing ecologic conditions or may be due to a decrease of host resistance. In the prevention of opportunistic infections due to overgrowth of indigenous organisms, continuous control of ecologic conditions regulating bacterial growth has high priority. The majority of microorganisms in periodontitis plaque can also be found occasionally in low proportions in health. These organisms may, therefore, be viewed as putative opportunistic pathogens. A small number of suspected pathogens, e.g. the Gram-negative anaerobe *Porphyromonas gingivalis*, are rare organisms in the mouth of healthy individuals. Some researchers have suggested that such bacteria may be considered exogenous pathogens. If some periodontal microorganisms were indeed exogenous pathogens, avoidance of exposure would become an important goal of prevention, and therapy should be aimed at the elimination of the microorganisms. Their mere presence would be an indication for intervention.

Dental plaque may accumulate supragingivally, i.e. on the clinical crown of the tooth, but also below the gingival margin, i.e. in the subgingival area of the sulcus or pocket. Differences in the composition of the subgingival microbiota have been attributed in part to the local availability of blood products, pocket depth, redox potential and pO_2. Therefore, the question of whether the presence of specific microorganisms in patients or distinct sites may be the cause or the consequence of disease continues to be a matter of dispute (Socransky et al. 1987). Many microorganisms considered to be periodontopathogens are fastidious, strict anaerobes and, as such, may contribute little to the initiation of disease in shallow gingival pockets. If their preferred habitat were the deep periodontal pocket, they would be linked to the progression in sites with preexisting disease, rather than to the initiation of disease in shallow sites. These microbiologic aspects are to be put in perspective with the host response. Further discussions are presented in Chapter 4.

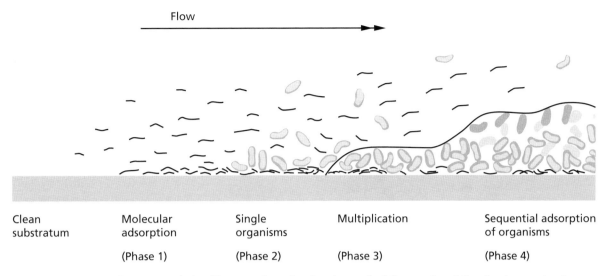

Flow

Clean substratum	Molecular adsorption	Single organisms	Multiplication	Sequential adsorption of organisms
	(Phase 1)	(Phase 2)	(Phase 3)	(Phase 4)

Fig. 3-2. Stages in the formation of a biofilm on a clean, hard and non-shedding surface following immersion into a fluid environment. Phase 1: Molecular adsorption to condition the biofilm formation. Phase 2: Bacterial adhesion by single organisms. Phase 3: Growth of extracellular matrix production and multiplication of the adhering bacteria. Phase 4: Sequential adsorption of further bacteria to form a more complex and mature biofilm. Adapted from Marshall (1992).

GENERAL INTRODUCTION TO PLAQUE FORMATION

Growth and maturation patterns of bacterial plaque have been studied on natural hard oral surfaces, such as enamel and dentin, or artificial surfaces, such as metal or acrylic, using light and electron microscopy and bacterial culture (Theilade & Theilade 1985). Despite differences in surface roughness, free energy and charge, the most important features of initial plaque development are similar on all these materials (Siegrist et al. 1991).

The ability to adhere to surfaces is a general property of almost all bacteria. It depends on an intricate, sometimes exquisitely specific, series of interactions between the surface to be colonized, the microbe and an ambient fluid milieu (Mergenhagen & Rosan 1985).

Immediately upon immersion of a solid substratum into the fluid media of the oral cavity, or upon cleaning of a solid surface in the mouth, hydrophobic and macromolecules begin to adsorb to the surface to form a conditioning film (Fig. 3-2, Phase 1), termed the acquired pellicle. This film is composed of a variety of salivary glycoproteins (mucins) and antibodies. The conditioning film alters the charge and free energy of the surface, which in turn increases the efficiency of bacterial adhesion. Bacteria adhere variably to these coated surfaces. Some possess specific attachment structures such as extracellular polymeric substances and fimbriae, which enable them to attach rapidly upon contact (Fig. 3-2, Phase 2). Other bacteria require prolonged exposure to bind firmly. Behaviors of bacteria change once they become attached to surfaces. This includes active cellular growth of previously starving bacteria and synthesis of new outer membrane components. The bacterial mass increases due

to continued growth of the adhering organisms, adhesion of new bacteria (Fig. 3-2, Phase 4), and synthesis of extracellular polymers. With increasing thickness, diffusion into and out of the biofilm becomes more and more difficult. An oxygen gradient develops as a result of rapid utilization by the superficial bacterial layers and poor diffusion of oxygen through the biofilm matrix. Completely anaerobic conditions eventually emerge in the deeper layers of the deposits. Oxygen is an important ecologic determinant because bacteria vary in their ability to grow and multiply at different levels of oxygen. Diminishing gradients of nutrients supplied by the aqueous phase, i.e. the saliva, are also created. Reverse gradients of fermentation products develop as a result of bacterial metabolism.

Dietary products dissolved in saliva are an important source of nutrients for bacteria in the supragingival plaque. Once a deepened periodontal pocket is formed, however, the nutritional conditions for bacteria change because the penetration of substances dissolved in saliva into the pocket is very limited. Within the deepened pocket, the major nutritional source for bacterial metabolism comes from the periodontal tissues and blood. Many bacteria found in periodontal pockets produce hydrolytic enzymes with which they can break down complex macromolecules from the host into simple peptides and amino acids. These enzymes may be a major factor in destructive processes of periodontal tissues.

Primary colonization is dominated by facultatively anaerobic Gram-positive cocci. They adsorb onto the pellicle-coated surfaces within a short time after mechanical cleaning. Plaque collected after 24 h consists mainly of streptococci; S. sanguis is the most prominent of these organisms. In the next phase, Gram-positive rods, which are present in very low numbers

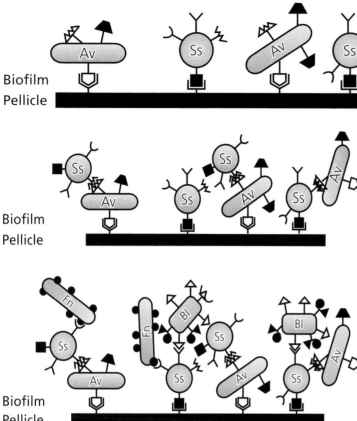

Fig. 3-3. Primary colonization by predominantly Gram-positive facultative bacteria. Ss: *Streptococcus sanguis* is most dominant. Av: *Actinomyces spp.* are also found in 24 h plaque.

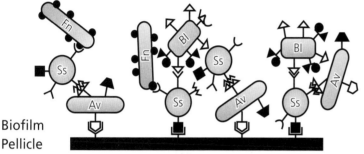

Fig. 3-4. Gram-positive facultative cocci and rods co-aggregate and multiply.

Fig. 3-5. Surface receptors on the Gram-positive facultative cocci and rods allow the subsequent adherence of Gram-negative organisms, which have a poor ability to directly adhere to the pellicle. Fn: *Fusobacterium nucleatum*. Bl: *Prevotella intermedia*.

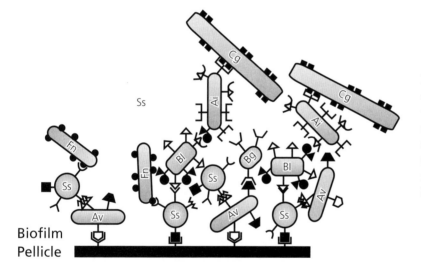

Fig. 3-6. The heterogeneity increases as plaque ages and matures. As a result of ecologic changes, more Gram-negative strictly anaerobic bacteria colonize secondarily and contribute to an increased pathogenicity of the biofilm.

initially, gradually increase and eventually outnumber the streptococci (Fig. 3-3). Gram-positive filaments, particularly *Actinomyces* spp., are the predominating species in this stage of plaque development (Fig. 3-4). Surface receptors on the deposited Gram-positive cocci and rods allow subsequent adherence of Gram-negative organisms with poor ability to attach directly to pellicle. *Veillonella*, fusobacteria and other anaerobic Gram-negative bacteria can attach in this way (Fig. 3-5). The heterogeneity of plaque thus gradually increases and, with time, includes large numbers of Gram-negative organisms. A complex array of interrelated bacterial species is the result of this development. Exchange of nutrients between different species, but also negative interactions, e.g. the

production of bacteriocins, play a role in the establishment of a stable bacterial community (Fig. 3-6). Due to the influences of local environmental factors, structurally different types of plaque evolve at different locations. Protection of the growing plaque from shear forces and local availability of certain nutrients are most important. A distinct composition of mature bacterial deposits can eventually be recognized at specific sites and under specific clinical conditions. Examples are the plaque on smooth enamel surface versus fissure plaque, or the plaque in shallow and less shallow gingival crevices.

Accumulation of plaque along the gingival margin leads to an inflammatory reaction of the soft tissues. The presence of this inflammation has a profound influence on the local ecology. The availability of blood and gingival fluid components promotes growth of Gram-negative bacterial species with an increased periodontopathic potential. Bacterial samples from established gingivitis lesions have increased numbers of these bacteria. Because of the capability enzymatically to digest proteins, many of these organisms do not depend upon a direct availability of dietary carbohydrates. Such bacteria do not produce extracellular polymers and develop only loosely adherent plaque in the developing periodontal pocket. Cultivation of samples from advanced periodontal lesions reveals a predominance of Gram-negative anaerobic rods. Under the microscope, particularly high numbers of anaerobic uncultivable spirochetes can be demonstrated. Further details on the microbial ecology of subgingival plaque are discussed in Chapter 4.

In summary, immediately following immersion of hard, non-shedding surfaces into the fluid environment of the oral cavity, adsorption of macromolecules will lead to the formation of a *biofilm*. Bacterial adhesion to this glycoprotein layer will first involve primary plaque formers, such as Gram-positive facultative cocci and rods. Subsequent colonization onto receptors of these organisms will involve Gram-negative, strictly anaerobic bacteria, while the primary plaque formers also multiply to form colonies. The heterogeneity of the complex biofilm increases with time, as the ecologic conditions gradually change.

DENTAL PLAQUE AS A BIOFILM

The term *biofilm* describes the relatively undefinable microbial community associated with a tooth surface or any other hard, non-shedding material (Wilderer & Charaklis 1989). In the lower levels of most biofilms a dense layer of microbes is bound together in a polysaccharide matrix with other organic and inorganic materials. On top of this layer is a looser layer, which is often highly irregular in appearance and may extend into the surrounding medium. The fluid layer bordering the biofilm may have a rather "stationary" sublayer and a fluid layer in motion. Nutrient components may penetrate this fluid medium by molecular diffusion. Steep diffusion gradients, especially for oxygen, exist in the more compact lower regions of biofilms. The ubiquity with which anaerobic species are detected from these areas of biofilms provides evidence for these gradients (Ritz 1969).

Accumulation of bacteria on solid surfaces is not an exclusive dental phenomenon. Biofilms are ubiquitous; they form on virtually all surfaces immersed in natural aqueous environments. Biofilms form particularly fast in flow systems where a regular nutrient supply is provided to the bacteria. Rapid formation of visible layers of microorganisms due to extensive bacterial growth accompanied by excretion of copious amounts of extracellular polymers is typical for biofilms. Biofilms effectively protect bacteria from antimicrobial agents. Treatment with antimicrobial substances is often unsuccessful unless the deposits are mechanically removed. Adhesion-mediated infections that develop on permanently or temporarily implanted materials such as intravascular catheters, vascular prostheses or heart valves are notoriously resistant to antibiotics and tend to persist until the device is removed. Similar problems are encountered in water conduits, wherein potentially pathogenic bacteria may be protected from chlorination, or on ship hulls, where biofilms increase frictional resistance and turbulence (Gristina 1987, Marshall 1992).

In summary, *dental plaque* as a naturally occurring microbial deposit *represents a true biofilm* which consists of bacteria in a matrix composed mainly of extracellular bacterial polymers and salivary and/or gingival exudate products.

STRUCTURE OF DENTAL PLAQUE

Supragingival plaque

Supragingival plaque has been examined in a number of studies by light and electron microscopy to gain information on its internal structure (Mühlemann & Schneider 1959, Turesky et al. 1961, Theilade 1964, Frank & Brendel 1966, Leach & Saxton 1966, Frank & Houver 1970, Schroeder & De Boever 1970, Theilade & Theilade 1970, Eastcott & Stallard 1973, Saxton 1973, Rönström et al. 1975, Tinanoff & Gross 1976, Lie 1978). The introduction of the electron microscope in dental research was a significant development for studies of dental plaque, both because the size of many bacteria approaches the ultimate resolving power of the light microscope, and because the resins used for embedding allowed for sections thinner than the smallest bacterial dimension. Hereby the substructure of plaque could be identified.

In studies of the internal details of plaque, samples are required in which the deposits are kept in their original relation to the surface on which they have formed. This may be accomplished by removing the deposits with the tooth. If plaque of known age is the object of study, the tooth surfaces are cleaned at a predetermined time before removal (McDougall 1963, Frank & Houver 1970, Schroeder & De Boever 1970). Pieces of natural teeth or artificial surfaces may also be attached to solid structures in the mouth and removed after a given interval. This method of plaque collection was already used at the beginning of the last century by Black (1911). The systematic use of artificial surfaces for collection of plaque was reintroduced during the 1950s. Thin plastic foils of Mylar® were attached to mandibular incisor teeth for known periods, after which they were removed for histologic, histochemical and electron microscopic examination of the deposited material (Mandel et al. 1957, Mühle-

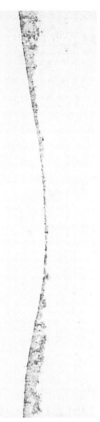

Fig. 3-7. Electron micrographic illustration of a 4-h dental pellicle. The pellicle has formed on an artificial surface of plastic, which was painted on to the surface of the tooth. The plastic surface was exposed to the environment for a 4-h period. A thin condensed layer of organic material is covering the film. The material has a relatively homogeneous appearance but varies in thickness over the surface. From Brecx et al. (1981).

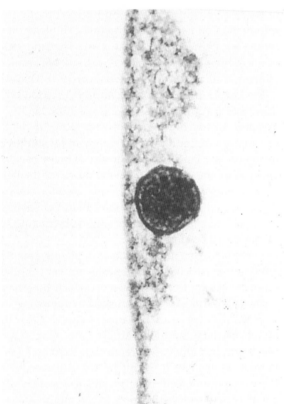

Fig. 3-8. Electron micrographic illustration of a 4-h dental pellicle with a single bacterium included in the film. The microbe appears attached to the surface. The dental pellicle varies in thickness but has a homogeneous morphology. From Brecx et al. (1981).

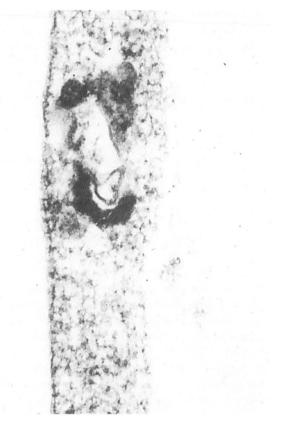

Fig. 3-9. Electron micrographic illustration of a 4-h dental pellicle, formed on a plastic surface attached to the buccal surface of a tooth. A condensed layer of organic material is observed on the surface and cell remnants are embedded in the film. From Brecx et al. (1981).

mann & Schneider 1959, Zander et al. 1960, Schroeder 1963, Theilade 1964). Other types of plastic materials such as Westopal®, Epon®, Araldite®, and *spray plast* have since been employed for this purpose (Berthold

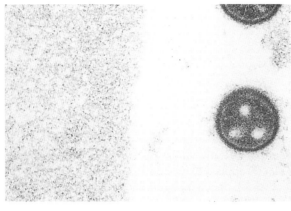

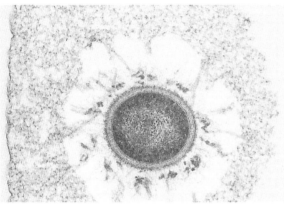

Fig. 3-10. High power electron micrographic illustration of a 4-h pellicle with bacteria residing in the pellicle at a distance of around one micron from the condensed organic material. The pellicle is rather even in composition and, at the oral side, an irregular condensed organic material is seen close to the bacteria. From Brecx et al. (1981).

Fig. 3-11. High power electron micrographic illustration of a 4-h pellicle with an embedded bacterium. The bacterium is deposited on the film surface together with the dental pellicle. Around the bacterium empty spaces are observed representing the radius of extrusions of filaments radiating from the microorganisms. From Brecx et al. (1981).

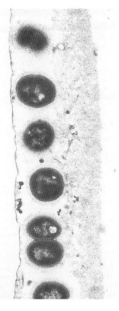

Fig. 3-12. Electron micrographic illustration of a 4-h dental pellicle with bacteria attached to a plastic surface, which had been adhering to a buccal tooth surface and was exposed to the oral environment. A single row of bacteria attached to the surface is seen to the left. On top of the bacteria, a layer of condensed organic material representing the oral lateral portion of the dental pellicle is noted. From Brecx et al. (1981).

et al. 1971, Kandarkar 1973, Lie 1975, Listgarten et al. 1975, Rönström et al. 1975). Results from several such studies indicate that plaque formed on natural or artificial surfaces does not differ significantly in structure or microbiology (Hazen 1960, Berthold et al. 1971, Nyvad et al. 1982, Theilade et al. 1982a, b), indicating that at least some of the principal mechanisms involved in plaque formation are unrelated to the nature of the solid surface colonized. However, there are small, but important, differences in the chemical composition of the first layer of organic material formed on these artificial surfaces compared with that formed on natural tooth surfaces (Sönju & Rölla 1973, Sönju & Glantz 1975, Öste et al. 1981). Tooth surfaces, enamel

as well as exposed cementum, are normally covered by a thin acquired pellicle of glycoproteins (Fig. 3-7). If removed, e.g. by mechanical instrumentation, it reforms within minutes. The pellicle is believed to play an active part in the selective adherence of bacteria to the tooth surface (Fig. 3-8). For details of the proposed mechanisms, see Chapter 4.

The first cellular material adhering to the pellicle on the tooth surface or other solid surfaces consists of coccoid bacteria with numbers of epithelial cells and polymorphonuclear leukocytes (Fig. 3-9). The bacteria are encountered either on (Fig. 3-10) or within the pellicle as single organisms (Fig. 3-11) or as aggregates of microorganisms (Fig. 3-12). Larger numbers of mi-

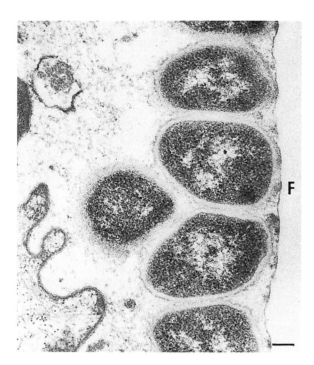

Fig. 3-13. Thin section of plaque colony consisting of morphologically similar bacteria deposited on plastic film (F) applied to the buccal surface of a premolar during an 8-h period. Magnification × 35 000. Bar: 0.2 μm. From Brecx et al. (1980).

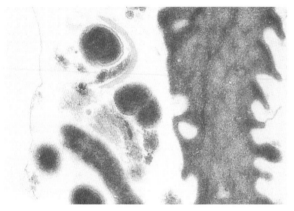

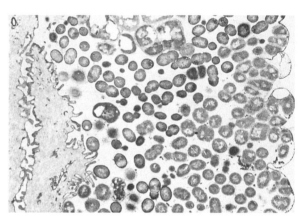

Fig. 3-14. Electron micrographic illustration of early plaque formation. The film surface on which the pellicle and bacteria adhere is located to the left. Bacteria of varying morphology are attached to the film. They are surrounded by organic pellicle material. An epithelial cell remnant is seen in close vicinity to the microbes. From Brecx et al. (1981).

Fig. 3-15. Electron micrographic illustration of 24-h dental plaque formed on a plastic film surface attached to the buccal surface of the tooth. A multilayer bacterial plaque is noted. A remnant of an epithelial cell has been trapped in the microbial mass. From Brecx et al. (1981).

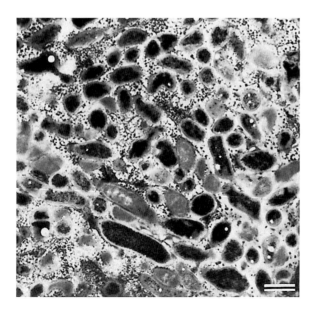

Fig. 3-16. Thin section of old plaque stained for the demonstration of polysaccharides by reacting them with electron-dense material appearing dark in the illustration. Many bacteria contain large amounts of intracellular polysaccharide, and the intermicrobial matrix contains extracellular polysaccharides. Magnification × 7000. Bar: 1 μm. From Theilade & Theilade (1970).

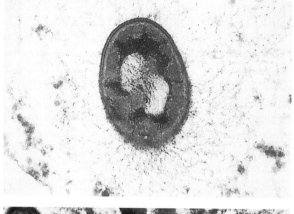

Fig. 3-17. High power electron micrographic illustration of a single bacterium attached to the pellicle by filaments which extend from the bacterial surface to the tooth surface. The surface had been exposed to the oral environment for an 8-h period. From Brecx et al. (1981).

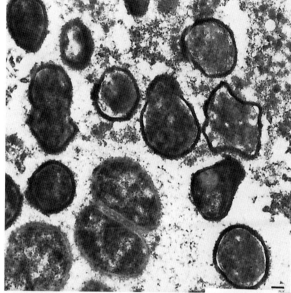

Fig. 3-18. Thin section of plaque with granular or homogeneous intermicrobial matrix. Magnification × 20 000. Bar: 0.1 µm. From Theilade & Theilade (1970).

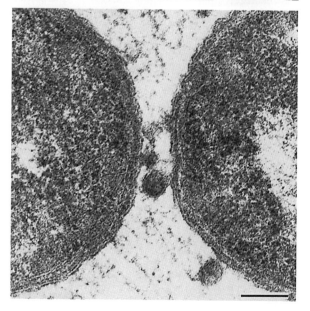

Fig. 3-19. Thin section of plaque with a region predominated by Gram-negative bacteria. Between them, vesicles are surrounded by a trilaminar membrane (two thin electron-dense layers with an electron-lucent layer in between). This substructure is also seen in the outermost endotoxin containing cell wall layer of the adjacent Gram-negative bacteria. Magnification × 110 000. Bar: 0.1 µm. From Theilade & Theilade (1970).

croorganisms may be carried to the tooth surface by epithelial cells.

The number of bacteria found on the surface a few hours after cleaning depends on the procedures applied to the sample before examination, the reason being that adherence to the solid surface is initially very weak. If no special precautions are taken during the preparatory processing, the early deposits are easily lost (Brecx et al. 1980). Apparently the adherence

of microorganisms to solid surfaces takes place in two steps:

1. a reversible state in which the bacteria adhere loosely, and later
2. an irreversible state, during which their adherence becomes consolidated (Gibbons & van Houte 1980).

Another factor which may modify the number of bacteria in early plaque deposits is the presence of gingivitis, which increases the plaque formation rate so that the more complex bacterial composition is attained earlier (Saxton 1973, Hillam & Hull 1977, Brecx et al. 1980). Plaque growth may also be initiated by microorganisms harbored in minute irregularities in which they are protected from the natural cleaning of the tooth surface.

During the first few hours, bacteria that resist detachment from the pellicle may start to proliferate and form small colonies of morphologically similar organisms (Fig. 3-13). However, since other types of organisms may also proliferate in an adjacent region, the pellicle becomes easily populated by a mixture of different microorganisms (Fig. 3-14). In addition, some organisms seem able to grow between already established colonies (Fig. 3-15). Finally, it is likely that clumps of organisms of different species will become attached to the tooth surface or to the already attached microorganism, contributing to the complexity of the plaque composition after a few days. At this time, different types of organisms may benefit from each other. One example is the corncob configurations resulting from the growth of cocci on the surface of a filamentous microorganism (Listgarten et al. 1973). Another feature of older plaque is the presence of dead and lysed bacteria which may provide additional nutrients to the still viable bacteria in the neighborhood (Theilade & Theilade 1970).

The material present between the bacteria in dental plaque is called the intermicrobial matrix and accounts for approximately 25% of the plaque volume. Three sources may contribute to the intermicrobial matrix: the plaque microorganisms, the saliva, and the gingival exudate.

The bacteria may release various metabolic products. Some bacteria may produce various extracellular carbohydrate polymers, serving as energy storage or as anchoring material to secure their retention in plaque (Fig. 3-16). Degenerating or dead bacteria may also contribute to the intermicrobial matrix. Different bacterial species often have distinctly different metabolic pathways and capacity to synthesize extracellular material. The intermicrobial matrix in plaque, therefore, varies considerably from region to region. A fibrillar component is often seen in the matrix between Gram-positive cocci (Fig. 3-17) and is in accordance with the fact that several oral streptococci synthesize levans and glucans from dietary sucrose. In other regions, the matrix appears granular or homogeneous (Fig. 3-18). In parts of the plaque with the presence of Gram-negative organisms, the intermicrobial matrix is regularly characterized by the presence of small vesicles surrounded by a trilaminar membrane, which is similar in structure to that of the outer envelope of the cell wall of the Gram-negative microorganisms (Fig. 3-19). Such vesicles probably contain endotoxins and proteolytic enzymes, and may also be involved in adherence between bacteria (Hofstad et al. 1972, Grenier & Mayrand 1987).

It must be remembered, however, that the transmission electron microscope does not reveal all organic components of the intermicrobial matrix. The more soluble constituents may be lost during the procedures required prior to sectioning and examination of the plaque sample. Biochemical techniques may be used to identify such compounds (Silverman & Kleinberg 1967, Krebel et al. 1969, Kleinberg 1970, Hotz et al. 1972, Rölla et al. 1975, Bowen 1976). Such studies indicate that proteins and carbohydrates constitute the bulk of the organic material while lipids appear in much lower amounts.

The carbohydrates of the matrix have received a great deal of attention, and at least some of the polysaccharides in the plaque matrix are well characterized: fructans (levans) and glucans. Fructans are synthesized in plaque from dietary sucrose and provide a storage of energy which may be utilized by microorganisms in time of low sugar supply. The glucans are also synthesized from sucrose. One type of glucan is dextran, which may also serve as energy storage. Another glucan is mutan, which is not readily degraded, but acts primarily as a skeleton in the matrix in much the same way as collagen stabilizes the intercellular substance of connective tissue. It has been suggested that such carbohydrate polymers may be responsible for the change from a reversible to an irreversible adherence of plaque bacteria.

The small amount of lipids in the plaque matrix are as yet largely uncharacterized. Part of the lipid content is found in the small extracellular vesicles, which may contain lipopolysaccharide endotoxins of Gram-negative bacteria.

Subgingival plaque

Owing to the difficulty of obtaining samples with subgingival plaque preserved in its original position between the soft tissues of the gingiva and the hard tissues of the tooth, there are only a limited number of studies on the detailed internal structure of human subgingival plaque (Schroeder 1970, Listgarten et al. 1975, Listgarten 1976, Westergaard et al. 1978). From these it is evident that in many respects subgingival plaque resembles the supragingival variety, although the predominant types of microorganisms found vary considerably from those residing coronal to the gingival margin.

Between subgingival plaque and the tooth an electron-dense organic material is interposed, termed a *cuticle* (Fig. 3-20). This cuticle probably contains the remains of the epithelial attachment lamina originally connecting the junctional epithelium to the tooth, with the addition of material deposited from the gingival exudate (Frank & Cimasoni 1970, Lie & Selvig 1975, Eide et al. 1983). It has also been suggested that the cuticle represents a secretory product of the adjacent

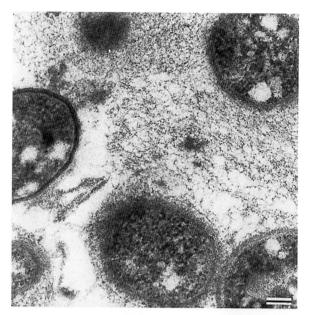

Fig. 3-20. Semithin section of subgingival plaque. An electron-dense cuticle bordering the enamel space is visible to the left. Filamentous bacteria are less than in supragingival plaque. The surface toward the gingival tissue contains many spirochetes (between arrows). Various host tissue cells can be seen on the right side. Magnification × 775. Bar: 10 µm. From Listgarten (1976).

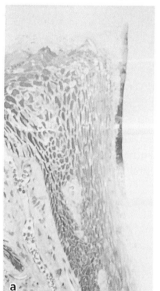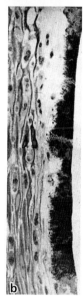

Fig. 3-21. (a) Light microscopic image of the dentogingival region of a dog with experimental gingivitis. A thin layer of dentogingival plaque can be seen, extending from the supragingival region approximately ½ mm into the gingival sulcus. (b) Higher magnification of a region of the plaque shown in (a). The subgingival plaque has a varying thickness and the epithelial cells are separated from the surface by a layer of leukocytes. There are also numerous leukocytes in the superficial portion of the sulcus epithelium. The apical termination of the plaque is bordered by leukocytes separating the epithelium from direct contact with the plaque bacteria.

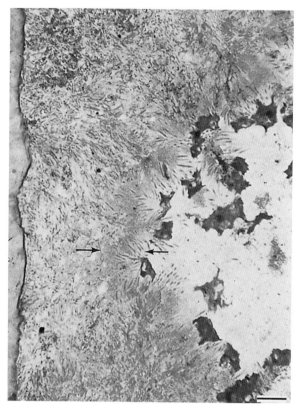

Fig. 3-22. Semithin section of supragingival plaque with layer of predominantly filamentous bacteria adhering to the enamel (to the left). Lighter staining indicates calcification of part of the plaque close to the tooth. Magnification × 750. Bar: 10 µm. From Listgarten (1976).

epithelial cells (Schroeder & Listgarten 1977). Information is lacking concerning its chemical composition, but its location in the subgingival area makes it unlikely that salivary constituents contribute to its formation.

The subgingival plaque structurally resembles supragingival plaque, particularly with respect to plaque associated with gingivitis without the forma-tion of deep pockets (Fig. 3-21a). A densely packed accumulation of microorganisms is seen adjacent to the cuticular material covering the tooth surface (Fig. 3-22). The bacteria comprise Gram-positive and Gram-negative cocci, rods and filamentous organisms. Spirochetes and various flagellated bacteria may also be encountered, especially at the apical extension of the plaque. The surface layer is often less densely

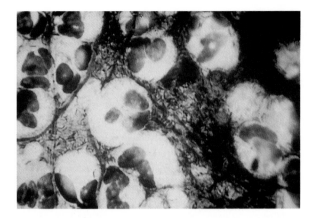

Fig. 3-23. Light microscopic image of a smear sample taken from the dentogingival region in a subject who had abstained from mechanical oral hygiene during 3 weeks. Numerous leukocytes can be observed embedded in a dense accumulation of bacteria.

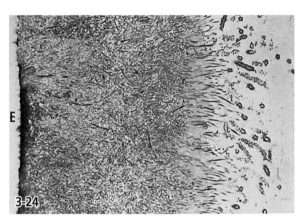

Fig. 3-24, 3-25. Semithin section of supragingival plaque on enamel (E), which has been dissolved prior to sectioning. Filamentous organisms predominate. At the surface some of these organisms are surrounded by cocci. This configuration resembles a corncob. Magnification × 750 and × 1400. Bars: 10 μm and 1 μm. From Listgarten (1976).

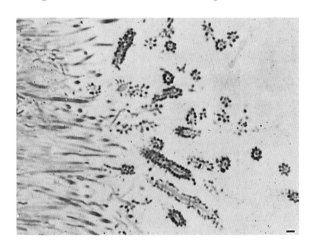

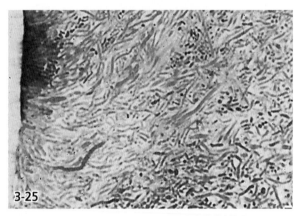

Fig. 3-26. The corncob formations seen at the plaque surface in Fig. 3-24 and 3-25. Magnification × 1300. Bar: 1 μm. From Listgarten (1976).

packed and leukocytes are regularly interposed between the plaque and the epithelial lining of the gingival sulcus (Fig. 3-23).

When a periodontal pocket has formed, the appearance of the subgingival bacterial deposit becomes much more complex. In this case the tooth surface may either represent enamel or cementum from which the periodontal fibers are detached. Plaque accumulation on the portion of the tooth previously covered by periodontal tissues does not differ markedly from that observed in gingivitis (Fig. 3-24). In this layer, filamentous microorganisms dominate (Figs. 3-25, 3-26, 3-27), but cocci and rods also occur. However, in the deeper parts of the periodontal pocket, the filamentous or-

ganisms become fewer in number, and in the apical portion they seem to be virtually absent. Instead, the dense, tooth-facing part of the bacterial deposit is dominated by smaller organisms without particular orientation (Listgarten 1976) (Fig. 3-28).

The surface layers of microorganisms in the periodontal pocket facing the soft tissue are distinctly different from the adherent layer along the tooth surface, and no definite intermicrobial matrix is apparent (Figs. 3-28, 3-29). The microorganisms comprise a larger number of spirochetes and flagellated bacteria. Gram-negative cocci and rods are also present. The multitude of spirochetes and flagellated organisms are motile bacteria and there is no intermicrobial ma-

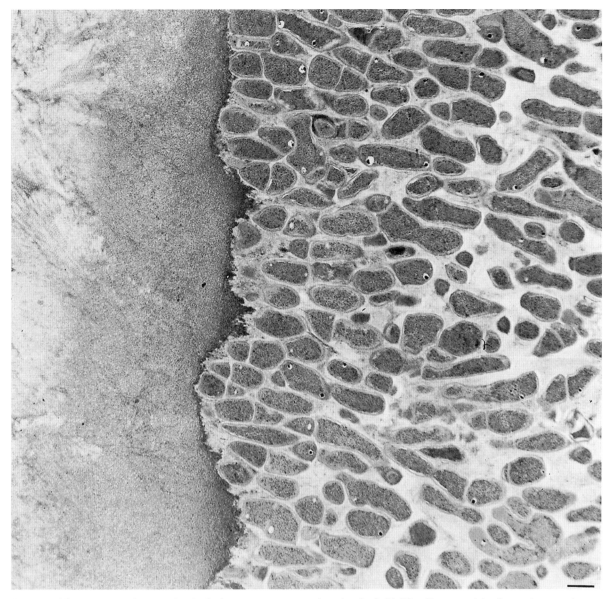

Fig. 3-27. Thin section of supragingival plaque on a root surface (to the left). The Gram-positive bacteria are oriented in a palisading arrangement. Magnification × 6400. Bar: 1 μm. From Listgarten (1976).

trix between them. This outer part of the microbial accumulation in the periodontal pocket adheres loosely to the soft-tissue pocket wall (Listgarten 1976).

In cases of juvenile periodontitis (Listgarten 1976, Westergaard et al. 1978) the bacterial deposits in deep pockets are much thinner than those found in adult forms of periodontal disease. Areas of the tooth surface in the periodontal pocket may sometimes even be devoid of adherent microbial deposits. The cuticular material has an uneven thickness (Figs. 3-30, 3-31). The adherent layer of microorganisms varies considerably in thickness and shows considerable variation in arrangement. It may exhibit a palisaded organization of the bacteria (Fig. 3-32). The microorganisms in this layer are mainly cocci, rods or filamentous bacteria, primarily of the Gram-negative type (Fig. 3-33). A surface layer with some Gram-positive cocci, frequently associated with filamentous organisms in the typical corncob configuration, may also be found.

Subgingivally located bacteria appear to have the capacity to invade dentinal tubules, the openings of which have become exposed as a consequence of inflammatory driven resorptions of the cementum (Adriaens et al. 1988). Such a habitat might serve as the source for bacterial recolonization of the subgingival space following treatment of periodontal disease. The mechanisms involved in such reversed invasion of the subgingival space are unknown.

The sequential events taking place during the development of subgingival plaque have not been studied in man. However, in dogs, subgingival plaque may develop in the gingival sulcus within a few days, if oral hygiene is discontinued (Matsson & Attström 1979, Ten Napel et al. 1983). From these studies it has been established that early dental plaque in the dog has many structural similarities with that occurring in man. This applies to the supragingival plaque (Fig. 3-21a) as well as to the subgingival accumulation (Fig. 3-21b). The deposits may either appear as an apical continuation of the supragingival plaque, or as dis-

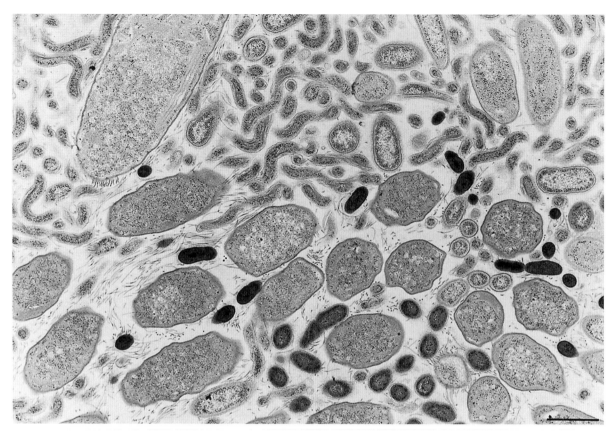

Fig. 3-28. Thin section of subgingival plaque from a deep periodontal pocket. Small microorganisms predominate, many of which are spirochetes. Magnification × 13 000. Bar: 1 µm. From Listgarten (1976).

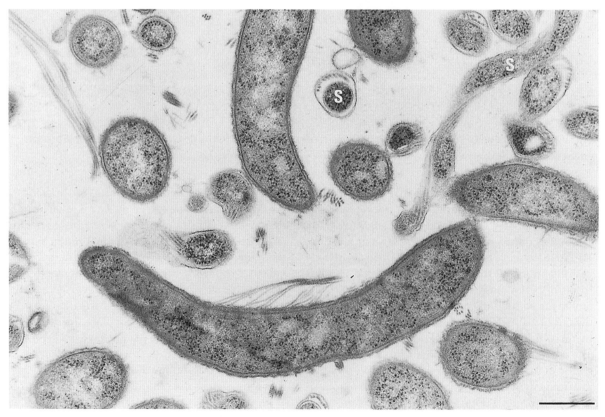

Fig. 3-29. Thin section of subgingival plaque from a deep periodontal pocket with many spirochetes (S), which are recognized by their axial filaments. In the lower part of the figure is a curved organism with flagella at its concave surface. Magnification × 25 000. Bar: 0.5 µm. From Listgarten (1976).

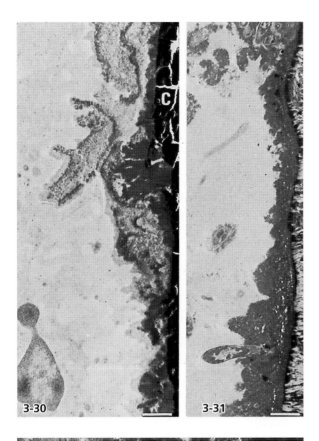

Fig. 3-30. Thin section of deposit in deep pocket of patient with juvenile periodontitis. The cementum (C) is covered with cuticular material and cellular remnants. Magnification × 5500. Bar: 1 µm. From Westergaard et al. (1978).

Fig. 3-31. Thin section of deposit in deep pocket of patient with juvenile periodontitis. A cuticle of uneven thickness is seen to the right on the cementum. A small colony of degenerating bacteria adheres to the cuticle in the upper part of the illustration, and below a single rod-shaped microorganism is partly embedded in the cuticle. Magnification × 5500. Bar: 1 µm. From Westergaard et al. (1978).

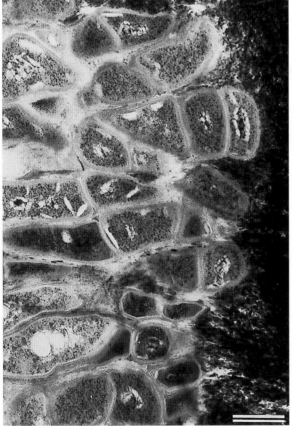

Fig. 3-32. Thin section of plaque in deep pocket of patient with juvenile periodontitis. Densely packed Gram-positive rods grow perpendicular to the cementum to the right in the illustration. Magnification × 23 000. Bar: 0.5 µm. From Westergaard et al. (1978).

crete aggregates at some distance from the supragingival deposit. Old established subgingival plaque shows considerable variation in bacterial composition between dogs: in some, a subgingival microbiota dominated by spirochetes is seen; in others, colonies of Gram-negative cocci and rods are found in the gingival crevice, whereas spirochetes are virtually absent (Soames & Davies 1975, Theilade & Attström 1985). A characteristic feature of subgingival plaque is the presence of leukocytes interposed between the surfaces of the bacterial deposit and the gingival sulcular epithelium (Fig. 3-34). Some bacteria may be

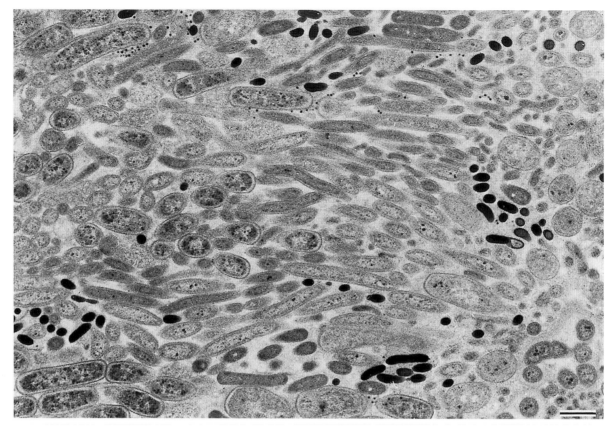

Fig. 3-33. Thin section of plaque in deep pocket of patient with juvenile periodontitis. The bacterial flora is characterized by cocci, rods or filamentous organisms, primarily of the Gram-negative type. Magnification × 9200. Bar: 1 μm. From Westergaard et al. (1978).

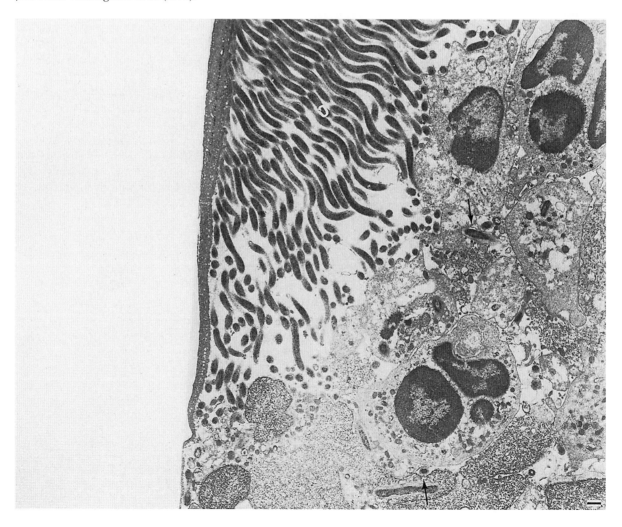

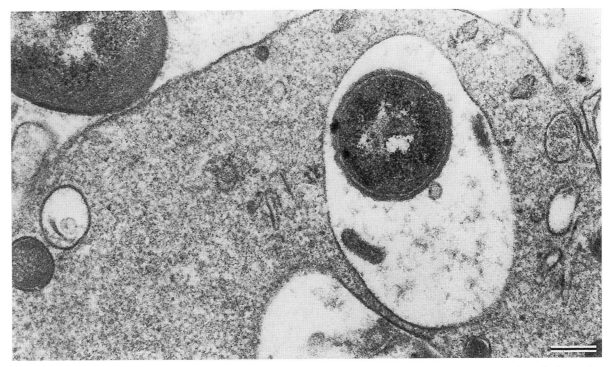

Fig. 3-35. Thin section of part of a leukocyte situated between subgingival plaque and the junctional epithelium of the dog. The large membrane bound compartment of the leukocyte cytoplasm contains a phagocytized Gram-negative microorganism. Another bacterium is in close apposition to the cytoplasmic membrane of the leukocyte. Magnification × 21 500. Bar: 0.5 μm. From Theilade & Attström (1985).

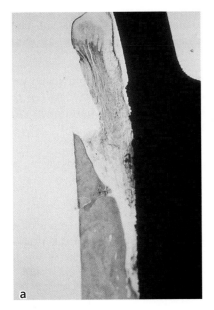 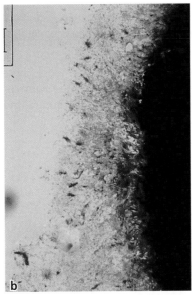

Fig. 3-36. Peri-implant infection. (a) Human explant of an ITI® dental implant affected by a peri-implantitis with an infrabony lesion. Adhering plaque closely resembles the structure of subgingival microbiota encountered in advanced periodontitis. (b) Higher magnification of plaque adhering to the implant surface.

found between the epithelial cells. Evidence of phagocytosis (by polymorphonuclear leukocytes) is frequently encountered (Fig. 3-35).

Although subgingival plaque formation in the dog may not develop identically to that in man, the dog may still serve as a convenient model for investigating the basic phenomena governing the formation of subgingival plaque (Schroeder & Attström 1979).

In summary, there are four distinct subgingival ecologic niches which are probably different in their composition:

1. the tooth (or implant) surface
2. the gingival exudate fluid medium
3. the surface of epithelial cells and
4. the superficial portion of the pocket epithelium.

← Fig. 3-34. Thin section of old subgingival plaque in a dog with long-standing gingivitis. The most apical colony consists primarily of spirochetes attached to a dense cuticle and surrounded by migrated leukocytes. Single microorganisms are seen between them (arrows). Magnification × 2800. Bar: 1 μm. From Theilade & Attström (1985).

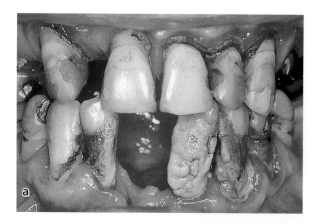
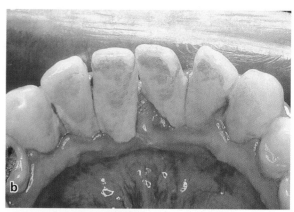
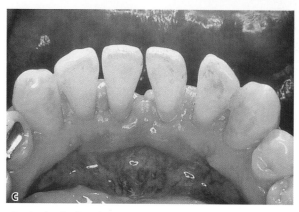

Fig. 3-37. Abundance of supragingival calculus deposits. (a) Gross deposits as a result of long-term neglect of oral hygiene. Two mandibular incisors have been exfoliated. (b) Supragingival plaque usually covering the lingual aspect of mandibular incisors. Note the intense inflammatory reaction adjacent to the deposits. (c) Same patient and region as in Fig. 3-37b following removal of the calculus. The gingival tissues demonstrate healing.

The composition of the bacteria in these niches has still not been completely investigated. The influence of the different bacterial compartments on the pathogenesis of the disease process is generally unknown.

Peri-implant plaque

Biofilms form not only on natural teeth, but also on artificial surfaces exposed to the oral environment. As a consequence, the formation of bacterial plaque on oral implants deserves some attention. Although a number of studies have characterized the plaque deposits of the human peri-implant sulcus or pocket using either dark field microscopy (Mombelli et al. 1988, Quirynen & Listgarten 1990) or microbiologic culturing techniques (Rams et al. 1984, Mombelli et al. 1987, 1988, Apse et al. 1989, Leonhardt et al. 1992), no studies have attempted to document the structure of the supramucosal or the peri-implant (submucosal) microbiota. However, the similarities between peri-implant and subgingival microbial deposits have clearly been demonstrated in cross-sectional (Mombelli et al. 1987, 1995) and longitudinal studies (Mombelli et al. 1988, Pontoriero et al. 1994), and it may be anticipated that the structure of peri-implant plaque deposits may resemble that encountered in the subgingival environment. Micrographs from an implant

retrieved because of a peri-implant infection may provide some evidence for the similarity between the structural image of the submucosal peri-implant microbiota (Fig. 3-36).

DENTAL CALCULUS

Although calculus formation has been reported to occur in germ-free animals as a result of calcification of salivary proteins, dental calculus or tartar usually represents mineralized bacterial plaque.

Clinical appearance, distribution and clinical diagnosis

Supragingivally, calculus can be recognized as a creamy-whitish to dark yellow or even brownish mass of moderate hardness (Fig. 3-37). The degree of calculus formation is not only dependent on the amount of bacterial plaque present but also on the secretion of the salivary glands. Hence, supragingival calculus is predominantly found adjacent to the excretion ducts of the major salivary glands, such as the lingual aspect of the mandibular anterior teeth and the buccal aspect of the maxillary first molars, where the parotid gland

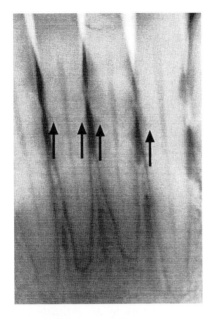

Fig. 3-38. Subgingival calculus may be visible (arrows) on radiographs if abundant deposits are present.

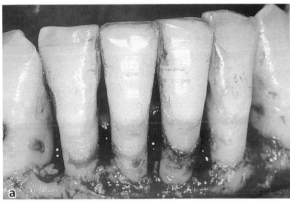

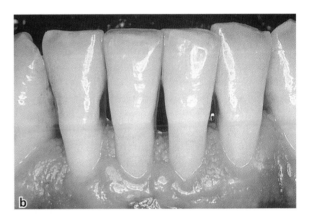

Fig. 3-39. Subgingival calculus presents as a black-brownish hard mass if the gingival margin is retracted or reflected during a surgical procedure (a). Healing of the site following removal of all hard deposits (b).

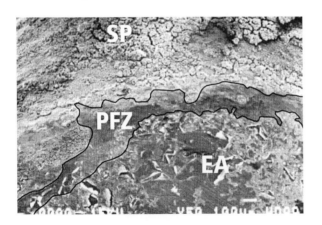

Fig. 3-40. Plaque- and calculus-free zone coronal to the epithelial attachment. SP: Subgingival plaque bacteria. PFZ: Plaque-free zone. EA: Remnants of junctional epithelium.

ducts open into the oral vestibule. The duct openings of the submandibular glands are located in the former region. It should be noted that calculus continually harbors a viable bacterial plaque (Zander et al. 1960, Theilade 1964, Schroeder 1969).

Subgingivally, calculus may be found by tactile exploration only, since its formation occurs apical to the gingival margin and, hence, is usually not visible to the naked eye. Occasionally, subgingival calculus may be visible in dental radiographs provided that the deposits present an adequate mass (Fig. 3-38). Small

deposits or residual deposits following root instrumentation may barely be visualized radiographically. If the gingival margin is pushed open by a blast of air or retracted by a dental instrument, a brownish to black calcified hard mass with a rough surface may become visible (Fig. 3-39). Again, this mineralized mass reflects predominantly bacterial accumulations mixed with products from gingival crevicular fluid and blood. Consequently, subgingival calculus is found in most periodontal pockets, usually extending from the cemento-enamel junction and reaching close

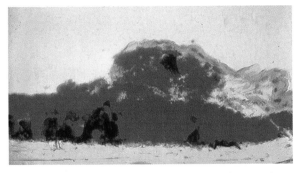

Fig. 3-41. Seven-day-old calcified plaque. Observe the isolated calcification centers indicated by the black areas (van Kossa stain).

to the bottom of the pocket. However, a band of approximately 0.5 mm is usually found coronal to the apical extension of the periodontal pocket (Fig. 3-40). This zone appears to be free from mineralized deposits owing to the fact that gingival crevicular fluid is exudating from the periodontal soft tissues and acting as a gradient against the microbial accumulation. Like supragingival calculus, subgingival calculus also provides an ideal environment for bacterial adhesion (Zander et al. 1960, Schroeder 1969).

Plaque mineralization varies greatly between and within individuals and – as indicated above – also within the different regions of the oral cavity. Not only the formation rate for bacterial plaque (amount of bacterial plaque per time and tooth surface), but also the formation rate for dental calculus (time period during which newly deposited supragingival plaque with an ash weight of 5-10% becomes calcified and yields an ash weight of approximately 80%) is subject to great variability. In some subjects, the time required for the formation of supragingival calculus is 2 weeks, at which time the deposit may already contain approximately 80% of the inorganic material found in mature calculus (Fig. 3-41) (Mühlemann & Schneider 1959, Mandel 1963, Mühlemann & Schroeder 1964). In fact, evidence of mineralization may already be pre-

sent after a few days (Theilade 1964). Nevertheless, the formation of dental calculus with the mature crystalline composition of old calculus may require months to years (Schroeder & Baumbauer 1966). Supragingival plaque becomes mineralized saliva and subgingival plaque in the presence of the inflammatory exudate in the pocket. It is, therefore, evident that subgingival calculus represents a secondary product of infection and not a primary cause of periodontitis.

Attachment to tooth surfaces and implants

Dental calculus generally adheres tenaciously to tooth surfaces. Hence, the removal of subgingival calculus may be expected to be rather difficult. The reason for this firm attachment to the tooth surface is the fact that the pellicle beneath the bacterial plaque also calcifies. This, in turn, results in an intimate contact with enamel (Fig. 3-42), cementum (Fig. 3-43) or dentin crystals (Fig. 3-44) (Kopczyk & Conroy 1968, Selvig 1970). In addition, the surface irregularities are also penetrated by calculus crystals and, hence, calculus is virtually locked to the tooth. This is particularly the case on exposed root cementum, where small pits and irregularities occur at the sites of the previous insertion of Sharpey's fibers (Bercy & Frank 1980). Uneven root surfaces may be the result of carious lesions and small areas of cementum may have been lost due to resorption, when the periodontal ligament was still invested into the root surface (Moskow 1969). Under such conditions it may become extremely difficult to remove all calculus deposits without sacrificing some hard tissues of the root.

Although some irregularities may also be encountered on oral implant surfaces, the attachment to commercially pure titanium generally is less intimate than to root surface structures. This in turn, would mean that calculus may be chipped off from oral implants (Fig. 3-45) without detriment to the implant surface (Matarasso et al. 1996).

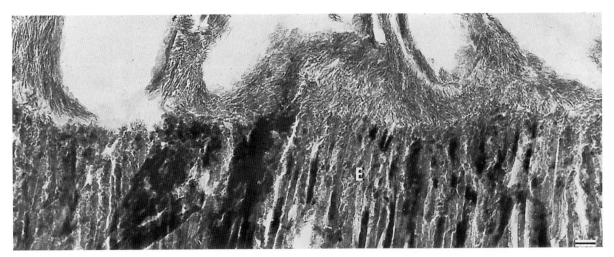

Fig. 3-42. Thin section of enamel surface (E) with overlying calculus. The enamel and calculus crystals are in intimate contact, and the latter extends into the minute irregularities of the enamel. Magnification × 37 500. Bar: 0.1 µm. From Selvig (1970).

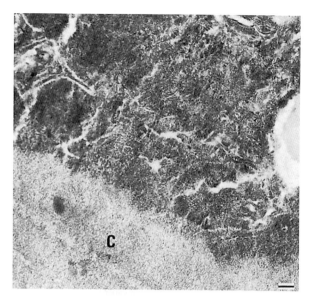

Fig. 3-43. Thin section of cementum surface (C) with overlying calculus. The calculus is closely adapted to the irregular cementum and is more electron-dense and therefore harder than the adjacent cementum. To the right in the illustration, part of an uncalcified microorganism. Magnification × 32 000. Bar: 0.1 µm. From Selvig (1970).

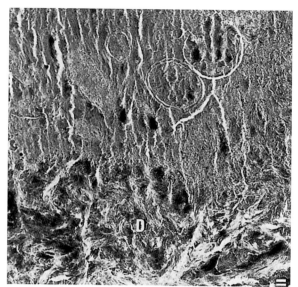

Fig. 3-44. Thin section of dentin (D) surface with overlying calculus. The interface between the calculus and dentin cannot be precisely determined because the calculus crystals fill the irregularities of the dentin surface, which is devoid of cementum as a result of a previous scaling of the root surface. The circular profiles in the calculus completely surround calcified bacteria. Magnification × 19 000. Bar: 1 µm. From Selvig (1970).

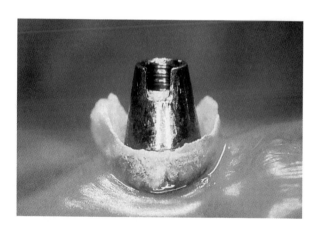

Fig. 3-45. Calculus deposit on an oral implant in a patient without regular maintenance care.

Mineralization, composition and structure

The mineralization starts in centers which arise intracellularly in bacterial colonies (Fig. 3-46) or extracellularly from matrix with crystallization nuclei (Fig. 3-47). Recent and old calculus consists of four different crystals of calcium phosphate (for review see Schroeder 1969):

1. $CaH(PO_4) \times 2\,H_2O$ = Brushite (**B**)
2. $Ca_4H(PO_4)_3 \times 2\,H_2O$ = Octa calcium phosphate (**OCP**)
3. $Ca_5(PO_4)_3 \times OH$ = Hydroxyapatite (**HA**)
4. $\beta\text{-}Ca_3(PO_4)_2$ = Whitlockite (**W**)

Supragingival calculus is clearly built up in layers and yields a great heterogeneity from one layer to another with regard to mineral content. On average, the mineral content is 37%, but ranges from 16% to 51%, with some layers yielding a maximal density of minerals of up to 80% exceptionally (Kani et al. 1983, Friskopp & Isacsson 1984). The predominant mineral in exterior layers is **OCP**, while **HA** is dominant in inner layers of old calculus. **W** is only found in small proportions (Sundberg & Friskopp 1985). **B** is identified in recent calculus, not older than 2 weeks, and appears to form the basis for supragingival calculus formation. The appearance of the crystals is characteristic for **OCP** as forming platelet-like crystals, for **HA** as forming sandgrain or rod-like crystals, while **W** presents with hexagonal (cuboidal, rhomboidal) crystals (Kodaka et al. 1988).

Subgingival calculus appears somewhat more homogeneous since it is built up in layers with an equally high density of minerals. On average the density is 58% and ranges from 32% to 78%. Maximal values of 60-80% have been found (Kani et al. 1983, Friskopp & Isacsson 1984). The predominant mineral is always **W**,

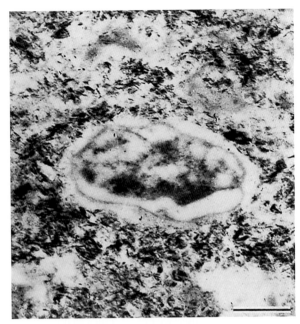

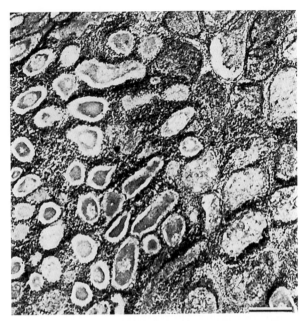

Fig. 3-46. Thin section of old plaque. A degenerating organism is surrounded by intermicrobial matrix in which initial mineralization has started by the deposition of small needle-shaped electron-dense apatite crystals. Magnification × 26 500. Bar: 0.5 µm. From Zander et al. (1960).

Fig. 3-47. Thin section of old mineralizing plaque. The intermicrobial matrix is totally calcified, and many microorganisms show intracellular crystal deposition. Magnification × 9500. Bar: 1 µm. From Theilade (1964).

although **HA** has been found (Sundberg & Friskopp 1985). **W** contains small proportions (3%) of magnesia (McDougall 1985).

In the presence of a relatively low plaque-pH and a concomitant high Ca/P-ratio in saliva, **B** is formed which may later on develop into **HA** and **W**. When supragingival plaque mineralizes, **OCP** forms and is gradually changed into **HA**. In the presence of alkaline and anaerobic conditions and concomitant presence of magnesia (or Zn and CO₃), large amounts of **W** are formed, which are a stable form of mineralization.

Clinical implications

Although strong associations between calculus deposits and periodontitis have been demonstrated in experimental (Wærhaug 1952, 1955) and epidemiologic studies (Lövdal et al. 1958), it has to be realized that calculus is always covered by an unmineralized layer of viable bacterial plaque. It has been debated whether or not calculus may exert a detrimental effect on the soft tissues owing to its rough surface. However, it has clearly been established that surface roughness alone does not initiate gingivitis (Wærhaug 1956). On the contrary, in monkeys a normal epithelial attachment with the junctional epithelial cells forming hemidesmosomes and a basement membrane on calculus could be established (Listgarten & Ellegaard 1973) if the calculus surface had been disinfected using chlorhexidine (Fig. 3-48). Furthermore, it has been demonstrated that autoclaved calculus may be encapsulated in connective tissue without inducing marked

inflammation or abscess formation (Allen & Kerr 1965).

These studies clearly exclude the possibility of dental calculus being a primary cause of periodontal diseases. The effect of calculus seems to be secondary by providing an ideal surface configuration conducive to further plaque accumulation and subsequent mineralization.

Nevertheless, calculus deposits may have developed in areas with difficult access for oral hygiene or may – by the size of the deposits – jeopardize proper oral hygiene practices. Calculus may also amplify the effects of bacterial plaque by keeping the bacterial deposits in close contact with the tissue surface, thereby influencing both bacterial ecology and tissue response (Friskopp & Hammarström 1980).

Well-controlled animal (Nyman et al. 1986) and clinical (Nyman et al. 1988, Mombelli et al. 1995) studies have shown that the removal of subgingival plaque on top of subgingival calculus will result in healing of periodontal lesions and the maintenance of healthy gingival and periodontal tissues, provided that the supragingival deposits are meticulously removed on a regular basis. One of these studies (Mombelli et al. 1995) clearly demonstrated that the diligent and complete removal of subgingival plaque on top of mineralized deposits after chipping off gross amounts of calculus showed almost identical results in the composition of the microbiota and the clinical parameters to those obtained with routine removal of subgingival calculus by root surface instrumentation. Again, it has to be realized that meticulous supragingival plaque control guarantees the depletion of the supragingival

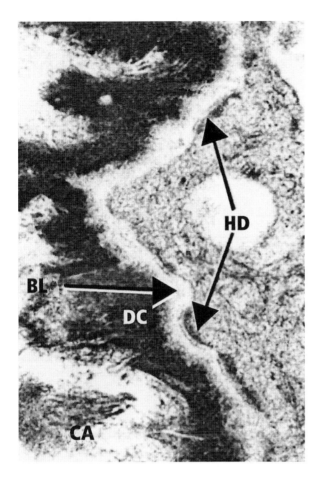

Fig. 3-48. Hemidesmosomal attachment of junctional epithelium on dental calculus in the absence of bacteria following application of chlorhexidine. CA: Calculus, HD: Hemidesmosomes, BL: Basement lamina, DC: Dental cuticle. × 32 000. Data from Listgarten & Ellegaard (1973).

bacterial reservoir for subgingival recolonization. These studies have clearly elucidated the role of subgingival calculus as a plaque-retaining factor.

In summary, dental calculus represents mineralized bacterial plaque. It is always covered by unmineralized viable bacterial plaque, and hence, does not directly come into contact with the gingival tissues.

Calculus, therefore, is a secondary etiologic factor for periodontitis. Its presence, however, makes adequate plaque removal impossible and prevents patients from performing proper plaque control. It is the most prominent plaque-retentive factor which has to be removed as a basis for adequate periodontal therapy and prophylactic activities.

REFERENCES

Adriaens, P.A., De Boever, J.A. & Loesche, W.J. (1988). Bacterial invasion in root cementum and radicular dentin of periodontally diseased teeth in humans. A reservoir of periodontopathic bacteria. *Journal of Periodontology* **59**, 222-230.

Allen, D.L. & Kerr, D.A. (1965). Tissue response in the guinea pig to sterile and non-sterile calculus. *Journal of Periodontology* **36**, 121-126.

Apse, P., Ellen, R.P., Overall, C.M. & Zarb, G.A. (1989). Microbiota and crevicular fluid collagenase activity in the osseointegrated dental implant sulcus: a comparison of sites in edentulous and partially edentulous patients. *Journal of Periodontal Research* **24**, 96-105.

Bercy, P. & Frank, R.M. (1980). Microscopie electronique à balayage de la surface du cément humain normal et carié. *Journal de Biologie Buccale* **8**, 331-352.

Berthold, C.H., Berthold, P. & Söder, P.O. (1971). The growth of dental plaque on different materials. *Svensk Tandläkare Tidsskrift* **64**, 863-877.

Black, G.V. (1911). Beginnings of pyorrhea alveolaris – treatment for prevention. *Dental Items of Interest* **33**, 420-455.

Bowen, W.H. (1976). Nature of plaque. *Oral Sciences Reviews* **9**, 3-21.

Brecx, M., Theilade, J. & Attström, R. (1980). Influence of optimal and excluded oral hygiene on early formation of dental plaque on plastic films. A quantitative and descriptive light and electron microscopic study. *Journal of Clinical Periodontology* **7**, 361-373.

Brecx, M., Theilade, J. & Attström, R. (1981). Ultrastructural estimation of the effect of sucrose and glucose rinses on dental plaque formed on plastic films. *Scandinavian Journal of Dental Research* **89**, 157-164.

Eastcott, A.D. & Stallard, R.E. (1973). Sequential changes in developing human dental plaque as visualized by scanning electron microscopy. *Journal of Periodontology* **44**, 218-244.

Eide, B., Lie, T. & Selvig, K.A. (1983). Surface coatings on dental cementum incident to periodontal disease. I. A scanning electron microscopic study. *Journal of Clinical Periodontology* **10**, 157-171.

Frank, R.M. & Brendel, A. (1966). Ultrastructure of the approximal dental plaque and the underlying normal and carious enamel. *Archives of Oral Biology* **11**, 883-912.

Frank, R.M. & Cimasoni, G. (1970). Ultrastructure de l'epithelium cliniquement normal du sillon et de jonction gingivodentaires. *Zeitschrift für Zellforschung und Mikroskopische Anatomie* **109**, 356-379.

Frank, R.M. & Houver, G. (1970). An ultrastructural study of human supragingival dental plaque formation. In: McHugh, W.D., ed. *Dental plaque*. Edinburgh: Livingstone, pp. 85-108.

Friskopp, J. & Hammarström, L. (1980). A comparative scanning electron microscopic study of supragingival and subgingival calculus. *Journal of Periodontology* **51**, 553-562.

Friskopp, J. & Isacsson, G. (1984). Mineral content of supragingival and subgingival dental calculus. A quantitative microradiographic study. *Scandinavian Journal of Dental Research* **92**, 417-423.

Gibbons, R.J. & van Houte, J. (1980). Bacterial adherence and the formation of dental plaques. In: Beachey, E.H., ed. *Bacterial adherence*. Receptors and recognition, series B, Vol. 6. London: Chapman, pp. 60-104.

Grenier, D. & Mayrand, D. (1987). Functional characterization of vesicular vesicles produced by *Bacteroides gingivalis*. *Infection and Immunity* **55**, 111-117.

Gristina, A.G. (1987). Biomaterial-centered infection: Microbial adhesion versus tissue integration. *Science* **237**, 1588-1595.

Hazen, S.P. (1960). A study of four week old *in vivo* calculus formation. Thesis. Rochester, NY: University of Rochester.

Hillam, D.G. & Hull, P.S. (1977). The influence of experimental gingivitis on plaque formation. *Journal of Clinical Periodontology* **4**, 56-61.

Hofstad, T., Kristoffersen. T. & Selvig, K.A. (1972). Electron microscopy of endotoxic lipopolysaccharide from *Bacteroides*, *Fusobacterium* and *Sphaerophorus*. *Acta Pathologica and Microbiologica Scandinavia*, Sec B **80**, 413-419.

Hotz, P., Guggenheim, B. & Schmid, R. (1972). Carbohydrates in pooled dental plaque. *Caries Research* **6**, 103-121.

Kandarkar, S.V. (1973). Ultrastructure of dental plaque and acquired pellicle formed on the artificial tooth surface (araldite plate). *Journal of the Indian Dental Association* **45**, 122-129.

Kani, T., Kani, M., Moriwaki, Y. & Doi, Y. (1983). Microbeam x-ray diffraction analysis of dental calculus. *Journal of Dental Research* **62**, 92-95.

Kleinberg, I. (1970). Biochemistry of the dental plaque. *Archives of Oral Biology* **4**, 43-90.

Kodaka, T., Debari, K. & Higashi, S. (1988). Magnesium-containing crystals in human dental calculus. *Journal of Electronic Microscopy* **37**, 73-80.

Kopczyk, R.A. & Conroy, C.W. (1968). The attachment of calculus to root-planed surfaces. *Periodontics* **6**, 78-83.

Krebel, J., Frank, R.M. & Deluzarche, A. (1969). Fractionation of human dental plaque. *Archives of Oral Biology* **14**, 563-565.

Leach, S.A. & Saxton, C.A. (1966). An electron microscopic study of the acquired pellicle and plaque formed on the enamel of human incisors. *Archives of Oral Biology* **11**, 1081-1094.

Leonhardt, Å., Bergenlundh, T., Ericsson, I. & Dahlén, G. (1992). Putative periodontal pathogens on titanium implants and teeth in experimental gingivitis and periodontitis in beagle dogs. *Clinical Oral Implants Research* **3**, 112-119.

Lie, T. (1975). Growth of dental plaque on hydroxy-apatite splints. A method of studying early plaque morphology. *Journal of Periodontal Research* **9**, 137-145.

Lie, T. (1978). Ultrastructural study of early dental plaque formation. *Journal of Periodontal Research* **13**, 391-409.

Lie, T. & Selvig, K.A. (1975). Formation of an experimental dental cuticle. *Scandinavian Journal of Dental Research* **83**, 145-152.

Listgarten, M.A. (1976). Structure of the microbial flora associated with periodontal health and disease in man. A light and electron microscopic study. *Journal of Periodontology* **47**, 1-18.

Listgarten, M.A. & Ellegaard, B. (1973). Electron microscopic evidence of a cellular attachment between junctional epithelium and dental calculus. *Journal of Periodontal Research* **8**, 143-150.

Listgarten, M.A., Mayo, H. & Amsterdam, M. (1973). Ultrastructure of the attachment device between coccal and filamentous microorganisms in "corn cob" formations in dental plaque. *Archives of Oral Biology* **8**, 651-656.

Listgarten, M.A., Mayo, H. & Tremblay, R. (1975). Development of dental plaque in epoxy resin crowns in man. A light and electron microscopic study. *Journal of Periodontology* **46**, 10-26.

Löe, H., Theilade, E. & Jensen, S.B. (1965). Experimental gingivitis in man. *Journal of Periodontology* **36**, 177-187.

Loesche, W.J. (1979). Clinical and microbiological aspects of chemotherapeutic agents used according to the specific plaque hypothesis. *Journal of Dental Research* **58**, 2404-2414.

Lövdal, A., Arnö, A. & Wærhaug, J. (1958). Incidence of clinical manifestations of periodontal disease in light of oral hygiene and calculus formation. *Journal of the American Dental Association* **56**, 21-33.

Mandel, I.D. (1963). Histochemical and biochemical aspects of calculus formation. *Periodontics* **1**, 43-52.

Mandel, I.D., Levy, B.M. & Wasserman, B.H. (1957). Histochemistry of calculus formation. *Journal of Periodontology* **28**, 132-137.

Marshall, K.C. (1992). Biofilms: An overview of bacterial adhesion, activity, and control at surfaces. *American Society of Microbiology News* **58**, 202-207.

Matarasso, S., Quaremba, G., Coraggio, F., Vaia, E., Cafiero, C. & Lang, N.P. (1996). Maintenance of implants: an *in vitro* study of titanium implant surface modifications subsequent to the application of different prophylaxis procedures. *Clinical Oral Implants Research* **7**, 64-72.

Matsson, L. & Attström, R. (1979). Histologic characteristics of experimental gingivitis in the juvenile and adult beagle dog. *Journal of Clinical Periodontology* **6**, 334-350.

McDougall, W.A. (1963). Studies on dental plaque. II. The histology of the developing interproximal plaque. *Australian Dental Journal* **8**, 398-407.

McDougall, W.A. (1985). Analytical transmission electron microscopy of the distribution of elements in human supragingival dental calculus. *Archives of Oral Biology* **30**, 603-608.

Mergenhagen, S.E. & Rosan, B. (1985). *Molecular basis of oral microbial adhesion*. Washington: American Society of Microbiology.

Mombelli, A., Buser, D. & Lang, N.P. (1988). Colonization of osseointegrated titanium implants in edentulous patients: early results. *Oral Microbiology and Immunology* **3**, 113-120.

Mombelli, A., Marxer, M., Gaberthüel, T., Grunder, U. & Lang, N.P. (1995). The microbiota of osseointegrated implants in patients with a history of periodontal disease. *Journal of Clinical Periodontology* **22**, 124-130.

Mombelli, A., Nyman, S., Brägger, N., Wennström, J. & Lang, N.P. (1995). Clinical and microbiological changes associated with an altered subgingival environment induced by periodontal pocket reduction. *Journal of Clinical Periodontology* **22**, 780-787.

Mombelli, A., van Oosten, M.A.C., Schürch, E. & Lang, N.P. (1987). The microbiota associated with successful or failing osseointegrated titanium implants. *Oral Microbiology and Immunology* **2**, 145-151.

Moskow, B.S. (1969). Calculus attachment in cemental separations. *Journal of Periodontology* **40**, 125-130.

Mühlemann, H.R. & Schneider, U.K. (1959). Early calculus formation. *Helvetica Odontologica Acta* **3**, 22-26.

Mühlemann, H.R. & Schroeder, H.E. (1964) Dynamics of supragingival calculus. In: Staple, P.H., ed. *Advances in oral biology*. New York: Academic Press, pp. 175-203.

Nyman, S., Sarhed, G., Ericsson, I., Gottlow, J. & Karring, T. (1986). Role of "diseased" root cementum in healing following treatment of periodontal disease. An experimental study in the dog. *Journal of Periodontal Research* **21**, 496-503.

Nyman, S., Westfelt, E., Sarhed, G., & Karring, T. (1988). Role of "diseased" root cementum in healing following treatment of periodontal disease. A clinical study. *Journal of Clinical Periodontology* **15**, 464-468.

Nyvad, B., Fejerskov, O., Theilade, J., Melsen, B., Rölla, G. & Karring, T. (1982). The effect of sucrose or casein on early microbial colonization on Mylar and tooth surfaces in monkeys. *Journal of Dental Research* **61**, 570.

Öste, R., Rönström, A., Birkhed, D., Edwardsson, S. & Stenberg, M. (1981). Gas-liquid chromatographic analysis of amino acids in pellicle formed on tooth surface and plastic film *in vitro*. *Archives of Oral Biology* **26**, 635-641.

Pontoriero, R., Tonelli, M.P., Carnevale, G., Mombelli, A., Nyman, S.R. & Lang, N.P. (1994). Experimentally induced peri-implant mucositis. A clinical study in humans. *Clinical Oral Implants Research* **5**, 254-259.

Quirynen, M. & Listgarten, M.A. (1990). The distribution of bacterial morphotypes around natural teeth and titanium implants *ad modum* Brånemark. *Clinical Oral Implants Research* **1**, 8-12.

Rams, T.E., Roberts, T.W., Taum, H.Jr., Keyes, P.H. (1984). The subgingival microbial flora associated with human dental implants. *Clinical Oral Implants Research* **51**, 529-534.

Ritz, H.L. (1969). Fluorescent antibody staining of Neisseria, Streptococcus and Veillonella in frozen sections of human dental plaque. *Archives of Oral Biology* **14**, 1073-1083.

Rölla, G., Melsen, B. & Sönju, T. (1975). Sulphated macromolecules in dental plaque in the monkeys *Macaca irus*. *Archives of Oral Biology* **20**, 341-343.

Rönström, A., Attström, R. & Egelberg, J. (1975). Early formation of dental plaque on plastic films. 1. Light microscopic observations. *Journal of Periodontal Research* **10**, 28-35.

Saxton, C.A. (1973). Scanning electron microscope study of the formation of dental plaque. *Caries Research* **7**, 102-119.

Schroeder, H.E. (1963). Inorganic content and histology of early calculus in man. *Helvetica Odontologica Acta* **7**, 17-30.

Schroeder, H.E. (1969). *Formation and inhibition of dental calculus.* Berne: Hans Huber Publishers.

Schroeder, H.E. (1970). The structure and relationship of plaque to the hard and soft tissues: electron microscopic interpretation. *International Dental Journal* **20**, 353-381.

Schroeder, H.E. & Attström, R. (1979). Effects of mechanical plaque control on development of subgingival plaque and initial gingivitis in neutropenic dogs. *Scandinavian Journal of Dental Research* **87**, 279-287.

Schroeder, H.E. & Baumbauer, H.U. (1966). Stages of calcium phosphate crystallization during calculus formation. *Archives of Oral Biology* **11**, 1-14.

Schroeder, H.E. & De Boever, J. (1970). The structure of microbial dental plaque. In: McHugh, W.D., ed. *Dental plaque.* Edinburgh: Livingstone, pp. 49-74.

Schroeder, H.E. & Listgarten, M.A. (1977). *Fine structure of the developing epithelial attachment of human teeth.* Basel: S. Karger.

Selvig, K.A. (1970). Attachment of plaque and calculus to tooth surfaces. *Journal of Periodontal Research* **5**, 8-18.

Siegrist, B.E., Brecx, M.C., Gusberti, F.A., Joss, A. & Lang, N.P. (1991). *In vivo* early human dental plaque formation on different supporting substances. A scanning electron microscopic and bacteriological study. *Clinical Oral Implants Research* **2**, 38-46.

Silverman, G. & Kleinberg, T. (1967). Fractionation of human dental plaque and the characterization of its cellular and acellular components. *Archives of Oral Biology* **12**, 1387-1405.

Soames, J.V. & Davies, R.M. (1975). The structure of subgingival plaque in a beagle dog. *Journal of Periodontal Research* **9**, 333-341.

Socransky, S.S., Haffajee, A.D., Smith, G.L.F. & Dzink, J.L. (1987). Difficulties encountered in the search for the etiologic agents of destructive periodontal disease. *Journal of Clinical Periodontology* **14**, 588-593.

Sönju, T. & Glantz, P.-O. (1975). Chemical composition of salivary integuments formed *in vivo* on solids with some establ-

ished surface characteristics. *Archives of Oral Biology* **20**, 687-691.

Sönju, T. & Rölla, G. (1973). Chemical analysis of the acquired pellicle formed in two hours on cleaned human teeth. *Caries Research* **7**, 30-38.

Sundberg, J.R. & Friskopp, J. (1985). Crystallography of supragingival and subgingival human dental calculus. *Scandinavian Journal of Dental Research* **93**, 30-38.

Ten Napel, J., Theilade, J., Matsson, L. & Attström, R. (1983). Ultrastructure of developing subgingival plaque in beagle dogs. *Journal of Clinical Periodontology* **12**, 507-524.

Theilade, E. (1986). The non-specific theory in microbial etiology of inflammatory periodontal diseases. *Journal of Clinical Periodontology* **13**, 905-911.

Theilade, E. & Theilade, J. (1970). Bacteriological and ultrastructural studies of developing dental plaque. In: McHugh, W.D., ed. *Dental plaque.* Edinburgh: Livingstone, pp. 27-40.

Theilade, E. & Theilade, J. (1985). Formation and ecology of plaque at different locations in the mouth. *Scandinavian Journal of Dental Research* **93**, 90-95.

Theilade, E., Theilade, J. & Mikkelsen, L. (1982a). Microbiological studies on early dentogingival plaque on teeth and Mylar strips in humans. *Journal of Periodontal Research* **17**, 12-25.

Theilade, E., Wright, W.H., Jensen, B.S. & Löe, H. (1966). Experimental gingivitis in man. II. A longitudinal clinical and bacteriological investigation. *Journal of Periodontal Research* **1**, 1-13.

Theilade, J. (1964). Electron microscopic study of calculus attachment to smooth surfaces. *Acta Odontologica Scandinavia* **22**, 379-387.

Theilade, J. & Attström, R. (1985). Distribution and ultrastructure of subgingival plaque in beagle dogs with gingival inflammation. *Journal of Periodontal Research* **20**, 131-145.

Theilade, J., Fejerskov, O., Karring, T., Rölla, G. & Melsen, B. (1982b). TEM of the effect of sucrose on plaque formation on Mylar and tooth surfaces in monkeys. *Journal of Dental Research* **61**, 570.

Tinanoff, N. & Gross, A. (1976). Epithelial cells associated with the development of dental plaque. *Journal of Dental Research* **55**, 580-583.

Turesky, S., Renstrup, G. & Glickman, I. (1961). Histologic and histochemical observations regarding early calculus formation in children and adults. *Journal of Periodontology* **32**, 7-14.

Wærhaug, J. (1952). The gingival pocket. *Odontologisk Tidskrift* **60**, Suppl. 1.

Wærhaug, J. (1955). Microscopic demonstration of tissue reaction incident to removal of dental calculus. *Journal of Periodontology* **26**, 26-29.

Wærhaug, J. (1956). Effect of rough surfaces upon gingival tissues. *Journal of Dental Research* **35**, 323-325.

Westergaard, J., Frandsen, A. & Slots, J. (1978). Ultrastructure of the subgingival flora in juvenile periodontitis. *Scandinavian Journal of Dental Research* **86**, 421-429.

Wilderer, P.A. & Charaklis, W.G. (1989). Structure and function of biofilms. In: Charaklis, W.G., Wilderer, P.A., eds. *Structure and function of biofilms.* Chichester, UK: John Wiley, pp. 5-17.

Zander, H.A., Hazen, S.P. & Scott, D.B. (1960). Mineralization of dental calculus. *Proceedings of the Society of Experimental Biology and Medicine* **103**, 257-260.

Chapter 4

Microbiology of Periodontal Disease

Sigmund S. Socransky and Anne D. Haffajee

Introduction

Periodontal diseases are infections that are caused by microorganisms that colonize the tooth surface at or below the gingival margin. It is estimated that about 500 different species are capable of colonizing the mouth and any individual may typically harbor 150 or more different species. Counts in subgingival sites range from about 10^3 in healthy, shallow sulci to $> 10^8$ in deep periodontal pockets. Numbers in supragingival plaque can exceed 10^9 on a single tooth surface. Thus, while hundreds of millions or even billions of bacteria continually colonize the tooth at or below the gingival margin throughout life, most periodontal sites in most individuals are not exhibiting new loss of the supporting structures of the teeth at any given time. This recognition is critical. The ecological relationships between the periodontal microbiota and its host by and large are benign in that damage to the supporting structures of the tooth is infrequent. Occasionally, a subset of bacterial species are either introduced, overgrow or exhibit new properties that lead to the destruction of the periodontium. The resulting stressed equilibrium is usually spontaneously corrected, or corrected by therapy. In either instance, microbial species continue to colonize above and below the gingival margin, hopefully in a new and "peaceful" equilibrium.

Similarities of periodontal diseases to other infectious diseases

Our concepts of infectious diseases often appear to be influenced by our experiences with acute infections, particularly upper respiratory infections. In acute infections, an agent is acquired by exposure to an individual harboring that agent or from the environment. The agent establishes within tissues or on mucous membranes or skin. Within a short time, signs or symptoms of a disease appear at the site of introduction or elsewhere in the individual. A "battle" occurs between the parasite and the host resulting in increasingly obvious clinical signs and symptoms. This host-bacterial interaction is often resolved within a short time, usually, but not always, in favor of the host. Thus, daily experience suggests that colonization by a pathogen is rapidly followed by expression of disease. While certain infections follow this pattern, more commonly, colonization by a pathogenic species does not lead to overt disease, at least immediately. For example, 15% of the American population is colonized by *Neisseria meningitidis* (Caugant et al. 1988), but only 1–2 cases of meningitis occur per 100 000 of the population (*Morbidity and Mortality Weekly Report*, 1996). *Mycobacterium tuberculosis* colonizes about 5% of Americans (Sudre et al. 1992), but only 8–10 new cases of tuberculosis per 100 000 are reported each year (*Morbidity and Mortality Weekly Report*, 1996). Finally, about one third of the adult population is colonized by *Hemophilus influenzae* (Kilian & Frederiksen 1981) but only a tiny fraction exhibit disease. Even the highly virulent HIV virus may be detected in individuals for years prior to the development of clinical symptoms.

In a similar fashion, individuals may be colonized continuously by periodontal pathogens at or below the gingival margin and yet not show evidence of ongoing or previous periodontal destruction. Many of the organisms that colonize such sites are members of species thought to be periodontal pathogens. In spite of their presence, periodontal tissue damage does not take place. This is not an anomaly. This phenomenon is consistent with other infectious diseases in which it may be observed that a pathogen is necessary but not sufficient for a disease to occur.

Infectious diseases in a given organ system are caused by one or more of a relatively finite set of pathogens. Further, different species have different tissue specificities and cause diseases in different sites in the body. Lung infections may be caused by a wide range of species that include *Streptococcus pneumoniae*, *M. tuberculosis*, *Klebsiella pneumoniae*, *Legionella pneumophilia* and others. Infections of the intestine are caused by *Salmonella typhi*, *Shigella dysenteriae*, *Vibrio cholera*, *Escherichia coli* and *Campylobacter* species. In a similar fashion periodontal diseases appear to be caused by a relatively finite group of periodontal pathogens acting alone or in combination. Such species include *Actinobacillus actinomycetemcomitans*, *Bacteroides forsythus*, *Campylobacter rectus*, *Eubacterium nodatum*, *Fusobacterium nucleatum*, *Peptostreptococcus micros*, *Porphyromonas gingivalis*, *Prevotella intermedia*, *Prevotella nigrescens*, *Streptococcus intermedius* and *Treponema* sp. (Haffajee & Socransky 1994).

There are a number of other common themes observed in different infectious diseases, particularly those that affect mucous membranes, such as the need to attach to one or more surfaces, the need to "sense" the environment and turn on or off various virulence factors and the need to overcome or evade host defense mechanisms. Infectious agents have evolved a set of common strategies to perform these tasks and the host has developed a series of responses to combat these infections. Thus, periodontal diseases are infectious diseases that have many properties that are similar to bacterial infections in other parts of the body and to a large extent can be combatted in similar fashions.

Unique features of periodontal infections

Although periodontal diseases have certain features in common with other infectious diseases, there are a number of features of these diseases that are quite different. In certain ways, periodontal diseases may be among the most unusual infections of the human. The major reason for this uniqueness is *the unusual anatomic feature that a mineralized structure, the tooth, passes through the integument, so that part of it is exposed to the external environment while part is within the connective tissues.* The tooth provides a surface for the

colonization of a diverse array of bacterial species. Bacteria may attach to the tooth itself, to the epithelial surfaces of the gingiva or periodontal pocket, to underlying connective tissues, if exposed, and to other bacteria which are attached to these surfaces. In contrast to the outer surface of most parts of the body, the outer layers of the tooth do not "shed" and thus microbial colonization (accumulation) is facilitated. Thus, a situation is set up in which microorganisms colonize a relatively stable surface, the tooth, and are continually held in immediate proximity to the soft tissues of the periodontium. This poses a potential threat to those tissues and indeed to the host itself.

The organisms that cause periodontal diseases reside in biofilms that exist on tooth or epithelial surfaces. The biofilm provides a protective environment for the colonizing organisms and fosters metabolic properties that would not be possible if the species existed in a free-living (planktonic) state. Periodontal infections and another biofilm induced disease, dental caries, are arguably the most common infectious diseases affecting the human. The onset of these diseases is usually delayed for prolonged periods after initial colonization by the pathogen(s). The course of these diseases typically runs for years. The etiologic agents in most instances appear to be members of the indigenous microbiota and, thus, the infections might be thought of as endogenous. The source of the infecting agents for any given individual is usually unknown although transfer from parents or significant others is thought to play a primary role (Petit et al. 1993a,b, Saarela et al. 1993, van Steenbergen et al. 1993, Preus et al. 1994). The major characteristics of these diseases are that they are caused by organisms that reside in biofilms outside the body. Their treatment is complex in that physical, antimicrobial and ecological approaches are required.

The presence of a tooth increases the complexity of the host parasite relationship in a number of ways. The bacteria colonizing the tooth are by and large outside the body where they are less able to be controlled by the potent mechanisms which operate within the tissues. The environment within a plaque may be conducive for microbial survival, but it is unlikely to be a particularly effective environment for the host to seek out and destroy microorganisms. Factors such as *hydrogen ion concentration (pH), oxidation reduction potential (Eh), and proteolytic enzymes*, can affect the performance of host defense mechanisms. In addition, the tooth provides "sanctuaries" in which microorganisms can hide, persist at low levels during treatment and then re-emerge to cause further problems. Bacteria in dentinal tubules, flaws in the tooth, or areas that were demineralized by bacteria are not easily approached by the much larger host cells. In a similar fashion, non-cellular host factors must face diffusion barriers, lytic enzymes and absorption by the mineral structure of the tooth. Mechanical debridement other than vigorous removal of tooth material cannot reach organisms within the tooth. Chemotherapeutic agents will also have difficulty in reaching the organisms.

Taken together, the infections which affect the tooth and its supporting structures present a formidable problem for both the host and the therapist. The unique anatomical features of this "organ system" must be borne in mind as we attempt to unravel the etiology and pathogenesis of periodontal diseases and plan treatment or prevention strategies for their control.

HISTORICAL PERSPECTIVE

The search for the etiologic agents of periodontal diseases has been in progress for over a century. The search started in the "golden age of microbiology" (approx. 1880-1920), when the etiologic agents of many medically important infections were determined. It is not surprising that parallel investigations of the etiology of periodontal diseases were initiated in this era. However, these investigations were not as successful as some of the investigations of extraoral infectious diseases. It seems worthwhile to briefly review the findings of the early era and to understand the effect that the inconclusive nature of many of the studies had on the concepts of etiology and treatment of disease. The references for this section may be found in Socransky & Haffajee (1994).

The early search

Investigators in the period from 1880 to 1930 suggested four distinct groups of microorganisms as possible etiologic agents: amoeba, spirochetes, fusiforms and streptococci. The basis of this determination was primarily the seeming association of these organisms with periodontal lesions. The identification of a suspected pathogen was heavily influenced by the nature of the techniques available. The major techniques at that time were wet mount or stained smear microscopy and limited cultural techniques. The different techniques suggested different etiologic agents. This is a situation not unlike that found today. While a greater variety of improved techniques are available, different techniques can emphasize the importance of different organisms.

Amoeba
Certain groups of investigators used stained smears to seek amoeba in bacterial plaque. They found higher proportions of amoebae in lesions of destructive periodontal diseases than in samples taken from sites from healthy mouths or mouths with gingivitis. Local therapies for this organism included the use of dyes or other antiseptic agents to decrease the numbers of amoebae in the oral cavity. Other approaches employed agents such as the emitic, emitin, administered

systemically or locally. The role of amoeba in periodontal disease was questioned by some authors because amoeba were found in sites with minimal or no disease and could not be detected in many sites with destructive disease, and because of the failure of emitin to ameliorate the symptoms of the disease.

Spirochetes
Other investigators used wet mount preparations or specific stains for spirochetes when they examined dental plaque. They reported higher proportions of spirochetes and other motile forms in lesions of destructive disease when compared with control sites in the same or other individuals. This finding led to the suggestion that spirochetes may be etiologic agents of destructive periodontal disease. Therapies were proposed that sought to control disease by the elimination or suppression of these microorganisms including the systemic administration of Neosalvarsan (compound 606), the anti-spirochetal agent used to treat syphilis, coupled with the use of subgingival scaling to control destructive periodontal disease. Other investigators employed bismuth compounds to treat oral spirochetal infections. Many investigators claimed success in controlling advanced destructive periodontal disease by combining local and systemic therapy. Others questioned the relationship of spirochetes to periodontal diseases.

Fusiforms
The third group of organisms which were frequently suggested to be etiologic agents of destructive periodontal diseases, including Vincent's infection, were the spindle-shaped fusiforms. These organisms were originally recognized on the basis of their frequent appearance in microscopic examination of subgingival plaque samples. The organisms were first related to periodontal disease by Plaut (1894). Vincent (1899) distinguished certain pseudomembraneous lesions of the oral cavity and throat from diphtheria and recognized the important role of fusiforms and spirochetes in this disease. In honor of this investigator the infection became known as Vincent's infection. The important role of spirochetes and fusiforms in Vincent's infection was widely recognized in the succeeding two decades.

As a footnote to this section, it is worth noting that ANUG appears to have been declining in many "first world countries" for many decades. Many older practitioners can remember periods when they would see several cases of ANUG a month or even a week. Detection of this disease is much less common today. In reviewing the earlier literature, we were struck with how common the disease appeared to be from about 1915 to 1930. Most of us are aware of the devastation this disease caused in the combat troops of World War I, when the disease was commonly called Trench mouth (due to its frequent occurrence in troops stationed in the trenches of the battlegrounds). What we are less aware of is how common the disease became in countries out of the war zone (e.g. the US) after World War I. For example, Daley (1927a,b) examined over 1000 patients who came to Tufts Dental College in Boston for operative dentistry (not periodontal problems). He found Vincent's infection in one in three people using clinical criteria and stained smears seeking the presence of fusiforms and spirochetes. Daley carefully described the lesions in terms acceptable today; i.e. as an ulcerated lesion that bled easily on probing and had a distinctive fetid odor. He further pointed out that the disease was rare in Boston prior to 1917, at which time the troops began to return home. He described an outbreak stemming from a local barracks, which led to 75 cases being treated at Tufts within 48 hours. Daley and others in the era felt that the severe outbreak after the war was due to the transmission of more virulent bacteria among an unprotected (not immune) population. Assuming that the disease described in this era was ANUG, it is interesting to note that there was a virtual epidemic. This is particularly intriguing in that it supports the notion that periodontal pathogens can be readily transmitted from one person to another, as modern molecular techniques are documenting today.

Streptococci

The fourth group of microorganisms which were proposed as etiologic agents of periodontal diseases in this era were the streptococci. These microorganisms were proposed on the basis of cultural examination of samples of plaque from subgingival sites of periodontal disease. The selection of the streptococci may have been predicated upon the fact that these were the only species that could be consistently isolated from periodontitis lesions using the cultural techniques of that era. Among this group, the streptococci would have been most prominent. Since there were no methods available at that time for the specific control of streptococci, workers turned to non-specific agents such as intramuscular injection of mercury or to the use of vaccines for the control of periodontal diseases.

Vaccines

For the first three decades of the twentieth century, vaccines were commonly employed by physicians and dentists in attempts to control bacterial infections. Three types of vaccines were employed for the control of periodontal diseases. These included vaccines prepared from pure cultures of streptococci, and other oral organisms, autogenous vaccines and stock vaccines such as Van Cott's vaccine, Goldenberg's vaccine or Inava Endocorps vaccine. These vaccines were administered systemically or locally in the periodontal tissues.

Autogenous vaccines were prepared from the dental plaque of patients with destructive periodontal diseases. Plaque samples were removed from the diseased site, "sterilized" by heat and/or by immersion in iodine or formalin solutions, then re-injected into the same patient, either in the local periodontal lesion or systemically. Proponents of all three techniques claimed great efficacy for the vaccination methods employed, while others using the same techniques were more skeptical.

Other forms of therapy directed against oral microorganisms

The difficulty in controlling microorganisms in the absence of specific antimicrobial agents gave rise to a series of rather remarkable treatment procedures. For example, ultraviolet light was widely used to attempt to control the oral microbiota and to improve the well-being of the local tissue (for review see Rasmussen 1929). Other measures were somewhat more dramatic and in some instances rather frightening. Dental practitioners used electrochemical techniques, caustic agents such as phenol, sulfuric, trichloracetic or chromic acids, nascent copper and castor oil soap (sodium ricolineate), and even radium was used to combat root canal infections. In the last instance radium at levels of up to 0.135 millicuries was placed in canals to "sterilize" them. As might be expected, the reports were glowing. The recent interest in controlling the epithelium in order to maximize re-attachment had antecedents in this era. One technique which appears to have been commonly employed was the use of sodium sulfide to "dissolve" the epithelial lining of the pocket and permit reattachment.

Invasion – the early years

One of the more interesting phenomena of research is the fact that research workers keep rediscovering the same phenomena in a cyclical fashion. Invasion of the periodontal tissues by bacteria was thought to be important in the pathogenesis of periodontal diseases in the early 1900s, was forgotten and then re-discovered.

Beckwith et al. (1925) used stains specific for bacteria to study biopsy specimens from prisoners at San Quentin who had periodontitis. They regularly observed bacteria both within the epithelium and in the underlying tissues. Bacteria in the epithelium were usually streptococci or "diptheroids". Gram-negative rods were observed in the connective tissue. They noted the rare occurrence of spiral forms in the tissues, although they were routinely detected in the plaque overlying the tissues. Other investigators also showed invasion into periodontal tissues. Invasion of spirochetes deep into the lesions of Vincent's infection was clearly documented. It was thought that the spirochetes moved into the connective tissues first and were followed by fusiform-shaped species.

Comment

Over this period, literally hundreds of papers were published which suggested certain specific etiologic agents of periodontal diseases or advocated specific therapies directed at microbial control. In spite of this enthusiasm, the concept of the infectious nature of periodontal diseases and the recognition that treatment should be directed at the causative agents, disappeared. Reasons for the demise of this promising area of research could have included the possibility of incorrect etiologic agents, inadequate therapies, multiplicity of diseases and competing theories. A more likely scenario was the failure of early researchers (and this is still true today) to recognize that periodontal diseases represent an array of infections each requiring different specific therapies. Indeed, a similar situation exists today where a given adjunctive antibiotic therapy is effective in some individuals and not others. Finally, competing theories of the etiology of periodontal diseases in this era appeared to, temporarily at least, gain popularity, due primarily to their nebulous and untestable nature. Such hypotheses as "diffuse alveolar atrophy", and "continuing eruption", "lack of function" and "constitutional defects" became acceptable alternatives (to some) to the recognition of the infectious nature of periodontal diseases.

The decline of interest in microorganisms

The initial enthusiasm for the hunt for the etiologic agents of destructive periodontal diseases slowly subsided and by the mid-1930s there were virtually no workers involved in this quest. This state was eloquently described by Belding & Belding (1936) in the aptly titled "Bacteria – Dental Orphans". During the period from the mid-1920s to the early 1960s, the attitude toward the etiology of periodontal disease changed. In the first two decades of this period it was thought that periodontal disease was due to some constitutional defect on the part of the patient, to trauma from occlusion, to disuse atrophy or to some combination of these factors. Bacteria were thought to be merely secondary invaders in this process or at most, contributors to the inflammation observed in periodontal destruction.

Non-specific plaque hypothesis

Treatment of patients based on the notion of constitutional defects or trauma from occlusion was not effective in controlling periodontal diseases. Clinicians recognized that plaque control was essential in the satisfactory treatment of periodontal patients. During the late 1950s, a group of clinicians, sometimes referred to as "plaque evangelists", heavily emphasized the need for plaque control in the prevention and treatment of periodontal diseases. Thus, once again bacteria were thought to play a role in the etiology of destructive periodontal disease, but as non-specific causative agents. According to this "non-specific plaque" hypothesis, any accumulations of microorganisms at or below the gingival margin would produce irritants leading to inflammation. The inflammation in turn was responsible for the periodontal tissue destruction. The specific species of microorganisms that accumu-

lated on the teeth was not considered to be particularly significant providing that their numbers were sufficiently large to trigger a destructive process.

Mixed anaerobic infections

Beginning in the late 1920s, a series of oral and medical microbiologists believed that periodontal disease was the result of "mixed infections". This hypothesis had been considered since the late 1800s when microscopic observations by Vincent in France suggested that certain forms of periodontal disease, particularly acute necrotizing ulcerative gingivitis (ANUG), were due to a complex of microorganisms dominated by fusiforms and spirochetes. These infections were known as fuso-spirochetal infections. In the early 1930s, investigators found that mixtures of microorganisms taken from lung infections or subgingival plaque would induce lesions when subcutaneously injected into various experimental animals. A combination of a fusiform, a spirochete, an anaerobic vibrio and an alpha hemolytic streptococcus could cause transmissible infections in the guinea pig. Later investigators failed to reproduce their results either with the above combination of microorganisms or with many other combinations they tested. They did demonstrate, however, that mixed infections were due to bacteria (rather than a virus).

Macdonald and co-workers (1956) were later able to produce transmissible mixed infections in the guinea pig groin using combinations of pure cultures. The critical mixture of four organisms included a *Bacteroides melaninogenicus* strain, a Gram-positive anaerobic rod and two other Gram-negative anaerobic rods. This combination of organisms was completely different from those used by earlier investigators to cause transmissible infections. These results led to the concept that mixed infections might be "bacteriologically non-specific but biochemically specific". In other words, any combination of microorganisms capable of producing an array of destructive metabolites could lead to transmissible infections in animals and, by extension, to destructive periodontal infections in humans. Later experiments suggested that members of the *B. melaninogenicus* group were the key species in these infections.

Return to specificity in microbial etiology of periodontal diseases

In the 1960s, interest in the specific microbial etiology of periodontal disease was rekindled by two groups of experiments. The first demonstrated that periodontal disease could be transmitted in the hamster from animals with periodontal disease to animals without periodontal disease by caging them together. Swabs of plaque or feces from diseased animals were effective in transmitting the disease to animals free of disease. It was demonstrated that a pure culture of an organism that later became known as *Actinomyces viscosus* was capable of causing destructive periodontal disease in animals free of disease. Other species isolated from the plaques of hamsters with periodontal disease did not have this capability.

At about the same time, it was demonstrated that spirochetes with a unique ultrastructural morphology could be detected in practically pure cultures in the connective tissue underlying lesions of ANUG and within the adjacent epithelium. Control tissue taken from healthy individuals and individuals with other forms of disease did not exhibit a similar tissue invasion. To date, the spirochete associated with ANUG has not been cultivated.

Such findings suggested that there might be more specificity to the microbial etiology of periodontal disease than had been accepted for the previous four decades. However, the emphasis in the 1960s was on the mechanical control of plaque accumulation. This approach was consistent with the prevailing concept that periodontal disease was due to a non-specific accumulation of bacteria on tooth surfaces. This concept is very much in evidence today and still serves as the basis of preventive techniques in most dental practices. It is also clear that non-specific plaque control is not able to effectively prevent all forms of periodontal disease.

The transmissibility studies stimulated a new concept of periodontal diseases. The organisms which were responsible for the periodontal destruction observed in the hamster clearly differed from other organisms by their ability to form large amounts of bacterial plaque both in the hamster and in *in vitro* test systems. A concept emerged that microorganisms that were capable of forming large amounts of plaque *in vivo* and *in vitro* should be considered as prime suspects in the etiology of periodontal diseases. Human isolates of *Actinomyces* species were shown to have this ability *in vitro* and led to plaque formation and periodontal destruction in animal model systems. These findings reinforced the notion that organisms that formed abundant plaque were responsible for destructive periodontal disease. Unfortunately, later research findings revealed major discrepancies in this hypothesis.

Changing concepts of the microbial etiology of periodontal diseases

By the end of the 1960s it was generally accepted that dental plaque was in some way associated with human periodontal disease. It was believed that the presence of bacterial plaque initiated a series of as yet undefined events that led to the destruction of the periodontium. The composition of plaque was thought to be relatively similar from patient to patient and from site to site within patients. Variability was recognized, but the true extent of differences in bacterial composition was not appreciated. It was thought that the major event triggering destructive periodontal disease was an increase in mass of bacterial plaque, possibly accompanied by a diminution of host resistance. Indeed, in the mid 1960s the classic studies of Löe, Theilade and co-workers (Löe et al. 1965, 1967, Theilade et al. 1966) convincingly demonstrated that plaque accumulation directly preceded and initiated gingivitis. Many investigators believed that gingivitis was harmful and led to the eventual destruction of the periodontal tissues, probably by host-mediated events.

Yet, certain discrepancies continued to baffle clinicians and research workers alike. If all plaques were more or less alike and induced a particular systemic response in the host, why was periodontal destruction localized, taking place adjacent to one tooth but not another? If plaque mass was a prime trigger for periodontal destruction, why did certain subjects accumulate much plaque, frequently accompanied by gingivitis, but fail, even after many years, to develop destruction of the supporting structures? On the other hand, why did some individuals with little detectable plaque or clinical inflammation develop rapid periodontal destruction? If inflammation was the main mediator of tissue destruction, why were so many teeth retained in the presence of continual gingivitis? One explanation may have been that there were inconsistencies in the host response, or disease required the superimposition of local factors such as trauma from occlusion, overhanging fillings, etc. Other explanations can be derived from more recent studies of the microbiology of periodontal diseases.

The recognition of differences in the composition of bacterial plaque from subject to subject and site to site within subjects led to a series of investigations. Some studies attempted to determine whether specific microorganisms were found in lesion sites as compared to healthy sites. Other studies sought differences in the microorganisms in subgingival plaque samples taken from subjects with clinically different forms of periodontal disease. Newman and co-workers (1976, 1977) and Slots (1976) demonstrated that the microbial composition of subgingival plaque taken from diseased sites differed substantially from the samples taken from healthy sites in subjects with localized juvenile periodontitis (LJP). Tanner et al. (1979) and Slots (1977) demonstrated that the microbiota recovered from lesion sites from subjects with adult periodontitis differed from the microbiota from healthy sites in the same subjects and also from lesion sites in LJP subjects. These studies along with the demonstration that subjects with LJP could be treated successfully with local debridement and systemic antibiotics provided the initial impetus to perform larger scale studies attempting to relate specific microorganisms to the etiology of different periodontal diseases.

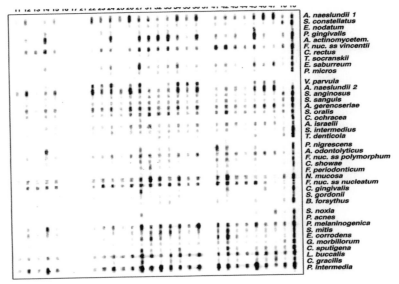

Fig. 4-1. Example of checkerboard DNA–DNA hybridization being used to detect 40 bacterial species in 28 subgingival plaque samples from a single patient. The vertical lanes are the plaque samples numbered from 11 (upper right central incisor) to 47 (lower right second molar). In this subject, teeth 16, 17, 21 and 37 were missing. The two vertical lanes on the right are standards containing either 10^5 or 10^6 cells of each test species. The horizontal lanes contained the indicated DNA probes in hybridization buffer. A signal at the intersection of the vertical and horizontal lanes indicates the presence of a species. The intensity of the signal is related to the number of organisms of that species in the sample. In brief, samples of plaque were placed into individual Eppendorf tubes and the DNA released from the microorganisms by boiling in NaOH. After neutralization, the released DNA was transferred to the surface of a nylon membrane using the 30 channels of a Minislot device (Immunetics, Cambridge, MA). The DNA was fixed to the membrane by UV light and baking and placed in a Miniblotter 45 (Immunetics) with the lanes of DNA at right angles to the 45 channels of the Miniblotter device. Whole genomic DNA probes labelled with digoxigenin were placed in hybridization buffer into 40 of the lanes and hybridized overnight. After stringency washing, the signals were detected using phosphatase-conjugated antibody to digoxigenin and chemifluorescence substrates. Signals were compared to the standards using a Storm Fluorimager and converted to counts.

CURRENT SUSPECTED PATHOGENS OF DESTRUCTIVE PERIODONTAL DISEASES

Criteria for defining periodontal pathogens

For more than a century, the classical "Koch's postulates" have been used to define a causal relation between an infectious agent and a disease. These postulates were: (1) the agent must be isolated from every case of the disease, (2) it must not be recovered from cases of other forms of disease or non-pathogenically, and (3) after isolation and repeated growth in pure culture, the pathogen must induce disease in experimental animals (Carter 1987). The criteria for defining pathogens of destructive periodontal diseases initially were based on Koch's postulates but have been amended and extended in recent years. These criteria include association, elimination, host response, virulence factors, animal studies and risk assessment. The discrimination of a pathogen from a non-pathogenic species is not based on a single criterion but rather on a "weight of evidence" evaluation.

The criterion of association is really the same as Koch's first two postulates; i.e. the species should be found more frequently and in higher numbers in cases of the infection than in individuals without overt disease or with different forms of disease. However, periodontal microbiologists do not expect to find the pathogen in "all cases of the disease" because they currently cannot distinguish "all cases of the disease". The criterion of elimination is based on the concept that elimination of a species should be accompanied by a parallel remission of disease. If a species is eliminated by treatment and the disease progresses, or if the level of a species remains high or increases in a site and the disease stops, doubt would be cast on that species' role in pathogenesis. This criterion (like all of the others) has certain problems in that therapy rarely (if ever) eliminates only one species at a time. The criterion of host response, particularly the immunological response, appears to be of value in defining periodontal pathogens. If a species (or its antigens) gains access to underlying periodontal tissues and causes damage, it seems likely that the host will produce antibodies or a cellular immune response that is directed specifically to that species. Thus, the host response could act as a pointer to the pathogen(s). Biochemical determinants (virulence factors) may also provide valuable clues to pathogenicity. Potentially damaging metabolites produced, or properties

Table 4-1. Summary of some of the types of data that suggest that *Actinobacillus actinomycetemcomitans* may be an etiologic agent of destructive periodontal diseases (for literature citations see text and Haffajee & Socransky 1994)

Association	Elevated in lesions of localized juvenile periodontitis, pre-pubertal or adolescent periodontal disease
	Lower in health, gingivitis and edentulous subjects or sites
	Elevated in some adult periodontitis lesions
	Elevated in active lesions of juvenile periodontitis
	Detected in prospective studies
	Detected in apical areas of pocket or in tissues from LJP lesions
Elimination	Elimination or suppression resulted in successful therapy
	Recurrent lesions harbored the species
Host response	Elevated antibody in serum or saliva of LJP patients
	Elevated antibody in serum or saliva of chronic periodontitis patients
	Elevated local antibody in LJP sites
Virulence factors	Leukotoxin; collagenase; endotoxin; epitheliotoxin; fibroblast inhibitory factor; bone resorption inducing factor; induction of cytokine production from macrophages; modification of neutrophil function; degradation of immunoglobulins; cytolethal distending toxin (Cdt); induces apoptotic cell death
	Invades epithelial and vascular endothelial cells *in vitro* and buccal epithelial cells *in vivo*
Animal studies	Induced disease in gnotobiotic rats
	Subcutaneous abscesses in mice

Table 4-2. Summary of some of the types of data that suggest that *Porphyromonas gingivalis* may be an etiologic agent of destructive periodontal diseases (for literature citations see text and Haffajee & Socransky 1994)

Association	Elevated in lesions of periodontitis
	Lower in sites of health, gingivitis and edentulous subjects
	Elevated in actively progressing lesions
	Elevated in subjects exhibiting periodontal disease progression
	Detected in cells or tissues of periodontal lesions
	Presence indicates increased risk for alveolar bone loss and attachment level loss
Elimination	Elimination resulted in successful therapy
	Recurrent lesions harbored the species
	Successful treatment lowered level and/or avidity of antibody
Host response	Elevated antibody in serum or saliva in subjects with various forms of periodontitis
	Altered local antibody in periodontitis
Virulence factors	Collagenase; endotoxin; proteolytic trypsin-like activity; fibrinolysin; hemolysin; other proteases including gingipain; Phospholipase A; degrades immunoglobulin; fibroblast inhibitory factor; H2S; NH3; fatty acids; factors that adversely affect PMNs; capsular polysaccharide; bone resorption inducing factor; induction of cytokine production from various host cells; generates chemotactic activities; inhibits migration of PMNs across epithelial barriers; invades epithelial cells *in vitro*
Animal studies	Important in experimental pure or mixed subcutaneous infections
	Induced disease in gnotobiotic rats
	Studies in sheep, monkeys and dogs
	Immunization diminished disease in experimental animals

possessed, by certain species may be suggestive that that species could play a role in the disease process.

Animal model systems provide suggestive evidence that a microbial species may play a role in human disease. Particularly noteworthy are studies of experimentally induced disease in dogs or monkeys, which can be manipulated to favor selection of single or subsets of species that may or may not induce pathology. These models usually suggest a possible etiologic role of a species indigenous to the test animal that may have analogues in the human subgingival microbiota. Finally, technological developments, such as checkerboard DNA–DNA hybridization (Fig. 4-1) and PCR, now permit assessment of specific microorganisms in large numbers of subgingival plaque samples. This allows prospective studies to be performed

Table 4-3. Summary of some of the types of data that suggest that *Bacteroides forsythus* may be an etiologic agent of destructive periodontal diseases (for literature citations see text and Haffajee & Socransky 1994)

Association	Elevated in lesions of periodontitis
	Lower in sites of health or gingivitis
	Elevated in actively progressing lesions
	Elevated in periodontal abscesses
	Increased in subjects with refractory periodontitis
	Detected in epithelial cells of periodontal pockets
	Presence indicates increased risk for alveolar bone loss, tooth and attachment level loss
Elimination	Elimination resulted in successful therapy
	Recurrent lesions harbored the species
	Reduced in successfully treated peri-implantitis
Host response	Elevated antibody in serum of periodontitis subjects and very high in a subset of subjects with refractory periodontitis
Virulence factors	Endotoxin; fatty acid and methylglyoxal production; induces apoptotic cell death; cytokine production from various host cells; invades epithelial cells *in vitro* and *in vivo*
Animal studies	Increased levels in ligature-induced periodontitis and peri-implantitis in dogs
	Induced disease in gnotobiotic rats

in which the risk of periodontal disease progression conferred by the presence of an organism at given levels may be assessed.

Periodontal pathogens

The World Workshop in Periodontology (Consensus report 1996) designated *A. actinomycetemcomitans*, *P. gingivalis* and *B. forsythus* as periodontal pathogens. Tables 4-1 to 4-3 summarize some of the data that indicate an etiologic role of these species in periodontal diseases, categorized according to the criteria defined above. The summary is by no means exhaustive but does indicate that a growing literature suggests some reasonable candidates as etiologic agents of destructive periodontal diseases.

Actinobacillus actinomycetemcomitans
One of the strongest associations between a suspected pathogen and destructive periodontal disease (at least in terms of number of publications) is provided by *A. actinomycetemcomitans*. This is a small, non-motile, Gram-negative, saccharolytic, capnophilic, round-ended rod that forms small, convex colonies with a "star-shaped" center when grown on blood agar plates (Fig. 4-2). This species was first recognized as a possible periodontal pathogen by its increased frequency of detection and higher numbers in lesions of localized juvenile periodontitis (Newman et al. 1976, Slots 1976, Newman & Socransky 1977, Slots et al. 1980, Mandell & Socransky 1981, Zambon et al. 1983a, Chung et al. 1989) when compared with numbers in plaque samples from other clinical conditions including periodontitis, gingivitis, and health. Soon after, it was demonstrated that the majority of subjects with LJP had an enormously elevated serum antibody re-

sponse to this species (Genco et al. 1980, Listgarten et al. 1981, Tsai et al. 1981, Altman et al. 1982, Ebersole et al. 1982, 1987) and that there was local synthesis of antibody to this species (Schonfeld & Kagan 1982, Ebersole et al. 1985, Smith et al. 1985, Tew et al. 1985a). When subjects with this form of disease were treated successfully, the species was eliminated or lowered in level, while treatment failures were associated with failure to lower the numbers of the species in treated sites (Slots & Rosling 1983, Haffajee et al. 1984, Christersson et al. 1985, Kornman & Robertson 1985, Mandell et al. 1986, Preus 1988, Shiloah et al. 1998, Tinoco et al. 1998). The species produced a number of potentially damaging metabolites including a leukotoxin (Baehni et al. 1979), a cytolethal distending toxin (Saiki et al. 2001, Shenker et al. 2001) and induced disease in experimental animals (Irving et al. 1978). *A. actinomycetemcomitans* has been shown, *in vitro*, to have the ability to invade cultured human gingival epithelial cells (Blix et al. 1992, Sreenivasan et al. 1993), human vascular endothelial cells (Schenkein et al. 2000) and buccal epithelial cells *in vivo* (Rudney et al. 2001). Further, studies have shown that *A. actinomycetemcomitans* induced apoptotic cell death (Arakawa et al. 2000, Kato et al. 2000).

Perhaps the strongest association data came from studies of "active lesions" in which the species was elevated in actively progressing periodontal lesions when compared with non-progressing sites (Haffajee et al. 1984, Mandell 1984, Mandell et al. 1987) and in prospective studies of as yet undiseased siblings of LJP subjects (DiRienzo et al. 1994). *A. actinomycetemcomitans* was also elevated in studies of disease progression in young Indonesian subjects (Timmerman et al. 2001). Collectively, the data suggest that *A. actinomycetemcomitans* is a probable pathogen of LJP. However, this should not be interpreted as meaning

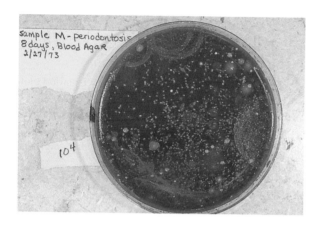

sample M-periodontosis
8 days, Blood Agar
2/27/73

10⁴

Fig. 4-2. Photograph of a primary isolation plate of a subgingival plaque sample from a diseased site in a subject with LJP. A dilution of the plaque sample was grown for 7 days at 35°C on an enriched blood agar plate in an atmosphere of 80% N_2, 10% H_2 and 10% CO_2. The majority of the small, round, convex colonies on this plate are isolates of *Actinobacillus actinomycetemcomitans*.

that it is the sole cause of this clinical condition since a subset of subjects with LJP did not exhibit this species in samples of their subgingival plaque and had no elevated antibody response to the species (Loesche et al. 1985, Moore 1987).

The possibility that only a subset of *A. actinomycetemcomitans* clonal types is responsible for localized juvenile periodontitis was raised by recent studies. Strains of *A. actinomycetemcomitans* were isolated from members of 18 families with at least one member with active LJP as well as from 32 control subjects. Restriction fragment length polymorphisms (RFLP) indicated 13 distinct RFLP groups of *A. actinomycetemcomitans* (DiRienzo & McKay 1994). Isolates from LJP subjects fell into predominantly RFLP pattern II, while RFLP patterns XIII and XIV were seen exclusively in isolates from periodontally healthy subjects. Further, disease progression was related strongly to the presence of RFLP group II (DiRienzo et al. 1994).

Haubek et al. (1996) demonstrated that strains of *A. actinomycetemcomitans* isolated from families of African origin living in geographically different areas were characterized by a 530 base pair deletion in the leukotoxin gene operon leading to a significantly increased production of leukotoxin. They speculated that this virulent clonal type found in individuals of African origin may account for an increased prevalence of LJP in African-Americans and other individuals of African descent. The same investigators found a strong association between the presence of *A. actinomycetemcomitans* with the 530 bp deletion and early onset periodontitis in Moroccan school children, but no association between the presence of *A. actinomycetemcomitans* without the deletion and early onset periodontitis (Haubek et al. 2001). This deletion was not detected in any strains of *A. actinomycetemcomitans* isolated from adult Chinese subjects (Mombelli et al. 1999, Tan et al. 2001) or Asian subjects in the US (Contreras et al. 2000). Subjects harboring *A. actinomycetemcomitans* with the 530 bp deletion were 22.5 times more likely to convert to LJP than subjects who had *A. actinomycetemcomitans* variants containing the full length leukotoxin promoter region (Bueno et al. 1998).

A. actinomycetemcomitans has also been implicated in adult forms of destructive periodontal disease, but its role is less clear. The species has been isolated from

adult periodontitis lesions, but less frequently and in lower numbers than from lesions in LJP subjects (Rodenburg et al. 1990, Slots et al. 1990a). In addition, its numbers in plaque samples from adult lesions were often not as high as those observed for other suspected pathogens in the same plaque samples. The most frequently isolated serotype of *A. actinomycetemcomitans* from lesions of LJP in American subjects was serotype b (Zambon et al. 1983b), whereas serotype a was more commonly detected in samples from adult subjects (Zambon et al. 1983a). This finding was corroborated indirectly by examination of serum antibody levels to the two serotypes. Most elevated responses to *A. actinomycetemcomitans* in LJP subjects were to serotype b while elevated responses to serotype a were more common in subjects with adult periodontal disease (Listgarten et al. 1981). Some subjects in each group exhibited elevated serum antibody responses to both serotypes. In Finnish subjects, serotypes a and b were more frequently isolated from subjects with periodontal disease and serotype c from periodontally healthy subjects (Asikainen et al. 1991). However, this pattern of serotype distribution was not observed in Korea (Chung et al. 1989) or Japan (Saito et al. 1993) where *A. actinomycetemcomitans* serotype c was frequently observed in plaque samples from sites of periodontal pathology. Recently, two other serotypes, d and e, have been recognized (Dogan et al. 1999, Mombelli et al. 1999).

Antibody data and data from the treatment of *A. actinomycetemcomitans* infected patients with adult or refractory periodontitis provide the most convincing evidence of a possible etiological role of *A. actinomycetemcomitans* in adult forms of periodontal disease. 36 of 56 adults with destructive periodontal disease examined at multiple time periods at The Forsyth Institute exhibited an elevated serum antibody response to *A. actinomycetemcomitans* serotypes a and/or b. Elevated responses to other suspected periodontal pathogens were far less common. van Winkelhoff et al. (1992) treated 50 adult subjects with "severe generalized periodontitis" and 40 subjects with refractory periodontitis who were culture-positive for *A. actinomycetemcomitans* using mechanical debridement and systemically administered amoxicillin and metronidazole. Only 1 of 90 subjects was culture posi-

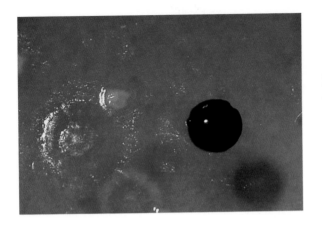

Fig. 4-3. Photograph of part of a primary isolation plate of a subgingival plaque sample from a subject with adult periodontitis. The medium and growth conditions were as described in Fig. 4-2. The black-pigmented colony is an isolate of *Porphyromonas gingivalis*.

tive for *A. actinomycetemcomitans* 3-9 months post-therapy (van Winkelhoff et al. 1992) and 1 of 48 subjects was culture positive 2 years post-therapy (Pavicic et al. 1994). There was a significant gain in attachment level and decrease in probing pocket depth in virtually all patients after therapy.

Porphyromonas gingivalis

P. gingivalis is a second consensus periodontal pathogen. Isolates of this species are Gram-negative, anaerobic, non-motile, asaccharolytic rods that usually exhibit coccal to short rod morphologies. *P. gingivalis* is a member of the much investigated "black-pigmented *Bacteroides*" group (Fig. 4-3). Organisms of this group form brown to black colonies (Oliver & Wherry 1921) on blood agar plates and were initially grouped into a single species, *B. melaninogenicus* (*Bacterium melaninogenicum*, Burdon (1928)). The black-pigmented *Bacteroides* have a long history of association with periodontal diseases since the early efforts of Burdon (1928) through the mixed infection studies of Macdonald and co-workers (1960) to the current intense interest. In the late 1970s, it was recognized that the black-pigmented *Bacteroides* contained species that were asaccharolytic (eventually *P. gingivalis*), and either had an intermediate level of carbohydrate fermentation (which eventually led to a group of species including *P. intermedia*) or were highly saccharolytic (leading to the group that includes *Prevotella melaninogenica*).

Early interest in *P. gingivalis* and other black-pigmented *Bacteroides* arose primarily because of their essential role in certain experimental mixed infections (Macdonald et al. 1956, 1963, Socransky & Gibbons 1965) and their production of an unusually large array of virulence factors (Table 4-2, Haffajee & Socransky 1994, Deshpande & Khan 1999). Members of these species produce collagenase, an array of proteases (including those that destroy immunoglobulins), hemolysins, endotoxin, fatty acids, NH3, H2S, indole etc. *P. gingivalis* can inhibit migration of PMNs across an epithelial barrier (Madianos et al. 1997) and has been shown to affect the production or degradation of cytokines by mammalian cells (Darveau et al. 1998, Fletcher et al. 1998, Sandros et al. 2000). Studies initiated in the late 1970s and extending to date strength-

ened the association of *P. gingivalis* with disease and demonstrated that the species was uncommon and in low numbers in health or gingivitis but more frequently detected in destructive forms of disease (Table 4-2, Haffajee & Socransky 1994, O'Brien-Simpson et al. 2000). This species has also been shown to be increased in numbers and/or frequency of detection in deteriorating periodontal sites (Dzink et al. 1988, Lopez 2000, Kamma et al. 2001) or in subjects exhibiting periodontal disease progression (Albandar et al. 1997). The species has been shown to be reduced in successfully treated sites but is commonly encountered in sites that exhibit recurrence of disease or persistence of deep periodontal pockets post-therapy (Bragd et al. 1987, Haffajee et al. 1988a, van Winkelhoff et al. 1988, Berglundh et al. 1998, Shiloah et al. 1998, Winkel et al. 1998, Takamatsu et al. 1999, Chaves et al. 2000, Mombelli et al. 2000). *P. gingivalis* has been associated with an increased risk of periodontal disease severity and progression (Beck et al. 1990, 1992, 1997, Grossi et al. 1994, 1995).

P. gingivalis has been shown to induce elevated systemic and local immune responses in subjects with various forms of periodontitis (Table 4-2, Mahanonda et al. 1991, Haffajee & Socransky 1994, O'Brien-Simpson et al. 2000). Indeed, there has been a remarkably intense effort in many laboratories in the last few years, not only to compare the level of antibody response in subjects with and without disease, but to examine relative avidities of antibody (Lopatin & Blackburn 1992, Whitney et al. 1992, Mooney et al. 1993), subclass of antibody (Lopatin & Blackburn 1992, Wilton et al. 1992), the effect of treatment (Chen et al. 1991, Johnson et al. 1993) and the nature of the antigens which elicit the elevated responses (Ogawa et al. 1989, Yoshimura et al. 1989, Curtis et al. 1991, Papaioannou et al. 1991, Duncan et al. 1992, Schifferle et al. 1993). Noteworthy in this regard are the observations of Ogawa et al. (1989), which indicate that an average of approximately 5% of plasma cells in lesions of advanced periodontitis form antibody to the fimbriae of *P. gingivalis*. The consensus of the antibody studies is that many, but not all, subjects who have experienced periodontal attachment loss exhibit elevated levels of antibody to antigens of *P. gingivalis* suggesting that this species gained access to the underlying tissues and may have initiated or contributed to the observed pathology.

P. gingivalis-like organisms are also strongly related to destructive periodontal disease in naturally occurring or ligature-induced disease in dogs, sheep or monkeys (Table 4-2). The species or closely related organisms were higher in number in lesion sites than in non-lesion sites in naturally occurring disease. When disease was induced by ligature in dogs or monkeys, the level of the species rose at the diseased sites concomitant with the detection of disease. Of great interest were the observations of Holt et al. (1988) who demonstrated that a microbiota suppressed by systemic administration of rifampin (and without detectable *P. gingivalis*) would not cause ligature-induced disease, but the reintroduction of *P. gingivalis* to the microbiota resulted in initiation and progress of the lesions. Ligature-induced periodontitis and peri-implantitis in dogs were also accompanied by a significant increase in the detection of *P. gingivalis* (Nociti et al. 2001). Like *A. actinomycetemcomitans*, *P. gingivalis* has been shown to be able to invade human gingival epithelial cells *in vitro* (Lamont et al. 1992, Duncan et al. 1993, Sandros et al. 1993) and buccal epithelial cells *in vivo* (Rudney et al. 2001) and has been found in higher numbers on or in epithelial cells recovered from the periodontal pocket than in associated plaque (Dzink et al. 1989). Attachment to and invasion of epithelial cells appears to be mediated by the *P. gingivalis* fimbriae (Njoroge et al. 1997, Weinberg et al. 1997). Finally, studies in monkeys and gnotobiotic rats have indicated that immunization with whole organisms or specific antigens affected the progress of the periodontal lesions. In most instances, periodontal breakdown was decreased (Evans et al. 1992, Persson et al. 1994). However, in one study the disease severity was increased after immunization (Ebersole et al. 1991). The differences in results may have been due to differences in animal species, the protocol used for induction of periodontal disease, antigen preparation or method of immunization. From the viewpoint of this section, the studies demonstrate that altering the host–*P. gingivalis* equilibrium by raising the level of specific antibodies to *P. gingivalis* antigens markedly affected disease outcome. Such data reinforce the importance of this bacterial species in periodontal disease, at least in the animal model systems employed.

Bacteroides forsythus

The third consensus periodontal pathogen, *B. forsythus*, was first described in 1979 (Tanner et al. 1979) as a "fusiform" *Bacteroides*. This species was difficult to grow, often requiring 7–14 days for minute colonies to develop. The organism is a Gram-negative, anaerobic, spindle-shaped, highly pleomorphic rod. The growth of the organism was shown to be enhanced by co-cultivation with *F. nucleatum* and indeed commonly occurs with this species in subgingival sites (Socransky et al. 1988). The species was shown to have an unusual requirement for N-acetylmuramic

acid (Wyss 1989). Inclusion of this factor in culture media markedly enhanced growth. The organism was found in higher numbers in sites of destructive periodontal disease or periodontal abscesses than in gingivitis or healthy sites (Lai et al. 1987, Herrera et al. 2000, Papapanou et al. 2000). In addition, *B. forsythus* was detected more frequently and in higher numbers in active periodontal lesions than inactive lesions (Dzink et al. 1988) (Table 4-3). Further, subjects who harbored *B. forsythus* were at greater risk for alveolar bone loss, attachment loss and tooth loss compared with subjects in whom this species was not detected (Machtei et al. 1999). This species has been shown to produce trypsin-like proteolytic activity (BANA test positive, Loesche et al. 1992), methylglyoxal (Kashket et al. 2002) and induce apoptotic cell death (Arakawa et al. 2000).

Initially, *B. forsythus* was thought to be a relatively uncommon subgingival species. However, the studies of Gmur et al. (1989) using monoclonal antibodies to enumerate the species directly in plaque samples, suggested the species was more common than previously found in cultural studies and its levels were strongly related to increasing pocket depth. Lai et al. (1987) corroborated these findings using fluorescent-labelled polyclonal antisera and demonstrated that *B. forsythus* was much higher in subgingival than supragingival plaque samples. Data of Tanner et al. (1998) suggested that *B. forsythus* was a major species found at sites that converted from periodontal health to disease. *B. forsythus* was found at higher levels at sites which showed breakdown after periodontal therapy than sites which remained stable or gained attachment (Shiloah et al. 1998). *B. forsythus* has also been shown to be decreased in frequency of detection and counts after successful periodontal therapy including SRP (Haffajee et al. 1997, Takamatsu et al. 1999, Darby et al. 2001), periodontal surgery (Levy et al. 2002), or systemically administered antibiotics (Winkel et al. 1998, 2001, Feres et al. 2000,). Successful treatment of peri-implantitis with local delivery of tetracycline was accompanied by a significant decrease in the frequency of detection of *B. forsythus* (Mombelli et al. 2001). Ligature-induced periodontitis and peri-implantitis in dogs were accompanied by a significant increase in the frequency of detection of *B. forsythus* (Nociti et al. 2001). Finally, the persistent presence of *B. forsythus* at sites in subjects with low severity of chronic periodontitis indicated a 5.3 times greater chance of having at least one site in their mouths losing attachment compared with subjects with occasional or no presence of this species (Tran et al. 2001).

Studies using checkerboard DNA–DNA hybridization techniques to examine subgingival plaque samples confirmed the high levels of *B. forsythus* detected using fluorescent-labelled antisera and demonstrated that *B. forsythus* was the most common species detected on or in epithelial cells recovered from periodontal pockets (Dibart et al. 1998). It was infrequently detected in epithelial cell samples from

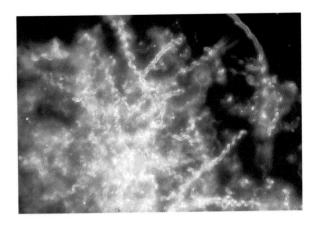

Fig. 4-4. Photomicrograph of a sample of subgingival plaque from subjects with advanced adult periodontitis viewed by darkfield microscopy. The sample is dominated by large spirochetes with the typical corkscrew appearance.

healthy subjects. Double-labelling experiments demonstrated that *B. forsythus* was both on and in periodontal pocket epithelial cells indicating the species ability to invade. Listgarten et al. (1993) found that the species most frequently detected in "refractory" subjects was *B. forsythus*. Serum antibody to *B. forsythus* has been found to be elevated in a number of periodontitis patients (Taubman et al. 1992) and was often extremely elevated in a subset of refractory periodontal disease subjects.

The role of this species in periodontal diseases has been clarified by studies in numerous laboratories involving non-cultural methods of enumeration such as DNA probes, PCR or immunologic methods. For example, Grossi et al. (1994, 1995) considered *B. forsythus* to be the most significant microbial risk factor that distinguished subjects with periodontitis from those who were periodontally healthy.

Spirochetes

Spirochetes are Gram-negative, anaerobic, helical-shaped, highly motile microorganisms that are common in many periodontal pockets (Fig. 4-4). The role of spirochetes in the pathogenesis of destructive periodontal diseases deserves extended comment. Clearly, a spirochete has been implicated as the likely etiologic agent of acute necrotizing ulcerative gingivitis by its presence in large numbers in tissue biopsies from affected sites (Listgarten & Socransky 1964, Listgarten 1965). The role of spirochetes in other forms of periodontal disease is less clear. The organisms have been considered as possible periodontal pathogens since the late 1800s and in the 1980s enjoyed a resurgence of interest for use as possible diagnostic indicators of disease activity and/or therapeutic efficacy (Keyes & Rams 1983, Rams & Keyes 1983). The major reason for the interest in this group of organisms has been their increased numbers in sites with increased pocket depth. Healthy sites exhibit few, if any, spirochetes, sites of gingivitis but no attachment loss exhibit low to moderate levels, while many deep pockets harbor large numbers of these organisms.

The major difficulty encountered in defining the role of spirochetes has been the difficulty in distinguishing individual species. At least 15 species of subgingival spirochetes have been described, but in most studies of plaque samples, spirochetes are combined in a single group or groups based on cell size; i.e. small, medium or large. Thus, while there may be pathogens among the spirochetes, their role may have been obscured by unintentionally pooling their numbers with non-pathogenic spirochetes. This would be similar to combining in a single count, organisms with coccal morphologies, such as *P. gingivalis, Veillonella parvula* and *Streptococcus sanguis*. In spite of the limitations of combining spirochetes into a single morphogroup, spirochetes have been related with increased risk at a site for the development of gingivitis (Riviere & DeRouen 1998) and periodontitis (Riviere et al. 1997). The need to evaluate the role of individual species of spirochetes in periodontal diseases is reinforced by studies of serum antibody responses to different species. When antibody responses to individual species were examined in subjects with adult or juvenile periodontitis or a healthy periodontium, different responses were observed to different species. Certain spirochetal species elicited an elevated response in one or more of the groups with destructive periodontal disease (Mangan et al. 1982, Tew et al. 1985c, Lai et al. 1986), while others were related to depressed antibody responses in certain patient groups (Steinberg & Gershoff 1968, Tew et al. 1985c). Such data suggest that pooling spirochete species into a collective group may obscure meaningful host–parasite interactions.

More recently, specific species of spirochetes have been related to periodontal breakdown. *Treponema denticola* was found to be more common in periodontally diseased than healthy sites, more common in subgingival than supragingival plaque (Simonson et al. 1988, Riviere et al. 1992, Albandar et al. 1997, Haffajee et al. 1998, Yuan et al. 2001) and more common in healthy sites that progressed to gingivitis (Riviere & DeRouen 1998). *T. denticola* was shown to decrease in successfully treated periodontal sites, but not change or increase in non-responding sites (Simonson et al. 1992). Cultural studies suggested that *T. denticola* and a "large treponeme" were found more frequently in patients with severe periodontitis than in healthy or gingivitis sites (Moore et al. 1982). Riviere et al. (1991a,b,c, 1992) employed a monoclonal antibody directed against *Treponema pallidum*, the etiologic agent of syphilis, to examine supra and subgingival

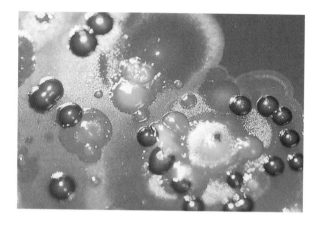

Fig. 4-5. Photograph of part of a primary isolation plate of a subgingival plaque sample from a subject with adult periodontitis. The medium and growth conditions were as described in Fig. 4-2. The dark-pigmented colonies are isolates of *Prevotella intermedia*.

plaque samples and/or tissues from healthy, periodontitis and ANUG subjects. This antibody cross-reacted with antigens of uncultivated spirochetes in many of the plaque samples. These "pathogen-related oral spirochetes" (PROS) were the most frequently detected spirochetes in supra and subgingival plaques of periodontitis patients and were the most numerous spirochetes in periodontitis lesion sites. Their presence in periodontally healthy sites related to an increased risk of development of periodontitis (Riviere et al. 1997). The PROS were also detected in plaque samples from ANUG (Riviere et al. 1991c) and tissue biopsies from ANUG lesions using immunohistochemical techniques (Riviere et al. 1991a). PROS were also shown to have the ability to penetrate a tissue barrier in *in vitro* systems (Riviere et al. 1991b). This property was shared with *T. pallidum* but not with other cultivated species of oral spirochetes such as *T. denticola, Treponema socranskii, Treponema pectinovorum* or *Treponema vincentii*. These studies and others suggest that certain species of spirochetes are important in the pathogenesis of ANUG and certain forms of periodontitis. Precise evaluation of the role of individual spirochete species appears to be realistic based on their detection in plaque samples by immunologic, PCR or DNA probe techniques. Indeed, enumeration of even uncultivable spirochete taxa is possible using oligonucleotide probes (Tanner et al. 1994) or specific antibody as described above. Studies performed using such techniques permit better distinction of species of spirochetes and a clearer understanding of their possible role in disease.

Prevotella intermedia/Prevotella nigrescens

Table 4-3 summarizes some of the data that suggest a possible role of other subgingival species in the pathogenesis of destructive periodontal diseases. At present the data for other species are more limited, but these organisms appear to merit further investigation (Zambon 1996). *P. intermedia* is the second black-pigmented *Bacteroides* to receive considerable interest (Fig. 4-5). The levels of this Gram-negative, short, round-ended anaerobic rod have been shown to be particularly elevated in acute necrotizing ulcerative gingivitis (Loesche et al. 1982), in certain forms of periodontitis (Tanner et al. 1979, Dzink et al. 1983, Moore et al. 1985,

Maeda et al. 1998, Herrera et al. 2000, Papapanou et al. 2000), and in progressing sites in chronic periodontitis (Tanner et al. 1996, Lopez 2000), and has been detected by immunohistological methods in the intercellular spaces of periodontal pocket biopsies from rapidly progressive periodontitis subjects (Hillmann et al. 1998). Isolates of this species can induce alveolar bone loss in rats (Yoshida-Minami et al. 1997). Persistence of *P. intermedia/nigrescens* after standard mechanical therapy has been shown to be associated with a large proportion of sites exhibiting bleeding on probing (Mombelli et al. 2000). Berglundh et al. (1998) demonstrated that improved clinical parameters after the use of mechanical therapy and systemically administered amoxicillin and metronidazole were associated with a decrease of periodontal pathogens including *P. intermedia*. Successful treatment of peri-implantitis with local delivery of tetracycline also significantly decreased the frequency of detection of *P. intermedia/nigrescens* (Mombelli et al. 2001).

This species appears to have a number of the virulence properties exhibited by *P. gingivalis* and was shown to induce mixed infections on injection in laboratory animals (Hafstrom & Dahlen 1997). It has also been shown to invade oral epithelial cells *in vitro* (Dorn et al. 1998). Elevated serum antibodies to this species have been observed in some but not all subjects with refractory periodontitis (Haffajee et al. 1988b). Strains of "*P. intermedia*" that show identical phenotypic traits have been separated into two species, *P. intermedia* and *P. nigrescens* (Shah & Gharbia 1992). This distinction makes earlier studies of this "species" difficult to interpret since data from two different species may have been inadvertently pooled. However, new studies which discriminate the species in subgingival plaque samples might strengthen the relationship of one or both species to periodontal disease pathogenesis.

Fusobacterium nucleatum

F. nucleatum is a Gram-negative, anaerobic, spindle-shaped rod that has been recognized as part of the subgingival microbiota for over 100 years (Plaut 1894, Vincent 1899). This species is the most common isolate found in cultural studies of subgingival plaque samples comprising approximately 7–10% of total isolates from different clinical conditions (Dzink et al. 1985, 1988, Moore et al. 1985). *F. nucleatum* is prevalent in subjects with periodontitis (Papapanou et al. 2000, Socransky et al. 2002) and periodontal abscesses (Herrera et al. 2000). Successful treatment of peri-implantitis with local delivery of tetracycline was associated with a significant reduction in frequency of detection in several species including *F. nucleatum* (Mombelli et al. 2001). Invasion of this species into human gingival epithelial cells *in vitro* was accompanied by an increased secretion of IL-8 from the epithelial cells (Han et al. 2000). The species can induce apoptotic cell death in mononuclear and polymorphonuclear cells (Jewett et al. 2001) and cytokine, elastase and oxygen radical release from leukocytes (Sheikhi et al. 2000).

Although there were differences detected in levels of this species between active and inactive periodontal lesions (Dzink et al. 1988), the differences may have been minimized by the inadvertent pooling of subspecies of *F. nucleatum*. Support for this contention may be derived from the antibody responses in subjects with different forms of periodontal disease to different homology groups of *F. nucleatum* (Tew et al. 1985b). It is anticipated that a clearer understanding of the role of *F. nucleatum* will be achieved when subspecies such as *F. nucleatum ss nucleatum, F. nucleatum ss polymorphum, F. nucleatum ss vincentii* and *F. periodonticum* are individually evaluated for their association with disease status and progression.

Campylobacter rectus

C. rectus is a Gram-negative, anaerobic, short, motile vibrio. The organism is unusual in that it utilizes H_2 or formate as its energy source. It was first described as a member of the "vibrio corroders", a group of short nondescript rods that formed small convex, "dry spreading" or "corroding" (pitting) colonies on blood agar plates. These organisms were eventually shown to include members of a new genus *Wolinella* (most species have been redefined as *Campylobacter*), and *Eikenella corrodens*. *C. rectus* has been shown to be present in higher numbers in disease sites as compared with healthy sites (Moore et al. 1983, 1985, Lippke et al. 1991, Lai et al. 1992, Papapanou et al. 1997, Macuch & Tanner 2000) and it was found in higher numbers and more frequently in sites exhibiting active periodontal destruction (Dzink et al. 1985, 1988, Tanner & Bouldin 1989, Rams et al. 1993) or converting from periodontal health to disease (Tanner et al. 1998). In addition, *C. rectus* was found less frequently and in lower numbers after successful periodontal therapy (Tanner et al. 1987, Haffajee et al. 1988a, Levy et al. 2002) or treatment of peri-implantitis with local delivery of tetracycline (Mombelli et al. 2001). *C. rectus* was also found in combination with other suspected pathogens in sites of subjects with refractory periodontal diseases (Haffajee et al. 1988b). Like *A. actinomycetemcomitans*, *C. rectus* has been shown to produce a leukotoxin. These are the only two oral species known to possess this characteristic

(Gillespie et al. 1992). The species is also capable of stimulating human gingival fibroblasts to produce IL-6 and IL-8 (Dongari-Bagtzoglou & Ebersole 1996). The role of *C. rectus* has been somewhat difficult to determine because of the presence in plaque samples of a number of very closely related organisms such as *Campylobacter showae* and *Wolinella* X (Etoh et al. 1993).

Eikenella corrodens

E. corrodens is a Gram-negative, capnophilic, asaccharolytic, regular, small rod with blunt ends. It has been recognized as a pathogen in other forms of disease, particularly osteomyelitis (Johnson & Pankey 1976), infections of the central nervous system (Emmerson & Mills 1978, Brill et al. 1982) and root canal infections (Goodman 1977). This species was found more frequently in sites of periodontal destruction as compared with healthy sites (Savitt & Socransky 1984, Muller et al. 1997, Yuan et al. 2001). In addition, *E. corrodens* was found more frequently and in higher levels in active sites (Dzink et al. 1985, Tanner et al. 1987) and in sites of subjects who responded poorly to periodontal therapy (Haffajee et al. 1988b). Successfully treated sites harbored lower proportions of this species (Tanner et al. 1987). *E. corrodens* has also been found in association with *A. actinomycetemcomitans* in some lesions of LJP (Mandell 1984, Mandell et al. 1987). In tissue culture systems, *E. corrodens* has been shown to stimulate the production of matrix metalloproteinases (Dahan et al. 2001) and IL-6 and IL-8 (Yumoto et al. 1999). While there is some association of this species with periodontal disease, to date it has not been particularly strong (Chen et al. 1989).

Peptostreptococcus micros

P. micros is a Gram-positive, anaerobic, small, asaccharolytic coccus. It has long been associated with mixed anaerobic infections in the oral cavity and other parts of the body (Finegold 1977). Two genotypes can be distinguished with the smooth genotype being more frequently associated with periodontitis lesions than the rough genotype (Kremer et al. 2000). *P. micros* has been detected more frequently and in higher numbers at sites of periodontal destruction as compared with gingivitis or healthy sites (Moore et al. 1983, 1985, Herrera et al. 2000, Papapanou et al. 2000, Riggio et al. 2001) and was elevated in actively breaking down sites (Dzink et al. 1988). The levels and frequency of detection of the species were decreased at successfully treated periodontal sites (Haffajee et al. 1988a). Studies of systemic antibody responses to suspected periodontal pathogens indicated that subjects with severe generalized periodontitis had elevated antibody levels to this species when compared with healthy subjects or subjects with LJP (Tew et al. 1985a). In a mouse skin model system, it was shown that *P. micros* in combination with either *P. intermedia* or *P. nigrescens* could produce transmissible abscesses (van Dalen et al. 1998).

Selenomonas species

Selenomonas species have been observed in plaque samples using light microscopy for many decades. The organisms may be recognized by their curved shape, tumbling motility and, in good preparations, by the presence of a tuft of flagella inserted in the concave side. The *Selenomonas* spp. are Gram-negative, curved, saccharolytic rods. The organisms have been somewhat difficult to grow and speciate. However, Moore et al. (1987) described six genetically and phenotypically distinct groups isolated from the human oral cavity. *Selenomonas noxia* was found at a higher proportion of shallow sites (PD < 4 mm) in chronic periodontitis subjects compared with similar sites in periodontally healthy subjects (Haffajee et al. 1998). Further, *S. noxia* was found to be associated with sites that converted from periodontal health to disease (Tanner et al. 1998).

Eubacterium species

Certain *Eubacterium* species have been suggested as possible periodontal pathogens due to their increased levels in disease sites, particularly those of severe periodontitis (Moore et al. 1982, 1985, Uematsu & Hoshino 1992, Papapanou et al. 2000). *E. nodatum, Eubacterium brachy* and *Eubacterium timidum* are Gram-positive, strictly anaerobic, small, somewhat pleomorphic rods. They are often difficult to cultivate, particularly on primary isolation, and appear to grow better in roll tubes than on blood agar plates. Some of these species elicited elevated antibody responses in subjects with different forms of destructive periodontitis (Tew et al. 1985a,b, Vincent et al. 1986, Martin et al. 1988). The *Eubacterium* species appear to be promising candidates as periodontal pathogens; however, difficulty in their cultivation has slowed assessment of their contribution. It seems likely that the role of the *Eubacterium* species will be clarified when non-cultural methods are routinely employed for their detection, as discussed for *B. forsythus*.

The "milleri" streptococci

Streptococci were frequently implicated as possible etiologic agents of destructive periodontal diseases in the early part of the last century. Cultural studies of the last two decades have also suggested the possibility that some of the streptococcal species are associated with and may contribute to disease progression. At this time, evidence suggests that the "milleri" streptococci, *Streptococcus anginosus, S. constellatus* and *S. intermedius* might contribute to disease progression in subsets of periodontal patients. The species was found to be elevated at sites which demonstrated recent disease progression (Dzink et al. 1988). Walker and co-workers (1993) found *S. intermedius* to be elevated in a subset of patients with refractory disease at periodontal sites which exhibited disease progression. Colombo et al (1998) found that subjects exhibiting a poor response to SRP and then to periodontal surgery with systemically administered tetracycline had higher levels and proportions of *S. constellatus,* than subjects who responded well to periodontal therapy. The data on streptococci are somewhat limited, but a continued examination of their role in disease seems warranted.

Other species

Obviously all periodontal pathogens have not yet been identified. Interest has grown in groups of species not commonly found in the subgingival plaque as initiators or possibly contributors to the pathogenesis of periodontal disease, particularly in individuals who have responded poorly to periodontal therapy. Species not commonly thought to be present in subgingival plaque can be found in a proportion of such subjects or even in subjects who have not received periodontal treatment. Emphasis has been placed on enteric organisms, staphylococcal species as well as other unusual mouth inhabitants. Slots et al. (1990b) examined plaque samples from over 3000 chronic periodontitis patients and found that 14% of these patients harbored enteric rods and pseudomonads. *Enterobacter cloaceae, K. pneumoniae, Pseudomonas aeruginosa, Klebsiella oxytoca* and *Enterobacter agglomerans* comprised more than 50% of the strains isolated. This group of investigators also examined 24 subjects with periodontal disease in the Dominican Republic and found that the prevalence of enteric rods in these subjects was higher than levels found in subjects in the US (Slots et al. 1991). In the 16 of 24 subjects in which this group of organisms was detected, they averaged 23% of the cultivable microbiota. Rams et al. (1990, 1992) identified a number of species of staphylococci and enterococci in subjects with various forms of periodontal disease. The presence of unusual species in periodontal lesions suggests the possibility that they may play a role in the etiology of periodontal diseases. However, such roles must be evaluated in the same manner as the species discussed earlier in this section. It is worth noting that systemically administered ciprofloxacin improved the treatment response of patients whose periodontal pockets were heavily infected with enteric rods (Slots et al. 1990a).

More recently, viruses including cytomegalo, Epstein Barr, papilloma and herpes simplex have been proposed to play a role in the etiology of periodontal diseases, possibly by changing the host response to the local subgingival microbiota (Contreras & Slots 1996, 2000, Parra & Slots 1996, Contreras et al. 1997, 1999a,b, Velazco et al. 1999, Hanookai et al. 2000, Ting et al. 2000). Human cytomegalo, Epstein Barr and herpes simplex virus were found more frequently in deteriorating periodontal sites than in control, stable periodontitis sites in the same subject (Kamma et al. 2001).

Mixed infections

To this point, attention has been paid to the possible role of individual species as risk factors for destructive periodontal diseases. However, microbial complexes colonizing the subgingival area can provide a spectrum of relationships with the host, ranging from beneficial – the organisms prevent disease, to harmful – the organisms cause disease. At the pathogenic end of the spectrum, it is conceivable that different relationships exist between pathogens. The presence of two pathogens at a site could have no effect or diminish the potential pathogenicity of one or other of the species. Alternatively, pathogenicity could be enhanced either in an additive or synergistic fashion. It seems likely that mixed infections occur in subgingival sites since so many diverse species inhabit this habitat. Evidence to support this concept has been derived mainly from studies in animals in which it was shown that combinations of species were capable of inducing experimental abscesses, even though the components of the mixtures could not (Smith 1930, Proske & Sayers 1934, Cobe 1948, Rosebury et al. 1950, Macdonald et al. 1956, Socransky & Gibbons 1965). It is not clear whether the combinations suggested in the experimental abscess studies are pertinent to human periodontal diseases. The relationship of microbial complexes to periodontal diseases will be discussed in detail below.

THE NATURE OF DENTAL PLAQUE – THE BIOFILM WAY OF LIFE

Biofilms colonize a widely diverse set of moist surfaces including the oral cavity, the bottom of boats and docks, and the inside of pipes, as well as rocks in streams. Infectious disease investigators are interested in biofilms that colonize a wide array of artificial devices that have been implanted in the human including catheters, hip and voice prostheses and contact lenses. Biofilms consist of one or more communities of microorganisms, embedded in a glycocalyx, that are attached to a solid surface. The reason for the existence of a biofilm is that it allows microorganisms to stick to and to multiply on surfaces. Thus, attached bacteria (sessile) growing in a biofilm display a wide range of characteristics which provide a number of advantages over single cell (planktonic) bacteria. References to pertinent biofilm literature may be found in Socransky & Haffajee (2001) and Newman & Wilson (1999).

The nature of biofilms

Biofilms are fascinating structures. They are the preferred method of growth for many, perhaps most, species of bacteria. This method of growth provides a number of advantages to colonizing species. A major advantage is the protection that the biofilm provides to colonizing species from competing microorganisms, from environmental factors such as host defense mechanisms, and from potentially toxic substances in the environment, such as lethal chemicals or antibiotics. Biofilms also can facilitate processing and uptake of nutrients, cross-feeding (one species providing nutrients for another), removal of potentially harmful metabolic products (often by utilization by other bacteria) as well as the development of an appropriate physico chemical environment (e.g. a properly reduced oxidation reduction potential).

A crude analogy to the development of a biofilm might be the development of a city. Successful human colonization of new environments requires several important factors including a stable nutrient supply, an environment conducive to proliferation and an environment with limited potential hazards. Cities (like biofilms) develop by an initial "attachment" of humans to a dwelling site followed by multiplication of the existing inhabitants and addition of new inhabitants. Cities and biofilms typically spread laterally and then in a vertical direction, often forming columnar habitation sites. Cities and biofilms offer to their inhabitants many benefits. These include shared resources and interrelated activities. Inhabitants of cities or biofilms are capable of "metabolic processes" and synthetic capabilities that could not be performed by individuals in an unattached (planktonic) or nomadic state. An important benefit provided by a city or biofilm is protection both from other potential colonizers of the same species, from exogenous species and from sudden harmful changes in the environment. Individuals in the "climax community" of a flourishing city/biofilm can facilitate joint activities and live in a far more stable environment than individuals who live in isolation. Cities, like biofilms, require a means to bring in nutrients and raw materials, and to remove waste products. In cities, these are usually roads, water or sewage pipes; in biofilms they may be water channels such as those described below. Cities have maximum practical sizes based on physical constraints and nutrient/waste limits; so do biofilms. Cities that are mildly perturbed, e.g. by a snow storm or a local fire, usually reform a climax community that is similar to that which was present in the first place; as do biofilms. However, major perturbations in the environment such as prolonged drought or a radioactive cloud can lay waste to a city. Major perturbations in the environment such as a toxic chemical can severely affect the composition or existence of a biofilm. Communication between individuals in a city is essential to allow inhabitants to interact optimally. This is usually performed by vocal, written or pictorial means. Communication between bacterial cells within a biofilm is also necessary for optimum community development and is performed by production of signaling molecules such as those found in "quorum sensing" or perhaps by the exchange of genetic information. The long-term survival of the human species as well as a species in a biofilm becomes more likely if that species (or the human) colonizes multiple sites. Thus, detachment of cells from biofilms and establishment in new sites is as important for survival of biofilm-dwellers as the migration of individuals and establishment of new cities is for human beings. Thus, we may regard mixed species biofilms as primitive precursors to the more complex organizations observed for eukaryotic species.

Properties of biofilms

Structure

Biofilms are composed of microcolonies of bacterial cells (15–20% by volume) that are non-randomly distributed in a shaped matrix or glycocalyx (75–80% volume). Earlier studies of thick biofilms (> 5 mm) that develop in sewage treatment plants indicated the presence of voids or water channels between the microcolonies that were present in these biofilms. The water channels permit the passage of nutrients and other agents throughout the biofilm, acting as a primitive "circulatory" system. Nutrients make contact with the sessile (attached) microcolonies by diffusion from the water channel to the microcolony rather than from the matrix. Microcolonies occur in different shapes in biofilms which are governed by shear forces due to the passage of fluid over the biofilm. At low shear force, the colonies are shaped liked towers or mushrooms, while at high shear force, the colonies are elongated and capable of rapid oscillation. Individual microcolonies can consist of a single species, but more frequently are composed of several different species.

Exopolysaccharides – the backbone of the biofilm

The bulk of the biofilm consists of the matrix or glycocalyx and is composed predominantly of water and aqueous solutes. The "dry" material is a mixture of exopolysaccharides, proteins, salts and cell material. Exopolysaccharides (EPS), which are produced by the bacteria in the biofilm, are the major components of the biofilm making up 50–95% of the dry weight. They play a major role in maintaining the integrity of the biofilm as well as preventing desiccation and attack by harmful agents. In addition, they may also bind essential nutrients such as cations to create a local nutritionally rich environment favoring specific microorganisms. The EPS matrix could also act as a buffer and assist in the retention of extracellular enzymes (and their substrates) enhancing substrate utili-

zation by bacterial cells. The EPS can be degraded and utilized by bacteria within the biofilm. One distinguishing feature of oral biofilms is that many of the microorganisms can both synthesize and degrade the EPS.

Physiological heterogeneity within biofilms

Cells of the same microbial species can exhibit extremely different physiologic states in a biofilm even though separated by as little as 10 microns. Typically, DNA indicating the presence of bacterial cells is detected throughout the biofilm, but protein synthesis, respiratory activity and RNA are detected primarily in the outer layers.

The use of micro-electrodes has shown that pH can vary quite remarkably over short distances within a biofilm. Two-photon excitation microscopy of in vitro plaque made up of 10 intra-oral species showed that, after a sucrose challenge, microcolonies with a pH < 3.0 could be detected adjacent to microcolonies with pH values > 5.0. The number of metal ions can differ sufficiently in different regions of a biofilm so that difference in ion concentration can produce measurable potential differences. Bacterial cells within biofilms can produce enzymes such as β lactamase against antibiotics or catalases, or superoxide dismutases against oxidizing ions released by phagocytes. These enzymes are released into the matrix producing an almost impregnable line of defense. Bacterial cells in biofilms can also produce elastases and cellulases which become concentrated in the local matrix and produce tissue damage. Measurement of oxygen and other gases has demonstrated that certain microcolonies are completely anaerobic even though composed of a single species and grown in ambient air. Carbon dioxide and methane can reach very high concentrations in specific microcolonies in industrial biofilms. Thus, studies to date indicate that sessile cells growing in mixed biofilms can exist in an almost infinite range of chemical and physical microhabitats within microbial communities.

Quorum sensing

Some of the functions of biofilms are dependent on the ability of the bacteria and microcolonies within the biofilm to communicate with one another. Quorum sensing in bacteria "involves the regulation of expression of specific genes through the accumulation of signaling compounds that mediate inter cellular communication" (Prosser 1999). Quorum sensing is dependent on cell density. With few cells, signaling compounds may be produced at low levels; however, auto induction leads to increased concentration as cell density increases. Once the signaling compounds reach a threshold level (quorum cell density), gene expression is activated. Quorum sensing may give biofilms their distinct properties. For example, expression of genes for antibiotic resistance at high cell densities may provide protection. Quorum sensing also has the potential to influence community structure by encouraging the growth of beneficial species (to the biofilm) and discouraging the growth of competitors. It is also possible that physiological properties of bacteria in the community may be altered through quorum sensing. Quorum-sensing signaling molecules produced by putative periodontal pathogens such as *P. gingivalis, P. intermedia* and *F. nucleatum* have been detected (Frias et al. 2001).

Signaling is not the only way of transferring information in biofilms. The high density of bacterial cells growing in biofilms facilitates exchange of genetic information between cells of the same species and across species or even genera. Conjugation, transformation, plasmid transfer and transposon transfer have all been shown to occur in naturally occurring or *in vitro* prepared mixed species biofilms. Of particular interest was the demonstration of transfer of a conjugative transposon conferring tetracycline resistance from cells of one genus, *Bacillus subtilis*, to a *Streptococcus* species present in dental plaque grown as a biofilm in a constant depth film fermenter.

Attachment of bacteria

The key characteristic of a biofilm is that the microcolonies within the biofilm attach to a solid surface. Thus, adhesion to a surface is the essential first step in the development of a biofilm. In the mouth, there are a wide variety of surfaces to which bacteria can attach including the oral soft tissues, the pellicle-coated teeth and other bacteria. Many bacterial species possess surface structures such as fimbriae and fibrils that aid in their attachment to different surfaces. Fimbriae have been detected on a number of oral species including *Actinomyces naeslundii, P. gingivalis*, and some strains of streptococci such as *Streptococcus salivarius, Streptococcus parasanguis* and members of the *Streptococcus mitis* group. Fibrils can also be found on a number of oral bacterial species. They are morphologically different and shorter than fimbriae and may be densely or sparsely distributed on the cell surface. Oral species that possess fibrils include *S. salivarius, S. mitis* group, *P. intermedia, P. nigrescens* and *Streptococcus mutans*.

Mechanisms of increased antibiotic resistance of organisms in biofilms

As will be discussed elsewhere in this book, antibiotics have been and continue to be used effectively in the treatment of periodontal infections. However, the indiscriminate use of antimicrobials and biocides has the potential of leading to the development of resistant bacteria. It has also been suggested that resistance from one type of antimicrobial such as a biocide can be transferred to a different type of antimicrobial such as an antibiotic. Thus, it is important to understand the factors leading to antimicrobial resistance in biofilms such as dental plaque.

It has been recognized for considerable periods of time that organisms growing in biofilms are more resistant to antibiotics than the same species growing in a planktonic (unattached) state. While the mechanisms of resistance to antibiotics of organisms growing in biofilms are not entirely clear, certain general principles have been described. Almost without exception, organisms grown in biofilms are more resistant to antibiotics than the same cells grown in a planktonic state. Estimates of 1000 to 1500 times greater resistance for biofilm-grown cells than planktonic grown cells have been suggested, although these estimates have been considered too high by some investigators. The mechanisms of increased resistance in biofilms differ from species to species, from antibiotic to antibiotic and for biofilms growing in different habitats. One important mechanism of resistance appears to be the slower rate of growth of bacterial species in biofilms, which makes them less susceptible to many but not all antibiotics. It has been shown in many studies that the resistance of bacteria to antibiotics, biocides or preservatives is affected by their nutritional status, growth rate, temperature, pH and prior exposure to subeffective concentrations of antimicrobials. Variations in any of these parameters can lead to a varied response to antibiotics within a biofilm. The matrix performs a "homeostatic function", such that cells deep in the biofilm experience different conditions such as hydrogen ion concentration or redox potentials than cells at the periphery of the biofilm or cells growing planktonically. Growth rates of these deeper cells will be decreased allowing them to survive better than faster growing cells at the periphery when exposed to antimicrobial agents. In addition, the slower growing bacteria often overexpress "non-specific defense mechanisms" including shock proteins and multidrug efflux pumps and demonstrate increased exopolymer synthesis.

The exopolymer matrix of a biofilm, although not a significant barrier in itself to the diffusion of antibiotics, does have certain properties that can retard diffusion. For example, strongly charged or chemically highly reactive agents can fail to reach the deeper zones of the biofilm because the biofilm acts as an ion-exchange resin removing such molecules from solution. In addition, extracellular enzymes such as β lactamases, formaldehyde lyase and formaldehyde dehydrogenase may become trapped and concentrated in the extracellular matrix, thus inactivating susceptible, typically positively charged, hydrophilic antibiotics. Some antibiotics such as the macrolides, which are positively charged but hydrophobic, are unaffected by this process. Thus, the ability of the matrix to act as a physical barrier is dependent on the type of antibiotic, the binding of the matrix to that agent and the levels of the agent employed. Since reaction between the agent and the matrix will reduce the levels of the agent, a biofilm with greater bulk will deplete the agent more readily. Further, hydrodynamics and the turnover rate of the microcolonies will also impact on antibiotic effectiveness.

Alteration of genotype and/or phenotype of the cells growing within a biofilm matrix is receiving

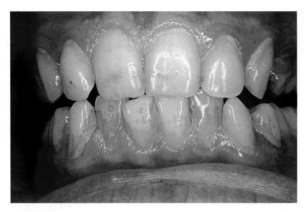

Fig. 4-6. Clinical photograph of a subject exhibiting tooth stain and supragingival dental plaque.

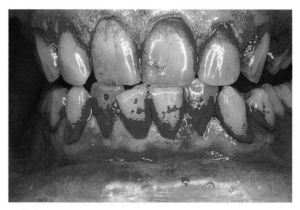

Fig. 4-7. Clinical photograph of the subject in Fig. 4-6 after staining with disclosing solution.

increased attention. Cells growing within a biofilm express genes that are not observed in the same cells grown in a planktonic state and they can retain this resistance for some time after being released from the biofilm. For example, it was demonstrated that cells of *P. aeruginosa* liberated from biofilms were considerably more resistant to tobramycin than planktonic cells, suggesting that the cells became intrinsically more resistant when growing in a biofilm and retained some of this resistance even outside the biofilm.

The presence of a glycocalyx, a slower growth rate and development of a biofilm phenotype cannot provide a total explanation for the phenomenon of antibiotic resistance. These features probably delay elimination of the target bacteria, allowing other selection events to take place. Recently, the notion of a subpopulation of cells within a biofilm, that are "super-resistant", was proposed. Such cells could explain remarkably elevated levels of resistance to certain antibiotics that have been suggested in the literature.

The oral biofilms that lead to periodontal diseases

The section on biofilm biology presented above provides a background to help understand the ecology of the incredibly complex community of organisms that colonize the tooth surface and lead to periodontal diseases. Fig. 4-6 presents a clinical photograph of a subject with less than optimal home care. Evident in this photograph is stain on the tooth surfaces that may have resulted from smoking, coffee or tea drinking. Of greater concern is the occurrence of a thin film of bacterial plaque on many of the tooth surfaces, along with the quite obvious plaque formation in regions such as the mesial buccal surfaces of the upper left and lower right canines. These biofilm (plaque) regions are highlighted in Fig. 4-7, which shows the same dentition after staining with a disclosing solution. The thin films such as those on the lower incisors might consist of biofilm communities that are 50 to 100 cells in thickness. Thicker plaques such as those on the upper left and lower right canines might consist of biofilms

that are 300 or more cell layers in thickness. The number of organisms that reside on the mesial surface of the upper left or lower right canine probably exceeds 300 million. This number is remarkable in that it exceeds the entire population of the US. These microbial communities are very complex. About 500 bacterial taxa have been detected in subgingival samples from the oral cavity (Paster et al. 2001). In any given plaque sample, it is not uncommon to detect 30 or more bacterial species. Thus, the biofilms that colonize the tooth surface may be among the most complex biofilms that exist in nature. This complexity is due in large part to the non-shedding surface of the tooth, which permits persistent colonization and the opportunity for very complex ecosystems to develop. In addition, the relatively high nutrient abundance as well as the remarkable ability of oral species to coaggregate with one another, as discussed earlier, may facilitate this complexity.

Fig. 4-8 is a section of human supragingival dental plaque grown on an epon crown in a human volunteer (Listgarten et al. 1975, Listgarten 1976, 1999). The section demonstrates many of the features of biofilms outlined earlier. Bacterial species adhered to the solid surface, multiplied and, in this section, formed columnar microcolonies. The heterogeneity of colonizing species is evident even at a morphological level and would be emphasized if the cells within the section had been characterized by cultural or molecular techniques. The surface of the biofilm exhibits morphotypes that are not evident in deeper layers and emphasizes the role that coaggregation plays in the development of biofilms. Not evident in this section are the water channels in biofilms described earlier. This might be due to preparation or fixation artifacts (Costerton et al. 1999) or it might be because the plaque is typical of a "dense" bacterial model. Water channels have been observed in plaque grown in the human oral cavity by confocal microscopy (Wood et al. 2000). This dental biofilm has all of the properties of biofilms in other habitats in nature. It has a solid substratum, in this case an epon crown but more typically a tooth, it has the mixed microcolonies growing in a glycoca-

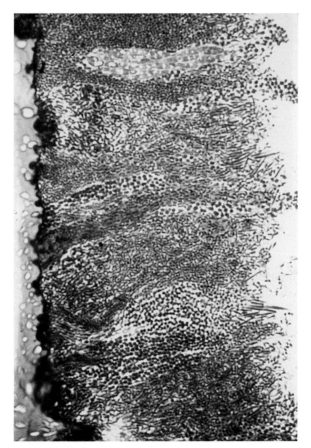

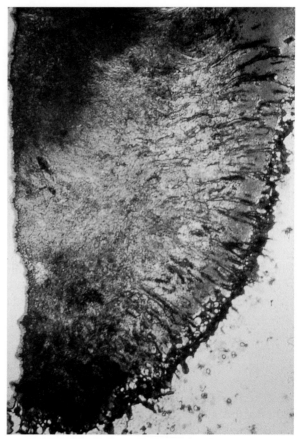

Fig. 4-8. Histological section of human supragingival plaque stained with toluidine blue-methylene blue. The supragingival plaque was allowed to develop for 3 days on an epon crown in a human volunteer. The crown surface is at the left and the saliva interface is towards the right. (Courtesy of Dr. Max Listgarten, University of Pennsylvania.)

Fig. 4-9. Histological section of human subgingival dental plaque stained with toluidine blue-methylene blue. The tooth surface is to the left and the epithelial lining of the periodontal pocket is to the right. Bacterial plaque attached to the tooth surface is evident towards the upper left of the section, while a second zone of organisms can be observed lining the periodontal pocket wall. (Courtesy of Dr Max Listgarten, University of Pennsylvania.)

lyx and it has the bulk fluid interface provided by saliva.

A second biofilm ecosystem is shown in Fig 4-9. This is a section of human subgingival plaque. The section is at lower magnification than Fig. 4-8 to permit visualization of regions within the biofilm. The plaque attached to the tooth surface is evident in the upper left portion of the section. This tooth-associated biofilm is an extension of the biofilm found above the gingival margin and may be quite similar in microbial composition. A second, possibly epithelial cell-associated biofilm, may be observed lining the epithelial surface of the pocket. This biofilm contains primarily spirochetes and Gram-negative bacterial species (Listgarten et al. 1975, Listgarten 1976, 1999). *P. gingivalis* and *T. denticola* have been detected in large numbers in periodontal pocket, epithelial cell-associated biofilms by immunocytochemistry (Kigure et al. 1995). *B. forsythus* might also be numerous in this zone, since high levels of this species have been detected, using DNA probes, in association with the epithelial cells lining the periodontal pocket (Dibart et al. 1998). Between the tooth-associated and epithelial cell-asso-

ciated biofilms, a less dense zone of organisms may be observed. These organisms may be "loosely attached" or they might be in a planktonic state. The critical feature of Fig. 4-9 is that there appears to be tooth-associated and epithelial cell-associated regions in subgingival plaque as well as a possible third weakly or unattached zone of microorganisms. It is strongly suspected that these regions differ markedly in microbial composition, physiological state and their response to different therapies.

Microbial complexes

The association of bacteria within mixed biofilms is not random, rather there are specific associations among bacterial species. Socransky et al. (1998) examined over 13 000 subgingival plaque samples from 185 adult subjects and used cluster analysis and community ordination techniques to demonstrate the presence of specific microbial groups within dental plaque (Fig. 4-10). Six closely associated groups of bacterial species were recognized. These included the *Acti-*

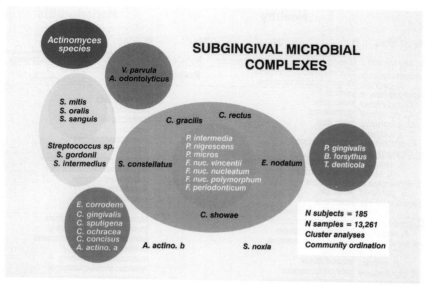

Fig. 4-10. Diagram of the association among subgingival species (adapted from Socransky et al. 1998). The data were derived from 13 321 subgingival plaque samples taken from the mesial aspect of each tooth in 185 adult subjects. Each sample was individually analyzed for the presence of 40 subgingival species using checkerboard DNA–DNA hybridization. Associations were sought among species using cluster analysis and community ordination techniques. The complexes to the left are comprised of species thought to colonize the tooth surface and proliferate at an early stage. The orange complex becomes numerically more dominant later and is thought to bridge the early colonizers and the red complex species which become numerically more dominant at late stages in plaque development.

nomyces, a yellow complex consisting of members of the genus *Streptococcus*, a green complex consisting of *Capnocytophaga* species, *A. actinomycetemcomitans* serotype a, *E. corrodens* and *Campylobacter concisus* and a purple complex consisting of *V. parvula* and *Actinomyces odontolyticus*. These groups of species are early colonizers of the tooth surface whose growth usually precedes the multiplication of the predominantly Gram-negative orange and red complexes (Fig. 4-10). The orange complex consists of *Campylobacter gracilis*, *C. rectus*, *C. showae*, *E. nodatum*, *F. nucleatum* subspecies, *F. periodonticum*, *P. micros*, *P. intermedia*, *P. nigrescens* and *S. constellatus*, while the red complex consists of *B. forsythus*, *P. gingivalis* and *T. denticola*. These two complexes are comprised of the species thought to be the major etiologic agents of periodontal diseases.

Similar relationships have been demonstrated in *in vitro* studies examining interactions between different oral bacterial species (Kolenbrander et al. 1999). These studies of oral bacteria have indicated that cell to cell recognition is not random but that each strain has a defined set of partners. Further, functionally similar adhesins found on bacteria of different genera may recognize the same receptors on other bacterial cells. Most human oral bacteria adhere to other oral bacteria. This cell to cell adherence is known as coaggregation.

Factors that affect the composition of subgingival biofilms

Although this chapter emphasizes the effect that microorganisms have on their habitat, periodontal tissues, it is important to understand that the habitat has a major effect on the composition, metabolic activities and virulence properties of the colonizing microorganisms. The importance of this axiom that the microorganisms affect the habitat and the habitat affects the microorganisms has recently begun to be fully appreciated. Thus, modifications of the supra and subgingival microbiota certainly affect the outcome, periodontal health or disease; but changes in the host or local habitat also affect the composition and activities of the microbiota. Understanding this relationship should help to lead us into better approaches to diagnosing the etiology and contributing factors of a patient's disease and to optimizing appropriate therapy. In this section we will provide examples of some of the factors that are known to modify subgingival microbial composition.

Periodontal disease status

Perhaps the most influential factor on the composition of the subgingival microbiota is the periodontal disease status of the host. Fig. 4-11 presents the percentage of sites colonized and counts of 40 subgingival taxa in subjects with chronic periodontitis or periodontal health (Haffajee et al. 1998). Clearly, the major difference between health and disease was the increased prevalence and counts of the red complex

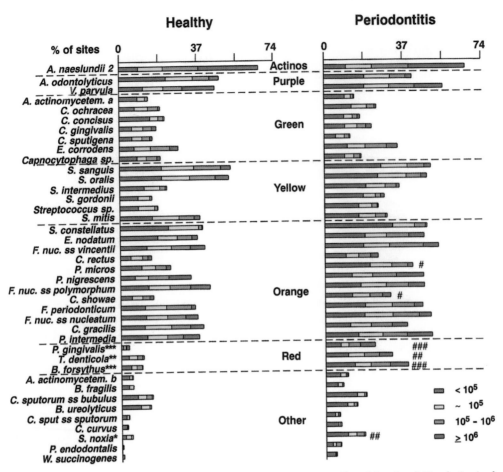

Fig. 4-11. Stacked bar charts of the mean prevalence (% of sites colonized) and levels of 40 subgingival species evaluated in 27 periodontally healthy and 115 untreated periodontitis subjects. The species were ordered according to the microbial complexes described by Socransky et al. (1998). The percentage of sites colonized at different levels by each of the 40 species examined was computed for each subject and then averaged across subjects in the two groups. Significance of differences in mean counts and prevalence between groups was evaluated using the Mann-Whitney test. For counts: * = p < 0.05, ** = p < 0.01 and *** = p < 0.001; for prevalence, # = p < 0.05, ## = p < 0.01 and ### = p < 0.001 after adjusting for multiple comparisons (Socransky et al. 1991).

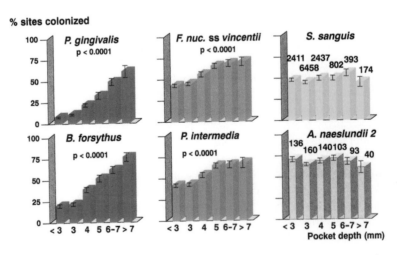

Fig. 4-12. Bar charts of the mean counts ($\times 10^5 \pm$ SEM) of six subgingival species at selected pocket depths. *B. forsythus* and *P. gingivalis* are representative of the red complex, *F. nucleatum* ss *vincentii* and *P. intermedia* are representative of the orange complex species, and *S. sanguis* and *A. naeslundii* genospecies 2 are typical of the remaining cluster groups. The mean counts of each species at each pocket depth category were computed for each subject and then averaged across subjects. Significance of differences among pocket depth categories was tested using the Kruskal-Wallis test.

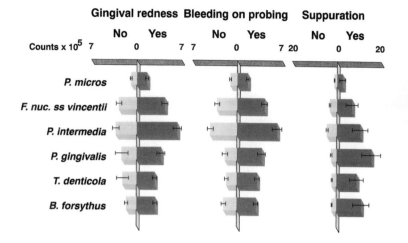

Fig. 4-13. Bar charts of the mean counts ($\times 10^5 \pm$ SEM) of six subgingival species at sites positive or negative for gingival redness, BOP and suppuration. *B. forsythus*, *P. gingivalis* and *T. denticola* are representative of the red complex, while *F. nucleatum* ss *vincentii*, *P. micros* and *P. intermedia* are representative of the orange complex species. The mean counts of each species at positive or negative sites for each parameter were computed for each subject and then averaged across subjects. The left bars (yellow) represent the sites negative for the clinical parameters and the right bars (red) represent the positive sites. These six species were significantly higher at positive sites for all three clinical parameters using the Wilcoxon signed ranks test.

species, *B. forsythus*, *P. gingivalis* and *T. denticola*, in subjects with periodontal disease. In addition, other putative periodontal pathogens including *P. micros* and *C. showae*, members of the orange complex, were also more prevalent in periodontitis subjects.

The local environment
One host factor that influences the subgingival environment is pocket depth. Fig. 4-12 indicates that the prevalence and levels of subgingival species may differ at sites of different pocket depths. Red complex species, *B. forsythus*, *P. gingivalis* and *T. denticola* (data not shown), increased strikingly in prevalence and numbers with increasing pocket depth. All orange complex species also demonstrated this relationship. *S. sanguis* and *A. naeslundii* genospecies 2 were typical of the majority of species in the other four complexes that showed little relationship to pocket depth. Thus, red and orange complex species are not only related to periodontal disease status in a subject, but to disease status at the periodontal site. The species of the red and orange complexes are also elevated at sites exhibiting gingival inflammation, as measured by gingival redness, bleeding on probing and suppuration (Fig. 4-13). Other species did not show this relationship.

Transmission
In planning control of periodontal pathogens, it is essential to clarify their source. If an individual were fortunate enough not to encounter virulent periodontal pathogens, he or she would exhibit minimal periodontal disease even if susceptible. However, most individuals have acquired strains of suspected periodontal pathogens at some time in their lives. For the most part, it appears that subgingival species found

in humans are unique to that environment. The subgingival species, by and large, are not commonly encountered in the environment (e.g. soil, air, water) or indeed in the subgingival microbiota of other animal species. (There are exceptions, such as the detection of the same strain of *A. actinomycetemcomitans* in a patient with LJP and in the family dog (Preus & Olsen 1988).) Thus, the typical pattern requires the transmission of periodontal pathogens from the oral cavity of one individual to the oral cavity of another. Two types of transmission are recognized: "vertical", that is transmission from parent to offspring, and "horizontal", i.e. passage of an organism between individuals outside the parent–offspring relationship.

Evidence for both forms of transmission has been provided using molecular epidemiology techniques. The usual approach of these techniques is to isolate DNA from strains of a given species recovered from different individuals. The DNA is cut with restriction endonucleases, run on agarose gel electrophoresis and the resulting fingerprint patterns compared, either directly or with the help of various DNA probes. When these techniques were employed on isolates from subgingival plaque, it was demonstrated that *A. actinomycetemcomitans* and *P. gingivalis* strains isolated from parents and children within the same family exhibited identical restriction endonuclease patterns. Different patterns were found for strains isolated from different families (DiRienzo & Slots 1990, Alaluusua et al. 1993, Petit et al. 1993a,b). In other studies it was found that *A. actinomycetemcomitans* and *P. gingivalis* strains isolated from husband and wife had the same restriction endonuclease patterns or ribotypes indicating that these species could be transmitted within married couples (Saarela et al. 1993, van Steenbergen et al. 1993).

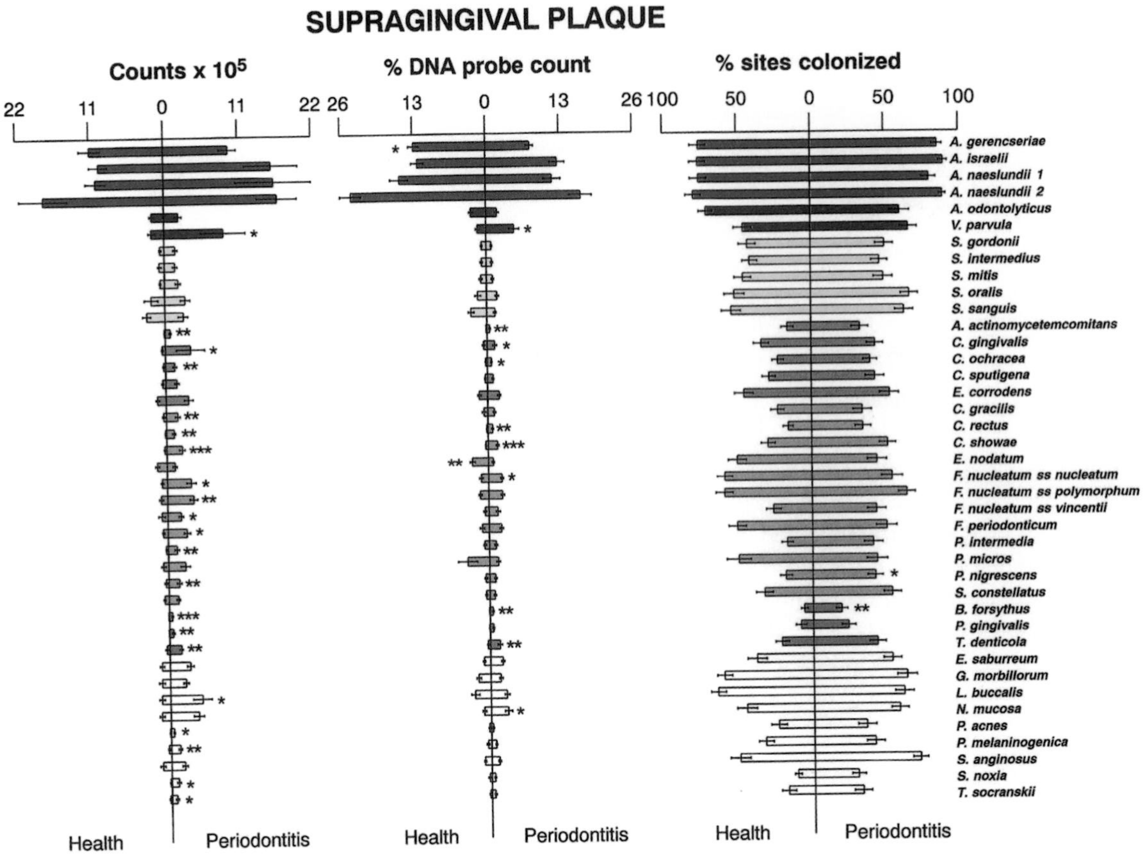

SUPRAGINGIVAL PLAQUE

Fig. 4-14. Bar charts of the counts ($\times 10^5$), proportions and percentage of sites colonized in supragingival plaque samples taken from 22 periodontally healthy and 23 subjects with adult periodontitis. The bars represent the mean values and the whiskers the SEM. Supragingival plaque samples were taken from the mesial surface of each tooth, excluding third molars and individually processed for their content of 40 bacterial species using checkerboard DNA–DNA hybridization. The left bars represent health and the right bars disease. The species are arranged within microbial complexes described by Socransky et al. (1998) and are color coded accordingly. Significance of difference between health and disease was determined using the Mann-Whitney test and adjusted for multiple comparisons (Socransky et al. 1991).

The above data should not be surprising in view of the fact that periodontal pathogens have to come from somewhere, and the most likely source would appear to be a family member, whether spouse, sibling or parent. However, while intra-family transmission has been demonstrated, it appears likely that transmission of pathogens also occurs between unrelated individuals. Earlier, the transmission of ANUG was described both within troops in trenches in World War I and in communities outside the war zone after World War I. If such reports are accurate, then it appears that periodontal pathogens can be transmitted rather readily, perhaps even on casual contact. Thus, while there has been an intuitive feeling that the oral microbiota is relatively stable within an individual, it seems likely that new species or different clonal types of the same species can be introduced into an individual at various stages of his or her life. For example, in the experiments outlined above, one spouse acquired *A. actinomycetemcomitans* or *P. gingivalis* from their spouse. This species might not have been present in the recipient and thus its introduction represented the acquisition of a new species. Alternatively, the new clonal type might have replaced or been added to a previously existing clonal type of the same species. In any of these events, the studies demonstrated that acquisition of new strains of pathogenic species can occur at both young and older ages. If the newly acquired strain is more virulent than the pre-existing strain of that species, then a change in disease pattern could occur.

The recognition that transmission of pathogens may occur relatively frequently in both younger and older individuals must influence our approach to therapy. If a species were established in young individuals only and were maintained throughout life, then treatment would involve "battling" that organism(s) and possibly repeated recurrences due to that organism over a lifetime. If pathogens are readily transmitted from person to person, at any age, then new infections may prove to be the rule and therapeutic approaches altered to reflect this situation. Molecular fingerprinting techniques should be invaluable in distinguishing recurrences from new infections and guiding approaches to therapy.

SUBGINGIVAL PLAQUE

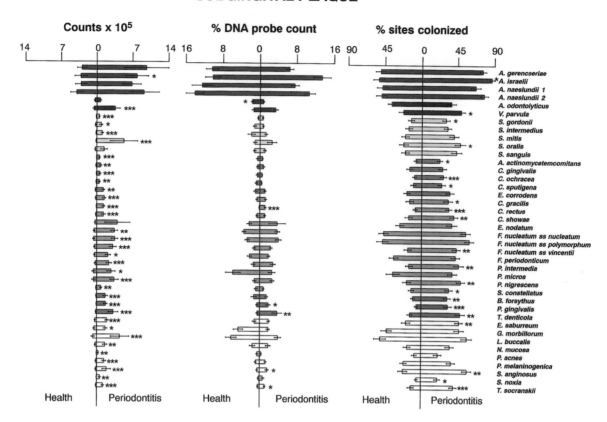

Fig. 4-15. Bar charts of the counts ($\times 10^5$), proportions and percentage of sites colonized in subgingival plaque samples taken from 22 periodontally healthy and 23 subjects with adult periodontitis. The format of the figure is as described for Fig. 4-14.

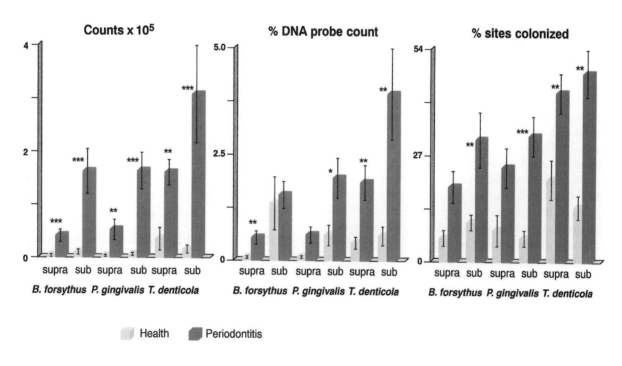

Fig. 4-16. Bar charts of the counts ($\times 10^5$), proportions and percentage of sites colonized by the red complex species, *B. forsythus*, *P. gingivalis* and *T. denticola* in supra and subgingival plaque samples taken from 22 periodontally healthy and 23 subjects with adult periodontitis. Significance of difference between health and disease was determined using the Mann-Whitney test and adjusted for multiple comparisons (Socransky et al. 1991).

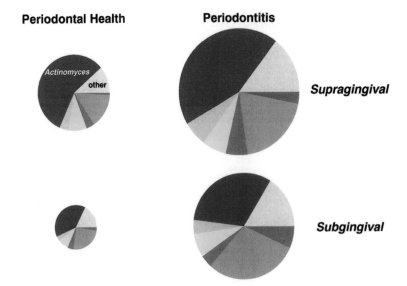

Fig. 4-17. Pie charts of the mean percentage DNA probe count of microbial groups in supra and subgingival plaque samples from 22 periodontally healthy and 23 periodontitis subjects. The species were grouped into seven microbial groups based on the description of Socransky et al. (1998). The areas of the pies were adjusted to reflect the mean total counts at each of the sample locations. The significance of differences in mean percentages of the supra and subgingival complexes in health and disease was tested using the Kruskal Wallis test. The "red", "orange" and *Actinomyces* species were significantly different at p < 0.001 and the "green" complex species differed at p < 0.05 after adjusting for seven comparisons. The "other" category represents probes to species that did not fall into a complex as well as probes to new species whose relationships with other species have not yet been ascertained.

Microbial composition of supra and subgingival biofilms

The bacteria associated with periodontal diseases reside within biofilms both above and below the gingival margin. The supragingival biofilm is attached to the tooth surface and is predominated by *Actinomyces* species in most plaque samples. Fig. 4-14 provides the counts, proportions and prevalence (% of sites colonized) of 40 taxa grouped according to microbial complexes (Socransky et al. 1998) in supragingival plaque samples from periodontally healthy and periodontitis subjects (Ximenez-Fyvie et al. 2000). The *Actinomyces* predominate in both health and disease irrespective of the method of enumeration. Further, all taxa examined could be found (on average) in both health and disease although counts and proportions of periodontal pathogens were significantly higher in the periodontally diseased subjects.

As described above, the nature of subgingival biofilms is more complex with both a tooth-associated and tissue-associated biofilm separated by loosely bound or planktonic cells. Fig. 4-15 presents the counts, proportions and prevalence of 40 taxa in subgingival plaque samples from periodontally diseased and periodontally healthy individuals (Ximenez-Fyvie et al. 2000). Similar to supragingival plaque, the dominant species subgingivally are the *Actinomyces*, but significantly higher counts, proportions and prevalence of red and orange complex species were found in the samples from the periodontitis subjects. Data for the red complex species are provided in Fig. 4-16, which highlights the increased levels, propor-

tions and prevalence of these species in both supra and subgingival plaque of periodontitis subjects when compared with similar samples from periodontally healthy individuals. Fig. 4-17 summarizes the major differences in microbial complexes between supra and subgingival plaque in health and periodontitis. As one moves from the supragingival to the subgingival environment and from health to disease, there is a significant decrease in the *Actinomyces* species and an increase in the proportion of members of the red complex (*B. forsythus, P. gingivalis* and *T. denticola*). Knowledge of the differences between health and disease should help the therapist to define microbial endpoints in the treatment of periodontal infections.

PREREQUISITES FOR PERIODONTAL DISEASE INITIATION AND PROGRESSION

It is a common feature of many infectious diseases that a pathogenic species may colonize a host and yet the host may not manifest clinical features of that disease for periods of time varying from weeks to decades or ever. Thus, it appears that periodontal disease progression is dependent on the simultaneous occurrence of a number of factors (Socransky & Haffajee 1992, 1993). The host must be susceptible both systemically and locally. The local environment has to contain bacterial species which enhance the infection or at very least do not inhibit the pathogen's activity. The environment also must be conducive to the expression of virulence factors by the pathogen. This might take the form of affecting the regulation of virulence factor expression or stressing the organism so that it manifests properties which lead to tissue damage. The pathogen(s) must achieve sufficient numbers to initiate or cause progression of the infection in that particular individual in the given local environment. Fortunately, the simultaneous occurrence of all these factors does not happen frequently or else periodontal disease would be more prevalent and severe in the population.

The virulent periodontal pathogen

Detection of suspected periodontal pathogens in plaque samples from periodontally healthy mouths (Dahlen et al. 1989, McNabb et al. 1992, Haffajee et al. 1998) or healthy sites in periodontally diseased mouths (Socransky et al. 1991) raises the question as to whether all strains of a pathogenic species are virulent. A major recognition of the last decade was that all clonal types of a pathogenic species are not equally virulent. For many medically important pathogenic species, a very small proportion of clonal types account for the majority of the disease that is observed (briefly reviewed in Socransky & Haffajee 1991, 1992). Studies of the pathogenic potential of different strains of *P. gingivalis* in animal model systems support the notion of strain differences in virulence (Grenier & Mayrand 1987a, van Steenbergen et al. 1987, Marsh et al. 1989, Neiders et al. 1989, Sundqvist et al. 1991, Baker et al. 2000). Certain clonal types of *P. gingivalis* were detected more frequently in samples from periodontitis subjects than control periodontally healthy subjects, suggesting an association of more virulent clonal types with disease (Griffen et al. 1999). These studies highlight the fact that there are major differences in virulence of different isolates of *P. gingivalis* and suggest that in some instances when suspected pathogens are found in periodontally healthy sites, the strains may be avirulent. *P. gingivalis fimA* gene encoding fimbrillin, a subunit of fimbriae, has been classified into five genotypes (Types I-V) based on their nucleotide sequences. Amano et al. (2000) examined the *P. gingivalis fimA* genotypes in dental plaque samples from 380 periodontally healthy adults and 139 periodontitis patients. Type I and Type V genotypes were most common in *P. gingivalis*-positive healthy adults, while Type II and Type IV were far more common in subjects with periodontitis. Such data suggest that *fimA* genotype may be an important factor influencing the pathogenicity of *P. gingivalis*.

Another requirement for a pathogen to express virulence is that the organism possesses all of the necessary genetic elements. Some of these elements might be missing in a strain inhabiting the gingival crevice area, but could be received from other strains of that species (or possibly other species) via phage, plasmids or transposons. Thus, periodontally healthy sites might be colonized with periodontal pathogens without a full complement of genes needed to lead to tissue destruction.

Finally, the pathogen must be in the right location in a site (e.g. at the apical area of the pocket or adjacent to the epithelium) in sufficient numbers to initiate disease. There are probably minimum numbers of a pathogen needed to initiate disease.

The local environment

If periodontal disease progression is a comparatively infrequent phenomenon, most of the resident species are likely to be host-compatible and in some instances may be actively beneficial to the host. Thus, microbial interactions play a role in the nature of species that colonize a site and ultimately on the outcome of health or disease. Some interactions might be harmful, leading to mixed infections as discussed earlier. Others might be more beneficial to the host. Host-compatible species could colonize sites that otherwise would be colonized by pathogens. They might "dilute" the number of pathogens in a pocket, compete for or alter binding sites for pathogens or destroy virulence factors produced by pathogens (Socransky & Haffajee 1991).

One carefully studied interbacterial antagonism has implications for our understanding of the ecology of destructive periodontal diseases. Hillman and co-workers (1982, 1985, 1987) became interested in the long-term stability of LJP lesions after treatment with surgery and systemic tetracycline. They surmised that a microbiota was established after treatment that was antagonistic to the return of the presumed pathogen *A. actinomycetemcomitans*. Such proved to be the case. It was shown that certain species such as *S. sanguis*, *Streptococcus uberis* and *A. naeslundii* genospecies 2 produced factors that were inhibitory to the growth of *A. actinomycetemcomitans* (Hillman et al. 1985). These species were absent or in low numbers in lesion sites of LJP prior to therapy but in elevated numbers after therapy. The mechanism of inhibition was shown to be hydrogen peroxide formation by the "beneficial" species (Hillman & Socransky 1987), which either directly, or via a host peroxidase system (Tenovuo & Pruitt 1984), inhibited the pathogen. Stevens et al. (1987) and Hammond et al. (1987) demonstrated the reverse antagonism. *A. actinomycetemcomitans* was shown to specifically inhibit the growth of *S. sanguis*, *S. uberis* and *A. naeslundii* genospecies 2 (but not other species) by the production of a bacteriocin. This mutual antagonism is highly specific and its outcome may strongly influence whether a subject or a site will exhibit disease due to *A. actinomycetemcomitans*. Such interactions demonstrate the potent role that resident microbial species play in permitting or preventing the establishment or spread of pathogenic species. The tremendous controlling pressure of the resident microbiota is reinforced when an investigator attempts to implant a human oral isolate into the microbiota of a conventional animal or purposely attempts to implant strains isolated from one human into the subgingival plaque of another.

The local subgingival environment can affect disease pathogenesis in other ways. One of the more intriguing ways centers around the recognition that virulent strains of pathogenic species do not always express their virulence factors (Socransky & Haffajee 1991). Often, a global "regulon" simultaneously turns on or off the production of multiple virulence factors. The "regulon" is affected by specific factors in the local environment such as temperature, osmotic pressure, or the concentration of iron, magnesium or calcium. The effect of environment on protein expression has been shown in subgingival species. For example, the level of iron in the environment will affect the expression of outer membrane proteins of *P. gingivalis* and will also affect virulence of the strain in animal model systems (McKee et al. 1986, Barua et al. 1990, Bramanti & Holt 1990). Even the presence of specific other species might lead to expression of virulence genes by pathogenic species. For example, the production of a surface protein by *Streptococcus cristatus* caused repression of the *P. gingivalis fim*A gene, possibly influencing the development a pathogenic plaque (Xie et al. 2000). The effect of environment on virulence factor expression seems a fertile area for investigation. It may help to explain the long lag phase that occurs prior to disease initiation. Conceivably, a pathogen may reside quietly in an area for years as a compatible member of the microbiota. However, some stress generated by a change in the environment might influence that organism to express long-hidden, rather damaging factors.

Host susceptibility

For a period of time considerably longer than the search for microbial etiologic agents of periodontal diseases, dental practitioners have hypothesized that differences in disease pattern or severity may be due to differences in host susceptibility (in earlier years termed resistance). In spite of these hypotheses, it is remarkable how few "host susceptibly factors" have been identified. With increased research in this area and better methods for comparing populations, a number of host or environmental factors have been suggested that impact on the initiation and rate of progression of periodontal diseases. Such factors include defects in polymorphonuclear leukocyte levels or function, a poorly regulated immunological response, smoking, diet and various systemic diseases (Genco et al. 1986, Bergstrom & Eliasson 1987, Greenspan et al. 1989, Williams et al. 1990, de Pommereau et al. 1992, Greenspan & Greenspan 1993, Seppala et al. 1993, Thorstensson & Hugoson 1993).

HIV infection

Debilitating systemic illness can alter the host's ability to cope with infections and may exacerbate existing infections. In early studies, it appeared that periodontal diseases were more prevalent and severe in HIV positive individuals than patients who were not infected with HIV (Greenspan et al. 1989, Williams et al. 1990, Greenspan & Greenspan 1993). In some HIV positive subjects, unusual necrotic, rapidly destructive periodontal lesions were observed. These observations led to speculation that either unusual pathogenic species were involved or that the modification of host resistance was so severe that it led to extreme tissue destruction. Examination of plaque samples taken from periodontitis sites in HIV positive individuals indicated that the subgingival microbiota was very similar to that seen in non-HIV infected periodontitis subjects, except that occasionally unusual organisms were encountered (Murray et al. 1989, 1991, Zambon et al. 1990, Rams et al. 1991, Moore et al. 1993). Further, suspected periodontal pathogens including *P. gingivalis, P. intermedia, F. nucleatum* and *A. actinomycetemcomitans* were found more frequently in periodontitis sites in HIV infected subjects than in either gingivitis and in particular healthy sites in these subjects (Murray et al. 1989). Rams et al. (1991) in a study of 14 HIV infected individuals with periodontitis found that *A. actinomycetemcomitans, C. rectus, P. micros* and *P. intermedia* each averaged 7–16% of the cultivable microbiota in patients positive for the species. In addition, levels of spirochetes were high, while levels of *Candida albicans* and Gram-negative enteric rods were low. Thus, the microbiota of lesions in HIV positive individuals was quite similar to that in HIV negative subjects. However, not all HIV positive subjects exhibit periodontal disease, and certainly not the extremely rapid form of disease. In addition, patients with the mild or rapid forms of disease are successfully treated using conventional periodontal therapies including local debridement, antiseptic mouthwashes and local and/or systemically administered antimicrobial agents (Williams et al. 1990, Winkler & Robertson 1992, Greenspan & Greenspan 1993).

Diabetes

Another systemic illness which has been associated with increased prevalence and incidence of periodontal disease is diabetes. Many studies (de Pommereau et al. 1992, Seppala et al. 1993, Thorstensson & Hugoson 1993), but not all (Barnett et al. 1984, Rylander et al. 1987) indicated that periodontitis is more severe in juvenile or adult diabetic subjects than non-diabetic controls. Microbiological studies of diabetic subjects have indicated that similar periodontal pathogens were found in diseased sites of diabetic subjects as in non-diabetic periodontal patients. *A. actinomycetemcomitans, Capnocytophaga* sp. and "anaerobic vibrios" were found to be elevated in subgingival plaque samples from juvenile diabetic subjects (Mashimo et al. 1983), while Sastrowijoto et al. (1989) found that *A.*

actinomycetemcomitans, P. gingivalis and *P. intermedia* were elevated in diseased sites of adult diabetic subjects. Mandell et al. (1992) found that a number of suspected periodontal pathogens were elevated at disease sites in poorly controlled insulin-dependent diabetics including *P. intermedia, P. melaninogenica, C. gracilis, E. corrodens, F. nucleatum* and *C. rectus,* when compared with healthy sites in the same subject. Similar species were found in adult periodontitis patients with non-insulin-dependent diabetes. *P. intermedia* was the most frequently detected species, while *C. rectus* and *P. gingivalis* were also very common (Zambon et al. 1988).

The intriguing aspect of the studies of HIV positive and diabetic subjects, is that periodontal lesions, for the most part, appeared to be related to already suspected periodontal pathogens and not to some novel species. Studies such as these suggest that altered host susceptibility may change the rate of disease progression in affected individuals, but by and large the periodontal pathogens are likely to be the same as those found in uncompromised subjects.

Smoking

The deleterious effects of cigarette smoking on the periodontium have been reported in numerous studies (briefly reviewed in Haffajee & Socransky (2000)). It has been shown that cigarette smokers have more bone loss, attachment loss, deeper periodontal pockets and less gingival bleeding than non-smokers. As described in an earlier section, suspected or known periodontal pathogens were more prevalent, i.e. colonized a larger proportion of sites, in current smokers than in past or never smokers. On average, this increased extent of colonization was from 10–25%, i.e. 3 to 7 teeth (of 28) in each subject. The species that differed significantly between smokers and non-smokers were primarily species of the red and orange complexes. The increased extent of colonization appeared to occur primarily at shallow periodontal pockets (< 4 mm) rather than deeper pockets. The difference in prevalence of these species helps to explain the greater severity of periodontal destruction in smokers than in non-smokers, since more sites are at risk (colonized by potential pathogens) in subjects who smoke. The reason for this difference in colonization pattern is not clear. Cigarette smoke could directly affect the pathogens or their local habitats. Tobacco usage also could affect the host's ability to control the infection by diminishing the local and systemic immune response. Whatever the reason, the widespread colonization of potential pathogens even at clinically healthy sites is likely to lead to future tissue damage at these sites. Further, the greater extent of colonization by periodontal pathogens, could complicate periodontal therapy since elimination or control of species would be more difficult.

MECHANISMS OF PATHOGENICITY

Essential factors for colonization of a subgingival species

For a periodontal pathogen to cause disease, it is essential that the pathogen be able to (1) colonize the subgingival area and (2) produce factors that either directly damage the host tissue or lead to the host tissue damaging itself. To colonize subgingival sites, a species must be able to (1) attach to one or more of the available surfaces, (2) multiply, (3) compete successfully against other species desiring that habitat, and (4) defend itself from host defense mechanisms.

Adhesins

To establish in a periodontal site, a species must be able to attach to one or more surfaces including the tooth (or host-derived substances binding to the tooth), the sulcular or pocket epithelium or other bacterial species attached to these surfaces. Studies of bacterial adhesion have demonstrated specificity in the involved mechanisms. At the simplest level there are one or more specific receptors on the host cell or other surfaces to which specific "adhesin" molecule(s) on the bacterial surface may attach. It has been demonstrated that there is a multiplicity of receptors on tooth surfaces, epithelial or other mammalian cells and other bacteria. Some of the adhesins that have been identified on subgingival species include fimbriae (Cisar et al. 1984, Clark et al. 1986, Sandberg et al. 1986, 1988, Isogai et al. 1988) and cell associated proteins (Murray et al. 1986, 1988, Mangan et al. 1989, Weinberg & Holt 1990). Receptors on tissue surfaces include galactosyl residues (Cisar et al. 1984, Murray et al. 1988, Sandberg et al. 1988, Mangan et al. 1989), sialic acid residues (Murray et al. 1986), proline rich proteins or statherin (Clark et al. 1986) and Type I or IV collagens (Naito & Gibbons 1988, Winkler et al. 1988).

Coaggregation

While many species attach directly to host surfaces, other species attach to bacteria attached to such surfaces. This phenomenon is called coaggregation. It has been shown that there is specificity in the attachment of one species to another in *in vitro* systems and *in vivo* (Kolenbrander & Andersen 1989, Kolenbrander et al. 1989, Kaufman & DiRienzo 1989). In some instances, coaggregation between non-coaggregating species may be mediated by cellular constituents (e.g. vesicles) of a third species (Grenier & Mayrand 1987b, Ellen & Grove 1989). Further, the mechanism of attachment of cells of a given pair of species appears to be mediated by specific receptor–adhesin interactions. Many of these interactions are lectin-like in that they are based on the attachment of a specific protein on the surface of one species to a specific carbohydrate on the surface of the other (Kinder & Holt 1989, Kolenbrander & Andersen 1989, Kolenbrander et al. 1989, Abeygunawardana et al. 1990), but other mechanisms exist (Kolenbrander et al. 1989, Kolenbrander & Andersen 1990). For example, the *S. sanguism–A. naeslundii* genospecies 2 interaction was shown to be due to the attachment of a fimbrial-associated lectin on *A. naeslundii* genospecies 2 to a polysaccharide with a repeating heptasaccharide on *S. sanguis* (Abeygunawardana et al. 1990). In certain instances more than one type of adhesin–receptor interaction has been detected between a species pair. It is of interest that the same galactose-binding adhesin of *F. nucleatum* to *P. gingivalis* and *A. actinomycetemcomitans* also binds the cell to human epithelial cells and fibroblasts (Weiss et al. 2000).

Multiplication

The gingival crevice and/or periodontal pocket might be considered a lush area for microbial growth, but is in fact a rather stringent environment for a bacterial species to live. The mean temperature of the area averages about 35°C and ranges from 30°–38°C (Haffajee et al. 1992), eliminating whole classes of potential colonizing organisms such as thermophiles and psychrophiles. The pH is rather restricted (pH 7.0–8.5) (Forscher et al. 1954, Kleinberg & Hall 1969, Cimasoni 1983) and numerous microbial species find this range unacceptable. Oxidation reduction potential measurements vary from an Eh of about –300 to +310 mv at pH 7.0 (Onisi et al. 1960, Kenney & Ash 1969). The wide range of Eh provides suitable microenvironments for numerous bacterial species, although extremes of Eh in a local environment could be limiting to certain species.

The selective physical environment of the gingival crevice area is accompanied by limited nutritional availability. Three sources of nutrient are available to subgingival organisms (diet, host and other subgingival species). Certain nutrients essential to some bacterial species must be formed by other species in that area (e.g. vitamin K analogues) (Gibbons & Macdonald 1960). However, the precursors to such substances and certain specific growth factors such as hemin (Evans 1951, Gibbons & Macdonald 1960) must be derived from the host. Gingival crevice fluid is not particularly rich in nutrients, creating a major competition for the small amounts available. In addition, nutrients delivered in relative abundance to the outer layers of plaque may not reach deeper layers.

Interbacterial relationships

Bacterial interactions play important roles in species survival. Some inter-species relationships are favorable, in that one species provides growth factors for, or facilitates attachment of, another. Other relationships are antagonistic due to competition for nutrients and binding sites or to the production of substances which limit or prevent growth of a second species.

A number of types of inter-species interactions have been described. The inter-species agglutinations described above are an important means of bacterial attachment for some species. Bacterial attachment may also be influenced by the production of extracellular enzymes by one set of organisms which uncover binding sites fostering the attachment of a second set of organisms. For example *S. mitis* and *S. sanguis* bind in comparable levels to intact epithelial cells, as do strains of *P. gingivalis* and *P. intermedia*. However, if epithelial cells are exposed to bacterial neuraminidase the attachment of the streptococci is diminished, but attachment of the *P. gingivalis* and *P. intermedia* strains is enhanced (Gibbons 1989). It is suspected that removal of sialic acid reveals galactosyl residues that foster attachment of the suspected pathogens. This mechanism may account for the greater level of such species on cells from periodontal pockets than from healthy sulci (Dzink et al. 1989).

Other beneficial interactions are mediated by one species providing growth conditions favorable to another. Such conditions include altered physico-chemical parameters such as *Eh* (Socransky et al. 1964), *pH* (Kleinberg & Hall 1969), or *temperature* (Haffajee et al. 1992). One of the more important environmental parameters is the oxygen level. Subgingival species differ in their ability to grow in the presence or absence of oxygen. Obligate aerobes require oxygen for growth and cannot multiply in its absence. Obligately anaerobic species are killed by even low levels of oxygen, while facultative species can grow in either situation. Dental plaque provides a spectrum of environments with high levels of oxygen available on outer surfaces and adjacent to periodontal tissues, but low levels of oxygen and a low oxidation reduction potential within the plaque. The differences in microenvironments are due in part to location within the periodontal pocket and in part due to the intense reducing abilities of many subgingival species. The survival of some anaerobic species may be due to the presence of facultative or aerobic species that utilize oxygen and or detoxify its potentially cell damaging activated radicals such as the hydroxyl radicals. Subgingival species also provide specific growth factors utilized by other species including branched chain fatty acids and polyamines (Socransky et al. 1964), analogues of vitamin K (Gibbons & Macdonald 1960), lactate (Rogosa 1964), formate or hydrogen (Tanner & Socransky 1984).

Colonization of a pathogenic species in the presence of a species that produces substances antagonistic to its survival presents a different challenge to a pathogen. Antagonistic substances vary from those that affect binding (e.g. the enzymes that favored *P. intermedia* above probably adversely affected *S. mitis*) to those that kill the species. Factors that kill other species include bacteriocins (Rogers et al. 1979, Hammond et al. 1987, Stevens et al. 1987), H_2O_2 (Holmberg & Hallander 1973, Hillman et al. 1985) and organic acids (Mashimo et al. 1985). These factors may be considered as virulence factors since they suppress the growth of competing species or different clonal types of the same species (Hillman & Socransky 1989). Defense against such factors varies. The simplest way to avoid such factors is to find sites that are not colonized by antagonistic species. A second method is to produce factors that destroy the antagonistic species. For example, *S. sanguis* produces H_2O_2 which inhibits the growth of *A. actinomycetemcomitans* (Hillman et al. 1985), while *A. actinomycetemcomitans* produces a bacteriocin that inhibits *S. sanguis* (Hammond et al. 1987, Stevens et al. 1987). Thus, the bacteriocin that protects the suspected pathogen *A. actinomycetemcomitans* from the deleterious effect of the more commonly detected *S. sanguis* must be considered to be a virulence factor.

Overcoming host defense mechanisms

Subgingival plaque microorganisms appear to overgrow and lead to severe disease in immune-compromised hosts, particularly those with neutrophil disorders (Genco et al. 1986, Shenker 1987, Winkler et al. 1989). Such findings suggest that host defense mechanisms are important in limiting the numbers of bacteria in subgingival plaque and preventing tissue damage.

A bacterial species has a number of host-derived obstacles to overcome when colonizing a subgingival site. These include the flow of saliva and gingival crevice fluid and mechanical displacement by chewing and speaking. Substances in saliva and gingival crevice fluid may aid in the prevention of colonization by blocking the binding of bacterial cells to mammalian surfaces. Such factors include specific antibodies, salivary glycoproteins, mucins and proline rich proteins, which may act as non-specific blocking agents (Gibbons 1984).

Once a bacterial cell has successfully attached to a surface in the subgingival area, other host mechanisms come into play. Desquamation of epithelial cells presents a new cleansing mechanism, which is overcome by certain species by their ability to bind to underlying epithelial cells (Freter 1985). Other species are able to invade the epithelial cells (Finlay & Falkow 1989) and may multiply intracellularly and spread to adjacent cells.

Specific antibody in the subgingival area could act by preventing bacterial attachment or, in some instances, by making the bacterial cell susceptible to various phagocytic or killing mechanisms. A number of subgingival species have evolved mechanisms for evading the effect of specific antibody. Species including *P. gingivalis, P. intermedia, P. melaninogenica* and *Capnocytophaga* species possess IgG and IgA proteases that can destroy antibody (Kilian 1981, Saito et al. 1987, Grenier et al. 1989). Other species are capable of evading antibody by changing their surface antigens (Gibbons & Quereshi 1980) or possibly by mimicking the host's antigens (Ellen 1985).

Polymorphonuclear leukocytes affect subgingival species in at least two ways: by phagocytosing and ultimately killing bacterial cells or by releasing their lysosomal enzymes into the crevice or pocket. A number of bacterial mechanisms exist that might counteract these effects, including the production of leukotoxin by *A. actinomycetemcomitans* (Baehni et al. 1979) and capsules by *P. gingivalis* and other species that inhibit phagocytosis (Okuda & Takazoe 1988). In addition, a number of species have developed strategies to interfere with the killing mechanisms of the polymorphonuclear leukocytes (Boehringer et al. 1986, Seow et al. 1987, 1989, Sela et al. 1988, Yoneda et al. 1990).

If a species enters the underlying connective tissue, it has moved into the area where the host's defense mechanisms are the most formidable. Polymorphonuclear leukocytes and antibodies are joined by macrophages and various types of lymphocytes, completing an awesome array of antagonistic cells and their biologically active substances. To be successful in this area a species would have to have evolved sophisticated mechanisms to evade, hide from or destroy opposition. Some of the periodontal pathogens may have devised such mechanisms. For example, it has been shown that *A. actinomycetemcomitans* leukotoxin affects not only polymorphonuclear leukocytes and monocytes (Baehni et al. 1979) but also kills mature T and B lymphocyte cell lines (Simpson et al. 1988) or facilitates a non-lethal suppression of immune cells (Rabie et al. 1988). Other species such as *P. intermedia, Porphyromonas endodontalis* and *T. denticola* have been shown to produce substances that suppress immune mechanisms (Shenker et al. 1984, Ochiai et al. 1989, Shenker & Slots 1989).

Finally, artificial agents including antiseptics and antibiotics have been developed that augment the host's natural defense mechanisms against bacterial pathogens. In turn the microorganisms have evolved mechanisms of resistance to these agents and added insult to injury by having the ability to pass these resistance factors to one another even across species (Guiney & Bouic 1990).

Factors that result in tissue damage

The set of properties that result in a species causing periodontal tissue loss in destructive periodontal diseases is poorly understood. Some or all tissue damage may result from an immunopathologic reaction triggered by a species which is sustained until the species is eliminated or suppressed. However, the fact that disease progression is rare and is associated with specific species, and that inflammation without attachment loss is common, suggests specificity in the properties of organisms that lead to tissue damage. Two general mechanisms of pathogenesis have been hypothesized. The first involves invasion by subgingival species. The second suggests a "long-range" attack where cells of the pathogenic species remain in the pocket but fragments of cells as well as other "virulence factors" enter the underlying periodontal tissues and either directly damage the tissues or cause "immune pathology" (Allenspach-Petrzilka & Guggenheim 1982, Fillery & Pekovic 1982, Gillett & Johnson 1982, Sanavi et al. 1985, Saglie et al. 1986, 1988, Christersson et al. 1987, Liakoni et al. 1987, Listgarten 1988).

Invasion

The possibility of invasion in periodontal infections gained credence with the unequivocal demonstration of invasion by a spirochete with a unique ultrastructural morphology during active episodes of acute necrotizing ulcerative gingivitis (Listgarten & Socransky 1964, Listgarten 1965). Other instances of invasion have been reported in tissues obtained from advanced periodontitis (Frank & Voegel 1978), LJP (Gillett & Johnson 1982, Christersson et al. 1987) and progressing periodontal lesions (Saglie et al. 1988).

As discussed earlier, strains of *A. actinomycetemcomitans* and *P. gingivalis* have been shown to be capable of invading epithelial cells derived from human periodontal pockets or gingival sulci. Other studies demonstrated that *B. forsythus* was present in high numbers in preparations of human periodontal pocket epithelial cells, and cells of this species could be detected within the epithelial cells. The property of invasion of epithelial cells is a common property of a wide range of mucosal pathogens including members of the genera *Salmonella*, *Shigella*, *Yersinia*, *Escherichia* and *Listeria*. The mechanisms of attachment to and subsequent entry differ from species to species. However, the ability to enter into and survive within human cells confers an advantage to potential pathogens in that they are protected from many of the host's defense mechanisms.

Adherence to underlying tissues such as basement membrane and various types of collagen has been demonstrated (Winkler et al. 1987, 1988, Naito & Gibbons 1988). Strains of *F. nucleatum* and *P. gingivalis* adhere well to preparations of basement membrane and Type IV collagen. *P. gingivalis* also adheres well to Type I collagen, a property that may be useful in invasion of deeper tissues.

Deeper invasion may be important in progression of disease and could be facilitated by the property of motility. The flexible, sinuous spirochete has the physical tools to move through amorphous jelly-like intercellular matrix. If other virulence factors were present, it is likely that spirochetes and other motile forms such as *Selenomonas* and *Campylobacter* would have unique invasive capacities.

Factors that cause tissue damage

The microbial substances that lead to damage of the periodontal tissues are poorly understood, in large part because so many potential "virulence factors" have been described for subgingival species and their roles inadequately evaluated. Virulence factors can be arbitrarily divided into three categories: substances that damage tissue cells (e.g. H_2S), substances that cause cells to release biologically active substances (e.g. lipopolysaccharide) and substances that affect the intercellular matrix (e.g. collagenase). There is an unfortunate overlap in this categorization, since some substances elicit more than one response. Further, factors that affect the cells involved in host defense mechanisms may inhibit protective responses and/or lead to the production of substances that can directly damage the tissues.

Some of the suspected virulence factors produced by three periodontal pathogens are summarized in Tables 4-1 to 4-3. Enzymes produced by subgingival species appear to be able to degrade virtually all of the macromolecules found in periodontal tissues. The periodontal pathogen, *P. gingivalis*, produces an unusually wide array of proteases including those that degrade collagen (Gibbons & Macdonald 1961, Smalley et al. 1988, Winkler et al. 1988, Jin et al. 1989), immunoglobulins (Kilian 1981, Saito et al. 1987, Grenier et al. 1989) and fibronectin (Wikstrom & Linde 1986, Smalley et al. 1988, Lantz et al. 1990). Of particular interest are the cysteine proteinases commonly referred to as ARG-gingipain and LYS-gingipain, which are important to the organism in order to break down proteins to peptides and amino acids necessary for its growth (Kadowaki et al. 2000). These proteinases are also important in the processing/maturation of cell surface proteins of *P. gingivalis* such as *fim*A fimbrillin. Other species produce additional or other lytic enzymes. It might be argued that enzymes produced by bacterial species might not be necessary to the pathogenesis of periodontal diseases since similar enzymes can be derived from host tissue. However, if a specific lytic enzyme is essential to disease progression, current data suggest that some subgingival species would form it.

A wide variety of cell preparations or substances has been shown to adversely affect the growth and/or metabolism of mammalian cells in tissue culture. Some of the substances are low molecular weight end-products of metabolism such as H_2S, NH_3, fatty acids or indole (Socransky 1970, Singer & Buckner 1981, van Steenbergen et al. 1986). Other factors are less defined and constitute factors present in the extracellular milieu of bacterial cultures or extracts of the bacterial cells themselves. The importance of this group of inhibitory factors in the pathogenesis of disease is unclear. However, even minor inhibitions of cell metabolism might adversely affect structural integrity of the periodontal tissues.

It has been known for some time that certain bacterial products can induce organ cultures or tissue cells, including cells involved in host defense, to elaborate biologically active substances. One such factor derived from cultured white blood cells was initially described as osteoclast activating factor, since it accelerated bone resorption in tissue culture systems (Horton et al. 1972), but was later recognized as interleukin-1β (Dewhirst et al. 1985). Production of this factor was shown to be induced in a number of ways including stimulation by bacterial lipopolysaccharides or whole cells (Uchida et al. 2001). Numerous other biologically active mediators including prostaglandins, tumor necrosis factor, thymocyte activating factor, IL-8 (Uchida et al. 2001) and chemotactic factors have been shown to be formed in response to the addition of bacterial cells or their products to mammalian cells in tissue culture (Bom-van Noorloos et al. 1986, Millar et al. 1986, Garrison et al. 1988, Hanazawa et al. 1988, Lindemann 1988, Lindemann et al. 1988, Takada et al. 1988, Sismey-Durrant et al. 1989, Uitto et al. 1989). *P. gingivalis* can perturb the cytokine network not only by stimulating the release of cytokines from host cells, but by removing them from its local environment (Fletcher et al. 1997).

FINAL COMMENTS

Infections of any organ system are caused by a relatively finite set of pathogens sometimes working individually, occasionally in small mixtures. For example, lung infections may be caused by any of a variety of organisms including *M. tuberculosis, S. pneumoniae* and *K. pneumoniae*. No single therapy is effective against all lung infections. Each of these infections requires the use of a different chemotherapeutic agent and the selection of the agent is based on the findings of diagnostic tests. The analogy to periodontal infections is clear. There is no single cause to these infections, no one treatment can control the infections, and the choice of treatment should be guided by the nature of the infecting microbiota. Obviously a great deal of additional research is needed to define precisely the contribution of each periodontal pathogen to periodontal disease progression, to devise tests for their presence and to determine the best therapy for each pathogen's suppression. However, when the most appropriate anti-infective therapy is applied to a given subject or site, disease progression should, at minimal, be stopped and the potential for long-term periodontal stability markedly enhanced. The effects of different therapies on the composition of the subgingival microbiota will be discussed in Chapter 26.

REFERENCES

Abeygunawardana, C., Bush, C.A. & Cisar, J.O. (1990). Complete structure of the polysaccharide from *Streptococcus sanguis* J22. *Biochemistry* **29**, 234-248.

Alaluusua, S., Saarela, M., Jousimies-Somer, H. & Asikainen, S. (1993). Ribotyping shows intrafamilial similarity in *Actinobacillus actinomycetemcomitans* isolates. *Oral Microbiology and Immunology* **8**, 225-229.

Albandar, J.M., Brown, L.J. & Löe, H. (1997). Putative periodontal pathogens in subgingival plaque of young adults with and without early-onset periodontitis. *Journal of Periodontology* **68**, 973-981.

Allenspach-Petrzilka, G.E. & Guggenheim, B. (1982). *Bacteroides melaninogenicus* subsp. *intermedius* invades rat gingival tissue. *Journal of Dental Research* **61**, 259.

Altman, L.C., Page, R.C., Ebersole, J.L. & Vandesteen, E.G. (1982). Assessment of host defenses and serum antibodies to suspected periodontal pathogens in patients with various types of periodontitis. *Journal of Periodontal Research* **17**, 495-497.

Amano, A. Kuboniwa, M., Nakagawa, I., Akiyama, S., Morisaki, I. & Hamada, S. (2000). Prevalence of specific genotypes of *Porphyromonas gingivalis* fimA and periodontal health status. *Journal of Dental Research* **79**, 1664-1668.

Arakawa, S., Nakajima, T., Ishikura, H., Ichinose, S., Ishikawa, I. & Tsuchida, N. (2000). Novel apoptosis-inducing activity in *Bacteroides forsythus*: a comparative study with three serotypes of *Actinobacillus actinomycetemcomitans*. *Infection and Immunity* **68**, 4611-4615.

Asikainen, S., Lai, C.H., Alaluusua, S. & Slots, J. (1991). Distribution of *Actinobacillus actinomycetemcomitans* serotypes in periodontal health and disease. *Oral Microbiology and Immunology* **6**, 115-118.

Baehni, P., Tsai, C.C., McArthur, W.P., Hammond, B.F. & Taichman, N.S. (1979). Interaction of inflammatory cells and oral microorganisms. VIII. Detection of leukotoxic activity of a plaque-derived Gram-negative microorganism. *Infection and Immunity* **24**, 233-243.

Baker, P.J., Dixon, M., Evans, R.T. & Roopenian, D.C. (2000). Heterogeneity of *Porphyromonas gingivalis* strains in the induction of alveolar bone loss in mice. *Oral Microbiology and Immunology* **15**, 27-32.

Barnett, M.L., Baker, R.L., Yancey, J.M., MacMillan, D.R. & Kotoyan, M. (1984). Absence of periodontitis in a population of insulin-dependent diabetes mellitus (IDDM) patients. *Journal of Periodontology* **55**, 402-405.

Barua, P.K., Dyer, D.W. & Neiders, M.E. (1990). Effect of iron limitation on *Bacteroides gingivalis*. *Oral Microbiology and Immunology* **5**, 263-268.

Beck, J.D., Cusmano, L., Green-Helms, W., Koch, G.G. & Offenbacher, S. (1997). A 5-year study of attachment loss in community-dwelling older adults: incidence density. *Journal of Periodontal Research* **32**, 506-515.

Beck, J.D., Koch, G.G., Rozier, R.G. & Tudor G.E. (1990). Prevalence and risk indicators for periodontal attachment loss in a population of older community-dwelling blacks and whites. *Journal of Periodontology* **61**, 521-528.

Beck, J.D., Koch, G.G., Zambon, J.J., Genco, R.J. & Tudor, G.E. (1992). Evaluation of oral bacteria as risk indicators for periodontitis in older adults. *Journal of Periodontology* **63**, 93-99.

Beckwith, T.D., Simonton, F.V. & Williams, A. (1925). A histologic study of the gum in pyorrhea. *Journal of the American Dental Association* **12**, 129-153.

Belding, P.H. & Belding, L.J. (1936). Bacteria – dental orphans. *Dental Cosmos* **78**, 506-513.

Berglundh, T., Krok, L., Liljenberg, B., Westfelt, E., Serino, G. & Lindhe, J. (1998). The use of metronidazole and amoxicillin in the treatment of advanced periodontal disease. A prospective, controlled clinical trial. *Journal of Clinical Periodontology* **25**, 354-362.

Bergstrom J. & Eliasson S. (1987). Noxious effect of cigarette smoking on periodontal health. *Journal of Periodontal Research* **22**, 513-517.

Blix, I.J., Hars, R., Preus, H.R. & Helgeland, K. (1992). Entrance of *Actinobacillus actinomycetemcomitans* into HEp-2 cells in vitro. *Journal of Periodontology* **63**, 723-728.

Boehringer, H.R., Berthold, P.H. & Taichman, N.S. (1986). Studies on the interaction of human neutrophils with plaque spirochetes. *Journal of Periodontal Research* **21**, 195-209.

Bom-van Noorloos, A.A., Schipper, C.A., van Steenbergen, T.J.M., de Graaf, J, & Burger, E.H. (1986). *Bacteroides gingivalis* activates mouse spleen cells to produce a factor that stimulates resorptive activity of osteoclasts in vitro. *Journal of Periodontal Research* **21**, 440-444.

Bragd, L., Dahlen, G., Wikstrom, M. & Slots J. (1987). The capability of *Actinobacillus actinomycetemcomitans, Bacteroides gingivalis* and *Bacteroides intermedius* to indicate progressive periodontitis; a retrospective study. *Journal of Clinical Periodontology* **14**, 95-99.

Bramanti, T.E. & Holt, S.C. (1990). Iron-regulated outer membrane proteins in the periodontopathic bacterium, *Bacteroides gingivalis*. *Biochemistry & Biophysics Research Communications* **166**, 1146-1154.

Brill, C.B., Pearlstein, L.S., Kaplan, M. & Mancall, E.L. (1982). CNS infections caused by *Eikenella corrodens*. *Achives of Neurology* **39**, 431-432.

Bueno, L.C., Mayer, M.P. & DiRienzo, J.M. (1998). Relationship between conversion of localized juvenile periodontitis-susceptible children from health to disease and *Actinobacillus actinomycetemcomitans* leukotoxin promoter structure. *Journal of Periodontology* **70**, 998-1007.

Burdon K.L. (1928). *Bacterium melaninogenicum* from normal and pathologic tissues. *Journal of Infectious Diseases* **42**, 161-171.

Carter, K.C. (1987). *Essays of Robert Koch*. New York: Greenwood Press, pp. xvii-xix, 161.

Caugant, D.A., Kristiansen, B-E., Froholm, L.O., Bovre, K. & Selander, R.K. (1988). Clonal diversity of *Neisseria meningitidis* from a population of asymptomatic carriers. *Infection and Immunity* **56**, 2060-2068.

Chaves, E.S., Jeffcoat, M.K., Ryerson, C.C. & Snyder, B. (2000). Persistent bacterial colonization of *Porphyromonas gingivalis, Prevotella intermedia* and *Actinobacillus actinomycetemcomitans* in periodontitis and its association with alveolar bone loss after 6 months of therapy. *Journal of Clinical Periodontology* **27**, 897-903.

Chen, C.K., Dunford, P.G., Reynolds, H.S. & Zambon J.J. (1989). *Eikenella corrodens* in the human oral cavity. *Journal of Periodontology* **60**, 611-616.

Chen, H.A., Johnson, B.D., Sims, T.J., Darveau, R.P., Moncla, B.J., Whitney, C.W., Engel, D. & Page, R.C. (1991). Humoral immune responses to *Porphyromonas gingivalis* before and following therapy in rapidly progressive periodontitis patients. *Journal of Periodontology* **62**, 781-791.

Christersson, L.A., Albini, B., Zambon, J.J., Wikesjo, U.M.E. & Genco, R.J. (1987). Tissue localization of *Actinobacillus actinomycetemcomitans* in human periodontitis. I. Light, immunofluorescence and electron microscopic studies. *Journal of Periodontology* **58**, 529-539.

Christersson, L.A, Slots, J., Rosling, B.G. & Genco R.J. (1985). Microbiological and clinical effects of surgical treatment of localized juvenile periodontitis. *Journal of Clinical Periodontology* **12**, 465-476.

Chung, H-J., Chung, C-P., Son, S-H. & Nisengard R.J. (1989). *Actinobacillus actinomycetemcomitans* serotypes and leukotoxicity in Korean localized juvenile periodontitis. *Journal of Periodontology* **60**, 506-511.

Cimasoni, G. (1983). *Crevicular fluid updated*. Monographs in Oral Science 12. Basel: Karger, p. 71.

Cisar, J.O., Sandberg, A.L. & Mergenhagen, S.E. (1984). The function and distribution of different fimbriae on strains of *Actinomyces viscosus* and *Actinomyces naeslundii*. *Journal of Dental Research* **63**, 393-396.

Clark, W.B., Wheeler, T.T., Lane, M.D. & Cisar, J.O. (1986). *Actinomyces* adsorption mediated by Type-1 fimbriae. *Journal of Dental Research* **65**, 1166-1168.

Cobe H.M. (1948). Vincent's infection: experimental reproduction of lesions and the role of streptococci. *Journal of American Dental Association* **37**, 317-324.

Colombo, A.P., Haffajee, A.D., Dewhirst, F.E., Paster, B.J., Smith, C.M., Cugini, M.A. & Socransky, S.S. (1998). Clinical and microbiological features of refractory periodontitis. *Journal of Clinical Periodontology* **25**, 169-180.

Consensus report for periodontal diseases pathogenesis and microbial factors (1996). *Annals of Periodontology* **1**, 926-932.

Contreras, A., Falkler, W.A. Jr., Enwonwu, C.O., Idigbe, E.O., Savage, K.O., Afolabi, M.B., Onwujekwe, D., Rams, T.E. & Slots, J. (1997). Human Herpesviridae in acute necrotizing ulcerative gingivitis in children in Nigeria. *Oral Microbiology and Immunology* **12**, 259-265.

Contreras, A., Rusitanonta, T., Chen, C., Wagner, W.G., Michalowicz, B.S. & Slots, J. (2000). Frequency of 530-bp deletion in *Actinobacillus actinomycetemcomitans* leukotoxin promoter region. *Oral Microbiology and Immunology* **15**, 338-340.

Contreras, A. & Slots, J. (1996). Mammalian viruses in human periodontitis. *Oral Microbiology and Immunology* **11**, 381-386.

Contreras, A. & Slots, J. (2000). Herpesviruses in human periodontal disease. *Journal of Periodontal Research* **35**, 3-16.

Contreras, A., Umeda, M., Chen, C., Bakker, I., Morrison, J.L. & Slots. J. (1999a). Relationship between herpesviruses and adult periodontitis and periodontopathic bacteria. *Journal of Periodontology* **70**, 478-484.

Contreras, A., Zadeh, H.H., Nowzari, H. & Slots, J. (1999b). Herpesvirus infection of inflammatory cells in human periodontitis. *Oral Microbiology and Immunology* **14**, 206-212.

Costerton, J.W., Cook, G. & Lamont, R. (1999). The community architecture of biofilms: dynamic structures and mechanisms. In: Newman, H.N. & Wilson, M., eds. *Dental Plaque Revisited*. Cardiff: Bioline, pp. 5-14.

Curtis, M.A., Slaney, J.M., Carman, R.J. & Johnson, N.W. (1991). Identification of the major surface protein antigens of *Porphyromonas gingivalis* using IgG antibody reactivity of periodontal case-control serum. *Oral Microbiology and Immunology* **6**, 321-326.

Dahan M., Nawrocki, B., Elkaim, R., Soell, M., Bolcato-Bellemin, A.L., Birembaut, P. & Tenenbaum, H. (2001). Expression of matrix metalloproteinases in healthy and diseased human gingiva. *Journal of Clinical Periodontology* **28**, 128-136.

Dahlen, G., Manji, F., Baelum, V. & Fejerskov O. (1989). Black-pigmented Bacteroides species and *Actinobacillus actinomycetemcomitans* in subgingival plaque of adult Kenyans. *Journal of Clinical Periodontology* **16**, 305-310.

Daley, F.H. (1927a). Vincent's gingivitis in Boston in 1926. *Apollonium* **2**, 69-83.

Daley, F.H. (1927b). Vincent's gingivitis in Boston; report no. II. *Apollonium* **2**, 203-206.

Darby, I.B., Mooney, J. & Kinane, D.F. (2001). Changes in subgingival microflora and humoral immune response following periodontal therapy. *Journal of Clinical Periodontology* **28**, 796-805.

Darveau, R.P., Belton, C.M., Reife, R.A. & Lamont, R.J. (1998). Local chemokine paralysis, a novel pathogenic mechanism for *Porphyromonas gingivalis*. *Infection and Immunity* **66**, 1660-1665.

de Pommereau, V., Dargent-Pare, C., Robert, J.J. & Brion M. (1992). Periodontal status in insulin-dependent diabetic adolescents. *Journal of Clinical Periodontology* **19**, 628-632.

Deshpande, R.G. & Khan, M.B. (1999). Purification and characterization of hemolysin from *Porphyromonas gingivalis* A7436. *FEMS Microbiology Letters* **176**, 387-394.

Dewhirst, F.E., Stashenko, P.P., Mole, J.E. & Tsurumachi, T. (1985). Purification and partial sequence of human osteoclast-activating factor: identity with interleukin 1β. *Journal of Immunology* **135**, 2562-2568.

Dibart, S, Skobe, Z., Snapp, K.R., Socransky, S.S., Smith, C. & Kent, R. (1998). Identification of bacterial species on or in crevicular epithelial cells from healthy and periodontally diseased patients using DNA-DNA hybridization. *Oral Microbiology and Immunology,* **13**, 30-35.

DiRienzo, J.M. & McKay, T.L. (1994). Identification and characterization of genetic cluster groups of *Actinobacillus actinomycetemcomitans* isolated from the human oral cavity. *Journal of Clinical Microbiology* **32**, 75-81.

DiRienzo, J.M. & Slots, J. (1990). Genetic approach to the study of epidemiology and pathogenesis of *Actinobacillus actinomycetemcomitans* in localized juvenile periodontitis. *Archives of Oral Biology* **35**, (suppl.) 79S-84S.

DiRienzo, J.M., Slots, J., Sixou, M., Sol, M-A., Harmon, R. & McKay, T.L. (1994). Specific genetic variants of *Actinobacillus actinomycetemcomitans* correlate with disease and health in a regional population of families with localized juvenile periodontitis. *Infection and Immunity* **62**, 3058-3065.

Dogan, B., Saarela, M.H., Jousimies-Somer, H., Alaluusua, S. & Asikainen, S. (1999). *Actinobacillus actinomycetemcomitans* serotype e-biotypes, genetic diversity and distribution in relation to periodontal status. *Oral Microbiology and Immunology* **14**, 98-103.

Dongari-Bagtzoglou, A.I. & Ebersole, J.L. (1996). Production of inflammatory mediators and cytokines by human gingival fibroblasts following bacterial challenge. *Journal of Periodontal Research* **31**, 90-98.

Dorn, B.R., Leung, K.L. & Progulske-Fox, A. (1998). Invasion of human oral epithelial cells by Prevotella intermedia. *Infection and Immunity* **66**, 6054-6057.

Duncan, A.J., Carman, R.J., Harper, F.H., Griffiths, G.S. & Curtis, M.A. (1992). *Porphyromonas gingivalis*: presence of a species-specific antigen which is discriminatory in chronic inflammatory adult periodontal disease. *Microbial Ecology in Health and Disease* **5**, 15-20.

Duncan, M.J., Nakao, S., Skobe, Z. & Xie, H. (1993). Interactions of *Porphyromonas gingivalis* with epithelial cells. *Infection and Immunity* **61**, 2260-2265.

Dzink, J.L., Gibbons, R.J., Childs, III, W.C. & Socransky, S.S. (1989). The predominant cultivable microbiota of crevicular epithelial cells. *Oral Microbiology and Immunology* **4**, 1-5.

Dzink, J.L., Socransky, S.S., Ebersole, J.L. & Frey, D.E. (1983). ELISA and conventional techniques for identification of black-pigmented *Bacteroides* isolated from periodontal pockets. *Journal of Periodontal Research* **18**, 369-374.

Dzink, J.L., Socransky, S.S. & Haffajee, A.D. (1988). The predominant cultivable microbiota of active and inactive lesions of destructive periodontal diseases. *Journal of Clinical Periodontology* **15**, 316-323.

Dzink, J.L., Tanner, A.C.R., Haffajee, A.D. & Socransky, S.S. (1985). Gram-negative species associated with active destructive periodontal lesions. *Journal of Clinical Periodontology* **12**, 648-659.

Ebersole, J.L, Brunsvold, M., Steffensen, B., Wood, R. & Holt, S.C. (1991). Effects of immunization with *Porphyromonas gingivalis* and *Prevotella intermedia* on progression of ligature-induced periodontitis in the nonhuman primate Macaca fascicularis. *Infection and Immunity* **59**, 3351-3359.

Ebersole, J.L. & Taubman, M.A. (1994). Immunology of periodontal diseases. *Periodontology 2000* **5**, 112-141.

Ebersole, J.L., Taubman, M.A. & Smith, D.J. (1985). Gingival crevicular fluid antibody to oral microorganisms. II. Distribution and specificity of local antibody responses. *Journal of Periodontal Research* **20**, 349-356.

Ebersole, J.L., Taubman, M.A., Smith, D.J., Frey, D.E., Haffajee, A.D. & Socransky, S.S. (1987). Human serum antibody responses to oral microorganisms. IV. Correlation with homologous infection. *Oral Microbiology and Immunology* **2**, 53-59.

Ebersole, J.L., Taubman, M.A., Smith, D.J., Genco, R.J. & Frey D.E. (1982). Human immune responses to oral microorganisms. I. Association of localized juvenile periodontitis (LJP) with serum antibody responses to *Actinobacillus actinomycetemcomitans*. *Clinical Experimental Immunology* **47**, 43-52.

Ellen, R.P. (1985). Specificity of attachment as a tissue-tropic influence on oral bacteria. In: Mergenhagen, S.E. & Rosan, B., eds. *Molecular basis of oral microbial adhesion*. Washington: American Society for Microbiology, pp. 33-39.

Ellen, R.P. & Grove, D.A. (1989). *Bacteroides gingivalis* vesicles bind to and aggregate Actinomyces viscosus. *Infection and Immunity* **57**, 618-620.

Emmerson, A.M. & Mills, F. (1978). Recurrent meningitis and brain abscess caused by *Eikenella corrodens*. *Postgraduate Medical Journal* **54**, 343-345.

Etoh, Y., Dewhirst, F.E., Paster, B.J., Yamamoto, A. & Goto, N. (1993). *Campylobacter showae* sp. nov., isolated from the human oral cavity. *International Journal of Systematic Bacteriology* **43**, 631-639.

Evans, R.J. (1951). Haematin as a growth factor for a strict anaerobe *Fusiformis melaninogenicus*. *Proceedings of the Society for General Microbiology* **5**, XIX.

Evans, R.T., Klausen, B., Sojar, H.T., Bedi, G.S., Sfintescu, C., Ramamurthy, N.S. & Genco, R.J. (1992). Immunization with *Porphyromonas (Bacteroides) gingivalis* fimbriae protects against periodontal destruction. *Infection and Immunity* **60**, 2926-2935.

Feres, M., Haffajee, A.D., Allard, K.A., Som, S. & Socransky, S.S. (2000). Change in subgingival microbial profiles in adult periodontitis subjects receiving either systemically administered amoxicillin or metronidazole. *Journal of Clinical Periodontology* **28**, 597-609.

Fillery, E.D. & Pekovic, D.D. (1982). Identification of microorganisms in immunological mechanisms on human gingivitis. *Journal of Dental Research* **61**, 253.

Finegold, S.M. (1977). Anaerobic bacteria and human disease. New York: Academic Press, p. 44.

Finlay, B.B. & Falkow, S. (1989). Common themes in microbial pathogenicity. *Microbiological Reviews* **53**, 210-230.

Fletcher, J., Nair, S., Poole, S., Henderson, B. & Wilson, M. (1998). Cytokine degradation by biofilms of *Porphyromonas gingivalis*. *Current Microbiology* **36**, 216-219.

Fletcher, J., Reddi, K., Poole, S., Nair, S., Henderson, B., Tabona, P. & Wilson, M. (1997). Interactions between periodontopathogenic bacteria and cytokines. *Journal of Periodontal Research* **32**, 200-205.

Forscher, B.K., Paulsen, A.G. & Hess, W.C. (1954). The pH of the periodontal pocket and the glycogen content of the adjacent tissue. *Journal of Dental Research* **33**, 444-453.

Frank, R.M. & Voegel, J.C. (1978). Bacterial bone resorption in advanced cases of human periodontitis. *Journal of Periodontal Research* **13**, 251-261.

Freter, R. (1985). Bacterial adherence, physiological state, and nutrition as interdependent determinants of colonizing ability. In: Mergenhagen, S.E. & Rosan, B., eds. *Molecular basis of oral microbial adhesion*. Washington: American Society for Microbiology, pp. 61-66.

Frias, J., Olle, E. & Alsina M. (2001). Periodontal pathogens produce quorum sensing molecules. *Infection and Immunity* **69**, 3431-3434.

Garrison, S.W., Holt, S.C. & Nichols, F.C. (1988). Lipopolysaccharide-stimulated PGE2 release from human monocytes. Comparison of lipopolysaccharide prepared from suspected periodontal pathogens. *Journal of Periodontology* **59**, 684-687.

Genco, R.J, Slots, J. & Mouton, C. (1980). Systemic immune responses to oral anaerobic organisms. In: Lambe, D.W. Jr., Genco, R.J. & Mayberry-Carson, K.J., eds. *Anaerobic bacteria: selected topics*. New York: Plenum Press, pp. 277-293.

Genco, R.J., Van Dyke, T.E., Levine, M.J., Nelson, R.D. & Wilson, M.E. (1986). 1985 Kreshover lecture. Molecular factors influencing neutrophil defects in periodontal disease. *Journal of Dental Research* **65**, 1379-1391.

Gibbons, R.J. (1984). Adherent interaction which may affect microbial ecology in the mouth. *Journal of Dental Research* **63**, 378-385.

Gibbons, R.J. (1989). Bacterial adhesion to oral tissues: A model for infectious diseases. *Journal of Dental Research* **68**, 750-760.

Gibbons, R.J. & Macdonald, J.B. (1960). Hemin and vitamin K compounds as required factors for the cultivation of certain strains of *Bacteroides melaninogenicus*. *Journal of Bacteriology* **80**, 164-170.

Gibbons, R.J. & Macdonald, J.B. (1961). Degradation of collagenous substrates by *Bacteroides melaninogenicus*. *Journal of Bacteriology* **81**, 614-621.

Gibbons, R.J. & Quereshi, J.V. (1980). Virulence-related physiological changes and antigenic variation of *Streptococcus mutans* colonizing gnotobiotic rats. *Infection and Immunity* **29**, 1082-1091.

Gillespie, J., De Nardin, E., Radel, S., Kuracina, J., Smutko, J. & Zambon, J.J. (1992). Production of an extracellular toxin by the oral pathogen *Campylobacter rectus*. *Microbial Pathogenesis* **12**, 69-77.

Gillett, R. & Johnson, N.W. (1982). Bacterial invasion of the periodontium in a case of juvenile periodontitis. *Journal of Clinical Periodontology* **9**, 93-100.

Gmur, R., Strub, J.R. & Guggenheim, B. (1989). Prevalence of *Bacteroides forsythus* and *Bacteroides gingivalis* in subgingival plaque of prosthodontically treated patients on short recall. *Journal of Periodontal Research* **24**, 113-120.

Goodman, A.D. (1977). *Eikenella corrodens* isolated in oral infections of dental origin. *Oral Surgery, Oral Medicine, Oral Pathology* **44**, 128-134.

Greenspan, D. & Greenspan, J.S. (1993). Oral manifestations of human immunodeficiency virus infection. *Dental Clinics of North America* **37**, 21-32.

Greenspan, J.S., Greenspan, D., Winkler, J.R. & Murray, P.A. (1989). Acquired immunodeficiency syndrome; oral and periodontal changes. In: Genco, R.J., Goldman, H.M. & Cohen, D.W., eds. *Contemporary Periodontics*. Philadelphia: CV Mosby, pp. 298-322.

Grenier, D. & Mayrand, D. (1987a). Selected characteristics of pathogenic and nonpathogenic strains of *Bacteroides gingivalis*. *Journal of Clinical Microbiology* **25**, 738-740.

Grenier, D. & Mayrand, D. (1987b). Functional characterization of extracellular vesicles produced by *Bacteroides gingivalis*. *Infection and Immunity* **55**, 111-117.

Grenier, D., Mayrand, D. & McBride, B.C. (1989). Further studies on the degradation of immunoglobulins by black-pigmented *Bacteroides*. *Oral Microbiology and Immunology* **4**, 12-18.

Griffen, A.L., Lyons, S.R., Becker, M.R., Moeschberger, M.L. & Leys, E.J. (1999). *Porphyromonas gingivalis* strain variability and periodontitis. *Journal of Clinical Microbiology* **37**, 4028-4033.

Grossi, S.G., Genco, R.J., Machtei, E.E., Ho, A.W., Koch, G., Dunford, R.G., Zambon J.J. & Hausmann, E. (1995). Assessment of risk for periodontal disease. II. Risk indicators for bone loss. *Journal of Periodontology* **66**, 23-29.

Grossi, S.G., Zambon, J.J., Ho, A.W., Koch, G., Dunford, R.G., Machtei, E.E, Norderyd, O.M & Genco, R.J. (1994). Assessment of risk for periodontal disease. I. Risk indicators for attachment loss. *Journal of Periodontology* **65**, 260-267.

Guiney, D.G. & Bouic, K. (1990). Detection of conjugal transfer systems in oral, black-pigmented *Bacteroides* spp. *Journal of Bacteriology* **172**, 495-497.

Haffajee, A.D., Cugini, M.A., Dibart, S., Smith, C., Kent, R.L. Jr. & Socransky, S.S. (1997). The effect of SRP on the clinical and microbiological parameters of periodontal diseases. *Journal of Clinical Periodontology* **24**, 324-334.

Haffajee, A.D., Cugini, M.A., Tanner, A., Pollack, R.P., Smith, C., Kent, R.L. Jr. & Socransky, S.S. (1998). Subgingival microbiota in healthy, well-maintained elder and periodontitis subjects. *Journal of Clinical Periodontology* **25**, 346-353.

Haffajee, A.D., Dzink, J.L. & Socransky, S.S. (1988a). Effect of modified Widman flap surgery and systemic tetracycline on the subgingival microbiota of periodontal lesions. *Journal of Clinical Periodontology* **15**, 255-262.

Haffajee, A.D. & Socransky, S.S. (1994). Microbial etiological agents of destructive periodontal diseases. In: Socransky, S.S & Haffajee, A.D., eds. Microbiology and Immunology of periodontal diseases. *Periodontology 2000*, **5**, 78-111.

Haffajee, A.D. & Socransky, S.S. (2000). Relationship of cigarette smoking to attachment level profiles. *Journal of Clinical Periodontology* **28**, 283-295.

Haffajee, A.D., Socransky, S.S., Dzink, J.L., Taubman, M.A. & Ebersole, J.L. (1988b). Clinical, microbiological and immunological features of subjects with refractory periodontal diseases. *Journal of Clinical Periodontology* **15**, 390-398.

Haffajee, A.D., Socransky, S.S., Ebersole, J.L. & Smith, D.J. (1984). Clinical, microbiological and immunological features associated with the treatment of active periodontosis lesions. *Journal of Clinical Periodontology* **11**, 600-618.

Haffajee, A.D., Socransky, S.S. & Goodson, J.M. (1992). Subgingival temperature. (I). Relation to baseline clinical parameters. *Journal of Clinical Periodontology* **19**, 401-408.

Hafstrom, C. & Dahlen, G. (1997). Pathogenicity of *Prevotella intermedia* and *Prevotella nigrescens* isolates in a wound chamber model in rabbits. *Oral Microbiology and Immunology* **12**, 148-154.

Hammond, B.F., Lillard, S.E. & Stevens, R.H. (1987). A bacteriocin of *Actinobacillus actinomycetemcomitans*. *Infection and Immunity* **55**, 686-691.

Han, Y.W., Shi, W., Huang, G.T., Kinder Haake, S., Park, N.H., Kuramitsu, H. & Genco, R.J. (2000). Interactions between periodontal bacteria and human oral epithelial cells: *Fusobacterium nucleatum* adheres to and invades epithelial cells. *Infection and Immunity* **68**, 140-146.

Hanazawa, S., Hirose, K., Ohmori, Y., Amamo, S. & Kitano, S. (1988). *Bacteroides gingivalis* fimbriae stimulate production of thymocyte-activating factor by human gingival fibroblasts. *Infection & Immunity* **56**, 272-274.

Hanookai, D., Nowzari, H., Contreras, A., Morrison, J.L. & Slots, J. (2000). Herpesviruses and periodontopathic bacteria in Trisomy 21 periodontitis. *Journal of Periodontology* **71**, 376-384.

Haubek, D., Ennibi, O.K., Poulsen, K., Poulsen, S., Benzarti, N. & Kilian, M. (2001). Early-onset periodontitis in Morocco is associated with the highly leukotoxic clone of *Actinobacillus actinomycetemcomitans*. *Journal of Dental Research* **80**, 1580-1583.

Haubek, D., Poulsen, K., Westergaard, J., Dahlen, G. & Kilian M. (1996). Highly toxic clone of *Actinobacillus acinomycetemcomitans* in geographically widespread case of juvenile periodontitis. *Journal of Clinical Microbiology* **32**, 75-81.

Herrera, D., Roldan, S., Gonzalez, I. & Sanz, M. (2000). The periodontal abscess (I). Clinical and microbiological findings. *Journal of Clinical Periodontology* **27**, 387-394.

Hillman, J.D. & Socransky, S.S. (1982). Bacterial interference in the oral ecology of *Actinobacillus actinomycetemcomitans* and its relationship to human periodontosis. *Archives of Oral Biology* **27**, 75-77.

Hillman, J.D. & Socransky, S.S. (1987). Replacement therapy for the prevention of dental disease. *Advances in Dental Research* **1**, 119-125.

Hillman, J.D. & Socransky, S.S. (1989). The theory and application of bacterial interference to oral diseases. In: Myers, H.M., ed. *New Biotechnology in Oral Research*. Basel: Karger, pp. 1-17.

Hillman, J.D., Socransky, S.S. & Shivers, M. (1985). The relationships between streptococcal species and periodontopathic bacteria in human dental plaque. *Archives of Oral Biology* **30**, 791-795.

Hillmann, G., Dogan, S. & Geurtsen W. (1998). Histopathological investigation of gingival tissue from patients with rapidly progressive periodontitis. *Journal of Periodontology* **69**, 195-208.

Holmberg, K. & Hallander, H.O. (1973). Production of bacteriocidal concentrations of hydrogen peroxide by *Streptococcus sanguis*. *Archives of Oral Biology* **18**, 423-434.

Holt, S.C., Ebersole, J., Felton, J., Brunsvold, M. & Kornman, K.S. (1988). Implantation of *Bacteroides gingivalis* in nonhuman primates initiates progression of periodontitis. *Science* **239**, 55-57.

Horton, J.E., Raisz, L.G., Simmons, H.A., Oppenheim, J.J. & Mergenhagen, S.E. (1972). Bone resorbing activity in supernatant fluid from cultures of human peripheral blood leukocytes. *Science* **177**, 793-795.

Irving, J.T., Socransky, S.S. & Tanner, A.C. (1978). Histological changes in experimental periodontal disease in rats monoinfected with Gram-negative organisms. *Journal of Periodontal Research* **13**, 326-332.

Isogai, H., Isogai, E., Yoshimura, F., Suzuki, T., Kagota, W. &

Takano, K (1988). Specific inhibition of adherence of an oral strain of *Bacteroides gingivalis* 381 to epithelial cells by monoclonal antibodies against the bacterial fimbriae. *Archives of Oral Biology* **33**, 479-485.

Jewett, A. Hume, W.R., Le, H., Huynh, T.N., Han, Y.W., Cheng, G. & Shi, W. (2001). Induction of apoptotic cell death in peripheral blood mononuclear and polymorphonuclear cells by an oral bacterium, *Fusobacterium nucleatum*. *Infection and Immunity* **68**, 1893-1898.

Jin, K.C., Barua, P.K, Zambon, J.J. & Neiders, M.E. (1989). Proteolytic activity in black-pigmented bacteroides species. *Journal of Endodontics* **15**, 463-467.

Johnson, S.M. & Pankey, G.A. (1976). *Eikenella corrodens* osteomyelitis, arthritis, and cellulitis of the hand. *Southern Medical Journal* **69**, 535-539.

Johnson, V., Johnson, B.D., Sims, T.J., Whitney, C.W., Moncla, B.J. & Engel, L.D. (1993). Effects of treatment on antibody titer to *Porphyromonas gingivalis* in gingival crevicular fluid of patients with rapidly progressive periodontitis. *Journal of Periodontology* **64**, 559-565.

Kadowaki T., Nakayama, K., Okamoto, K., Abe, N., Baba, A., Shi, Y., Ratnayake, D.B. & Yamamoto, K. (2000). *Porphyromonas gingivalis* proteinases as virulence factors in progression of periodontal diseases. *Journal of Biochemistry* **128**, 153-159.

Kamma, J.J., Contreras, A. & Slots, J. (2001). Herpes virus and periodontopathic bacteria in early-onset periodontitis. *Journal of Clinical Periodontology* **28**, 879-885.

Kashket, S., Maiden, M., Haffajee, A. & Kasket, E.R. (2002). Accumulation of methylglyoxal in the gingival crevicular fluid of chronic periodontitis patients. *Journal of Clinical Periodontology*, submitted.

Kato, S., Nakashima, K., Inoue, M., Tomioka, J., Nonaka, K., Nishihar, T. & Kowashi, Y. (2000). Human epithelial cell death caused by *Actinobacillus actinomycetemcomitans* infection. *Journal of Medical Microbiology* **49**, 739-745.

Kaufman, J. & DiRienzo, J.M. (1989). Isolation of a corncob (coaggregation) receptor polypeptide from *Fusobacterium nucleatum*. *Infection and Immunity* **57**, 331-337.

Kenney, E.B. & Ash, M.M. (1969). Oxidation-reduction potential of developing plaque, periodontal pockets and gingival sulci. *Journal of Periodontology* **40**, 630-633.

Keyes, P.H. & Rams, T.E. (1983). A rationale for management of periodontal diseases: rapid identification of microbial 'therapeutic targets' with phase-contrast microscopy. *Journal of American Dental Association* **106**, 803-812.

Kigure, T., Saito, A., Seida, K., Yamada, S., Ishihara, K. & Okuda, K. (1995). Distribution of *Porphyromonas gingivalis* and *Treponema denticola* in human subgingival plaque at different periodontal pocket depths examined by immunohistochemical methods. *Journal of Periodontal Research* **30**, 332-341.

Kilian, M. (1981). Degradation of immunoglobulins A1, A2 and G by suspected principal periodontal pathogens. *Infection and Immunity* **34**, 757-765.

Kilian, M. & Frederiksen, W. (1981). Ecology of *Haemophilus*, *Pasteurella* and *Actinobacillus*. In: Kilian, M., Frederiksen, W. & Biberstein, E.L., eds. *Haemophilus, Pasteurella and Actinobacillus*. London: Academic Press Inc., pp. 11-38.

Kinder, S.A. & Holt, S.C. (1989). Characterization of coaggregation between *Bacteroides gingivalis* T22 and *Fusobacterium nucleatum* T18. *Infection and Immunity* **57**, 3425-3433.

Kleinberg, I. & Hall, G. (1969). pH and depth of gingival crevices in different areas of the mouth of fasting humans. *Journal of Periodontal Research* **4**, 109-117.

Kolenbrander, P.E. & Andersen, R.N. (1989). Inhibition of coaggregation between *Fusobacterium nucleatum* and *Porphyromonas (Bacteroides) gingivalis* by lactose and related sugars. *Infection and Immunity* **57**, 3204-3209.

Kolenbrander, P.E. & Andersen, R.N. (1990). Characterization of *Streptococcus gordonii* (*S. sanguis*) PK488 adhesin-mediated coaggregation with *Actinomyces naeslundii* PK606. *Infection and Immunity* **58**, 3064-3072.

Kolenbrander, P.E., Andersen, R.N., Clemans, D.L., Whittaker,

C.J. & Klier, C.M. (1999). Potential role of functionally similar coaggregation mediators in bacterial succession. In: Newman, H.N. & Wilson, M., eds. *Dental Plaque Revisited*. Cardiff: Bioline, pp. 171-186.

Kolenbrander, P.E., Andersen, R.N. & Moore, L.V. (1989). Coaggregation of *Fusobacterium nucleatum, Selenomonas flueggei, Selenomonas infelix, Selenomonas noxia,* and *Selenomonas sputigena* with strains from 11 genera of oral bacteria. *Infection and Immunity* **57**, 3194-3203.

Kornman, K.S. & Robertson, P.B. (1985). Clinical and microbiological evaluation of therapy for juvenile periodontitis. *Journal of Periodontology* **56**, 443-446.

Kremer, B.H., Loos, B.G., van der Velden, U., van Winkelhoff, A.J., Craandijk. J., Bulthuis, H.M., Hutter, J., Varoufaki, A.S. & van Steenbergen, T.J. (2000). *Peptostreptococcus micros* smooth and rough genotypes in periodontitis and gingivitis. *Journal of Periodontology* **71**, 209-218.

Lai, C-H., Listgarten, M.A., Evian, C.I. & Dougherty, P. (1986). Serum IgA and IgG antibodies to *Treponema vincentii* and *Treponema denticola* in adult periodontitis, juvenile periodontitis and periodontally healthy subjects. *Journal of Clinical Periodontology* **13**, 752-757.

Lai, C-H., Listgarten, M.A., Shirakawa, M. & Slots, J. (1987). *Bacteroides forsythus* in adult gingivitis and periodontitis. *Oral Microbiology and Immunology* **2**, 152-157.

Lai, C-H., Oshima, K., Slots, J. & Listgarten, M.A. (1992). *Wolinella recta* in adult gingivitis and periodontitis. *Journal of Periodontal Research* **27**, 8-14.

Lamont, R.J., Oda, D., Persson, R.E. & Persson, G.R. (1992). Interaction of *Porphyromonas gingivalis* with gingival epithelial cells maintained in culture. *Oral Microbiology and Immunology* **7**, 364-367.

Lantz, M.S., Allen, R.D., Bounelis, P., Switalski, L.M. & Hook, M. (1990). *Bacteroides gingivalis* and *Bacteroides intermedius* recognize different sites on human fibrinogen. *Journal of Bacteriology* **172**, 716-726.

Levy, R.M., Giannobile, W.V., Feres, M., Haffajee, A.D., Smith, C. & Socransky S.S. (2002). The effect of apically repositioned flap surgery on clinical parameters and the composition of the subgingival microbiota. 12 month data. *International Journal of Periodontics and Restorative Dentistry* **22**, 209-219.

Liakoni, H., Barber, P. & Newman, H.N. (1987). Bacterial penetration of pocket soft tissues in chronic adult and juvenile periodontitis cases. An ultrastructural study. *Journal of Clinical Periodontology* **14**, 22-28.

Lindemann, R.A. (1988). Bacterial activation of human natural killer cells: role of cell surface lipopolysaccharide. *Infection and Immunity* **56**, 1301-1308.

Lindemann, R.A., Economou, J.S. & Rothermel, H. (1988). Production of interleukin-1 and tumor necrosis factor by human peripheral monocytes activated by periodontal bacteria and extracted lipopolysaccharide. *Journal of Dental Research* **67**, 1131-1135.

Lippke, J.A., Peros, W.J., Keville, M.W., Savitt, E.D. & French, C.K. (1991). DNA probe detection of *Eikenella corrodens, Wolinella recta* and *Fusobacterium nucleatum* in subgingival plaque. *Oral Microbiology and Immunology* **6**, 81-87.

Listgarten, M.A. (1965). Electron microscopic observations of the bacterial flora of acute necrotizing ulcerative gingivitis. *Journal of Periodontology* **36**, 328-339.

Listgarten, M.A. (1976). Structure of the microbial flora associated with periodontal health and disease in man. A light and electron microscopic study. *Journal of Periodontology* **47**, 1-18.

Listgarten, M.A. (1988). Bacterial invasion of periodontal tissues (letter). *Journal of Periodontology* **59**, 412.

Listgarten, M.A. (1999). Formation of dental plaque and other oral biofilms. In: Newman, H.N. & Wilson, M., eds. *Dental Plaque Revisited*. Cardiff: Bioline, pp. 187-210.

Listgarten, M.A., Lai, C-H. & Evian, C.I. (1981). Comparative antibody titres to *Actinobacillus actinomycetemcomitans* in juvenile periodontitis, chronic periodontitis and periodontally healthy subjects. *Journal of Clinical Periodontology* **8**, 154-164.

Listgarten, M.A., Lai, C-H. & Young, V. (1993). Microbial composition and pattern of antibiotic resistance in subgingival microbial samples from patients with refractory periodontitis. *Journal of Periodontology* **64**, 155-161.

Listgarten, M.A., Mayo, H.E. & Tremblay, R. (1975). Development of dental plaque on epoxy resin crowns in man. A light and electron microscopic study. *Journal of Periodontology* **46**, 10-26.

Listgarten, M.A. & Socransky, S.S. (1964). Ultrastructural characteristics of a spirochete in the lesion of acute necrotizing ulcerative gingivostomatitis (Vincent's infection). *Archives of Oral Biology* **9**, 95-96.

Löe, H., Theilade, E. & Jensen, S.B. (1965). Experimental gingivitis in man. *Journal of Periodontology* **36**, 177-187.

Löe, H., Theilade, E., Jensen, S.B. & Schiott, C.R. (1967). Experimental gingivitis in man. III. The influence of antibiotics on gingival plaque development. *Journal of Periodontal Research* **2**, 282-289.

Loesche, W.J., Lopatin, D.E., Giordano, J., Alcoforado, G. & Hujoel, P.P. (1992). Comparison of the benzoyl-DL-arginine-naphthylamide (BANA) test, DNA probes, and immunological reagents for ability to detect anaerobic periodontal infections due to *Porphyromonas gingivalis*, *Treponema denticola* and *Bacteroides forsythus*. *Journal of Clinical Microbiology* **30**, 427-433.

Loesche, W.J., Syed, S.A., Laughon, B.E. & Stoll, J. (1982). The bacteriology of acute necrotizing ulcerative gingivitis. *Journal of Periodontology* **53**, 223-230.

Loesche, W.J., Syed, S.A., Schmidt, E. & Morrison, E.C. (1985). Bacterial profiles of subgingival plaques in periodontitis. *Journal of Periodontology* **56**, 447-456.

Lopatin, D.E. & Blackburn, E. (1992). Avidity and titer of immunoglobulin G subclasses to *Porphyromonas gingivalis* in adult periodontitis patients. *Oral Microbiology and Immunology* **7**, 332-337.

Lopez, N.J. (2000). Occurrence of *Actinobacillus actinomycetemcomitans*, *Porphyromonas gingivalis* and *Prevotella intermedia* in progressing adult periodontitis. *Journal of Periodontology* **71**, 948-954.

Macdonald, J.B., Gibbons, R.J. & Socransky, S.S. (1960). Bacterial mechanisms in periodontal disease. *Annals of the New York Academy of Sciences* **85**, 467-478.

Macdonald, J.B., Socransky, S.S. & Gibbons, R.J. (1963). Aspects of the pathogenesis of mixed anaerobic infections of mucous membranes. *Journal of Dental Research* **42**, 529-544.

Macdonald, J.B., Sutton, R.M., Knoll, M.L., Madlener, E.M. & Grainger, R.M. (1956). The pathogenic components of an experimental mixed infection. *Journal of Infectious Diseases* **98**, 15-20.

Machtei, E.E., Hausmann, E., Dunford, R., Grossi, S., Ho, A., Chandler, J., Zambon, J. & Genco, R.J. (1999). Longitudinal study of predictive factors for periodontal disease and tooth loss. *Journal of Clinical Periodontology* **26**, 374-380.

Macuch, P.J. & Tanner, A.C. (2000). *Campylobacter* species in health, gingivitis and periodontitis. *Journal of Dental Research* **79**, 785-792.

Madianos, P.N., Papapanou, P.N. & Sandros, J. (1997). *Porphyromonas gingivalis* infection of oral epithelium inhibits neutrophil transepithelial migration. *Infection and Immunity* **65**, 3983-3990.

Maeda, N., Okamoto, M., Kondo, K., Ishikawa, H., Osada, R., Tsurumoto, A. & Fujita, H. (1998). Incidence of *Prevotella intermedia* and *Prevotella nigrescens* in periodontal health and disease. *Microbiology and Immunology* **42**, 583-589.

Mahanonda, R., Seymour, G.J., Powell, L.W., Good, M.F. & Halliday, J.W. (1991). Effect of initial treatment of chronic inflammatory periodontal disease on the frequency of peripheral blood T-lymphocytes specific to periodontopathic bacteria. *Oral Microbiology and Immunology* **6**, 221-227.

Mandell, R.L. (1984). A longitudinal microbiological investigation of *Actinobacillus actinomycetemcomitans* and *Eikenella cor-*

rodens in juvenile periodontitis. *Infection and Immunity* **45**, 778-780.

Mandell, R.L., DiRienzo, J., Kent, R., Joshipura, K. & Haber, J. (1992). Microbiology of healthy and diseased periodontal sites in poorly controlled insulin dependent diabetics. *Journal of Periodontology* **63**, 274-279.

Mandell, R.L., Ebersole, J.L. & Socransky, S.S. (1987). Clinical immunologic and microbiologic features of active disease sites in juvenile periodontitis. *Journal of Clinical Periodontology* **14**, 534-540.

Mandell, R.L. & Socransky, S.S. (1981). A selective medium for *Actinobacillus actinomycetemcomitans* and the incidence of the organism in juvenile periodontitis. *Journal of Periodontology* **52**, 593-598.

Mandell, R.L., Tripodi, L.S., Savitt, E., Goodson, J.M. & Socransky, S.S. (1986). The effect of treatment on *Actinobacillus actinomycetemcomitans* in localized juvenile periodontitis. *Journal of Periodontology* **57**, 94-99.

Mangan, D.F., Laughon, B.E., Bower, B. & Lopatin, D.E. (1982). In vitro lymphocyte blastogenic responses and titers of humoral antibodies from periodontitis patients to oral spirochete isolates. *Infection and Immunity* **37**, 445-451.

Mangan, D.F., Novak, M.J., Vora, S.A., Mourad, J. & Kriger, P.S. (1989). Lectinlike interactions of *Fusobacterium nucleatum* with human neutrophiles. *Infection and Immunity* **57**, 3601-3611.

Marsh, P.D., McKee, A.S., McDermid, A.S. & Dowsett, A.B. (1989). Ultrastructure and enzyme activities of a virulent and an avirulent variant of *Bacteroides gingivalis* W50. *FEMS Microbiological Letters* **50**, 181-185.

Martin, S.A. Falkler, W.A. Jr., Vincent, J.W., Mackler, B.F. & Suzuki, J.B. (1988). A comparison of the reactivity of *Eubacterium* species with localized and serum immunoglobulins from rapidly progressive and adult periodontitis patients. *Journal of Periodontology* **59**, 32-39.

Mashimo, P.A., Yamamoto, Y., Nakanura, M., Reynolds, H.S. & Genco, R.J. (1985). Lactic acid production by oral *Streptococcus mitis* inhibits the growth of oral *Capnocytophaga*. *Journal of Periodontology* **56**, 548-552.

Mashimo, P.A., Yamamota, Y., Slots, J., Park, B.H. & Genco, R.J. (1983). The periodontal microflora of juvenile diabetics. Culture, immunofluorescence and serum antibody studies. *Journal of Periodontology* **54**, 420-430.

McKee, A.S., McDermid, A.S., Baskerville, A., Dowsett, A.B., Ellwood, D.C. (1986). Effect of hemin on the physiology and virulence of *Bacteroides gingivalis* W50. *Infection and Immunity* **52**, 349-355.

McNabb, H., Mombelli, A., Gmur, R., Mathey-Din, S. & Lang, N.P. (1992). Periodontal pathogens in the shallow pockets of immigrants from developing countries. *Oral Microbiology and Immunology* **7**, 267-272.

Millar, S.J., Goldstein, E.G., Levine, M.J. & Hausmann, E. (1986). Modulation of bone metabolism by two chemically distinct lipopolysaccharide fractions from *Bacteroides gingivalis*. *Infection and Immunity* **51**, 302-306.

Mombelli, A., Feloutzis, A., Bragger, U. & Lang, N.P. (2001). Treatment of peri-implantitis by local delivery of tetracycline. Clinical, microbiological and radiological results. *Clinical Oral Implants Research* **12**, 287-294.

Mombelli, A., Gmur, R., Lang, N.P., Corbert, E. & Frey, J. (1999). *Actinobacillus actinomycetemcomitans* in Chinese adults. Serotype distribution and analysis of the leukotoxin gene promoter locus. *Journal of Clinical Periodontology* **26**, 505-510.

Mombelli, A., Schmid, B., Rutar, A. & Lang, N.P. (2000). Persistence patterns of *Porphyromonas gingivalis*, *Prevotella intermedia/nigrescens*, and *Actinobacillus actinomycetemcomitans* after mechanical therapy of periodontal disease. *Journal of Periodontology* **71**, 14-21.

Mooney, J., Adonogianaki, E. & Kinane, D.F. (1993). Relative avidity of serum antibodies to putative periodontopathogens in periodontal disease. *Journal of Periodontal Research* **28**, 444-450.

Moore, W.E.C. (1987). Microbiology of periodontal disease. *Journal of Periodontal Research* **22**, 335-341.

Moore, W.E.C., Holdeman, L.V., Cato, E.P., Smibert, R.M., Burmeister, J.A., Palcanis, K.G. & Ranney, R.R. (1985). Comparative bacteriology of juvenile periodontitis. *Infection and Immunity* **48**, 507-519.

Moore, W.E.C., Holdeman, L.V., Cato, E.P., Smibert, R.M., Burmeister, J.A. & Ranney, R.R. (1983). Bacteriology of moderate (chronic) periodontitis in mature adult humans. *Infection and Immunity* **42**, 510-515.

Moore, W.E.C., Holdeman, L.V., Smibert, R.M., Hash, D.E., Burmeister, J.A. & Ranney, R.R. (1982). Bacteriology of severe periodontitis in young adult humans. *Infection and Immunity* **38**, 1137-1148.

Moore, L.V.H., Johnson, J.L. & Moore, W.E.C. (1987). *Selenomonas noxia* sp. nov., *Selenomonas flueggei* sp. nov., *Selenomonas infelix* sp. nov., *Selenomonas dianae* sp. nov. and *Selenomonas artemidis* sp. nov. from the human gingival crevice. *International Journal of Systematic Bacteriology* **36**, 271-280.

Moore, L.V.H., Moore, W.E.C., Riley, C., Brooks, C.N., Burmeister, J.A. & Smibert, R.M. (1993). Periodontal microflora of HIV positive subjects with gingivitis or adult periodontitis. *Journal of Periodontology* **64**, 48-56.

Morbidity and Mortality Weekly Report (1996). **45**, 1-28.

Muller, H.P., Heinecke, A., Borneff, M., Knopf, A., Kiencke, C. & Pohl, S. (1997). Microbial ecology of *Actinobacillus actinomycetemcomitans*, *Eikenella corrodens* and *Capnocytophaga* spp. in adult periodontitis. *Journal of Periodontal Research* **32**, 530-542.

Murray, P.A., Grassi, M. & Winkler, J.R. (1989). The microbiology of HIV-associated periodontal lesions. *Journal of Clinical Periodontology* **16**, 635-642.

Murray, P.A., Kern, D.G. & Winkler, J.R. (1988). Identification of a galactose-binding lectin on *Fusobacterium nucleatum* FN-2. *Infection and Immunity* **56**, 1314-1319.

Murray, P.A., Levine, M.J., Reddy, M.S., Tabak, L.A. & Bergey, E.J. (1986). Preparation of a sialic acid-binding protein from *Streptococcus mitis* KS32AR. *Infection and Immunity* **53**, 359-365.

Murray, P.A., Winkler, J.R., Peros, W.J., French, C.K. & Lippke, J.A. (1991). DNA probe detection of periodontal pathogens in HIV-associated periodontal lesions. *Oral Microbiology and Immunology* **6**, 34-40.

Naito, Y. & Gibbons, R.J. (1988). Attachment of *Bacteroides gingivalis* to collagenous substrata. *Journal of Dental Research* **67**, 1075-1080.

Neiders, M.E., Chen, P.B., Suido, H., Reynolds, H.S. & Zambon, J.J. (1989). Heterogeneity of virulence among strains of *Bacteroides gingivalis*. *Journal of Periodontal Research* **24**, 192-198.

Newman, H.N. & Wilson, M. (1999). *Dental Plaque Revisited*. Cardiff: Bioline.

Newman, M.G. & Socransky, S.S. (1977). Predominant cultivable microbiota in periodontosis. *Journal of Periodontal Research* **12**, 120-128.

Newman, M.G., Socransky, S.S., Savitt, E.D., Propas, D.A. & Crawford A. (1976). Studies of the microbiology of periodontosis. *Journal of Periodontology* **47**, 373-379.

Njoroge, T., Genco, R.J., Sojar, H.T., Hamada, N. & Genco, C.A. (1997). A role for the fimbriae in *Porphyromonas gingivalis* invasion of oral epithelial cells. *Infection and Immunity* **65**, 1980-1984.

Nociti, F.H. Jr., Cesco de Toledo, R., Machado, M.A., Stefani, C.M., Line, S.R. & Goncalves, R.B. (2001). Clinical and microbiological evaluation of ligature-induced peri-implantitis and periodontitis in dogs. *Clinical Oral Implants Research* **12**, 295-300.

O'Brien-Simpson, N.M., Black, C.L., Bhogal, P.S., Cleal, S.M., Slakeski, N., Higgins, T.J. & Reynolds, E.C. (2000). Serum immunoglobulin G (IgG) and IgG subclass responses to the RgpA-Kgp proteinase-adhesin complex of *Porphyromonas gingivalis* in adult periodontitis. *Infection and Immunity* **68**, 2704-2712.

Ochiai, K., Kurita, T., Nishimura, K. & Ikeda, O.T. (1989). Immu-noadjuvant effects of periodontitis-associated bacteria. *Journal of Periodontal Research* **24**, 322-328.

Ogawa, T., McGhee, M.L., Moldoveanu, Z., Hamada, S., Mestecky, J., McGhee, J.R. & Kiyono, H. (1989). *Bacteroides*-specific IgG and IgA subclass antibody-secreting cells isolated from chronically inflamed gingival tissues. *Clinical Experimental Immunology* **76**, 103-110.

Okuda, K. & Takazoe, I. (1988). The role of *Bacteroides gingivalis* in periodontal disease. *Advances in Dental Research* **2**, 260-268.

Oliver, W.W. & Wherry, W.B. (1921). Notes on some bacterial parasites of the human mucous membranes. *Journal of Infectious Diseases* **28**, 341-345.

Onisi, M., Condo, W., Horiuchi, I. & Uchiyama, Y. (1960). Preliminary report on the oxidation-reduction potentials obtained on surfaces of gingiva and tongue and in intradental space. *Bulletin Tokyo Medical Dental University* **7**, 161-164.

Papaioannou, S., Marsh, P.D. & Ivanyi, L. (1991). The immunogenicity of outer membrane proteins of haemin-depleted *Porphyromonas (Bacteroides) gingivalis* W50 in periodontal disease. *Oral Microbiology and Immunology* **6**, 327-331.

Papapanou, P.N., Baelum, V., Luan, W.M., Madianos, P.N., Chen, X., Fejerskov, O. & Dahlen G. (1997). Subgingival microbiota in adult Chinese: prevalence and relation to periodontal disease progression. *Journal of Periodontology* **68**, 651-656.

Papapanou, P.N., Neiderud, A.M., Papadimitriou, A., Sandros, J. & Dahlen, G. (2000). "Checkerboard" assessments of periodontal microbiota and their antibody responses: a case-control study. *Journal of Periodontology* **71**, 885-897.

Parra, B. & Slots, J. (1996). Detection of human viruses in periodontal pockets using polymerase chain reaction. *Oral Microbiology and Immunology* **11**, 289-293.

Paster, B.J., Boches, S.K., Galvin, J.L., Ericson, R.E., Lau, C.N., Levanos, V.A., Sahasrabudhe, A. & Dewhirst, F.E. (2001). Bacterial diversity in human subgingival plaque. *Journal of Bacteriology* **183**, 3770-3783.

Pavicic, M.J.A.M.P., van Winkelhoff, A.J., Douque, N.H., Steures, R.W.R. & de Graaff, J. (1994). Microbiological and clinical effects of metronidazole and amoxicillin in *Actinobacillus actinomycetemcomitans*-associated periodontitis: a 2-year evaluation. *Journal of Clinical Periodontology* **21**, 107-112.

Persson, G. R., Engel, D., Whitney, C., Darveau, R., Weinberg, A., Brunsvold, M., & Page, R.C. (1994). Immunization against *Porphyromonas gingivalis* inhibits progression of experimental periodontitis in nonhuman primates. *Infection and Immunity* **62**, 1026-1031.

Petit, M.D.A., Van Steenbergen, T.J.M., De Graaff, J. & Van der Velden, U. (1993a). Transmission of *Actinobacillus actinomycetemcomitans* in families of adult periodontitis patients. *Journal of Periodontal Research* **28**, 335-345.

Petit, M.D.A., Van Steenbergen, T.J.M., Scholte, L.M.H., Van der Velden, U. & De Graaff, J. (1993b). Epidemiology and transmission of *Porphyromonas gingivalis* and *Actinobacillus actinomycetemcomitans* among children and their family members. *Journal of Clinical Periodontology* **20**, 641-650.

Plaut, H.C. (1894). Studien zur bacteriellen Diagnostik der Diphtherie und der Anginen. *Deutsche Medicinische Wochenschrift* **20**, 920-923.

Preus, H.R. (1988). Treatment of rapidly destructive periodontitis in Papillon-Lefevre syndrome. Laboratory and clinical observations. *Journal of Clinical Periodontology* **15**, 639-643.

Preus, H.R. & Olsen, I. (1988). Possible transmittance of *A. actinomycetemcomitans* from a dog to a child with rapidly destructive periodontitis. *Journal of Periodontal Research* **23**, 68-71.

Preus, H.R., Zambon, J.J., Dunford, R.G. & Genco, R.J. (1994). The distribution and transmission of *Actinobacillus actinomycetemcomitans* in families with established adult periodontitis. *Journal of Periodontology* **65**, 2-7.

Proske, H.O. & Sayers, R.R. (1934). Pulmonary infections in pneumoconiosis. II. Fuso-spirochetal infection. Experiments in guinea pigs. *Public Health Reports* **29**, 1212-1217.

Prosser, J.I. (1999). Quorum sensing in biofilms. In: Newman,

H.N. & Wilson, M., eds. *Dental Plaque Revisited*. Cardiff: Bioline, pp. 79-88.

Rabie, G., Lally, E.T. & Shenker, B.J. (1988). Immunosuppressive properties of *Actinobacillus actinomycetemcomitans* leukotoxin. *Infection and Immunity* **56**, 122-127.

Rams, T.E., Andriola, M. Jr., Feik, D., Abel, S.N., McGiven, T.M. & Slots, J. (1991). Microbiological study of HIV-related periodontitis. *Journal of Periodontology* **62**, 74-81.

Rams, T.E., Feik, D. & Slots, J. (1990). Staphylococci in human periodontal diseases. *Oral Microbiology and Immunology* **5**, 29-32.

Rams, T.E., Feik, D. & Slots, J. (1993). *Campylobacter rectus* in human periodontitis. *Oral Microbiology and Immunology* **8**, 230-235.

Rams, T.E., Feik, D., Young, V., Hammond, B.F. & Slots, J. (1992). Enterococci in human periodontitis. *Oral Microbiology and Immunology* **7**, 249-252.

Rams, T.E. & Keyes, P.H. (1983). A rationale for the management of periodontal diseases: effects of tetracycline on subgingival bacteria. *Journal of American Dental Association* **107**, 37-41.

Rasmussen, A.T. (1929). Ultraviolet radiation in the treatment of periodontal diseases. *Journal of the American Dental Association* **16**, 3-17.

Riggio, M.P., Lennon, A. & Smith, A. (2001). Detection of peptostreptococcus micros DNA in clinical samples by PCR. *Journal of Medical Microbiology* **50**, 249-254.

Riviere, G.R. & DeRouen, T.A. (1998). Association of oral spirochetes from periodontally healthy sites with development of gingivitis. *Journal of Periodontology* **69**, 496-501.

Riviere, G.R., DeRouen, T.A., Kay, S.L., Avera, S.P., Stouffer, V.K & Hawkins, N.R. (1997). Association of oral spirochetes from sites of periodontal health with development of periodontitis. *Journal of Periodontology* **68**, 1210-1214.

Riviere, G.R., Elliot, K.S., Adams, D.F., Simonson, L.G., Forgas, L.B., Nilius, A.M. & Lukehart, S.A. (1992). Relative proportions of pathogen-related oral spirochetes (PROS) and *Treponema denticola* in supragingival and subgingival plaque from patients with periodontitis. *Journal of Periodontology* **63**, 131-136.

Riviere, G.R., Wagoner, M.A., Baker-Zander, S., Weisz, K.S., Adams, D.F., Simonson, L. & Lukehart, S.A. (1991a). Identification of spirochetes related to *Treponema pallidum* in necrotizing ulcerative gingivitis and chronic periodontitis. *New England Journal of Medicine* **325**, 539-543.

Riviere, G.R., Weisz, K.S., Simonson, L.G. & Lukehart, S.A. (1991b). Pathogen-related spirochetes identified within gingival tissue from patients with acute necrotizing ulcerative gingivitis. *Infection and Immunity* **59**, 2653-2657.

Riviere, G.R., Weisz, K.S., Adams, D.F. & Thomas, D.D. (1991c). Pathogen-related oral spirochetes from dental plaque are invasive. *Infection and Immunity* **59**, 3377-3380.

Rodenburg, J.P., van Winkelhoff, A.J., Winkel, E.G., Goene, R.J., Abbas, F. & de Graff, J. (1990). Occurrence of *Bacteroides gingivalis, Bacteroides intermedius* and *Actinobacillus actinomycetemcomitans* in severe periodontitis in relation to age and treatment history. *Journal of Clinical Periodontology* **17**, 392-399.

Rogers, A.H., van der Hoeven, J.S. & Mikx, F.H.M. (1979). Effect of bacteriocin production by *Streptococcus mutans* on the plaque of gnotobiotic rats. *Infection and Immunity* **23**, 571-576.

Rogosa, M. (1964). The genus *Veillonella* I. General, cultural, ecological and biochemical considerations. *Journal of Bacteriology* **87**, 162-170.

Rosebury, T., Clarke, A.R., Engel, S.G. & Tergis, F. (1950). Studies of fusospirochetal infection. I. Pathogenicity for guinea pigs of individual and combined cultures of spirochetes and other anaerobic bacteria derived from the human mouth. *Journal of Infectious Diseases* **87**, 217-225.

Rudney, J.D., Chen, R. & Sedgewick, G.J. (2001). Intracellular *Actinobacillus actinomycetemcomitans* and *Porphyromonas gingivalis* in buccal epithelial cells collected from human subjects. *Infection and Immunity* **69**, 2700-2707.

Rylander, H., Ramberg, P., Blohme, G. & Lindhe, J. (1987). Prevalence of periodontal disease in young diabetics. *Journal of Clinical Periodontology* **14**, 38-43.

Saarela, M., von Troil-Linden, B., Torkko, H., Stucki, A-M., Alaluusua, S., Jousimies-Somer, H. & Asikainen, S. (1993). Transmission of oral bacterial species between spouses. *Oral Microbiology and Immunology* **8**, 349-354.

Saglie, F.R., Marfany, A. & Camargo, P. (1988). Intragingival occurrence of *Actinobacillus actinomycetemcomitans* and *Bacteroides gingivalis* in active destructive periodonta lesions. *Journal of Periodontology* **59**, 259-265.

Saglie, F.R., Smith, C.T., Newman, M.G., Carranza, F.A. Jr. & Pertuiset, J.J. (1986). The presence of bacteria in the oral epithelium in periodontal disease. II. Immunohistochemical identification of bacteria. *Journal of Periodontology* **57**, 492-500.

Saiki, K., Konishi, K., Gomi, T., Nishihara, T. & Yoshikawa, M. (2001). Reconstitution and purification of cytolethal distending toxin of *Actinobacillus actinomycetemcomitans*. *Microbiology and Immunology* **45**, 497-506.

Saito, A., Hosaka, Y., Nakagawa, T., Seida, K., Yamada, S., Takazoe, I. & Okuda, K. (1993). Significance of serum antibody against surface antigens of *Actinobacillus actinomycetemcomitans* in patients with adult periodontitis. *Oral Microbiology and Immunology* **8**, 146-153.

Saito, M., Otsuka, M., Maehara, R., Endo, J. & Nakamura, R. (1987). Degradation of human secretory immunoglobulin A by protease isolated from the anaerobic periodontopathogenic bacterium. *Bacteroides gingivalis*. *Archives of Oral Biology* **32**, 235-238.

Sanavi, F., Listgarten, M.A., Boyd, F., Sallay, K. & Nowotny, A. (1985). The colonization and establishment of invading bacterium in periodontium of ligature-treated immunosuppressed rats. *Journal of Periodontology* **56**, 273-280.

Sandberg, A.L., Mudrick, L.L., Cisar, J.O., Brennan, M.J., Mergenhagen, S.E. & Vatter, A.E. (1986). Type 2 fimbrial lectin-mediated phagocytosis of oral *Actinomyces* spp. bt polymorphonuclear leukocytes. *Infection and Immunity* **54**, 472-476.

Sandberg, A.L., Mudrick, L.L., Cisar, J.O., Metcalf, J.A. & Malech, H.L. (1988). Stimulation superoxide and lactoferrin from polymorphonuclear leukocytes by the Type 2 fimbrial lectin of *Actinomyces viscosus* T14V. *Infection and Immunity* **56**, 267-269.

Sandros, J., Karlsson, C., Lappin, D.F., Madianos, P.N., Kinane, D.F. & Papapanou, P.N. (2000). Cytokine responses of oral epithelial cells to *Porphyromonas gingivalis*. *Journal of Dental Research* **79**, 1808-1814.

Sandros, J., Papapanou, P. & Dahlen, G. (1993). *Porphyromonas gingivalis* invades oral epithelial cells in vitro. *Journal of Periodontal Research* **28**, 219-226.

Sastrowijoto, S.H., Hillemans, P., van Steenbergen, T.J.M., Abraham-Inpijn, L. & de Graaff J. (1989). Periodontal condition and microbiology of healthy and diseased periodontal pockets in type 1 diabetes mellitus patients. *Journal of Clinical Periodontology* **16**, 316-322.

Savitt, E.D. & Socransky, S.S. (1984). Distribution of certain subgingival microbial species in selected periodontal conditions. *Journal of Periodontal Research* **19**, 111-123.

Schenkein, H.A., Barbour, S.E., Berry, C.R., Kipps, B. & Tew, J.G. (2000). Invasion of human vascular endothelial cells by *Actinobacillus actinomycetemcomitans* via the receptor for platelet-activating factor. *Infection and Immunity* **68**, 5416-5419.

Schifferle, R.E., Wilson, M.E., Levine, M.J. & Genco, R.J. (1993). Activation of serum complement by polysaccharide-containing antigens of *Porphyromonas gingivalis*. *Journal of Periodontal Research* **28**, 248-254.

Schonfeld, S.E. & Kagan, J.M. (1982). Specificity of gingival plasma cells for bacterial somatic antigens. *Journal of Periodontal Research* **17**, 60-69.

Sela, M.N., Weinberg, A., Borinsky, R., Holt, S.C. & Dishon, T. (1988). Inhibition of superoxide production in human polymorphonuclear leukocytes by oral treponemal factors. *Infection and Immunity* **56**, 589-594.

Seppala, B., Seppala, M. & Ainamo, J. (1993). A longitudinal study on insulin-dependent diabetes mellitus and periodontal disease. *Journal of Clinical Periodontology* **20**, 161-165.

Seow, W.K., Bird, P.S., Seymour, G.J. & Thong, Y.H. (1989). Modulation of human neutrophil adherence by periodontopathic bacteria: reversal by specific monoclonal antibodies. *International Achives of Allergy and Applied Immunology* **90**, 24-30.

Seow, W.K., Seymour, G.J. & Thong, Y.H. (1987). Direct modulation of human neutrophil adherence by coaggregating periodontopathic bacteria. *International Achives of Allergy and Applied Immunology* **83**, 121-128.

Shah, H.N. & Gharbia, S.E. (1992). Biochemical and chemical studies on strains designated *Prevotella intermedia* and proposal of a new pigmented species, *Prevotella nigrescens* sp. nov. *International Journal of Systematic Bacteriology* **42**, 542-546.

Sheikhi, M., Gustafsson, A. & Jarstrand, C. (2000). Cytokine, elastase and oxygen radical release by *Fusobacterium nucleatum*-activated leukocytes: a possible pathogenic factor for periodontitis. *Journal of Clinical Periodontology* **27**, 758-762.

Shenker, B.J. (1987). Immunologic dysfunction in the pathogenesis of periodontal diseases. *Journal of Clinical Periodontology* **14**, 489-498.

Shenker, B.J., Hoffmaster, R.H., Zekavat, A., Yamaguchi, N., Lally, E.T. & Demuth, D.R. (2001). Induction of apoptosis in human T cells by *Actinobacillus actinomycetemcomitans* cytolethal distending toxin is a consequence of G(2) arrest of the cell cycle. *Journal of Immunology* **167**, 435-441.

Shenker, B.J., Listgarten, M.A. & Taichman, N.S. (1984). Suppression of human lymphocyte responses by oral spirochetes: a monocyte-dependent phenomenon. *Journal of Immunology* **132**, 2039-2045.

Shenker, B.J. & Slots, J. (1989). Immunomodulatory effects of *Bacteroides* products on in vitro human leukocyte functions. *Oral Microbiology and Immunology* **4**, 24-29.

Shiloah, J., Patters, M.R., Dean, J.W. 3rd., Bland, P. & Toledo, G. (1998) The prevalence of *Actinobacillus actinomycetemcomitans*, *Porphyromonas gingivalis* and *Bacteroides forsythus* in humans 1 year after four randomized treatment modalities. *Journal of Periodontology* **69**, 1364-1372.

Simonson, L.G., Goodman, C.H., Bial, J.J. & Morton, H.E. (1988). Quantitative relationship of *Treponema denticola* to severity of periodontal disease. *Infection and Immunity* **56**, 726-728.

Simonson, L.G., Robinson, P.J., Pranger, R.J., Cohen, M.E. & Morton, H.E. (1992). *Treponema denticola* and *Porphyromonas gingivalis* as prognostic markers following periodontal treatment. *Journal of Periodontology* **63**, 270-273.

Simpson, D.L., Berthold, P. & Taichma, N.S. (1988). Killing of human myelomonocytic leukemia and lymphocytic cell lines by *Actinobacillus actinomycetemcomitans* leukotoxin. *Infection and Immunity* **56**, 1162-1166.

Singer, R.E. & Buckner, B.A. (1981). Butyrate and propionate: important components of toxic dental plaque extracts. *Infection and Immunity* **32**, 458-463.

Sismey-Durrant, H.J., Atkinson, S.J., Hopps, R.M. & Heath, J.K. (1989). The effect of lipopolysaccharide from *Bacteroides gingivalis* and muramyl dipeptide on osteoblast collagenase release. *Calcified Tissue International* **44**, 361-363.

Slots, J. (1976). The predominant cultivable organisms in juvenile periodontitis. *Scandinavian Journal of Dental Research* **84**, 1-10.

Slots, J. (1977). The predominant cultivable microflora of advanced periodontitis. *Scandinavian Journal of Dental Research* **85**, 114-121.

Slots, J., Feik, D. & Rams, T.E. (1990a). *Actinobacillus actinomycetemcomitans* and *Bacteroides intermedius* in human periodontitis: age relationship and mutual association. *Journal of Clinical Periodontology* **17**, 659-662.

Slots, J., Feik, D. & Rams, T.E. (1990b). Prevalence and antimicrobial susceptibility of *Enterobacteriaceae*, *Pseudomonadaceae* and *Acinetobacter* in human periodontitis. *Oral Microbiology and Immunology* **5**, 149-154.

Slots, J., Rams, T.E., Feik, D., Taveras, H.D. & Gillespie, G.M. (1991). Subgingival microflora of advanced periodontitis in the Dominican Republic. *Journal of Periodontology* **62**, 543-547.

Slots, J., Reynolds, H.S. & Genco, R.J. (1980). *Actinobacillus actinomycetemcomitans* in human periodontal disease: a cross-sectional microbiological investigation. *Infection and Immunity* **29**, 1013-1020.

Slots, J. & Rosling, B.G. (1983). Suppression of the periodontopathic microflora in localized juvenile periodontitis by systemic tetracycline. *Journal of Clinical Periodontology* **10**, 465-486.

Smalley, J.W, Birss, A.J. & Shuttleworth, C.A. (1988). The degradation of type I collagen and human plasma fibronectin by the trypsin-like enzyme and extracellular membrane vesicles of *Bacteroides gingivalis* W50. *Archives of Oral Biology* **33**, 323-329.

Smith, D.T. (1930). Fusospirochetal disease of the lungs produced with cultures from Vincent's angina. *Journal of Infectious Diseases* **46**, 303-310.

Smith, D.J., Gadalla, L.M., Ebersole, J.L. & Taubman, M.A. (1985). Gingival crevicular fluid antibody to oral microorganisms. III. Association of gingival homogenate and gingival crevicular fluid antibody levels. *Journal of Periodontal Research* **20**, 357-367.

Socransky, S.S. (1970). Relationship of bacteria to the etiology of periodontal disease. *Journal of Dental Research* **49**, 203-222.

Socransky, S.S. & Gibbons, R.J. (1965). Required role of Bacteroides melaninogenicus in mixed anaerobic infections. *Journal of Infectious Diseases* **115**, 247-253.

Socransky, S.S. & Haffajee, A.D. (1991). Microbial mechanisms in the pathogenesis of destructive periodontal diseases: a critical assessment. *Journal of Periodontal Research* **26**, 195-212.

Socransky, S.S. & Haffajee, A.D. (1992). The bacterial etiology of destructive peridontal disease: current concepts. *Journal of Periodontology* **63**, 322-331.

Socransky, S.S. & Haffajee, A.D. (1993). Effect of therapy on periodontal infections. *Journal of Periodontology* **64**, 754-759.

Socransky, S.S & Haffajee, A.D. (1994). Evidence of bacterial etiology: a historical perspective. In: Socransky, S.S & Haffajee, A.D., eds. Microbiology and immunology of periodontal diseases. *Periodontology 2000* **5**, 7-25.

Socransky, S.S. & Haffajee, A.D. (2002). Dental biofilms: difficult therapeutic targets. *Periodontology 2000* **28**, 12-55.

Socransky, S.S., Haffajee, A.D., Cugini, M.A., Smith, C. & Kent, R.L. Jr. (1998). Microbial complexes in subgingival plaque. *Journal of Clinical Periodontology* **25**, 134-144.

Socransky, S.S., Haffajee, A.D. & Dzink, J.L. (1988). Relationship of subgingival microbial complexes to clinical features at the sampled sites. *Journal of Clinical Periodontology* **15**, 440-444.

Socransky, S.S., Haffajee, A.D., Smith, C. & Dibart, S. (1991). Relation of counts of microbial species to clinical status at the site. *Journal of Clinical Periodontology* **18**, 766-775.

Socransky, S.S., Loesche, W.J., Hubersack, C. & Macdonald, J.B. (1964). Dependency of *Treponema microdentium* on other oral organisms for isobutyrate, polyamines, and a controlled oxidation-reduction potential. *Journal of Bacteriology* **88**, 200-209.

Socransky, S.S., Smith, C. & Haffajee, A.D. (2002). Subgingival microbial profiles in refractory periodontal disease. *Journal of Clinical Periodontology* **29**, 260-268.

Sreenivasan, P.K., Meyer, D.H. & Fives-Taylor, P.M. (1993). Requirements for invasion of epithelial cells by *Actinobacillus actinomycetemcomitans*. *Infection and Immunity* **61**, 1239-1245.

Steinberg, A.I. & Gershoff, S.N. (1968). Quantitative differences in spirochetal antibody observed in periodontal disease. *Journal of Periodontology* **39**, 286-289.

Stevens, R.H., Lillard, S.E. & Hammond, B.F. (1987). Purification and biochemical properties of a bacteriocin from *Actinobacillus actinomycetemcomitans*. *Infection and Immunity* **55**, 686-691.

Sudre, P., ten Dam, G. & Kochi, A. (1992). Tuberculosis: a global overview of the situation today. *Bulletin of the World Health Organization* **70**, 149-159.

Sundqvist, G., Figdor, D., Hanstrom, L., Sorlin, S. & Sandstrom, G. (1991). Phagocytosis and virulence of different strains of *Porphyromonas gingivalis*. *Scandinavian Journal of Dental Research* **99**, 117-129.

Takada, H., Ogawa, T., Yoshimura, F., et al. (1988). Immunobiological activities of a porin fraction isolated from *Fusobacterium nucleatum* ATCC10953. *Infection and Immunity* **56**, 855-863.

Takamatsu, N., Yano, K., He, T., Umeda, M. & Ishikawa, I. (1999). Effect of initial periodontal therapy on the frequency of detecting *Bacteroides forsythus*, *Porphyromonas gingivalis* and *Actinobacillus actinomycetemcomitans*. *Journal of Periodontology* **70**, 574-580.

Tan, K.S., Woo, C.H., Ong, G. & Song, K.P. (2001). Prevalence of *Actinobacillus actinomycetemcomitans* in an ethnic adult Chinese population. *Journal of Clinical Periodontology* **28**, 886-890.

Tanner, A. & Bouldin, H. (1989). The microbiology of early periodontis lesions in adults. *Journal of Clinical Periodontology* **16**, 467-471.

Tanner, A.C.R., Dzink, J.L., Ebersole, J.L. & Socransky, S.S. (1987). *Wolinella recta, Campylobacter concisus, Bacteroides gracilis*, and *Eikenella corrodens* from periodontal lesions. *Journal of Periodontal Research* **22**, 327-330.

Tanner, A.C.R., Haffer, C., Bratthall, G.T., Visconti, R.A. & Socransky, S.S. (1979). A study of the bacteria associated with advancing periodontitis in man. *Journal of Clinical Periodontology* **6**, 278-307.

Tanner, A., Kent, R., Maiden, M.F. & Taubman, M.A. (1996). Clinical, microbiological and immunological profile of health, gingivitis, and putative active periodontal subjects. *Journal of Periodontal Research* **31**, 195-204.

Tanner, A., Maiden, M.F., Macuch, P.J., Murray, L.L. & Kent, R.L. Jr. (1998). Microbiota of health, gingivitis and initial periodontitis. *Journal of Clinical Periodontology* **25**, 85-98.

Tanner, A., Maiden, M.F.J., Paster, B.J. & Dewhirst, F.E. (1994). The impact of 16S ribosomal RNA-based phylogeny on the taxonomy of oral bacteria. In: Socransky, S.S & Haffajee, A.D., eds. Microbiology and immunology of periodontal diseases. *Periodontology 2000* **5**, 26-51.

Tanner, A.C.R. & Socransky, S.S. (1984). Genus *Wolinella*. In: Buchanan, N. & Gibbons. N., eds. *Bergey's Manual of Determinative Bacteriology*, 8th edn. Baltimore: The Williams and Wilkins Co, pp. 646-650.

Taubman, M.A., Haffajee, A.D., Socransky, S.S., Smith, D.J. & Ebersole, J.L. (1992). Longitudinal monitoring of humoral antibody in subjects with destructive periodontal diseases. *Journal of Periodontal Research* **27**, 511-521.

Tenovuo, J. & Pruitt, K.M. (1984). Relationship of the human salivary peroxidase system to oral health. *Journal of Oral Pathology* **13**, 573-584.

Tew, J.G., Marshall, D.R., Burmeister, J.A. & Ranney, R.R. (1985a). Relationship between gingival crevicular fluid and serum antibody titers in young adults with generalized and localized periodontitis. *Infection and Immunity* **49**, 487-493.

Tew, J.G., Marshall, D.R., Moore, W.E,. Best, A.M., Palcanis, K.G. & Ranney, R.R. (1985b). Serum antibody reactive with predominant organisms in the subgingival flora of young adults with generalized severe periodontitis. *Infection and Immunity* **48**, 303-311.

Tew, J.G., Smibert, R.M., Scott, E.A., Burmeister, J.A. & Ranney, R.R. (1985c). Serum antibodies in young adult humans reactive with periodontitis associated treponemes. *Journal of Periodontal Research* **20**, 580-590.

Theilade, E., Wright, W.H., Jensen, S.B. & Löe, H. (1966). Experimental gingivitis in man. II. A longitudinal clinical and bacteriological investigation. *Journal of Periodontal Research* **1**, 1-13.

Thorstensson, H. & Hugoson, A. (1993). Periodontal disease experience in adult long-duration insulin-dependent diabetics. *Journal of Clinical Periodontology* **20**, 352-358.

Timmerman, M.F., van der Weijden, G.A., Arief, E.M., Armand, S., Abbas, F., Winkel, E.G., van Winkelhoff, A.J. & van der Velden, U. (2001). Untreated periodontal disease in Indonesian adolescents: Subgingival microbiota in relation to experienced progression of periodododontis. *Journal of Clinical Periodontology* **28**, 617-627.

Ting, M., Contreras, A. & Slots, J. (2000). Herpesvirus in localized juvenile periodontitis. *Journal of Periodontal Research* **35**, 17-25.

Tinoco, E.M., Beldi, M.I., Campedelli, F., Lana, M., Loureiro, C.A., Bellini, H.T., Rams, T.E., Tinoco, N.M., Gjermo, P. & Preus, H.R. (1998). Clinical and microbiological effects of adjunctive antibiotics in the treatment of localized juvenile periodontitis. A controlled clinical trial. *Journal of Periodontology* **69**, 1355-1363.

Tran, S.D., Rudney, J.D., Sparks, B.S. & Hodges, J.S. (2001). Persistent presence of *Bacteroides forsythus* as a risk factor for attachment loss in a population with low prevalence and severity of adult periodontitis. *Journal of Periodontology* **72**, 1-10.

Tsai, C-C., McArthur, W.P., Baehni, P.C., Evian, C., Genco, R.J. & Taichman, N.S. (1981). Serum neutralizing activity against *Actinobacillus actinomycetemcomitans* leukotoxin in juvenile periodontitis. *Journal of Clinical Periodontology* **8**, 338-348.

Uchida, Y., Shiba, H., Komatsuzawa, H., Takemoto, T., Sakata, M., Fujita, T., Kawaguchi, H., Sugai, M. & Kurihara, H. (2001). Expression of IL-1 beta and IL-8 by human gingival epithelial cells in response to *Actinobacillus actinomycetemcomitans*. *Cytokine* **7**, 152-161.

Uematsu, H. & Hoshino, E. (1992). Predominant obligate anaerobes in human periodontal pockets. *Journal of Periodontal Research* **27**, 15-19.

Uitto, V.J., Larjava, H., Heino, J. & Sorsa, T. (1989). A protease of *Bacteroides gingivalis* degrades cell surface and matrix glycoproteins of cultured gingival fibroblasts and induces secretion of collagenase and plasminogen activator. *Infection and Immunity* **57**, 213-218.

van Dalen, P.J., van Deutekom-Mulder, E.C., de Graaff, J. & van Steenbergen, T.J. (1998). Pathogenicity of *Peptostreptococcus micros* morphotypes and *Prevotella* species in pure and mixed cultures. *Journal of Medical Microbiology* **47**, 135-140.

van Steenbergen, T.J.M., Delemarre, F.G., Namavar, F. & de Graaff, J. (1987). Differences in virulence within the species *Bacteroides gingivalis*. *Antonie Van Leeuwenhoek* **53**, 233-244.

van Steenbergen, T.J., Petit, M.D., Scholte, L.H., Van der Velden, U. & de Graaff, J. (1993). Transmission of *Porphyromonas gingivalis* between spouses. *Journal of Clinical Periodontology* **20**, 340-345.

van Steenbergen, T.J.M., van der Mispel, L.M.S. & de Graaff, J. (1986). Effects of ammonia and volatile fatty acids produced by oral bacteria on tissue culture cells. *Journal of Dental Research* **65**, 909-912.

van Winkelhoff, A.J., Rams, T.E. & Slots, J. (1996). Systemic antibiotic therapy in periodontics. *Periodontology 2000* **10**, 45-78.

van Winkelhoff, A.J., Tijhof, C.J. & de Graaff, J. (1992). Microbiological and clinical results of metronidazole plus amoxicillin therapy in *Actinobacillus actinomycetemcomitans*-associated periodontitis. *Journal of Periodontology* **63**, 52-57.

van Winkelhoff, A.J., van der Velden, U. & de Graaf, J. (1988). Microbial succession in recolonizing deep periodontal pockets after a single course of supra- and subgingival debridement. *Journal of Clinical Periodontology* **15**, 116-122.

Velazco, C.H., Coelho, C., Salazar, F., Contreras, A., Slots, J. & Pacheco, J.J. (1999). Microbiological features of Papillon-Lefevre syndrome periodontitis. *Journal of Clinical Periodontology* **26**, 622-627.

Vincent, J.W., Falkler, W.A. Jr. & Suzuki, J.B. (1986). Systemic antibody response of clinically characterized patients with antigens of *Eubacterium brachy* initially and following periodontal therapy. *Journal of Periodontology* **57**, 625-631.

Vincent, M.H. (1899). Recherches bacteriologiques sur l'angine a bacilles fusiformes. *Annales de L'Institut Pasteur* **8**, 609-620.

Walker, C., Gordon, J., Magnusson, I. & Clark, W.B. (1993). A role for antibiotics in the treatment of refractory periodontitis. *Journal of Periodontology* **64**, 772-781.

Weinberg, A., Belton, C.M., Park, Y. & Lamont R.J. (1997). Role of fimbriae in *Porphyromonas gingivalis* invasion of gingival epithelial cells. *Infection and Immunity* **65**, 313-316.

Weinberg, A. & Holt, S.C. (1990). Interaction of *Treponema denticola* TD-4, GM-1, and MS25 with human gingival fibroblasts. *Infection and Immunity* **58**, 1720-1729.

Weiss, E.I., Shaniztki, B., Dotan, M., Ganeshkumar, N., Kolenbrander, P.E. & Metzger, Z. (2000). Attachment of *Fusobacterium nucleatum* PK1594 to mammalian cells and its coaggregation with periodontopathic bacteria are mediated by the same galactose-binding adhesin. *Oral Microbiology and Immunology* **15**, 371-377.

Whitney, C., Ant, J., Moncla, B., Johnson, B., Page, R.C. & Engel, D. (1992). Serum immunoglobulin G antibody to *Porphyromonas gingivalis* in rapidly progressive periodontitis: titer, avidity, and subclass distribution. *Infection and Immunity* **60**, 2194-2200.

Wikstrom, M. & Linde, A. (1986). Ability of oral bacteria to degrade fibronectin. *Infection and Immunity* **51**, 707-711.

Williams, C.A., Winkler, J.R., Grassi, M. & Murray, P.A. (1990). HIV-associated periodontitis complicated by necrotizing stomatitis. *Oral Surgery, Oral Medicine, Oral Pathology* **69**, 351-355.

Wilton, J.M., Hurst, T.J. & Austin, A.K. (1992). IgG subclass antibodies to *Porphyromonas gingivalis* in patients with destructive periodontal disease. A case control study. *Journal of Clinical Periodontology* **19**, 646-651.

Winkel, E.G., van Winkelhoff, A.J., Timmerman, M.F., van der Velden, U. & nan der Weijden, G.A. (2001). Amoxicillin plus metronidazole in the treatment of adult periodontitis patients. A double-blind placebo-controlled study. *Journal of Clinical Periodontology* **28**, 296-305.

Winkel, E.G., van Winkelhoff, A.J. & van der Velden, U. (1998). Additional clinical and microbiological effects of amoxicillin and metronidazole after initial periodontal therapy. *Journal of Clinical Periodontology* **25**, 857-864.

Winkler, J.R., John, S.R., Kramer, R.H., Hoover, C.I. & Murray, P.A. (1987). Attachment of oral bacteria to a basement-membrane-like matrix and to purified matrix proteins. *Infection and Immunity* **55**, 2721-2726.

Winkler, J.R., Matarese, V., Hoover, C.I., Kramer, R.H. & Murray, P.A. (1988). An in vitro model to study bacterial invasion of periodontal tissues. *Journal of Periodontology* **59**, 40-45.

Winkler, J.R., Murray, P.A., Grassi, M. & Hammerle, C. (1989). Diagnosis and management of HIV-associated periodontal lesions. *Journal of the American Dental Association* **119**, 25S-34S.

Winkler, J.R. & Robertson, P.B. (1992). Periodontal disease associated with HIV infection. *Oral Surgery, Oral Medicine, Oral Pathology* **73**, 145-150.

Wood, S.R., Kirkham, J., Marsh, P.D., Shore, R.C., Nattress, B. & Robinson, C. (2000). Architecture of intact natural human plaque biofilms studied by confocal lasers canning microscopy. *Journal of Dental Research* **79**, 21-27.

Wyss, C. (1989). Dependence of proliferation of *Bacteroides forsythus* on exogenous N-acetylmuramic acid. *Infection and Immunity* **57**, 1757-1759.

Xie, H., Cook, G.S., Costerton, J.W., Bruce, G., Rose, T.M. & Lamont, R.J. (2000). Intergeneric communication in dental plaque biofilms. *Journal of Bacteriology* **182**, 7067-7069.

Ximenez-Fyvie, L.A., Haffajee, A.D. & Socransky, S.S. (2000). Comparison of the microbiota of supra- and subgingival plaque in subjects in health and periodontitis. *Journal of Clinical Periodontology* **27**, 648-657.

Yoneda, M., Maida, K. & Aono, M. (1990). Suppression of bactericidal activity of human polymorphonuclear leukocytes by *Bacteroides gingivalis*. *Infection and Immunity* **58**, 406-411.

Yoshida-Minami, I., Suzuki, A., Kawabata, K., Okamoto, A., Nishihara, Y., Nagashima, S., Morisaki, I. & Ooshima, T. (1997). Alveolar bone loss in rats infected with a strain of *Prevotella intermedia* and *Fusobacterium nucleatum* isolated from a child with prepubertal periodontitis. *Journal of Periodontology* **68**, 12-17.

Yoshimura, F., Watanabe, K., Takasawa, T., Kawanami, M. & Kato, H. (1989). Purification and properties of a 75-kilodalton major protein, an immunodominant surface antigen, from the oral anaerobe *Bacteroides gingivalis*. *Infection and Immunity* **57**, 3646-3652.

Yuan, K., Chang, C.J., Hsu, P.C., Sun, H.S., Tseng, C.C. & Wang, J.R. (2001). Detection of putative periodontal pathogens in non-insulin-dependent diabetes mellitus and non-diabetes mellitus by polymerase chain reaction. *Journal of Periodontal Research* **36**, 18-24.

Yumoto, H., Nakae, H., Fujinaka, K., Ebisu, S. & Matsuo, T. (1999). Interleukin-6 (IL-6) and IL-8 are induced in human oral epithelial cells in response to exposure to periodontopathic *Eikenella corrodens*. *Infection and Immunity* **67**, 384-394.

Zambon, J.J. (1996). Periodontal diseases: microbial factors. *Annals of Periodontology* **1**, 879-925.

Zambon, J.J., Christersson, L.A. & Slots, J. (1983a). *Actinobacillus actinomycetemcomitans* in human periodontal disease. Prevalence in patient groups and distribution of biotypes and serotypes within families. *Journal of Periodontology* **54**, 707-711.

Zambon, J.J., Reynolds, H., Fisher, J.G., Shlossman, M., Dunford, R. & Genco, R.J. (1988). Microbiological and immunological studies of adult periodontitis in patients with noninsulin-dependent diabetes mellitus. *Journal of Periodontology* **59**, 23-31.

Zambon, J.J., Reynolds, H.S. & Genco, R.J. (1990). Studies of the subgingival microflora in patients with acquired immunodeficiency syndrome. *Journal of Periodontology* **61**, 699-704.

Zambon, J.J., Slots, J. & Genco, R.J. (1983b). Serology of oral *Actinobacillus actinomycetemcomitans* and serotype distribution in human periodontal disease. *Infection and Immunity* **41**. 19-27.

Chapter 5

Host-Parasite Interactions in Periodontal Disease

Denis F. Kinane, Tord Berglundh and Jan Lindhe

INITIATION AND PROGRESSION OF PERIODONTAL DISEASE

Introduction

Current concepts regarding the etiology and patho-genesis of periodontal disease are derived mainly from the results of epidemiological studies, analyses of autopsy and biopsy material, clinical trials and animal experimentation. Findings from epidemiological studies have consistently revealed that the experience and extent of periodontal disease increases with age and with inadequate oral hygiene (see Chapter 3). Studies on the extent and severity of periodontal disease involvement have changed our view on the prevalence and progression of destructive periodontal disease. Relatively few subjects in each age group suffer from advanced periodontal destruction and these few subjects account for most of the sites which are severely periodontally involved (Löe et al. 1986, Papapanou et al. 1988, Yoneyama et al. 1988, Jenkins & Kinane, 1989). In addition, longitudinal studies using large thresholds for declaring disease detection have shown that relatively few sites undergo extensive periodontal destruction within a given observation period and these are found in only a small subset of the population (Haffajee et al. 1983a,b, Lindhe et al. 1983, Jenkins et al. 1988). Socransky et al. (1984) suggested that periodontitis progresses in episodes of exacerbation and remission (the burst hypothesis). More recent studies have suggested that the progression may be more continuous than episodic and that

detection of "bursts" may be due to an inadequate resolution of clinical measurements (Jeffcoat & Reddy 1991).

- In summary, periodontal disease is subject related; only a few individuals experience advanced destruction affecting several teeth; and the progression of the disease is probably continuous with brief episodes of localized exacerbation and remission.

Initiation of periodontal disease

Most normal subjects maintaining a high standard of oral hygiene are not likely to develop advanced periodontal disease. Experimental, short-term clinical studies have shown that microorganisms quickly start to colonize clean tooth surfaces once an individual abstains from mechanical tooth cleaning; within a few days microscopical and clinical signs of gingivitis are then apparent. These inflammatory alterations are resolved or reversed when adequate tooth-cleaning measures are resumed (Löe et al. 1965). Thus, microorganisms which form the dental biofilm contain or release components which induce gingivitis. Consistent with this conclusion is the finding that topical applications of soluble plaque extracts produce inflammatory alterations in gingival tissues (Helldén & Lindhe 1973). Long-term clinical trials have underlined the importance of removing the subgingival biofilm in order to successfully treat periodontal disease in humans (Ramfjord et al. 1968, Lindhe & Nyman 1975, 1984, Axelsson & Lindhe 1978, 1981).

Furthermore, animal experiments (especially in

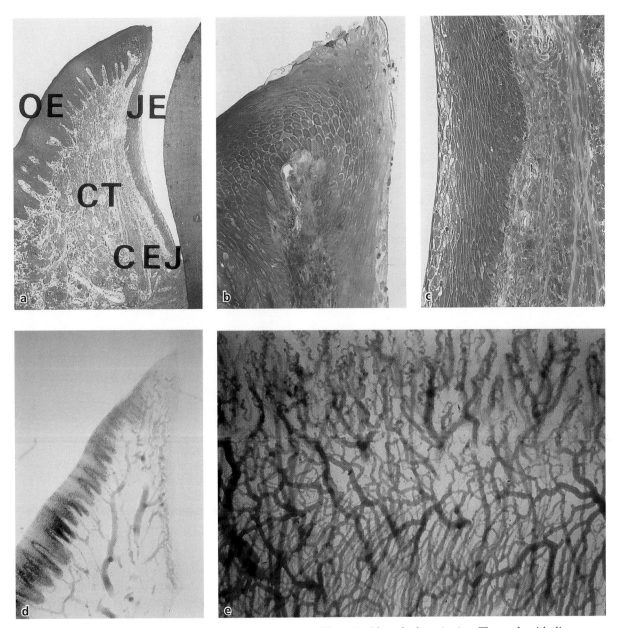

Fig. 5-1. (a) Overview of a buccal-lingual section of a normal (pristine) beagle dog gingiva. The oral epithelium (OE) is continuous with the junctional epithelium (JE), which is facing the enamel surface. CT = connective tissue; CEJ = cemento-enamel junction. (b) Detail of 5-1a. The oral epithelium is continuous with a thin junctional epithelium. Note the presence of neutrophils in the outer portion of the junctional epithelium. (c) The junctional epithelium is only 10-15 cell layers thick and permeable for bacterial products. (d) Micrograph of a buccal-lingual section of a normal (pristine) beagle dog gingiva illustrating the vasculature of the gingival unit. A thin vascular network is present beneath the junctional epithelium. (e) The thin vascular network (plexus) is shown in a mesial-distal section.

dogs and non-human primates) have confirmed the infectious etiology of gingival/periodontal lesions. Long-term observations in beagles, for example, indicate that gingivitis develops only in animals that accumulate plaque. The inflammatory changes may remain confined to the gingival area for several years, but at some sites gingivitis eventually shifts to destructive periodontal disease resulting in loss of connective tissue attachment and alveolar bone (Saxe et al. 1967, Lindhe et al. 1975).

It is implied that most forms of periodontal disease are plaque-associated disorders which start as an overt inflammation of the gingiva. If left untreated, in certain susceptible individuals, inflammation may spread to involve deeper portions of the periodontium. It is not presently understood why, in some patients, lesions remain localized to the marginal portion of the gingival tissues, whilst in others they progress to involve the loss of connective tissue attachment and supporting alveolar bone. The same arguments are true for individual sites within a susceptible individual. Clearly some imbalance of the host-microbial relationship is occurring in the destructive lesions, which may be unique to that site and to periodontally susceptible individuals generally.

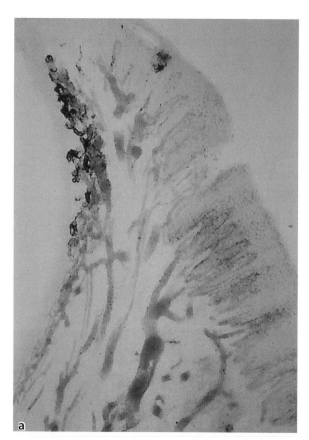

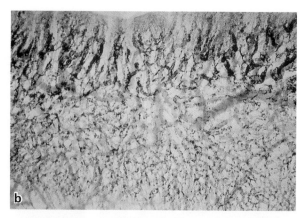

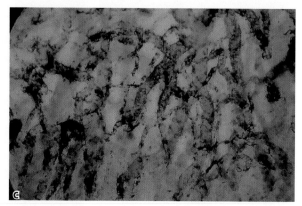

Fig. 5-2. (a) Microphotograph of a buccal-lingual section of a normal beagle dog gingiva. A filter paper-strip has been introduced between the junctional epithelium and the tooth. An increased permeability of the gingival vessels has occurred. The increased vascular permeability is in this case identified by the presence of carbon particles which prior to biopsy were injected intravenously. The carbon particles have become trapped in the open endothelial junctions, and so-called vascular labelling has occurred. (b) A mesio-distal section of the same gingival unit as in Fig. 5-2a. (c) Higher magnification of Fig. 5-2b (from Egelberg 1967).

Normal "clinically healthy" gingiva and "experimental gingivitis"

Normal gingiva is characterized clinically by its pink color and firm consistency and the gingival margin exhibits a scalloped outline. The interdental papillae are firm, do not bleed on gentle probing and fill the space below the contact areas. The gingiva often exhibits a stippled appearance and there is a knife edge margin between tooth and soft tissue. Normal gingivae are theoretically free from histological inflammation but this "ideal" condition can only be established experimentally in humans after supervised meticulous daily plaque control for several weeks. Such fastidious and time consuming oral hygiene measures are uncommon and thus the gingivae we would routinely classify as "clinically healthy gingivae" are not as histologically perfect as the "normal gingivae" described. Clinically healthy gingivae would be typically that level of health which could be attained by patients regularly practising a good standard of plaque control.

Normal gingiva which is free from "significant" accumulations of inflammatory cells may be better described as "pristine gingiva". Thus, in the research literature we have to deal with two types of healthy gingivae, a super healthy or "pristine" state which histologically has little or no inflammatory infiltrate, and the "clinically healthy" gingiva which looks similar clinically but histologically features an inflammatory infiltrate, and is the healthy gingiva we would see clinically in everyday situations. The oral surface of "clinically healthy gingivae" consists of keratinized oral epithelium that is continuous with the junctional epithelium (Fig. 5-1a) and is firmly attached to the tooth surface by hemidesmosomes. Neutrophils and macrophages can be seen in the junctional epithelium. Supporting the oral and junctional epithelia is connective tissue containing prominent collagen fibers which maintain the form of the tissues in health and assist the relatively weak hemidesmosomal attachment of the junctional epithelium to the tooth. Below the junctional epithelium is a vascular network which supplies the epithelium with various nutrients and defense cells and molecules (Fig. 5-1d).

The clinically healthy gingiva features an infiltrate of inflammatory cells, predominantly neutrophils associated with the junctional epithelium and lymphocytes in the subjacent connective tissue (Page & Schroeder 1976). Even in this very early stage of inflammation, which is not clinically detectable, collagen depletion within the infiltrated area is noted along with an increase in vascular structures. Exudative and

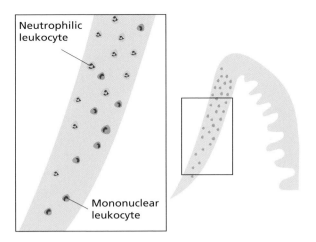

Neutrophilic leukocyte

Mononuclear leukocyte

Fig. 5-3. Leukocytes in the junctional epithelium. Observe that the volume of leukocytes decreases in apical direction and approaches 0 in the most apical portion. Within the junctional epithelium, the mononuclear leukocytes are located in more basal layers, while the neutrophilic granulocytes are present primarily in the superficial portions of the junctional epithelium.

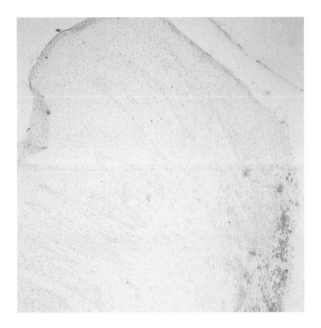

Fig. 5-4. Immunostained section showing neutrophils in the junctional epithelium of healthy gingiva.

transudative fluid and plasma proteins arrive in the gingival crevice region having left the vessels and travelled through the tissues to create the gingival crevicular fluid (GCF) (Egelberg 1967, Cimasoni 1983) (Figs. 5-1 and 5-2). The infiltrate at this stage may occupy as much as 5% of the connective tissue volume and is composed of monocytes, macrophages, lymphocytes and neutrophils. These cells are found in the junctional epithelium as well as in the connective tissue of clinically healthy gingivae (Fig. 5-3). Neutrophils predominate in the crevice region and appear to migrate continuously through the junctional epithelium into the sulcus (Fig. 5-4). The recruitment of leukocytes (predominantly PMNs) from the tissues to the crevice is due both to the chemoattractant actions of the host systems (interleukin-8, complement component C5a, leukotriene B4 etc., see below) and products derived from the biofim (formyl methionyl leucyl phenylalanine, lipopolysaccharide etc). With further deposition of plaque and the development of overt gingivitis, there is a marked increase in leukocytes recruited to the area (Attström, 1971, Moughal et al.1992). One additional effect of the inflammation

which encourages rapid accumulation of leukocytes is the pro-inflammatory cytokine-mediated upregulation of adhesion molecules on the endothelial cells. This encourages leukocytes, particularly PMNs, in the early stages to adhere to postcapillary venules and begin migrating through the vessel and chemotacting to the gingival crevice. This upregulation of adhesion molecules (ICAM-1 and ELAM-1) occurs during "experimental gingivitis" (Löe et al. 1965) with a concomitant increase in leukocyte infiltration which corresponds with days of plaque accumulation (Kinane et al. 1991, Moughal et al. 1992) (Fig. 5-5).

Clinically healthy gingiva appears to deal with microbial challenges without progressing to a diseased state, probably because of several defensive factors which include:

1. Regular shedding of epithelial cells into the oral cavity
2. Intact epithelial barrier
3. Positive fluid flow of the gingival crevice which may remove non-attached microorganisms and noxious products

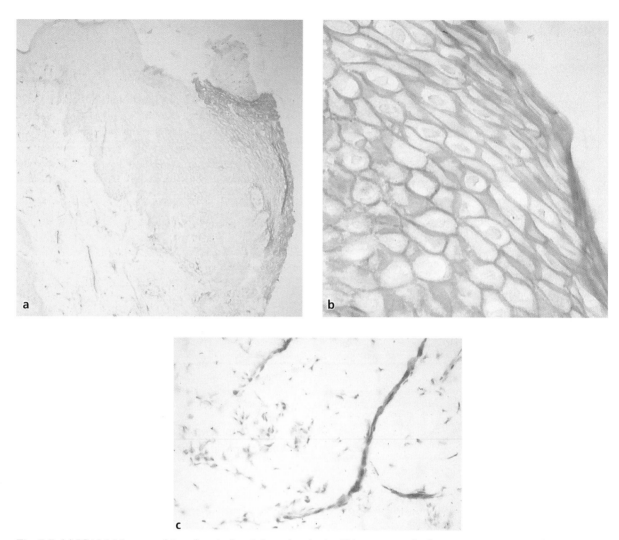

Fig. 5-5. (a) ICAM-1 immunohistochemical staining of a gingival biopsy sample during an experimental gingivitis study in humans after day 7. ICAM-1 positive blood vessels and junctional epithelium can be clearly seen.
(b) Higher magnification of Fig 5-5a showing the extensive junctional epithelium staining. (c) Higher magnification of Fig 5-5a showing the ICAM-1 positive vessels within the connective tissue.

4. Antimicrobial effect of antibodies
5. Phagocytic function of neutrophils and macrophages
6. Detrimental effect of complement on the microbiota.

All of these factors may operate at the same time to reduce the bacterial load and thus prevent an over-response of the tissue defense systems which could result in the formation of a lesion. The host-microbial interplay which constitutes the clinically healthy situation must clearly change if gingivitis and periodontitis is to follow. Gingivitis will follow if there is sufficient plaque accumulation such that microbial products will initiate a substantive inflammatory response. This response can be modified by hormones as in the case of puberty or pregnancy (resulting in edematous gingivitis) or by drugs such as phenytoin, cyclosporin or nidefipine (which induce gingival overgrowth). Gingivitis lesions are accompanied by more pronounced loss of collagen albeit in discrete areas. The gingivitis response will also initiate and perpetuate

immune responses to the oral microorganisms but the level of this early response, particularly at the local site, will be considerably less than the gross tissue destruction and bone loss seen in more advanced periodontitis lesions. Gingivitis may persist at sites for many years without appreciable loss of periodontal attachment, destruction of periodontal ligament or evidence of bone loss. Clearly certain individuals (and sites) go on to develop periodontitis from gingivitis lesions whilst others remain resistant and merely exhibit gingivitis responses to the accumulating plaque microorganisms. Investigations of periodontal manifestations of systemic disease suggest that individuals with obvious defects of the inflammatory system, e.g. neutrophil depletion or dysfunction, may rapidly develop severe periodontitis. In addition, there appears to be a genetic predisposition to both aggressive and chronic forms of periodontitis (Michalowicz et al. 2000, Hodge & Michalowicz 2001). There is an accumulating body of evidence which suggests that the host's immune response to periodontopathogens may be quite different in those affected by chronic perio-

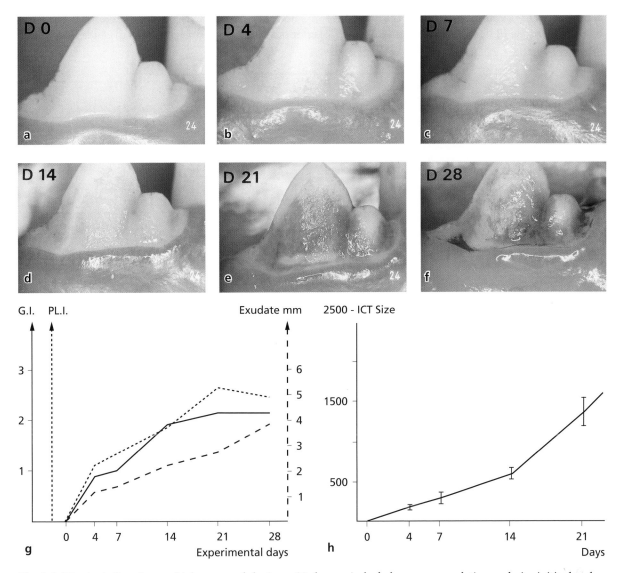

Fig. 5-6. Gingival alterations which occurred during a 28-day period of plaque accumulation and gingivitis development in beagles. (a) Normal gingival. (b) Day 4. (c) Day 7. (d) Day 14. (e) Day 21. (f) Day 28 of undisturbed plaque accumulation. Note the gradually developing plaque on the tooth surfaces and the inflammatory changes in the gingiva. The vascular reaction is illustrated by a gradually increasing number of vessels in the gingival margin. (g) Gingival index (GI), plaque index (PLI) and gingival exudate alterations (exudate) that occurred during the experimental gingivitis period. (h) In gingival biopsies obtained at various time intervals it can be seen that the inflammatory cell infiltrate (ICT) in the gingiva gradually increased in size.

dontitis and those resistant to this disease, who would not progress beyond gingivitis. There is also evidence that "protective" antibodies increase following a course of initial periodontal therapy, whereas those individuals with a poor outcome following periodontal therapy have antibodies which are less functional (Mooney et al. 1995).

Initial, early, established and advanced lesions

Introduction
Within 10-20 days of plaque accumulation, clinical signs of gingivitis are established in most individuals, although this varies greatly with some individuals being intrinsically more resistant and others more prone to overt gingivitis (Van der Weijden et al. 1993). This gingivitis appears as gingival redness, swelling and an increased tendency of the soft tissue to bleed on gentle probing (Fig. 5-6). Even at this stage clinical signs are reversible following removal of microbial plaque by effective plaque control measures (Löe et al. 1965, Lindhe & Rylander 1975).

Histopathological features of gingival inflammation
The clinical changes may appear subtle in the early stages of gingivitis but the underlying histopathological changes are quite marked. Alterations in the vascular network occur with many capillary beds being opened up. Exudative fluid and proteins swell the tissues and an influx of inflammatory cells in the connective tissue occurs subjacent to the junctional epithelium. The inflammatory cell infiltrate mainly

Table 5-1. Size (% volume) of various components of the normal connective tissue (NCT) and the infiltrated connective tissue (ICT) at various days (4, 14 and 28) after onset of plaque formation (from Lindhe & Rylander 1975)

Parameter	Normal connective tissue (NCT) %	Infiltrated connective tissue (ICT) %		
	(Day 0)	Day 4	Day 14	Day 28
Size of infiltrate	0	5	15	37
Collagen filters	60	20	24	30
Fibroblasts	13	8	7	7
Vessels	7	22	14	16
Residual tissue	20	40	45	36
Neutrophils	0.5	8	4	1
Plasma cells Lymphocytes Macrophages	0.1	3	0.1	3

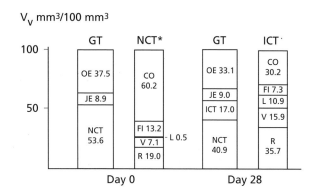

V_v mm3/100 mm3

Fig. 5-7. Composition of the gingiva (GT), non-infiltrated (NCT) and infiltrated (ICT) gingival connective tissue on day 0 (normal gingiva) and on day 28 of gingivitis in beagles. Note that the infiltrated connective tissue portion amounts to 17% of the free gingival margin on day 28 and that the collagen content is reduced from approximately 60% on day 0 to 30% on day 28 in the area where the inflammatory infiltrate has become established. Note also that in this area (on day 28) a reduction in fibroblast proportion has occurred, as well as an increase of vessels and residual tissue. OE: oral epithelium, JE: junctional epithelium, NCT: non-infiltrated connective tissue, ICT: infiltrated connective tissue, CO: collagen fibers, FI: fibroblasts, V: vascular structures, L: leukocytes, R: residual tissue. (From Lindhe & Rylander 1975)

comprises lymphocytes, macrophages and neutrophils. As the cellular infiltrate develops, the structural and cellular composition of the tissues changes. An experimental gingivitis study in dogs has compared the cellular and structural composition of the affected area before and during the development of gingivitis over a period of 28 days (Lindhe & Rylander 1975). Plaque was allowed to accumulate on the teeth of dogs with initially normal gingiva, and biopsy samples were taken at various times. The normal tissue (Day 0) is referred to below as non-infiltrated connective tissue (NCT) and the altered area as the infiltrated connective tissue (ICT) (Table 5-1).

At Day 0 of this dog experiment the normal gingival unit has virtually no inflammatory cells (Fig. 5-7) and is comprised of approximately 40-45% epithelium and 55-60% connective tissue. The NCT zone consists of collagen (60%), fibroblasts (13%), vessels (7%) and other tissue constituents, such as intercellular matrix and nerves (20%). Following plaque accumulation, neutrophils and mononuclear leukocytes readily mi-

grate to this area and the ICT begins to form and increase in volume over the 28-day period. At this 28-day interval the ICT is comprised of lymphocytes, plasma cells and macrophages (Fig. 5-7) which adhere to the collagen matrix and remain in the tissue, whereas neutrophils continue to migrate into the gingival sulcus. With the extensive influx of leukocytes, a marked reduction in the amount of collagen and fibroblasts occurs and the volume of residual tissue (intercellular matrix, degraded collagen, exudate material, degenerated or dead cells) and small blood vessels increases.

In 1976, Page and Schroeder classified the progression of gingival and periodontal inflammation on the basis of the then available clinical and histopathological evidence. They divided the progressing lesion into four phases: *initial, early, established* and *advanced* stages or lesions. The initial and early lesion descriptions were thought to reflect the histopathology of clinically early stages of gingivitis, while the established lesion reflected the histopathology of more

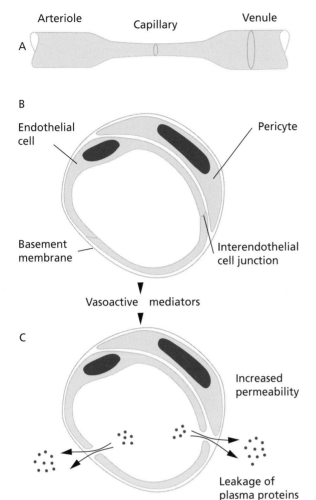

Fig. 5-8. Schematic illustrations depicting the terminal vascular bed and the mechanisms of increased vascular permeability. Under normal conditions the terminal vessels are freely permeable to small molecules, salt and water. The intercellular junctions between the endothelial cells are closed. Via the influence of vasoactive mediators the endothelial cells become separated and increased vascular permeability occurs. Large molecules and plasma proteins leak into surrounding tissue. A number of inflammatory mediators present in plasma are activated when they enter the perivascular tissue.

"chronic" gingivitis. The description of the histopathology of the advanced lesion was considered to reflect the progression of gingivitis to periodontitis. The evidence on which these descriptions were based was the prevailing information gleaned predominantly from animal biopsy material and some human adolescent samples. Therefore the following account by Page and Schroeder (1976) of lesion progression is based very much on data from non-human experiments.

The classical phases of "acute" and "chronic" inflammation are not easily applied in periodontal disease, probably because in most clinically healthy situations a lesion similar to an acute lesion occurs. Subsequently, chronic inflammatory changes become superimposed so that both acute and chronic elements co-exist in early, established and advanced lesions. It is important to repeat that in most clinically "normal" human gingival biopsies a similar infiltrate can be seen to that noted in the initial and early gingival lesions of dogs. The Page and Schroeder system will be utilized as a framework to outline the histopathogenesis of periodontal disease and modern conflicting views will be outlined. A rational synthesis of opinions will be attempted and a new classification based on our current understanding of lesion progression will be presented (Table 5-2).

Table 5-2. A new classification is outlined

Clinical condition	Histopathologic condition
Pristine gingiva	Histologic perfection
Normal health gingiva	Initial lesion of Page & Schroeder
Early gingivitis	Early lesion of Page & Schroeder (few plasma cells)
Established gingivitis	Established lesion with no bone loss nor apical epithelial migration (plasma cell density between 10% and 30% of leukocyte infiltrate)
Periodontitis	Established lesion with bone loss and apical epithelial migration from the amelocemental junction (plasma cell density > 50%)

The initial lesion

Inflammation quickly develops as plaque is deposited on the tooth. Within 24 hours marked changes are evident in the microvascular plexus beneath the junctional epithelium as more blood is brought to the area. Dilation of the arterioles, capillaries and venules of the dentogingival plexus is evident histopathologically. Hydrostatic pressure within the microcirculation increases and intercellular gaps form between adjacent

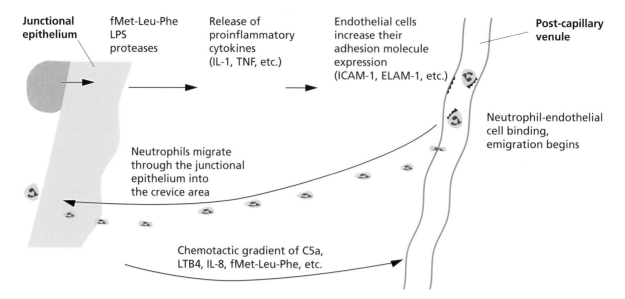

Fig. 5-9. Schematic illustration of the process whereby neutrophils are attracted into the junctional epithelium and crevice region.

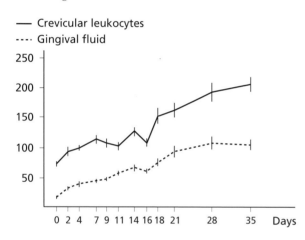

Fig. 5-10. Alterations in number of crevicular leukocytes and in gingival fluid during a period of developing gingivitis in beagles. Note the gradual increase of leukocytes and fluid flow during the experimental period. (From Attström & Egelberg 1970.)

capillary endothelial cells. An increase in the permeability of the microvascular bed results, so that fluids and proteins exude into the tissues (Fig. 5-8).

As the lesion enlarges, and gingival crevicular fluid flow increases, noxious substances from microbes will be diluted both in the tissue and the crevice. Bacteria and their products may thus be flushed from the sulcus. Plasma proteins escaping from the microcirculation include defensive proteins such as antibodies, complement and protease inhibitors and other macromolecules with numerous functions, which will be discussed below. This gingival crevicular fluid (GCF) can be readily sampled by placing filter strips at the gingival margin to absorb the exudate. The volume of the exudate is proportional to the severity of the gingival inflammation present (Fig. 5-6). The absolute amounts and the concentration of various plasma proteins, tissue proteases, inhibitors and breakdown products and leukocyte enzymes in the gingival sulcus have been studied extensively. GCF components are considered as very useful markers of the inflammatory process and are currently being developed as diagnostic markers of periodontal disease.

Simultaneously with these vascular alterations,

PMN cell migration from the dentogingival vascular system is enhanced by the adhesion molecules, intercellular adhesion molecule-1 (ICAM-1) and endothelial leukocyte adhesion molecule-1 (ELAM-1) and other adhesins. These molecules assist PMNs binding to the post capillary venules and help the cells to leave the blood vessel (Fig. 5-9). The leukocytes migrate up a chemoattractant gradient to the crevice and are probably further assisted in their movement by the adhesion molecules uniquely present on the junctional epithelial cells (Fig. 5-5) (Moughal et al. 1992) and by the presence of host and microbial chemotactic factors. Lymphocytes may be retained in tissues on contact with antigens, cytokines or adhesion molecules and thus are not so readily lost through the junctional epithelium and into oral cavity, as are PMNs. Most lymphocytes have the ability to produce CD44 (CD = cluster determinant) receptors on their surfaces, which permit binding of the cell to the connective tissue framework. This is consistent with the T and B cell requirement to remain within the tissues and to perform cell mediated and humoral immune functions locally.

Probably within 2-4 days of plaque build-up the

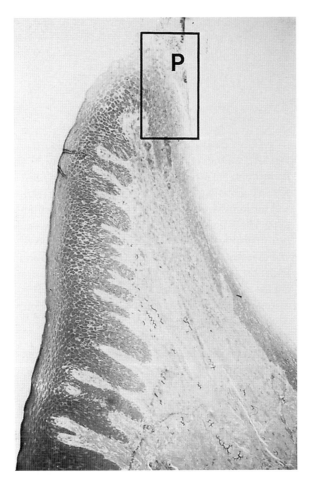 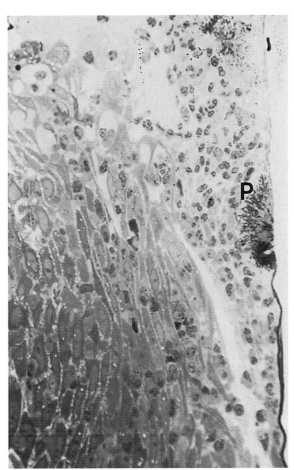

Fig. 5-11. Buccolingual section of the gingiva on day 4 of developing gingivitis in a beagle. Note plaque (P) in the sulcus region and increased cellularity in the coronal part of the connective tissue below the junctional epithelium. Note the presence of leukocytes in the coronal part of the junctional epithelium and at the surfaces of the subgingival plaque.

cellular response is well established and is helped by chemotactic substances originating from the plaque microbiota as well as from host cells and secretions. PMNs move through the connective tissue and the majority seem to accumulate in the junctional epithelium and gingival sulcus region (Figs 5-9 and 5-10).

The early lesion

The early gingival lesion occurs after approximately one week of plaque accumulation (Fig. 5-11). Only an approximation of the time required can be given as marked subject variation occurs in humans although this may well be less variable in animal models. The variation seen amongst humans could be due to differences in plaque accumulation, both at the site and subject level, or to differences between individuals in features such as hormonal levels. Histologically the vessels below the junctional epithelium remain dilated, but their numbers increase due to the opening up of previously inactive capillary beds (compare Fig. 5-1 and 5-12). The course, size and quantity of microvasculature units are reflected in the clinical appearance of the gingival margin during this phase (Egelberg 1967, Lindhe & Rylander 1975).

Lymphocytes and PMNs are the predominant infiltrating leukocytes at this stage and very few plasma

cells are noted within the lesion (Listgarten & Ellegaard 1973, Payne et al. 1975, Seymour et al. 1983, Brecx et al. 1987). The inflammatory cell infiltrate may at this stage comprise as much as 15% of the connective tissue volume. Within the lesion fibroblasts degenerate. This probably occurs by apoptosis and serves to remove fibroblasts from the area, thus permitting more leukocyte infiltration (Page & Schroeder 1976, Takahashi et al. 1995). Similarly collagen destruction occurs in the infiltrated area and is necessary in order that the tissues can be pushed apart to accommodate the infiltrating cells and thus could be considered as a space creating process. Inflammatory changes are detectable clinically at this stage and nearing the end of the second week of plaque accumulation, a subgingivally located biofilm can be found.

The basal cells of the junctional and sulcular epithelium have now proliferated. This represents an attempt by the body to enhance the innate barrier to plaque (Fig. 5-13). Epithelial rete pegs can be seen invading the coronal portion of the lesion (Schroeder 1970, Schroeder et al. 1973).

The duration of the early lesion in humans has not been determined. The early lesion may persist for much longer than previously thought and the variability in time required to produce an established

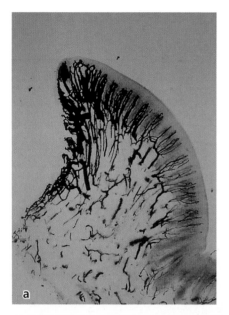

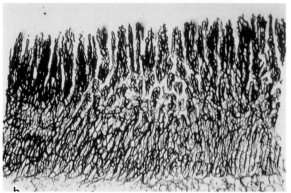

Fig. 5-12. (a) Buccolingual section of chronically inflamed gingiva in a dog. The vessels have been filled with a contrasting carbon suspension. Note the wide and tortuous vessels below the junctional epithelium to the left in the illustration. Compare with the vasculature in healthy gingiva in Fig. 5-10. The pronounced vascular reaction in this area is a result of plaque accumulation. (b) Mesiodistal section of a gingiva illustrating the vessels below the junctional epithelium of chronically inflamed gingiva. Note vascular dilation and proliferation at the level of the gingival margin (GM). Note also that vascular proliferation has occurred in the apical part of the vascular plexus (from Egelberg 1967).

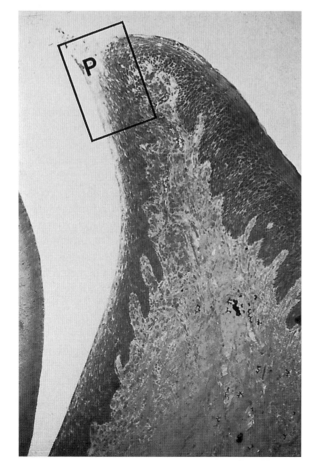

Fig. 5-13. Buccolingual section of the gingiva on day 7 of developing gingivitis in a beagle. Note the subgingival extension of plaque (P), as well as the increased number of inflammatory cells in the connective tissue below the dentogingival epithelium.

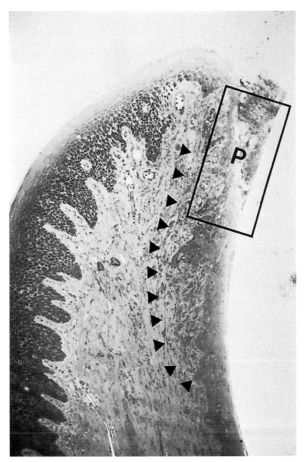

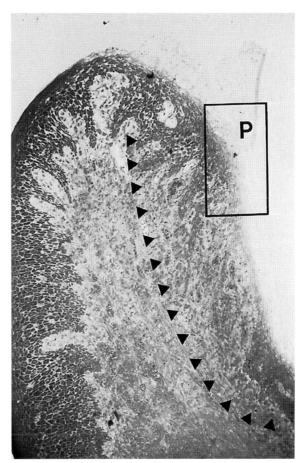

Fig. 5-14. Buccolingual section of the gingiva on day 21 of developing gingivitis in a beagle. Compare with Fig. 5-15. Note the extension of the subgingival plaque (P) as well as the apical extension of the infiltrate (the lesion) in the connective tissue.

Fig. 5-15. Buccolingual section of the gingiva on day 28 of gingivitis development in a beagle. Note the extension of the subgingival plaque (P) and the increased number of leukocytes in the connective tissue below the junctional epithelium. Note rete pegs in the dentogingival epithelium.

lesion may reflect susceptibility variance within and between subjects.

The established lesion

Generally there is a further enhancement of the inflammatory state as exposure to plaque continues. There is increased fluid exudation and leukocyte migration into the tissues and the gingival crevice. Clinically this lesion will exhibit more edematous swelling than the "early gingivitis" lesion and could be considered as "established gingivitis".

The established lesion as defined by Page and Schroeder is one dominated by plasma cells. This conclusion was based mainly on data from animal experiments. However, Brecx et al. (1988) demonstrated that even following 6 months of oral hygiene neglect, the plasma cell fraction in human biopsies comprised only 10% of the cellular infiltrate and was clearly not the dominant cell type. Thus, the human established lesion apparently requires much more time to "mature" than its animal counterparts.

In the established lesion described by Page and Schroeder (1976), plasma cells are seen situated primarily in the coronal connective tissues as well as

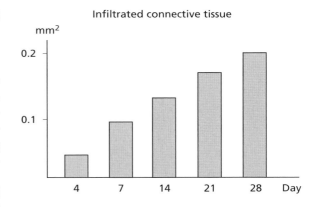

Fig. 5-16. Diagram showing the increase in size of the infiltrated connective tissue during the development of gingivitis in beagles (from Mattsson & Attström 1979).

around vessels. Collagen loss continues in both lateral and apical directions as the inflammatory cell infiltrate expands, resulting in collagen depleted spaces extending deeper into the tissues which are then available for leukocytic infiltration (Figs. 5-14, 5-15, 5-16). During this time the dentogingival epithelium contin-

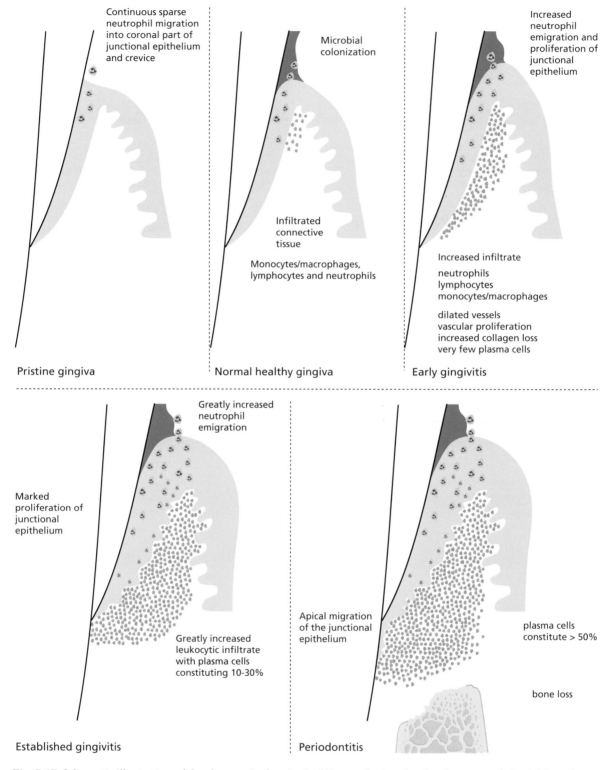

Fig. 5-17. Schematic illustration of the changes in the gingival tissues during the development of gingivitis and periodontitis. The most significant differences are in the extent and composition of the inflammatory infiltrate and the epithelial proliferation in gingivitis, and the apical migration of epithelium and bone loss seen in periodontitis lesions.

ues to proliferate and the rete pegs extend deeper into the connective tissue in an attempt to maintain epithelial integrity and a barrier to microbial entry. The junctional epithelium is changed and is no longer closely attached to the tooth surface. The pocket epithelium that now has formed has a heavy leukocyte infiltrate, predominantly of PMNs which eventually

migrate across the epithelium into the gingival pocket. In comparison to the original junctional epithelium, the pocket epithelium is more permeable to the passage of substances into and out of the underlying connective tissues and may in places be temporarily ulcerated. Fig. 5-17 schematically illustrates the alterations which occur in the epithelium and the connective tissue during the development of gingivitis and periodontitis.

Two types of established lesion appear to exist: one remains stable and is not progressing for months or years (Lindhe et al. 1975, Page et al. 1975), while the second becomes more active and converts to a progressive and destructive advanced lesion.

The advanced lesion

The final stage in this process is known as the advanced lesion. As the pocket deepens, probably due to the epithelium spreading apically in response to plaque irritation and further short-lived and microscopic destructive episodes, plaque continues its apical downgrowth and flourishes in this anaerobic ecological niche. The inflammatory cell infiltrate extends laterally and further apically into the connective tissues. The advanced lesion has all the characteristics of the established lesion but differs importantly in that alveolar bone loss occurs, fiber damage is extensive, the junctional epithelium migrates apically from the cemento-enamel junction, and there are widespread manifestations of inflammatory and immunopathological tissue damage. The lesion is no longer localized to the gingival, and the inflammatory cell infiltrate extends laterally and apically into the connective tissue of the true attachment apparatus. It is generally accepted that plasma cells are the dominant cell type in the advanced lesion (Garant & Mulvihill 1972). There are major similarities between the established lesion of "chronic gingivitis" and the advanced lesion of "chronic periodontitis".

- In summary, in the progression from health to gingivitis and on to periodontitis there are many unknown factors related to timing. In addition, there is extensive subject and site variability in both exacerbating factors and innate susceptibility.

HOST-PARASITE INTERACTIONS

Introduction

Inflammatory and immune reactions to microbial plaque are the predominant features of gingivitis and periodontitis. The inflammatory reaction is visible both microscopically and clinically in the affected periodontium and represents the host's response to the plaque microbiota and its products.

Inflammatory and immune processes operate in the gingival tissues to protect against local microbial attack and prevent microorganisms from spreading or invading into the tissues. In some cases these host defense reactions may be harmful to the host in that inflammation can damage surrounding cells and connective tissue structures. Furthermore, inflammatory and immune reactions extending deeper into the connective tissue beyond the base of the pocket may also include alveolar bone loss in this destructive process. Thus, these "defensive" processes may paradoxically account for much of the tissue injury observed in gingivitis and periodontitis.

Whilst inflammatory and immune reactions within the periodontal tissues may appear similar to those seen elsewhere in the body, there are significant differences. To some extent this is a consequence of the anatomy of the periodontium (see Chapter 1), i.e. the permeable junctional epithelium that has remarkable cell and fluid dynamics and that at all times seeks to preserve epithelial continuity across the hard and soft tissue interface. In addition, inflammatory and immune processes in periodontal tissues are a response, not simply to one microbial species, but to large numbers of microbes – that reside outside the soft tissue – and their products acting over a long period.

Periodontal disease has sometimes been referred to as a "mixed bacterial infection" to denote that more than one microbial species contributes to the development of disease. Microbial species interact, and although some may not be overtly pathogenic they may still influence the disease process, promoting the virulence potential of other microbes by providing specific growth or defensive factors for them. The microbiota in periodontal pockets is in a state of continual flux; species which are relevant at one stage of disease may not be important at another. In other words, periodontal destruction may result from combinations of bacterial factors which vary over time. This contrasts with most other classical infectious diseases (e.g. tuberculosis, syphilis, gonorrhea) where the host contends with one organism and the diagnosis of the disease state is indicated by the presence of this pathogen.

The pathogenicity of microorganisms relates as much to the particular host's innate and/or inflammatory and/or immune capability, as to the virulence of the bacteria themselves. For example, periodontal destruction could result from microbial enzymes that directly digest the tissue or from inflammation and/or from immune reponses to these enzymes. In addition, destructive responses might result from the host's inflammatory or immune reaction to normal physiological components of the bacteria such as the lipopolysaccharides found in the outer membrane of Gram-negative bacteria.

Epidemiological studies have shown that even within the same individual, the severity of periodontal tissue injury often varies from tooth to tooth and from one tooth surface to another. Thus, whilst many teeth within an individual mouth may exhibit advanced loss of connective tissue attachment and alveolar bone, other teeth or tooth surfaces (sites) may be almost unaffected and surrounded by a normal periodontium. Hence, a patient who is susceptible to, and exhibiting, periodontal disease is not afflicted with a "homogenous" condition. Each affected site in his/her mouth represents an "individualized" or "specific" microenvironment. In some sites, the inflammatory lesion may be contained within the gingiva (gingivitis) for prolonged periods of time without any apparent progression of the disease into deeper tissues. In other sites, active periodontal destruction (periodontitis) may occur and may be a consequence of a variety of host and parasite factors, a discussion of which now follows.

Microbial virulence factors

Periodontal disease is initiated and sustained by factors (substances) produced by the subgingival microbiota (the biofilm). Some of these substances can directly injure host cells and tissues. Other microbial constituents may activate inflammatory or cellular and humoral immune systems which secondarily damage the periodontium. It is the latter pathway which accounts for most periodontal injury.

In this context, however, *microbial invasion* of the soft tissues should be considered. Invasion of the dentogingival epithelium by spirochetes was conclusively documented in lesions of necrotizing ulcerative gingivitis (Listgarten 1965). Although there have been numerous reports of microbial invasion in other forms of periodontitis, the significance of these observations is unclear. In terms of *in vivo* and *in vitro* demonstrations of invasion the evidence is conflicting with no clear understanding emerging. Even if bacteria enter into the tissues, it is not known whether this represents true invasion (i.e. microbial colonization and proliferation within the tissues) or displacement or translocation of the bacteria from the biofilm into the soft tissues during late stages of disease. Thus, it is not known whether microbial invasion presents an important challenge to the host or is merely artifactual, or whether the process may actually benefit the host by early exposure of microbial antigens to the host immune system so that an effective immune response can be developed.

Microorganisms produce a variety of soluble enzymes in order to digest extracellularly host proteins and other molecules and thereby produce nutrients for their growth. They also release numerous metabolic waste products, such as ammonia, indole, hydrogen sulfide and butyric acid.

Amongst the enzymes released by bacteria are *proteases* (proteinases) capable of digesting collagen, elastin, fibronectin, fibrin and various other components of the intercellular matrix of epithelial and connective tissues. One protease that has attracted much attention is the Arg1-protease produced by *P. gingivalis* for which high potency is claimed. This protease, in addition, has the capability to induce a strong humoral immune response (Aduse-Opoku et al. 1995). *Leukotoxin* was in the focus of interest for many years, but as yet no *in vivo* evidence exists for its claimed role in periodontal tissue destruction (Haubek et al. 1995). This leukotoxin has been researched in both America and Europe but it appears that the strains investigated differ (Haubek et al. 1995). It appears that the more

virulent form of *A. actinomycetemcomitans* which produces leukotoxin in excess and thus has great capacity to kill leukocytes, is common in the US but virtually absent in European strains.

Lipopolysaccharides (LPS) (endotoxins) of Gram-negative microorganisms are capable of invoking both the inflammatory and immune responses as they interact with host cells. Many of the functions attributed to LPS in the past were associated with their cytokine stimulating actions but also with the many outer membrane molecules, proteins and enzymes, bound in the LPS molecules. LPS has also been shown to have profound effects on the blood coagulation system and the complement system resulting in altered hemostasis and the formation of various pro-inflammatory peptides. The reported properties of LPS and of *lipoteichoic acids* (LTA) of Gram-positive organisms are numerous and may be due to the many other molecules associated with these outer membrane structures. LPS, LTA and the specific proteins or polysaccharides produced and released from subgingival microorganisms activate chemical mediators of inflammation to produce vascular permeability and encourage, through chemotactic actions, inflammatory cells to move into the tissues and invoke defense cells to release pro-inflammatory agents and cytokines.

Immune responses to microorganisms will mainly be directed against outer membrane proteins and polysaccharides and against extracellularly released enzymes and toxins. These immune reactions will result in further release of cytokines and proinflammatory mediators which in turn will increase the inflammation and thus be more harmful to the host. Currently interest in specific molecules is increased, particularly molecules from *P. gingivalis*, which may be capable of generating a strong immunological reaction. These so called immunodominant molecules include Arg1-protease, fimbrillin (types I and II), heat shock proteins and various other surface antigens thought to be capable of inducing an excessive antibody response. If these molecules prove to be truly immunodominant, this could suggest that they are important pathogenic factors in periodontitis and thus may be worth targeting in immunological based therapeutic strategies. One major difficulty in designing and developing an effective periodontal disease vaccine is the multiplicity of putative periodontopathogens, i.e. although one microbial species or strain may be successfully eradicated, other members of the extensive flora may replace them and take over their role in the pathogenic process.

- In summary, microbes are capable of producing a variety of substances which either directly or indirectly harm the host. The main detrimental effect may be the host's own immune response to the foreign antigens which the microbes present.

Host defense processes

Host parasite reactions can be divided into innate (non-specific) and adaptive (specific) responses. Innate reactions include the inflammatory response and do not involve immunological mechanisms. Adaptive reactions that include immunological responses tend to be more effective as the host response is specifically "tailored" to the offending pathogen(s).

The innate defense systems
Innate immune mechanisms operate without any previous contact with the disease-causing microorganism. These mechanisms include the *physical barriers* of the oral mucosal epithelial surfaces and *vascular* and *cellular* aspects of the *inflammatory responses*.

The *epithelial surface* is the first region of the periodontium which comes into contact with and responds to bacteria attaching and colonizing the dento-gingival region. Prevention of attachment and colonisation is important for the host defenses and this is achieved through multiple innate mechanisms which include the washing effect of the *saliva* and *gingival crevicular fluid (GCF)*, the *constituents* of these fluids such as antibodies and proteases, complement, salivary antibacterial agents and lactoferrin and other salivary proteins which are detrimental to bacterial growth and can be bactericidal. The oral mucosa itself is not simply a barrier but has a chemical composition which may be detrimental to bacteria. Furthermore, the cells of the epithelium can respond to the bacteria by (1) producing and/or releasing cytokines and other molecules that kill the microbes and (2) releasing other molecules (such as IL-1) capable of inducing or enhancing the inflammatory reaction. The epithelium can also respond by increasing expression of surface molecules such as cell adhesion molecules which can function with cytokines and chemoattractants to bring leukocytes to the region.

Molecules in saliva such as *lactoferrin* have several detrimental effects on bacteria, which include the binding and restriction of iron in the environment that prevents microbial growth. In addition, lactoferrin is also highly cidal for bacteria. Molecules present in the GCF include *complement*, which can kill bacteria directly or together with antibodies, and can bring PMNs to the region (via chemotaxis). The presence of PMNs may be further detrimental to the bacteria.

The concept that epithelial and other non-leukocytic cells such as endothelial cells and even fibroblasts are not involved in specific immune or inflammatory reactions has been disproved as we continually uncover specificity in what we previously viewed as innate defense systems. Toll-like receptors on epithelial and endothelial cells which bind microbial lipopolysaccharides and molecules such as *defensins* (from serum) have specificity to particular bacteria. This indicates that even innate responses of the host can be tailored to particular bacteria. These findings have further influenced the way we currently view host-microbe interactions in infectious disease. Host and pathogens have developed together over millions of years and have learned to mimic and utilize each other's systems in highly sophisticated ways.

Inflammatory processes
The host has an extensive repertoire of defensive responses to ward off invasion by pathogens. Effective responses either result in a rapidly resolving lesion (e.g. a staphylococcal abscess which heals) or no lesion at all (e.g. smallpox infection in a successfully vaccinated host). An ineffective response may result in a chronic lesion which does not resolve (e.g. tuberculosis) or if excessively deployed, in a lesion in which the host responses contribute significantly to the destructive process (e.g. rheumatoid arthritis or asthma).

In the classical description of inflammation an area is presented which appears macroscopically red, swollen, hot and painful, and with possible loss of function in specific sites. Redness and heat are due to vasodilatation and increased blood flow. Swelling is a result of increased vascular permeability and leakage of plasma proteins which create an osmotic potential that draws fluid into the inflamed tissues. Related to the vascular changes there is an accumulation of inflammatory cells infiltrating the lesion. Pain is rarely experienced in periodontal disease, particularly in the early stages, but could theoretically occur due to stimulation of afferent nerves by chemical mediators of inflammation (necrotizing ulcerative gingivitis where rapid tissue destruction is typical) and pressure from vastly increased tissue tension (typical of periodontal abscesses). Impairment of function is classically illustrated in arthritically swollen joints. An oral example of impaired function is the reduced opening or trismus of the mandible sometimes associated with pericoronitis in the third molar region. A periodontal example of loss of function would be the reduced masticatory efficiency of mobile teeth following advanced tissue destruction in periodontitis.

Molecules, cells and processes

Proteinases (proteases)
Periodontal disease results in tissue degradation, and thus proteases, both host and microbial, are central to the destructive processes. Proteinases, or proteases, cleave proteins by hydrolyzing peptide bonds and may be classified into two major classes, *endopeptidases* and *exopeptidases*, depending on the location of activity of the enzyme on its substrate. Endopeptidases cleave bonds in their substrate within the polypeptide chain, whereas the exopeptidases cleave their substrate near the end of the polypeptide chain. Numerous studies have been conducted in order to assess endopeptidase activity and concentrations in gingival crevicular fluid. These studies include both experimental gingivitis (where volunteers abstain from toothbrushing for several weeks), cross-sectional studies (of periodontitis patients) and longitudinal

studies before and after periodontal treatment. In most cases assessment of proteases has been by their enzyme activity, although immunoassays have also been used. A reduction of protease levels following treatment has been obtained in most studies. Endopeptidase activity, including collagenase, elastase-like and trypsin-like, as well as serine and cysteine proteinases, has also been detected in homogenates of gingival tissue.

Proteinase inhibitors

Release of proteases in the gingivae and the crevicular area promotes inflammatory reactions and contributes to connective tissue damage via several pathways. In contrast, *proteinase inhibitors* would serve as modulators of protease function in the area and would dampen the inflammatory process. All the host derived endopeptidases known to be released into the gingival crevice can be inhibited by the combined function of alpha-2 macroglobulin (A2-M) and alpha-1 antitrypsin (A1-AT). In fact, gingival collagenase inhibition by A2-M has been demonstrated and polymorphonuclear leukocyte (PMN) collagenase is in addition inhibited by A1-AT. Bacterial collagenases can also be inhibited by human proteinase inhibitors but there are also possibilities that potent proteinases from microorganisms such as *P. gingivalis* (Arg-1 protease or gingipain) are capable of degrading these inhibitors.

- In summary, many host and microbial enzymes are likely to be present in the crevice at any one time. Realizing the potentially destructive features of such enzymes, consideration should be given to the source of these enzymes, their relative proportions and the inhibitory mechanisms available within the crevice. The main enzyme activity is host derived and specific and non-specific inhibitors are plentiful within the crevice and thus enzyme activity will be localized and short-lived.

Matrix metalloproteinases (MMP)

Fullmer and Gibson (1966) showed that both epithelial cells and cells in the inflamed gingival connective tissue are capable of producing collagenase in tissue culture. The periodontium is structurally comprised of fibrous elements including collagen, elastin and glycoproteins (laminin, fibronectin, proteoglycans), minerals, lipids, water and tissue-bound growth factors. In addition there exists a large variety of extracellular matrix components including tropocollagen, proteoglycans and other proteins (elastin, fibronectin, laminin, osteocalcin, osteopontin, bone sialoprotein, osteonectin and tenascin). All of these matrix components are constantly in a state of turnover and thus there is much matrix enzyme activity in both health, disease and tissue repair and remodeling (Kinane 2001). Matrix metalloproteinases (MMP) are responsible for remodeling and degradation of matrix components. MMPs also degrade interstitial and base-

ment membrane collagens, fibronectin, elastin, laminin, and the proteoglycan core protein. MMPs are made in a proenzyme form, and activation is extracellular.

One of the MMPs receiving much attention is the *neutrophil (PMN) collagenase* which is found in higher concentrations in inflamed gingival specimens than in clinically healthy gingivae. Immunolocalization of tissues for collagenase demonstrated that gingival biopsies taken from patients with periodontal disease indicated the presence of the enzyme, whereas gingival specimens obtained from treated subjects had no enzyme present. The increased presence of these MMP enzymes in diseased over healthy sites (Ohlsson et al. 1973), their increase during experimental gingivitis (Kowashi et al. 1979) and decrease after periodontal treatment (Haerian et al. 1995, 1996) suggest that MMPs are involved in periodontal tissue breakdown. Among the MMPs both PMN and fibroblast collagenase have the unique ability of cleaving the triple helix of type I, II and III collagens, thus initiating extracellular matrix degradation which is not shared by the other members of the family.

The periodontal ligament is one of the most metabolically active tissues in the body, and collagen metabolism represents most of this activity. The biological reason for this activity probably relates to its ability to adapt to occlusal forces generated during function. An important feature of connective tissues in general and the periodontal ligament in particular, is the process of constant renewal of the extracellular matrix components involving matrix metalloproteinase (MMP). The breakdown of collagen occurs during inflammation, tissue breakdown, remodeling, tissue repair or wound healing. This process can occur by either an intracellular or extracellular route. In periodontal lesions, the balance between synthesis and degradation is disrupted. Even during early gingivitis many of the collagen fibers in the overt gingiva are broken down, to make space for the infiltrating inflammatory cells. This process changes a firm, pink gingiva into a swollen, loose and reddish tissue which has lost its integrity. When this condition becomes chronic, progression of the lesion into deeper periodontal structures may occur and then the collagen fibers of the periodontal ligament are broken down, together with the supporting alveolar bone. This occurs via an MMP-mediated extracellular digestion.

- In summary, it is evident that the activity of MMPs and their inhibitors is associated with tissue turnover as well as with gingivitis, destructive periodontitis and with the healing of the periodontal tissues following therapy.

Cytokines

Cytokines are soluble proteins, secreted by cells, which act as messenger molecules that transmit signals to other cells. They have numerous actions which include initiation and maintenance of immune and inflammatory responses and regulation of growth and differentiation of cells. The interleukins are important members of the cytokine group and are primarily involved in communication between leukocytes and other cells, such as epithelia, endothelia and fibroblasts, involved in both immune and inflammatory processes. These molecules are released in small amounts and have a variety of actions on cells which carry the specific receptor for the particular interleukin. Cytokines are numerous, many have overlapping functions and they are interlinked forming an active network which controls the host response. Control of cytokine release and action is complex and involves inhibitors and receptors. Many cytokines are capable of acting back on the cell which produced them so as to stimulate their own production and the production of other cytokines.

Pro-inflammatory cytokines: Cytokines such as *interleukin (IL)-1a, IL-1b* and *tumour necrosis factor (TNF)-α* stimulate bone resorption and inhibit bone formation *in vitro* and *in vivo*. Studies on the mechanism of IL-1 action on fibroblasts *in vitro*, suggest that IL-1 can act on the fibroblasts to promote cellular matrix repair or destruction.

Chemotactic cytokines: A series of more than 20 molecules have been identified, among which the most famous and best characterized is interleukin 8 (IL-8), which has powerful chemotactic functions for leukocytes particulary for neutrophils but also for lymphocytes and macrophages. These molecules act to recruit defense cells to areas where they are needed and are important in cell mediated responses. The term chemokine is used to describe these molecules and is an abridged form of the term "chemotactic cytokine".

Lymphocyte signaling cytokines: T helper cells are lymphocytes within the tissues which regulate both the humoral and cell mediated immune responses via cytokines. The humoral immune response is promoted by a T helper cell type 2 (TH-2) which produces characteristic cytokines namely Il-4, IL-5, IL-10 and IL-13. The TH-1 lymphocytes release IL-2 and interferon (IFN)-γ which enhance cell mediated responses (Fig. 5-18). These cytokines provide a precise mechanism for the control of the immune response so that a sufficient response is produced to deal with the offending pathogen.

Cytokines can influence the immune response through determining the class of immunoglobulin being produced, which may have quite a profound effect on antibody function. For example IgM molecules are more effective at bacteriolysis and IgG molecules are more effective at opsonization. The IgG antibodies exist as four distinct subclasses (IgG1, IgG2, IgG3 and IgG4) based on differences in the Fc portion of these molecules. The antibody subclass influences antibody function, IgG2 being less strong in binding antigen than IgG1. Several researchers have found IgG2 to be elevated over IgG1 in patients with severe

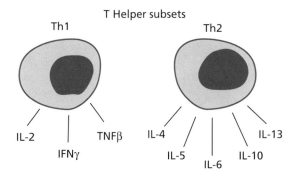

Fig. 5-18. Diagram illustrating the cytokines produced by type 1 (TH1) and type 2 (TH2) T helper cells.

periodontitis and propose that IgG subclass levels are important factors in susceptibility to periodontitis (Wilson et al. 1995).

Prostaglandins

Prostaglandins are arachidonic acid derivatives which are important mediators of inflammation. Not surprisingly therefore they have been implicated in the pathogenesis of periodontal disease (Offenbacher et al. 1993a). The pro-inflammatory cytokines are capable of inducing macrophages and other cells to produce copious amounts of prostaglandins, particularly PGE2 which are potent vasodilators and inducers of cytokine production by various cells. PGE2 acts on fibroblasts and osteoclasts, together with cytokines, to induce MMP production, which is relevant to tissue turnover and in the destructive process in peridontitis. Many studies have examined the association of PGE2 with periodontal disease and suggest that its concentration in gingival crevicular fluid increases in gingivitis relative to health and is at very high concentrations during periods of periodontal disease progression (Offenbacher et al. 1993b).

Polymorphonuclear leukocytes (PMNs)

The PMN is the predominant leukocyte within the gingival crevice/pocket in both health and disease. PMNs from the circulation are attracted to the area via chemotactic stimuli elicited from microorganisms in the biofilm, and histologically PMNs can be seen traversing the gingival connective tissue in inflammation. PMNs are, however, also present in clinically healthy gingiva and are recruited to this tissue in response to chemotactic factors in the gingival crevice region. Attström and Egelberg (1970), in an experiment on dogs, showed that carbon labeled peripheral blood neutrophils from the circulation migrated into the gingival crevice and that their migration rate was higher in inflamed than in healthy crevices. PMN numbers increase in the gingival crevice with the development of gingivitis and more PMNs are found in periodontitis compared to gingivitis sites.

As in other tissues, migration of leukocytes from the vessels into the gingival connective tissue, and

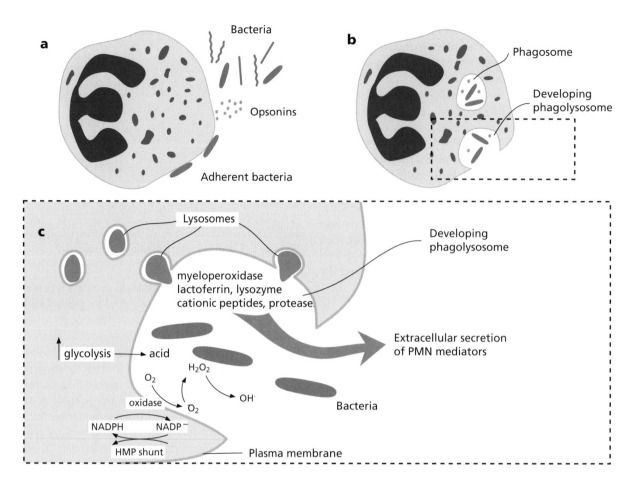

Fig. 5-19. Major events in the encounter between PMNs and invading microorganisms: (a) Once PMNs emigrate from the microcirculation, they migrate toward bacteria under the influence of chemotactic factors. Upon contact PMNs adhere to the organisms (many types of bacteria must be opsonized to facilitate PMN adherence and phago-cytosis). (b) Coincident with adhesion, PMNs begin to phagocytose these organisms. This is accomplished as the plasma membrane flows around and then invaginates to internalize attached organisms which are now contained within phagosomes. Several bacteria can be phagocytosed simultaneously by the PMN. (c) As these events occur PMNs demonstrate dramatic metabolic alterations including: an elevation in glycolysis, a marked rise in oxygen consumption and increased glucose utilization by the hexose monophosphate shunt. Glycolytic metabolism of glu-cose provides the energy required by phagocytosis and also results in a drop in intracellular pH due to the forma-tion of lactate. The oxidative burst is largely the result of NADPH oxidase activity (an enzyme associated with the cell membrane), which oxidizes NADPH to NADP and results in the reduction of oxygen to various free radicals. These oxidants are released into the phagosome to kill bacteria. The hexose monophosphate shunt provides for the regeneration of NADPH. At the same time, lysosomes are mobilized toward the developing phagosome and fuse with the phagosome membrane, giving rise to a phagolysosome. Lysosomal antimicrobial compounds (myeloper-oxidase, lysozyme, lactoferrin, cationic proteins, etc.) are discharged into the vacuole. The combination of oxidative and non-oxidative (acid pH, lysosomal agents) pathways explains how PMNs kill ingested organisms. Lysozyme and neutral proteases (particularly elastase) derived from lysosomes digest and dispose of the dead organisms. Be-fore invagination is completed, biologically-active products can be released from the phagosome into the external environment. These agents play a role in extracellular killing of microorganisms but also may adversely affect sur-rounding host cells and tissue structures.

through the junctional epithelium into the gingival crevice, is controlled via *adhesion molecules* (Fig. 5-9). Moughal et al. (1992), in a study in which volunteers were asked to stop normal hygiene practices for sev-eral weeks (an experimental gingivitis study), showed that vessels in the gingival connective tissue express ELAM-1 and ICAM-1 both in health and in gingivitis. Furthermore, PMNs were found in great abundance in areas expressing intense ELAM-1 and ICAM-1 staining. In addition, the junctional epithelium

stained strongly positive for ICAM-1, suggesting the importance of this adhesion molecule in allowing PMN migration through this epithelium into the gin-gival crevice.

PMNs in the gingival crevice form the first line of defense against periodontal pathogens. This is illus-trated by the fact that qualitative and quantitative deficiencies, as found in cyclic neutropenia and Chediak Higashi syndrome, result in gross periodon-tal tissue destruction.

Elastase, a serine protease, is contained in the primary granules of the PMN. Elastase may cause tissue breakdown and is present with increased activity at sites of gingival inflammation. Murray et al. (1995) showed that although there is an increase in the concentration of elastase with increasing severity of gingivitis (and periodontitis), the enzyme may not be in an active form.

Lactoferrin is contained in the secondary granules of the PMN, is released during PMN migration and is correlated with PMN activation. Differences in the relative amounts of elastase (primary granule constituent) and lactoferrin (secondary granule constituent) were found in periodontal sites with varying degree of inflammation. A greater proportion of lactoferrin to elastase was found in periodontitis than in gingivitis sites. This variation in the release by PMNs, of primary and secondary granule enzymes, may indicate alterations in PMN function in different disease environments.

- In summary, PMNs seem to play a central role in the pathogenesis of periodontal disease. They play a primary role in the inflammatory process which, if effective, may stop the disease process and prevent the consequent antigenic challenge and the more destructive immune processes (Fig. 5-19). Tissue damage from PMNs may be superficial to the underlying attachment apparatus and may be preferable to the stimulation of the immune system that could cause deeper and more long-term destruction.

Interaction between endothelial cells and leukocytes
The endothelium which lines the vasculature, structurally and functionally, separates the blood elements from extravascular tissue. During a local inflammatory response, injury to a tissue site results in release of chemical mediators of inflammation which change vascular proteins, and cells of the blood accumulate at the site of the injury; and localized adhesion of peripheral blood leukocytes to the endothelial cell lining occurs. Adhesion of leukocytes is an essential step in a variety of pathophysiological processes and a key event in the pathogenesis of certain vascular diseases. Cellular migration involves three main structures: the endothelial cells, the cell adhesion molecules (receptors and their ligands) and the extravasating cells. Adhesion of leukocytes appears to be essential in controlling cellular traffic into inflamed areas and it has been proposed that cytokines may play an important role in regulation of this traffic. This may be mediated in part by effects of cytokines on endothelial cells, both in promoting the expression of endothelial cell adhesion molecules for leukocytes and in stimulating endothelial cells to facilitate leukocyte migration through the vessel wall.

The immune or adaptive defense system

Introduction
The hallmark of any immune response is specificity and is based on the specific antigen-antibody interaction of both the cellular and humoral immune responses. Immunology has developed rapidly in the last few years. Advances have occurred in molecular genetics, cloning of immunogenic cells, studies on cell surface receptors and their biological functions, regulatory mechanisms, effector mechanisms and effector mediators. Many recent developments in immunology have influenced research into immune inflammatory diseases such as periodontal disease.

The humoral immune response
In considering the specific humoral immune response in periodontal disease, i.e. antibodies directed against particular oral microorganisms, there are several issues which must be addressed. First, microorganisms play a decisive role in the development of gingivitis and periodontitis (see Chapter 4). Second, several microorganisms in the biofilm may provoke an immune response but not fulfill other aspects of Socransky's extended Koch's postulates (Socransky et al. 1984). Third, species such as *P. gingivalis* and *A. actinomycetemcomitans* require particular attention because of their current strong association with both chronic and aggressive periodontitis.

It is also important to consider antibody function, i.e. the ability of an antibody to opsonize bacteria and to bind strongly (binding strength = avidity) to fimbriae and hereby prevent bacterial colonization. Consideration should be given to whether local antibody levels in the gingival crevicular fluid (GCF) or in serum or both are of importance; and whether local levels are merely a reflection of serum levels, or whether significant antibody production by gingival plasma cells is taking place. This is important in the determination of subject and site susceptibility to disease onset and progression. In addition, there is evidence that the subclass of immunoglobulin produced has a bearing on aspects of its function such as complement fixation and opsonization. Certain studies have reported a preponderance of IgG2 production over IgG1 in localized aggressive periodontitis. This means that the functionally (binding strength; avidity) less effective IgG2 may have some role in rendering these patients more susceptible to periodontal tissue destruction (Wilson et al. 1995). Several studies suggest that assessments of the titer and avidity (the binding strength) of a patient's antibody to various microorganisms in the subgingival biofilm may be useful in the differential diagnosis and classification of periodontal diseases (Mooney et al. 1993).

IgG has four subclasses and IgA has two subclasses. Antibodies of different subclasses have different properties. Thus, IgG2 antibodies are effective against carbohydrate antigens (LPS) whereas the other subclasses are mainly directed against proteins. Kinane et

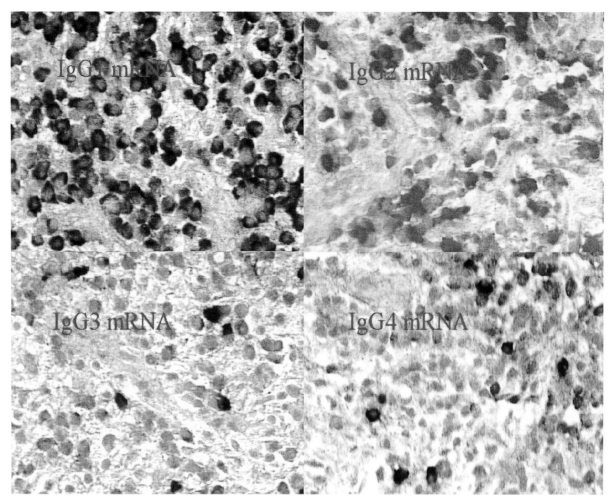

Fig. 5-20. Plasma cells within the periodontal gingiva. The mRNA for immunoglobulin production is noted in abundance within the plasma cell cytoplasms indicating that gingival plasma cells have the ability to produce antibodies locally (Kinane et al. 1997).

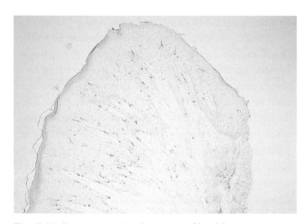

Fig. 5-21. Immunostained section of healthy gingiva showing Langerhans cells in the junctional epithelium.

al. (1997) studied the immunoglobulin subclasses (IgG1-4 and IgA1-2) produced by plasma cells in the gingival lesion of periodontitis patients (Fig. 5-20). The proportions of plasma cells producing IgG and IgA subclasses were similar to the proportions of these immunoglobulin subclasses in serum. IgG1-producing plasma cells were predominant (mean 63%) in the gingival; 23% of all IgG-producing plasma cells produced IgG2 antibodies, while IgG3 and IgG4-produc-

ing cells were present in much smaller numbers (3% and 10% respectively). Similar proportions of IgG subclass proteins were detected in crevicular fluid of the same patients.

• In summary, measurement of specific microbial antibodies in longitudinal studies may provide information on the relationship between antibody titer and avidity at both subject and site levels and prognosis.

The cell mediated immune response
Generally cell mediated immunity is initiated when antigen from subgingival plaque penetrates into the connective tissue through the junctional epithelium. Antigen presenting cells, such as the Langerhans cells within the epithelium (Fig. 5-21), process the antigen and alter it to a form that is recognizable by the immune system, i.e. the antigenic peptide binds to the class II major histocompatibility complex (MHC). The T-helper cell recognizes this binding between the *foreign antigen* and the *self MHC* and becomes stimulated. The T-helper cell proliferates and starts to release cytokines. The cytokines should be regarded as signals which act on other cell types (i.e. macrophages, B

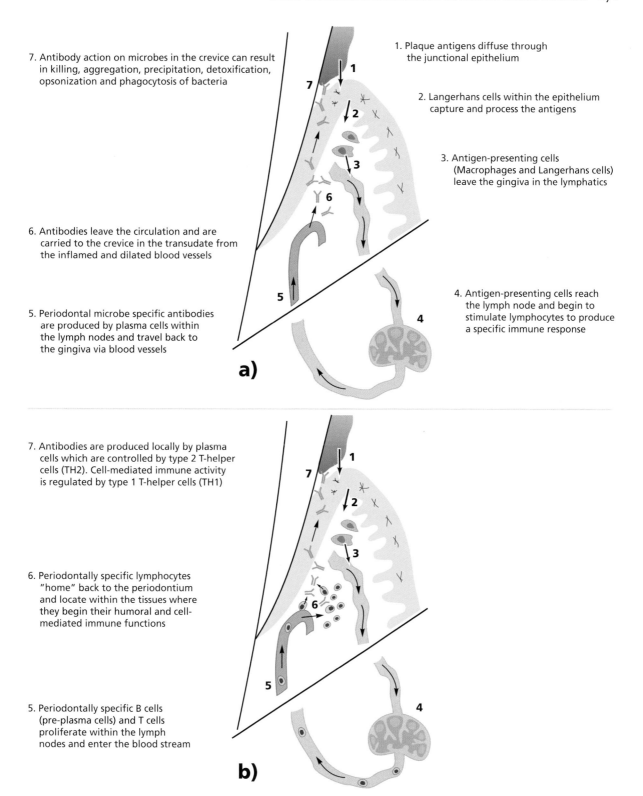

7. Antibody action on microbes in the crevice can result in killing, aggregation, precipitation, detoxification, opsonization and phagocytosis of bacteria

1. Plaque antigens diffuse through the junctional epithelium

2. Langerhans cells within the epithelium capture and process the antigens

3. Antigen-presenting cells (Macrophages and Langerhans cells) leave the gingiva in the lymphatics

6. Antibodies leave the circulation and are carried to the crevice in the transudate from the inflamed and dilated blood vessels

4. Antigen-presenting cells reach the lymph node and begin to stimulate lymphocytes to produce a specific immune response

5. Periodontal microbe specific antibodies are produced by plasma cells within the lymph nodes and travel back to the gingiva via blood vessels

a)

7. Antibodies are produced locally by plasma cells which are controlled by type 2 T-helper cells (TH2). Cell-mediated immune activity is regulated by type 1 T-helper cells (TH1)

6. Periodontally specific lymphocytes "home" back to the periodontium and locate within the tissues where they begin their humoral and cell-mediated immune functions

5. Periodontally specific B cells (pre-plasma cells) and T cells proliferate within the lymph nodes and enter the blood stream

b)

Fig. 5-22. (a) Schematic illustration of the systemic humoral immune response to microbial antigens within the gingival crevice region. (b) Schematic illustration of the local cellular immune response within the gingival crevice region and how this is invoked by microbial antigens and the mechanism by which pertinent periodontal immune cells traffic to the periodontium.

cells and other T cells) to stimulate, inhibit or even kill. Through this action inflammation and tissue damage may result.

The T-helper cells are following the first exposure to the foreign material sensitized, and upon re-exposure to the same antigen they respond promptly by proliferating and synthesizing cytokines. They may also produce cytokines when stimulated by mitogenic substances released either by the subgingival microbiota or by other cells in the inflammatory reaction.

The protective role of the immune responses

Understanding of the function of the humoral immune responses of the periodontium is incomplete. For example, it is not known if the plasma cells of the gingival tissue are producing relevant or totally nonspecific antibodies to the microorganism within the biofilm.

It is possible that Langerhans cells and other antigen presenting cells are setting up humoral immune responses within peripheral lymph nodes and that the antibodies produced in the lymph nodes are arriving at the gingiva to begin their function (Fig. 5-22a). It is also possible that a homing mechanism, and/or a local proliferation of B cells into periodontally relevant plasma cells, within the gingival tissue can occur (Fig. 5-22b). Evidence for homing of both cellular and humoral immune cells is emerging (Kinane et al. 1993a).

Recruitment of leukocytes into areas of injury or infection is essential for an effective host defense. The constant migration of T cells and other leukocytes to sites throughout the body allows the immune system to protect the tissues from a variety of antigenic challenges.

Leukocyte migration into tissues is particularly prominent during inflammatory responses and results from the cytokine-induced expression of adhesion molecules on the surface of vascular endothelial cells (Kinane et al. 1991) (Fig. 5-9). Endothelial leukocyte adhesion molecule-1 (ELAM-1) and intercellular adhesion molecule-1 (ICAM-1) are two adhesion molecules which appear to be crucial for cellular trafficking (Fig. 5-5). The changes in vascular adhesion molecule expression and numbers of infiltrating leukocytes during a 21-day experimental gingivitis episode were investigated immunohistochemically (Moughal et al. 1992). ELAM-1 and ICAM-1 positive vessels and T cells and neutrophils were identified within gingival biopsies taken on days 0, 7, 14 and 21. Vascular endothelium expressed ELAM-1 and ICAM-1 both in clinically "healthy" tissue (day 0) and in experimentally inflamed tissue (day 7 to 21). Positive vessels were found mainly in the connective tissue subjacent to the junctional epithelium where the highest numbers of T cells and neutrophils were also seen. A gradient of ICAM-1 was found to exist in the junctional epithelium, with the strongest staining on the crevicular aspect. This observation, together with the vascular expression of ELAM-1 and ICAM-1 in both clinically "healthy" and inflamed tissue, suggests that the adhesion molecules are crucial and that they direct leukocyte migration towards the gingival crevice (Fig. 5-9). The importance of these mechanisms is highlighted by the rapid and severe periodontitis that is found in patients suffering from leukocyte adhesion deficiency syndrome (LAD).

Specific antibody responses

P. gingivalis and *A. actinomycetemcomitans* are considered to be important pathogens in various types of periodontal disease (Chapter 4). Several studies have demonstrated that the antibody titers to these two organisms are increased in patients with periodontitis compared with subjects without disease (Kinane et al. 1993b, Mooney & Kinane 1994, Kinane et al. 1999).

Furthermore, Naito et al. (1987) and Aukhil et al. (1988) demonstrated that the serum titer to *P. gingivalis* was *reduced* in subjects with advanced periodontitis following successful treatment. In this regard a study by Mooney et al. (1995) must be recognized. They reported on specific antibody titer and avidity to *P. gingivalis* and *A. actinomycetemcomitans* in chronic periodontitis patients before and after periodontal therapy. The authors observed that *IgG avidities* (the binding strength of the antibodies) to *P. gingivalis* increased significantly and specific *IgA levels* more than doubled as a result of treatment. Interestingly, only patients who had high levels of antibody before treatment showed a significant increase in antibody avidity. In addition, patients who originally had high levels of IgG and IgA to *P. gingivalis* also had better treatment outcomes – in terms of a reduced number of deep pockets and sites which bled on probing – than patients with initially lower titers.

Initial serostatus (i.e. antibody levels) is probably dependent on a number of factors including previous exposure to the subgingival microbiota and the host's ability to respond to a particular antigen. The effect of treatment on antibody level and avidity may be the result of an inoculation (transient bacteremia) effect that occurs during scaling and root planing. The reduction in the amount of bacteria, i.e. the antigen load, which occurs after subgingival scaling and root planing, results in the activation of B-cell clones that produce antibodies of high avidity (binding strength).

The findings described above suggest that periodontal therapy affects the magnitude and quality of the humoral immune response to periodontal pathogens, that this effect is dependent on initial serostatus, and that, thus, initial serostatus may have a bearing on treatment outcome.

• In conclusion, the humoral immune response, especially IgG and IgA, is considered to have a protective role in the pathogenesis of periodontal disease but the precise mechanisms are still unknown. Periodontal therapy may improve the magnitude and quality of the humoral immune response through a process of immunization.

Immune regulation processes

The host response to factors released by microbial plaque in periodontal diseases involves a series of different effector mechanisms that are activated by the *innate* immune response. The effector mechanisms in this first line of defense may be insufficient to eliminate a given pathogen (e.g. from *P. gingivalis*). The *adaptive* immune response, which is a second line of defense, is then activated. The adaptive response improves the host's ability to recognize the pathogen.

Immune memory and *clonal expansion* of immune

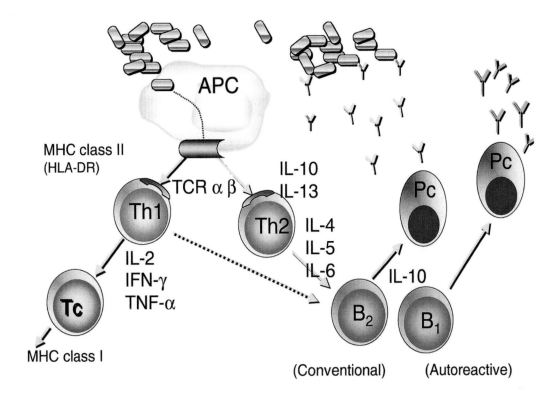

Fig. 5-23. Immune regulation in periodontal diseases.

cells are the hallmarks of adaptive immunity. Although the effector mechanisms activated by the adaptive system appear to be similar to those of the innate system, the antimicrobial activities in adaptive immunity are specialized functions regulated by lymphocytes. This means that the defense mechanisms in the gingiva are synchronized by the communication through signals (cytokines) between specific groups of cells.

The cell types involved in the adaptive response and which reside in the inflammatory lesion in sites with periodontitis have been described in several studies that included a histopathological analysis of the tissue composition (e.g. Zappa 1995, Berglundh et al. 1998). It was observed that plasma cells and lymphocytes were the most common cell types in the lesions and that they occupied similar volumes of the inflammatory cell infiltrate. The lymphocytes in such lesions were further divided into T cells and B cells and it was reported that T cells and B cells also occurred in similar proportions.

The following outline provides an overview of T cell and B cell characteristics and immunoregulatory mechanisms of importance in periodontitis (Fig. 5-23).

Antigen presentation

The biofilm present in the subgingival niche is consistently challenging the host. The antigens produced include proteins from Gram-positive bacteria and lipopolysaccharides (LPS) (endotoxins) from Gram-negative microorganisms. Antigen-presenting cells (APCs) (Fig. 5-21) have a unique ability to internalize and process antigens. Different APCs, such as Langer-hans cells, dendritic cells, macrophages (and, in the presence of LPS-containing antigens, also B cells) may serve as APCs. The processed antigen (a peptide) inside the APC binds to an important carrying molecule. This molecule, termed *class-II* molecule of the major histocompatibility complex (*MHC*), transports the peptide to the cell surface. The peptide will thus, together with the MHC class-II molecule, become identifiable (i.e. presented) to T cells.

TCRs

The presentation of the processed antigen involves interactions with receptors on the T cells; TCRs = T cell receptors. It is in this context important to realize that the resulting immune response from this presentation varies with the build up of the TCR. The TCR is comprised of two glycoprotein chains, mainly and (Fig. 5-23). The external portion of these γ and δ chains contains a variable segment which has many features in common with the antigen-binding site at immunoglobulins. This means that the composition of the variable segment in the γ or the δ chain determines the type of immune reaction that will occur.

It is well known that the composition – or expression – of the variable chains of TCR – TCR γ/δ phenotype or genes – is of importance in several autoimmune diseases (Bröker et al. 1993) and also in periodontal disease (Nakajima et al. 1996, Yamazaki et al. 1997, Geatch et al. 1997, Berglundh et al. 1998). The results reported on TCR in periodontitis have consistently revealed that the TCR repertoire of T cells in the local periodontitis lesions differs from that of T cells in peripheral blood. In other words, factors present at the local site, i.e. antigens released from microorganisms in the subgingival biofilm, may influence the expression of TCR in the periodontitis lesion (Mathur et al. 1995). This fact also explains the differences observed in the distribution of TCR in gingival tissues (1) before and after periodontal therapy (Berglundh et al. 1999) and (2) between adult subjects with advanced chronic periodontitis and children with aggressive periodontitis (Berglundh et al. 2001).

T cell dependent (mediated) processes

Cytokines produced by T-helper (Th) cells regulate most systems within adaptive immunity of periodontal disease. T-helper cells occur as Th-1 and Th-2 cells. Both Th-1 and Th-2 cells express the CD4 marker but are distinguished from each other by their cytokine production (cytokine profiles) (Fig. 5-23).

Th-1 cells produce *interleukin (IL)-2, interferon (IFN)-γ* and *tumor necrosis factor (TNF)-α*. These cytokines have several functions and may activate other T cells, including the so-called cytotoxic T cells.

Cytotoxic T cells (Tc) express the CD8 marker and serve as guards against microorganisms that are capable of invading host cells, i.e. virus and invasive bacteria. In the infected host cells the antigen (peptide) produced by the intracellularly located pathogen binds to *MHC class-I molecules* which carry the peptide to the surface of the infected host cell. The cytotoxic T cell has the ability to recognize this alteration in the MHC class-I molecules and exerts its host defense action by destroying the cell membrane of the infected host cell and by activating its nucleases. This cell-mediated host response orchestrated by the Tc also includes activation of macrophages.

It is well established that CD8-positive cells are found in smaller numbers in periodontitis lesions than CD4-positive cells (Yamazaki et al. 1995, Berglundh et al. 2002a). It may therefore be anticipated that viruses and other invasive microorganisms do not constitute a major part of the antigens in periodontitis.

B cell regulation processes

The large amounts of soluble and accessible antigens occurring in the periodontal environment require the involvement of host defense systems different from those involved in cell-mediated immunity. Specific antibodies (immunoglobulins), occurring in fluids such as plasma or gingival crevicular fluid, have the ability to bind to the antigen. This type of host defense is called *humoral immune response*. By the process of binding to the antigen the antibody activates different effector systems, e.g. *complement*. The activation of the complement system in turn mediates PMN and macrophage migration and phagocytosis. The process in which the antibody contributes to the elimination of antigens by enhancing phagocytosis is termed *opsonization*.

Antibodies are produced by plasma cells that represent the final stage in B cell proliferation. The activation and differentiation of B cells require the presence of certain cytokines, IL-4, IL-5 and IL-6, that are mainly produced by Th-2 cells (Gemmell & Seymour 1998). Since plasma cells and B cells constitute a major part of the leukocytes in advanced periodontitis lesions, it is reasonable to assume that Th-2 functions may dominate over those dependent on Th-1. In early studies it was indeed suggested that the immunoregulatory mechanisms in the advanced periodontitis lesions involve Th-2 cells to a larger extent than Th-1 cells (Seymour et al. 1993, 1996). Several later studies have, however, failed to confirm this observation (Yamazaki et al. 1994, 1997, Fujihashi et al. 1996, Prabhu et al. 1996, Yamamoto et al. 1997). Berglundh et al. (2002a) reported that the soft tissue lesions in advanced periodontitis contained similar proportions of cells expressing cytokine profiles characteristic for Th-1 (IFN-g + IL-2) and Th-2 (IL-4 + IL-6). Current data thus suggest that chronic periodontitis lesions are regulated by a combined Th-1 and Th-2 function.

The immunoglobulins produced by plasma cells in the gingival lesions are mainly directed towards antigens present in the subgingival biofilm. Data have been presented, however, which indicate that antibodies directed against host tissue components, i.e. *auto-antibodies*, may also occur in the gingival lesion (Hirsch et al. 1988, 1989, Jonsson et al. 1991). *Auto-reactive B cells*, also referred to as *B-1 cells*, are associated with the production of auto-antibodies. Large amounts of B-1 cells are present in the peripheral blood of patients with autoimmune disease, such as rheumatoid arthritis and Sjögren's syndrome (Youinou et al. 1988). The presence of circulating auto-reactive B cells in periodontitis patients has also been described. Thus, Afar et al. (1992) and Berglundh et al. (1998, 2002b) reported that B-1 cells occur in large numbers in the peripheral blood of patients with advanced periodontitis. The gingival lesion in patients with chronic periodontitis also contains a substantial number of B cells out of which about 30% exhibit auto-reactive characteristics (Sugawara et al. 1992, Berglundh et al. 2002b).

In this context it should be recognized that clinically successful, non-surgical periodontal therapy (i.e. reduction of sites with deep pockets and that exhibited bleeding on probing) failed to alter the proportion of B-1 cells in peripheral blood (Berglundh et al. 1999). It was suggested that the elevated levels of B-1 cells in peripheral blood may not entirely reflect a response to microorganisms in the subgingival biofilm. Rather, it appears that the effector systems in the humoral immune response in periodontitis may include production of antibodies harmful to the gingival tissues.

Homing – recruitment of specific inflammatory and immune cells to the periodontium

As explained previously, the recruitment of leukocytes into areas of injury or infection (homing) is essential for an effective host defense and the constant migration of leukocytes into the inflamed periodontal tissues results from the cytokine-induced expression of adhesion molecules on the surface of vascular endothelial cells. It has been suggested that Langerhans cells and other antigen presenting cells set up humoral immune response functions within peripheral lymph nodes. Evidence exists, however, that homing of cells involved in both humoral and cellular immune responses is pronounced in diseased periodontal tissues. Thus, local proliferation of such leukocytes seems to play a minor role (Koulouri et al 1999). In other words, the large number of T cells and B cells that occur in the periodontitis lesion are attracted to the diseased site through selective homing and are not the result of local T and B cell proliferation.

In summary

1. Homing of relevant immune cells takes place within the periodontal lesion
2. Th-2 cells outnumber Th-1 cells in chronic periodontal lesions
3. Plasma cells are among the most active secretory cells in the advanced periodontal lesions
4. The ratio of IgG subclasses are similar in serum and gingival crevicular fluid
5. An individual's ability to mount a specific antibody response to microorganisms present in the subgingival biofilm may indicate his/her susceptibility to the disease and his/her ability to respond to treatment.

OVERALL SUMMARY

Biofilm formation on the surface of teeth adjacent to the gingival tissues brings the oral sulcular and junctional epithelial cells into contact with enzymes, waste products, and surface components of the colonizing bacteria. The epithelial cells are triggered by the microbial substances to produce pro-inflammatory cytokines and other chemical mediators of inflammation. These mediators induce an inflammatory response within the gingival tissues, which follows the classical pathway of inflammation. Thus, the gingiva becomes edematous as fluid accumulates and cell infiltration commences. Clinical signs of gingivitis develop. In the early stages, the PMNs predominate due to the mobility and flexibility of these cells, and due to the effects of adhesion molecules on the blood vessels which preferentially bind PMNs. In addition, a chemotactic gradient of bacterial products is established – from the gingival crevice into the connective tissue – and thus PMNs are attracted towards the gingival crevice. Chemotactic factors include microbial proteins and peptides as well as host factors such as the chemokines (particularly IL-8), neutrophil produced molecules such as leukotriene B4 and molecules derived from the complement system (C5a).

PMNs are attracted into the area along with other leukocytes such as monocytes, macrophages and lymphocytes. The macrophages are probably the only type of cell other than the PMN that have a useful function in the gingival crevice area; they can phagocytose dead and dying PMNs and thus remove them from the crevice. This is helpful to the host since dying PMNs will degranulate and release their enzymes in an uncontrolled manner, and may thus cause more damage to the host tissues and amplify inflammation. The scavenging function of the macrophage is therefore useful in dampening down inflammation. The other main function of the macrophage, i.e. the antigen presenting role, cannot operate in the crevice area since it is not possible for these cells to return to the host tissues and to the lymphatic system where they could have exercised this particular function.

The antigen presenting role of macrophages and the immune functions of B cells and T cells take place within the connective tissue of the gingiva. Through the function of certain adhesion molecules, such as CD44, these immune cells are anchored within the tissues and are not lost into the crevice (Murakami et al. 1991). These adhesion molecules are upregulated (increased in number) during inflammation by various pro-inflammatory cytokines produced by a variety of cells. Leukocytes such as B cells and T cells which need to remain in the connective tissue to perform their functions express large numbers of tissue adhesion molecules, whereas cells such as the PMNs, which function in close proximity to the microorganisms, express only few adhesion molecules.

In addition, the role of specific adhesion molecules such as ICAM-1 in the junctional epithelium may assist the PMNs' movements into the crevice and are in fact upregulated by bacterial products and by cytokines produced by the PMNs. Thus PMNs arrive in large numbers to the gingival crevice and begin their function of phagocytosing bacteria, aided by complement and antibody (opsonins). The process of phagocytosis is dependent on Fc receptors that are present on the PMN cell membrane.

As inflammation ensues, the immune process is either initiated (if this is the very first response to these antigens) or reawakened (typical response). In the initiation of the immune response, the Langerhans cells within the epithelium take up microbially derived antigenic material and take it to lymphoid tissue where antigen presentation to lymphocytes occurs. This antigen presentation results in committed lymphocytes returning to the site of microbial exposure where B cells transform to plasma cells and produce antibodies, or T cells become engaged in aiding this humoral response and developing cell mediated immune responses to the microbial antigens. Antibodies may be produced locally or systemically and act by (1) aggregating or clumping microorganisms, (2) preventing bacteria from adhering to the epithelium, (3) working with complement to lyse the microbes, and (4) in conjunction with PMNs, permit efficient phagocytosis (opsonization). Our current understanding is that antibody number and function are important such that individuals who can mount an effective antibody response may be more resistant to periodontitis than those with antibody responses deficient in quantity or quality.

PMN cell accumulation and activity in the gingival crevice results in many enzymes being released which have detrimental effects on bacteria as well as on host tissues. The inflammatory cell infiltrate that forms in the gingiva needs space to begin its function. Therefore structural components (fibroblasts, collagen, matrix) must be lost to create physical room for the infiltrating leukocytes. Furthermore, as layers of the junctional epithelium are broken down and the contact to the tooth surface is lost, a pocket is formed. The environment hereby created invites the colonization of anaerobic and facultative microorganisms. As the infiltrate extends apically, bone is resorbed in order to make more room for the defense cells. Granulation tissue forms which is rich in vascular structures and full of plasma cells that produce antibodies. This granulation tissue gradually occupies more space. Many cells within the inflammatory cell infiltrate produce matrix degrading enzymes and cytokines which directly and indirectly further degrade the connective tissue and bone. Ultimately, if left unchecked, the microbes will continue to produce products detrimental to the host, the host will continue its frustrated response to these products, the pocket will deepen, granulation tissue will extend, bone and ligament will erode and eventually sufficient supporting structures of the tooth will disappear such that the tooth is lost.

REFERENCES

Aduse-Opoku, J., Muir, J., Slaney, J.M., Rangarajan, M. & Curtis, M.A. (1995). Characterisation, genetic analysis, and expression of a protease antigen (PrpPI) of Porphyromonas gingivalis W50. *Infection and Immunity* **63**, 4744-4754.

Afar, B., Engel, D. & Clark, E.A. (1992). Activated lymphocyte subsets in adult periodontitis. *Journal of Periodontal Research* **2**, 126-133.

Attström, R. (1971). Studies on neutrophil polymorphonuclear leukocytes at the dento-gingival junction in gingival health and disease. *Journal of Periodontal Research*, Supplement 8.

Attström, R. & Egelberg, J. (1970). Emigration of blood neutrophils and monocytes into the gingival crevices. *Journal of Periodontal Research* **5**, 48-55.

Aukhil, I., Lopatin, D.E., Syed S.A., Morrison E.C., & Kowalski, C.J. (1988). The effects of periodontal therapy on serum antibody (IgG) levels to plaque microorganisms. *Journal of Clinical Periodontology* **15**, 544-550.

Axelsson, P. & Lindhe, J. (1978). Effect of controlled oral hygiene procedures on caries and periodontal disease in adults. *Journal of Clinical Periodontology* **5**, 133-151.

Axelsson, P. & Lindhe, J. (1981). The significance of maintenance care in the treatment of periodontal disease. *Journal of Clinical Periodontology* **8**, 281-295.

Berglundh, T., Liljenberg, B. & Lindhe, J. (1999) Some effects of periodontal therapy on local and systemic immunological parameters. *Journal of Clinical Periodontology* **2**, 91-98.

Berglundh, T., Liljenberg, B. & Lindhe, J. (2002a). Some cytokine profiles of T-helper cells in lesions of advanced periodontitis. *Journal of Clinical Periodontology* (accepted for publication).

Berglundh, T., Liljenberg, B., Tarkowski, A. & Lindhe, J. (1998). Local and systemic TCR V gene expression in advanced periodontal disease. *Journal of Clinical Periodontology* **25**, 125-133.

Berglundh, T., Liljenberg, B., Tarkowski, A. & Lindhe, J. (2002b). The presence of local and circulating autoreactive B cells in patients with advanced periodontitis. *Journal of Clinical Periodontology* **29**, 281-286.

Berglundh, T., Wellfelt, B., Liljenberg, B. & Lindhe, J. (2001). Some local and systemic immunological features of prepubertal periodontitis. *Journal of Clinical Periodontology* **28**, 113-121.

Brecx, M.C., Fröhlicher, I., Gehr, P. & Lang, N.P. (1988). Stereological observations on long-term experimental gingivitis in man. *Journal of Clinical Periodontology* **15**, 621-627.

Brecx, M.C., Gautschi, M., Gehr, P. & Lang, N.P. (1987). Variability of histologic criteria in clinically healthy human gingiva. *Journal of Periodontal Research* **22**, 468-472.

Bröker, B.M., Korthauer, U., Heppt, P., Weseloh, G., de la Camp, R., Kroczek, R.A. & Emmrich, F. (1993). Biased T cell receptor V gene usage in rheumatoid arthritis. Oligoclonal expansion of T cells expressing Va2 genes in synovial fluid but not in peripheral blood. *Arthritis and Rheumatism* **36**, 1234-1243.

Cimasoni, G. (1983). *Crevicular Fluid Updated*. Basel: Karger.

Egelberg, J. (1967). The topography and permeability of vessels at the dentogingival junction in dogs. *Journal of Periodontal Research* **20**, Supplement 1.

Fujihashi, K., Yamamoto, M., Hiroi, T., Bamberg, T.V., McGhee, J.R. & Kiyono, H. (1996). Selected Th1 and Th2 cytokine mRNA expression by CD4(+) T cells isolated from inflamed human gingival tissues. *Clinical and Experimental Immunology* **103**(3), 422-428.

Fullmer, H.M. & Gibson, W. (1966). Collagenolytic activity in gingivae of man. *Nature* **209**, 728-729.

Garant P.R. & Mulvihill J.E. (1972). The fine structure of gingivitis in the beagle. III. Plasma cell infiltration of the subepithelial connective tissue. *Journal of Periodontal Research* **7**, 161-172.

Geatch, D.R., Ross, D.A., Heasman, P.A. & Taylor, J.J. (1997). Expression of T-cell receptor Vbeta2, 6 and 8 gene families in chronic adult periodontal disease. *European Journal of Oral Science* **105**, 397-404.

Gemmell, E. & Seymour, G.J. (1998). Cytokine profiles of cells extracted from humans with periodontal diseases. *Journal of Dental Research* **77**, 16-26.

Haerian, A., Adonogianaki, E., Mooney, J., Docherty, J. & Kinane, D.F. (1995). Gingival crevicular stromelysin, collagenase and tissue inhibitor of metalloproteinases levels in healthy and diseased sites. *Journal of Clinical Periodontology* **22**, 505-509.

Haerian, A., Adonogianaki, E., Mooney, J., Manos, A. & Kinane, D.F. (1996). Effects of treatment on gingival crevicular collagenase, stromelysin and tissue inhibitor of metalloproteinases and their ability to predict response to treatment. *Journal of Clinical Periodontology* **23**, 83-91.

Haffajee, A.D., Socransky, S.S. & Goodson, J.M. (1983a). Clinical parameters as predictors of destructive periodontal disease activity. *Journal of Clinical Periodontology* **10**, 257-265.

Haffajee, A.D., Socransky, S.S. & Goodson, I.M. (1983b). Comparison of different data analyses for detecting changes in attachment level. *Journal of Clinical Periodontology* **10**, 298-310.

Haubek, D., Poulsen, K. & Kilian, M. (1995). Evidence for absence in northern Europe of especially virulent clonal types of Actinobacillus actinomycetemcomitans. *Journal of Clinical Microbiology* **33**, 395-401.

Helldén, L. & Lindhe, J. (1973). Enhanced emigration of crevicular leucocytes mediated by factors in human dental plaque. *Scandinavian Journal of Dental Research* **81**, 123-129.

Hirsch, H.Z., Tarkowski, A., Koopman, W.J. & Mestecky, J. (1989). Local production of IgA- and IgM-rheumatoid factors in adult periodontal disease. *Journal of Clinical Immunology* **9**(4), 273-278.

Hirsch, H.Z., Tarkowski, A., Miller, E.J., Gay, S., Koopman, W.J. & Mestecky, J. (1988). Autoimmunity to collagen in adult periodontal disease. *Journal of Oral Pathology* **17**(910), 456-459.

Hodge, P. & Michalowicz, B. (2001). Genetic predisposition to periodontitis in children and young adults. *Periodontology 2000* **26**,113-134.

Jeffcoat, M.K., & Reddy, M.S. (1991). Progression of probing attachment loss in adult periodontitis. *Journal of Periodontology* **62**, 185-189.

Jenkins, W.M.M. & Kinane, D.F. (1989). The "high risk" group in periodontitis. *British Dental Journal* **167**, 168-171.

Jenkins, W.M.M., MacFarlane, T.W. & Gilmour, W.H. (1988). Longitudinal study of untreated periodontitis: (I). Clinical findings. *Journal of Clinical Periodontology* **15**, 324-330.

Jonsson, R., Pitts, A., Lue, C., Gay, S. & Mestecky, J. (1991). Immunoglobulin isotype distribution of locally produced autoantibodies to collagen type I in adult periodontitis. *Journal of Clinical Periodontology* **18**, 703-707.

Kinane, D.F. (2001). Regulators of tissue destruction and homeostasis as diagnostic aids in periodontology. *Periodontology 2000* **24**, 215-225.

Kinane, D.F., Adonogianaki, E., Moughal, N., Mooney, J. & Thornhill, M. (1991). Immunocytochemical characterisation of cellular infiltrate, related endothelial changes and determination of GCF acute phase proteins during human experimental gingivitis. *Journal of Periodontal Research* **26**, 286-288.

Kinane, D.F., Goudie, R.B., Karim, S.N., Garioch, J.J., Moughal, N.A. & Al Badri, A. (1993a). Heterogeneity and selective localisation of T cell clones in human skin and gingival mucosa. *Journal of Periodontal Research* **28**, 497-499.

Kinane, D.F., Lappin, D.F., Koulouri, O. & Buckley, A. (1999). Humoral immune responses in periodontal disease may have mucosal and systemic immune features. *Clinical and Experimental Immunology* **115**, 534-541.

Kinane D.F., Mooney, J., MacFarlane, T.W. & McDonald, M. (1993b). Local and systemic antibody response to putative periodontopathogens in patients with chronic periodontitis: correlation with clinical indices. *Oral Microbiology and Immunology* **8**, 65-68.

Kinane, D.F., Takahashi, K. & Mooney, J. (1997). Crevicular fluid and serum IgG subclasses and corresponding mRNA expressing plasma cells in periodontal lesions. *Journal of Periodontal Research* **32**, 176-178.

Koulouri, O., Lappin, D.F., Radvar, M. & Kinane, D.F. (1999). Cell division, synthetic capacity and apoptosis in periodontal lesions analysed by in situ hybridisation and immunohistochemistry. *Journal of Clinical Periodontology* **26**, 552-559.

Kowashi, Y., Jaccard, F. & Cimasoni, G. (1979). Increase of free collagenase and neutral protease activities in the gingival crevice during experimental gingivitis in man. *Archives of Oral Biology* **34**, 645-650.

Lindhe, J., Haffajee, A.D. & Socransky, S.S. (1983). Progression of periodontal disease in adult subjects in the absence of periodontal therapy. *Journal of Clinical Periodontology* **10**, 433-442.

Lindhe, J., Hamp, S-E. & Löe, H. (1975). Plaque-induced periodontal disease in beagle dogs. A 4-year clinical, roentgenographical and histometric study. *Journal of Periodontal Research* **10**, 243-255.

Lindhe, J., Liljenberg, B. & Listgarten, M. (1980). Some microbiological and histopathological features of periodontal disease in man. *Journal of Periodontology* **51**, 267-269.

Lindhe, J. & Nyman, S. (1975). The effect of plaque control and surgical pocket elimination on the establishment and maintenance of periodontal health. A longitudinal study of periodontal therapy in cases of advanced disease. *Journal of Clinical Periodontology* **2**, 67-79.

Lindhe, J. & Nyman, S. (1984). Long-term maintenance of patients treated for advanced periodontal disease. *Journal of Clinical Periodontology* **11**, 504-514.

Lindhe, J. & Rylander, H. (1975). Experimental gingivitis in young dogs. *Scandinavian Journal of Dental Research* **83**, 314-326.

Listgarten, M.A. (1965). Electron microscopic observations on the bacterial flora of acute necrotizing ulcerative gingivitis. *Journal of Periodontology* **36**, 328-339.

Listgarten, M.A. & Ellegaard, B. (1973). Experimental gingivitis in the monkey. Relationship of leucocyte in junctional epithelium, sulcus depth and connective tissue inflammation scores. *Journal of Periodontology* **8**, 199-214.

Löe, H., Anerud, A., Boysen, H. & Morrison, E. (1986). Natural history of periodontal disease in man. Rapid, moderate and no loss of attachment in Sri Lankan labourers 14 to 46 years of age. *Journal of Clinical Periodontology* **13**, 431-440.

Löe, H., Theilade, E. & Jensen, S.B. (1965). Experimental gingivitis in man. *Journal of Periodontology* **36**, 177-187.

Mathur, A., Michalowicz, B., Yang, C. & Aeppli, D. (1995). Influence of periodontal bacteria and disease status on Vb expression in T cells. *Journal of Periodontal Research* **30**, 369-373.

Matsson, L. & Attström, R. (1979). Histologic characteristics of experimental gingivitis in the juvenile and adult beagle dog. *Journal of Clinical Periodontology* **6**, 334-350.

Michalowicz, B.S., Diehl, S.R., Gunsolley, J.C., Sparks, B.S., Brooks, C.N., Koertge, T.E., Califano, J.V., Burmeister, J.A. & Schenkein, H.A. (2000). Evidence of a substantial genetic basis for risk of adult periodontitis. *Journal of Periodontology* **71**, 1699-1707.

Mooney, J., Adonogianaki, E. & Kinane, D.F. (1993). Relative avidity of serum antibodies to putative periodontopathogens in periodontal disease. *Journal of Periodontal Research* **28**, 444-450.

Mooney J., Adonogianaki, E., Riggio, M., Takahashi, K., Haerian, A. & Kinane D.F. (1995). Initial serum antibody titer to Porphyromonas gingivalis influences development of antibody avidity and success of therapy for chronic periodontitis. *Infection and Immunity* **63**, 3411-3416.

Mooney, J. & Kinane, D.F. (1994). Humoral immune responses to Porphyromonas gingivalis and Actinobacillus actinomycetemcomitans in adult periodontitis and rapidly progressive periodontitis. *Oral Microbiology and Immunology* **9**, 321-326.

Moughal, N.A., Adonogianaki, E., Thornhill, M.H. & Kinane D.F. (1992). Endothelial cell leukocyte adhesion molecule-1 (ELAM-1) and intercellular adhesion molecule-1 (ICAM-1) expression in gingival tissue during health and experimentally induced gingivitis. *Journal of Periodontal Research* **27**, 623-630.

Murakami, S., Miayake, K., Kincade, P.W. & Hodes, R.J. (1991). Functional role of CD44 (Pgp-1) on activated B cells. *Immunology Research* **10**, 15-27.

Murray, M.C., Mooney, J. & Kinane, D.F. (1995). The relationship between elastase and lactoferrin in healthy, gingivitis and periodontitis sites. *Oral Diseases* **1**, 106-109.

Naito, Y., Okuda, K. & Takazoe, I. (1987). Detection of specific antibody in adult human periodontitis sera to surface antigens of Bacteroides gingivalis. *Infection and Immunity* **55**, 832-834.

Nakajima, T., Yamazaki, K. & Hara, K. (1996). Biased T cell receptor V gene usage in tissues with periodontal disease. *Journal of Periodontal Research* **31**, 2-10.

Offenbacher, S., Collins, J.G. & Heasman, P.A. (1993a). Diagnostic potential of host response mediators. *Advances in Dental Research* **7**, 175-181.

Offenbacher, S., Heasman, P.A. & Collins, J.G. (1993b). Modulation of host PG2 secretion as a determinant of periodontal disease expression. *Journal of Periodontology* **64**, 432-444.

Ohlsson, K., Olsson I. & Tynelius-Brathall, G. (1973). Neutrophil leukocyte collagenase, elastase and serum protease inhibitors in human gingival crevices. *Acta Odontologica Scandinavica* **31**, 51-59.

Page, R.C. & Schroeder, H.E. (1976). Pathogenesis of inflammatory periodontal disease. A summary of current work. *Laboratory Investigation* **33**, 235-249.

Page, R.C., Simpson, D.M. & Ammons, W.F. (1975). Host tissue response in chronic inflammatory periodontal disease. IV. The periodontal and dental status of a group of aged great apes. *Journal of Periodontology* **46**, 144-155.

Papapanou, P.N., Wennstrom, J.L., Gröndahl, K. (1988). Periodontal status in relation to age and tooth type. A cross-sectional radiographic study. *Journal of Clinical Periodontology* **15**, 469-478.

Payne, W.A., Page, R.C., Ogilvie, A.L. & Hall, W.B. (1975). Histopathologic features of the initial and early stages of experimental gingivitis in man. *Journal of Periodontal Research* **10**, 51-64.

Prabhu, A., Michalowicz, B.S. & Mathur, A. (1996). Detection of local and systemic cytokines in adult periodontitis. *Journal of Periodontology* **67**, 515-22.

Ramfjord, S.P., Nissle, R.R., Shick, R.A. & Cooper, H. Jr. (1968). Subgingival curettage versus surgical elimination of periodontal pockets. *Journal of Periodontology* **39**, 167-175.

Saxe, S.R., Greene, J.C., Bohannan, H.M. & Vermillion, J.R. (1967). Oral debris, calculus and periodontal disease in the beagle dog. *Periodontics* **5**, 217-224.

Schroeder, H.E., Münzel-Pedrazzoli, S. & Page, R.C. (1973). Correlated morphometric and biochemical analysis of gingival tissue in early chronic gingivitis in man. *Archives of Oral Biology* **18**, 899-923.

Schroeder, H.E. (1970). Quantitative parameters of early human gingival inflammation. *Archives of Oral Biology* **15**, 383-400.

Seymour, G.J., Gemmell, E., Kjeldsen, M., Yamazaki, K., Nakajima, T. & Hara, K. (1996). Cellular immunity and hypersensitivity as components of periodontal destruction. *Oral Diseases* **2**, 96-101.

Seymour, G.J., Gemmell, E., Reinhardt, R.A., Eastcotyt, J. & Taubman, M.A. (1993). Immunopathogenesis of chronic inflammatory periodontal disease: cellular and molecular mechanisms. *Journal of Periodontal Research* **28**, 478-486.

Seymour, G.J., Powell, R.N., Cole, K.L., Aitken, J.F., Brooks, D., Beckman, I., Zola, H., Bradley, J. & Burns, G.F. (1983). Experimental gingivitis in humans. A histochemical and immunological characterisation of the lymphoid cell subpopulations. *Journal of Periodontal Research* **18**, 375-385.

Socransky, S.S., Haffajee, A.D., Goodson, J.M. & Lindhe, J. (1984). New concepts of destructive periodontal disease. *Journal of Clinical Periodontology* **11**, 21-32.

Sugawara, M., Yamashita, K., Yoshie, H. & Hara, K. (1992). Detection of, and anti-collagen antibody produced by, CD5 positive B cells in inflamed gingival tissues. *Journal of Periodontal Research* **27**, 489-498.

Takahashi, K., Poole, I. & Kinane, D.F. (1995). Detection of IL-1 MRNA-expressing cells in human gingival crevicular fluid by in situ hybridization. *Archives of Oral Biology* **40**, 941-947.

Van der Weijden, G.A., Timmerman, M.F., Danser, M.M., Nijboer, A., Saxton, C.A., Van der Welden, U. (1994). Effect of pre-experimental maintenance care duration on the development of gingivitis in a partial mouth experimental gingivitis model. *Journal of Periodontal Research* **29**, 168-173.

Wilson, M.E., Bronson, P.M. & Hamilton, R.G. (1995). Immunoglobulin G2 antibodies promote neutrophil killing of Actinobacillus actinomycetemcomitans. *Infection and Immunity* **63**, 1070-1075.

Yamamoto, M., Fujihashi, K., Hiroi, T., McGhee, J.R., Van Dyke, T.E. & Kiyono, H. (1997). Molecular and cellular mechanisms for periodontal diseases: role of Th1 and Th2 type cytokines in induction of mucosal inflammation. *Journal of Periodontal Research* **32**, 115-119.

Yamazaki, K., Nakajima, T., Gemmell, E., Polak, B., Seymour, G.J. & Hara, K. (1994). IL-4 and IL-6 producing cells in human periodontal disease tissue. *Journal of Oral Pathology and Medicine* **23**, 347-353.

Yamazaki, K., Nakajima, T. & Hara, K. (1995). Immunohistological analysis of T cell functional subsets in chronic inflammatory periodontal disease. *Clinical Experimental Immunology* **99**, 384-391.

Yamazaki, K., Nakajima, T., Kubota, Y., Gemmell, E., Seymour, G.J. & Hara, K. (1997). Cytokine messenger RNA expression in chronic inflammatory periodontal disease. *Oral Microbiology and Immunology* **12**, 281-287.

Yoneyama, T., Okamoto, H., Lindhe, J., Socransky, S.S. & Haffajee, A.D. (1988). Probing depth, attachment loss and gingival recession. Findings from a clinical examination, Ushiku, Japan. *Journal of Clinical Periodontology* **15**, 581-591.

Youinou, P., Mackenzie, L., le Masson, G., Papadopoulos, N.M., Jouguan, J., Pennec, Y.L., Angelidis, P., Katsakis, P., Moutsopoulos, H.M. & Lydyard, P.M. (1988). CD5-expressing B lymphocytes in the blood and salivary glands of patients with primary Sjögren's syndrome. *Journal of Autoimmunology* **1**(2),185-194.

Zappa, U. (1995). Histology of the periodontal lesion: implications for diagnosis. *Periodontology 2000* **7**, 22-38.

CHAPTER 6

Modifying Factors: Diabetes, Puberty, Pregnancy and the Menopause and Tobacco Smoking

RICHARD PALMER AND MENA SOORY

Diabetes mellitus
  Oral and periodontal effects
  Association of periodontal infection and diabetic control
  Modification of the host/bacteria relationship

Puberty, pregnancy and the menopause
  Periodontal treatment during pregnancy

Menopause and osteoporosis
Hormonal contraceptives

Tobacco smoking
  Periodontal disease in smokers
  Modification of the host/bacteria relationship in smoking

Diabetes, pregnancy and tobacco smoking have profound and far reaching effects on the host, including effects on the:

1. Physiological response
2. Vascular system
3. Inflammatory response
4. Immune system
5. Tissue repair

They therefore have the potential to modify the:

1. Susceptibility to disease
2. Plaque microbiota
3. Clinical presentation of periodontal disease
4. Disease progression
5. Response to treatment

Diabetes and smoking were cited as risk factors for periodontitis in Chapter 2 and the epidemiological evidence for their association with periodontitis was dealt with. Both factors are particularly important because they may affect the individual over a great many years, usually decades, and challenge the host to varying degrees. In contrast, pregnancy is of rela-

tively short duration (although possibly with multiple episodes) but should be considered in relation to other hormonal changes which occur at puberty, menopause and in women on hormonal contraceptives.

These three modifying factors are extremely important in many other disease processes, for example cardiovascular disease, which also affects people to varying degrees. Much of this variation in susceptibility is probably due to genetic interactions, and there is increasing evidence of important associations with many genetic polymorphisms. There will undoubtedly be emerging genetic evidence to link periodontal disease susceptibility to modifying factors considered in this chapter.

DIABETES MELLITUS

Diabetes mellitus is a complex disease with varying degrees of systemic and oral complications, depending on the extent of metabolic control, presence of infection and underlying demographic variables. This has led to conflicting results in epidemiological studies, with regard to periodontal disease presentation in

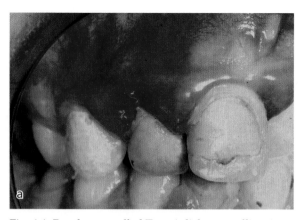 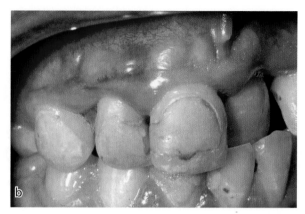

Fig. 6-1. Poorly-controlled Type 1 diabetes mellitus in a young female aged 19 years. (a) Very inflamed and swollen gingival tissues; early attachment loss was present. (b) The same patient after responding to a course of non-surgical periodontal treatment and improved oral hygiene.

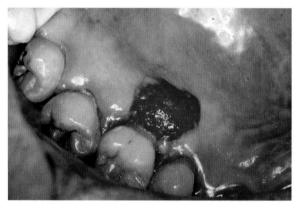

Fig. 6-2. A localized palatal periodontal abscess associated with a periodontal pocket in a 42-year-old poorly-controlled diabetic patient.

diabetic patients and their response to treatment. This section deals with diabetes and its implications on the host response to bacterial plaque, in the context of clinical and laboratory data pertaining to periodontal disease.

Type 1 and Type 2 diabetes mellitus

Diabetes mellitus (DM) is categorized as Type 1 and Type 2 DM. Type 1 DM develops due to impaired production of insulin, while Type 2 DM is caused by deficient utilization of insulin. Type 1 DM results from destruction of the insulin producing β-cells of the pancreas. This can occur when genetically predisposed individuals succumb to an inducing event such as a viral infection or other factors that trigger a destructive autoimmune response (Szopa et al.1993). Approximately 10-20% of all diabetics are insulin-dependent or Type 1. They usually have a rapid onset of symptoms associated with a deficiency or total lack of insulin and the condition may be difficult to control. Nearly 90% are diagnosed before the age of 21years.

Type 2 DM results from insulin resistance which also contributes to cardiovascular and other metabolic disturbances (Murphy & Nolan 2000). However, insu-

lin production may decrease later in the disease process and require supplementation (Slavkin 1997), in addition to controlling diet or using oral hypoglycemic agents. The onset of symptoms in Type 2 DM is more gradual and less severe, usually presenting after the age of 40 years.

Clinical symptoms

The typical signs and symptoms of diabetes are polyuria, polydipsia, polyphagia, pruritus, weakness and fatigue. These features are more pronounced in Type 1 than in Type 2 DM, and are a result of hyperglycemia. The complications of DM include retinopathy, nephropathy, neuropathy, macrovascular disease and impaired wound healing (Lalla et al. 2000, Soory 2000a). In view of these findings, the treatment of DM is aimed at reducing blood glucose levels to prevent such complications.

There is conclusive evidence of the importance of glycemic control in the prevention of diabetic complications. Patients regularly use blood glucose monitors to provide effective feedback for adjustment of insulin dosage to meet individual requirements (Mealey 1998). Recent studies have shown significant improvement in reducing complications associated with Type 2 DM with controlled blood glucose levels (UKPDS 1998a,b). In these studies of over 5000 Type 2 DM patients, the risk of retinopathy and nephropathy was reduced by 25% with effective glycemic control, using sulfonyl ureas, metformin or insulin. The risk of developing hypoglycemia needs to be monitored in these patients on intensive treatment regimes, particularly those on insulin.

Oral and periodontal effects

Poorly-controlled diabetic subjects may complain of diminished salivary flow and burning mouth or tongue. Diabetic subjects on oral hypoglycemic agents may suffer from xerostomia, which could predispose

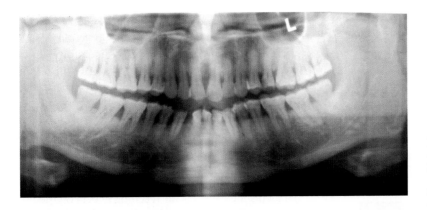

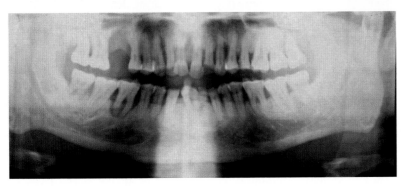

Fig. 6-3 (a,b). Radiographs of a 50-year-old male who developed Type 2 diabetes mellitus in the period between the two radiographs, which were taken 3 years apart. There has been rapid bone loss and tooth loss associated with recurrent multiple periodontal abscesses.

to opportunistic infections with *Candida albicans*. Candidiasis has been reported in patients with poorly-controlled diabetes (Ueta et al. 1993), associated with suppressed free oxygen radical release by PMNs and reduced phagocytosis.

There is good evidence to support the concept that there is an association between poorly-controlled diabetes mellitus and periodontitis (Fig. 6-1). Any differences in periodontal health between Type 1 DM and Type 2 DM patients may relate to differences in management of glycemic control, age, duration of disease, utilization of dental care, periodontal disease susceptibility and habits such as smoking. The Type 1 DM patients have an increased risk of developing periodontal disease with age, and with the severity and duration of their diabetes.

Periodontal attachment loss has been found to occur more frequently in moderate and poorly-controlled diabetic patients, of both Type 1 DM and Type 2 DM, than in those under good control (Westfelt et al. 1996). In addition, diabetics with more advanced systemic complications present with a greater frequency and severity of periodontal disease (Karjalainen et al. 1994). Conversely, initial phase periodontal treatment comprising motivation and debridement of periodontal pockets in Type 2 diabetic patients resulted in improved metabolic control of diabetes (Stewart et al. 2001). Insulin resistance can develop in response to chronic bacterial infection seen in periodontal disease, resulting in worse metabolic control in diabetic patients (Grossi et al. 1996).

Probably the most classic description of the undiagnosed or poorly-controlled diabetic is the patient presenting with multiple periodontal abscesses, leading to rapid destruction of periodontal support (Figs.

6-2 and 6-3). Harrison et al. (1983) reported a case of deep neck infection of the submental, sublingual and submandibular spaces, secondary to periodontal abscesses involving the mandibular incisors, in a poorly-controlled diabetic patient. In a population study Ueta et al. (1993) demonstrated that diabetes mellitus was a predisposing factor for periodontal and periapical abscess formation due to suppression of neutrophil function. The effects on the host response, and in particular neutrophil function may account for this finding (Ueta et al. 1993).

Association of periodontal infection and diabetic control

The presence of acute infection can predispose to insulin resistance (Atkinson & Maclaren 1990). This can occur independently of a diabetic state and persist for up to 3 weeks after resolution of the infection (Yki-Jarvien et al. 1989). In a longitudinal study of subjects with Type 2 DM, it was demonstrated that subjects with severe periodontal disease demonstrated significantly worse control of their diabetic condition than those with minimal periodontal involvement (Taylor et al. 1996) (Fig. 6-4). The incidence of proteinuria and cardiovascular complications, as a result of uncontrolled diabetes, was found to be significantly greater in diabetics with severe periodontal disease than those with gingivitis or early periodontal disease (Thorstensson et al. 1996). Some studies have shown that stabilization of the periodontal condition with mechanical therapy, in combination with systemic tetracycline, improves the diabetic condition in such patients (Grossi et al. 1997). Reduced insulin dosage in

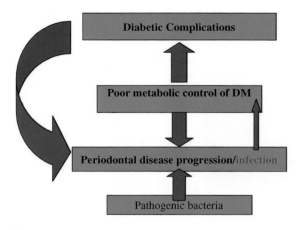

Fig. 6-4. Diabetes control and periodontal disease progression.

Type 1 diabetics following periodontal treatment has also been reported (Sastrowijoto et al. 1990). However, other studies have not shown improvement in diabetic control following non-surgical periodontal treatment (Aldridge et al. 1995). These effects of periodontal therapy may be more pronounced in poorly-controlled diabetic patients with severe periodontal disease.

Modification of the host/bacteria relationship in diabetes

Effects on microbiota
Hyperglycemia in uncontrolled diabetics has implications on the host response (Gugliucci 2000) and affects the regional microbiota. This can potentially influence the development of periodontal disease and caries, in poorly-controlled Type 1 and Type 2 DM patients. *Capnocytophaga* species have been isolated as the predominant cultivable organisms from periodontal lesions in Type 1 diabetics, averaging 24% of the cultivable flora (Mashimo et al. 1983). A similar distribution of the predominant putative pathogens *Prevotella intermedia, Campylobacter rectus, Porphyromonas gingivalis, A. actinomycetemcomitans* and *P. gingivalis,* to those associated with chronic adult periodontal dis-

ease was detected in periodontal lesions of Type 2 diabetics (Zambon et al. 1988), with potential for disease activity during poor metabolic control. In an insulin dependent diabetic population with a large proportion of poorly-controlled diabetics, Seppala & Ainamo (1996) showed significantly increased percentages of spirochetes, motile rods and decreased levels of cocci in periodontal lesions, compared with well-controlled patients.

Effects on the host response
Diabetes mellitus has far reaching effects on the host response (Fig. 6-5). These are dealt with in the following sections.

Polymorphonuclear leucocytes (PMNs)
Reduced PMN function (Marhoffer et al. 1992) and defective chemotaxis in uncontrolled diabetics can contribute to impaired host defenses and progression of infection (Ueta et al. 1993). Crevicular fluid collagenase activity, originating from PMNs, was found to be increased in diabetic patients and this could be inhibited *in vitro* by tetracycline through its enzyme inhibitory effects (Sorsa et al. 1992). The PMN enzymes beta-glucuronidase (Oliver et al. 1993) and elastase in association with diabetic angiopathy (Piwowar et al. 2000) have been detected at significantly higher levels in poorly-controlled diabetic patients.

Cytokines, monocytes and macrophages
Diabetic patients with periodontitis have significantly higher levels of IL-1β and PGE$_2$ in crevicular fluid compared to non-diabetic controls with a similar degree of periodontal disease (Salvi et al. 1997). In addition, the release of these cytokines (IL-1β, PGE$_2$, TNF-α) by monocytes has been shown to be significantly greater in diabetics than in non-diabetic controls. Chronic hyperglycaemia results in non-enzymatic glycosylation of numerous proteins, leading to the accumulation of advanced glycation end products (AGE), which play a central role in diabetic complications (Brownlee 1994). Increased binding of AGEs to macrophages and monocytes (Brownlee 1994) can result in a destructive cell phenotype with increased sensitivity

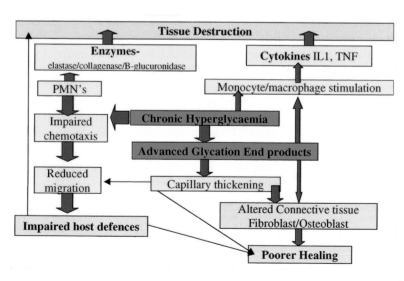

Fig. 6-5. Effects of diabetes mellitus on the host response.

to stimuli, resulting in excessive release of cytokines. Altered macrophage phenotype due to cell surface binding with AGE, prevents the development of macrophages associated with repair. This could contribute to delayed wound healing seen in diabetic patients (Iacopino 1995).

Connective tissue

A hyperglycemic environment, due to decreased production or utilization of insulin, can reduce growth, proliferation and matrix synthesis by gingival and periodontal ligament fibroblasts and osteoblasts. The formation of AGE results in reactive oxygen species, which are damaging to cellular function in gingival tissues, due to oxidative stress (Schmidt et al. 1996). The accumulation of AGE in tissues alters the function of several intercellular matrix components, including vascular wall collagen, resulting in deleterious complications (Ulrich & Cerami 2001). This has adverse effects on cell-matrix interactions and vascular integrity, potentially affecting periodontal disease presentation and treatment responses in uncontrolled diabetics. Vascular changes such as thickening of the capillary basement membrane in a hyperglycemic environment can impair oxygen diffusion, metabolic waste elimination, PMN migration and diffusion of antibodies. Binding of AGE to vascular endothelial cells can trigger responses that induce coagulation, leading to vasoconstriction and microthrombus formation (Esposito et al. 1992), resulting in impaired perfusion of tissues.

Effects on healing and treatment response

Wound healing is impaired due to the cumulative effects on cellular functions as described above. In summary, these factors include:

1. Decreased synthesis of collagen by fibroblasts
2. Increased degradation by collagenase
3. Glycosylation of existing collagen at wound margins
4. Defective remodeling and rapid degradation of newly synthesized, poorly cross-linked collagen.

Periodontal treatment

The treatment of well-controlled DM patients would be similar to that of non-diabetic patients for most routine dental procedures. The short-term non-surgical treatment response of stable diabetics has been found to be similar to that of non-diabetic controls, with similar trends in improved probing depths, attachment gain and altered sub-gingival microbiota (Christgau et al. 1998). Well-controlled diabetics with regular supportive therapy have been shown to maintain treatment results 5 years after a combination of non-surgical and surgical treatment (Westfelt et al. 1996). However, a less favorable treatment outcome may occur in long-term maintenance therapy of poorly-controlled diabetics, who may succumb to more rapid recurrence of initially deep pockets (Tervonen & Karjalainen 1997).

Puberty, pregnancy and the menopause

The hormonal variations experienced by women during physiological and non-physiological conditions (such as hormone replacement therapy and use of hormonal contraceptives) result in significant changes in the periodontium, particularly in the presence of pre-existing, plaque-induced gingival inflammation. Periods of hormonal flux are known to occur during puberty, menstruation, pregnancy and the menopause. Changes in hormone levels occur when the anterior pituitary secretes follicle stimulating hormone (FSH) and luteinizing hormone (LH), resulting in the maturation of the ovary and cyclical production of estrogen and progesterone.

The gingiva is a target tissue for the actions of steroid hormones. Clinical changes in the tissues of the periodontium have been identified during periods of hormonal fluctuation. The effects of estrogen and progesterone on the periodontium have received significant research attention. The main potential effects of these hormones on the periodontal tissues can be summarized as:

- Estrogen affects salivary peroxidases, which are active against a variety of microorganisms (Kimura et al. 1983), by changing the redox potential.
- Estrogen has stimulatory effects on the metabolism of collagen and angiogenesis (Sultan et al. 1986).
- Estrogen can trigger autocrine or paracrine polypeptide growth factor signaling pathways, whose effects may be partially mediated by the estrogen receptor itself (Chau et al. 1998).
- Estrogen and progesterone can modulate vascular responses and connective tissue turnover in the periodontium, associated with interaction with inflammatory mediators (Soory 2000b).

The interaction of estrogen and progesterone with inflammatory mediators may help to explain the increased levels of inflammation seen during periods of hormonal fluctuation. For example, when cultured human gingival fibroblasts were incubated with progesterone concentrations common in late pregnancy, there was a 50% reduction in the formation of the inflammatory mediator IL-6, compared with control values (Lapp et al. 1995). IL-6 induces the synthesis of tissue inhibitor of metallo-proteinases (TIMP) in fibroblasts (Lotz & Guerne 1991), reduces the levels of TNF and enhances the formation of acute phase proteins (Le & Vilcek 1989). A progesterone-induced reduction in IL-6 levels could result in less TIMP, more proteolytic enzyme activity and higher levels of TNF

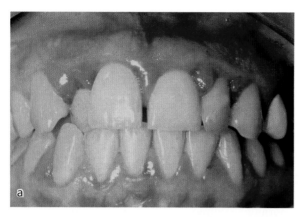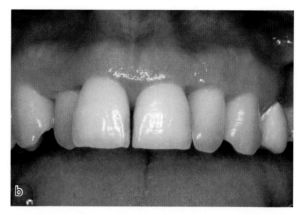

Fig. 6-6. Gingivitis associated with pregnancy. (a) A patient in the last trimester of pregnancy with very inflamed edematous gingival tissue which tended to bleed with the slightest provocation. (b) The improvement in gingival health 6 months after birth of the baby and an intensive course of non-surgical periodontal treatment.

at the affected sites, due to less inhibition, resulting in inflammation and obvious clinical manifestations.

Puberty and menstruation

During puberty, there are raised levels of testosterone in males and estradiol in females. Several studies have demonstrated an increase in gingival inflammation in children of circum-pubertal age, with no change in plaque levels (Sutcliffe 1972). In a longitudinal study, Mombelli et al. (1989) reported that the mean papillary bleeding scores and percentage of interdental bleeding sites correlated with the development of secondary sexual characteristics at puberty, while other studies did not find a significant correlation between the onset of puberty and gingival changes in parapubescent women (Tiainen et al. 1992). These discrepancies may be attributed to factors such as the oral hygiene status of the population and study design.

The prevalence of certain periodontal pathogens reported during puberty may have a direct association with the hormones present and their utilization by selected pathogens. For example *Prevotella intermedia* is able to substitute progesterone and estrogen for menadione (vitamin K) as an essential nutrient (Kornman & Loesche 1979). An association between pubertal gingivitis, *Prevotella intermedia* and serum levels of testosterone, estrogen and progesterone has been reported in a longitudinal study (Nakagawa et al. 1994).

Pre-existing plaque-induced gingivitis may be an important factor in detecting hormone-induced changes during the menstrual cycle. Holm-Pedersen & Loe (1967) demonstrated that women with gingivitis experienced increased inflammation with an associated increase in crevicular fluid exudate during menstruation compared with healthy controls. Most female patients are not aware of any changes in their gingivae during the menstrual cycle (Amar & Chung 1994), while a few experience enlarged hemorrhagic gingivae in the days preceding menstrual flow. This has been associated with more gingivitis, increased crevicular fluid flow and tooth mobility (Grant et al.

1988). Early studies demonstrated similar findings during the menstrual cycle in a population with pre-existing gingivitis, in response to fluctuations in the levels of estrogen and progesterone (Lindhe & Attstrom 1967).

Pregnancy

During pregnancy, the increased levels of sex steroid hormones are maintained from the luteal phase which results in implantation of the embryo, until parturition. Pregnant women, near or at term, produce large quantities of estradiol (20 mg/day), estriol (80 mg/day) and progesterone (300 mg/day). Gingival inflammation initiated by plaque, and exacerbated by these hormonal changes in the second and third trimester of pregnancy, is referred to as pregnancy gingivitis. Parameters such as gingival probing depths (Hugoson 1970, Miyazaki et al. 1991), bleeding on probing (Miyazaki et al. 1991) and crevicular fluid flow (Hugoson 1970) were found to be increased. These inflammatory features can be minimized by maintaining good plaque control.

According to early reports, the prevalence of pregnancy gingivitis ranges from 35% (Hasson 1966) to 100% (Lundgren et al. 1973). In a study of 130 pregnant women, Machuca et al. (1999) demonstrated gingivitis in 68% of the population, ranging from 46% in technical executives to 88% in manual workers. Cross-sectional studies examining pregnant and postpartum women have shown that pregnancy is associated with significantly more gingivitis than at postpartum, despite similar plaque scores (Silness & Loe 1963). Further observations were made by Hugoson (1970) in a longitudinal study of 26 women during and following pregnancy, which also demonstrated that the severity of gingival inflammation correlated with the gestational hormone levels during pregnancy (Fig. 6-6). A more recent study of a rural population of Sri Lankan women (Tilakaratne et al. 2000a) showed increased gingivitis of varying degrees of significance amongst all the pregnant women investigated, compared with

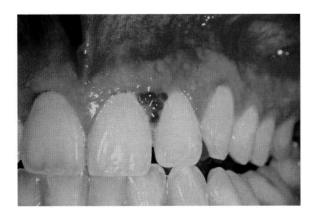

Fig. 6-7. Multilobulated appearance of an early pregnancy epulis, demonstrating vascular elements and tissue edema.

matched non-pregnant controls. There was a progressive increase in inflammation with advancing pregnancy which was more significant in the second and third trimester of pregnancy, despite the plaque levels remaining unchanged. At the third month after parturition, the level of gingival inflammation was similar to that observed in the first trimester of pregnancy. This suggests a direct correlation between gingivitis and sustained, raised levels of gestational hormones during pregnancy, with regression during the postpartum period. In investigations by Cohen et al. (1969) and Tilakaratne et al. (2000a), the values for loss of attachment remained unchanged during pregnancy and three months postpartum.

Effects on the microbiota

There is an increase in the selective growth of periodontal pathogens such as *Prevotella intermedia* in subgingival plaque during the onset of pregnancy gingivitis at the third to fourth month of pregnancy. The gestational hormones act as growth factors, by satisfying the naphthoquinone requirement for bacteria (Di Placido et al. 1998). These findings were also confirmed by Muramatsu & Takaesu (1994) who showed that from the third to fifth month of pregnancy, the number of gingival sites which bled on probing corresponded with the percentage increase in *Prevotella intermedia*. During pregnancy, progesterone is less actively catabolized to its inactive products, resulting in higher levels of the active hormone (Ojanotko-Harri et al. 1991). A 55-fold increase in the proportion of *P. intermedia* has been demonstrated in pregnant women compared with non-pregnant controls (Jensen et al. 1981), implying a role for gestational hormones in causing a change in microbial ecology in the gingival pocket. Although an overall association has been demonstrated, a cause and effect relationship may be less clear.

Effects on the tissues and host response

The increase in severity of gingivitis during pregnancy has been partly attributed to the increased circulatory levels of progesterone and its effects on the capillary vessels (Lundgren et al. 1973). Elevated progesterone levels in pregnancy enhance capillary permeability and dilatation, resulting in increased gingival exudate. The effects of progesterone in stimulating prostaglandin synthesis can account for some of the vascular changes (Miyagi et al. 1993).

The elevated levels of estrogen and progesterone in pregnancy affect the degree of keratinization of the gingival epithelium and alter the connective tissue ground substance. The decreased keratinization of the gingivae, together with an increase in epithelial glycogen, are thought to result in decreased effectiveness of the epithelial barrier in pregnant women (Abraham-Inpijn et al. 1996). Hormonal factors that affect the epithelium and increase vascular permeability can contribute to an exaggerated response to bacterial plaque during pregnancy.

The influence of gestational hormones on the immune system can contribute further to the initiation and progression of pregnancy gingivitis. High levels of progesterone and estrogen associated with pregnancy (and the use of some oral contraceptives) have been shown to suppress the immune response to plaque (Sooriyamoorthy & Gower 1989). Neutrophil chemotaxis and phagocytosis, along with antibody and T-cell responses have been reported to be depressed in response to high levels of gestational hormones (Raber-Durlacher et al. 1993).

Pregnancy granuloma or epulis

A pedunculated, fibro-granulomatous lesion can sometimes develop during pregnancy and is referred to as a pregnancy granuloma or epulis. A combination of the vascular response induced by progesterone and the matrix stimulatory effects of estradiol, contribute to the development of pregnancy granulomas, usually at sites with pre-existing gingivitis (Fig. 6-7). The vascular effects result in a bright red, hyperemic and edematous presentation. The lesions often occur in the anterior papillae of the maxillary teeth and usually do not exceed 2 cm in diameter. They can bleed when traumatized and their removal is best deferred until after parturition, when there is often considerable regression in their size (Wang et al. 1997). Surgical removal of the granuloma during pregnancy can result in recurrence due to a combination of poor plaque control and hormone mediated growth of the lesion. Careful oral hygiene and debridement during preg-

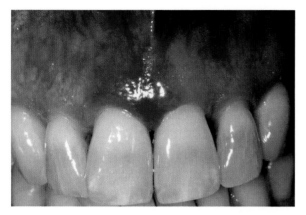

Fig. 6-8. Clinical appearance of anterior maxillary gingiva with pronounced desquamation in a woman during menopause.

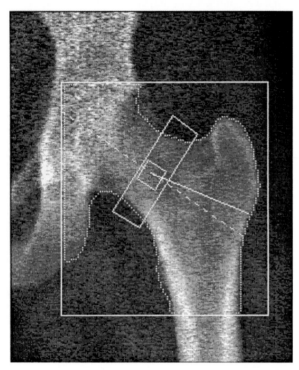

Fig. 6-9. A DEXA scan used to measure mineral bone density in the hip. This is not routinely applied to the jaws.

nancy are important in preventing its occurrence (Wang et al. 1997).

Periodontal treatment during pregnancy

Pregnant women need to be educated on the consequences of pregnancy on gingival tissues and thoroughly motivated in plaque control measures, with professional treatment as required. They are likely to be more comfortable to receive dental treatment during the second trimester than in the first or third trimester of pregnancy, although emergency treatment is permissible at any stage during pregnancy (Amar & Chung 1994). Since most medications cross the placental barrier and organogenesis occurs mainly in the first trimester, pregnant women are best treated in the second trimester, to avoid the occurrence of developmental defects. Any form of medication during pregnancy must only be used if the gravity of the condition being treated outweighs the consequences. Amongst the antibiotics, tetracycline, vancomycin and streptomycin can contribute to staining of teeth and ototoxic and nephrotoxic effects during 4-9 months of pregnancy; erythromycin, penicillins and cephalosporins are relatively safer, but any medication must only be administered in consultation with the patient's obstetrician (Lynch et al. 1991).

Menopause and osteoporosis

During menopause there is a decline in hormonal levels due to decreased ovarian function. This is characterized by tissue changes such as desquamation of gingival epithelium (Fig. 6-8) and osteoporosis (Fig. 6-9) which may be attributed to hormone deficiency. It has been demonstrated that women with early onset of menopause have a higher incidence of osteoporosis and significantly lower bone mineral density (Kritz-Silverstein & Barrett-Connor 1993).

A third of women over age 60 are affected by postmenopausal osteoporosis (Baxter 1987). The changes involved are a reduction in bone density, affecting its mass and strength without significantly affecting its chemical composition. An alteration in the calcium-phosphate equilibrium due to deficient absorption of dietary calcium and increased excretion due to diminished estrogen levels can account for some of the bone changes seen in postmenopausal women (Shapiro et al. 1985), usually involving the mandible more than the maxilla.

Estrogen replacement therapy has been shown to prevent osteoporosis and maintain bone mineral content at several sites throughout the skeleton (Moore et al. 1990), with a 5% increase in bone mineral content in the region of the head compared to those taking placebo (Gotfredsen at al. 1986). The influence of estrogen on bone mineral density has been demonstrated in these studies, but a cause and effect relationship with periodontal disease is less clear.

A 2-year follow-up study of 42 171 postmenopausal women (Grodstein et al. 1996) showed that the risk of tooth loss was significantly lower amongst hormone users. These findings reinforce those of Paganini-Hill (1995), who showed a 36% decrease in tooth loss in estrogen users compared with non-users. There is evidence to suggest that use of estrogen is necessary to protect against bone loss (Grady et al. 1992). Although osteoporosis in postmenopausal women may not be the cause of periodontal disease, it may affect the severity of pre-existing disease. The circulating levels of estrogen have been shown to have an influence on alveolar bone density in postmenopausal women (Payne et al. 1997).

Effect of smoking on osteoporosis

A negative association between smoking and bone density has been demonstrated by Krall & Dawson-Hughes (1991). Smokers can differ from non-smokers in weight, caffeine intake, age at menopause and alcohol consumption (Rigotti 1989, Lindquist & Bengtsson 1979); all these factors can potentially confound an association between smoking and bone density. A study on female twins by Hopper & Seeman (1994) showed that in the 20 pairs who varied most, by 20 or more pack years, the differences in bone density within pairs were 9.3% at the lumbar spine, 5.8% at the femoral neck and 6.5% at the femoral shaft. This study also demonstrated increased serum levels of follicle stimulating hormone and luteinizing hormone in smokers, implying reduced circulating levels of estrogen, leading to increased bone resorption. Other investigators have demonstrated the effects of smoking on the synthesis and degradation of estrogen (Jensen et al. 1985). The study by Jensen et al. (1985) investigated 136 postmenopausal women who were treated with three different doses of estrogen-progesterone or placebo. They showed reduced levels of estrogen in smokers (range of 1-30 cigarettes/day in the previous 6 months, mean 12.4), compared with non-smokers (not smoked in the previous 3 months). There was also a significant inverse correlation between the number of cigarettes smoked per day and the serum levels of estrogen, suggestive of increased hepatic metabolism of estrogen in postmenopausal smokers, resulting in lower serum levels of these hormones.

Treatment of osteoporosis

In osteoporotic patients, the rate of bone loss during the early postmenopausal period increases to 3-4% per year. Estrogen replacement therapy, which slows bone turnover, results in increased bone density in the trabecular spaces during remodeling (Frost 1989). The increased skeletal bone mass which occurs in response to estrogen replacement therapy is apparent in the first 2 years of treatment and maintained with continuation of treatment (Kimmel et al. 1994). The effects of estrogen in regaining bone mass to premenopausal levels and in preventing/reversing postmenopausal osteoporotic changes in the long bones and spine have been demonstrated in several studies (Takahashi et al. 1994, Armamento-Villareal et al. 1992).

There is some controversy with regard to the benefits of hormone replacement due to the risk factors involved. Fractures due to osteoporosis and heart disease in postmenopausal women can be reduced by 50% with estrogen replacement therapy. However, hormone replacement with estrogen alone exposes such patients to the risk of endometrial cancer. Long-term hormone replacement therapy has been shown to correlate with an increased risk of breast cancer. Modern formulations utilize combined therapy with a suitable dose of progesterone in combination with estrogen in order to minimize some of these risk factors (Whitehead & Lobo 1988).

Hormonal contraceptives

Contraceptives utilize synthetic gestational hormones (estrogen and progesterone), to reduce the likelihood of ovulation/implantation (Guyton 1987). Less dramatic but similar effects to pregnancy are sometimes observed in the gingivae of hormonal contraceptive users. The most common oral manifestation of elevated levels of ovarian hormones is an increase in gingival inflammation with an accompanying increase in gingival exudate (Mariotti 1994).

There are reported systemic risk factors associated with long-term use of hormonal contraceptives. The correlation between hormonal contraceptive use and significant cardiovascular disease associated with arterial and venous thromboembolic episodes has been reviewed by Westhoff (1996). Estrogen is responsible for both arterial and venous effects, while progesterone affects arterial changes. Women using oral contraceptives show elevated plasma levels of several clotting factors, related to the dose of estrogen. Raised levels of factors VIIc and XIIc are significant, since they increase the likelihood of coagulation and in men these factors have a strong positive correlation with ischemic heart disease. However, the relative risk is dependent on the contraceptive formulation used and there may not be a consistent biological plausibility to explain this association (Davis 2000).

There are several different formulations of hormonal contraceptives (Davis 2000) including:

1. Combined oral contraceptives containing artificial analogues of estrogen and progesterone
2. Progesterone based mini-pill
3. Slow release progesterone implants placed subdermally that last up to 5 years (e.g Norplant)
4. Depo Provera, a very effective progestin injection given by a doctor every 3 months.

Current combined oral contraceptives consist of low doses of estrogens of 50 µg/day and/or progestins of 1.5 mg/day (Mariotti 1994). The formulations used in the early periodontal studies contained higher concentrations of gestational hormones, e.g. 50 µg estrogen with 4 mg progestin (El-Ashiry et al. 1971), 100 µg estrogen with 5 mg progestin (Lindhe & Bjorn 1967). The results obtained in these studies would partly reflect the contraceptive preparation used. In one early study (Knight & Wade 1974) women who were on hormonal contraceptives for more than 1.5 years exhibited greater periodontal destruction compared to the control group of comparable age and oral hygiene. This could partly reflect higher dose of gestagens used in older contraceptive preparations. However, a recent study on a population of rural Sri Lankan women confirmed these findings (Tilakaratne et al. 2000b), showing significantly higher levels of gingivitis in contraceptive users (0.03 mg estradiol and 0.15 mg of a progestin), than non-users, despite similar plaque scores. There was also significant periodontal breakdown in those who used the progesterone injection (a depot preparation of 150 mg progesterone) 3 monthly for 2-4 years, compared with those who used it for less than 2 years. These findings may be attributed to the duration of use, and the effects of progesterone in promoting tissue catabolism, resulting in increased periodontal attachment loss. However, if low plaque levels are established and maintained for the duration of use, these effects could be minimized.

Effect on tissue response

Both estrogen and progesterone are known to cause increased gingival exudate, associated with inflammatory edema (Lindhe & Bjorn 1967). A 53% increase in crevicular fluid volume has been demonstrated in hormonal contraceptive users compared with controls. El-Ashiry et al. (1971) observed that the most pronounced effects on the gingiva occurred in the first 3 months of contraceptive treatment, but the dose of gestational hormones was higher in the older formulations compared with those used currently (Davis 2000), accounting for a more florid response in the tissues.

It has been suggested that the interaction of estrogen with progesterone results in the mediation of the effects characteristic of progesterone. Human gingiva has receptors for progesterone and estrogen (Vittek et al. 1982, Staffolani et al. 1989), providing evidence that gingiva is a target tissue for both gestational hormones. In *in vitro* studies of cultured gingival fibroblasts, estrogen enhanced the formation of anabolic androgen metabolites, while progesterone caused a diminished response. The combined effect of both gestational hormones on the yield of androgens was less pronounced than with estrogen alone, implying a more catabolic role for progesterone (Tilakaratne & Soory 1999).

Progesterone causes increased vascular permeability, resulting in the infiltration of polymorphonuclear leukocytes and raised levels of prostaglandin E_2 in the sulcular fluid (Miyagi et al. 1993). Increased capillary permeability may be induced by estrogen by stimulating the release of mediators such as bradykinin, prostaglandins and histamine. However, the main effects of estrogen are in controlling blood flow. Hence the combination of estrogen and progesterone in the contraceptive pill can contribute to vascular changes in the gingivae. The resultant gingivitis can be minimized by establishing low plaque levels at the beginning of oral contraceptive therapy (Zachariasen 1993).

TOBACCO SMOKING

Tobacco smoking is very common, with cigarettes being the main product smoked. In the European Union, an average of 29% of the adult population smoke. The figure is higher for men (34%) than for women (24%). Most smokers start the habit as teenagers, with the highest prevalence in the 20-24 year old age group. Socio-economic differences also exist with higher smoking in the lower socio-economic groups. These data are similar for the US population (Garfinkel 1997), but reported smoking rates for third world countries are even higher. Smoking is associated with a wide spectrum of disease including stroke, coronary artery disease, peripheral artery disease, gastric ulcer and cancers of the mouth, larynx, esophagus, pancreas, bladder and uterine cervix. It is also a major cause of chronic obstructive pulmonary disease and a risk factor for low birth weight babies. Approximately 50% of regular smokers are killed by their habit and smoking causes 30% of cancer deaths.

Cigarette smoke is a very complex mixture of substances with over 4000 known constituents. These include carbon monoxide, hydrogen cyanide, reactive oxidizing radicals, a high number of carcinogens and the main psychoactive and addictive molecule – nicotine (Benowitz 1996). Many of these components could modify the host response in periodontitis. In most of the *in vitro* studies considered in the latter parts of this chapter the experimenters utilized simple models with nicotine alone. Tobacco smoke has a gaseous phase and solid phase which contains tar droplets. The tar and nicotine yields of cigarettes have been reduced due to physical characteristics of the filters. However, there has been little change in the tar and nicotine content of the actual tobacco and the dose an individual receives is largely dependent upon the way in which they smoke (Benowitz 1989). Inter subject smoking variation includes: frequency of inhalation, depth of inhalation, length of the cigarette stub left, presence or absence of a filter and the brand of cigarette (Benowitz 1988). The patient's exposure to tobacco smoke can be measured in a number of ways including interviewing the subject using simple questions or more sophisticated questionnaires and biochemical analyses (Scott et al. 2001). The latter tests include exhaled carbon monoxide in the breath, which is commonly measured in smoking cessation clinics, and cotinine (a metabolite of nicotine) in saliva, plasma/serum or urine (Wall et al. 1988). Cotinine measurements are more reliable in determining a subject's exposure to tobacco smoke because the half-life is 14-20 hours compared with the shorter half-life of nicotine which is 2-3 hours (Jarvis et al. 1988). The mean plasma and salivary cotinine concentrations of regular smokers are approximately 300 ng/ml and

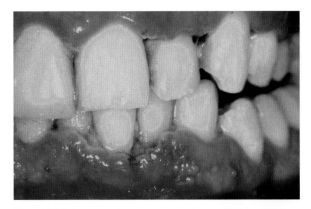

Fig. 6-10. The typical appearance of necrotizing ulcerative gingivitis in a heavy smoker with poor oral hygiene.

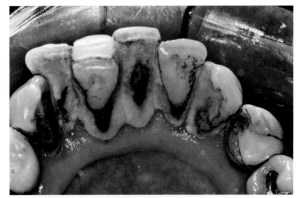

Fig. 6-11. The lingual aspects of the lower incisors showing gross supragingival calculus formation and relatively little gingival inflammation in a female patient who has smoked 20 cigarettes per day for over 20 years.

urine concentrations are about 1500 ng/ml. Non-smokers typically have plasma/saliva concentrations under 2 ng/ml, but this may be raised slightly due to environmental exposure (passive smoking).

Inhalation of tobacco smoke allows very rapid absorption of nicotine into the blood and transport to the brain, which is faster than an intravenous infusion. Nicotine in tobacco smoke from most cigarettes is not well absorbed through the oral mucosa because the nicotine is in an ionized form as a result of the pH (5.5). In contrast cigar and pipe smoke is more alkaline (pH 8.5), which allows good absorption of un-ionized nicotine through the buccal mucosa (Benowitz 1988). Nicotine is absorbed rapidly in the lung where the smoke is well buffered. The administration of nicotine causes a rise in the blood pressure, an increase in heart rate, an increase in respiratory rate and decreased skin temperature due to peripheral vasoconstriction. However, at other body sites, such as skeletal muscle, nicotine produces vasodilatation. These differing actions of nicotine have led to some controversy over its action in the periodontal tissues. Clarke and co-workers (1981) showed that the infusion of nicotine resulted in a transient decrease in gingival blood flow in a rabbit model. However, Baab and Öberg (1987) using laser Doppler flowmetry to monitor relative gingival flow in 12 young smokers, observed an immediate but transient increase in relative gingival blood flow during smoking, compared to the presmoking or resting measurements. The authors hypothesized that the steep rise in heart rate and blood pressure due to smoking could lead to an increase in the gingival circulation during smoking. These results were confirmed by Meekin et al. (2000) who showed that subjects who smoked only very occasionally experienced an increase in blood flow to the head, whereas regular smokers showed no change in blood flow, demonstrating tolerance in the regular smoker.

Periodontal disease in smokers

Pindborg (1947) was one of the first investigators to study the relationship between smoking and periodontal disease. He discovered a higher prevalence of acute necrotizing ulcerative gingivitis, a finding that was confirmed in many subsequent studies of this condition (Pindborg 1949, Kowolik & Nisbet 1983, Johnson & Engel 1984) (Fig. 6-10). Early studies showed that smokers had higher levels of periodontitis but they also had poorer levels of oral hygiene (Brandzaeg & Jamison 1984) and higher levels of calculus (Alexander 1970, Sheiham 1971) (Fig. 6-11). Later studies which took account of oral hygiene status and employed more sophisticated statistical analyses showed that smokers had more disease regardless of oral hygiene (Ismail et al. 1983, Bergstrom 1989, Bergstrom & Preber 1994).

A large number of studies have established that in comparing smokers and non-smokers with periodontitis, smokers have:

1. Deeper probing depths and a larger number of deep pockets (Feldman et al. 1983, Bergstrom & Eliasson 1987a, Bergstrom et al. 2000a)
2. More attachment loss including more gingival recession (Grossi et al. 1994, Linden & Mullally 1994, Haffajee & Socransky 2001a)
3. More alveolar bone loss (Bergstrom & Floderus Myhred 1983, Bergstrom & Eliasson 1987b, Feldman et al. 1987, Bergstrom et al. 1991, 2000b, Grossi et al. 1995)
4. More tooth loss (Osterberg & Mellstrom 1986, Krall et al. 1997)
5. Less gingivitis and less bleeding on probing (Feldman et al. 1983, Preber & Bergstrom 1985, Bergstrom & Preber 1986, Haffajee & Socransky 2001a)
6. More teeth with furcation involvement (Mullally & Linden 1996)

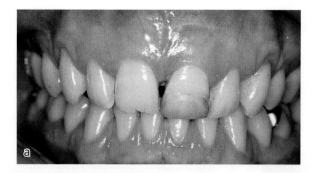

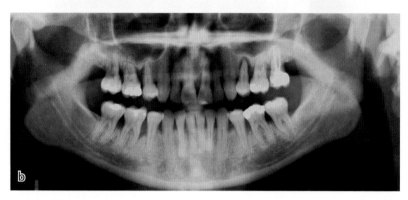

Fig. 6-12. A 30-year-old female smoker with advanced periodontitis. (a) The clinical appearance shows marginal gingiva with little signs of inflammation. Probing depths greater than 6 mm were present at most interproximal sites, but with little bleeding on probing. (b) The generalized advanced bone loss in this patient.

The finding of less gingival bleeding on probing is associated with less inflamed marginal tissue and lower bleeding scores when probing the depth of the pockets. The typical clinical appearance of the smoker's gingival tissue is shown in Fig. 6-12, which demonstrates relatively low levels of marginal inflammation and a tendency to a more fibrotic appearance with little edema. Despite the clinical appearance of the gingival tissue, the patient has deep pockets, advanced attachment loss and bone loss as shown in Fig. 6-12b.

Modification of the host/bacteria relationship in smoking

There are a number of theories as to why smokers have more periodontal disease than non-smokers, involving both bacterial aspects and the host response.

Effects on plaque bacteria

Smokers may have higher levels of plaque than non-smokers, which may be accounted for by poorer levels of oral hygiene rather than higher rates of supragingival plaque growth (Bergstrom 1981, Bergstrom & Preber 1986). Several studies have shown that smokers harbor more bacterial species which are associated with periodontitis including *Porphyromonas gingivalis, Actinobacillus actinomycetemcomitans, Bacteroides forsythus* (Zambon et al. 1996), *Prevotella intermedia, Peptostreptococcus micros, Fusobacterium nucleatum, Campylobacter rectus* (van Winkelhoff et al. 2002), *Staphylococcus aureus, Eschericia coli* and *Candida albicans* (Kamma et al. 1999) than non-smokers. Smokers may have a higher proportion of sites harboring these putative periodontal pathogens, in particular the palatal

aspects of the maxillary teeth and the upper and lower incisor regions (Haffajee & Socransky 2001a,b).

Effects on the host response

The relationship between plaque accumulation and development of inflammation in smokers has been studied in classical experimental gingivitis studies (Bergstrom & Preber 1986). They demonstrated that there is no difference in plaque accumulation when comparing smokers and non-smokers. However, the development of inflammation was very much retarded in the smoking group with less sites exhibiting redness or bleeding on probing. They also showed lower amounts of gingival crevicular fluid during the development of gingivitis. The reduced bleeding has been proposed to be caused by nicotine induced vasoconstriction, but as previously described in this chapter, more recent evidence has failed to show a reduction in blood flow to the gingiva following smoking a cigarette in regular smokers (Meekin et al. 2000). The reduced bleeding on the other hand may be due to long-term effects on the inflammatory lesion. Histological comparisons of the lesions from smokers and non-smokers has shown fewer blood vessels in the inflammatory lesions of smokers (Rezavandi et al. 2001).

Smoking has a profound effect on the immune and inflammatory system (reviewed by Barbour et al. 1997). Smokers have an increased number of leukocytes in the systemic circulation, but fewer cells may migrate into the gingival crevice/pocket. Smoking is associated with chronic obstructive pulmonary disease (Barnes 2000) and many of the mechanisms indicated are paralleled in findings related to periodontal disease. It is thought that the main cell type responsible for destruction of lung parenchyma is the neutrophil, which is delayed in its transit through the pulmonary vasculature (McNee et al. 1989) where it is stimulated to release proteases including elastase, cathepsins and matrix metalloproteases (Barnes 2000). These destructive molecules are balanced by inhibitors such as α-1-antitrypsin and tissue inhibitors of matrix metalloproteases.

Studies *in vitro* have shown a direct inhibition of neutrophil and monocyte-macrophage defensive functions by high concentrations of nicotine that may be achieved in patients using smokeless tobacco (Pabst et al. 1995). MacFarlane and co-workers (1992) examined patients with refractory periodontitis and found a high proportion of smokers in this diagnostic group. These investigators demonstrated abnormal PMN phagocytosis associated with a high level of cigarette smoking.

The PMN is a fundamental defense cell in the periodontal tissue. There is a constant traffic of PMNs from the gingival vasculature through the connective tissue and junctional epithelium into the gingival sulcus/pocket. This is described in some detail in Chapter 5. The PMN is the first line of defense and is chemotactically attracted to bacterial challenge at the dento-gingival junction. The PMN contains a powerful battery of enzymes including elastase and other collagenases that have been implicated in tissue destruction in periodontitis and pulmonary disease. Eichel and Shahrik (1969) suggested decreased PMN migration into the oral cavity of smokers. Subsequently, PMNs harvested from the gingival sulcus of smokers were shown to have reduced phagocytic capacity compared to PMNs from non-smokers (Kenney et al. 1977). Neutrophil defects have been associated with an increased susceptibility to periodontitis, including cyclic neutropenia where there is a reduction in the number of neutrophils, and conditions such as leukocyte adhesion deficiency (LAD 1 and LAD 2), which may be responsible for cases of generalized prepubertal periodontitis as described by Page et al. (1983). It is proposed that smoking causes alterations to PMN function which could be considered to be minor variations of these more profound defects.

The normal passage of the PMN from the microvasculature to the periodontal tissues involves a classic series of events including capture, rolling on the endothelium, firm adhesion to the endothelium and transmigration through the vessel wall into the connective tissue (Ley 1996). This involves a complex interaction between receptors and ligands on the leukocyte surface and endothelium including selectins, ICAM-1 and LFA1 (CD18, CD11b) (Crawford & Watanabe 1994, Gemmel et al. 1994). Defects in the functional ligands for the selectins have been implicated in LAD 2 and mutations in the gene encoding CD18 resulting in absence of the β 2 integrins with LAD 1. Subjects with LAD are susceptible to serious and life-threatening infections and have tremendous destruction of the periodontal tissues, often leading to total tooth loss in the deciduous dentition. These serious and rare conditions illustrate the overwhelming importance of the adhesion molecules and suggest that minor defects in them may also give rise to more subtle conditions that could lead to increased susceptibility to periodontal destruction. In this respect, it has been shown that smokers are affected by upregulation of molecules such as ICAM-1 on the endothelium and they have higher levels of circulating soluble ICAM-1 which could interfere with the normal receptor ligand binding and function of the leukocyte in the defense of the periodontal tissue (Koundouros et al. 1996, Palmer et al. 1999, Scott et al. 2000a). A potential destructive mechanism is the release of elastase from neutrophils following binding of ICAM with CD18 (Mac 1 and LFA 1) (Barnett et al. 1996). Lower levels of elastase detected in the gingival fluid of smokers compared to non-smokers, may indicate more elastase release within the tissues (Alavi et al. 1995), and this is especially important considering the effects of smoking on protease inhibitors.

Tobacco smoking has a chronic effect on the elevated levels of sICAM and there is evidence that the subject may return to more normal levels after quitting smoking (Scott et al. 2000b). These molecules can be detected in the serum and in the gingival crevicular fluid. It has also been shown that cotinine is present in the gingival crevicular fluid in about the same concentration as it appears in serum, but the levels of sICAM are much lower in smokers despite very much higher serum levels than non-smokers (Fraser et al. 2001).

The effects of smoking on lymphocyte function and antibody production are very complex, with the various components having the potential to cause immunosuppression or stimulation. The leukocytosis observed in smokers results in increased numbers of circulating T and B lymphocytes (reviewed in Sopori & Kozak 1998). Smoking appears to affect both B and T cell function, inducing functional unresponsiveness in T cells. Smoking has been shown to reduce most of the immunoglobulin classes except for IgE and to inhibit pro-inflammatory cytokines (Barbour et al. 1997, Quinn et al. 1998).

The clinical change in the tissues of smokers was described above. It is not surprising that histological evaluation of smokers' tissues has shown that there is a decrease in the vascularity of the tissues (Rezavandi et al. 2001). This is a chronic effect due to smoking and may also be associated with alterations in the expression of adhesion molecules within the endothelium. The effect of tobacco smoking on the expression of adhesion molecules on leukocytes, within the inflammatory lesion, in the junctional epithelium and cells of the pocket epithelium could have important implications on the progression of periodontitis in smokers. The effect of smoking on macrovasular disease is well documented (Powell 1998) and its effects on microvascular disease could also be of importance in the periodontal disease and in healing.

Effects on healing and treatment response

The healing potential of tissues has important implications in any chronic inflammatory lesion and in repair following treatment. Smoking has been identified as an important cause of impaired healing in orthopedic surgery, plastic surgery, dental implant surgery (Bain & Moy 1993) and in all aspects of periodontal treatment including non-surgical treatment, basic periodontal surgery, regenerative periodontal surgery and mucogingival plastic periodontal surgery (Preber & Bergstrom 1986, Miller 1987, Grossi et al. 1996, 1997, Kaldahl et al. 1996, Tonetti et al. 1995, Bostrom et al. 1998).

In non-surgical treatment, smoking is associated with poorer reductions in probing depth and gains in clinical attachment. In most studies the smokers at baseline have a lower level of bleeding, and following treatment bleeding scores are reduced in smokers in a similar manner to non-smokers. The poorer reductions in probing depths and gains in attachment level amount to a mean of approximately 0.5 mm. Much of this may be due to less recession of the marginal tissues in smokers as there is less edema and more fibrosis in the gingiva. The same may be true for the deeper tissues of the periodontium where there is less of an inflammatory infiltrate and vascularity at the depth of the pocket. These differences in the tissues between smokers and non-smokers in the untreated state may largely account for the differences in treatment response in non-surgical treatment. It has been proposed that these differences may be manifest by differences in probe penetration in smokers and non-smokers, particularly in deep pockets (Biddle et al. 2001).

The poor response to treatment in smokers in non-surgical treatment may also apply to those treated with adjunctive antibiotics (Kinane & Radvar 1997, Palmer et al. 1999). Response to non-surgical treatment may be seen merely as resolution of inflammation, improvement of the epithelial attachment together with some formation of collagen. However, the response following periodontal surgery is more complex and involves an initial inflammatory reaction followed by organization of the clot, formation of granulation tissue consisting of capillary buds and fibroblasts laying down collagen. The surgical flaps have to revascularize and the epithelial attachment has to reform on the surface. In regenerative surgery there also has to be formation of a connective tissue attachment and cementogenesis. Tobacco smoke and nicotine undoubtedly affect the microvasculature, the fibroblasts and connective tissue matrix, the bone and also the root surface itself. It has been shown in *in vitro* studies that fibroblasts are affected by nicotine in that they demonstrate reduced proliferation, reduced migration and matrix production and poor attachment to surfaces (Raulin et al. 1988, Tipton & Dabbous 1995, James et al. 1999). The root surfaces in smokers are additionally contaminated by products of smoking such as nicotine and cotinine and these molecules may affect the attachment of cells (Raulin et al. 1988). Smoking has a direct effect on bone and is an established risk factor in osteoporosis. It has also been proposed that it may have a direct affect on bone loss in periodontitis (Bergstrom et al. 1991) and it undoubtedly delays healing of bone in fracture wound repair. It is not surprising therefore that tobacco smoking has been implicated in poorer responses to periodontal surgical treatment.

Smoking cessation

All patients should be assessed for smoking status and given advice to quit the habit. About 70% of people who smoke would like to quit and should be assisted. They should be referred to specialist cessation services if the treating practitioner does not feel confident in this area. They can be advised about nicotine replacement therapy. People's success with quitting is considerably improved using nicotine replacement therapy and drugs such as buproprion hydrochloride. Former smokers more closely resemble non-smokers in their periodontal health status and response to treatment, but the time required to revert to this status has not been defined.

REFERENCES

Abraham-Inpijn, L., Polsacheva, D.V. & Raber-Durlacher, J.E. (1996). The significance of endocrine factors and microorganisms in the development of gingivitis in pregnant women. *Stomatolgiia* **75**, 15-18.

Alavi, A.L., Palmer, R.M., Odell, E.W., Coward, P.Y. & Wilson, R.F. (1995). Elastase in gingival crevicular fluid from smokers and non-smokers with chronic inflammatory periodontal disease. *Oral Diseases* **1**, 103-105.

Aldridge, J.P., Lester, V., Watts, T.L., Collins, A., Viberti, G. & Wilson, R.F. (1995). Single blind studies on the effects of improved periodontal health on metabolic control in type 1 diabetes mellitus. *Journal of Clinical Periodontology* **22**, 271-275.

Alexander, A.G. (1970). The relationship between tobacco smoking, calculus and plaque accumulation and gingivitis. *Dental Health* **9**, 6-9.

Amar, S. & Chung, K.M. (1994). Influence of hormonal variation on the periodontium in women. *Periodontology 2000* **6**, 79-87.

Armamento-Villareal, R., Villareal, D.T., Avioli, L.V. & Civitelli, R. (1992). Estrogen status and heredity are major determinants of premenopausal bone mass. *Journal of Clinical Investigation* **90**, 2464-2471.

Atkinson, M.A. & Maclaren, N.K. (1990). What causes diabetes? *Scientific American* **263**, 62-63, 66-71.

Baab, D.A. & Öberg, P.A. (1987). The effect of cigarette smoking on gingival blood flow in humans. *Journal of Clinical Periodontology* **14**, 418-424.

Bain, C.A. & Moy, P.K. (1993). The association between the failure of dental implants and cigarette smoking. *International Journal Oral & Maxillofacial Implants* **8**, 609-615.

Barbour, S.E., Nakashima, K., Zhang, J.B. et al. (1997). Tobacco and smoking: environmental factors that modify the host response (immune system) and have an impact on periodontal health. *Critical Reviews in Oral Biology & Medicine* **8**, 437-460.

Barnes, P.J. (2000). Chronic obstructive pulmonary disease. *New England Journal of Medicine* **343**, 269-280.

Barnett, C.C, Moore, E.E, Moore, F.A., Biffl, W.L. & Partrick D.A. (1996). Soluble intercellullar adhesion molecule-1 provokes polymorphonuclear leukocyte elastase release by CD18. *Surgery* **120**, 395-402.

Baxter, J.C. (1987). Osteoporosis: oral manifestations of a systemic disease. *Quintessence International* **18**, 472-479.

Benowitz, N.L. (1988). Pharmacological aspects of cigarette smoking and nicotine addiction. *New England Journal of Medicine* **319**, 1318-1330.

Benowitz, N.L. (1989). Health and public policy implications of the low yield cigarette. *New England Journal of Medicine* **320**, 1619-1621.

Benowitz N.L. (1996). Pharmacology of nicotine: addiction and therapeutics. *Annual Reviews in Pharmacology Toxicology* **36**, 597-613.

Bergstrom J. (1981). Short-term investigation on the influence of cigarette smoking upon plaque accumulation. *Scandinavian Journal of Dental Research* **89**, 235-238.

Bergstrom, J. (1989). Cigarette smoking as a risk factor in chronic periodontal disease. *Community Dentistry and Oral Epidemiology* **17**, 245-247.

Bergstrom, J. & Eliasson, S. (1987a). Noxious effect of cigarette smoking on periodontal health. *Journal of Periodontal Research* **22**, 513-517.

Bergstrom, J. & Eliasson, S. (1987b). Cigarette smoking and alveolar bone height in subjects with high standard of oral hygiene. *Journal of Clinical Periodontology* **14**, 466-469.

Bergstrom, J., Eliasson, S. & Dock, J. (2000a). A 10-year prospective study of tobacco smoking and periodontal health. *Journal of Periodontology* **71**, 1338-1347.

Bergstrom, J., Eliasson, S. & Dock, J. (2000b). Exposure to smoking and periodontal health. *Journal of Clinical Periodontology* **27**, 61-68.

Bergstrom, J., Eliasson, S. & Preber, H. (1991). Cigarette smoking and periodontal bone loss. *Journal of Periodontology* **62**, 244-246.

Bergstrom, J. & Floderus Myrhed, B. (1983). Co-twin control study of the relationship between smoking and some periodontal disease factors. *Community Dentistry and Oral Epidemiology* **11**, 113 -116.

Bergstrom, J., Persson, L. & Preber, H. (1988). Influence of cigarette smoking on vascular reaction during experimental gingivitis. *Scandinavian Journal of Dental Research* **96**, 34-39.

Bergstrom, J. & Preber, H. (1986). The influence of tobacco smoking on the development of experimental gingivitis. *Journal of Periodontal Research* **21**, 668-676.

Bergstrom, J. & Preber, H. (1994). Tobacco use as a risk factor. *Journal of Periodontology* **65**, 545-550.

Biddle, A., Palmer, R.M., Wilson, R.F. & Watts, T.L.P. (2001). Comparison of periodontal probing measurements in smokers and non-smokers. *Journal of Clinical Periodontology* **28**, 806-812.

Bostrom, L., Linder, L.E. & Bergstrom, J. (1998). Influence of smoking on the outcome of periodontal surgery. A 5-year follow-up. *Journal of Clinical Periodontology* **25**, 194-201.

Brandzaeg, P. & Jamison, H.C. (1984). A study on periodontal health and oral hygiene in Norwegian army recruits. *Journal of Periodontology* **35**, 303-307.

Brownlee, M. (1994). Glycation and diabetic complications. *Diabetes* **43**, 836-841.

Chau, D., Mancoll, J.S., Lee, S., Zhao, J., Phillips, L.G., Gittes, G.K. & Longaker, M.T. (1998). Tamoxifen downregulates TGFβ-

production in keloid fibroblasts. *Annals of Plastic Surgery* **40**, 490-493.

Christgau, M., Palitzsch, K.D., Schmalz, G., Kreiner, U. & Frenzel, S. (1998). Healing response to non-surgical periodontal therapy in patients with diabetes mellitus: Clinical, microbiological and immunological results. *Journal of Clinical Periodontology* **25**, 112-124.

Clarke, N.G., Shepherd, B.C. & Hirsch, R.S. (1981). The effects of intra-arterial epinephrine and nicotine on gingival circulation. *Oral Surgery, Oral Medicine, Oral Pathology* **52**, 577-582.

Cohen, D.W., Friedman, L., Shapiro, J. & Kyle, G.C. (1969). A longitudinal investigation of the periodontal changes during pregnancy. *Journal of Periodontology* **40**, 563-570.

Crawford, J.M. & Watanabe K. (1994). Cell adhesion molecules in inflammation and immunity: relevance to periodontal diseases. *Critical Reviews in Oral Biology & Medicine* **5**, 91-123.

Davis, A.J. (2000). Advances in contraception (review). *Obstetrics and Gynaecology Clinics of North America* **27**, 597-610.

Di Placido, G., Tumini, V., D'Archivio, D. & Peppe, G. (1998). Gingival hyperplasia in pregnancy II. Aetiopathogenic factors and mechanisms. *Minerva Stomatologica* **47**, 223-229.

Eichel, G. & Shahrik, H.A. (1969). Tobacco smoke toxicity: loss of human oral leucocyte function and fluid cell metabolism. *Science* **166**, 1424-1428.

El-Ashiry, G.M., El- Kafrawy, A.H., Nasr, M.F. et al. (1971). Effects of oral contraceptives on the gingiva. *Journal of Periodontology* **56**, 18-20.

Esposito, C., Gerlach, H., Brett, J., Stern, D. & Vlassara, H. (1992). Endothelial receptor mediated binding of glucose-modified albumin is associated with increased monolayer permeability and modulation of cell-surface coagulant properties. *Journal of Experimental Medicine* **170**, 1387-1407.

Feldman, R.S., Alman, J.E. & Chauncey, H.H. (1987). Periodontal disease indexes and tobacco smoking in healthy ageing men. *Gerodontics* **1**, 43-46.

Feldman, R.S., Bravacos, J.S. & Rose, C.L. (1983). Association between smoking different tobacco products and periodontal disease indexes. *Journal of Periodontology* **54**, 481-487.

Fraser, H.S., Palmer, R.M., Wilson, R.F., Coward, P.Y. & Scott, D.A. (2001). Elevated systemic concentrations of soluble ICAM-1 are not reflected in the gingival crevicular fluid of smokers with periodontitis. *Journal of Dental Research* **80**, 1643-1647.

Frost, H.M. (1989). Some effects of basic multicellular unit-based remodelling on photon absorptiometry of trabecular bone. *Bone and Mineral* **7**, 47-65.

Garfinkel (1997). Trends in cigarette smoking in the United States. *Preventive Medicine* **26**, 447-450.

Gemmell, E., Walsh, L.J., Savage, N.W. & Seymour, G.J. (1994). Adhesion molecule expression in chronic inflammatory periodontal disease tissue. *Journal of Periodontal Research* **29**, 46-53.

Gotfredsen, A., Nilas, L., Riis, B.J., Thomsen, K. & Christiansen, C. (1986). Bone changes occurring spontaneously and caused by oestrogen in early post-menopausal women: a local or generalised phenomenon? *British Medical Journal* **292**, 1098-1100.

Grady, D., Rubin, S.M., Petitti, D.B. et al. (1992). Hormone therapy to prevent disease and prolong life in post-menopausal women. *Annals of Internal Medicine* **117**, 1016-1037.

Grant, D., Stern, J. & Listgarten, M. (1988). The epidemiology, etiology and public health aspects of periodontal disease. In: Grant, D., Stern, J. and Listgarten, M., eds. *Periodontics*. St. Louis: CV Mosby Co, pp.229, 332-335.

Grodstein, F., Colditz, G.A. & Stampfer, M.J. (1996). Post-menopausal hormone use and tooth loss: A prospective study. *Journal of the American Dental Association* **127**, 370-377.

Grossi, S.G., Genco, R.J., Machtei, E.E. et al. (1995). Assessment of risk for periodontal disease. II. Risk indicators for alveolar bone loss. *Journal of Periodontology* **66**, 23-29.

Grossi, S.G., Skrepcinski, F.B., DeCaro, T., Zambon, J.J., Cummin, D. & Genco, R.J. (1996). Response to periodontal therapy in diabetics and smokers. *Journal of Periodontology* **67**, 1094-1102.

Grossi, S.G., Skrepcinski, F.B., DeCaro, T., Zambon, J.J., Cummin, D. & Genco, R.J. (1997). Treatment of periodontal disease in diabetics reduces glycated haemoglobin. *Journal of Periodontology* **68**, 713-719.

Grossi, S.G., Zambon, J.J., Ho, A.W. et al. (1994). Assessment of risk for periodontal disease. I. Risk indicators for attachment loss. *Journal of Periodontology* **65**, 260-267.

Grossi, S.G., Zambon, J., Machtei, E.E. et al. (1997). Effects of smoking and smoking cessation on healing after mechanical therapy. *Journal of the American Dental Association* **128**, 599-607.

Gugliucci, A. (2000). Glycation as the glucose link to diabetic complications (review). *Journal of the American Osteopathic Association* **100**, 621-634.

Guyton, A.C. (1987). *Human Physiology and Mechanisms of Disease*, 4th edn. Philadelphia: W.B. Saunders Co.

Haber, J., Wattles, J., Crowley, M., Mandell, R., Joshipura, K. & Kent, R.L. (1993). Evidence for cigarette smoking as a major risk factor for periodontitis. *Journal of Periodontology* **64**, 16-23.

Haffajee, A.D. & Socransky, S.S. (2001a). Relationship of cigarette smoking to attachment level profiles. *Journal of Clinical Periodontology* **28**, 283-295.

Haffajee, A.D. & Socransky, S.S. (2001b). Relationship of cigarette smoking to the subgingival microbiota. *Journal of Clinical Periodontology* **28**, 377-388.

Harrison, G.A., Schultz, T.A. & Schaberg, S.J. (1983). Deep neck infection complicated by diabetes mellitus. *Oral Surgery* **55**, 133-137.

Hasson, E. (1996). Pregnancy gingivitis. *Harefuah* **58**, 224-230.

Holm-Pedersen, P. & Loe, H. (1967). Flow of gingival exudate as related to menstruation and pregnancy. *Journal of Periodontal Research* **2**, 13-20.

Hopper, J.L. & Seeman, E. (1994). The bone density of female twins discordant for tobacco use. *New England Journal of Medicine* **330**, 387-392.

Hugoson, A. (1970). Gingival inflammation and female sex hormones. *Journal of Periodontal Research* **5**, (suppl.) 9.

Iacopino, A.M. (1995). Diabetic periodontitis: possible lipid induced defect in tissue repair through alteration of macrophage phenotype function. *Oral Diseases* **1**, 214-229.

Ismail A.I., Burt, B.A. & Eklund, S.A. (1983). Epidemiologic patterns of smoking and periodontal disease in the United States. *Journal of the American Dental Association* **106**, 617-621.

James, J.A., Sayers, N.S., Drucker, D.B. & Hull, P.S. (1999). Effects of tobacco products on the attachment and growth of periodontal ligament fibroblasts. *Journal of Periodontology* **70**, 518-525.

Jarvis, M.J., Russell, M.A.H., Benowitz, N.L. & Feyerabend, C. (1988). Elimination of cotinine from body fluids: Implications for non-invasive measurement of tobacco smoke exposure. *American Journal of Public Health* **78**, 696-698.

Jarvis, M.J., Tunstall-Pedoe, H., Feyerabend, C., Vesey, C. & Saloojee, Y. (1987). Comparison of tests used to distinguish smokers from non-smokers. *American Journal of Public Health* **77**, 1435-1438.

Jensen, J., Christiansen, C. & Rodbro, P. (1985). Cigarette smoking, serum oestrogens and bone loss during hormone-replacement therapy early after menopause. *New England Journal of Medicine* **313**, 973-975.

Jensen, J., Liljemark, W. & Bloomquist, C. (1981). The effect of female sex hormones on subgingival plaque. *Journal of Periodontology* **52**, 599-602.

Johnson, B.D. & Engel, D. (1986). Acute necrotizing ulcerative gingivitis. A review of diagnosis, etiology and treatment. *Journal of Periodontology* **57**, 141-150.

Kaldahl, W.B, Johnson, G.K, Patil, K. & Kalkwarf, K.L. (1996). Levels of cigarette consumption and response to periodontal therapy. *Journal of Periodontology* **67**, 675-681.

Kamma, J.J., Nakou, M. & Baehni, P.C. (1999). Clinical and microbiological characteristics of smokers with early onset periodontitis. *Journal of Periodontal Research* **34**, 25-33.

Karjalainen, , K.M., Knuuttila, M.L. & von Dickhoff, K.J. (1994). Association of the severity of periodontal disease with organ complications in type 1 diabetic patients. *Journal of Periodontology* **65**, 1067-1072.

Kenney, E.B., Kraal, J.H., Saxe, S.R. & Jones, J. (1977). The effect of cigarette smoke on human oral polymorphonuclear leukocytes. *Journal of Periodontal Research* **12**, 227-234.

Kimmel, D.B., Slovik, D.M. & Lane, N.E. (1994). Current and investigational approaches for reversing established osteoporosis. *Rheumatoid Disease Clinics of North America* **20**, 735-758.

Kimura, S., Elce, J.S. & Jellinek, P.H. (1983). Immunological relationship between peroxidases in eosinophils, uterus and other tissues of the rat. *Biochemical Journal* **213**, 165-169.

Kinane D.F. & Radvar M. (1997). The effect of smoking on mechanical and antimicrobial periodontal therapy. *Journal of Periodontology* **68**, 467-472.

Knight, G.M. & Wade, A.B. (1974). The effects of hormonal contraceptives on the human periodontium. *Journal of Periodontal Research* **9**, 18-22.

Kornman, K.S. & Loesche, W.J. (1979). Effects of oestradiol and progesterone on Bacteroides melaninogenicus. *Journal of Dental Research* **58A**, 107.

Koundouros, E., Odell, E., Coward, P.Y., Wilson, R.F. & Palmer, R.M. (1996). Soluble adhesion molecules in serum of smokers and non-smokers, with and without periodontitis. *Journal of Periodontal Research* **31**, 596-599.

Kowolik, M.J. & Nisbet, T. (1983). Smoking and acute ulcerative gingivitis. *British Dental Journal* **154**, 241-242.

Kraal, J.H. & Kenney, R.B. (1979). The response of polymorphonuclear leucocytes to chemotactic stimulation for smokers and non-smokers. *Journal of Periodontal Research* **14**, 383-389.

Krall, E.A. & Dawson-Hughes, B. (1991). Smoking and bone loss among post-menopausal women. *Journal of Bone and Mineral Research* **6**, 331-338.

Krall, E.A., Dawson-Hughes, B., Garvey, A.J. & Garcia, R.I. (1997). Smoking, smoking cessation and tooth loss. *Journal of Dental Research* **76**, 1653-1659.

Kritz-Silverstein, D. & Barrett-Connor, E. (1993). Early menopause, number of reproductive years and bone mineral density in postmenopausal women. *American Journal of Public Health* **83**, 983-988.

Lalla, E., Lamster, I.B., Drury, S., Fu, C. & Schmidt, A.M. (2000). Hyperglycaemia, glycooxidation and receptor for advanced glycation end products: potential mechanisms underlying diabetic complications, including diabetes-associated periodontitis (review). *Periodontology 2000* **23**, 50-62.

Lapp, C.A., Thomas, M.E. & Lewis, J.B. (1995). Modulation by progesterone of interleukin-6 production by gingival fibroblasts. *Journal of Periodontology* **66**, 279-284.

Le, J. & Vilcek, J. (1989). Interleukin-6: A multifunctional cytokine regulating immune reactions and the acute phase response. *Laboratory Investigation* **61**, 588-602.

Ley, K. (1996). Molecular mechanisms of leukocyte recruitment in the inflammatory process. *Cardiovascular Research* **32**, 733-742.

Linden, G.J. & Mullally, B.H. (1994). Cigarette smoking and periodontal destruction in young adults. *Journal of Periodontology* **65**, 718-723.

Lindhe, J. & Attstrom, R. (1967). Gingival exudation during the menstrual cycle. *Journal of Periodontal Research* **2**, 194-198.

Lindhe, J. & Bjorn, A.L. (1967). Influence of hormonal contraceptives on the gingivae of women. *Journal of Periodontal Research* **2**, 1-6.

Lindquist, O. & Bengtsson, C. (1979). Menopausal age in relation to smoking. *Acta Med Scandinavia* **205**, 73-77.

Lotz, M. & Guerne, P-A. (1991). Interleukin-6 induces the synthesis of tissue inhibitor of metalloproteinase-1/erythroid potentiating activity (TIMP-1/EPA). *Journal of Biological Chemistry* **266**, 2017-2020.

Lundgren, D., Magnussen, B. & Lindhe, J. (1973). Connective tissue alterations in gingiva of rats treated with oestrogens and progesterone. *Odontological Revy* **24**, 49-58.

Lynch, C.M., Sinnott, J.T., Holt, D.A. & Herold, A.H. (1991). Use of antibiotics during pregnancy. *American Family Physician* **43**, 1365-1368.

MacFarlane, G.D., Herzberg, M.C., Wolff, L.F. & Hardie, N.A. (1992). Refractory periodontitis associated with abnormal polymorphonuclear leukocyte phagocytosis and cigarette smoking. *Journal of Periodontology* **63**, 908-913.

Machuca, G., Khoshfeiz, O., Lacalle, J.R., Machuca, C. & Bullon, P. (1999). The influence of general health and socio-cultural variables on the periodontal condition of pregnant women. *Journal of Periodontology* **70**, 779-785.

Marhoffer, W., Stein, M., Maeser, E. & Federlin, K. (1992). Impairment of polymorphonuclear leucocyte function and metabolic control of diabetes. *Diabetes care* **15**, 156-260.

Mariotti, A. (1994). Sex steroid hormones and cell dynamics in the periodontium. *Critical Reviews in Oral Biology and Medicine* **5**, 27-53.

Mashimo, P.A., Yamamoto, Y., Slots, J., Park, B.H. & Genco, R.J. (1983). The periodontal microflora of juvenile diabetics. Culture, immunofluorescence, and serum antibody studies. *Journal of Periodontology* **54**, 420-430.

McNee, W., Wiggs, B., Belzberg, A.S. & Hogg, J.C. (1989). The effect of cigarette smoke on neutrophil kinetics in human lungs. *New England Journal of Medicine* **321**, 924-928.

Mealey, B.L. (1998). Impact of advances in diabetes care on dental treatment of the diabetic patient. *Compendium of Continuing Education in Dentistry* **19**, 41-58.

Meekin, T.N., Wilson, R.F., Scott, D.A., Ide, M. & Palmer, R.M. (2000). Laser Doppler flowmeter measurement of relative gingival and forehead skin blood flow in light and regular smokers during and after smoking. *Journal of Clinical Periodontology* **23**, 236-242.

Miller, P.D. (1987). Root coverage with free gingival grafts. Factors associated with incomplete coverage. *Journal of Periodontology* **58**, 674-681.

Miyagi, M., Morishita, M. & Iwamoto, Y. (1993). Effects of sex hormones on production of prostaglandin E_2 by human peripheral monocytes. *Journal of Periodontology* **64**, 1075-1078.

Miyazaki, H., Yamashita, Y., Shirahama, R., Goto-Kimura, K., Shimada, N., Sogame, A. & Takehara, T. (1991). Periodontal condition of pregnant women assessed by CPITN. *Journal of Clinical Periodontology* **18**, 751-754.

Mombelli, M., Gusberti, F.A., van Oosten, M.A.C. & Lang, N.P. (1989). Gingival health and gingivitis development during puberty. *Journal of Clinical Periodontology* **16**, 451-456.

Moore, M., Bracker, M., Sartoris, D., Saltman, P. & Strause, L. (1990). Long-term oestrogen replacement therapy in post-menopausal women sustains vertebral bone mineral density. *Journal of Bone and Mineral Research* **5**, 659-664.

Mullally, B.H. & Linden, G.J. (1996). Molar furcation involvement associated with cigarette smoking in periodontal referrals. *Journal of Clinical Periodontology* **23**, 658-661.

Muramatsu, Y. & Takaesu, Y. (1994). Oral health status related to subgingival bacterial flora and sex hormones in saliva during pregnancy. *Bulletin of the Tokyo Dental College* **35**, 139-151.

Murphy, E. & Nolan, J.J. (2000). Insulin sensitiser drugs (review). *Expert Opinion on Investigational Drugs* **9**, 347-361.

Nakagawa, S., Fujii, H., Machida, Y. & Okuda, K. (1994). A longitudinal study from prepuberty to puberty of gingivitis. Correlation between the occurrence of *Prevotella intermedia* and sex hormones. *Journal of Clinical Periodontology* **21**, 658-665.

Ojanotko-Harri, A.O., Harri, M.P., Hurttia, H.M. & Sewon, L.A. (1991) Altered tissue metabolism of progesterone in pregnancy gingivitis and granuloma. *Journal of Clinical Periodontology* **18**, 262-266.

Oliver, R.C., Tervonen, T., Flynn, D.G. & Keenan, K.M. (1993). Enzyme activity in crevicular fluid in relation to metabolic control of diabetes and other periodontal risk factors. *Journal of Periodontology* **64**, 358-362.

Osterberg, T. & Mellstrom, D. (1986). Tobacco smoking: A major risk factor for loss of teeth in three 70-year-old cohorts. *Community Dentistry and Oral Epidemology* **14**, 367-370.

Pabst, M.J., Pabst, K.M., Collier, J.A. et al. (1995). Inhibition of neutrophil and monocyte defensive functions by nicotine. *Journal of Periodontology* **66**, 1047-1055.

Paganini-Hill, A. (1995). The benefits of oestrogen relacement therapy on oral health. *Archives of Internal Medicine* **155**, 325-329.

Page, R.C., Bowen, T., Altman, L., Vandesteen, E., Ochs, H., Mackenzie, P., Osterberg, S., Engel, L.D. & Williams, B.L. (1983). Prepubertal periodontitis I. Definition of a clinical disease entity. *Journal of Periodontology* **54**, 257-271.

Palmer, R.M, Matthew, J.P. & Wilson, R.F. (1999). Non-surgical periodontal treatment with and without adjunctive metronidazole in smokers and non-smokers. *Journal of Clinical Periodontology* **26**, 158-163.

Palmer, R.M, Scott, D.A, Meekin, T.N, Wilson, R.F., Poston, R.N. & Odell E.W. (1999). Potential mechanisms of susceptibility to periodontitis in tobacco smokers. *Journal of Periodontal Research* **34**, 363-369.

Payne, J.B., Zachs, N.R., Reinhardt, R.A., Nummikoski, P.V. & Patil, K. (1997). The association between oestrogen status and alveolar bone density changes in post-menopausal women with a history of periodontitis. *Journal of Periodontology* **68**, 24-31.

Pindborg, J.J. (1947). Tobacco and gingivitis. 1. Statistical examination of the significance of tobacco in the development of ulceromembranous gingivitis and in the formation of calculus. *Journal of Dental Research* **26**, 261-264.

Pindborg, J.J. (1949). Tobacco and gingivitis. II Correlation between consumption of tobacco, ulceromembranous gingivitis and calculus. *Journal of Dental Research* **28**, 460-463.

Piwowar, A., Knapik-Kordecka, M. & Warwas, M. (2000). Concentrations of leukocyte elastase in plasma and polymorphonuclear neutrophil extracts in type 2 diabetes. *Clinical Chemistry & Laboratory Medicine* **38**, 1257-1261.

Powell J.T. (1998). Vascular damage from smoking: disease mechanisms at the arterial wall. *Vascular Medicine* **3**, 21-28.

Preber, H. & Bergstrom, J. (1985). Occurrence of gingival bleeding in smoker and non-smoker patients. *Acta Odontologica Scandinavica* **43**, 315-320.

Preber, H. & Bergstrom, J. (1986). The effect of non-surgical treatment on periodontal pockets in smokers and non-smokers. *Journal of Clinical Periodontology* **13**, 319-323.

Quinn, S.M., Zhang, J.B., Gunsolley, J.C., Schenkein, H.A. & Tew, J.G. (1998). The influence of smoking and race on adult periodontitis and serum 1gG2 levels. *Journal of Periodontology* **69**, 171-177.

Raber-Durlacher, J.E., Leene, W., Palmer-Bouva, C.C.R., Raber, J. & Abraham-Inpijn, L. (1993). Experimental gingivitis during pregnancy and post-partum: Immunological aspects. *Journal of Periodontology* **64**, 211-218.

Raulin, L.A., McPherson, J.C., McQuade, M.J. & Hanson, B.S. (1988). The effect of nicotine on the attachment of human fibroblasts to glass and human root surfaces in vitro. *Journal of Periodontology* **59**, 318-325.

Rezavandi, K., Palmer, R.M., Odell, E.W., Scott, D.A. & Wilson, R.F. (2001). Expression of E-Selectin and ICAM-1 in gingival tissues of smokers and non-smokers with periodontitis. *Journal of Oral Pathology and Medicine* **31**, 59-64.

Rigotti, N.A. (1989). Cigarette smoking and body weight. *New England Journal of Medicine* **320**, 931-933.

Salvi, G.E., Yalda, B., Collins, J.G., Jones, B.H., Smith, F.W., Arnold, R.R. & Offenbacher, S. (1997). Inflammatory mediator response as a potential risk marker for periodontal diseases in insulin-dependent diabetes mellitus patients. *Journal of Periodontology* **68**, 127-135.

Sastrowijoto, S.H., van der Velden, U., van Steenbergen, T.J.M. et al. (1990). Improved metabolic control, clinical periodontal status and subgingival microbiology in insulin-dependent diabetes mellitus. A prospective study. *Journal of Clinical Periodontology* **17**, 233-242.

Schmidt, A.M., Weidman, E., Lalla, E. et al. (1996). Advanced glycation end products (AGEs) induce oxidant stress in the gingiva: A potential mechanism underlying accelerated periodontal disease associated with diabetes. *Journal of Periodontal Research* **31**, 508-515.

Scott, D.A., Palmer, R.M. & Stapleton, J.A. (2001). Validation of smoking status in clinical research into inflammatory periodontal disease: a review. *Journal of Clinical Periodontology* **28**, 712-722.

Scott, D.A., Stapleton, J.A., Wilson, R.F. et al. (2000b). Dramatic decline in circulating intercellular adhesion molecule-1 concentration on quitting tobacco smoking. *Blood Cells Molecules Diseases* **26**, 255-258.

Scott, D.A., Todd, D.H., Wilson, R.F. et al. (2000a). The acute influence of tobacco smoking on adhesion molecule expression on monocytes and neutrophils and on circulating adhesion molecule levels in vivo. *Addiction Biology* **5**, 195-205.

Seppala, B. & Ainamo, J. (1996). Dark field microscopy of the subgingival microflora in insulin-dependent diabetes. *Journal of Clinical Periodontology* **23**, 63-67.

Shapiro, S., Bomberg, J., Benson, B.W. et al. (1985). Postmenopausal osteoporosis: dental patients at risk. *Gerodontics* **1**, 220-225.

Sheiham, A. (1971) Periodontal disease and oral cleanliness in tobacco smokers. *Journal of Periodontology* **42**, 259-263.

Silness, J. & Loe, H. (1963). Periodontal disease in pregnancy. II. Correlation between oral hygiene and periodontal condition. *Acta Odontologica Scandinavica* **22**, 121-135.

Slavkin, H.C. (1997). Diabetes, clinical dentistry and changing paradigms. *Journal of the American Dental Association* **128**, 638-644.

Sooriyamoorthy, M. & Gower, D.B. (1989). Hormonal influences on gingival tissue: relationship to periodontal disease. *Journal of Clinical Periodontology* **16**, 201-208.

Soory, M. (2000a). Hormonal factors in periodontal disease. *Dental Update* **27**, 380-383.

Soory, M. (2000b). Targets for steroid hormone mediated actions of periodontal pathogens, cytokines and therapeutic agents: some implications on tissue turnover in the periodontium. *Current Drug Targets* **1**, 309-325.

Sopori, M.L. & Kozak, W. (1998). Immunomodulatory effects of cigarette smoke. *Journal of Neuroimmunology* **83**, 148-156.

Sorsa, T., Ingman, T., Suomalainen, K. et al. (1992). Cellular source and tetracycline inhibition of gingival crevicular fluid collagenase of patients with labile diabetes mellitus. *Journal of Clinical Periodontology* **19**, 146-149.

Staffolani, N., Guerra, M. & Pugliese, M. (1989). Hormonal receptors in gingival inflammation. *Minerva Stomatologica* **38**, 823-826.

Stewart, J.E., Wager, K.A., Friedlander, A.H. & Zadeh, H.H. (2001). The effect of periodontal treatment on glycaemic control in patients with type 2 diabetes mellitus. *Journal of Clinical Periodontology* **28**, 306-310.

Sultan, C., Loire, C. & Kern, P. (1986). Collagen and hormone steroids. *Annals of Biological Clinics* **44**, 285-288.

Sutcliffe, P. (1972). A longitudinal study of gingivitis and puberty. *Journal of Periodontal Research* **7**, 52-58.

Szopa, T.M., Titchener, P.A., Portwood, N.D. & Taylor, K.W. (1993). Diabetes mellitus due to viruses – some recent developments. *Diabetologia* **36**, 687-695.

Takahashi, K., Tsuboyama, T., Matsushita, M. et al. (1994). Effective intervention of low peak bone mass and bone remodelling in the spontaneous murine model of senile osteoporosis, SAM-P/6, by Ca supplement and hormone treatment. *Bone* **15**, 209-215.

Taylor, G.W., Burt, B.A., Becker, M.P. et al. (1996). Severe periodontitis and risk for poor glycemic control in patients with non-insulin-dependent diabetes mellitus. *Journal of Periodontology* **67,** (suppl.) 1085-1093.

Tervonen, T. & Karjalainen, K. (1997). Periodontal disease related to diabetic status. A pilot study of the response to periodontal therapy in Type 1 diabetes. *Journal of Clinical Periodontology* **24**, 505-510.

Tervonen, T. & Oliver, R. (1993). Long-term control of diabetes mellitus and periodontitis. *Journal of Clinical Periodontology* **20**, 431-435.

Thorstensson, H., Kuylenstierna, J. & Hugoson, A. (1996). Medical status and complications in relation to periodontal disease experience in insulin-dependent diabetics. *Journal of Clinical Periodontology* **23**, 194-202.

Tiainen, L., Asikainen, S. & Saxen, L. (1992). Puberty-associated gingivitis. *Community Dentistry & Oral Epidemiology* **20**, 87-89.

Tilakaratne, A. & Soory, M. (1999). Modulation of androgen metabolism by oestradiol-17β and progesterone, alone and in combination, in human gingival fibroblasts in culture. *Journal of Periodontology* **70**, 1017-1025.

Tilakaratne, A., Soory, M., Ranasinghe, A.W., Corea, S.M.X., Ekanayake, S.L. & De Silva, M. (2000a). Periodontal disease status during pregnancy and 3 months post-partum in a rural population of Sri-Lankan women. *Journal of Clinical Periodontology* **27**, 787-792.

Tilakaratne, A., Soory, M., Ranasinghe, A.W., Corea, S.M.X., Ekanayake, S.L. & De Silva, M. (2000b). Effects of hormonal contraceptives on the periodontium in a population of rural Sri-Lankan women. *Journal of Clinical Periodontology* **27**, 753-757.

Tipton, D.A. & Dabbous, M.K. (1995). Effects of nicotine on proliferation and extracellular matrix production of human gingival fibroblasts in vitro. *Journal of Periodontology* **66**, 1056-1064.

Tonetti, M.S., Pini-Prato, G. & Cortellini, P. (1995). Effect of cigarette smoking on periodontal healing following GTR in infrabony defects. A preliminary retrospective study. *Journal of Clinical Periodontology* **22**, 229-234.

Ueta, E., Osaki, T., Yoneda, K. & Yamamoto, T. (1993). Prevalence of diabetes mellitus in odontogenic infections and oral candidiasis: an analysis of neutrophil suppression. *Journal of Oral Pathology and Medicine* **22**, 168-174.

UKPDS (1998a). UK Prospective Diabetes Study Group. Intensive blood-glucose control with sulfonylureas or insulin compared with conventional treatment and risk of complications in patients with Type 2 diabetes. *Lancet* **352**, 837-853.

UKPDS (1998b). UK Prospective Diabetes Study Group. Effect of intensive blood-glucose control with metformin on complications in overweight patients with Type 2 diabetes. *Lancet* **352**, 854-865.

Ulrich, P. & Cerami, A. (2001). Protein glycation, diabetes and aging. *Recent Progress in Hormone Research* **56**, 1-21.

van Winkelhoff. A.J., Bosch-Tijhof, C.J., Winkel, E.G. & van der Reijden, W.A. (2001). Smoking affects the subgingival microflora in periodontitis. *Journal of Periodontology* **72**, 666-671.

Vittek, J., Munnangi, P.R., Gordon, G.G., Rappaport, S.G. & Southren, A.L. (1982). Progesterone receptors in human gingiva. IRCS, *Medical Science* **10**, 381.

Wall, M.A., Johnson, J., Jacob, P. & Benowitz, NL (1988). Cotinine in the serum, saliva and urine of nonsmokers, passive smokers and active smokers. *American Journal of Public Health* **78**, 699-701.

Wang, P.H., Chao, H.T., Lee, W.L., Yuan, C.C. & Ng, H.T. (1997). Severe bleeding from a pregnancy tumour. A case report. *Journal of Reproductive Medicine* **42**, 359-362.

Westfelt, E., Rylander, H., Blohme, G., Joanasson, P. & Lindhe, J. (1996). The effect of periodontal therapy in diabetes. *Journal of Clinical Periodontology* **23**, 92-100.

Westhoff, C.L. (1996). Oral contraceptives and venous thromboembolism: should epidemiological associations drive clinical decision making? *Contraception* **54**, 1-3.

Whitehead, M.I. & Lobo, R.A. (1988). Progestogen use in postmenopausal women. Consensus conference. *Lancet* **ii**, 1243-1244.

Yki-Jarvien, H., Sammalkorpi, K., Koivisto, V.A. & Nikkila, E.A. (1989). Severity, duration and mechanisms of insulin resistance during acute infections. *Journal of Clinical Endocrinology and Metabolism* **69**, 317-323.

Zachariasen, R.D. (1993). The effect of elevated ovarian hormones on periodontal health: oral contraceptives and pregnancy. *Women and Health* **20**, 21-30.

Zambon, J.J., Grossi, S.G., Machtei, E.E., Ho, A.W., Dunford, R. & Genco, R.J. (1996). Cigarette smoking increases the risk for subgingival infection with periodontal pathogens. *Journal of Periodontology* **67**, 1050-1054.

Zambon, J.J., Reynolds, H., Fisher, J.G., Shlossman, M., Dunford, R. & Genco, R.J. (1988). Microbiological and immunological studies of adult periodontitis in patients with non-insulin dependent diabetes mellitus. *Journal of Periodontology* **59**, 23-31.

CHAPTER 7

Plaque Induced Gingival Disease

NOEL CLAFFEY

Histopathologic features of gingivitis

Gingivitis associated with local contributing factors

Treatment of plaque induced gingivitis

Gingival diseases modified by endocrine factors

Gingival diseases modified by malnutrition

Gingival diseases modified by systemic conditions

Gingival diseases modified by medications

Necrotizing ulcerative gingivitis

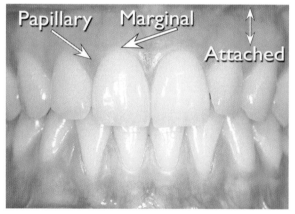

Fig. 7-1. Clinical photograph to demonstrate the different zones of the gingivae for clinical descriptive purposes.

Table 7-1. Characteristics common to all gingival diseases. From Mariotti (1999)

1. Signs and symptoms that are confined to the gingiva.

2. The presence of dental plaque to initiate and/or exacerbate the severity of the lesion.

3. Clinical signs of inflammation (enlarged gingival contours due to edema or fibrosis, color transition to a red and/or bluish-red hue, elevated sulcular temperature, bleeding upon stimulation, increased gingival exudate).

4. Clinical signs and symptoms associated with stable attachment levels on a periodontium with no loss of attachment or on a stable but reduced periodontium.

5. Reversibility of the disease by removing the etiology(ies).

6. Possible role as a precursor to attachment loss around teeth.

This chapter will describe the clinical manifestations, sequalae and treatment of gingival diseases induced by bacterial dental plaque. The characteristics of gingival diseases in general have been described by Mariotti (1999) and are presented in Table 7-1.

Although most, if not all, pathological conditions of the gingiva are affected to greater or lesser extents by bacterial activity, this section concentrates on: (1) Those inflammatory conditions whose etiology is solely attributable to bacteria within dental plaque, excluding gingival inflammation associated with active destructive periodontitis. (2) Those gingival conditions which, although primarily plaque induced, are modified by systemic disease or medication.

For clinical descriptive purposes, the gingiva may be divided into three zones (Fig. 7-1):

1. *Marginal gingiva*: The tissue at the junction of a tooth. Thus, for example, an inflammation confined only to this area may be termed a marginal gingivitis.
2. *Papillary gingiva*: The tissue in the interproximal area. Inflammation confined to this area may be termed papillary gingivitis.
3. *Attached gingiva*: The remaining gingival tissue extending from the marginal/papillary areas to the mucogingival junction. Changes throughout the

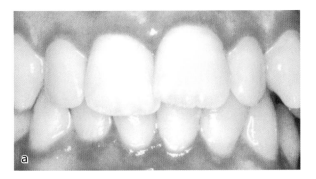

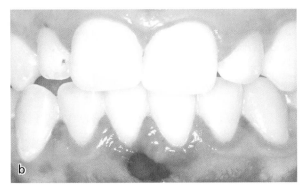

Fig. 7-2. (a) Typical generalized marginal and papillary gingivitis. (b) Marginal and papillary gingivitis in the mandibular anterior buccal segment with an area of diffuse gingivitis in the lower central incisor area.

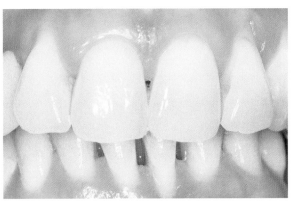

Fig. 7-3. A treated periodontitis case displaying relative lack of inflammation. If such a case developed inflammation and no further loss of attachment could be demonstrated, the term plaque induced gingival inflammation could be applied.

Table 7-2. Characteristics of plaque-induced gingivitis. From Mariotti (1999).

1.	Plaque present at gingival margin
2.	Disease begins at the gingival margin
3.	Change in gingival color
4.	Change in gingival contour
5.	Sulcular temperature change
6.	Increased gingival exudate
7.	Bleeding upon provocation
8.	Absence of attachment loss*
9.	Absence of bone loss*
10.	Histological changes including an inflammatory lesion
11.	Reversible with plaque removal

* In the case of gingivitis superimposed on a reduced periodontium following treatment for periodontitis, both attachment loss and bone loss are most probably present (Fig. 7-3).

vertical extent of the attached gingiva can be termed diffuse (Glickman 1953).

The use of the terms localized and generalized provides a useful descriptor of location for gingival changes within the mouth. For example, a subject may be characterized as having an area of diffuse gingivitis localized to the lower incisor area that is superimposed on a generalized marginal and papillary gingivitis (Fig. 7-2).

Exposure of the gingival tissues to dental plaque results in inflammation within the tissues which manifests as clinical signs of gingivitis (Table 7-2). Table 7-3 describes typical alterations from health to disease commonly seen clinically. There are changes in color, size, shape, consistency and tendency for

Table 7-3. Common clinical changes from health to gingivitis

	Normal gingiva	Gingivitis
Color	Pale pink (melanin pigmentation common in certain groups)	Reddish/bluish red
Size	Papillary gingiva fills interdental spaces; marginal gingiva forms knife edge with tooth surface; sulcus depth ≤ 3 mm	Swelling both coronally and bucco/lingually; false pocket formation
Shape	Scalloped – troughs in marginal areas rise to peaks in interdental areas	Edema which blunts the marginal and papillary tissues leads to loss of knife edge adaptation. Marginal swelling leads to less accentuated scalloping
Consistency	Firm	Soft; pressure induced pitting due to edema
Tendency to bleed	No bleeding to normal probing	Bleeding on probing

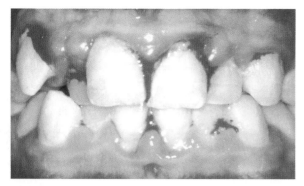

Fig. 7-4. Severe bleeding following brushing. This is often a useful indicator for patients in self-monitoring their oral hygiene efforts.

bleeding from the gingival sulcus. Patients may complain of bleeding on brushing and halitosis (Fig. 7-4). Pain is generally not a feature of dental plaque induced gingivitis although tenderness when brushing may be a complaint. Raised sulcus temperature has also been shown to be a feature of plaque induced gingival inflammation (Haffajee et al. 1992, Wolff et al. 1997, Löe et al. 1965, Mühlemann & Son 1971, Polson & Goodson 1985, Engelberger et al. 1983).

The primary etiological factor, dental plaque, may be encouraged to accumulate by local factors facilitating its retention in marginal and papillary areas. Calculus, vertical or horizontal marginal deficiencies in restorations and rough surfaces on teeth or restorations are examples of such factors (Mariotti 1999).

The reversibility of the condition is worth particular note. Löe et al. (1965) demonstrated a causal effect of dental bacterial plaque on the development of gingivitis. Subjects who were relatively plaque free at baseline were instructed to discontinue their oral hygiene regime. Increasing levels of inflammation developed in association with increasing plaque formation. Abatement of these inflammatory levels to baseline levels followed the re-introduction of effective plaque control measures.

HISTOPATHOLOGIC FEATURES OF GINGIVITIS

Upon exposure to the organisms within dental plaque, changes occur in the gingival vascular complex, the cellular content of the connective tissue and in the junctional epithelium. These underlying alterations are largely responsible for the clinical changes described above (Egelberg 1966).

Vascular changes include substantial increases in the number of patent vessels. Dilation of the vessels is also a feature. Alterations in permeability of the vessel walls and in the hydrostatic pressure within these vessels give rise to fluid and cellular exchange between blood and gingival connective tissue. Edema and color changes to a more red or reddish blue are

consequences of these underlying changes. The junctional epithelium shows infiltration with migrating leucocytes and up to 70% of the volume of the affected region of the junctional epithelium may be made up of bacteria and their products as well as cellular, fluid and molecular products of the inflammatory lesion in the underlying connective tissue. This disrupted junctional epithelium, together with the increased number of patent vessels in the plexus of vessels contiguous to the junctional epithelium, is responsible for the tendency for inflamed gingiva to bleed on gentle stimulation. There is an increase in sulcular fluid flow and a concomitant increase in the number of leukocytes found in the gingival fluid (Payne et al. 1975, Page & Schroeder 1976, Greenstein et al. 1981).

GINGIVITIS ASSOCIATED WITH LOCAL CONTRIBUTING FACTORS

Tooth abnormalities such as enamel pearls and cemental tears

There are several factors related to tooth anatomy such as enamel projections and enamel pearls that modify or predispose to plaque induced gingival disease (Blieden 1999) (Fig. 7-5). Enamel pearls are ectopic deposits of enamel and various shapes, usually associated with furcation areas on molars (Moskow & Canut 1990). Enamel pearls are found in 1.1-5.7% of molar teeth and the maxillary second molars are most commonly involved (Loh 1980).

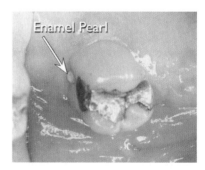

Fig. 7-5. Enamel pearl associated with distal furcation on an upper molar.

Dental restorations

Subgingival margin discrepancies of restorations and violation of the biologic width can affect the health of the adjacent gingival tissues (Björn et al. 1969, Garguilo et al. 1961) (Fig. 7-6). Subgingival margins of restorations can cause greater inflammation when compared with subgingival restorative margins (Nevins & Skurow 1984). The severity of the marginal discrepancy, the amount of time it is present and the ability of the patient to maintain the area free of plaque are important factors in determining the extent of damage to the periodontium.

Root fractures

Root fractures are often associated with inflammation of the gingivae because of the enhanced plaque accumulation in the fracture line (Meister et al. 1980) (Fig. 7-7).

Cervical root resorption

Cervical root resorption may result in inflammation particularly when a communication is established with the gingival sulcus leading to enhanced plaque formation (Fig. 7-8).

TREATMENT OF PLAQUE INDUCED GINGIVITIS

The treatment of plaque induced gingivitis is primarily self-administered plaque control. Although mechanical plaque control remains the mainstay for plaque control, chemical control of plaque is an effective option for those individuals who, because of physical or mental disability, cannot effectively apply mechanical means. However, the presence of plaque retaining factors, such as dental calculus or inadequate restorations, may result in either method being ineffective. Professional intervention is needed to eliminate these as an adjunct to self-administered plaque control. The important sequela of gingivitis is progression of the inflammatory process to involve the underlying connective tissue attachment and periodontal ligament which, in a proportion of susceptible individuals (currently thought to be approximately 10%), leads to major destruction of most of the supporting structures of the dentition (see Chapter 2).

The data currently available would suggest that periodontitis can be successfully halted in the majority of individuals by elimination of the causative bacteria and their products, thereby reducing the levels of inflammation. The return of inflammation to sites treated for periodontitis is not uncommon in susceptible patients. The possibility exists that this recurrent inflammation may be confined to the gingival tissues and may not lead to further periodontal attachment loss. However, as there are currently no reliable methods to confirm such a phenomenon, the return of inflammation is viewed by clinicians as a recurrence of periodontitis and not as a gingivally contained inflammation that is reversible with oral hygiene methods alone (Mariotti 1999, Sheiham 1997).

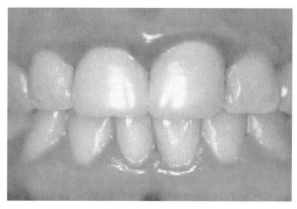

Fig. 7-6. Gingival inflammation associated with violation of biologic width and overhanging restorations retaining plaque.

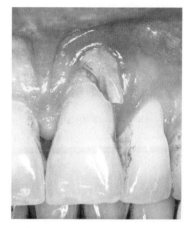

Fig. 7-7. Root fracture with associated periodontal destruction and gingival inflammation.

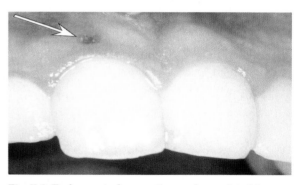

Fig. 7-8. Early cervical resorption and associated inflammation.

GINGIVAL DISEASES MODIFIED BY ENDOCRINE FACTORS

(see also Chapter 6)

Pregnancy associated gingivitis

Pregnancy is associated with an exaggerated response of the gingiva to local irritants. The gingivae show levels of inflammation, often characterized by edema, color and contour change and propensity to bleed on

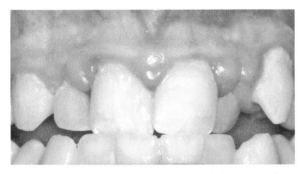

Fig. 7-9. Gingival inflammation in an adolescent with a malocclusion which is more pronounced in the anterior of the mouth perhaps associated with mouth-breathing.

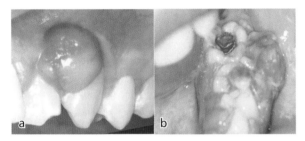

Fig. 7-10. (a) Pyogenic granuloma of pregnancy. (b) Large pyogenic granuloma of pregnancy interfering with function.

gentle stimulation, which are not usually commensurate with the plaque levels present. The plaque microbiota involved is characteristic of gingivitis (see Chapter 3) and the condition seems to be an exaggerated localized host response which is modulated by levels of endogenous hormones such as androgens, estrogens and progesterone. These changes often appear during the second trimester of pregnancy and regress upon parturition. The condition can be reversed with suitably high levels of plaque control (Eiselt 1840, Pinard 1877, Mariotti 1994, Hugoson 1971, Arafat 1974).

Puberty associated gingivitis

As with pregnancy associated gingivitis, puberty associated gingivitis appears to be an exaggerated response of the gingival tissues to plaque mediated by high levels of hormones, perhaps most importantly estrogens and testosterone (Mariotti 1994). This effect seems to be transient and can be reversed with oral hygiene measures. The gingival changes appear relatively non-specific, with color and contour changes, and bleeding to mild stimulation the most commonly seen. Mariotti (1994) proposed that the diagnosis of pubertal gingivitis should apply only to the exaggerated response seen in those cases for which hormone levels at least reached those designated by Tanner as stage 2 (girls with estradiol levels ≥ 26 pmol/L; boys

with testosterone levels ≥ 8.7 nmol/L). Mouth breathing, which often accompanies Angle's classification 2 division 1 malocclusion, is considered by some to be an exacerbating factor in children and adolescents (Fig. 7-9). A differentiation between the effects of mouth breathing and hormonal influences on gingival inflammation can therefore be difficult.

Menstrual cycle associated gingivitis

Although bright red hemorrhagic lesions have been described prior to the onset of menses, clinically detectable changes do not seem to be associated with the menstrual cycle. However, an increase in gingival fluid by 20% has been described in 75% of women during ovulation (Mühlemann 1948, Hugoson 1971).

Pyogenic granuloma of pregnancy

This is a localized mass of highly vascularized tissue arising as an exaggerated response to plaque in pregnancy. It commonly arises from the proximal gingival tissues and has a pedunculated base (Fig. 7-10a). It may show ulceration of its thin epithelial lining, and bleeding, especially upon mastication or even spontaneously, may be a presenting complaint. The lesion is more common in the maxilla and although it can arise in the first trimester of pregnancy, the usual presentation is in the second or third trimester. The histological features are those of a pyogenic granuloma: a highly vascularized mass of granulation tissue. The lesion may regress or completely disappear following parturition. Occasionally the lesion may be so large as to interfere with normal speech or mastication, whereupon its removal is necessitated (Fig. 7-10b). As with the common pyogenic granuloma, excision should be accompanied by thorough debridement of the contiguous crown and root surfaces or recurrence may result.

GINGIVAL DISEASES MODIFIED BY MALNUTRITION

Deficiency in vitamin C results in scurvy, one of the manifestations of which is gingival changes including redness, swelling, tendency towards bleeding upon minimal stimulation and an alteration towards a spongy consistency (Hodges et al. 1971). Improvements in living standards have resulted in scurvy being a rare condition in the modern era, but it may persist in countries of the developing world and in such severely undernourished individuals as alcoholics (Fig. 7-11). Although it is generally accepted that various nutritional deficiencies may alter the response

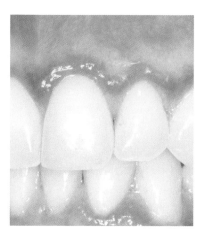

Fig. 7-11. Gingival changes associated with vitamin C deficiency. Note the relative absence of dental plaque and the distance of the color changes from the marginal gingivae.

of the gingiva to bacterial plaque, there is little direct evidence to directly implicate nutritional factors in the gingival response to dental plaque. There are suggestions that lack of vitamins A, B_2 and vitamin B_{12} complex may be associated with changes in the gingiva (Mariotti 1999).

GINGIVAL DISEASES MODIFIED BY SYSTEMIC CONDITIONS

Diabetes mellitus

There is evidence to suggest that Type 1 diabetes in children is associated with exaggerated response of the gingival tissues to dental plaque (Cianciola et al. 1982, Gusberti et al. 1983, Ervasti et al. 1985). It would appear that when this type of diabetes is under good control the gingival inflammation is less exaggerated. In adults it is generally accepted that poorly controlled Type 1 diabetes may be associated with increased levels of periodontitis (see also Chapter 6). However, no convincing evidence exists that gingivitis is exacerbated in such adult patients.

Leukemias and other blood dysplasias

The leukemias have been associated with gingival changes. Perhaps the leukemia most commonly associated with gingival changes is acute myeloid leukemia (Fig. 7-12). Although dental plaque can exacerbate the changes brought about, which include gingival swelling, redness/blueness, sponginess and a glazed appearance, it may not be necessary for the development of these signs. However, oral manifestations vary widely, particularly with leukemias other than myeloid leukemias (Fig. 7-13). Persistent and otherwise unexplained gingival bleeding may indicate an

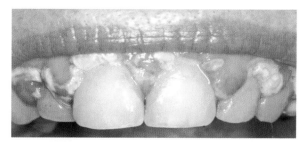

Fig. 7-12. Gingival changes associated with acute monocytic leukemia. Note the acute candidiasis superimposed upon the infiltrative gingival changes. Distressing oral symptoms lessened when antiseptic mouthwashes were administered.

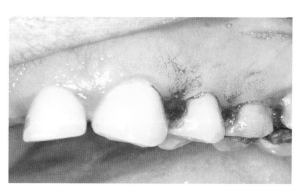

Fig. 7-13. Spontaneous bleeding in a patient who was then diagnosed with chronic lymphocytic leukemia. The bleeding ceased when the patient was treated by conventional periodontal therapy.

underlying thrombocytopenia associated with, for instance, a leukemic condition or with any condition affecting platelet deficiency (Fig. 7-14a and 7-14b).

Cyclic neutropenia, a condition characterized by fluctuations in neutrophil counts with a periodicity of 14-36 days, is associated with oral ulceration, an exaggerated inflammatory response to dental plaque bacteria and aggressive periodontitis of early onset (Spencer & Flemming 1985, Long et al. 1983, Pernu et al. 1996) (Fig. 7-15). Systemic treatment with granulocyte colony stimulating factor G-CSF can be used to regulate the blood cell deficit although its effectiveness on the periodontal manifestations is unclear.

GINGIVAL DISEASES MODIFIED BY MEDICATIONS

There are three commonly used drug types that are associated with gingival overgrowth: phenytoin sodium or epinutin – an anticonvulsant used for the treatment of epilepsy; cyclosporin A – an immunosuppressant used in order to avoid host rejection of grafted tissues and as a treatment for conditions such as severe psoriasis; and calcium channel blocking agents such as nifedipine – antihypertensive drugs.

The clinical manifestations of the drug induced gingival changes are similar for the three medication

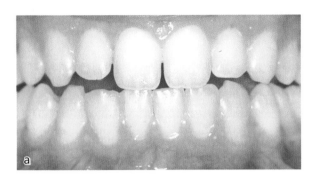

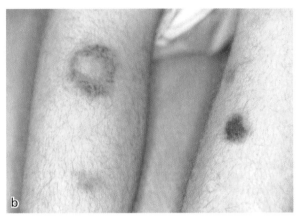

Fig. 7-14. Acute B-cell leukemia. (a) Intra-oral photograph shows relatively normal gingivae. However, the gingivae bled for a prolonged period following probing and (b) bruising was evident on the limbs. The chief complaint was a feeling of tightness in the anterior dentition, perhaps due to infiltration of the mental foramina with leukemic cells.

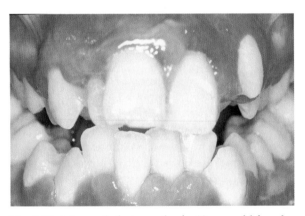

Fig. 7-15. Intra-oral photograph of a 10-year-old female with cyclic neutropenia. In addition to the florid gingival inflammation, attachment loss was present.

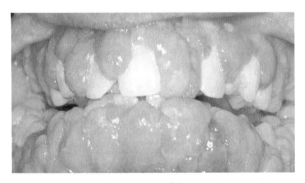

Fig. 7-16. Severe enlargement of the gingivae associated with cyclosporin medication in a kidney transplant patient.

types (Fig. 7-16). Some transplant patients have both cyclosporin A and nifedipine prescribed and the combined effect of these medications may result in greater gingival enlargement than the use of either medication alone (Santi & Brai 1998). Gingival inflammation and the presence of dental plaque have been reported as significant risk factors in the development of gingival enlargement in individuals using phenytoin or calcium channel blocking drugs (Majola et al. 2000,

Brunet et al. 2001, Miranda et al. 2001). Enlargement of gingival tissues associated with these drugs may be more common in the anterior region of the mouth and younger age groups may be more susceptible. The typical early clinical signs include a shape and size change in the papilla regions. As the process develops, the papillae may become grossly enlarged and the marginal and attached gingiva may also become involved. There is no evidence that attachment loss is a sequela to the condition although drug induced enlargement may be superimposed on a pre-existing periodontitis. The histological characteristics of the enlarged tissue may be similar to that of normal gingiva (Hassell 1981, Seymour et al. 1996).

In hyperplasia associated with the use of phenytoin, the presence of dental plaque does not seem necessary to initiate the enlargement. The role of dental plaque in the initiation of enlargement associated with cyclosporin and calcium blocking agents has not been established. However, plaque and resultant inflammation often exacerbate the lesions associated with all medication types. Animal studies suggest that thorough plaque removal can prevent or reverse the enlargement associated with calcium blockers. Additional animal studies focusing on phenytoin have demonstrated that oral hygiene measures may limit the severity of the lesions but are unable alone to lead to a reversal of the condition (Hassell 1981, Steinberg & Steinberg 1982, Hassell et al. 1984, Nishikawa et al. 1996, Barclay et al. 1992, Heijl & Sundin 1989, Angelopoulos & Goaz 1972). Treatment of gingival enlargement induced by medication is achieved by a combination of a rigorous oral hygiene regime, debridement and in those cases where aesthetics, function or speech are compromised, surgical excision. Recurrence following treatment can take place and is more likely in those patients with less than optimal plaque control (Hall 1997). When patients taking cyclosporin have their medication changed to, for example, tacrolimus, another anti-graft rejection drug, their gingival enlargement may undergo partial or com-

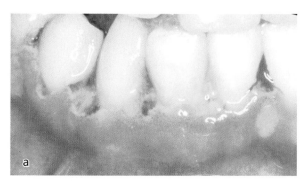 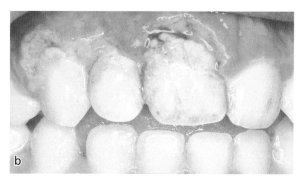

Fig. 7-17. Necrotizing ulcerative gingivitis showing (a) destruction of the interdental papillae, pseudomembrane and spontaneous bleeding. Although usually confined to the papilla, occasionally the marginal tissues are involved (b).

plete reversal (Hernández et al. 2000, James et al. 2000).

NECROTIZING ULCERATIVE GINGIVITIS

(see also Chapter 10)

Microbiology, host response and predisposing factors

Necrotizing ulcerative gingivitis (NUG) can be defined as an acute and sometimes recurring gingival infection of complex etiology, characterized by rapid onset of gingival pain, interdental gingival necrosis, and bleeding (Rowland 1999) (Fig. 7-17a and 7-17b). It has been called many names: Vincent's disease, trench mouth, acute necrotizing ulcerative gingivitis (ANUG) and fusospirochetal gingivitis being the more common examples. This form of gingivitis is relatively rare (Loesche et al. 1982). The patients affected are typically adolescents or young adults, may be cigarette smokers (Kirkpatrick & Clements 1934, Dean & Singleton 1945, Stevens et al. 1984) and are often psychologically stressed (Goldberg et al. 1956, Formicola et al. 1970, Cohen-Cole et al. 1983). Pain, ulceration and necrosis of the interdental papillae and bleeding, either spontaneous or to gentle manipulation, are cardinal clinical signs of the disease (Grant 1955, Stevens et al. 1984).

Perhaps the most important differential diagnosis of NUG is that from primary herpetic gingivostomatitis. The contrasting features of the two disease entities are presented in Table 7-4.

On microscopic examination the lesion appears as a non-specific acute inflammatory process, covered by a slough or pseudomembrane. The pseudomembrane contains dead epithelial cells, inflammatory cells, a fibrin meshwork and various microorganisms. The connective tissue displays dilated capillaries and a marked acute inflammatory cell infiltrate. The mononuclear inflammatory cells seem to be the most active cells in the phagocytosis of microorganisms (Listgarten 1965).

The borders of the lesion show hydropic degeneration of the epithelium. Spirochetes are seen invading the underlying connective tissue. The histopathology of ANUG lesions was investigated using electron microscopy and has been described by dividing the lesion into four zones (Listgarten 1965):

Table 7-4. Important characteristics for differential diagnosis between necrotizing ulcerative gingivitis and primary herpetic gingivostomatitis

	NUG	PHS
Etiology	Bacteria	Herpes simplex virus
Age	15-30 years	Frequently children
Site	Interdental papillae	Gingiva and the entire dental mucosa
Symptoms	Ulceration and necrotic tissue and a yellowish-white plaque	Multiple vesicles which burst leaving small round fibrin-covered ulcers which tend to coalesce
Duration	1-2 days if treated	1-2 weeks
Contagious	No	Yes
Immunity	No	Partial
Healing	Destruction of periodontal tissue remains	No permanent destruction

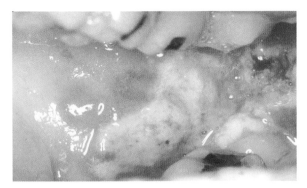

Fig. 7-18. Necrotizing ulcerative stomatitis resulting from a spread of NUG to the buccal tissues.

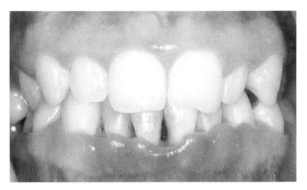

Fig. 7-19. Cratering as a result of previous NUG.

1. *The bacterial zone*: This is the most superficial layer consisting of multifarious types of bacteria.
2. *The neutrophil-rich zone*: This zone is rich in leucocytes and bacteria.
3. *Necrotic zone*: Dead cells and a fibrin meshwork predominate in this zone. Numerous spirochetes of various types are seen.
4. *Zone of spirochetal infiltration*: This zone is characterized by connective tissue displaying an acute inflammatory response with infiltrating spirochetes of various sizes.

Quantitative analysis of the bacteria associated with NUG has been limited to bacterial smear techniques. When the flora of NUG was studied using quantitative anaerobic culturing techniques, the following organisms and their relative proportions were found: Treponema species 32%; Selenomonas species 6%; Bacteroides intermedius 24%; Fusobacterium species 3% (Loesche et al.1982).

It must be stressed that no bacteriological experiment has produced the typical lesion of NUG in animals or humans. The organisms can be isolated from the oral lesions of NUG and grown in pure culture, thereby satisfying the first two of Koch's postulates. However, the third postulate remains unsatisfied as the typical disease pattern cannot be produced in animals or humans. King (1943) traumatized his own gingiva and introduced to the area of trauma debris from the lesion of a patient with NUG. The experiment proved negative until he became ill a short time afterwards, whereupon the characteristic lesions of NUG appeared in the experimental area.

Although it has not been possible to implicate bacteria directly in the causation of the disease, the prompt resolution of the disease process with the antibiotic penicillin or the antibacterial agent metronidazole is of interest (Schinn 1977, Emslie 1967, Duckworth et al. 1966). It has been suggested that the characteristic bacterial flora of NUG develops as a consequence of altered host response (Loesche et al. 1982).

Host response in acute necrotizing ulcerative gingivitis

Attempts have been made to identify some altered host response mechanisms in patients suffering from NUG. It has been suggested that systemic disease, for example ulcerative colitis, blood dyscrasias and nutritional deficiency states, predispose to the development of NUG (Goldberger & Wheeler 1928, Cautley 1943). The rate of lymphocyte transformation has been found to be reduced in patients with NUG (Wilton et al. 1971). There are two studies reported in which no significant rises in antibody titers were found for NUG patients against the characteristic bacteria (Lehner & Clarry 1966, Dolby 1972).

Abnormalities of white blood cell function have also been reported (Wilton et al. 1971, Cogen et al. 1983, Claffey et al. 1986). It has been suggested that patients suffering from acquired immune deficiency syndrome (AIDS) may have an increased incidence of ANUG (Pindborg et al. 1986). It has also been reported that malnutrition is a predisposing factor in the onset of necrotizing ulcerative gingivitis (Johnson & Engel 1986, Armitage 1980). Very young children can be affected by NUG in developing countries (Osuji 1990, Taiwo 1995) and this seems to be related to viral infections such as measles, protozoal infections (Osuji 1990), or most commonly insufficient protein intake as a result of a very poor diet (Enwonwu 1972). Poor nutritional habits seem to be the reason why NUG affects young adults in Europe and the United States (Osuji 1990, Taiwo 1995).

Although its nomenclature indicates necrotizing ulcerative gingivitis to be a gingivally contained lesion, it has been suggested that it is associated with periodontal attachment loss (MacCarthy & Claffey 1991). Necrotizing ulcerative gingivitis may progress to a fulminating oro-facial infection called noma or cancrum oris (Johnson & Engel 1986, Armitage 1980). Noma may develop when the initial gingival necrosis progresses to a necrotizing periodontitis and thereafter to necrotizing stomatitis when the infection spreads to other soft tissues and the bone (Fig. 7-18). It is often lethal and it affects mainly malnourished children or otherwise compromised patients (Enwonwu 1972, Osuji 1990, Taiwo 1995).

Treatment of NUG

Treatment includes oral hygiene instructions, mechanical debridement of the teeth and systemic antimicrobial therapy (Johnson & Engel 1986). Debridement would appear to be the mainstay of treatment, but adjunctive prescription of antibiotics from the penicillin group or metranidazole may be indicated if gingival destruction is severe, if there is an accompanying involvement of the local lymph nodes or if systemic symptoms such as pyrexia or malaise are present. Changes in gingival architecture following NUG, in particular interdental cratering, may require surgical correction in order to facilitate plaque control procedures (Fig. 7-19).

References

Angelopoulos, A.P. & Goaz, P.W. (1972). Incidence of diphenylhydantoin gingival hyperplasia. *Oral Surgery, Oral Medicine, Oral Pathology* **34**, 898-906.

Arafat, A. (1974). The prevalence of pyogenic granuloma in pregnant women. *Journal of the Baltimore College Dental Surgery* **29**, 64-70.

Armitage, G.C. (1980). Acute periodontal lesions. In: *Biologic basis of periodontal maintenance therapy.* Berkeley, CA: Praxis Publishing Company, pp.145-164.

Barclay, S. Thomanson, J.M., Idle, J.R. & Seymour, R.A. (1992). The incidence and severity of nifedipine-induced gingival overgrowth. *Journal of Clinical Periodontology* **60**, 104-112.

Björn, A.L., Bjorn H. & Girkovic, B. (1969). Marginal fit of restorations and its relation to periodontal bone levels. I. Metal fillings. *Odontology Revy* **20**, 311-321.

Blieden, T.M (1999). Tooth-related issues. *Annals of Periodontology* **4**, 91-96.

Brunet, L., Miranda, J., Roset, P., Berini, L., Farré, M. & Mendieta, C. (2001). Prevalence and risk of gingival enlargement in patients treated with anticonvulsant drugs. *European Journal of Clinical Investigation* **31**, 781-788.

Cautley, R.L. (1943). Vincent's infection. *British Dental Journal* **74**, 34-37.

Cianciola, L.J., Park, B.H., Bruck, E., Moscovich, L. & Genco, R.J. (1982). Prevalence of periodontal disease in insulin-dependent diabetes mellitus (juvenile diabetes*). Journal of the American Dental Association* **104**, 653-660.

Claffey, N., Russell, R. & Shanley, D. (1986). Peripheral blood phagocyte function in acute necrotizing ulcerative gingivitis. *Journal of Periodontal Research* **21**, 288-297.

Cogen, R.B., Stevens, A.W. Jr., Cohen-Cole, S., Kirk, K. & Freeman, A. (1983). Leukocyte function in the etiology of acute necrotizing ulcerative gingivitis. *Journal of Periodontology* **54**, 402-207.

Cohen-Cole, S., Cogen, R.B., Stevens, A.W. Jr., Kirk, K. & Freeman, A. (1983). Psychiatric, psychosocial and endocrine correlates of acute necrotizing ulcerative gingivitis (trench mouth): A preliminary report. *Psychiatric Medicine* **1**, 215-225.

Dolby, A.E. (1972). Acute ulcerative gingivitis. Immune complex. *Journal of Dental Research* **51**, 1639-1641.

Duckworth, R., Waterhouse, J.P., Britton, D.E., Nmuke, K., Sheiham, A., Winter, R. & Blake, G.C. (1966). Acute ulcerative gingivitis: a double blind controlled trial of metronidazole. *British Dental Journal* **120**, 599-602.

Egelberg, J. (1966). Permeability of the dento-gingival blood vessels. I. Application of the vascular labelling method and gingival fluid measurements. *Journal of Periodontal Research* **1**, 180-191.

Eiselt, P. (1840). Gingival hypertrophy during pregnancy. *Medizinische Jahrbucher des Osterr Staates* **21**, 560.

Emslie, R.D. (1967). Treatment of acute necrotizing ulcerative gingivitis. A clinical trial using chewing gums containing metronizazole or penicillin. *British Dental Journal* **122**, 307-308.

Engelberger, T., Hefti, A. & Rateitschack K-H. (1983). Correlations among papilla bleeding index, other clinical indices and histologically determined inflammation of gingival papilla. *Journal of Clinical Periodontology* **10**, 579-589.

Enwonwu, C.O. (1972). Epidemiological and biochemical studies of necrotizing ulcerative gingivitis and noma (cancrum oris) in Nigerian children. *Archives of Oral Biology* **17**, 1357-1371.

Ervasti, T., Knuuttila, M., Pohjamo, L. & Haukipuro, K. (1985). Relation between control of diabetes and gingival bleeding. *Journal of Periodontology* **56**, 154-157.

Formicola, A.J., Witte, E.T. & Curran, P.M. (1970). A study of personality traits and acute necrotizing gingivitis. *Journal of Periodontology* **41**, 36-38.

Garguilo, A.W., Wentz, F.M. & Orban, B. (1961). Dimensions and relations of the dentogingival junction in humans. *Journal of Periodontology* **32**, 261-267.

Glickman, I. (1953). *Clinical Periodontology.* Philadelphia & London: W.B. Saunders, p.92.

Goldberg, H., Ambinder, W.G., Copper, I. & Abrams, A.L. (1956). Emotional status of patients with acute gingivitis. *New York Dental Journal* **22**, 308-318.

Goldberger, J. & Wheeler, G.A. (1928). In: Carranza, F.A., ed. *Glickman's Clinical Periodontology,* 5th edn, Chapter 11, pp.133-147.

Grant, D.A. (1955). Necrotizing ulcerative gingivitis. *Journal of Southern Californian Dental Association* **23**, 21-29.

Greenstein, G., Caton J. & Polson, A.M. (1981). Histologic characterisics associated with bleeding after probing and visual signs of inflammation. *Journal of Periodontology* **52**, 420-425.

Gusberti, F.A., Syed, S.A., Bacon, G., Grossman, N. & Loesche, W.J. (1983). Puberty gingivitis in insulin-dependent diabetic children. I. Cross-section observations. *Journal of Periodontology* **54**, 714-720.

Haffajee, A.D., Socransky, S.S. & Goodson, G.M. (1992). Subgingival temperature (I) Relation to baseline clinical parameters. *Journal of Clinical Periodontology* **19**, 401-408.

Hall, E.E. (1997). Prevention and treatment considerations in patients with drug-induced gingival enlargement. *Current Opinion Periodontology* **4**, 59-63.

Hassell, T.M. (1981). Phenytoin: gingival overgrowth. In: Myers, H.M., ed. *Epilepsy and the Oral Manifestations of Phenytoin Therapy*, vol. 9. Basel: S. Karger A.G., pp.116-202.

Hassell, T., O'Donnell, J., Pearlman, J., Tesini, D., Murphy, T. & Best, T. (1984). Phenytoin induced gingival overgrowth in institutionalised epileptics. *Journal of Clinical Periodontology* **11**, 242-253.

Heijl, L. & Sundin, Y. (1989). Nifedipine-induced gingival overgrowth in dogs. *Journal of Periodontology* **19**, 311-314.

Hernández, G., Arriba, L., Lucas, M. & Andrés, A. (2000). Reduction of severe gingival overgrowth in a kidney transplant by replacing Cyclosporin A with tacrolimus. *Journal of Periodontology* **71**, 1630-1636.

Hodges, R.E., Hood, J., Canham, J.E., Sauberlich, H.E. & Baker, E.M. (1971). Clinical manifestations of ascorbic acid deficiency in man. *American Journal of Clinical Nutrition* **24**, 432-443.

Hugoson, A. (1971). Gingivitis in pregnant women. A longitudinal clinical study. *Odontologisk Revy* **22**, 65-84.

James, J. A., Boomer, S., Maxwell, A.P., Hull, P.S., Short, C.D., Campbell, B.A., Johnson, R. W., Irwin, C.R., Marley, J.J., Spratt, H. & Linden, G.J. (2000). Reduction of gingival overgrowth associated with conversion from cyclosporin A to tacrolimus. *Journal of Clinical Periodontology* **27**, 144-148.

Johnson, B.D. & Engel, D. (1986). Acute necrotizing ulcerative gingivitis. A review of diagnosis, aetiology and treatment. *Journal of Periodontology* **57**, 141-150.

King, J.E. (1943). Nutritional and other factors in trench mouth, with special reference to nicotinic acid component of the Vitamin B$_2$ complex. *British Dental Journal* **74**, 113-122.

Kirkpatrick, R.M. & Clements, F.W. (1934). Diet in relation to Vincent's infection. *Dental Journal of Australia* **6**, 317-372.

Lehner, T. & Clarry, E.D. (1966). Acute ulcerative gingivitis. *British Dental Journal* **121**, 366-370.

Listgarten, M.A. (1965). Electron microscopic observation on the bacterial flora of acute necrotizing ulcerative gingivitis. *Journal of Periodontology* **36**, 223-230.

Löe, H., Theilande, E. & Jensen, S.B. (1965). Experimental gingivitis in man. *Journal of Periodontology* **36**, 177-187.

Loesche, W.J., Syed, S.A., Laughon, B.E. & Stall, J. (1982). The bacteriology of acute necrotizing ulcerative gingivitis. *Journal of Periodontology* **53**, 223-230.

Loh, H.S. (1980). A local study of enamel pearls. *Singapore Dental Journal* **5**, 55-59.

Long, L.M., Jacoway, J.R. & Bawden, J.W. (1983). Cyclic neutropenia. Case report of two siblings. *Paediatric Dentistry* **5**, 142-144.

MacCarthy, D. & Claffey, N. (1991). Acute necrotizing ulcerative gingivitis is associated with attachment loss. *Journal of Clinical Periodontology* **18** (10), 776-779.

Majola, M.P., McFadyen, M.L., Connolly, C., Nair, Y.P., Govender, M. & Laher, M.H. (2000). Factors influencing phenytoin-induced gingival enlargement. *Journal of Clinical Periodontology* **27**, 506-512.

Mariotti, A. (1994). Sex steroid hormones and cell dynamics in the periodontium. *Critical Reviews in Oral Biological Medicine* **5**, 27-53.

Mariotti, A. (1999). Dental plaque-induced gingival diseases. *Annals of Periodontology* **4**, 7-19.

Meister, F. Jr., Lommel, T.J. & Gerstein, H. (1980). Diagnosis and possible causes of vertical root fractures. *Oral Surgery Oral Medicine and Oral Pathology* **49**, 243-253.

Miranda, J., Brunet, L., Roset, P., Berini, L., Farré, M. & Mendieta, C. (2001). Prevalence and risk of gingival enlargement in patients treated with nifedipine. *Journal of Periodontology* **72**, 605-611.

Moskow, B.S. & Canut, P.M. (1990). Studies on root enamel (2). Enamel pearls. A review of their morphology, localization, nomenclature, occurrence, classification, histogenesis and incidence. *Journal of Clinical Periodontology* **17**, 275-281.

Mühlemann, H.R (1948). Gingivitis intermenstrualis. *Schneizer Monatsschrift für Zahmeidizin. jn.* **58**, 865-885.

Mühlemann, H.R. & Son, S. (1971). Gingival sulcus bleeding – a leading symptom in initial gingivitis. *Helvetica Odontologica Acta* **15**, 107-113.

Nevins, M., & Skurow, H. (1984). The intracravicular restorative margin, the biologic width, and the maintenance of the gin-gival margin. *International Journal of Periodontics and Restorative Dentistry* **3**, 31-49.

Nishikawa, S., Nagata, T., Morisaki, I., Oka, T. & Ishida, H. (1996). Pathogenesis of drug-induced gingival overgrowth. A review of studies in the rat model. *Journal of Periodontology* **67**, 463-471.

Osuji, O.O. (1990). Necrotizing ulcerative gingivitis and cancrum oris (noma) in Ibaban, Nigeria. *Journal of Periodontology* **61**, 769-772.

Page, R.C. & Schroeder, H.E. (1976). Pathogenesis of inflammatory periodontal disease. *Laborarory Investigation* **33**, 235-249.

Payne, W.A., Page, R.C., Ogilvie, A.L. & Hall, W.B. (1975). Histopathologic features of the initial and early stages of experimental gingivitis in man. *Journal of Periodontal Research* **10**, 51-64.

Pernu, H.E., Pajara, U.H. & Lanning, M. (1996). The importance of regular dental treatment in patients with cyclic neutropenia. Follow-up of two cases. *Journal of Periodontology* **67**, 454-459.

Pinard, A. (1877). Gingivitis in pregnancy. *Dental Register* **31**, 258-259.

Pindborg, J.J., Thorn, J.J., Schiodt, M., Gaub, J. & Black, F.T. (1986). Acute necrotizing gingivitis in AIDS patient. *Tandlaegebladet* **90**, 450-453.

Polson, A.M. & Goodson, J.M. (1985). Periodontal diagnosis. Current status and future needs. *Journal of Periodontology* **56**, 25-34.

Rowland, R.W. (1999). Necrotizing ulcerative gingivitis. *Annals of Periodontology* **4**(1), 65-73.

Santi, E. & Brai, M. (1998). Effect of treatment on cyclosporine- and nifedipine-induced gingival enlargement: clinical and histologic results. *International Journal of Periodontics and Restorative Dentistry* **18**, 80-85.

Schinn, D.L. (1977). Vincent's disease and its treatment with metranidozale. Finegold (ed.) 334 *Excerpta Medica.*

Seymour, R.A, Thomason, J.M. & Ellis, J.S. (1996). The pathogenesis of drug-induced gingival overgrowth. *Journal of Clinical Periodontology* **23**, 165-175.

Sheiham, A. (1997). Is the chemical prevention of gingivitis necessary to prevent severe periodontitis? *Periodontology 2000* **15**, 15-24.

Spencer, P. & Flemming, J.E. (1985). Cyclic neutropenia: A literature review and report of case. *Journal of Dentistry for Children* **52**, 108-144.

Steinberg, S.C & Steinberg, A.D. (1982). Phenytoin-induced gingival overgrowth control in severely retarded children. *Journal of Periodontology* **53**, 429-433.

Stevens, A.W. Jr., Cogen-Cole, S. & Freeman, A. (1984). Demographic and clinical data associated with acute necrotizing ulcerative gingivitis in a dental school population. (ANUG-Demographic and clinical data) *Journal of Clinical Periodontology* **11**, 487-493.

Taiwo, J.O. (1995). Severity of necrotizing ulcerative gingivitis in Nigerian children. *Periodontal Clinical Investigations* **17**, 24-27.

Wilton, J.M.A., Ivanyi, A. & Lehner, T. (1971). Cell mediated immunity and humeral antibodies in acute ulcerative gingivitis. *Journal of Periodontal Research* **6**, 9-16.

Wolff, L.F., Koller, N.J., Smith, Q.T., Mathur, A. & Aeppli, D. (1997). Subgingival temperature: relation to gingival crevicular fluid enzymes, cytokines, and subgingival plaque microorganisms. *Journal of Clinical Periodontology* **24**, 900-906.

CHAPTER 8

Chronic Periodontitis

DENIS F. KINANE AND JAN LINDHE

Risk factors or susceptibility to chronic periodontitis
  Bacterial risk factors
  Age
  Smoking
  Host response related
    Systemic disease

Stress
Genetics

Scientific basis for periodontal therapy

Effect of surgical treatment

Comparisons of surgical and non-surgical therapy

The clinical features of chronic periodontitis are gingival inflammation (color and texture alterations), bleeding on probing (BOP) from the gingival pocket area, reduced resistance of the periodontal tissues to probing (periodontal pocketing), loss of clinical attachment and loss of alveolar bone. Variable features include enlargement or recession of the gingiva, root furcation exposure, increased tooth mobility, drifting and eventually exfoliation of teeth.

Figs. 8-1 (a-c) illustrate the clinical status of a 55-year-old male with chronic periodontitis and Fig. 8-2 presents the radiographic status of the same patient. Note the presence of gingival recession at a large number of buccal and interproximal sites. A number of teeth can be identified from the radiographs, around which there is extensive alveolar bone loss. At teeth 16, 26, 27 and 47 the furcation areas have lost their periodontal tissue support and are open for "through and through" probing.

Chronic periodontitis is initiated as gingivitis at or soon after puberty but symptoms such as bone and attachment loss are not observed until later. Although chronic periodontitis is initiated and sustained by microbial plaque, host defense mechanisms have a crucial role to play in its pathogenesis and the inherent susceptibility of a patient to the disease (see Chapter 5). Chronic periodontitis is generally a slowly progressing form of periodontitis which at any stage may undergo an acute exacerbation with associated attachment loss. From prevalence studies, chronic periodontitis is the most commonly occurring form of periodontitis. Varying levels of severity of chronic periodontitis exist. Advanced forms of chronic periodontitis are seen in only a subset of the population (Chapter 2).

Chronic periodontitis is variable in that it does not affect all teeth evenly, but has both a subject and site predilection. When considering changes in attachment level over time, it is also peculiar that only relatively few sites actually undergo extensive periodontal destruction during any given observation period. Socransky et al. (1984) have suggested that periodontitis progresses in episodes of exacerbation and remission and they termed this the "burst hypothesis". Further studies have suggested that the progression may actually be continuous rather than following an episodic pattern. The consensus is that the progression of chronic periodontitis is a continuous process that undergoes periods of acute exacerbation. Clinically, the progressive nature of the disease can only be confirmed by repeated examinations but it is a safe assumption that untreated lesions will progress.

In summary
Chronic periodontitis: (1) is subject-related with only a few individuals experiencing advanced destruction, (2) affects specific teeth and (3) the progression of this inflammatory disease is continuous with brief episodes of localized exacerbation and occasional remission.

The histopathology of chronic periodontitis has been discussed in Chapter 5 and it is likely that the lesion in many aspects is similar to that of aggressive periodontitis.

Local and systemic risk factors (as discussed later) may have a bearing on the rate of progression of the lesions and may in fact determine whether an individual will actually manifest as advanced disease. Local risk factors include any feature which would increase

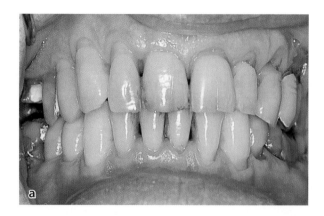

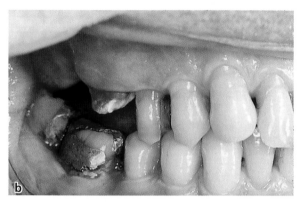

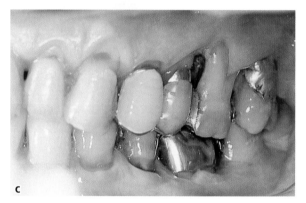

Fig. 8-1 (a-c). Clinical status of a 55-year-old male with periodontitis.

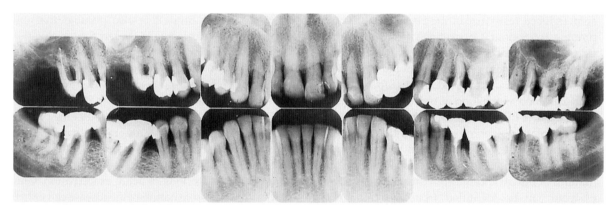

Fig. 8-2. Radiographic status of the patient presented in Fig. 8-1.

Table 8-1. Prevalence of chronic periodontitis expressed in percentage terms of subjects with clinical attachment loss (CAL) across various age groups (modified from Flemmig 1999)

Age (years)	CAL 3-4 mm	CAL ≥ 5 mm
18-35	9-35	0.3-6
36-35	18-70	12-27
> 55	44-81	35-51

plaque accumulation or plaque retention (e.g. overhanging restorations) in an area, or predispose the local tissues to be more susceptible to the inflammatory effects of microbial plaque, for example clasps of partial dentures, traumatic occlusions, local smoking effects etc.

Clinical attachment loss (CAL) of 1 mm or 2 mm can be found in nearly all members of an adult population. The prevalence of subjects with one or more sites with CAL 3 mm or greater increases with age (Table 8-1). Furthermore the number of diseased sites in any one individual increases with age. Also the population prevalence, extent and severity of chronic periodontitis increase with age. Age of onset and rate of progression, however, vary between individuals and are probably related to both genetic and environmental risk factors.

In untreated populations additional CAL of 3 mm or more that occurred over a one-year period was found in up to 27% of subjects (Flemmig 1999). On a site basis, the overall annualized incidence ranged

Table 8-2. Summary of clinical features and characteristics of chronic periodontitis

1. Chronic periodontitis is more prevalent in adults but can also be found in children and adolescents.

2. The amount of periodontal destruction is commensurate with oral hygiene or plaque levels, local predisposing factors and systemic risk factors including smoking, stress, diabetes, HIV and inherent host defense capabilities of the patient.

3. The composition of microbial plaque is complex and varies greatly within and between patients and subgingival calculus is a common finding.

4. Chronic periodontitis can be classified as localized when fewer than 30% of sites are affected, and generalized when this level is exceeded.

5. Further classification of the disease is based on the extent and severity of the clinically evident periodontal destruction.

6. Although chronic periodontitis is initiated and sustained by microbial plaque, host factors influence the pathogenesis and progression of the disease.

7. Progression can only be confirmed by repeated clinical examinations and is considered likely to occur in diseased sites that are left untreated.

from 0.3% to 4.2% (Flemmig 1999), which indicates that the number of sites which actually exhibit progression within a given time is very variable. The mean annual CAL and bone loss (BL) has been reported to range from 0.04 to 1.04 mm. The distribution of this annual progression indicates that only a small proportion of the population show a high mean rate of disease progression. Factors which influence disease progression are factors also associated with the initiation of chronic periodontitis. Furthermore, the current extent of disease within an individual, i.e. number of sites with CAL, BL and/or deep pockets (PPD), is a predictor of future disease occurrence. In fact the best predictor of disease progression is the previous disease experience.

Chronic periodontitis is often classified according to extent and severity of diseased sites. For the extent of disease the low category would involve 1 to 10 sites, medium 11 to 20 and high would be greater than 20 sites affected. Severity can be differentiated according to clinical attachment loss into mild (1-2 mm CAL), moderate (3-4 mm CAL) or severe (to ≥ 5 mm CAL). The extent and severity of chronic periodontitis, as stated previously, are useful predictors of future disease progression, and taken together with the patient's age may be clinically valuable in predicting disease progression and thus the need for therapy and maintenance. Table 8-2 provides a summary of the clinical features of chronic periodontitis.

RISK FACTORS OR SUSCEPTIBILITY TO CHRONIC PERIODONTITIS

The term "risk factor" means an aspect of lifestyle, or an environmental exposure, or an inborn or inherited characteristic, which on the basis of epidemiological evidence is known to be associated with a given disease. Risk factors may be part of the causal chain of a disease and/or may predispose the host to develop a disease. An individual presenting with one or more risk factors has an increased probability of contracting the disease or of the disease being made worse.

Bacterial risk factors

These aspects are dealt with in previous chapters and from these the reader can ascertain that a cumulative risk for a given microbiota can be estimated. It is not clear however if the specific microbiota is the principal disease causing factor or whether it reflects the disease process. Specific microorganisms have been considered as potential periodontal pathogens but it is clear that although pathogens are necessary, their mere presence may not be enough for disease activity to occur. Microbial plaque (biofilm) is a crucial factor in inflammation of the periodontal tissues, but the progression of gingivitis to periodontitis is largely governed by host-based risk factors. Microbial biofilms of particular compositions will initiate chronic periodontitis (see Chapter 4) in certain individuals whose host response and cumulative risk factors predispose them to periodontal destruction rather than to gingivitis.

Age

Although the prevalence of periodontal disease increases with age it is unlikely that becoming older in itself greatly increases susceptibility to periodontal disease. It is more likely that the cumulative effects of disease over a lifetime, i.e. deposits of plaque and calculus, and the increased number of sites capable of harboring such deposits, as well as attachment and bone loss experience, explain the increased prevalence of disease in older people.

Smoking

The association between periodontal disease and smoking is dealt with in detail in Chapter 6. Only a brief discussion of smoking as a risk factor for chronic periodontitis is thus given here. The literature consistently indicates a positive association between smoking and chronic periodontitis across the many cross-sectional and longitudinal studies performed over the years (Kinane & Chestnutt 2000) and the risk attributable to tobacco for chronic periodontitis is between 2.5 and 7.0. It is not only the risk of developing the disease that is enhanced by smoking, but also the response to periodontal therapy is impaired in smokers. A further feature in smokers is that their signs and symptoms of both gingivitis and chronic periodontitis, mainly gingival redness and bleeding on probing (BOP), are masked by the dampening of inflammation seen for smokers as compared to non-smokers.

Host response related

Systemic disease

It is difficult to determine the precise role any systemic disease may play in the pathogenesis of chronic periodontitis. There are several reasons for this. Firstly, in epidemiological studies attempting to evaluate the effect of systemic disease, control groups should be carefully matched in respect of age, sex, oral hygiene and socio-economic status. Many studies, particularly before the etiological importance of dental plaque was recognized, failed to include such controls. Secondly, because of the chronicity of periodontal disease, longitudinal studies spanning several years are preferable in individuals both with and without systemic disease. Unfortunately, most of the available data are derived from cross-sectional studies.

A reduction in number or function of polymorphonuclear leukocytes (PMNs) generally results in increased rate and severity of periodontal tissue destruction. Many drugs such as phenytoin, nifedipine and cyclosporin predispose to gingival overgrowth in response to plaque and thus may modify pre-existing chronic periodontitis. Changes in circulating hormone levels may increase severity of plaque induced gingival inflammation but typically do not result in any increased susceptibility to periodontitis. Hormonal changes following menopause have been associated with osteoporosis but studies are lacking to link this disease or an estrogen deficient state to a higher susceptibility to periodontal disease. Immuno-suppressive drug therapy and any disease resulting in suppression of inflammatory and immune processes (such as HIV infection) may predispose the individual to periodontal tissue destruction.

Nutritional deficiencies in animals have been shown to affect the periodontal tissues but epidemiological data do not support the suggestion that such deficiencies play an important role in chronic periodontal disease. Gingival bleeding is the most consistent oral feature of vitamin C deficiency or scurvy but there is also some evidence to suggest that avitaminosis-C may aggravate established chronic periodontitis.

The periodontal features of the histiocytoses group of diseases may present as necrotizing ulcerative periodontitis. Diabetes appears to be one of the most fascinating systemic diseases that interacts with periodontitis. On the one hand periodontitis severity and prevalence are increased in diabetics and more so in poorly-controlled diabetics, than non-diabetics. On the other hand, periodontitis may also exacerbate diabetes as it may decrease glycemic control (see Chapter 6).

Despite the paucity of high quality literature on individuals both with and without systemic disease the following general conclusions can be drawn:

1. The blood cells have a vital role in supplying oxygen, hemostasis and protection to the tissues of the periodontium. Systemic hematological disorders can thus have profound effects on the periodontium by denying any of these functions necessary for the integrity of the periodontium.

2. The polymorphonuclear leucocyte (PMN cell) is undoubtedly crucial to the defence of the periodontium. To exert this protective function several activities of PMNs must be integrated, namely chemotaxis, phagocytosis and killing or neutralization of the ingested organism or substance. Individuals with either quantitative (neutropenia) or qualitative (chemotactic or phagocytic) PMN deficiencies, exhibit severe destruction of the periodontal tissues, which is strong evidence that PMNs are an important component of the host's protective response to the subgingival biofilm. Quantitative deficiencies are generally accompanied by destruction of the periodontium of all teeth, whereas qualitative defects are often associated with localized destruction affecting only the periodontium of certain teeth (i.e. chronic periodontitis may be modified).

3. Leukemias which give excessive numbers of leucocytes in the blood and tissues also cause a greatly depleted bone marrow function with concomitant anemia, thrombocytopenia, neutropenia and reduced range of specific immune cells which give some characteristic periodontal features: anemic gingival pallor; gingival bleeding; gingival ulceration. Leukemic features are further complicated by the potential for the proliferating leucocytes to infiltrate the gingiva and result in gingival enlargement.

4. In broad terms leukemias result in gingival pathologies, whereas periodontal bone loss is the consequence of neutrophil functional defects or deficient numbers and other severe functional defects such as deficiency of leucocyte adhesion receptors.

5. There are numerous confounding variables, which must be considered in determining the true relationship between periodontitis and diabetes. The current consensus is that diabetics are at increased risk of periodontal disease, and whilst periodontitis can be successfully treated, both disease susceptibility and the outcome of therapy are influenced by poor metabolic control. Thus, it may be of benefit to the dentist to have knowledge of the control

status of diabetes in an individual patient, as in the longer term metabolic control could indicate the probable outcome of periodontal therapy. In addition, it is now accepted that periodontal therapy can improve metabolic control in diabetics, meaning that the relationship is two-way and periodontal therapy is beneficial to the control of both diseases.

6. Medications such as phenytoin, cyclosporin and nifedipine may predispose to gingival overgrowth in patients with gingivitis.

7. Genetic traits, which result in diseases that modify the periodontal structures or change the immune or inflammatory responses, can result in gross periodontal destruction in the affected individual and although the destruction seen may imitate periodontitis this is not etiopathologically chronic periodontitis.

Stress

Stress and other psychosomatic conditions may have direct anti-inflammatory and/or anti-immune effects and/or behavior mediated effects on the body's defenses. Hence both conditions may conceptually be relevant to the etiology of chronic periodontitis and necrotizing ulcerative conditions. Recent studies have suggested that academic stress and financial stress may be associated with an increased risk of periodontal disease. Most of the literature on stress and periodontal conditions is quite old, however, and reports of acute necrotizing ulcerative gingivitis (or trench mouth) were made on stressed soldiers on the front line during World War I. It is understood that stress may be immunosuppressive and that acute necrotizing ulcerative gingivitis may occur in the immunosuppressed (also in HIV patients), but there is insufficient data as yet to substantiate the assumption that psychosocial factors are indeed of etiological importance in chronic periodontitis.

Genetics

There is convincing evidence from twin studies for a genetic predisposition to the periodontal diseases. The twin studies have indicated that risk of chronic periodontitis has a high inherited component but that gingivitis is a general and common response which is unlikely to be linked with particular genes. A great deal of research is underway attempting to identify the genes and polymorphisms associated with all forms of periodontitis. It is likely that chronic periodontitis involves many genes, the composition of which may vary across individuals and races. Much attention has focused on polymorphisms associated with the genes involved in cytokine production. Such polymorphisms have been linked to an increased risk for chronic periodontitis but these findings have yet to be corroborated.

SCIENTIFIC BASIS FOR PERIODONTAL THERAPY

Periodontitis is initiated and sustained by microbes which are present in supra and subgingival plaque in the form of uncalcified and calcified (calculus) biofilms. Initial periodontal therapy or basic treatment of periodontitis involves the removal of both sub and supragingival plaque. The clinical outcome is largely dependent on the skill of the operator in removing subgingival plaque and the skill and motivation of the patient in practising adequate home care. A further variable is the innate susceptibility of the patient which is related to the way in which their innate, inflammatory and immune systems operate in response to the microbial challenge. In addition, local and systemic risk factors can influence the quantity and quality of both the microbial challenge and the host response to these pathogens. The relative contribution of these risk factors has yet to be fully determined but their influence would be negated if the periodontium was kept free of microbial plaque, and thus subgingival debridement and patient's home care are of vital importance.

Studies have been conducted which indicate the relative importance of operator and patient-based interventions (for further detail see Chapters 20 and 21) and only a brief summary is presented below.

Tooth loss

There is an established literature strongly supporting the concept that periodontal treatment of chronic periodontitis is effective, and numerous long term studies show low rates of tooth loss (≤ 0.1 tooth lost/year) in treated and well-maintained periodontitis patients (Lindhe & Nyman 1984, Nabers et al. 1988). Patients who, following treatment, were not complying with maintenance care had double the rate of tooth loss per year (0.2 teeth/year) (Becker et al. 1984), and untreated patients lost approximately 0.6 teeth/year (Becker et al. 1979). Thus there is substantial evidence supporting the concept that periodontal therapy and subsequent maintenance care are beneficial in maintaining the dentition.

Subgingival instrumentation and maintenance

The effects of cause related periodontal therapy were studied intensively during the 1980s and the work of Egelberg and his colleagues will be described now. Badersten et al. (1984) utilized patients with severe chronic periodontitis to study the effects of cause related periodontal therapy. The patients had a multitude of sites with deep pockets (up to 12 mm). Initial oral hygiene instruction was provided at two to three

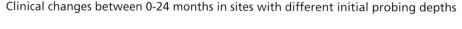

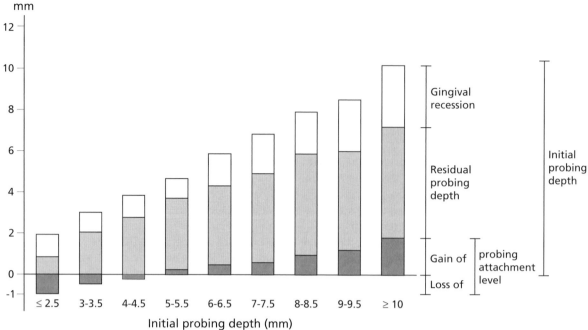

Fig. 8-3. Data from the Badersten et al. (1984) study showing the clinical changes at 2 years according to baseline pocket depth.

visits during the first month of the study. Additional instruction and reinforcement of self-performed plaque control was provided, as required, during the 2 years of the study. Subgingival debridement was performed at 3, 6 and 9 months and the results were evaluated over 2 years. Only minimal improvements in the periodontal indices occurred during the first 3 months in which no scaling and root planing was performed. Following supra and subgingival instrumentation, and gradually up until 12 months from baseline, the periodontal indices improved markedly. In the final 12 months of the 2-year period, no significant further improvements in the clinical condition occurred. These results demonstrate that chronic periodontitis can be treated successfully by intensive initial non-surgical periodontal therapy and this outcome can be maintained over time with supportive periodontal therapy (SPT).

Fig. 8-3 shows further data from the Badersten et al. (1984) study and reports the clinical changes at 2 years according to baseline pocket depth. It can be seen that pocket depth reduction after therapy is an arithmetic combination of gingival recession and gain or loss of clinical attachment. At the end of the study the mean pocket depth reduction was 1.5 mm although it is clear from Fig. 8-3 that the initially deeper pockets had the largest reduction in pocket depth over the 2 years and the greatest clinical attachment gain. An interesting feature is the fact that the sites with initially shallow pockets tended to lose clinical attachment over the study period. Several theories have been proposed to explain this fact. The most plausible explanation for the loss of clinical attachment at shallow sites is the trauma caused by subgingival instrumentation to the

supracrestal connective tissue attachment and the subsequent remodeling of the marginal tissues. The best predictor of further clinical attachment loss was residual deep pockets that occurred after treatment. Thus, Claffey and Egelberg (1995) found that at re-evaluation, patients with multiple sites with residual probing depth ≥ 6mm after active treatment had a greater risk for additional attachment loss than patients with mainly shallow sites.

Effect of surgical treatment

Surgical treatment of chronic periodontitis lesions permits visualization and access to the root surfaces and thus has clear advantages over a non-surgical approach for the cleaning of root surfaces. Tissues may also be manipulated and lesions modified, or granulation tissue surgically removed. The efficacy of surgical periodontal therapy compared within the various surgical treatment modalities and compared to non-surgical therapy has to be considered from the extensive scientific literature on these matters (for further detail see Chapter 25).

Comparisons of surgical and non-surgical therapy

Kaldahl et al. (1993) reviewed a large body of work on the advantages of different periodontal treatment modalities over others. Although the best assessment of clinical outcome is achieved from longer-term studies, actually following patients over the long term creates new confounding problems and these can reduce the benefit imparted by the longitudinal element of the investigation. For example, the patient drop-out increases over time which may increase the bias in the selection of the final group for analysis (usually the less motivated patients or less successfully treated patients will drop out). In addition, tooth loss may occur for which we do not know the reason and sites associated with such teeth are lost for longitudinal analysis. Nevertheless, useful long-term studies have been conducted over 5 to 8 years and have typically made intra-patient comparisons of different periodontal treatment modalities using split mouth designs. In the Kaldahl et al. (1993) review, some comprehensive summary statements were arrived at. In general:

1. Surgical and non-surgical periodontal therapy can improve periodontal clinical outcome measures.

2. Surgical therapy created greater short-term reductions in probing depth than non-surgical therapy although longer-term results varied between maintaining greater probing depth reduction or showing no differences with non-surgical therapy.

3. Flap surgery with and without osseous resection gave variable probing depth reductions in the short term. Some studies favored osseous resection whilst others showed no difference in probing depth reduction.

4. Flap surgery without osseous resection tended to produce greater better short and long-term gains in attachment levels.

5. In both short and long-term studies, surgery produced a greater loss of probing attachment in sites with initially shallow pockets. In sites with deeper pockets short and long-term studies reported no difference in attachment level change for non-surgical and surgical therapy.

6. Supragingival plaque control alone gave markedly inferior results to plaque control combined with subgingival root debridement.

REFERENCES

Badersten, A., Nilvéus, R. & Egelberg, J. (1984). Effect of non-surgical periodontal therapy. II. Severely advanced periodontitis. *Journal of Clinical Periodontology* **11**, 63-76.

Becker, W., Becker, B.E. & Berg, L.E. (1984). Periodontal treatment without maintenance. A retrospective study in 44 patients. *Journal of Periodontology* **55**, 505-509.

Becker, W., Berg, L. & Becker, B.E. (1979). Untreated periodontal disease: a longitudinal study. *Journal of Periodontology* **50**, 234-244.

Claffey, N. & Egelberg, J. (1995). Clinical indicators of probing attachment loss following initial periodontal treatment in advanced periodontitis patients. *Journal of Clinical Periodontology* **22**(9), 690-696.

Flemmig, T.F. (1999). Periodontitis. *Annal of Periodontology* **4**, 32-38.

Kaldahl, W.B., Kalkwarf, K.L. & Patil, K.D. (1993). A review of longitudinal studies that compared periodontal therapies. *Journal of Periodontology* **64**, 243-253.

Kinane, D.F. & Chestnutt, I. (2000). Smoking and Periodontal Disease. *Critical Reviews Oral Biological Medicine* **11**, 356-365.

Lindhe, J. & Nyman, S. (1984). Long-term maintenance of patients treated for advanced periodontal disease. *Journal of Clinical Periodontology* **11**(8), 504-514.

Nabers, C.L., Stalker, W.H., Esparza, D., Naylor, B. & Canales, S. (1988). Tooth loss in 1535 treated periodontal patients. *Journal of Periodontology* **59**(5), 297-300.

Socransky, S.S., Haffajee, A.D., Goodson, J.M. & Lindhe, J. (1984). New concepts of destructive periodontal disease. *Journal of Clinical Periodontology* **11**, 21-32.

CHAPTER 9

Aggressive Periodontitis

Maurizio S. Tonetti and Andrea Mombelli

Classification and clinical syndromes

Epidemiology

    Primary dentition and permanent dentition

    Screening

Etiology and pathogenesis

Diagnosis

    Clinical, microbiologic, genetic

Principles of therapeutic intervention

Periodontitis is an infection that can manifest itself with polymorph clinical presentations. This has led to the recognition of different clinical syndromes. Until recently, the question of whether or not these dissimilar clinical presentations represented different forms of disease has been open to discussion. Today several lines of evidence support the existence of truly different forms of periodontitis. These include:

1. The growing clinical consensus of differential prognosis and need for specific treatment approaches for the various syndromes
2. Heterogeneity in etiology with possible therapeutic implications
3. Heterogeneity in genetic and environmental susceptibility

At the 1999 international classification workshop, the different forms of periodontitis were reclassified into three major forms (chronic, aggressive and necrotizing forms of periodontitis) and into periodontal manifestations of systemic diseases. This chapter deals with aggressive, type 1, periodontitis. Until recently, this group of diseases was defined primarily based on the age of onset/diagnosis and was thus named early onset periodontitis (EOP). Features of this form of disease, however, can present themselves at any age and this form of periodontitis is not necessarily confined to individuals under the arbitrarily chosen age of 35.

Aggressive periodontitis (AgP) comprises a group of rare, often severe, rapidly progressive forms of periodontitis often characterized by an early age of clinical manifestation and a distinctive tendency for cases to aggregate in families. At the above mentioned classification workshop, AgP periodontitis was char-

acterized by the following major common features (Lang et al. 1999):

- Non-contributory medical history
- Rapid attachment loss and bone destruction
- Familial aggregation of cases

Frequently AgP presents early in the life of the individual; this implies that etiologic agents have been able to cause clinically detectable levels of disease over a relatively short time. This fact is central to the current understanding of these diseases, since it implies infection with a highly virulent microflora and/or a high level of subject susceptibility to periodontal disease. AgP, however, can occur at any age. Diagnosis of AgP requires exclusion of the presence of systemic diseases that may severely impair host defences and lead to premature tooth loss (periodontal manifestations of systemic diseases).

The existence of specific forms of AgP has also been recognized based on specific clinical and laboratory features: localized aggressive periodontitis (LAP, formerly known as localized juvenile periodontitis or LJP) and generalized aggressive periodontitis (GAP, formerly termed generalized juvenile periodontitis (GJP) or generalized early onset periodontitis, G-EOP) (Tonetti & Mombelli 1999).

In spite of its rare occurrence AgP has been the focus of many investigations aimed at understanding its etiology and pathogenesis. Difficulties in gathering sufficiently large populations, however, have resulted in few clinical studies addressing both diagnostic and therapeutic procedures for these subjects. Utilization of both clinical and advanced diagnostic procedures as well as of a variety of treatment approaches remains largely anecdotal and somehow based on the specific experience of individual clinicians rather than on well-documented scientific evidence.

CLASSIFICATION AND CLINICAL SYNDROMES

In the absence of an etiologic classification, aggressive forms of periodontal disease have been defined based on the following primary features (Lang et al. 1999):

- Non-contributory medical history
- Rapid attachment loss and bone destruction
- Familial aggregation of cases

Secondary features that are considered to be generally but not universally present are:

- Amounts of microbial deposits inconsistent with the severity of periodontal tissue destruction
- Elevated proportions of *Actinobacillus actinomycetemcomitans* and, in some Far East populations, *Porphyromonas gingivalis*
- Phagocyte abnormalities
- Hyper-responsive macrophage phenotype, including elevated production of PGE_2 and $IL-1\beta$ in response to bacterial endotoxins
- Progression of attachment loss and bone loss may be self-arresting

The international classification workshop identified clinical and laboratory features deemed specific enough to allow sub-classification of AgP into localized and generalized forms (Tonetti & Mombelli 1999, Lang et al. 1999). The following features were identified:

Localized aggressive periodontitis (LAP) (Fig. 9-1)
- Circumpubertal onset
- Localized first molar/incisor presentation with interproximal attachment loss on at least two permanent teeth, one of which is a first molar, and involving no more than two teeth other than first molars and incisors
- Robust serum antibody response to infecting agents

Generalized aggressive periodontitis (GAP) (Fig. 9-2)
- Usually affecting persons under 30 years of age, but patients may be older
- Generalized interproximal attachment loss affecting at least three permanent teeth other than first molars and incisors
- Pronounced episodic nature of the destruction of attachment and alveolar bone
- Poor serum antibody response to infecting agents

Diagnosis of one of these AgP forms requires the absence of systemic diseases that may severely impair host defences and lead to premature exfoliation of teeth. In such instances the appropriate clinical diagnosis will be periodontal manifestation of systemic diseases.

GAP represents the most heterogeneous group and includes the most severe forms of periodontitis. They comprise forms originally described as generalized juvenile periodontitis (emphasis on a possible relationship with LAP), severe periodontitis (emphasis on the advanced destruction in comparison with patient age), or rapidly progressing periodontitis (emphasis on the high rate of progression of lesions in these forms). Each of these GAP forms, however, remains highly heterogeneous in terms of clinical presentation and response to therapy. The European Workshop on Periodontology has therefore suggested that, while a better etiologic classification remains unavailable, these forms should be considered as a group to be further defined by the use of various clinical descriptors of the disease based on clinical, microbiological and immunologic parameters (Attström & Van der Velden 1993). Further rationale for an imprecise classification of these GAP forms comes from the fact that, given the severity of the disease and the heterogeneity of clinical presentation, each of these rare cases deserves individual consideration.

Often subjects present with attachment loss that does not fit the specific diagnostic criteria established for AgP or chronic periodontitis; this occurrence has been termed *incidental attachment loss*. It includes: recessions associated with trauma or tooth position, attachment loss associated with impacted third molars, attachment loss associated with removal of impacted third molars, etc. It may include initial clinical presentations of periodontitis. Patients with this clinical diagnosis should be considered as a high-risk group for AgP or chronic periodontitis.

Besides clinical presentation, a variety of radiographic, microbiologic and immunologic parameters are currently being used, along with the assessment of environmental exposures such as cigarette smoking, to further describe the AgP affecting the individual subject. These descriptors are important in treatment selection and to establish long-term prognosis. They will be further discussed in the section on diagnosis later in this chapter.

It is also important to underline that, in the present state of uncertainty regarding both the causative agents and the genetic and environmental susceptibility to AgP, it is possible that, in spite of the lines of evidence presented above, LAP and GAP may simply represent phenotypic variations of a single disease entity. Conversely, it is possible that different AgP forms may manifest themselves with a common clinical presentation. This aspect is of great diagnostic and therapeutic importance.

Some case reports have indicated that some subjects may experience periodontitis affecting the primary dentition, followed by LAP and later by GAP (Shapira et al. 1994). One investigation indicated that the primary dentition of LAP patients presented bone

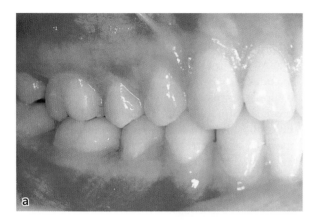

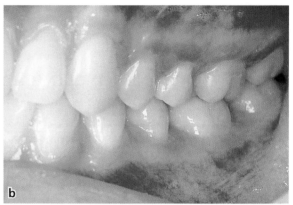

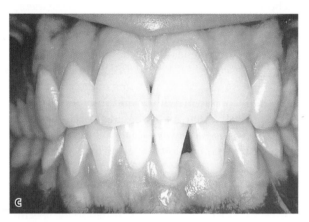

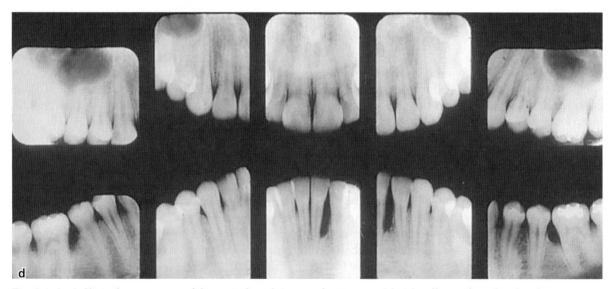

Fig. 9-1. (a-c) Clinical appearance of the periodontal tissues of a 15-year-old girl suffering from localized aggressive periodontitis. Note the proper oral hygiene conditions and the scalloped outline of the gingival margin. In the lower anterior region, the interdental papilla between teeth 31 and 32 has been lost. Intraoral radiographs (d) show the presence of localized angular bony defects, associated with clinical attachment level loss, at the mesial aspect of tooth 46, 36 and at the distal aspect of tooth 31. No significant bone loss and/or attachment loss was detectable in other areas of the dentition. Diagnosis: localized aggressive periodontitis (LAP).

loss at primary molars in 20-52% of the cases, suggesting that at least some LAP cases may initially affect the primary dentition (Sjodin et al. 1989, 1993). Furthermore, in LAP subjects an association between the number of lesions and the age of the subject has been described, suggesting an age-dependent shift from localized to generalized forms of AgP (Hormand & Frandsen 1979, Burmeister et al. 1984).

EPIDEMIOLOGY

Given the recent definition of AgP and the fact that it does not represent just a new term for the previously defined EOP, epidemiological studies available relate primarily to EOP. Relatively few investigations employing different epidemiological techniques have es-

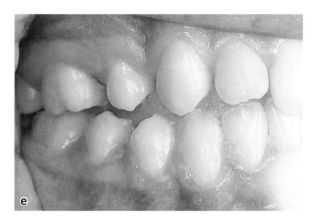

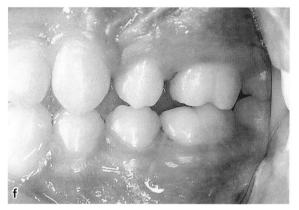

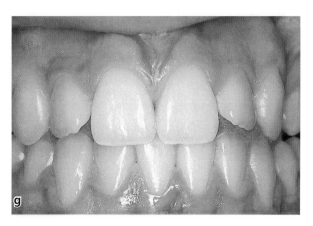

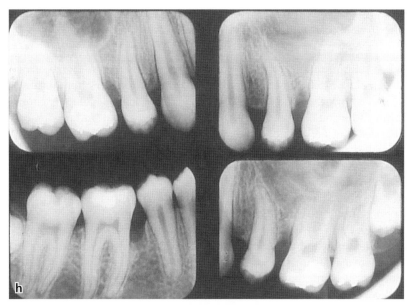

Fig. 9-1. (e-g) Clinical appearance of the 14-year-old sister of the proband depicted in (a-d). Note that in spite of the excellent oral hygiene status, bleeding on probing was provoked in the mesial of the molars, where deep pockets were present. (h) Angular bone loss is evident on the mesial of 16, 26 and 46.

timated the prevalence and the progression of EOP in the primary and permanent dentition(s) of children and young adults. All available investigations, however, indicate that early onset (aggressive) forms of periodontal diseases are detectable in all age and ethnic groups (Papapanou 1996). Wide variation in prevalence, however, has been reported, with some studies showing up to 51.5% affected individuals. These differences are probably due to differences in the employed epidemiological methodologies and definition of EOP.

Primary dentition

Little evidence is available concerning the prevalence of AgP affecting the primary dentition. In the few studies from industrialized countries, marginal alveo-

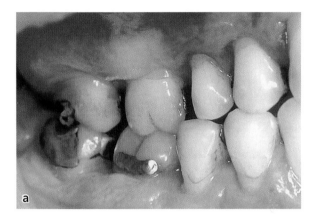
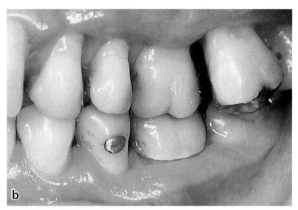
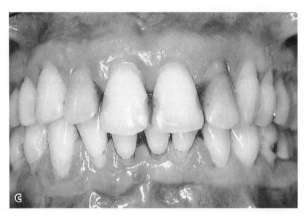

Fig. 9-2. (a-c) Clinical presentation in 1990 of a 32-year-old female with generalized severe bone loss and clinical attachment loss, recession of the gingival margin and presence of deep periodontal pockets. Presence of local factors, and intense inflammation and edema of the gingival margin are evident.

lar bone loss has been found to affect the primary dentition of 5 to 11 year olds with frequencies ranging from 0.9-4.5% of subjects (Sweeney et al. 1987, Bimstein et al. 1994, Sjodin & Mattson 1994). In this respect, it should be emphasized that periodontitis affecting the primary dentition does not necessarily mean presence of an aggressive form of periodontitis, but may indicate a chronic form of disease with relative abundance of local factors (plaque and calculus). A clinical case of localized periodontitis affecting the primary dentition is illustrated in Fig. 9-3. More severe cases affecting the primary dentition and leading to tooth exfoliation early in life are usually interpreted as periodontal manifestations of systemic (hematologic) diseases, such as leukocyte adhesion deficiency (see Chapter 2 and Fig. 9-4).

Permanent dentition

In the permanent dentition of 13 to 20-year-old individuals, the majority of studies have reported a prevalence of periodontitis of less than 1% (usually 0.1-0.2% in Caucasian populations). The risk of developing periodontitis at such an early age, however, does not seem to be shared equally in the population: among US schoolchildren 5-17 years of age, the prevalence of periodontitis has been estimated to range from about 0.2% for whites to about 2.6% for blacks (Löe & Brown

1991). Furthermore, in these young age groups higher prevalence of periodontitis has been reported in studies from some developing countries (see Chapter 2).

Longitudinal studies of disease progression in adolescents indicate that subjects with signs of destructive periodontitis at a young age are prone to further deterioration. Such deterioration appears to be more pronounced at initially affected sites, and in patients diagnosed with LAP and from low socio-economic classes. Deterioration of the periodontal status involves both an increase in extent (number of lesions within the dentition) and an increase in severity of lesions (further alveolar bone loss at initially diseased sites, Fig. 9-5) (Clerehugh et al. 1990, Lissau et al. 1990, Albandar et al. 1991a,b, 1993, Aass et al. 1994).

Some epidemiological investigations have reported high prevalence of attachment loss in adolescents and young adults that did not fit the characteristics of recognized periodontitis clinical syndromes. Such occurrences have been termed *incidental attachment loss*, and have been reported in 1.6-26% of the subjects. This group is thought to comprise both initial forms of periodontitis (including AgP) and a variety of defects such as recession due to traumatic tooth-brushing, attachment loss associated with removal of impacted third molars, etc.

Conclusion

A small but significant proportion of children and

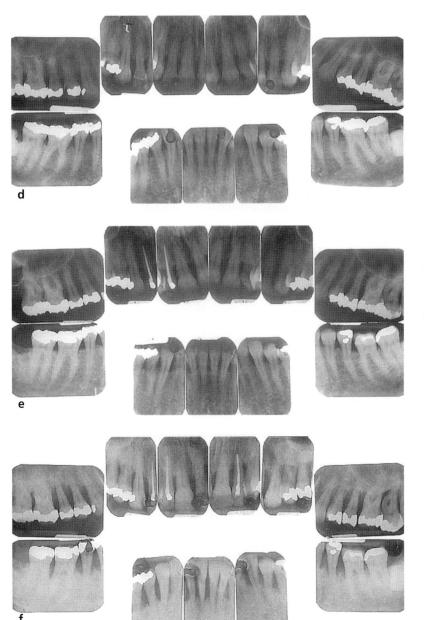

Fig. 9-2. (d-f). Previous radiographic examinations were available from 1984 and 1987. Comparison of the radiographs obtained over the 6-year period from 1984 to 1990 indicates that most of the periodontal destruction occurred during the last 3 years. The patient had been smoking 20 cigarettes/day for more than 10 years. Diagnosis: Generalized aggressive periodontitis (GAP) in a cigarette smoker.

young adults is affected by some form of periodontitis. A substantial proportion of these subjects is thought to be affected by AgP. Given the severity of these forms of periodontal diseases and their tendency to progress, early detection of periodontitis, and AgP in particular, should be a primary concern of both practitioners and public health officers. The whole population, including children and young adults, should receive a periodontal screening as part of their routine dental examination.

Screening

Given the low prevalence of AgP patients within the population, cost-effective detection of cases requires utilization of a sensitive screening approach, i.e. the application of a diagnostic approach able to correctly identify most of the cases with disease. The objective of screening is the detection in a population of possibly diseased subjects that would require a more comprehensive examination. In periodontology, the most sensitive diagnostic test for the detection of periodontitis is the measurement of attachment loss by probing. Application of this diagnostic procedure in the mixed dentition and in teeth that are not fully erupted, however, may be difficult.

In younger subjects, therefore, a currently utilized screening approach is the measurement of the distance between the alveolar crest and the cemento-enamel junction on bite-wing radiographs. An advantage of this approach relates to the fact that in most industrialized countries bite-wing radiographs of children and young adolescents in mixed dentition are routinely taken for caries prevention programs; these radiographs should therefore be screened not only for carious lesions but also for the presence of marginal alveolar bone loss.

Recent investigations have attempted to determine the "normal" distance between the cemento-enamel

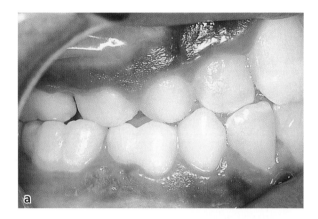
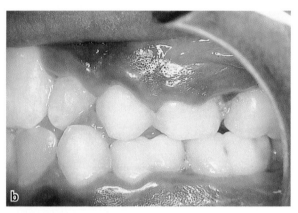

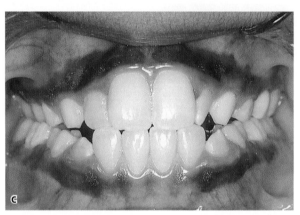

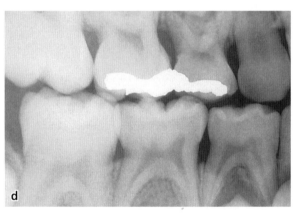
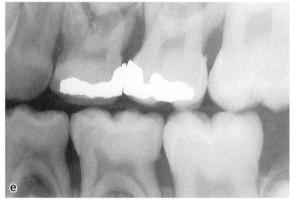

Fig. 9-3. Seven-year-old African-American female presenting with radiographic alveolar bone loss and probing attachment loss at the primary molars and permanent first molars and incisors: (a-c) clinical photographs, buccal view; (d-e) bite-wing radiographs. Clinical presentation shows moderate plaque accumulation, localized gingival inflammation, with ulceration of the gingival margin and loss of the interdental papilla mesial of #65. 4-6 mm pockets with bleeding on probing were present in the primary molar regions. Bone loss and attachment loss were limited to the molar region. The mesial aspects of the first permanent molars are also initially involved. Radiographic subgingival calculus is evident. Note that the upper left posterior sextant seems to be more severely affected than the other posterior segments. Diagnosis: localized aggressive (type 1) periodontitis.

junction and the alveolar crest of primary and permanent molars in 7 to 9-year-old children (Sjodin & Mattson 1992, Needleman et al. 1997). Median distances at primary molars were 0.8 to 1.4 mm. These values were in agreement with those previously reported for primary molars of 3 to 11-year-old children (Bimstein & Soskolne 1988). The cemento-enamel junction of permanent molars was 0 to 0.5 mm apical to the alveolar crest in 7 to 9 year olds. These values were age-dependent, and related to the state of erup-

tion of the tooth. In general, however, it should be noted that the majority of children present with distances significantly smaller than the 2-3 mm considered normal for the completely erupted dentitions of adults. In children, significantly greater distances have been detected at sites with caries, fillings or open contacts, indicating that these factors may contribute to bone loss in similar ways to in adult patients. Furthermore, presence of one of these local factors may suggest a local cause of bone loss, other than perio-

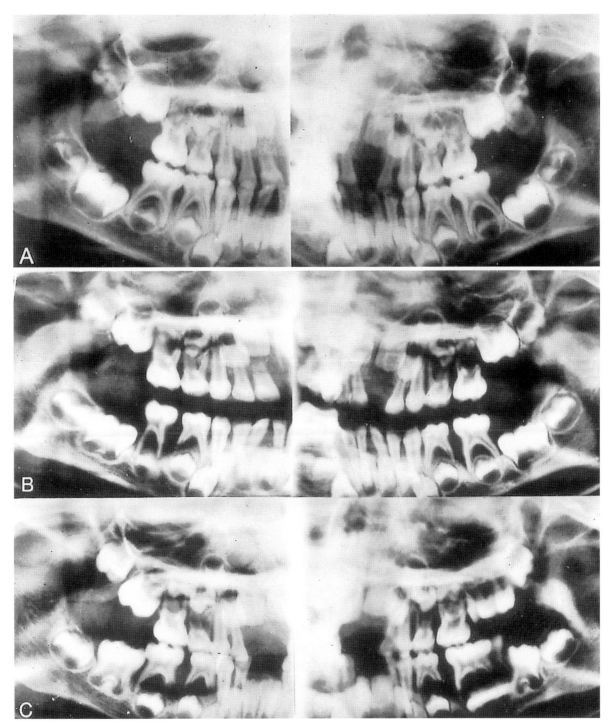

Fig. 9-4. Radiographs obtained from a Caucasian female with generalized pre-pubertal periodontitis. Radiographic situation in (A) April 1978 when she was 4-5 years old, (B) December 1978; and (C) August 1979. The radiographs illustrate the extent of alveolar bone loss that occurred over the 15-month period. Note the widespread bone loss. During infancy, this patient had severe, recurrent skin and ear infections sustained by *Staphylococcus aureus* and *Pseudomonas aeruginosa*, respectively. Delayed healing was also observed following minor injuries. White cell counts revealed a persistent leukocytosis, with absolute neutrophil counts always above $8000/mm^3$. Gingival biopsy indicated that the inflammatory infiltrate consisted almost completely of plasma cells and lymphocytes. No neutrophils were present, in spite of the abundance of these cells in the circulation. This history and clinical manifestation appears to be consistent with the diagnosis of periodontal manifestations of systemic disease in a subject with leukocyte adhesion deficiency (LAD). From Page et al. 1983.

dontitis. A distance of 2 mm between the cemento-enamel junction and the alveolar crest, in the absence of the above-mentioned local factors, argues therefore for a suspected diagnosis of periodontitis (Figs. 9-6 and 9-7) (Sjodin & Mattson 1992). This tentative diagnosis will have to be confirmed by a complete periodontal examination. In utilizing bite-wing radiographs for the screening of patients, clinicians should

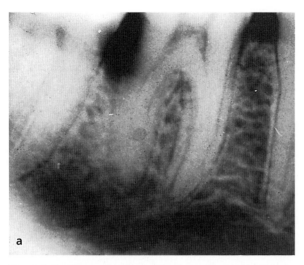
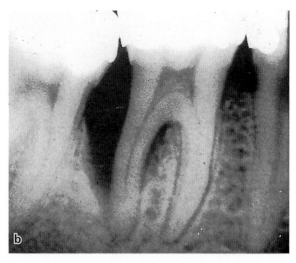

Fig. 9-5. Radiographs illustrating bone loss at the distal aspect of the mandibular first molar in a 15-year-old girl (a) and progression of disease 1 year later (b).

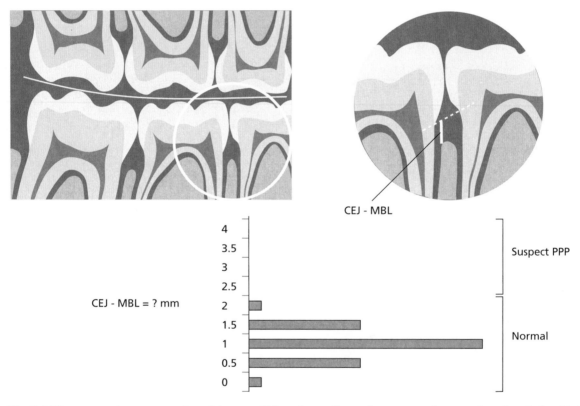

Fig. 9-6. Diagrammatic representation of the use of bite-wing radiographs to screen for prepubertal periodontitis in mixed dentition. The distance from the cemento-enamel junction (CEJ) and the marginal bone level (MBL) is measured from a line connecting the CEJ of the two adjacent teeth. Measurements are taken for each mesial and distal surface. Normal CEJ-MBL distances for 7-9 year olds are less than 2.0 mm. If the measurement exceeds this value, prepubertal periodontitis should be suspected, and a comprehensive periodontal examination should be performed.

be aware that radiographic marginal bone loss (in the presence of probing attachment loss) is a highly specific diagnostic sign of periodontitis. Its sensitivity, however, is lower than that of periodontal probing because initial intrabony lesions may not appear on radiographs as a result of the masking effects of intact cortical plates (Suomi et al. 1968, Lang & Hill 1977). Some initial cases of periodontitis may therefore remain undetected.

In older adolescents and adults, periodontal probing is a more appropriate screening examination than the use of radiographs. It is in this respect important to differentiate between clinical use of periodontal probing to perform a complete periodontal examination, and its use as a screening tool. Using probing to detect attachment loss during a screening examination requires circumferential probing to evaluate all sites around the tooth. In a screening examination,

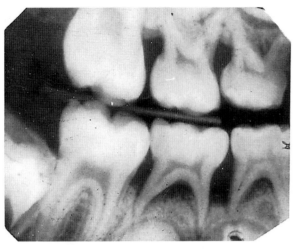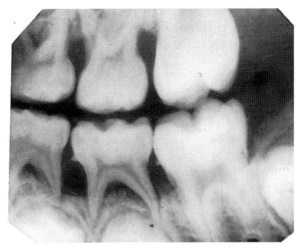

Fig. 9-7. Bite-wing radiographs illustrating advanced bone loss at primary molars, and initial involvement of the mesial aspect of the first molar in a child with early onset periodontitis. Note the marginal pattern of bone loss, which is significantly different from the pattern expected in association with the normal exfoliation of deciduous teeth. Subgingival calculus can also be observed.

however, attachment loss values for all sites are usually not recorded. Furthermore, the screening examination can be stopped once evidence of attachment loss has been detected, and therefore the need for a comprehensive examination has been established. The American Academy of Periodontology has recently endorsed a simplified screening examination for this purpose. This examination is based on a modification of the Community Periodontal Index of Treatment Needs (CPITN) (Ainamo et al. 1982, American Academy of Periodontology & American Dental Association 1992).

Once a case has been detected by a screening examination, a comprehensive periodontal examination will be necessary to establish a proper diagnosis. At this stage, once a case of periodontitis has been confirmed, a differential diagnosis between aggressive (type 1) periodontitis and chronic (type 2) periodontitis needs to be made in accordance with the criteria mentioned above and keeping in mind that cases which do not fit the AgP criteria should be diagnosed as chronic periodontitis.

Conclusion

Screening periodontal examinations should be performed as part of every dental visit. Marginal bone loss assessed on bite-wing radiographs, though less sensitive than periodontal probing, may be used as a screening tool in subjects with primary and mixed dentitions. Attachment loss evaluated by periodontal probing is the most sensitive screening approach currently available; it should be used in older adolescents and adults. Differential diagnosis between AgP and chronic periodontitis is made based on exclusion of AgP.

ETIOLOGY AND PATHOGENESIS

As a group, aggressive forms of periodontitis are characterized by severe destruction of the periodontal attachment apparatus at an early age. This short time of manifestation of clinically detectable lesions is generally interpreted as being the expression of highly virulent causative agents or high levels of susceptibility of the individual patient, or a combination of the two.

Bacterial etiology

The evidence implicating bacterial etiology in periodontitis has been described in Chapter 4. The most abundant evidence regarding the bacterial etiology of AgP comes from studies of LAP. Evidence relating to other forms of AgP (GAP) will be discussed only when specifically different from LAP.

Acceptance of bacterial etiology of aggressive forms of periodontitis has been particularly difficult since clinical presentation of cases frequently shows little visible plaque accumulation. Of great importance, in this respect, were microscopic studies demonstrating the presence of a layer of bacterial deposits on the root surface of advanced AgP lesions (Listgarten 1976, Westergaard et al. 1978). Early studies attempting the identification of the involved bacteria using culture techniques were performed by Newman et al. and by Slots (Newman et al. 1976, Slots 1976, Newman & Socransky 1977). In these studies, Gramnegative organisms comprised approximately two-thirds of the isolates from deep periodontal pockets. In contrast, these organisms averaged only about one-third of the isolates in control sites with normal gingiva. The dominant microorganisms in LJP included *Actinobacillus actinomycetemcomitans*, *Capnocytophaga* sp., *Eikenella corrodens*, *Prevotella intermedia*

Table 9-1. Classical studies on the distribution of *A. a.* in LAP, gingivitis, adult periodontitis and in normal non-diseased subjects

Study	Diagnosis	No. of subjects (sites)	% A.a. positive subjects	% A.a. positive sites
Slots et al. 1980	LAP	10 (34)	90	79
	Adult Periodontitis	12 (49)	50	35
	Normal Juveniles	10 (60)	20	3
	Normal Adults	11 (66)	36	17
Mandell & Socransky 1981	LAP	6 (18)	100	79
	Adult Periodontitis	25 (50)	0	–
	Gingivitis	23 (46)	0	–
Zambon et al. 1983	LAP	29	97	–
	Adult Periodontitis	134	21	–
	Normal Juveniles/Adults	142	17	–
Eisenmann et al. 1983	LAP	12 (12)	100	100
	Normal Juveniles	10 (10)	60	60
Moore et al. 1985	LAP	14 (31)	36	5
Asikainen et al. 1986	LAP	19 (38)	89	68

See text for a selection of more recent investigations.

and motile anaerobic rods, such as *Campylobacter rectus*. Gram-positive isolates were mostly streptococci, actinomycetes and peptostreptococci.

One of these organisms, *A. actinomycetemcomitans* (*A.a.*), has received particular attention in recent years and is regarded as being a key microorganism in LAP. This view is based on four lines of evidence (Socransky & Haffajee 1992):

1. *Association studies*, linking the organism to the disease: *A.a.* is generally isolated in periodontal lesions from more than 90% of LAP patients and is much less frequent in periodontally healthy individuals (Table 9-1) (for more recent investigations, see also Ashley et al. 1988, Van der Velden et al. 1989, Albandar et al. 1990, Gunsolley et al. 1990, Slots et al. 1990, Asikainen et al. 1991, Aass et al. 1992, Ebersole et al. 1994, Listgarten et al. 1995). In some studies it was possible to demonstrate elevated levels of *A.a.* in sites showing evidence of recent or ongoing periodontal tissue destruction (Haffajee et al. 1984, Mandell 1984, Mandell et al. 1987).

2. Demonstration of *virulence factors*: *A.a.* produces several potentially pathogenic substances, including a leukotoxin, and is capable of inducing disease in experimental animals and non-oral sites (for review see Zambon et al. 1988, Slots & Schonfeld 1991). Furthermore, it can translocate across epithelial membranes.

3. Findings of *immune responses* towards this bacte-

rium: investigators have repeatedly reported significantly elevated levels of serum antibodies to *A.a.* in LAP patients (Listgarten et al. 1981, Tsai et al. 1981, Altman et al. 1982, Ebersole et al. 1982, 1983, Genco et al. 1985, Vincent et al. 1985, Mandell et al. 1987, Sandholm et al. 1987). Such patients also locally produce antibodies against this organism at diseased sites (Schonfeld & Kagan 1982, Ebersole et al. 1985b, Tew et al. 1985).

4. Clinical studies showing a correlation between *treatment outcomes* and levels of *A.a.* after therapy: unsuccessful treatment outcomes have been linked to a failure in reducing the subgingival load of *A.a.* (Slots & Rosling 1983, Haffajee et al. 1984, Christersson et al. 1985, Kornman & Robertson 1985, Mandell et al. 1986, 1987, Preus 1988).

A.a. is one of the few oral microorganisms regarded as true infectious agents in periodontal disease. The acceptance of this concept has far-reaching consequences with regards to strategies for prevention and therapy of LAP or AgP. If *A.a.* is a real exogenous pathogen, (1) avoidance of exposure to the organism becomes a relevant issue in prevention, and (2) elimination of *A.a.* becomes a valid treatment goal. Thus, the mere presence of *A.a.* would have to be regarded as an indication for intervention. Consequently, highly sensitive tests to detect the bacterium would be useful diagnostic tools. Several studies have, in fact, provided evidence for transmission of *A.a.* between humans, e.g. from parent to child or between spouses

Table 9-2. Determinants of virulence and pathogenic potential of *A. actinomycetemcomitans*

Factor	Significance
Leukotoxin	Destroys human polymorphonuclear leukocytes and macrophages
Endotoxin	Activates host cells to secrete inflammatory mediators (prostaglandins, interleukin-1β, tumor necrosis factor-α)
Bacteriocin	May inhibit growth of beneficial species
Immunosuppressive factors	May inhibit IgG and IgM production
Collagenases	Cause degradation of collagen
Chemotactic inhibition factors	May inhibit neutrophil chemotaxis

(DiRienzo et al. 1990, 1994, Preus et al. 1992, Petit et al. 1993a,b, Poulsen et al. 1994, Von Troil-Lindén et al. 1995). Other studies have indicated that *A.a.* can be eliminated with appropriate mechanical treatment and adjunctive antibiotic therapy (Rams et al. 1992, Pavicic et al. 1994).

The view of LAP as an *A.a.* infection is, however, not undisputed. It has been opposed on the basis of cross-sectional studies, showing a high prevalence of this organism in certain populations, particularly from developing countries (Eisenmann et al. 1983, Dahlén et al. 1989, McNabb et al. 1992, Al-Yahfoufi et al. 1994, Gmür & Guggenheim 1994), and for the fact that there are patients with LJP who apparently neither show presence of *A.a.* in the oral flora nor have elevated antibody titers to the organism (Loesche et al. 1985, Moore 1987).

A.a. is a short, facultatively anaerobic, non-motile, Gram-negative rod. Using monoclonal antibody technology, five serotypes (a, b, c, d, e) of *A.a.* can be distinguished. Serotype-dependent variance in virulence has been suggested. Differences in serotype distribution have been noted between patients with periodontal disease and apparently non-affected carriers of *A.a.* Serotype b has been found particularly often in patients with LAP (Asikainen et al. 1991, Zambon et al. 1996).

Several properties of *A.a.* are regarded as important determinants of virulence and pathogenic potential (Table 9-2). Among them, leukotoxin production is considered highly significant since it may play an important role in *A.a.*'s evasion of local host defences. The leukotoxin produced by *A.a.* exhibits cytotoxic specificity and destroys human polymorphonuclear leukocytes and macrophages, but neither epithelial and endothelial cells nor fibroblasts. It belongs to the family of the RTX (Repeats in ToXin) toxins, which are pore-forming lytic toxins (for details the reader is referred to Lally et al. 1996). *A.a.* strains exhibit a wide range of variability in leukotoxin production. High leukotoxin-producing strains have been linked to the etiology of AgP. A substantially higher prevalence of highly leukotoxic strains has been reported in patients

with LAP than in chronic periodontitis patients or healthy subjects (Zambon et al. 1996).

All Gram-negative bacteria are enveloped by two membranes, of which the outer is rich in endotoxin. This identifying feature of Gram-negative bacteria consists of a lipid and a polysaccharide part and is therefore frequently termed lipopolysaccharide (LPS). LPS is set free when bacterial cells die or multiply. The LPS of *A.a.* can activate host cells, and macrophages in particular, to secrete inflammatory mediators such as prostaglandins, interleukin-1β and tumor necrosis factor-α. It is also highly immunogenic, since high titers of antibodies against its antigenic determinant are frequently detected in infected individuals.

A bacteriocin of *A.a.*, capable of inhibiting the growth of some streptococci and some actinomyces, has furthermore been detected (Hammond et al. 1987). Additional virulence factors interfering with fibroblast proliferation have been described for certain strains of *A.a.* Furthermore, immunosuppressive properties of *A.a.*, as well as collagenolytic activity and inhibition of neutrophil chemotaxis, have been demonstrated (for review see Fives-Taylor et al. 1996).

Secretion of membrane vesicles by *A.a.* has been observed. These vesicles may be important virulence factors since they may contain leukotoxin, endotoxin and other factors and may serve as a transport vehicle to spread pathogenic substances produced by the bacterium.

A.a., Capnocytophaga sputigena and *Prevotella intermedia* have also been shown to be the most prominent members of the subgingival microbiota of periodontitis lesions in the primary dentition. The microbial patterns observed in periodontal lesions of the primary dentition, however, seem to be more complex than the ones detected in LAP patients.

Generalized aggressive periodontitis (GAP), formerly named generalized early onset periodontitis (G-EOP) and rapidly progressive periodontitis (RPP), have been frequently associated with the detection of *Porphyromonas gingivalis, Bacteroides forsythus* and *A.a.* In contrast to *A.a.*, which is facultatively anaerobic, *P. gingivalis* and *B. forsythus* are fastidious strict anaerobes. *P. gingivalis* produces several potent enzymes, in

Table 9-3. Host defense mechanisms in the gingival sulcus

Intact epithelial barrier and epithelial attachment
Salivary flushing action, agglutinins, antibodies
Sulcular fluid flushing action, opsonins, antibodies, complement and other plasma components
Local antibody production
High levels of tissue turnover
Presence of normal flora or beneficial species
Emigrating PMNs and other leukocytes

Modified from Page (1990).

particular collagenases and proteases, endotoxin, fatty acids and other possibly toxic agents (Shah 1993). A relationship between the clinical outcome of therapy and bacterial counts has also been documented for *P. gingivalis*, and non-responding lesions often contain this organism in elevated proportions. High local and systemic immune responses against this bacterium have been demonstrated in patients with GAP (Tolo & Schenck 1985, Vincent et al. 1985, Ebersole et al. 1986, Murray et al. 1989).

Bacterial damage to the periodontium

Disease-associated bacteria are thought to cause destruction of the marginal periodontium via two related mechanisms: (1) the direct action of the microorganisms or their products on the host tissues, and/or (2) as a result of their eliciting tissue-damaging inflammatory responses (see Chapter 5 and Tonetti 1993). The relative importance of these two mechanisms in AgP remains speculative. Human investigations have indicated that *Actinobacillus actinomycetemcomitans* is able to translocate across the junctional epithelium and invade the underlying connective tissue (Saglie et al. 1988). These data support the hypothesis that direct bacterial invasion may be responsible for some of the observed tissue breakdown. Data from chronic periodontitis, however, seem to indicate that two-thirds of attachment loss and alveolar bone resorption is preventable through the action of non-steroidal anti-inflammatory drugs, and therefore tissue destruction seems to be driven by the inflammatory process (Williams et al. 1985, 1989). Apical spread of bacteria loosely adhering to the hard, non-shedding surface of the tooth is thought to be controlled through a first line of defense consisting of mechanisms such as the high turnover of junctional epithelium keratinocytes, the outward flow of crevicular fluid and the directed migration of polymorphonuclear leukocytes through the junctional epithelium; the efficiency of these innate immune mechanisms is highly enhanced by the presence in the gingival fluid of specific antibodies and complement fragments (Page 1990) (Table 9-3).

Host response to bacterial pathogens

Both local and systemic host responses to AgP-associated microflora have been described. Local inflammatory responses have been characterized by an intense recruitment of polymorphonuclear leukocytes both within the tissues and into the periodontal pocket. Such a preponderance of PMNs underlines the importance of these cells in the local defense against bacterial aggression and their potential role in host-mediated tissue destruction. B cells and antibody-producing plasma cells represent a significant component of the mononuclear cell-dominated connective tissue lesion (Liljenberg & Lindhe 1980). Plasma cells have been shown to be predominantly IgG-producing cells, with a lower proportion of IgA-producing cells (Mackler et al. 1977, 1978, Waldrop et al. 1981, Ogawa et al. 1989). Local IgG$_4$-producing cells, in particular, seem to be elevated. Another important component of the local inflammatory infiltrate are T cells. Subset analysis of local T cells has indicated a depressed T-helper to T-suppressor ratio as compared to both healthy gingiva and peripheral blood. These findings have been interpreted to suggest the possibility of altered local immune regulation (Taubman et al. 1988, 1991). Peripheral blood mononuclear cells from AgP patients have been reported to exhibit a reduced autologous mixed lymphocyte reaction, as well as a higher than normal response to B cell mitogens (for review see Engel 1996). Local inflammatory responses are characterized by high levels of prostaglandin E$_2$, interleukin-1α and interleukin-1β in both crevicular fluid and tissue (Masada et al. 1990, Offenbacher et al. 1993). Prostaglandin E$_2$ production, in particular, has been shown to be highly elevated in AgP subjects when compared to periodontally healthy individuals and chronic periodontitis patients.

Specific antibodies against AgP-associated microorganisms (Lally et al. 1980, Steubing et al. 1982, Ebersole et al. 1984, 1985a,b) and cleaved complement fragments (Schenkein & Genco 1977, Patters et al. 1989) have also been detected in crevicular fluid from AgP lesions. Of interest is the evidence indicating that crevicular fluid titers of antibodies against AgP-associated microorganisms are frequently higher than in the serum of the same patient (Ebersole et al. 1984,

(Fig. a)
Localized aggressive periodontitis in siblings of 22 families

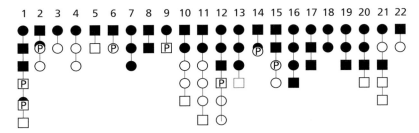

Prevalence of LAP
67% of siblings (> 12 yrs), uncorrected
34% of siblings (> 12 yrs), corrected for proband bias

Key:

○ Female, normal ℗ Pre-pubertal female

□ Male, normal P Pre-pubertal male

● Female, LAP ⓟ Pre-pubertal female, LAP developed during study

■ Male, LAP P Pre-pubertal male, LAP developed during study

(Fig. b)
Neutrophil chemotaxis in LAP families

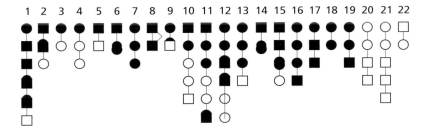

Fig. 9-8. (a) Patients suffering from LAP in 22 families are represented by solid black figures. In each family the proband is on the left. (b) Diagrammatic representation of sibships involved in study group. Numbers are the same as in (a). Solid black figures represent patients exhibiting depressed neutrophil chemotaxis. In this group, after correcting for sampling bias, 40% of subjects present with abnormal chemotaxis. Subjects in sibship 8 are identical twins. From Van Dyke et al. (1985).

1985a,b). This observation, together with substantial *in vitro* and *ex vivo* data, strongly suggests that substantial fractions of these antibodies are locally produced in the inflammatory infiltrate (Steubing et al. 1982, Hall et al. 1990, 1991, 1994). Substantial titers of antibodies against *A.a.* and *P. gingivalis* have also been detected in the serum of AgP patients. Furthermore, in some patients, titers of antibodies reactive with *A.a.* have been shown to be as high as the ones against *Treponema pallidum* present in tertiary syphilis (0.1-1 g/ml); this clearly indicates the extent of host response that can be mounted against these periodontal pathogens (for a review see Ebersole 1990, 1996).

Recent investigations have identified the immunodominant *A. actinomycetemcomitans* antigen to be the serotype specific carbohydrate; furthermore, it has been shown that the vast majority of antibodies reactive with this carbohydrate in AgP patients consist of IgG$_2$ (Califano et al. 1992). High titers and high avidity of *A.a.* specific IgG$_2$ have been demonstrated in LAP patients, where high antibody titers are thought to be associated with the host's ability to localize attach-

ment loss to few teeth; conversely, GAP patients are frequently seronegative for *A.a.* or display low titers and avidity. Anti *A.a.* serotype polysaccharide IgG$_2$, therefore, are considered to be protective against widespread AgP (Tew et al. 1996).

Of importance are findings reporting antibody response to *P. gingivalis* in GAP forms. Patients suffering from these forms of disease frequently show both low levels of serum antibodies against *P. gingivalis* and low levels of antibody avidity, indicating a specific inability of some GAP patients to effectively cope with these bacteria. Importantly, however, both titers and avidity of antibodies reacting with *P. gingivalis* can be improved as a result of therapy.

Another important aspect of host response towards AgP microorganisms has been the recognition that polymorphonuclear leukocytes (PMN) of some LAP and GAP patients present decreased migration and antibacterial functions (Genco et al. 1980, 1986, Van Dyke et al. 1982, 1986, 1988). These abnormalities are frequently minor in the sense that they are usually not associated with infections other than periodontitis. A

Major gene locus: AgP susceptibility gene **(Fig. a)**

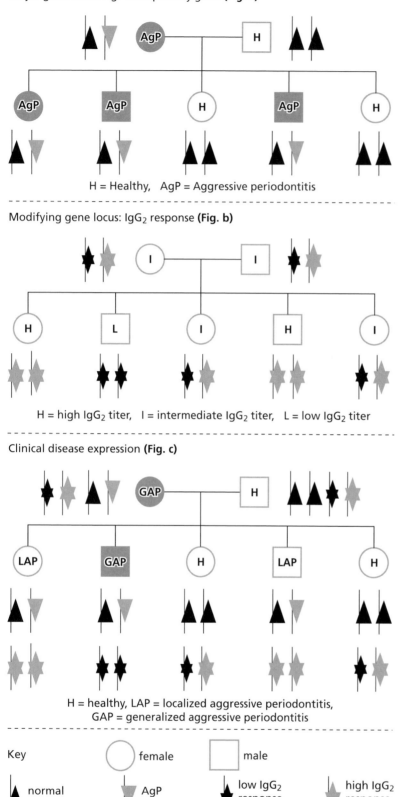

H = Healthy,   AgP = Aggressive periodontitis

Modifying gene locus: IgG$_2$ response **(Fig. b)**

H = high IgG$_2$ titer,   I = intermediate IgG$_2$ titer,   L = low IgG$_2$ titer

Clinical disease expression **(Fig. c)**

H = healthy, LAP = localized aggressive periodontitis,
GAP = generalized aggressive periodontitis

Key   ◯ female   □ male

▲ normal
allele

▽ AgP
allele

✦ low IgG$_2$
response
allele

✦ high IgG$_2$
response
allele

Fig. 9-9. (a) Genetic predisposition to AgP is determined by a single gene of major effect, inherited as an autosomal dominant trait. (b) Modifying genes may control immune responses that determine the clinical extent and severity of periodontal destruction in AgP. Here an allele controlling IgG$_2$ levels is inherited as a codominant trait. (c) Independent inheritance of major locus and modifying locus illustrating how LAP and GAP may segregate within the same family. The propensity to develop AgP is dependent upon inheritance of a major susceptibility gene. The clinical phenotype is dependent upon host ability to produce IgG$_2$ in response to periodontopathic bacteria. High IgG$_2$ titers limit disease extension. Intermediate and low IgG$_2$ titers are less effective in limiting intermediate disease progression. From Schenkein (1994), as modified by Hart (1996).

key report has indicated that PMN abnormalities in LAP patients seem to cluster in families much in the same way as AgP does (Van Dyke et al. 1985) (Fig. 9-8). This evidence has been interpreted as a suggestion that the LAP-associated PMN defect may be inherited. Other recent reports have indicated that PMN abnor-malities in LAP patients may be, at least in part, the result of a hyper-inflammatory state resulting in the presence of pro-inflammatory cytokines in the serum of some AgP patients (Shapira et al. 1994, Agarwal et al. 1996).

Genetic aspects of host susceptibility

Several family studies have indicated that the prevalence of AgP is disproportionately high among certain families, where the percentage of affected siblings may reach 40-50% (Saxen & Nevanlinna 1984, Beaty et al. 1987, Long et al. 1987, Boughman et al. 1992, Marazita et al. 1994). Such a dramatic familial aggregation of cases indicates that genetic factors may be important in susceptibility to AgP. Genetic studies in these families suggest that the pattern of disease transmission is consistent with mendelian inheritance of a gene of major effect (Saxen & Nevanlinna 1984, Beaty et al. 1987, Boughman et al. 1992, Hart et al. 1992, Marazita et al. 1994). This means that the observed familial pattern can be partly accounted for by one or more genes that could predispose individuals to de-

velop AgP. Segregation analyses have indicated that the likely mode of inheritance is autosomal dominant (Saxen & Nevanlinna 1984, Beaty et al. 1987, Hart et al. 1992, Marazita et al. 1994; Fig. 9-9a). Most of these investigations, however, were carried out in African-American populations; it is therefore possible that other modes of inheritance may exist in different populations. Segregation analysis can provide information about the mode of inheritance of a genetic trait but does not provide information about the specific gene(s) involved. The chromosomal location of a gene of major effect for a trait such as AgP susceptibility can be determined by linkage analysis. An investigation utilizing this methodology reported linkage of LAP to the vitamin D binding locus on region q of chromosome 4 in a large family of the Brandywine population (Boughman et al. 1986). These results, however, were

Table 9-4. Genes known to affect human PMN function or host response to LPS load and/or thought to be among the candidate genes of major effect in EOP susceptibility

Condition	OMIM*	Trans-mission	Chromo-some location	Comments
Bactericidal permeability increasing protein (BPIP)	109195	AD	20q11-12	BPIP is associated with PMN granules and is bactericidal to Gram organisms. It binds to LPS with high affinity. BPIP is 45% homologous to LPS binding protein.
Lipopolysaccharide binding protein (LBP)	151990	AD	20q11-12	Produced during acute phase of infection: binds to LPS and functions as a carrier for LPS; functions in monocyte response.
Monocyte differentiation antigen (CD14)	158126	AD	5q31	Receptor for LBP-LPS complex.
Prostaglandin synthase 2 (PTGS2)	600262	AR	1q25.2-3	Major role in regulation of prostaglandin synthesis. Dramatic induction of PTGS2 mRNA occurs in normal peripheral blood leukocytes in response to LPS.
PMN actin dysfunction (NAD)	257150	AR	?	Carriers (heterozygotes) have a 50% decrease in actin filament assembly; affected individuals (homozygotes) have recurrent bacterial infections. PMN severely defective in migration and particle ingestion; basic defect due to failure of PMN actin polymerization.
Myeloperoxidase deficiency (MPO)	254600	AR	17q12-21	Absence of MPO. MPO is a dimeric protein that catalyzes the production of oxidating agents with microbicidal activity against a wide range of microbes. Several variants have been described.
IgE elevation with PMN chemotaxis defect	147060	AD	?	Impaired lymphocyte response to Candida antigen; recurrent bacterial infections.
Fc receptor gamma IIA polymorphism (FCGR2A)	146790	AD	1q21-q23	Allelic variants of the Fc-gamma receptor 2A confer distinct phagocytic capacities providing a possible mechanism for hereditary susceptibility to infection. The H131 allele is the only FGR2A that recognizes IgG_2 efficiently, and optimal IgG_2 handling occurs only in the homozygous state for H131. The allelic variant R131 has low binding of IgG_2.
Immunoglobulin G2m allotypes	N/A	?	N/A	Specific allotypes associated with IgG_2 response to specific bacterial antigens. Subjects lacking specific allotypes may be selectively unable to mount efficient antibody response against specific antigens.

* Online Mendelian Inheritance in Man (OMIM). Modified from Hart (1996).

Table 9-5. Effect of smoking on extent and severity of GAP

	Smoking status	Mean % of sites with PAL ≥ 5 mm *	Mean PAL (mm) *
GAP	Smokers	49.0 ± 3.9	2.78 ± 0.2
	Non-smokers	36.8 ± 3.8	2.14 ± 0.2

* Values adjusted for age and mean plaque index, subject as unit of analysis. Smokers showed significantly greater extent and severity of periodontal disease than non-smokers after correcting for age and oral hygiene level.

Modified from Schenkein et al. (1995).

not confirmed in a subsequent study utilizing a different population (Hart et al. 1993). Such data are currently considered to support the existence of genetic heterogeneity in LAP forms, and of distinct forms of AgP. Therefore, it is currently maintained that although formal genetic studies of AgP support the existence of a gene of major effect, it is unlikely that all forms of AgP are due to the same genetic defect (Hart 1996). This notion is consistent with the fact that numerous diseases and syndromes with similar clinical appearance are known to result from different genetic polymorphisms. Based on current knowledge that AgP subjects present high prevalence of PMN function defects, and that they have been shown to produce high levels of inflammatory mediators in response to LPS stimulation, several loci have been proposed as genes conferring increased susceptibility to AgP. These genes are associated with neutrophil function and with the host ability to effectively deal with LPS exposure, and are listed in Table 9-4 (for review see Hart 1996).

Besides genes of major effect that may determine susceptibility to AgP, other genes may act as modifying genes and influence clinical expression of the disease. In this respect, particular interest has been focused on the impact of genetic control on antibody responses against specific AgP associated bacteria and against A.a. in particular. These studies have indicated that the ability to mount high titers of specific antibodies is race-dependent and probably protective (Gunsolley et al. 1987, 1988). This has been shown to be under genetic control as a co-dominant trait, independent of the risk for AgP. In individuals susceptible to AgP, therefore, the ability to mount high titers of antibodies (IgG_2 in particular) may be protective and prevent extension of disease to a generalized form (Schenkein 1994, Fig. 9-9b,c). Allelic variations in the Fc receptor for IgG_2 immunoglobulins have also been suggested to play a role in suboptimal handling of A.a. infections. PMN expressing the R131 allotype of FcγRIIa (i.e. an Fc receptor containing an arginine instead of a histidine at aminoacid 131) show decreased phagocytosis of A.a. (Wilson & Kalmar 1996).

Environmental aspects of host susceptibility

Recent evidence has indicated that, besides genetic influences, environmental factors may affect the clinical expression of AgP. In a large study, cigarette smoking was shown to be a risk factor for patients with generalized forms of AgP (Schenkein et al. 1995). Smokers with GAP had more affected teeth and greater mean levels of attachment loss than patients with GAP who did not smoke (Table 9-5). Environmental exposure to cigarette smoking, therefore, seems to add significant risk of more severe and prevalent disease to this group of already highly susceptible subjects. The mechanism(s) for this observation are not completely understood, but findings from the same group indicate that IgG_2 serum levels as well as antibody levels against A.a. are significantly depressed in subjects with GAP who smoked. Since these antibodies are considered to represent a protective response against A.a., it is possible that depression of IgG_2 in smokers may be associated with the observed increase in disease extent and severity in these subjects.

Current concepts

Aggressive forms of periodontitis are currently considered to be multifactorial diseases developing as a result of complex interactions between specific host genes and the environment. Inheritance of AgP susceptibility is probably insufficient for the development of disease: environmental exposure to potential pathogens endowed with specific virulence factors is also a necessary step. Host inability to effectively deal with the bacterial aggression and to avoid inflammatory tissue damage results in the initiation of the disease process. Interactions between the disease process and environmental (e.g. cigarette smoking) and genetically controlled (e.g. IgG_2 response to A.a.) modifying factors are thought to contribute to determining the specific clinical manifestation of disease (Figs. 9-9a-c and 9-10).

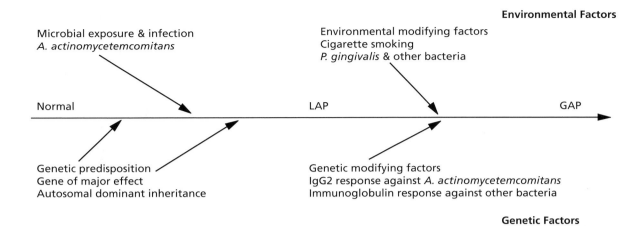

Fig. 9-10. Diagrammatic representation of the current understanding of the eco-genetic interactions leading to development of LAP and GAP in African-American populations. (See text for explanation.)

DIAGNOSIS

Clinical diagnosis

Clinical diagnosis is based on information derived from a specific medical and dental history and from the clinical examination of the periodontium. Limitations that will be discussed in this section, however, frequently require supplementation of clinical and anamnestic parameters with other, more advanced aids to properly diagnose, treatment plan and monitor these diseases. The purpose of clinical diagnosis is the identification of patients suffering from AgP and of factors that have an impact on how the case should be treated and monitored.

In the diagnosis of AgP the initial question that the clinician should ask is:

• Is there periodontitis?

This may sound like a trivial question, but in fact many cases of AgP are currently not identified because of a failure to detect signs of periodontitis. Conversely, some clinicians attribute to periodontitis pathological changes associated with other unrelated and sometimes self-limiting processes. Correctly answering this question requires systematic collection of clinical information regarding the following items:

• Is there loss of periodontal support (loss of clinical attachment and marginal resorption of alveolar bone)?
• Is the loss of attachment accompanied by pocket formation or mostly the result of recession?
• Is there a plausible cause for attachment loss other than periodontitis?
• Is there another process imitating periodontal disease by pseudopocket formation?

From a clinical standpoint, it is important to realize that clinically detectable loss of attachment may occur as a result of pathological events other than periodontitis. Examples are traumatic injuries, removal or presence of impacted teeth (Kugelberg 1992), tooth position, orthodontic tooth movement, advanced decay, subgingival margins of restorations, etc. This means that the clinician must recognize different causes for attachment loss and must rule out other causes of attachment loss by a combination of careful clinical examination and assessment of the dental history. Orthodontic considerations are necessary to evaluate attachment loss without pocket formation (recession). In such instances the appropriate clinical diagnosis may be the following.

Incidental attachment loss

After establishing the presence of periodontitis, the clinician should determine which clinical diagnosis best describes the disease in the individual patient: chronic, aggressive or necrotizing periodontitis. Since the current classification is based on the combination of clinical presentation, rate of disease progression, and pattern of familial aggregation of cases in the absence of a systemic cause for the clinical observations, the next questions should address these parameters:

• Does the patient have a systemic condition that would in itself explain the presence of periodontitis?

As indicated, the diagnosis of chronic, aggressive or necrotizing periodontitis implies presence of periodontal destruction in the absence of systemic diseases that may severely impair host defense. A well-constructed and well-taken medical history is fundamental for identifying the presence of systemic involvements accompanied with periodontitis (see Chapter 2). Careful questioning regarding recurrent infections, their familiarity, presence of severe diseases or their symptoms and signs should be part of the evaluation of all periodontal patients. Consultation with the attending physician and evaluation of laboratory parameters are frequently necessary. Understanding of the medical condition that may be associated with periodontitis is fundamental. Some conditions are relatively frequent disorders such as poorly-controlled diabetes mellitus; others are rare inherited disorders such as the palmo-plantar keratosis (Papillon-Lefèvre and Heim-Munk syndromes) or hypophosphatasia. Some are inborn defects such as the leukocyte adhesion deficiencies (LAD); others are acquired following exposure to pharmacological agents such as drug-induced granulocytopenia. Positive confirmed history of a significant systemic condition results in the diagnosis of the following.

Periodontal manifestation of systemic disease

In such instances, the periodontitis is likely to represent an oral manifestation of the systemic diseases. Examples of significant conditions are AIDS, leukemia, neutropenia, diabetes or rare genetic diseases such as histiocytosis X, the Papillon-Lefèvre syndrome or the Chediak-Steinbrinck-Higashi syndrome (see Chapter 5 and Fig. 9-4).

In the absence of significant systemic components, the next questions relate to the exclusion of the rare but clearly identified necrotizing/ulcerative forms. The question will then be:

• Does the patient have signs or symptoms of necrotizing periodontitis?

If the answer to both of the previous questions is negative, differential diagnosis between chronic or aggressive periodontitis will be required. In this respect it is important to observe that chronic periodontitis has been defined as the common form of periodontitis whose diagnosis is done by excluding the presence of aggressive periodontitis (Armitage 1999). Diagnosis of AgP is made by verification of the satisfaction by the individual cases of the primary and secondary features described in the international classification workshop (see discussion above).

In this respect it must be recognized that the features include both clinical and laboratory aspects. In the diagnosis of a case, clinical and history parameters are initially utilized to suspect the presence of AgP, while laboratory tests are frequently utilized to confirm the diagnosis. In this respect, it is important to realize that periodontal diagnosis based only on periodontal probing and dental radiography does not classify causes; rather, it describes destruction patterns.

A tentative clinical diagnosis of AgP is made based on the following criteria:

• Absence of significant systemic conditions
• Rapid attachment loss and bone destruction
• Familial aggregation of cases

• Lack of consistency between clinically visible bacterial deposits and severity of periodontal breakdown.

A rapid rate of destruction of the periodontium is a major criterion for the diagnosis of AgP. It is aimed at identifying subjects characterized by high virulence of the microflora and/or high levels of susceptibility. Although correct application of this criterion requires availability of clinical or radiographic data from more than one time point, presence of severe destruction in relation to the age of the subject is frequently considered to be sufficient information to infer rapid progression.

Establishing the presence of familial aggregation of cases is based on a combination of history and clinical examination of family members of the affected individual. At this stage there is inadequate evidence to establish the best approach to obtain a significant estimation of familial aggregation.

It is maintained that in the majority of AgP cases the amount of periodontal destruction seems to be higher than that expected from the mere accumulation of local factors. This observation, however, may not be true for all cases. In general, a discrepancy between local factors and the amount of periodontal tissue breakdown is considered to be an indication for either infection with particularly virulent microorganisms, or presence of a highly susceptible host. This information may be consequential in determining surgical goals of therapy, the impact of antibiotics, and the possible impact of sub-optimal hygiene as a risk factor for disease recurrence.

The international classification workshop consensus indicated that not all listed primary and secondary features need to be present in order to assign an AgP diagnosis and that the diagnosis may be based on clinical, radiographic and historical data alone. It also indicated that laboratory testing, although helpful, might not be essential in making an AgP diagnosis.

Once an AgP diagnosis has been made based on the criteria above, differential diagnosis between LAP and GAP needs to be made. In this respect specific clinical features have been suggested. A diagnosis of localized aggressive periodontitis (LAP) is made based on evidence of circumpubertal onset and localized first molar/incisor presentation with interproximal attachment loss on at least two permanent teeth, one of which is a first molar, and involving no more than two teeth other than first molars and incisors. A diagnosis of generalized aggressive periodontitis (GAP) takes into account the fact that this form of disease usually affects persons under 30 years of age (but patients may be older) and that it presents with generalized interproximal attachment loss affecting at least three permanent teeth other than first molars and incisors. Furthermore this pathology is characterized by a pronounced episodic nature of the destruction of attachment and alveolar bone. The differential diagnosis may benefit from additional laboratory investigations of the individual host response to the infecting organisms.

In order to properly describe the specific AgP case, modifying factors should also be explored by addressing the question of the presence of modifying or contributory factors such as smoking or drug abuse. Such additional information is relevant since these factors may explain a specific presentation of disease in terms of its extent and severity. Furthermore, these factors, unlike genetic factors, are amenable to modification through appropriate intervention. Therapy should therefore include an approach aimed at controling the impact of these factors.

Even though differential diagnosis between AgP and chronic periodontitis and differentiation between LAP and GAP is mostly based on history and clinical presentation, it must be emphasized that clinical parameters alone cannot further discriminate between forms of disease with similar clinical appearance. Inferences regarding a specific etiology are speculative under such circumstances and require further laboratory testing for confirmation.

In the previous classification system, age of onset or age at diagnosis was considered helpful to further characterize specific clinical syndromes. LAP, in particular, is thought to occur in adolescents 13-14 years old to 25 years, while GAP is generally found in adolescents or young adults of less than 30-35 years. It should be realized, however, that (1) some cases may present initial LAP at an earlier age, (2) LAP may start before puberty and affect the primary dentition, (3) patterns of periodontal destruction compatible with LAP may be initially detected at an age older than 25, and (4) there may be a tendency toward spreading from a localized to a generalized pattern of AgP in older subjects of these groups.

Another difficulty is related to the fact that periodontal destruction is often diagnosed when the attachment loss is already fairly advanced. In general, distinct alterations in the morphology of the periodontium and substantial tissue damage are necessary for establishing a clear diagnosis. Milder or initial stages of disease or sites at risk for future periodontal breakdown cannot be detected based on clinical parameters. This makes it difficult to intercept and treat initial forms of AgP. Furthermore, such difficulty makes it extremely important to examine the other members of the family of the proband as well: siblings may present with clinically undetectable disease in spite of the presence of the putative pathogens. A common strategy employed to overcome the insufficient ability of clinical parameters to detect early disease is to closely monitor high-risk patients such as the siblings of the probands. It is in this respect important to underline that "incidental attachment loss" may, in some cases, represent an initial manifestation of AgP. In such a case an isolated periodontal lesion characterized by attachment loss with pocketing may represent the only clinically evident AgP lesion. Such subjects should, therefore, be considered at high risk for the development of AgP and require close monitoring and possibly further microbiological diagnosis.

Microbiologic diagnosis

The international classification workshop indicated that the presence of specific microorganisms and *A.a.* in particular represent one of the secondary features of AgP. As such, microbiological diagnosis may be a useful laboratory addition to establish a differential diagnosis between aggressive and chronic forms of periodontitis.

Clinical studies have also indicated that successful treatment of LAP depends on the elimination of the bacterium *A.a.*, and that the elimination of this microorganism with conventional periodontal procedures is difficult. In the case of generalized forms of AgP it is important to know whether the specific condition is associated with *A.a.*, with other periodontal pathogens such as *P. gingivalis*, or a combination of several pathogenic microorganisms. This information has an impact on the need to supplement conventional therapy with antibiotics and on the choice of the antimicrobial drug (see Chapter 23).

Microbiologic diagnosis can be useful at different stages of the treatment plan, i.e. as a part of the initial diagnosis, at re-evaluation or during the recall phase. The need for microbiological information before therapy depends on the general strategy for treatment. Many clinicians prefer to remove bacterial deposits mechanically in a first treatment phase without the adjunctive use of systemic antibiotics. As microbiologic findings have no influence on the way this initial treatment is performed, microbiologic testing may be postponed until the first phase is completed. One should keep in mind, however, that the reduction in bacterial load might increase the possibility of false negative results when an insensitive microbiological test is used. If the specific clinical diagnosis is LAP, then the clinician can assume even without a microbiological test that the treatment should be directed towards a maximal suppression of *A.a.* This is due to the fact that the great majority of LAP patients are infected with this organism. This is different for all other forms of AgP, where such a close association of one microbial species with the disease cannot be assumed, and therefore microbial testing should be performed.

Since *A.a.* and *P. gingivalis* can be transmitted from periodontal patients to family members, microbial testing of spouses, children or siblings of AgP patients may be indicated to intercept early disease in susceptible individuals.

Evaluation of host defenses

Several forms of AgP have been associated with impairment of host defenses. Classic studies have indicated that in some populations both LAP and GAP forms are associated with high incidence of phagocyte

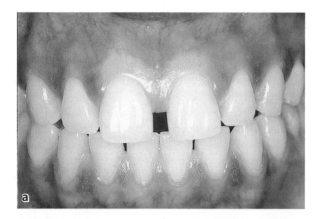

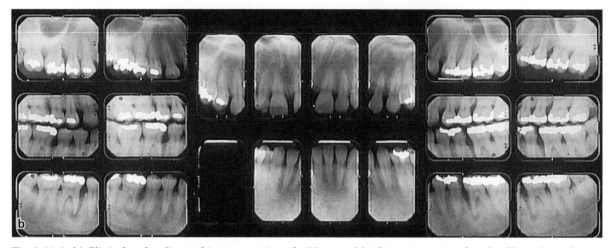

Fig. 9-11. (a-b) Clinical and radiographic presentation of a 22-year-old African-American female. Clinical attachment loss and alveolar bone loss are localized on the mesial aspect of the first molars, where deep, vertical defects are apparent. (c-e) Detailed views of the defect on the mesial aspect of 26. No other tooth appears to be affected. Microbiology (DNA probe analysis of *A. actinomycetemcomitans*, *P. gingivalis* and *P. intermedia*) confirmed the presence of high levels (> 10^4 bacteria/sample) of *A. actinomycetemcomitans* in all four deep lesions. *P. intermedia* was also detectable in three of four sites, while *P. gingivalis* was undetectable. The patient did not display abnormal leukocyte functions; furthermore, she had a non-contributory medical history, and did not smoke. She had a younger brother (15 years old) and an older sister (27 years old); on clinical examination, the periodontium of both of them appeared to be within normal limits. The following diagnosis was made: "LAP in a 22-year-old systemically healthy African-American female; associated with *A. actinomycetemcomitans* infection without clinically detectable levels of *P. gingivalis*; absence of demonstrable leukocyte defects; no known contributory factors; no cigarette smoking; no siblings displaying clinically detectable AgP".

functional disturbances such as depressed neutrophil chemotaxis and other phagocyte antibacterial dysfunctions. In many of these patients, AgP was the only infection that was associated with the reduced phagocyte function(s); this observation is important in two respects. First, AgP-associated phagocyte defects are frequently insignificant in terms of increasing susceptibility to infections other than periodontitis. Furthermore, it is likely that such "mild" leukocyte defects may go unnoticed until laboratory testing is performed in conjunction with periodontal diagnosis. Reports of such phagocyte defects relate mostly to AgP subjects from African-American groups; systematic evaluations of PMN and monocyte functions associated with clinical diagnosis of AgP in European Caucasians failed to confirm a high prevalence of abnormalities (Kinane et al. 1989a,b). Testing for these host-defense parameters, therefore, may be more re-

stricted to specific populations. Another important aspect is that, so far, no specific study has attempted to associate treatment response or incidence of recurrent disease with the presence of the above-mentioned abnormalities.

More recent investigations have indicated that specific patterns of host response to bacterial pathogens are associated with different forms of AgP; this early evidence may be extremely helpful for the development of clinically useful tests to estimate the risk of developing AgP. In this respect two findings deserve to be mentioned:

1. AgP patients present significantly higher levels of crevicular fluid prostaglandin E_2 than chronic periodontitis patients or healthy subjects. This finding may indicate that monocytes from these patients respond to bacterial and inflammatory stim-

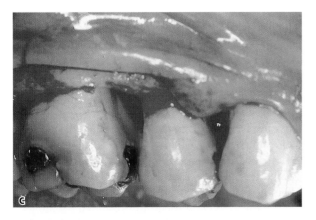

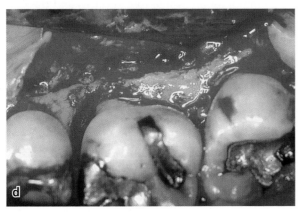

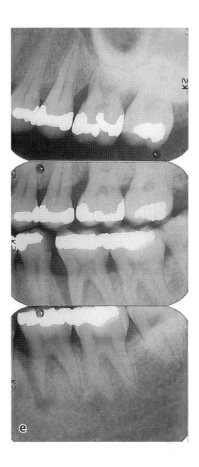

Fig. 9-11. (c-e).

uli with very high levels of local release of inflammatory mediators. These may induce an exuberant inflammatory reaction associated with high levels of activation of tissue-degrading matrix-metalloproteinases.

2. GAP patients have a decreased ability to mount high titers of specific IgG_2 antibodies to *A.a.* These subjects exhibit a tendency towards progressive periodontal destruction leading to tooth loss over a relatively short period of time. LAP patients, on the other hand, seem to have better prognosis and do not express this trait. Since there are indications that at least some LAP cases may progress into generalized forms, early detection of patients infected with *A.a.* but producing low levels of specific antibodies may allow early identification of a high-risk group for development of GAP. Serum antibody titers (IgG_2 in particular) and/or avidity to *A.a.* may be particularly useful in the differential diagnosis of GAP and LAP syndromes and in the early detection of the LAP cases with high risk for progression into the more widespread forms of disease.

Genetic diagnosis

Given the disproportionately high incidence of AgP in the families of affected individuals, evaluation of siblings of the proband and other family members is a requirement. Clinical determination of different dis-

ease forms in the family should be followed by construction of a pedigree of the AgP trait. Such diagnosis may bring considerable information regarding the level of risk eventually shared within the family. Furthermore, it helps to establish the need for monitoring clinically unaffected individuals.

All the evidence gathered during the diagnostic process should contribute to the definition of a specific diagnosis. An example of such diagnosis is illustrated in Fig. 9-11: LAP in a 22-year-old systemically healthy African-American female patient, associated with *A.a.* infection without detectable levels of *P. gingivalis*, inconsistency between local factors and amount of clinically detectable breakdown, absence of demonstrable leukocyte defects, no known contributory factors, and no siblings displaying clinically detectable periodontitis.

PRINCIPLES OF THERAPEUTIC INTERVENTION

Treatment of AgP should only be initiated after completion of a careful diagnosis by a specifically trained periodontist. The severity of some of the AgP forms suggests that specialists, possibly working in association with highly specialized centers, could best perform both diagnosis and treatment of these rare forms of periodontitis. The roles of the general practitioner, the pedodontist or the orthodontist, however, are fundamental in the detection of possible cases to be referred for further evaluation and therapy.

Successful treatment of AgP is considered to be dependent on early diagnosis, directing therapy towards elimination or suppression of the infecting microorganisms and providing an environment conducive to long-term maintenance. The differential element of treatment of AgP, however, relates to specific efforts to affect the composition and not only the quantity of the subgingival microbiota.

Elimination or suppression of the pathogenic flora

A.a. elimination has been associated with successful therapy; conversely, recurrent lesions have been shown to still harbor this organism. Several investigators have reported that scaling and root planing of juvenile periodontitis lesions could not predictably suppress *A.a.* below detection levels (Slots & Rosling 1983, Christersson et al. 1985, Kornman & Robertson 1985). Soft tissue curettage and access flap therapy also had limited success in eliminating *A.a.* (Christersson et al. 1985).

A.a. is also difficult to eliminate by conventional mechanical therapy in adult periodontitis patients, and it is therefore not surprising to observe the presence of this microorganism in the subgingival microflora of many non-responding periodontitis patients (Bragd et al. 1985, van Winkelhoff et al. 1989, Renvert et al. 1990a,b, Rodenburg et al. 1990, Mombelli et al. 1994). Similar, but less systematic observations have also been reported for the ability to suppress the microflora associated with some GAP forms, where high subgingival loads of *P. gingivalis, B. forsythus, A.a.* and other highly virulent bacteria are frequently detected.

Use of antibiotics has been suggested as a rational complement to mechanical debridement in these cases. Regimens including the adjunctive administration of tetracyclines or metronidazole, have been tested for the treatment of LAP and other forms of AgP (see Chapter 23). The choice of the antibiotic should be guided by information about the nature of the involved pathogenic microorganism(s). Metronidazole in combination with amoxicillin may suppress *A.a.* more effectively than single antibiotic regimes.

Substantial evidence indicates that subgingival *A.a.* can be eliminated or suppressed for a prolonged period by mechanical debridement supplemented with systemic metronidazole plus amoxicillin. Systemic antibiotics should only be administered as an adjunct to mechanical debridement because in undisturbed subgingival plaque the target organisms are effectively protected from the antibiotic agent due to the biofilm effect (see Chapter 23).

To incorporate antibiotics in the treatment of AgP a staged approach to the initial therapy is recommended. Treatment is started with an initial phase of mechanical therapy, including systematic scaling and planing of all accessible root surfaces and the introduction of meticulous oral hygiene. After a period of 4-6 weeks, the case is re-assessed clinically. Based on persistence of periodontal lesions, a second phase of therapy is planned. Decisions are made as to how to gain access to deep lesions with appropriate surgical procedures and concerning the administration of antimicrobial agents. Microbial samples from the deepest pocket in each quadrant provide proper information about the presence and relative importance of putative pathogens. Systemic antimicrobial therapy with the appropriate agent is usually initiated immediately upon completion of the surgical interventions or immediatedly after another round of mechanical instrumentation to ensure that subgingival plaque deposits have been reduced as much as possible and to disrupt the subgingival biofilm.

Microbiology testing may be repeated at 1-3 months after completion of therapy to verify the elimination or marked suppression of the putative pathogen(s). After resolution of the periodontal infection, the patient should be placed on an individually tailored maintenance care program including continuous evaluation of the occurrence and of the risk of disease progression. Optimal plaque control by the patient is of paramount importance for a favorable clinical and microbiologic response to therapy. Recurrence of disease is an indication for a repetition of microbiologic tests, for re-evaluation of the host immune response and re-assessment of the local and systemic modifying factors. Further therapy should be targeted against putative periodontal pathogens and should take into account the systemic immune responses of the subject.

References

Aass, A., Preus, H. & Gjermo, P. (1992). Association between detection of Oral Actinobacillus actinomycetemcomitans and radiographic bone loss in teenagers. *Journal of Periodontology* **63**, 682-685.

Aass, A., Tollefsen, T. & Gjermo, P. (1994). A cohort study of radiographic alveolar bone loss during adolescence. *Journal of Clinical Periodontology* **21**, 133-138.

Agarwal, S., Huang, J.P., Piesco, N., Suzuki, J.B. Riccelli, A.E. &

Johns, L.P. (1996). Altered neutrophil function in localized juvenile periodontitis: intrinsic or induced? *Journal of Periodontology* **67**, 337-344.

Ainamo, J., Barmes, D., Beagrie, B., Cutress, T., Martin, J. & Sardo-Infirri, J. (1982). Development of the World Health Organization (WHO) Community Periodontal Index of Treatment Needs (CPITN). *International Dental Journal* **32**, 281-291.

Al-Yahfoufi, Z., Mombelli, A., Wicki, A. & Lang, N.P. (1994). The occurrence of *Actinobacillus actinomycetemcomitans, Porphyromonas gingivalis* and *Prevotella intermedia* in an Arabic population with minimal periodontal disease. *Microbial Ecology in Health and Disease* **7**, 217-224.

Albandar, J., Olsen, I. & Gjermo, P. (1990). Associations between six DNA probe-detected periodontal bacteria and alveolar bone loss and other clinical signs of periodontitis. *Acta Odontologica Scandinavica* **48**, 415-423.

Albandar, J., Baghdady, V. & Ghose, L. (1991a). Periodontal disease progression in teenagers with no preventive dental care provisions. *Journal of Clinical Periodontology* **18**, 300-304.

Albandar, J.M., Buischi, Y.A. & Barbosa, M.F. (1991b). Destructive forms of periodontal disease in adolescents. A 3-year longitudinal study. *Journal of Periodontology* **62**, 370-376.

Albandar, J. M. (1993). Juvenile periodontitis – pattern of progression and relationship to clinical periodontal parameters. *Journal of Clinical Periodontology* **21**, 185-189.

Altman, L.C., Page, R.C. & Ebersole, J.L. (1982). Assessment of host defenses and serum antibodies to suspected periodontal pathogens in patients with various types of periodontitis. *Journal of Periodontal Research* **17**, 495-497.

American Academy of Periodontology (1996). Position Paper: Periodontal disease in children and adolescents. *Journal of Periodontology* **67**, 57-62.

American Academy of Periodontology & American Dental Association (1992). Periodontal screening and recording: an early detection system.

Armitage, G. (1999). Development of a classification system for periodontal diseases and conditions. *Annals of Periodontology* **4**, 1-6.

Ashley, F.P., Gallagher, J. & Wilson, R.F. (1988). The occurrence of *Actinobacillus actinomycetemcomitans, Bacteroides gingivalis, Bacteroides intermedius* and spirochaetes in the subgingival microflora of adolescents and their relationship with the amount of supragingival plaque and gingivitis. *Oral Microbiology and Immunology* **3**, 77-82.

Asikainen, S. (1986). Occurrence of *Actinobacillus actinomycetemcomitans* and spirochetes in relation to age in localized juvenile periodontitis. *Journal of Periodontology* **57**, 537-541.

Asikainen, S., Lai, C-H., Alaluusua, S. & Slots, J. (1991). Distribution of *Actinobacillus actinomycetemcomitans* serotypes in periodontal health and disease. *Oral Microbiology and Immunology* **6**, 115-118.

Attström, R. & Van der Velden, U. (1993). Summary of session 1. In: Lang, N. & Karring, T., eds. *Proceedings of the 1st European Workshop in Periodontology*. Berlin: Quintessence, pp. 120-126.

Baer, P. (1971). The case of periodontosis as a clinical entity. *Journal of Periodontology* **42**, 516-520.

Beaty, T.H., Boughman, J.A., Yang, P., Astemborski, J.A. & Suzuki, J.B. (1987). Genetic analysis of juvenile periodontitis in families ascertained through an affected proband. *American Journal of Human Genetics* **40**, 443-452.

Bimstein, E. & Soskolne, A. (1988). A radiographic study of interproximal alveolar bone crest between the primary molars in children. *ASDC Journal of Dentistry for Children* **55**, 348-350.

Bimstein, E., Treasure, E., Williams, S. & Dever, J. (1994). Alveolar bone loss in 5-year old New Zealand children: its prevalence and relationship to caries prevalence, socio-economic status and ethnic origin. *Journal of Clinical Periodontology* **21**, 447-450.

Boughman, J.A., Astemborski, J.A. & Suzuki, J.B. (1992). Phenotypic assessment of early onset periodontitis in sibships. *Journal of Clinical Periodontology* **19**, 233-239.

Boughman, J.A., Halloran, S.L., Roulston, D., Schwartz, S., Suzuki, J.B., Weitkamp, L.R., Wenk, R.E., Wooten, R. & Cohen, M.M. (1986). An autosomal-dominant form of juvenile periodontitis: its localization to chromosome 4 and linkage to dentinogenesis imperfecta and Gc. *Journal of Craniofacial Genetics and Developmental Biology* **6**, 341-350.

Bragd, L., Wikström, M. & Slots, J. (1985). Clinical and microbiological study of "refractory" adult periodontitis. *Journal of Dental Research* **64**, 234.

Burmeister, J.A., Best, A.M., Palcanis, K.G., Caine, F.A. & Ranney, R.R. (1984). Localized juvenile periodontitis and generalized severe periodontitis: clinical findings. *Journal of Clinical Periodontology* **11**, 181-192.

Califano, J.V., Schenkein, H.A. & Tew, J.G. (1992). Immunodominant antigens of *Actinobacillus actinomycetemcomitans* serotype b in early onset periodontitis patients. *Oral Microbiology and Immunology* **7**, 65-70.

Christersson, L.A., Slots, J., Rosling, B.G. et al. (1985). Microbiological and clinical effects of surgical treatment of localized juvenile periodontitis. *Journal of Clinical Periodontology* **12**, 465-476.

Clerehugh, V., Lennon, M. & Worthington, H. (1990). 5 year results of a longitudinal study of early onset periodontitis in 14 to 19-year old adolescents. *Journal of Clinical Periodontology* **17**, 702-708.

Dahlén, G., Firoze, M., Baelum, V. & Fejerskov, O. (1989). Black-pigmented *Bacteroides* species and *Actinobacillus actinomycetemcomitans* in subgingival plaque of adult Kenyans. *Journal of Clinical Periodontology* **16**, 305-310.

DiRienzo, J.M., Cornell, S., Kazoroski, L. & Slots, J. (1990). Probe-specific DNA fingerprinting applied to the epidemiology of localized juvenile periodontitis. *Oral Microbiology and Immunology* **5**, 49-56.

DiRienzo, J.M., Slots, J., Sixou, M., Sol, M.A., Harmon, R. & McKay, T. (1994). Specific genetic variants of *Actinobacillus actinomycetemcomitans* correlate with disease and health in a regional population of families with localized juvenile periodontitis. *Infection and Immunity* **62**, 3058-3065.

Ebersole, J.L. (1990). Systemic humoral immune response in periodontal disease. *Critical Reviews in Oral Biology and Medicine* **1**, 283-331.

Ebersole, J. (1996). Immune responses in periodontal diseases. In: Wilson, T. & Kornman, K., eds. *Fundamentals of Periodontics*. Chicago: Quintessence Publishing Co, pp. 109-158.

Ebersole, J., Cappelli, D. & Sandoval, M. (1994). Subgingival distribution of *A. actinomycetemcomitans* in periodontitis. *Journal of Clinical Periodontology* **21**, 65-75.

Ebersole, J., Taubman, M. & Smith, D. (1985a). Local antibody responses in periodontal diseases. *Journal of Periodontology* **56**, 51-56.

Ebersole, J. L., Taubman, M. A. & Smith, D. J. (1985b). Gingival crevicular fluid antibody to oral microorganisms. II. Distribution and specificity of local antibody responses. *Journal of Periodontal Research* **20**, 349-356.

Ebersole, J.L., Taubman, M.A., Smith, D.A. et al. (1983). Human immune response to oral microorganisms. II. Serum antibody responses to antigens from *Actinobacillus actinomycetemcomitans*. *Journal of Clinical Immunology* **3**, 321-331.

Ebersole, J.L., Taubman, M.A., Smith, D.J. & Frey, D.E. (1986). Human immune response to oral microorganisms: Patterns of antibody levels to *Bacteroides* species. *Infection and Immunity* **51**, 507-513.

Ebersole, J.L., Taubman, M.A., Smith, D.J., Genco, R.J. & Frey, D.E. (1982). Human immune responses to oral micro-organisms. I. Association of localized juvenile periodontitis (LJP) with serum antibody responses to *Actinobacillus actinomycetemcomitans*. *Clinical Experimental Immunology* **47**, 43-52.

Ebersole, J.L., Taubman, M.A., Smith, D.J. & Goodson, J.M. (1984). Gingival crevicular fluid antibody to oral microorganisms. I. Method of collection and analysis of antibody. *Journal of Periodontal Research* **19**, 124-132.

Eisenmann, A.C., Eisenmann, R., Sousa, O. & Slots, J. (1983). Microbiological study of localized juvenile periodontitis in Panama. *Journal of Periodontology* **54**, 712-713.

Engel, D. (1996). Lymphocyte function in early-onset periodontitis. *Journal of Periodontology* **67**, 332-336.

Fives-Taylor, P., Meyer, D. & Mintz, K. (1996). Virulence factors of the periodontopathogen *Actinobacillus actinomycetemcomitans*. *Journal of Periodontology* **67**, 291-297.

Genco, R.J., Van, D.T.E., Park, B., Ciminelli, M. & Horoszewicz, H. (1980). Neutrophil chemotaxis impairment in juvenile periodontitis: evaluation of specificity, adherence, deformability, and serum factors. *Journal of the Reticuloendothelial Society* **28**, 81s-91s.

Genco, R.J., VanDyke, T.E., Levine, M.J., Nelson, R.D. & Wilson, M.E. (1986). Molecular factors influencing neutrophil defects in periodontal disease (1985 Kreshover lecture). *Journal of Dental Research* **65**, 1379-1391.

Genco, R.J., Zambon, J.J. & Murray, P.A. (1985). Serum and gingival fluid antibodies as adjuncts in the diagnosis of *Actinobacillus actinomycetemcomitans*-associated periodontal disease. *Journal of Periodontology* **56**, 41-50.

Gmür, R. & Guggenheim, B. (1994). Interdental supragingival plaque – A natural habitat of *Actinobacillus actinomycetemcomitans, Bacteroides forsythus, Campylobacter rectus* and *Prevotella nigrescens*. *Journal of Dental Research* **73**, 1421-1428.

Gunsolley, J.C., Burmeister, J.A., Tew, J.G., Best, A.M. & Ranney, R.R. (1987). Relationship of serum antibody to attachment level patterns in young adults with juvenile periodontitis or generalized severe periodontitis. *Journal of Periodontology* **58**, 314-320.

Gunsolley, J.C., Ranney, R.R., Zambon, J.J., Burmeister, J.A. & Schenkein, H.A. (1990). *Actinobacillus actinomycetemcomitans* in families afflicted with periodontitis. *Journal of Periodontology* **61**, 643-648.

Gunsolley, J.C., Tew, J.G., Gooss, C.M., Burmeister, J.A. & Schenkein, H.A. (1988). Effects of race and periodontal status on antibody reactive with *Actinobacillus actinomycetemcomitans* strain. *Journal of Periodontal Research* **23**, 303-307.

Haffajee, A.D., Socransky, S.S. & Ebersole, J.L. (1984). Clinical, microbiological and immunological features associated with the treatment of active periodontosis lesions. *Journal of Clinical Periodontology* **11**, 600-618.

Hall, E.R., Falkler, W.A. Jr., Martin, S.A. & Suzuki, J.B. (1991). The gingival immune response to *Actinobacillus actinomycetemcomitans* in juvenile periodontitis. *Journal of Periodontology* **62**, 792-798.

Hall, E.R., Falkler, W.A. Jr. & Suzuki, J.B. (1990). Production of immunoglobulins in gingival tissue explant cultures from juvenile periodontitis patients. *Journal of Periodontology* **61**, 603-608.

Hall, E.R., Martin, S.A., Suzuki, J.B. & Falkler, W.A. Jr. (1994). The gingival immune response to periodontal pathogens in juvenile periodontitis. *Oral Microbiology and Immunology* **9**, 327-334.

Hammond, B.F., Lillard, S.E. & Stevens, R.H. (1987). A bacteriocin of *Actinobacillus actinomycetemcomitans*. *Journal of Periodontology* **55**, 686-691.

Hart, T. (1996). Genetic risk factors for early onset periodontitis. *Journal of Periodontology* **67**, 355-366.

Hart, T., Marazita, M., McCanna, K., Schenkein, H. & Diehl, S. (1993). Re-evaluation of the chromosome 4q candidate region for early onset periodontitis. *Human Genetics* **91**, 416-422.

Hart, T.C., Marazita, M.L., Schenkein, H.A. & Diehl, S.R. (1992). Re-interpretation of the evidence for X-linked dominant inheritance of juvenile periodontitis. *Journal of Periodontology* **63**, 169-173.

Hormand, J. & Frandsen, A. (1979). Juvenile periodontitis. Localization of bone loss in relation to age, sex, and teeth. *Journal of Clinical Periodontology* **6**, 407-416.

Kinane, D.F., Cullen, C.F., Johnston, F.A. & Evans, C.W. (1989a). Neutrophil chemotactic behaviour in patients with early onset forms of periodontitis. I. Leading front analysis in Boyden chambers. *Journal of Clinical Periodontology* **16**, 242-246.

Kinane, D.F., Cullen, C.F., Johnston, F.A. & Evans, C.W. (1989b). Neutrophil chemotactic behaviour in patients with early onset forms of periodontitis. II. Assessment using the under agarose technique. *Journal of Clinical Periodontology* **16**, 247-251.

Kornman, K.S. & Robertson, P.B. (1985). Clinical and microbiological evaluation of therapy for juvenile periodontitis. *Journal of Periodontology* **56**, 443-446.

Kugelberg, C.F. (1992). Third molar surgery. *Current Opinions in Oral and Maxillofacial Surgery and Infections* **2**, III, 9-16.

Lally, E., Baehni, P. & McArthur, W. (1980). Local immunoglobulin synthesis in periodontal disease. *Journal of Periodontal Research* **15**, 159-164.

Lally, E.T., Kieba, I.R., Golub, E.E., Lear, J.D. & Tanaka, J.C. (1996). Structure/function aspects of *Actinobacillus actinomycetemcomitans* leukotoxin. *Journal of Periodontology* **67**, 298-308.

Lang, N.P., Bartold, P.M., Cullinam, M., Jeffcoat, M., Mombelli, A., Murakami, S., Page, R., Papapanou, P., Tonetti, M. & Van Dyke, T. (1999). International Classification Workshop. Consensus report: Aggressive periodontitis. *Annals of Periodontology* **4**, 53.

Lang, N. & Hill, R. (1977). Radiographs in periodontics. *Journal of Clinical Periodontology* **4**, 16-28.

Liljenberg, B. & Lindhe, J. (1980). Juvenile periodontitis: some microbiological, histopathologic and clinical characteristics. *Journal of Clinical Periodontology* **7**, 748-761.

Lissau, I., Holst, D. & Friis-Hasché, E. (1990). Dental health behaviors and periodontal disease indicators in Danish youths. *Journal of Clinical Periodontology* **17**, 42-47.

Listgarten, M.A. (1976). Structure of the microbial flora associated with periodontal health and disease in man. *Journal of Periodontology* **47**, 1-18.

Listgarten, M.A., Lai, C.H. & Evian, C.I. (1981). Comparative antibody titers to *Actinobacillus actinomycetemcomitans* in juvenile periodontitis, chronic periodontitis, and periodontally healthy subjects. *Journal of Clinical Periodontology* **8**, 155-164.

Listgarten, M.A., Wong, M.Y. & Lai, C.H. (1995). Detection of *Actinobacillus actinomycetemcomitans, Porphyromonas gingivalis*, and *Bacteroides forsythus* in an *A. actinomycetemcomitans*-positive patient population. *Journal of Periodontology* **66**, 158-164.

Löe, H. & Brown, L.J. (1991). Early onset periodontitis in the United States of America. *Journal of Periodontology* **62**, 608-616.

Loesche, W.J., Syed, S.A., Schmidt, E. & Morrison, E.C. (1985). Bacterial profiles of subgingival plaques in periodontitis. *Journal of Clinical Periodontology* **56**, 447-456.

Long, J., Nance, W., Waring, P., Burmeister, J. & Ranney, R. (1987). Early onset periodontitis: a comparison and evaluation of two modes of inheritance. *Genetic Epidemiology* **4**, 13-24.

Mackler, B.F., Frostad, K.B., Robertson, R.B. & Levy, B.M. (1977). Immunoglobulin bearing lymphocytes and plasma cells in human periodontal disease. *Journal of Periodontal Research* **12**, 37-45.

Mackler, B.F., Waldrop, T.C., Schur, P., Robertson, P.B. & Levy, B.M. (1978). IgG subclasses in human periodontal disease. I. Distribution and incidence of IgG subclasses bearing lymphocytes and plasma cells. *Journal of Periodontal Research* **13**, 109-119.

Mandell, R.L. (1984). A longitudinal microbiological investigation of *Actinobacillus actinomycetemcomitans* and Eikenella corrodens in juvenile periodontitis. *Infection and Immunity* **45**, 778-780.

Mandell, R.L., Ebersole, L.J. & Socransky, S.S. (1987). Clinical immunologic and microbiologic features of active disease sites in juvenile periodontitis. *Journal of Clinical Periodontology* **14**, 534-540.

Mandell, R.L. & Socransky, S.S. (1981). A selective medium for *Actinobacillus actinomycetemcomitans* and the incidence of the organism in juvenile periodontitis. *Journal of Periodontology* **52**, 593-598.

Mandell, R.L., Tripodi, L.S., Savitt, E., Goodson, J.M. & Socransky, S.S. (1986). The effect of treatment on *Actinobacillus actinomycetemcomitans* in localized juvenile periodontitis. *Journal of Periodontology* **57**, 94-99.

Marazita, M., Burmeister, J. & Gunsolley, J. (1994). Evidence for autosomal dominant inheritance and race-specific heterogeneity in early-onset periodontitis. *Journal of Periodontology* **65**, 623-630.

Masada, M.P., Persson, R., Kenney, J.S., Lee, S.W., Page, R.C. & Allison, A.C. (1990). Measurement of interleukin-1 alpha and beta in gingival crevicular fluid: implications for pathogenesis of periodontal disease. *Journal of Periodontal Research* **25**, 156-163.

McNabb, H., Mombelli, A., Gmür, R., Mathey-Dinç, S. & Lang, N.P. (1992). Periodontal pathogens in shallow pockets in immigrants from developing countries. *Oral Microbiology and Immunology* **7**, 267-272.

Mombelli, A., Gmür, R., Gobbi, C. & Lang, N.P. (1994). *Actinobacillus actinomycetemcomitans* in adult periodontitis. II. Characterization of isolated strains and effect of mechanical periodontal treatment. *Journal of Periodontology* **65**, 827-834.

Moore, W.E.C. (1987). Microbiology of periodontal disease. *Journal of Periodontal Research* **22**, 335-341.

Moore, W.E.C., Holdeman, L.V., Cato, E.P., Good, I.J., Smith, E.P., Palcanis, K.G. & Ranney, R.R. (1985). Comparative bacteriology of juvenile periodontitis. *Infection and Immunity* **48**, 507-519.

Murray, P.A., Burstein, D.A. & Winkler, J.R. (1989). Antibodies to *Bacteroides gingivalis* in patients with treated and untreated periodontal disease. *Journal of Periodontology* **60**, 96-103.

Needleman, H., Nelson, L., Allred, E. & Seow, K. (1997). Alveolar bone height of primary and first permanent molars in healthy 7 to 9-year-old children. *ASDC Journal of Dentistry for Children* **64** (3), 188-196.

Newman, M.G. & Socransky, S.S. (1977). Predominant cultivable microbiota in periodontosis. *Journal of Periodontal Research* **12**, 120.

Newman, M.G., Socransky, S.S., Savitt, E.D., Propas, D.A. & Crawford, A. (1976). Studies of the microbiology of periodontosis. *Journal of Periodontology* **47**, 373-379.

Offenbacher, S., Heasman, P. & Collins, J. (1993). Modulation of host PGE$_2$ secretion as a determinant of periodontal disease. *Journal of Periodontology* **64**, 432-444.

Ogawa, T., Tarkowski, A., McGhee, M.L., Moldoveanu, Z., Mestecky, J., Hirsch, H.Z., Koopman, W.J., Hamada, S., McGhee, J.R. & Kiyono, H. (1989). Analysis of human IgG and IgA antibody secreting cells from localized chronic inflammatory tissue. *Journal of Immunology* **142**, 1140-1158.

Online Mendelian Inheritance in Man, OMIM. (1996). Center for Medical Genetics, Johns Hopkins University (Baltimore, MD) and National Center for Biotechnology Information, National Library of Medicine (Bethesda, MD). World Wide Web URL: http://www3.ncbi.nlm.nih.gov/omim/

Page, R.C. (1990). Risk factors involving host defense mechanisms. In: Bader, J.D., ed. *Risk assessment in dentistry.* Chapel Hill: University of North Carolina Dental Ecology, pp. 94-104.

Page, R.C., Altman, L.C., Ebersole, J.L., Vandesteen, G.E., Dahlberg, W.H., Williams, B.L. & Osterberg, S.K. (1983a). Rapidly progressive periodontitis. A distinct clinical condition. *Journal of Periodontology* **54**, 197-209.

Page, R.C., Bowen, T., Altman, L., Edward, V., Ochs, H., Mackenzie, P., Osterberg, S., Engel, L.D. & Williams, B.L. (1983b). Prepubertal periodontitis. I. Definition of a clinical disease entity. *Journal of Periodontology* **54**, 257-271.

Papapanou, P. (1996). Periodontal diseases: Epidemiology. *Annals of Periodontology* **1**, 1-36.

Patters, M., Niekrash, C. & Lang, N. (1989). Assessment of complement cleavage during experimental gingivitis in man. *Journal of Clinical Periodontology* **16**, 33-37.

Pavicic, M.J.A.M.P., van Winkelhoff, A.J., Douqué, N.H., Steures, R.W.R. & de Graaff, J. (1994). Microbiological and clinical effects of metronidazole and amoxicillin in *Actinobacillus actinomycetemcomitans*-associated periodontitis. *Journal of Clinical Periodontology* **21**, 107-112.

Petit, M.D.A., van Steenbergen, T.J.M., de Graaff, J. & van der Velden, U. (1993a). Transmission of *Actinobacillus actinomycetemcomitans* in families of adult periodontitis patients. *Journal of Periodontal Research* **28**, 335-345.

Petit, M.D.A., van Steenbergen, T.J.M., Scholte, L.H.M., van der Velden, U. & de Graaff, J. (1993b). Epidemiology and transmission of *Porphyromonas gingivalis* and *Actinobacillus actinomycetemcomitans* among children and their family members

– a report of four surveys. *Journal of Clinical Periodontology* **20**, 641-650.

Poulsen, K., Theilade, E., Lally, E.T., Demuth, D.R. & Kilian, M. (1994). Population structure of *Actinobacillus actinomycetemcomitans*: A framework for studies of disease-associated properties. *Microbiology* **140**, 2049-2060.

Preus, H.R. (1988). Treatment of rapidly destructive periodontitis in Papillon-Lefèvre syndrome. Laboratory and clinical observations. *Journal of Clinical Periodontology* **15**, 639-643.

Preus, H.R., Russell, D.T. & Zambon, J.J. (1992). Transmission of *Actinobacillus actinomycetemcomitans* in families of adult periodontitis patients. *Journal of Dental Research* **71**, 606.

Rams, T.E., Feik, D. & Slots, J. (1992). Ciprofloxacin/metronidazole treatment of recurrent adult periodontitis. *Journal of Dental Research* **71**, 319.

Renvert, S., Wikström, M., Dahlén, G., Slots, J. & Egelberg, J. (1990a). Effect of root debridement on the elimination of *Actinobacillus actinomycetemcomitans* and *Bacteroides gingivalis* from periodontal pockets. *Journal of Clinical Periodontology* **17**, 345-350.

Renvert, S., Wikström, M., Dahlén, G., Slots, J. & Egelberg, J. (1990b). On the inability of root debridement and periodontal surgery to eliminate *Actinobacillus actinomycetemcomitans* from periodontal pockets. *Journal of Clinical Periodontology* **17**, 351-355.

Rodenburg, J.P., van Winkelhoff, A.J., Winkel, E.G., Goene, R.J., Abbas, F. & de Graff, J. (1990). Occurrence of *Bacteroides gingivalis*, *Bacteroides intermedius* and *Actinobacillus actinomycetemcomitans* in severe periodontitis in relation to age and treatment history. *Journal of Clinical Periodontology* **17**, 392-399.

Saglie, F.R., Marfany, A. & Camargo, P. (1988). Intragingival occurrence of *Actinobacillus actinomycetemcomitans* and *Bacteroides gingivalis* in active destructive periodontal lesions. *Journal of Periodontology* **59**(4), 259-265.

Sandholm, L., Tolo, K. & Olsen, I. (1987). Salivary IgG, a parameter of periodontal disease activity? High responders to Actinobacillus actinomycetemcomitans Y4 in juvenile and adult periodontitis. *Journal of Clinical Periodontology* **14**, 289-294.

Saxen, L. & Nevanlinna, H.R. (1984). Autosomal recessive inheritance of juvenile periodontitis: test of a hypothesis. *Clinical Genetics* **25**, 332-335.

Schenkein, H. (1994). Genetics of early onset periodontal disease. In: Genco, R., Hamada, S., Lehner, T, McGhee, J. & Mergenhagen, S., eds. *Molecular pathogenesis of periodontal disease.* Washington, DC: American Society for Microbiology, pp. 373-383.

Schenkein, H.A. & Genco, R.J. (1977). Gingival fluid and serum in periodontal diseases. II. Evidence for cleavage of complement component C3, C3 proactivator (factor B) and C4 in gingival fluid. *Journal of Periodontology* **48**, 778-784.

Schenkein, H.A., Gunsolley, J.C., Koertge, T.E., Schenkein, J.G. & Tew, J.G. (1995). Smoking and its effects on early-onset periodontitis. *Journal of the American Dental Association* **126**, 1107-1113.

Schenkein, H. & Van-Dyke, T. (1994). Early onset periodontitis. Systemic aspects of etiology and pathogenesis. *Periodontology 2000* **6**, 7-25.

Schonfeld, S.E. & Kagan, J.M. (1982). Specificity of gingival plasma cells for bacterial somatic antigens. *Journal of Periodontal Research* **17**, 60-69.

Shah, H.N. (1993). Biology of the species *Porphyromonas gingivalis*. Boca Raton: CPC Press.

Shapira, L., Smidt, A., Van, D.T.E., Barak, V., Soskolne, A.W., Brautbar, C., Sela, M.N. & Bimstein, E. (1994). Sequential manifestation of different forms of early-onset periodontitis. A case report. *Journal of Periodontology* **65**, 631-635.

Shapira, L., Warbington, M. & Van Dyke, T.E. (1994). TNF-alpha and IL-1 beta in serum of LJP patients with normal and defective neutrophil chemotaxis. *Journal of Periodontal Research* **29**, 371-373.

Sjodin, B. & Mattson, L. (1992). Marginal bone level in the normal primary dentition. *Journal of Clinical Periodontology* **19**, 672-678.

Sjodin, B. & Mattson, L. (1994). Marginal bone loss in the primary dentition. A survey of 7 to 9 year olds in Sweden. *Journal of Clinical Periodontology* **21**, 313-319.

Sjodin, B., Crossner, C.G., Unell, L. & Ostlund, P. (1989). A retrospective radiographic study of alveolar bone loss in the primary dentition in patients with localized juvenile periodontitis. *Journal of Clinical Periodontology* **16**, 124-127.

Sjodin, B., Matsson, L., Unell, L. & Egelberg, J. (1993). Marginal bone loss in the primary dentition of patients with juvenile periodontitis. *Journal of Clinical Periodontology* **20**, 32-36.

Slots, J. (1976). The predominant cultivable organisms in juvenile periodontitis. *Scandinavian Journal of Dental Research* **84**, 1.

Slots, J., Feik, D. & Rams, T.E. (1990). *Actinobacillus actinomycetemcomitans* and *Bacteroides intermedius* in human periodontitis: age relationship and mutual association. *Journal of Clinical Periodontology* **17**, 659-662.

Slots, J., Reynolds, H.S. & Genco, R.J. (1980). *Actinobacillus actinomycetemcomitans* in human periodontal disease: a cross-sectional microbiological investigation. *Infection and Immunity* **29**, 1013-1020.

Slots, J. & Rosling, B.G. (1983). Suppression of the periodontopathic microflora in localized juvenile periodontitis by systemic tetracycline. *Journal of Clinical Periodontology* **10**, 465-486.

Slots, J. & Schonfeld, S.E. (1991). *Actinobacillus actinomycetemcomitans* in localized juvenile periodontitis. In: Hamada, S., Holt, S.C. & McGhee, J.R., eds. *Periodontal disease. Pathogens and host immune responses.* Tokyo: Quintessence, pp. 53-64.

Socransky, S.S. & Haffajee, A.D. (1992). The bacterial etiology of destructive periodontal disease: current concepts. *Journal of Periodontology* **63**, 322-331.

Steubing, P., MAckler, B., Schur, P. & Levy, B. (1982). Humoral studies of periodontal disease. I. Characterisation of immunoglobulins quantitated from cultures of gingival tissue. *Clinical Immunology and Immunopathology* **22**, 32-43.

Suomi, J., Plumbo, J. & Barbano, J. (1968). A comparative study of radiographs and pocket measurements in periodontal disease evaluation. *Journal of Periodontology* **39**, 311-315.

Sweeney, E.A., Alcoforado, G.A.P., Nyman, S. & Slots, J. (1987). Prevalence and microbiology of localized prepubertal periodontitis. *Oral Microbiology and Immunology* **2**, 65-70.

Taubman, M.A., Stoufi, E.D., Seymour, G.J., Smith, D.J. & Ebersole, J.L. (1988). Immunoregulatory aspects of periodontal diseases. *Advances in Dental Research* **2**, 328-333.

Taubman, M.A., Wang, H-Y., Lundqvist, C.A., Seymour, G.J., Eastcott, J.W. & Smith, D.J. (1991). The cellular basis of host responses in periodontal diseases. In: Hamada, S., Holt, S.C. & McGhee, J.R., eds. *Periodontal disease: pathogens and host immune responses.* Tokyo: Quintessence publishing Co, pp. 199-208.

Tew, J.G., Marshall, D.R. & Burmeister, J.A. (1985). Relationship between gingival crevicular fluid and serum antibody titers in young adults with generalized and localized periodontitis. *Infection and Immunity* **49**, 487-493.

Tew, J.G., Zhang, J.B., Quinn, S., Tangada, S., Nakashima, K., Gunsolley, J.C. Schenkein, H.A. & Califano, J.V. (1996). Antibody of the IgG$_2$ subclass, *Actinobacillus actinomycetemcomitans*, and early onset perioodontitis. *Journal of Periodontology* **67**, 317-322.

Tolo, K. & Schenck, K. (1985). Activity of serum immunoglobulins G, A, and M to six anaerobic, oral bacteria in diagnosis of periodontitis. *Journal of Periodontal Research* **20**, 113-121.

Tonetti, M. (1993). Etiology and Pathogenesis. *Proceedings of the 1st European Workshop on Periodontology,* Lang, N.P. & Karring, T., eds. Berlin: Quintessenz Verlags-GmbH, pp. 54-89.

Tonetti, M. & Mombelli, A. (1999). Early onset periodontitis. *Annals of Periodontology* **4**, 39-53.

Tsai, C.C., McArthur, W.P., Baehni, P.C. et al. (1981). Serum neutralizing activity against *Actinobacillus actinomycetem-*

comitans leukotoxin in juvenile periodontitis. *Journal of Clinical Periodontology* **8**, 338-348.

Van der Velden, U., Abbas, F., Van Steenbergen, T.J.M., De Zoete, O.J., Hesse, M., De Ruyter, C., De Laat, V.H.M. & De Graaff, J. (1989). Prevalence of periodontal breakdown in adolescents and presence of *Actinobacillus actinomycetemcomitans* in subjects with attachment loss. *Journal of Periodontology* **60**, 604-610.

Van Dyke, T.E., Horoszewicz, H.U. & Genco, R.J. (1982). The polymorphonuclear leukocyte (PMNL) locomotor defect in juvenile periodontitis. *Journal of Periodontology* **53**, 682-687.

Van Dyke, T.E., Offenbacher, S., Kalmar, J. & Arnold, R.R. (1988). Neutrophil defects and host-parasite interactions in the pathogenesis of localized juvenile periodontitis. *Advances in Dental Research* **2**, 354-358.

Van Dyke, T.E., Schweinebraten, M., Cianciola, L.J., Offenbacher, S. & Genco, R.J. (1985). Neutrophil chemotaxis in families with localized juvenile periodontitis. *Journal of Periodontal Research* **20**, 503-514.

Van Dyke, T.E., Zinney, W., Winkel, K., Taufiq, A., Offenbacher, S. & Arnold, R.R. (1986). Neutrophil function in localized juvenile periodontitis. Phagocytosis, superoxide production and specific granule release. *Journal of Periodontology* **57**, 703-708.

van Winkelhoff, A.J., Rodenburg, J.P., Goene, R.J., Abbas, F., Winkel, E.G. & de Graaff, J. (1989). Metronidazole plus amoxycillin in the treatment of *Actinobacillus actinomycetemcomitans* associated periodontitis. *Journal of Clinical Periodontology* **16**, 128-131.

Vincent, J.W., Suzuki, J.B., Falkler, W.A. & Cornett, W.C. (1985). Reaction of human sera from juvenile periodontitis, rapidly progressive periodontitis, and adult periodontitis patients with selected periodontopathogens. *Journal of Periodontology* **56**, 464-469.

Von Troil-Lindén, B., Torkko, H., Alaluusua, S., Wolf, J., Jousimies-Somer, H. & Asikainen, S. (1995). Periodontal findings in spouses: A clinical, radiographic and microbiological study. *Journal of Clinical Periodontology* **22**, 93-99.

Waldrop, T.C., Mackler, B.F. & Schur, P. (1981). IgG and IgG subclasses in human periodontosis (juvenile periodontitis). Serum concentrations. *Journal of Periodontology* **52**, 96-98.

Watanabe, K. (1990). Prepubertal periodontitis: a review of diagnostic criteria, pathogenesis, and differential diagnosis. *Journal of Periodontal Research* **25**, 31-48.

Westergaard, J., Frandsen, A. & Slots, J. (1978). Ultrastructure of the subgingival microflora in juvenile periodontitis. *Scandinavian Journal of Dental Research* **86**, 421-429.

Williams, R.C., Jeffcoat, M.K., Howell, T.H. et al. (1989). Altering the course of human alveolar bone loss with the nonsteroidal anti-inflammatory drug fluorbiprofen. *Journal of Periodontology* **60**, 485-490.

Williams, R.C., Jeffcoat, M.K., Kaplan, M.L., Goldhaber, P., Johnson, H.G. & Wechter, W.J. (1985). Fluorbiprofen: a potent inhibitor of alveolar bone resorption in beagles. *Science* **227**, 640-642.

Wilson, M.E. & Kalmar, J.R. (1996) FcRIIa (CD32): a potential marker defining susceptibility to localized juvenile periodontitis. *Journal of Periodontology* **67**, 323-331.

Zambon, J.J., Christersson, L.A. & Slots, J. (1983). *Actinobacillus actinomycetemcomitans* in human periodontal disease. Prevalence in patient groups and distribution of biotypes and serotypes within families. *Journal of Periodontology* **54**, 707-711.

Zambon, J.J., Haraszthy, V.I., Hariharan, G., Lally, E.T. & Demuth, D.R. (1996). The microbiology of early-onset periodontitis: association of highly toxic *Actinobacillus actinomycetemcomitans* strains with localized juvenile periodontitis. *Journal of Periodontology* **67**, 282-290.

Zambon, J.J., Umemoto, T., De Nardin, E., Nakazawa, F., Christersson, L.A. & Genco, R.J. (1988). *Actinobacillus actinomycetemcomitans* in the pathogenesis of human periodontal disease. *Advances in Dental Research* **2**, 269-274.

CHAPTER 10

Necrotizing Periodontal Disease

PALLE HOLMSTRUP AND JYTTE WESTERGAARD

NOMENCLATURE

Necrotizing gingivitis (NG), necrotizing periodontitis (NP) and necrotizing stomatitis (NS) are the most severe inflammatory periodontal disorders caused by plaque bacteria. The necrotizing diseases usually run an acute course and therefore the term acute is often included in the diagnoses. They are rapidly destructive and debilitating, and they appear to represent various stages of the same disease process (Horning & Cohen 1995). A distinction between NG and NP has not always been made in the literature, but parallel to the use of the term gingivitis, NG should be limited to lesions only involving gingival tissue with no loss of periodontal attachment (Riley et al. 1992). Most often, however, the disease results in loss of attachment (MacCarthy & Claffey 1991), and a more correct term in cases with loss of attachment is NP, provided the lesions are confined to the periodontal tissues including gingiva, periodontal ligament and alveolar bone. Further progression to include tissue beyond the mucogingival junction is characteristic of necrotizing stomatitis and distinguishes this disease from NP (Williams et al. 1990).

The necrotizing periodontal diseases have been mentioned under several names, some of which are: "Ulceromembranous gingivitis", "acute necrotizing ulcerative gingivitis" (ANUG) and "Vincent's gingivitis" or "Vincent's gingivostomatitis", "necrotizing gingivostomatitis", and "Trench mouth" (Pickard 1973, Johnson & Engel 1986, Horning & Cohen 1995). Vincent first described the mixed fusospirochetal microbiota of the so-called "Vincent's angina", characterized by necrotic areas in the tonsils (Vincent 1898). A similar mixed microbiota has been isolated from NG lesions, but Vincent's angina and NG usually occur independently of each other, and should be regarded as separate disease entities.

NS has features in common with the far more serious *cancrum oris*, also denoted noma. This is a destructive and necrotizing, frequently mortal, stomatitis in which the same mixed fusospirochetal flora dominates. It occurs almost exclusively in certain developing countries, mostly in children suffering from systemic diseases including malnutrition (Enwonwu 1972, 1985). It has been suggested that cancrum oris always develops from preexisting NG (Emslie 1963) but this connection has not been confirmed (Pindborg et al. 1966, 1967, Sheiham 1966).

In the literature, a distinction between NG, NP and NS is seldom made. However, the reader should be aware of this uncertainty and the consequences of the missing distinction between the three diagnoses in the referred reports. The uncertainty is reflected in the present chapter by the use of the term necrotizing periodontal disease (NPD) as a common denominator for necrotizing gingivitis, necrotizing periodontitis and necrotizing stomatitis.

PREVALENCE

During World War II, up to 14% of the Danish military personnel encountered NPD (Pindborg 1951a). Large numbers of civilians also suffered from the disease (King 1943, Stammers 1944). After World War II, the prevalence of NPD declined substantially and in industrialized countries NPD it is now rare. It occurs particularly among young adults. In the 1960s NPD was found in 2.5% of 326 US students during their first college year, but over the next year more students became affected, with a total of 6.7% demonstrating the disease during their first two college years (Giddon et al. 1964). More recent studies in industrialized countries have reported prevalences of 0.5% or less (Barnes et al. 1973, Horning et al. 1990). In Scandinavia, the disease is now very rare among otherwise healthy individuals, with a prevalence of 0.001% among young Danish military trainees (personal communication, Prætorius). NPD can be observed in all age groups but there are geographic differences in the age distribution. Among HIV-infected individuals the disease seems to occur slightly more often. Studies among groups of HIV-infected individuals have revealed prevalences of NPD between 0% and 11% (Holmstrup & Westergaard 1994). However, most studies have included cohorts of individuals connected with hospitals or dental clinics. Studies conducted outside these environments have shown relatively low prevalence figures. NP has been found in 1% of 200 HIV-seropositive individuals in Washington, D.C. (Riley et al. 1992), and the prevalence may not, in fact, differ so much from that of the general population (Drinkard et al. 1991, Friedman et al. 1991, Barr et al. 1992).

In developing countries, the prevalence of NPD is higher than in the industrialized countries, and the disease frequently occurs in children. This is practically never seen in western countries. In Nigerian villages, between 1.7% and 26.9% of 2-6-year-old children have been found with NPD (Sheiham 1966). In India, 54-68% of NPD cases occurred in children below 10 years of age (Migliani & Sharma 1965, Pindborg et al. 1966).

CLINICAL CHARACTERISTICS

Development of lesions

NG is an inflammatory destructive gingival condition, characterized by ulcerated and necrotic papillae and gingival margins resulting in a characteristic punched-out appearance. The ulcers are covered by a yellowish-white or grayish slough, which has been termed "pseudomembrane". However, the sloughed material has no coherence, and bears little resemblance to a membrane. It consists primarily of fibrin and necrotic tissue with leukocytes, erythrocytes and masses of bacteria. Consequently, the term is misleading and should be omitted. Removal of the sloughed material results in bleeding and ulcerated underlying tissue becomes exposed.

The necrotizing lesions develop rapidly and are painful, but in the initial stages, when the necrotic areas are relatively few and small, pain is usually moderate. Severe pain is often the chief reason for the patients to seek treatment. Bleeding is readily provoked. This is due to the acute inflammation and necrosis with exposure of the underlying connective tissue. Bleeding may start spontaneously as well as in response to even gentle touch. In early phases of the disease lesions are typically confined to the top of a few interdental papillae (Fig. 10-1). The first lesions are often seen interproximally in the mandibular anterior region, but they may occur in any interproximal space. In regions where lesions first appear, there are usually also signs of preexisting chronic gingivitis, but the papillae are not always edematous at this stage and gingival stippling may be maintained. Usually, however, the papillae rapidly swell and achieve a rounded contour, and this is particularly evident in the facial aspect. The zone between the marginal necrosis and the relatively unaffected gingiva usually exhibits a well-demarcated narrow erythematous zone, sometimes referred to as the linear erythema. This is an expression of hyperemia due to dilation of the vessels in the gingival connective tissue in the periphery of the necrotic lesions (Fig. 10-17a).

A characteristic and pronounced *foetor ex ore* is often associated with NPD, but can vary in intensity and in some cases is not very noticeable. Strong *foetor ex ore* is not pathognomonic of NPD as it can also be found in other pathologic conditions of the oral cavity such as chronic destructive periodontal disease.

Interproximal craters

The lesions are seldom associated with deep pocket formation, because extensive gingival necrosis often coincides with loss of crestal alveolar bone. The gingival necrosis develops rapidly and within a few days the involved papillae are often separated into one facial and one lingual portion with an interposed necrotic depression, a negative papilla, between them. The central necrosis produces considerable tissue destruction and a regular crater is formed. At this stage of the disease, the disease process usually involves the periodontal ligament and the alveolar bone, and loss of attachment is now established. The diagnosis of the disease process is consequently NP. Along with the papilla destruction, the necrosis usually extends laterally along the gingival margin at the oral and/or facial surfaces of the teeth. Necrotic areas originating from neighboring interproximal spaces frequently merge to form a continuous necrotic area (Figs. 10-2, 10-3). Superficial necrotic lesions only rarely cover a substantial part of the attached gingiva, which becomes reduced in width as the result of the disease progression. The palatal and lingual marginal gingiva is less frequently involved than the corresponding facial area. Frequently, gingiva of semi-impacted teeth and in the

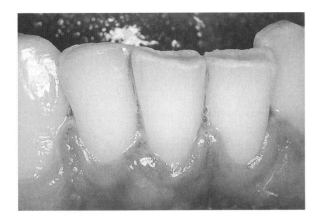

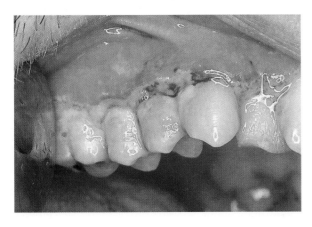

Fig. 10-1. Necrotizing gingivitis with initial punched-out defects at the top of the interdental papillae of the mandibular incisor region. Courtesy of Dr. Finn Prætorius.

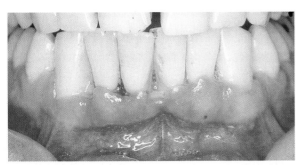

Fig. 10-2. Necrotizing gingivitis progressing along the gingival margin of the right maxilla. The interproximal necrotizing processes have merged.

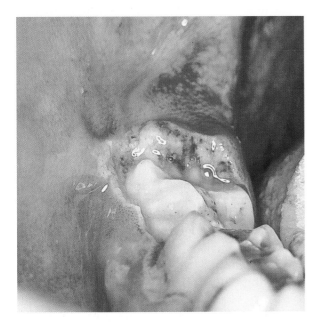

Fig. 10-3. Necrotizing periodontitis with more advanced lesions of interdental papillae and gingival margin. Note the irregular morphology of the gingival margin as determined by the progressive loss of the interdental papillae.

Fig. 10-4. Necrotizing gingivitis affecting gingiva of semi-impacted right mandibular third molar. Courtesy of Dr. Finn Prætorius.

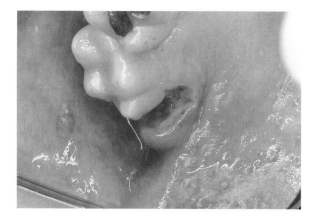

Fig. 10-5. Necrotizing periodontitis affecting right maxillary second molar periodontium. Note the extensive punch-out lesion.

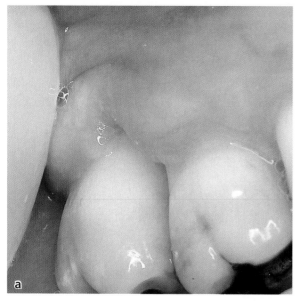

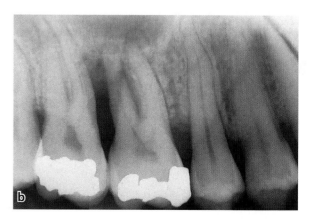

Fig. 10-6. (a) Necrotizing periodontitis often results in major loss of interdental tissue including alveolar bone of the molar regions as demonstrated in the radiograph (b).

posterior maxillary region are affected (Figs. 10-4, 10-5). Progression of the interproximal process often results in destruction of most interdental alveolar bone (Fig. 10-6a,b). In the more advanced cases, pain is often considerable and may be associated with a markedly increased salivary flow. As a result of pain it is often difficult for the patients to eat, and a reduced food intake may be critical to HIV-infected patients because they may already lose weight in association with their HIV infection.

Sequestrum formation

The disease progression may be rapid and result in necrosis of small or large parts of the alveolar bone. Such a development is particularly evident in severely immunocompromised patients including HIV-seropositive individuals. The necrotic bone, denoted a sequestrum, initially is irremovable but after some time becomes loosened, whereafter it may be removed with forceps. Analgesia may not be required. A sequestrum may not only involve interproximal bone

but also include adjacent facial and oral cortical bone (Fig. 10-7a,b).

Involvement of alveolar mucosa

When the necrotic process progresses beyond the mucogingival junction, the condition is denoted NS (Williams et al. 1990) (Figs. 10-8a,b & 10-9). The severe tissue destruction characteristic of this disease is related to seriously compromised immune functions typically associated with HIV infection and malnutrition (Fig. 10-10). Importantly, it may be life-threatening. NS may result in extensive denudation of bone, resulting in major sequestration with the development of oro-antral fistula and osteitis (SanGiacomo et al. 1990, Felix et al. 1991).

Swelling of lymph nodes

Swelling of the regional lymph nodes may occur in NPD but is particularly evident in advanced cases.

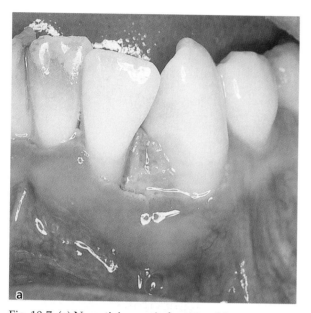
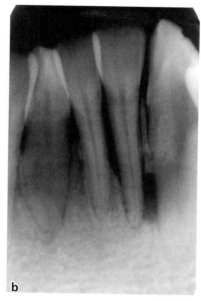

Fig. 10-7. (a) Necrotizing periodontitis with sequestration of alveolar bone between left mandibular lateral incisor and canine. The extension of the sequestrum as seen in the radiograph (b) covers the interdental septum almost to the apices of the roots.

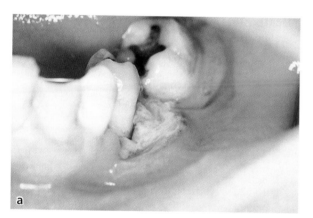
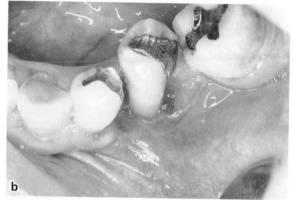

Fig. 10-8. (a) Necrotizing stomatitis affecting periodontium of left mandibular premolar region and adjacent alveolar mucosa. After treatment and healing, no attached gingiva remains (b).

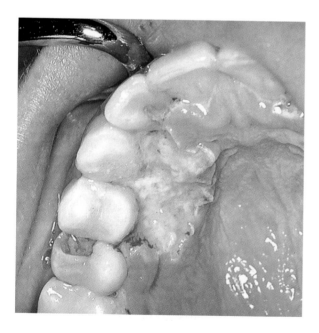

Fig. 10-9. Necrotizing stomatitis of right maxilla with extensive necrotic ulcer of palatal mucosa.

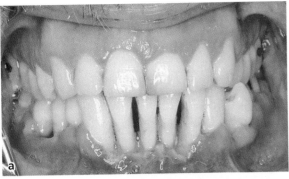
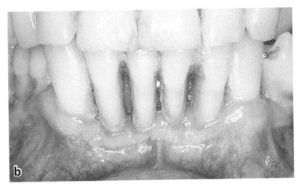

Fig. 10-10. (a) Necrotizing stomatitis affecting the mandible of an HIV-seropositive patient. Two years after treatment (b) the result of treatment is satisfactory, and there has been no recurrence.

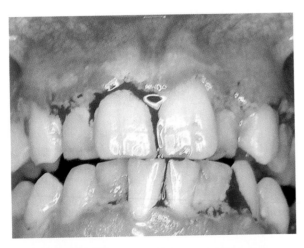

Fig. 10-11. A whitish film sometimes covers parts of the attached gingiva in patients with NPD as demonstrated in the maxillary gingiva. The film is composed of desquamated epithelial cells which have accumulated because the patient has not eaten or performed oral hygiene for days.

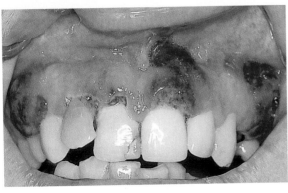

Fig. 10-12. Necrotizing periodontitis affecting Kaposi's sarcoma of left maxillary central incisor gingiva in HIV-infected patient. The sarcoma affected almost the entire maxillary gingiva after 9 months (Fig. 13-18(a)).

Such symptoms are usually confined to the submandibular lymph nodes, but the cervical lymph nodes may also be involved. In children with NPD, swelling of lymph nodes and increased bleeding tendency are often the most pronounced clinical findings (Jiménez & Baer 1975).

Fever and malaise

Fever and malaise is not a consistent characteristic of NPD. Some investigations indicate that elevated body temperature is not common in NG and that, when present, the elevation of body temperature is usually moderate (Grupe & Wilder 1956, Goldhaber & Giddon 1964, Shields 1977, Stevens et al. 1984). A small decrease in body temperature in NG has even been described. The disagreement on this point may, in fact, be due to misdiagnosis of primary herpetic gingivostomatitis as NG (see below).

Oral hygiene

The oral hygiene in patients with NPD is usually poor. Moreover, brushing of teeth and contact with the acutely inflamed gingiva is painful. Therefore, large amounts of plaque on the teeth are common, especially along the gingival margin. A thin, whitish film sometimes covers parts of the attached gingiva (Fig. 10-11). This film is a characteristic finding in patients who have neither eaten nor performed oral hygiene for days. It is composed of desquamated epithelial cells and bacteria in a meshwork of salivary proteins.

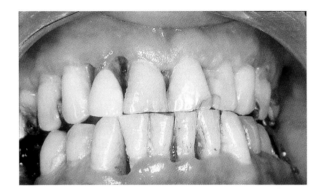

Fig. 10-13. Chronic necrotizing periodontitis with edematous gingiva particularly of mandible. The slightly active necrotizing processes at the bottom of the negative papillae are not visible.

It is easily removable. In general, the clinical characteristics of NPD in HIV-seropositive patients do not essentially differ from those in HIV-seronegative patients. However, the lesions in HIV-seropositive patients may not be associated with large amounts of plaque and calculus. Thus, the disease activity in these patients sometimes shows limited correlation with etiologic factors as determined by the amount of bacterial plaque (Holmstrup & Westergaard 1994). Further, lesions of NPD in HIV-seropositive patients have sometimes been revealed in gingival tissue affected by Kaposi's sarcoma (Fig. 10-12).

Acute and recurrent/chronic forms of necrotizing gingivitis and periodontitis

In most instances the course of the diseases is acute, as characterized by the rapid destruction of the periodontal tissue. However, if inadequately treated or left untreated, the acute phase may gradually subside. The symptoms then become less unpleasant to the patient, but the destruction of the periodontal tissues continues, although at a slower rate, and the necrotic tissues do not heal completely. Such a condition has been termed chronic necrotizing gingivitis, or periodontitis in the case of attachment loss (Fig. 10-13). The necrotizing lesions persist as open craters, frequently with a content of subgingival calculus and bacterial plaque. Although the characteristic ulcerative, necrotic areas of the acute phase usually disappear, acute exacerbations with intervening periods of quiescence

may also occur. In recurrent acute phases, subjective symptoms again become more prominent and necrotic ulcers reappear. Some authors prefer the term recurrent rather than chronic to describe this category of necrotizing disease (Johnson & Engel 1986). Plaque and necrotic debris are in these phases often less conspicuous than in the acute forms, because they are located in preexisting interdental craters. Several adjoining interdental craters may fuse, resulting in total separation of facial and oral gingivae, which form two distinct flaps. Recurrent forms of NG and NP may produce considerable destruction of supporting tissues. The most pronounced tissue loss usually occurs in relation to the interproximal craters.

DIAGNOSIS

The diagnosis of NG, NP and NS is based on clinical findings as described above. The patient has usually noticed pain and bleeding from the gingiva, particularly upon touch. The histopathology of the necrotizing diseases is not pathognomonic for NG, and biopsy is certainly not indicated in the heavily infected area.

Differential diagnosis

NPD may be confused with other diseases of the oral mucosa. Primary herpetic gingivostomatitis (PHG) is not infrequently mistaken for NPD (Klotz 1973). The

Table 10-1. Important characteristics for differential diagnosis between NPD and PHG

	NPD	PHG
Etiology	Bacteria	Herpes simplex virus
Age	15-30 years	Frequently children
Site	Interdental papillae. Rarely outside the gingiva	Gingiva and the entire oral mucosa
Symptoms	Ulcerations and necrotic tissue and a yellowish-white plaque	Multiple vesicles which disrupt, leaving small round fibrin-covered ulcerations
	Foetor ex ore	*Foetor ex ore*
	Moderate fever may occur	Fever
Duration	1-2 days if treated	1-2 weeks
Contagious	–	+
Immunity	–	Partial
Healing	Destruction of periodontal tissue remains	No permanent destruction

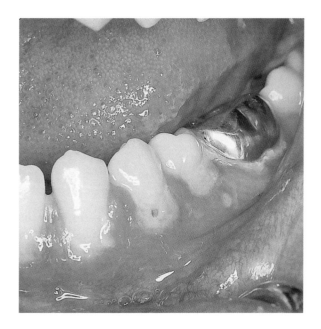

Fig. 10-14. Primary herpetic gingivostomatitis. Note that the ulcers affect the gingival margin but not primarily interdental papillae. A circular ulcer of the second premolar gingiva is highly suggestive of the diagnosis.

important differential diagnostic criteria for the two diseases have been listed in Table 10-1. It should be noted that in the USA and in northern Europe, NPD occurs very rarely in children, whereas PHG is most commonly found in children. If the body temperature is markedly raised, to 38°C or more, PHG should be suspected. NG and NP has a marked predilection for the interdental papillae, while PHG shows no such limitation and may occur anywhere on the free or the attached gingiva, or in the alveolar mucosa (Fig. 10-14). In PHG the erythema is of a more diffuse character and may cover the entire gingiva and parts of the alveolar mucosa. The vesicular lesions in PHG which disrupt and produce small ulcers surrounded by diffuse erythema, occur both on the lips and tongue as well as on the buccal mucosa. PHG and NPD may occur simultaneously in the same patient, and in such cases there may be mucosal lesions outside the gingiva, and fever and general malaise tend to occur more frequently than with NPD alone.

Among oral mucosal diseases that have been confused with NPD are desquamative gingivitis, benign mucous membrane pemphigoid, erythema multiforme exudativum, streptococcal gingivitis, gonococcal gingivitis, and others. All of these are clinically quite distinct from NPD.

In some forms of leukemia, especially acute leukemia, necrotizing ulcers may occur in the oral mucosa and are not infrequently seen in association with the gingival margin, apparently as an exacerbation of an existing chronic inflammatory condition. The clinical appearance can resemble NPD lesions, and the symptoms they produce may be the ones that first make the patient seek professional consultation. In acute leukemia the gingiva often appears bluish-red and edematous with varying degrees of ulceration and necrosis. Generally, the patient has more marked systemic symptoms than with ordinary NPD, but can for a while feel relatively healthy. The dentist should be aware of the possibility that leukemias present such

oral manifestations, which require medical examination of the patient, whereas biopsy is usually not indicated.

HISTOPATHOLOGY

Histopathologically, NG lesions are characterized by ulceration with necrosis of epithelium and superficial layers of the connective tissue and an acute, non-specific inflammatory reaction (Fig. 10-15a,b). An important aspect is the role of the microorganisms in the lesions, because they have been demonstrated not only in the necrotic tissue components but also in vital epithelium and connective tissue.

Sometimes the histologic findings demonstrate the formation of regular layers with certain characteristics (Listgarten 1965) but there may be variations in regularity. The surface cover of yellowish-white or grayish slough, which can be observed clinically, in the light microscope appears to be a meshwork of fibrin with degenerated epithelial cells, leukocytes and erythrocytes, and by bacteria and cellular debris. At the ultrastructural level, bacteria of varying sizes and forms including small, medium-sized and large spirochetes have been revealed between the inflammatory cells, the majority of which are neutrophilic granulocytes. Moreover, in presumably vital parts of the surface epithelium, compact masses of spirochetes and short, fusiform rods have been found intercellularly.

The vital connective tissue in the bottom of the lesion is covered by necrotic tissue, characterized by disintegrated cells, many large and medium-sized spirochetes, and other bacteria which, judging from their size and shape, may be fusobacteria. In the superior part of the vital connective tissue as characterized by intact tissue components, the tissue is infiltrated by large and medium-sized spirochetes, but no other microorganisms have been seen. In the vital connec-

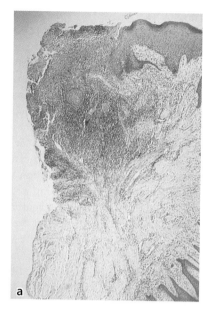
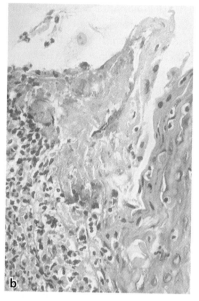

Fig. 10-15. Photomicrograph of gingival tissue affected by necrotizing gingivitis. (a) Upper right part of gingival biopsy shows gingival oral epithelium whereas upper left is ulcerated surface. Underneath the ulcer the connective tissue is heavily infiltrated by inflammatory cells. Higher magnification of margin of ulcer (b) shows necrotic tissue infiltrated with neutrophils. Right border is covered by epithelium. Courtesy of Dr. Finn Prætorius.

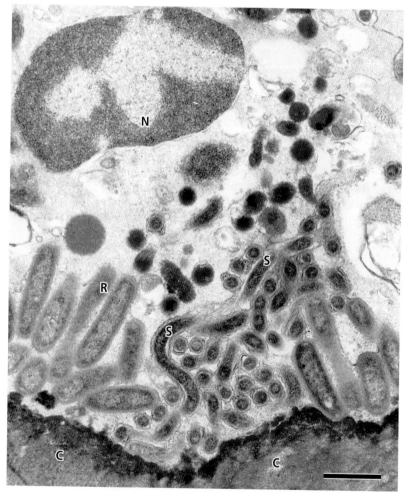

Fig. 10-16. Electronmicrograph demonstrating phagocytosing neutrophil (N) close to the surface of a sequestrum (C), covered by numerous microorganisms including spirochetes (S) and rods (R). Bar = 1 μm.

tive tissue the vessels are dilated. They also proliferate to form granulation tissue, and the tissue is heavily infiltrated by leukocytes. As always in acute processes the inflammatory infiltrate is dominated by neutrophils (Figs. 10-15b & 10-16). In the deeper tissue, the inflammatory process also comprises large numbers of monocytes and plasma cells (Listgarten 1965, Heylings 1967).

MICROBIOLOGY

Microorganisms isolated from necrotizing lesions

Microbial samples from NPD lesions have demonstrated a constant and a variable part of the flora. The "constant flora" primarily contained *Treponema sp.,*

Selenomonas sp., *Fusobacterium sp.* and *B. melaninogenicus ssp. intermedius (P. intermedia)*, and the "variable flora" consisted of a heterogeneous array of bacterial types (Loesche et al. 1982). Although the characteristic bacterial flora of spirochetes and fusobacteria has been isolated in large numbers from the necrotic lesions in several studies, their presence is no evidence of a primary etiologic importance. Their presence could equally well result from secondary overgrowth. Moreover, the microorganisms associated with NG are also harbored by healthy mouths and mouths with gingivitis or periodontitis (Johnson & Engel 1986). An important role for *Treponema sp.* and *B. intermedius (P. intermedia)* has been suggested by studies of antibodies in NPD patients to such bacteria, compared to levels in age- and sex-matched controls with healthy gingiva or simple gingivitis (Chung et al. 1983).

There is little available information about the microbiology of HIV-associated NPD. *Borrelia*, Gram-positive cocci, β-hemolytic streptococci and *C. albicans* have been isolated from the lesions (Reichart & Schiødt 1989). It has also been proposed that human cytomegalovirus (HCMV) may play a role in the pathogenesis of NPD (Sabiston 1986). This virus has been found in the digestive tract of HIV-patients (Kanas et al. 1987, Langford et al. 1990), and a case of oral HCMV-infection with similarities of necrotizing periodontitis has been reported (Dodd et al. 1993). An increased frequency of HCMV and other herpes viruses found in necrotizing lesions among Nigerian children supports a contributory role of the viruses (Contreras et al. 1997), although it remains to be demonstrated in future studies whether cytomegalovirus does play a causal role.

Pathogenic potential of microorganisms

Our knowledge of the pathogenic mechanisms by which the bacterial flora produces the tissue changes characteristic of NPD is limited. One reason is that it has been difficult to establish an acceptable animal experimental model. However, several of the pathogenic mechanisms which have been associated with chronic gingivitis and periodontitis may also be of etiologic importance in the necrotizing forms of the diseases.

An important aspect in the pathogenesis of periodontitis is the capacity of the microorganisms to invade the host tissues. Among the bacteria isolated from necrotizing lesions, spirochetes and fusiform bacteria can in fact invade the epithelium (Heylings 1967). The spirochetes can also invade the vital connective tissue (Listgarten 1965). The pathogenic potential is further substantiated by the fact that both fusobacteria and spirochetes can liberate endotoxins (Mergenhagen et al. 1961, Kristoffersen & Hofstad 1970).

A number of observations indicate that the effects of endotoxins are more prominent in NPD than in chronic gingivitis and periodontitis. The large masses of Gram-negative bacteria liberate endotoxins in close contact with connective tissue. Endotoxins may produce tissue destruction both by direct toxic effects and indirectly, by activating and modifying tissue responses of the host (Wilton & Lehner 1980). Through a direct toxic effect, endotoxins may lead to damage of cells and vessels. Necrosis is a prominent feature in the so-called "Shwartzman reaction", which is caused by endotoxins. Indirectly, endotoxins can contribute to tissue damage in several ways: they can function as antigens and elicit immune reactions, they can activate complement directly through the alternative pathway and thereby liberate chemotoxins, but they can also activate macrophages, B and T-lymphocytes, and influence the host's immune reactions by interfering with cytokines produced by these cells. Studies have in fact shown that endotoxins can stimulate catabolic processes with degradation of both connective tissue and bone induced by the released cytokines. The extent to which such reactions contribute to host defense or to tissue damage is not yet known.

An aspect which has been of major concern, especially in wartime, is the communicability of the disease. Several reports have considered this aspect but it has been concluded that the necrotizing diseases are not transmissible by ordinary means of contact (Johnson & Engel 1986). Attempts to transmit the disease from one animal to another, or to produce necrotic lesions in experimental animals, have failed to yield conclusive results (MacDonald et al. 1963). Several suspect microorganisms and several combinations of microorganisms can produce similar lesions in experimental animals. A combination of four different bacteria, none of them fusobacteria or spirochetes, has been found to possess such properties and there are indications that among the four bacterial species, *Bacteroides melaninogenicus* was the true pathogen (MacDonald et al. 1956, 1963). *B. melaninogenicus* may, under certain conditions, produce an enzyme which degrades native collagen (Gibbons & MacDonald 1961). It is still not clear, however, whether this microorganism is of particular importance in the pathogenesis of NPD. NG lesions have also been induced in dogs pretreated with steroids and inoculated with a fusiform-spirochete culture from dogs which had gingival lesions similar to the NG lesions seen in humans (Mikx & van Campen 1982). The lesions produced in experimental animals may not be identical to those which occur in humans. It is also important to note that even if necrotic lesions can be transmitted by transmission of infectious material or bacterial cultures, this does not necessarily mean that the disease is truly contagious.

It is obvious from the above observations and assumptions that a fundamental question remains to be answered, and at this point it may be stated that the necrotizing periodontal diseases belong to those diseases to which Pasteur referred when he said: "there are some bacteria that cause a disease, but there are some diseases that bring about a condition that is ideal for the growth of some bacteria" (Wilson 1952). If the microorganisms mentioned above play a role in the etiology of the disease, then, presumably, the disease is an opportunistic infection. Consequently, the pathogenic characteristics of the microorganisms are normally overcome by the host defense, and disease occurs when the host defense is impaired. The isolated microorganisms do possess biologic activities which may contribute to the pathogenesis, but the exact role of the various microorganisms has not yet been clarified (Johnson & Engel 1986).

HOST RESPONSE AND PREDISPOSING FACTORS

It is particularly evident for HIV-infected patients that the disease is associated with diminished host resistance but among other predisposing factors, the basic mechanism may appear to include altered host immunity. Changes in leukocyte function and immune system have been observed in some studies, although the biologic reason for, and significance of, these findings are unclear (Johnson & Engel 1986).

Significantly increased IgG and IgM antibody titers to intermediate-sized spirochetes and higher IgG titers to *B. melaninogenicus* ssp *intermedius* have been found in NG patients as compared to age- and sex-matched healthy and gingivitis control groups (Chung et al. 1983). These results, however, are in disagreement with other data showing no differences in serum antibody levels to bacterial antigens (Wilton et al. 1971).

Total leukocyte counts have been found to be similar for patients and controls. NG patients, however, displayed marked depression in polymorphonuclear leukocyte chemotaxis and phagocytosis as compared with control individuals. Reduced mitogen-induced proliferation of peripheral blood lymphocytes has also been found in NG patients. It was suggested that elevated blood steroids may account for the reduced chemotactic and phagocytic responses (Cogen et al. 1983).

For many years it has been known that a number of predisposing factors may interact with the host defense systems and render the patient susceptible to NPD. Usually, a single one of these factors is not sufficient to establish disease. The various factors, which have been focused upon, comprise systemic diseases, including HIV infection and malnutrition, poor oral hygiene, preexisting gingivitis and history of previous NPD, psychologic stress and inadequate sleep, smoking and alcohol use, Caucasian background and young age.

A recent analysis of suspected predisposing factors among American patients with NPD has shown that HIV seropositivity overwhelmed all other factors in importance when present (Horning & Cohen 1995).

Among the HIV-seronegative patients the ranked importance of the predisposing factors was: History of previous NPD, poor oral hygiene, inadequate sleep, unusual psychologic stress, poor diet, recent illness, social or greater alcohol use, smoking, Caucasian background and age under 21 years. The various predisposing factors mentioned below are obviously not equally important in industrialized and developing countries, but many of these factors are known to relate to impaired immunity.

Systemic diseases

Systemic diseases which impair immunity predispose to NPD. This is why NPD occurs more frequently in HIV-infected individuals and in patients with other leukocyte diseases including leukemia (Melnick et al. 1988). Examples of other diseases predisposing to NPD are measles, chicken pox, tuberculosis, herpetic gingivostomatitis and malaria, but malnutrition is also important. Whereas these examples of predisposing factors are rare in western patients, they are evident in the developing countries, where they often predispose to NPD and noma in children (Emslie 1963, Pindborg et al. 1966, 1967, Sheiham 1966, Enwonwu 1972, 1985). It is important to note that NPD is sometimes an early signal of impending serious illness (Enwonwu 1972).

HIV infection

In Africa, the general population shows a high HIV-seropositive prevalence rate, ranging up to 33% in some populations. In Europe, prevalence figures have been established for areas in Great Britain. The prevalence figures in patients attending London hospitals were below 0.7% in 1994 (Unlinked Anonymous HIV Surveys Steering Group 1995). In the industrialized countries, a significant part of patients with NPD are HIV-infected patients, and no characteristics have been revealed that distinguish NPD in HIV-seropositive from that in HIV-seronegative patients. A history of frequent relapses and poor response to traditional or drug therapy may be suggestive (Greenspan et al. 1986, Horning & Cohen 1995). Suspicion of HIV infection is also supported by the simultaneous presence of oral candidosis, "hairy leukoplakia", or Kaposi's tumor, but these lesions are far from always present in HIV-infected patients.

HIV infection attacks the T-helper cells of the body, causing a drastic change in the T-helper(CD4+)/T-suppressor(CD8+) ratio with severe impairment of the host's resistance to infection. Depleted peripheral helper T-lymphocyte counts correlate closely with the occurrence of NG as demonstrated in a study of 390 US HIV-seropositive soldiers (Thompson et al. 1992). Furthermore, a complete absence of T-cells in gingival tissue of HIV-infected patients with periodontitis has been reported (Steidley et al. 1992). The lack of local immune effector and regulatory cells in HIV-seropositive patients could in fact explain the characteristic and rapidly progressive nature of periodontitis in these patients. Moreover, a protective effect against HIV-associated gingivitis and periodontitis has been encountered with antiviral treatment of the HIV infection (Masouredis et al. 1992). NP has been revealed as a marker for immune deterioration, with a 95% predictive value that CD4+ cell counts were below 200 cells/mm^3, and, if untreated, a cumulative probability of death within 24 months (Glick et al. 1994). As a consequence of this finding, if possible all NPD patients may be recommended to be given a test for HIV infection.

Malnutrition

In developing countries with malnutrition, this has often been mentioned as a predisposing factor to NPD (Enwonwu 1972, Osuji 1990). Malnutrition results in lowered resistance to infection and protein malnutrition has been emphasized as the most common public health problem affecting underprivileged Nigerian children who are most often affected by NPD (Enwonwu 1985, 1994). In response to periodontal pathogens, phagocytes elaborate destructive oxidants, proteinases and other factors. Periodontal damage may occur as the result of the balance between these factors, the antioxidants and host-derived antiproteinases. Malnutrition is characterized by marked tissue depletion of the key antioxidant nutrients, and impaired acute-phase protein response to infections. This is due to impairment in the production and cellular action of the cytokines. Other features of malnutrition include inverted helper/suppressor T-lymphocyte ratio, histaminemia, hormonal imbalance with increased blood and saliva levels of free cortisol, and defective mucosal integrity. Malnutrition usually involves concomitant deficiencies of several essential macro- and micronutrients, and therefore has the potential to adversely influence the prognosis of periodontal infections (Enwonwu 1994).

Poor oral hygiene, preexisting gingivitis and history of previous NPD

Many of the early studies of NPD showed that a low standard of oral hygiene contributed to the establishment of the disease (Johnson & Engel 1986). This has been supported by recent studies in the USA and Nigeria (Taiwo 1993, Horning & Cohen 1995). Consequently, NPD is usually established on the basis of preexisting chronic gingivitis (Pindborg 1951b). It should be emphasized, however, that plaque accumulation as seen in NPD patients may also be enhanced by the discomfort experienced with oral hygiene practices due to the disease.

Based on questionnaires and personal interviews, 28% of NPD patients have been found with a history of previous painful gingival infection and 21% had

gingival scars suggestive of previous NPD (Horning & Cohen 1995).

Psychologic stress and inadequate sleep

Just as other ulcerative gastrointestinal conditions have been shown to have psychogenic origins, psychologic stress has often and for many years been mentioned as a predisposing factor (Johnson & Engel 1986). Epidemiologic investigations seem to indicate a more frequent occurrence of necrotizing diseases in periods when the individuals are exposed to psychologic stress (Pindborg 1951a,b, Giddon et al. 1963, Goldhaber & Giddon 1964). New recruits and deploying military personnel, college students during examination periods, patients with depression or other emotional disorders and patients feeling inadequate to handle life situations are more susceptible to NPD (Pindborg 1951a,b, Moulton et al. 1952, Giddon et al. 1963, Cohen-Cole et al. 1983). Urine levels of corticosteroids have been used as a physiologic measure of stress, and increased free cortisol levels in the urine of NPD patients as compared with controls have been encountered. The NPD patients showed significantly higher levels of trait anxiety, depression and emotional disturbance than did control individuals (Cohen-Cole et al. 1983). The role of anxiety and psychologic stress in the pathogenesis of NG has been borne out by both psychiatric and biochemical investigations (Moulton et al. 1952, Shannon et al. 1969, Maupin & Bell 1975). There are several ways by which psychologic stress factors may interfere with host susceptibility. Host tissue resistance may be changed by mechanisms acting through the autonomic nervous system and endocrine glands resulting in elevation of corticosteroid and catecholamine levels. This may reduce gingival microcirculation and salivary flow and enhance nutrition of *Prevotella intermedia*, but also depress neutrophil and lymphocyte functions which facilitate bacterial invasion and damage (Johnson & Engel 1986, Horning & Cohen 1995).

Inadequate sleep, often as the result of lifestyle choices or job requirements, has been mentioned by many patients with NPD (Horning & Cohen 1995).

Smoking and alcohol use

Smoking has been listed as a predisposing factor to NPD for many years and presumably predisposes to other types of periodontitis as well (The American Academy of Periodontology 1996).

Two studies from the 1950s found that 98% of the patients were smokers (Pindborg 1951a, Goldhaber 1957). More recent data have confirmed this by finding only 6% non-smokers among NPD patients in contrast to 63% in a matched control group (Stevens et al. 1984). The amount smoked also appears important since 41% of subjects with NG smoked more than 20 cigarettes daily whereas only 5% of controls smoked that much (Goldhaber & Giddon 1964).

The relationship between tobacco usage and NPD appears to be complex. It has often been stated that smokers in general have poorer oral hygiene than non-smokers but studies have shown that there is little difference in the level of plaque accumulation in smokers versus non-smokers. Also, there have been no conclusive studies to show that smoking adversely affects periodontal tissues by altering the microbial composition of plaque (The American Academy of Periodontology 1996). Smoking could lead to increased disease activity by influencing host response and tissue reactions. As examples, smokers have depressed numbers of T-helper lymphocytes, and tobacco smoke can also impair chemotaxis and phagocytosis of oral and peripheral phagocytes (Eichel & Shahrik 1969, Kenney et al. 1977, Ginns et al. 1982, Costabel et al. 1986, Lannan et al. 1992, Selby et al. 1992). Among further effects of tobacco, nicotine-induced secretion of epinephrine resulting in gingival vasoconstriction has been proposed as one possible mechanism by which smoking may influence tissue susceptibility (Schwartz & Baumhammers 1972, Kardachi & Clarke 1974, Bergström & Preber 1986). The exact mechanism of tobacco smoking predisposing to NPD, however, remains to be determined.

Social or heavy drinking has been admitted by NPD patients and its role as a predisposing factor has been accounted for by its numerous physiologic effects which add to other factors as general sources of debilitation (Horning & Cohen 1995).

Caucasian background

A number of American studies have demonstrated a 95% preponderance of Caucasian patients with NPD including a study in which the referring population was 41% African-American (Barnes et al. 1973, Stevens et al. 1984, Horning & Cohen 1995), but a proportion of 49% of African-Americans in another study casts doubt on race as a predisposing factor alone, and the mechanism for this factor is unknown.

Young age

In industrialized countries, young adults appear to be the most predisposed to NPD. The disease can occur at any age, the reported mean age for NPD being between 22 and 24 years. This may reflect a number of factors such as military population age, wartime stress and probably is related to the involvement of other factors such as smoking (Horning & Cohen 1995).

TREATMENT

The treatment of the necrotizing periodontal diseases is divided into two phases: acute and maintenance phase treatment.

Acute phase treatment

The aim of the acute phase treatment is to eliminate disease activity as manifest by ongoing tissue necrosis developing laterally and apically. A further aim is to avoid pain and general discomfort which may severely compromise food intake. Among patients suffering from systemic diseases resulting in loss of weight, further weight loss due to reduced food intake should be avoided by rapid therapeutic intervention.

At the first consultation scaling should be attempted, as thoroughly as the condition allows. Ultrasonic scaling may be preferable to the use of hand instruments. With minimal pressure against the soft tissues, ultrasonic cleaning may accomplish the removal of soft and mineralized deposits. The continuous water spray combined with adequate suction usually allows good visibility. How far it is possible to proceed with debridement at the first visit usually depends on the patient's tolerance of pain during instrumentation. Obviously toothbrushing in areas with open wounds does not promote wound healing. Therefore, patients should be instructed in substituting toothbrushing with chemical plaque control in such areas until healing is accomplished.

Hydrogen peroxide and other oxygen-releasing agents also have a long-standing tradition in the initial treatment of NPD. Hydrogen peroxide (3%) is still used for debridement in necrotic areas and as a mouthrinse (equal portions 3% H_2O_2 and warm water). It has been thought that the apparently favorable effects of hydrogen peroxide may be due to mechanical cleaning, and the influence on anaerobic bacterial flora of the liberated oxygen (Wennström & Lindhe 1979, MacPhee & Cowley 1981).

Twice daily rinses with a 0.2% chlorhexidine solution is a very effective adjunct to reduce plaque formation, particularly when toothbrushing is not performed. It also assists self-performed oral hygiene during the first weeks of treatment. Its effect is discussed elsewhere in this book. For an optimal effect of this medicament, it should be used only in conjunction with and in addition to systematic scaling and root planing. The chlorhexidine solution does not penetrate subgingivally and the preparation is readily inactivated by exudates, necrotic tissues and masses of bacteria (Gjermo 1974). The effectiveness of chlorhexidine mouthrinses therefore is dependent upon a simultaneous, thorough mechanical, debridement.

In some cases of NPD the patient's response to debridement is minimal or the general health is affected to such an extent that the supplementary use of

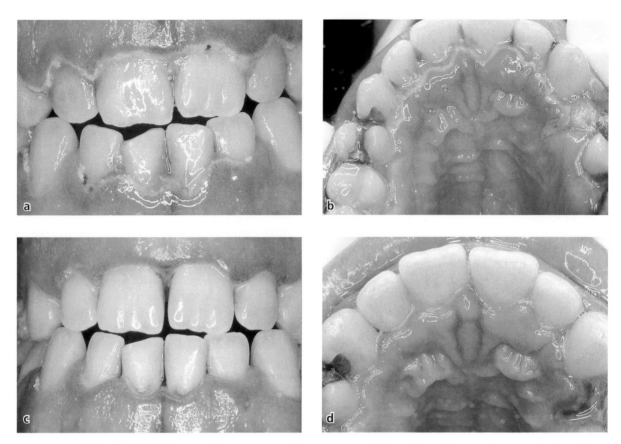

Fig. 10-17. Necrotizing periodontitis with severe pain. The entire gingival margin is the seat of a necrotic ulcer. (a) Facial aspect. (b) Palatal aspect. The patient was treated with scaling supplemented with metronidazole and the next day the patient was free of symptoms and the clinical features were significantly improved (c & d).

systemic antibiotics or chemotherapeutics is indicated. This also applies to patients with malaise, fever and lassitude. The choice of drug aims at a direct action on bacteria which are the cause of the inflammatory process in NPD.

Supplementary treatment with metronidazole 250 mg three times daily has been found effective against spirochetes and appears to be the first choice in the treatment of NPD (Proctor & Baker 1971, Shinn 1976, Loesche et al. 1982). The adjunctive use of metronidazole in HIV-associated NPD is reported to be extremely effective in reducing acute pain and promoting rapid healing (Scully et al. 1991). Acute pain usually disappears after a few hours (Figs. 10-17a-d).

Antibiotics such as penicillins and tetracyclines are also effective. Penicillin 1 mill i.u. three times daily should be used as an adjunct to scaling as for metronidazole until the ulcers are healed. Topical application of antibiotics is not indicated in the treatment of NPD, because intralesional bacteria are frequent, and topical application does not result in sufficient intralesional concentration of antibiotics.

It is important to emphasize that many HIV-seropositive patients with NPD at their initial visit are not aware of their serostatus. If HIV infection is a suspected predisposing factor, the patient can be referred to her or his physician for further examination. Some patients may prefer referral to a hospital department. Information on HIV-serostatus is frequently not available at initiation of therapy, but the lack of information has no serious implications for the choice of treatment or for the handling of the patient. As a consequence of a lack of information on HIV-serostatus of patients seeking dental treatment in general, all procedures in the dental office must always include precautions to protect against transmission of the virus to the dentist, to the dental auxiliaries and to other patients.

If the dentist asks the patient about his or her possible chance of having attracted HIV infection this should be done with great care, because HIV infection has serious implications for the patient. Consequently, a successful outcome depends on a confidential relationship between patient and dentist. In the case of a new patient, such a relationship is first established after at least a couple of appointments in the clinic.

Usually, in HIV-infected patients antibiotic prophylaxis in relation to scaling does not appear to be necessary. Bacteria recovered from venipuncture 15 min after scaling were not detectable in samples obtained at 30 min (Lucartoto et al. 1992). Neither does removal of sequestra always appear to require antibiotic cover (Robinson 1991). HIV-infected patients are susceptible to candidal infections (Holmstrup & Samaranayake 1990) and if oral candidosis is present or occurs throughout the period of antibiotic treatment, treatment with appropriate antimycotic drugs such as miconazole may be necessary.

Patients with NPD should be seen almost daily as

long as the acute symptoms persist. Appropriate treatment alleviates symptoms within a few days. Thereafter the patient should return in approximately 5 days. Systematic subgingival scaling should be continued with increasing intensity as the symptoms subside. Correction of restoration margins and polishing of restorations and root surfaces should be completed after healing of ulcers. When the ulcerated areas are healed, the local treatment is supplemented with oral hygiene instruction and patient motivation. Instruction in gentle but effective toothbrushing and approximal cleaning is mandatory. In many cases the extensive tissue destruction results in residual soft tissue defects that are difficult for the patient to keep clean. Oral hygiene in these areas often requires the use of interproximal devices and soft, smaller brushes. Sometimes healing is delayed in HIV-infected patients and intensive professional control may be necessary for prolonged periods of time.

Patients with NPD are not always easily motivated to carry out a proper program of oral hygiene. They frequently have poor oral hygiene habits and possibly a negative attitude to dental treatment in general. As a result, some patients discontinue treatment as soon as pain and other acute symptoms are alleviated. Motivation and instruction should be planned to prevent this happening, and should be reinforced during later visits. Patients with severely impaired immune functions, for instance due to HIV infection, may suffer from other infections or diseases during the period of treatment. This may complicate the treatment, because patients may be hospitalized.

Maintenance phase treatment

When the acute phase treatment has been completed, necrosis and acute symptoms in NPD have disappeared. The formerly necrotic areas are healed and the gingival craters are reduced in size, although some defects usually persist. In such areas bacterial plaque readily accumulates, and the craters, therefore, predispose to recurrence of NPD or to further destruction because of a persisting chronic inflammatory process, or both. These sites, therefore, may require surgical correction. Shallow craters can be removed by simple gingivectomy, while the elimination of deep defects may require flap surgery. Treatment of necrotizing gingivitis has not been completed until all gingival defects have been eliminated and optimal conditions for future plaque control have been established. If possible, elimination of predisposing factors is also very important to prevent recurrence. Due to delayed healing in HIV-infected patients, periodontal surgery is not recommended in these patients. Instead, intensive approximal cleaning is necessary to prevent recurrence of disease.

REFERENCES

The American Academy of Periodontology (1996). Tobacco use and the periodontal patient. *Journal of Periodontology* **67**, 51-56.

Barnes, G.P., Bowles, W.F. & Carter, H.G. (1973). Acute necrotizing ulcerative gingivitis: a survey of 218 cases. *Journal of Periodontology* **44**, 35-42.

Barr, C., Lopez, M.R. & Rua-Dobles, A. (1992). Periodontal changes by HIV serostatus in a cohort of homosexual and bisexual men. *Journal of Clinical Periodontology* **19**, 794-801.

Bergström, J. & Preber, H. (1986). The influence of cigarette smoking on the development of experimental gingivitis. *Journal of Periodontal Research* **21**, 668-676.

Chung, C.P., Nisengard, R.J., Slots, J. & Genco, R.J. (1983). Bacterial IgG and IgM antibody titers in acute necrotizing ulcerative gingivitis. *Journal of Periodontology* **54**, 557-562.

Cogen, R.B., Stevens, A.W.Jr., Cohen-Cole, S., Kirk, K. & Freeman, A. (1983). Leukocyte function in the etiology of acute necrotizing gingivitis. *Journal of Periodontology* **54**, 402-407.

Cohen-Cole, S.A., Cogen, R.B., Stevens, A.W.Jr., Kirk, K., Gaitan, E., Bird, J., Cooksey, A. & Freeman, A. (1983). Psychiatric, psychosocial and endocrine correlates of acute necrotizing ulcerative gingivitis (trench mouth): A preliminary report. *Psychiatric Medicine* **1**, 215-225.

Contreras, A., Falkler, W.A. Jr, Enwonwu, C.O., Idigbe, E.O., Savage, K.O., Afolabi, M.B., Onwujekwe, D., Rams, T.E. & Slots, J. (1997). Human Herpesviridae in acute necrotizing ulcerative gingivitis in children in Nigeria. *Oral Microbiology and Immunology* **12**, 259-265.

Costabel, U., Bross, K.J., Reuter, C., Rühle, K.H. & Matthys, H. (1986). Alterations in immunoregulatory T-cell subsets in cigarette smokers. A phenotypic analysis of bronchoalveolar and blood lymphocytes. *Chest* **90**, 39-44.

Dodd, C.L., Winkler, J.R., Heinic, G.S., Daniels, T.E., Yee, K. & Greenspan, D. (1993). Cytomegalovirus infection presenting as acute periodontal infection in a patient infected with the human immunodeficiency virus. *Journal of Clinical Periodontology* **20**, 282-285.

Drinkard, C.R., Decher, L., Little, J.W., Rhame, F.S., Balfour, H.H.Jr., Rhodus, N.L., Merry, J.W., Walker, P.O., Miller, C.E., Volberding, P.A. & Melnick, S.L. (1991). Periodontal status of individuals in early stages of human immunodeficiency virus infection. *Community Dentistry and Oral Epidemiology* **19**, 281-285.

Eichel, B. & Shahrik, H.A. (1969). Tobacco smoke toxicity: Loss of human oral leukocyte function and fluid cell metabolism. *Science* **166**, 1424-1428.

Emslie, R.D. (1963). Cancrum oris. *Dental Practitioner* **13**, 481-495.

Enwonwu, C.O. (1972). Epidemiological and biochemical studies of necrotizing ulcerative gingivitis and noma (cancrum oris) in Nigerian children. *Archives of Oral Biology* **17**, 1357-1371.

Enwonwu, C.O. (1985). Infectious oral necrosis (cancrum oris) in Nigerian children: a review. *Community Dentistry and Oral Epidemiology* **13**, 190-194.

Enwonwu, C.O. (1994). Cellular and molecular effects of malnutrition and their relevance to periodontal diseases. *Journal of Clinical Periodontology* **21**, 643-657.

Felix, D.H., Wray, D., Smith, G.L. & Jones, G.A. (1991). Oro-antral fistula: an unusual complication of HIV-associated periodontal disease. *British Dental Journal* **171**, 61-62.

Friedman, R.B., Gunsolley, J., Gentry, A., Dinius, A., Kaplowitz, L. & Settle, J. (1991). Periodontal status of HIV-seropositive and AIDS patients. *Journal of Periodontology* **62**, 623-627.

Gibbons, R.J. & MacDonald, J.B. (1961). Degradation of collagenous substrates by *Bacteroides melaninogenicus*. *Journal of Bacteriology* **81**, 614-621.

Giddon, D.B., Goldhaber, P. & Dunning, J.M. (1963). Prevalence of reported cases of acute necrotizing ulcerative gingivitis in a university population. *Journal of Periodontology* **34**, 366-371.

Giddon, D.B., Zackin, S.J. & Goldhaber, P. (1964). Acute necrotizing ulcerative gingivitis in college students. *Journal of the American Dental Association* **68**, 381-386.

Ginns, L.C., Goldenheim, P.D., Miller, L.G., Burton, R.C., Gillick, L., Colvin, R.B., Goldstein, G., Kung, P.C., Hurwitz, C. & Kazemi, H. (1982). T-lymphocyte subsets in smoking and lung cancer. Analyses of monoclonal antibodies and flow cytometry. *American Revue of Respiratory Diseases* **126**, 265-269.

Gjermo, P. (1974). Chlorhexidine in dental practice. *Journal of Clinical Periodontology* **1**, 143-152.

Glick, M., Muzyka, B.C., Salkin, L.M. & Lurie, D. (1994). Necrotizing ulcerative periodontitis: a marker for immune deterioration and a predictor for the diagnosis of AIDS. *Journal of Periodontology* **65**, 393-397.

Goldhaber, P. (1957). A study of acute necrotizing ulcerative gingivitis. *Journal of Dental Research* **35**, 18.

Goldhaber, P. & Giddon, D.B. (1964). Present concepts concerning the etiology and treatment of acute necrotizing ulcerative gingivitis. *International Dental Journal* **14**, 468-496.

Greenspan, D., Greenspan, J.S., Pindborg, J.J. & Schiödt, M. (1986). *Aids and the dental team*. Copenhagen: Munksgaard.

Grupe, H.E. & Wilder, L.S. (1956). Observations of necrotizing gingivitis in 870 military trainees. *Journal of Periodontology* **27**, 255-261.

Heylings, R.T. (1967). Electron microscopy of acute ulcerative gingivitis (Vincent's type). Demonstration of the fusospirochaetal complex of bacteria within prenecrotic gingival epithelium. *British Dental Journal* **122**, 51-56.

Holmstrup, P. & Samaranayake, L.P. (1990). Acute and AIDS-related oral candidoses. In: Samaranayake, L.P. & MacFarlane, T.W., eds. *Oral candidosis*. London: Wright, pp. 133-156.

Holmstrup, P. & Westergaard, J. (1994). Periodontal diseases in HIV-infected patients. *Journal of Clinical Periodontology* **21**, 270-280.

Horning, G.M. & Cohen, M.E. (1995). Necrotizing ulcerative gingivitis, periodontitis, and stomatitis: Clinical staging and predisposing factors. *Journal of Periodontology* **66**, 990-998.

Horning, G.M., Hatch, C.L. & Lutskus, J. (1990). The prevalence of periodontitis in a military treatment population. *Journal of the American Dental Association* **121**, 616-622.

Jiménez, M.L. & Baer, P.N. (1975). Necrotizing ulcerative gingivitis in children: a 9-year clinical study. *Journal of Periodontology* **46**, 715-720.

Johnson, B.D. & Engel, D. (1986). Acute necrotizing ulcerative gingivitis. A review of diagnosis, etiology and treatment. *Journal of Periodontology* **57**, 141-150.

Kanas, R.J., Jensen, J.L., Abrams, A.M. & Wuerker, R.B. (1987). Oral mucosal cytomegalovirus as a manifestation of the acquired immune deficiency syndrome. *Oral Surgery, Oral Medicine, Oral Pathology* **64**, 183-189.

Kardachi, B.J. & Clarke, N.G. (1974). Aetiology of acute necrotizing ulcerative gingivitis: A hypothetical explanation. *Journal of Periodontology* **45**, 830-832.

Kenney, E.B., Kraal, J.H., Saxe, S.R. & Jones, J. (1977). The effect of cigarette smoke on human oral polymorphonuclear leukocytes. *Journal of Periodontal Research* **12**, 227-234.

King, J.D. (1943). Nutritional and other factors in "trench mouth" with special reference to the nicotinic acid component of the vitamin B2 complex. *British Dental Journal* **74**, 113-122.

Klotz, H. (1973). Differentiation between necrotic ulcerative gingivitis and primary herpetic gingivostomatitis. *New York State Dental Journal* **39**, 283-294.

Kristoffersen, T. & Hofstad, T. (1970). Chemical composition of lipopolysaccharide endotoxins from oral fusobacteria. *Archives of Oral Biology* **15**, 909-916.

Langford, A., Kunze, R., Timm, H., Ruf, B. & Reichart, P. (1990).

Cytomegalovirus associated oral ulcerations in HIV-infected patients. *Journal of Oral Pathology & Medicine* **19**, 71-76.

Lannan, S., McLean, A., Drost, E., Gilloly, M., Donaldson, K., Lamb, D. & MacNee, W. (1992). Changes in neutrophil morphology and morphometry following exposure to cigarette smoke. *International Journal of Experimental Pathology* **73**, 183-191.

Listgarten, M.A. (1965). Electron microscopic observations on the bacterial flora of acute necrotizing ulcerative gingivitis. *Journal of Periodontology* **36**, 328-339.

Loesche, W.J., Syed, S.A., Laughon, B.E. & Stoll, J. (1982). The bacteriology of acute necrotizing ulcerative gingivitis. *Journal of Periodontology* **53**, 223-230.

Lucartoto, F.M., Franker, C.K. & Maza, J. (1992). Postscaling bacteremia in HIV-associated gingivitis and periodontitis. *Oral Surgery, Oral Medicine, Oral Pathology* **73**, 550-554.

MacCarthy, D. & Claffey, N. (1991). Acute necrotizing ulcerative gingivitis is associated with attachment loss. *Journal of Clinical Periodontology* **18**, 776-779.

MacDonald, J.B., Sutton, R.M., Knoll, M.L., Medlener, E.M. & Grainger, R.M. (1956). The pathogenic components of an experimental fusospirochaetal infection. *Journal of Infectious Diseases* **98**, 15-20.

MacDonald, J.B., Socransky, S.S. & Gibbons, R.J. (1963). Aspects of the pathogenesis of mixed anaerobic infections of mucous membranes. *Journal of Dental Research* **42**, 529-544.

MacPhee, T. & Cowley, G. (1981). *Essentials of periodontology*, 3rd edn. Oxford: Blackwell Science, pp. 157-177.

Masouredis, C.M., Katz, M.H., Greenspan, D., Herrera, C., Hollander, H., Greenspan, J.S. & Winkler, J.R. (1992). Prevalence of HIV-associated periodontitis and gingivitis and gingivitis in HIV-infected patients attending an AIDS clinic. *Journal of Acquired Immune Deficiency Syndromes* **5**, 479-483.

Maupin, C.C. & Bell, W.B. (1975). The relationship of 17-hydroxycorticosteroid to acute necrotizing ulcerative gingivitis. *Journal of Periodontology* **46**, 721-722.

Melnick, S.L., Roseman, J.M., Engel, D. & Cogen, R.B. (1988). Epidemiology of acute necrotizing ulcerative gingivitis. *Epidemiologic Reviews* **10**, 191-211.

Mergenhagen, S.E., Hampp, E.G. & Scherp, H.W. (1961). Preparation and biological activities of endotoxin from oral bacteria. *Journal of Infectious Diseases* **108**, 304-310.

Migliani, D.C. & Sharma, O.P. (1965). Incidence of acute necrotizing gingivitis and periodontosis among cases seen at the Government Hospital, Madras. *Journal of All India Dental Association* **37**, 183.

Mikx, F.H. & van Campen, G.J. (1982). Microscopical evaluation of the microflora in relation to necrotizing ulcerative gingivitis in the beagle dog. *Journal of Periodontal Research* **17**, 576-584.

Moulton, R., Ewen, S. & Thieman, W. (1952). Emotional factors in periodontal disease. *Oral Surgery, Oral Medicine, Oral Pathology* **5**, 833-860.

Osuji, O.O. (1990). Necrotizing ulcerative gingivitis and cancrum oris (noma) in Ibadan, Nigeria. *Journal of Periodontology* **61**, 769-772.

Pickard, H.M. (1973). Historical aspects of Vincent's disease. *Proceedings of the Royal Society of Medicine* **66**, 695-698.

Pindborg, J.J. (1951a). Gingivitis in military personnel with special reference to ulceromembranous gingivitis. *Odontologisk Revy* **59**, 407-499.

Pindborg, J.J. (1951b). Influence of service in armed forces on incidence of gingivitis. *Journal of the American Dental Association* **42**, 517-522.

Pindborg, J.J., Bhat, M., Devanath, K.R., Narayana, H.R. & Ramachandra, S. (1966). Occurrence of acute necrotizing gingivitis in South Indian children. *Journal of Periodontology* **37**, 14-19.

Pindborg, J.J., Bhat, M. & Roed-Petersen, B. (1967). Oral changes in South Indian children with severe protein deficiency. *Journal of Periodontology* **38**, 218-221.

Proctor, D.B. & Baker, C.G. (1971). Treatment of acute necrotizing ulcerative gingivitis with metronidazole. *Journal of the Canadian Dental Association* **37**, 376-380.

Reichart, P.A. & Schiødt, M. (1989). Non-pigmented oral Kaposi's sarcoma (AIDS): report of two cases. *International Journal of Oral & Maxillofacial Surgery* **18**, 197-199.

Riley, C., London, J.P. & Burmeister, J.A. (1992). Periodontal health in 200 HIV-positive patients. *Journal of Oral Pathology & Medicine* **21**, 124-127.

Robinson, P. (1991). The management of HIV. *British Dental Journal* **170**, 287.

Sabiston, C.B. Jr. (1986). A review and proposal for the etiology of acute necrotizing gingivitis. *Journal of Clinical Periodontology* **13**, 727-734.

SanGiacomo, T.R., Tan, P.M., Loggi, D.G. & Itkin, A.B. (1990). Progressive osseous destruction as a complication to HIV-periodontitis. *Oral Surgery, Oral Medicine, Oral Pathology* **70**, 476-479.

Schwartz, D.M. & Baumhammers, A. (1972). Smoking and periodontal disease. *Periodontal Abstracts* **20**, 103-106.

Scully, C., Laskaris, G., Pindborg, J J., Porter, S.R. & Reichardt, P. (1991). Oral manifestations of HIV infection and their management. I. More common lesions. *Oral Surgery, Oral Medicine, Oral Pathology* **71**, 158-166.

Selby, C., Drost, E., Brown, D., Howie, S & MacNee, W. (1992). Inhibition of neutrophil adherence and movement by acute cigarette smoke exposure. *Experimental Lung Research* **18**, 813-827.

Shannon, I.L., Kilgore, W.G. & O'Leary, T.J. (1969). Stress as a predisposing factor in necrotizing ulcerative gingivitis. *Journal of Periodontology* **40**, 240-242.

Sheiham, A. (1966). An epidemiological survey of acute ulcerative gingivitis in Nigerians. *Archives of Oral Biology* **11**, 937-942.

Shields, W.D. (1977). Acute necrotizing ulcerative gingivitis. A study of some of the contributing factors and their validity in an army population. *Journal of Periodontology* **48**, 346-349.

Shinn, D.L. (1976). Vincent's disease and its treatment. In: *Metronidazole*. Proceedings of the International Metronidazole Conference. pp. 334-340. Montreal, Quebec, Canada, May 26-28.

Stammers, A. (1944). Vincent's infection observations and conclusions regarding the etiology and treatment of 1017 civilian cases. *British Dental Journal* **76**, 147-209.

Steidley, K.E., Thompson, S.H., McQuade, M.J., Strong, S.L., Scheidt, M.J. & van Dyke, T.E. (1992). A comparison of T4:T8 lymphocyte ratio in the periodontal lesion of healthy and HIV-positive patients. *Journal of Periodontology* **63**, 753-756.

Stevens, A. Jr., Cogen, R.B., Cohen-Cole, S. & Freeman, A. (1984). Demographic and clinical data associated with acute necrotizing ulcerative gingivitis in a dental school population (ANUG-demographic and clinical data). *Journal of Clinical Periodontology* **11**, 487-493.

Taiwo, J.O. (1993). Oral hygiene status and necrotizing ulcerative gingivitis in Nigerian children. *Journal of Periodontology* **64**, 1071-1074.

Thompson, S.H., Charles, G.A. & Craig, D.B. (1992). Correlation of oral disease with the Walter Reed staging scheme for HIV-1-seropositive patients. *Oral Surgery, Oral Medicine, Oral Pathology* **73**, 289-292.

Vincent, H. (1898). Sur une forme particulière d'engine différoide (engine à bacilles fusiformes). *Archives Internationales de Laryngologie* **11**, 44-48.

Wennström, J. & Lindhe, J. (1979). Effect of hydrogen peroxide on developing plaque and gingivitis in man. *Journal of Clinical Periodontology* **6**, 115-130.

Williams, C.A., Winkler, J.R., Grassi, M. & Murray, P.A. (1990). HIV-associated periodontitis complicated by necrotizing stomatitis. *Oral Surgery, Oral Medicine, Oral Pathology* **69**, 351-355.

Wilson, J.R. (1952). Etiology and diagnosis of bacterial gingivitis including Vincent's disease. *Journal of the American Dental Association* **44**, 19-52.

Wilton, J.M.A., Ivanyi, L. & Lehner, T. (1971). Cell-mediated immunity and humoral antibodies in acute ulcerative gingivitis. *Journal of Periodontal Research* **6**, 9-16.

Wilton, J.M.A. & Lehner, T. (1980). Immunological and microbial aspects of periodontal disease. In: Thompson, R.A., ed. *Recent advances in clinical immunology*, No. 2. Edinburgh: Churchill Livingstone, pp. 145-181.

Chapter 11

The Periodontal Abscess

Mariano Sanz, David Herrera and Arie J. van Winkelhoff

Classification

Prevalence

Pathogenesis and histopathology

Microbiology

Diagnosis

Treatment

Complications

Odontogenic abscesses include a broad group of acute infections that originate from the tooth and/or the periodontium. Such abscesses are associated with an array of symptoms, including a localized purulent inflammation in the periodontal tissues that causes pain and swelling. Abscesses are one of the main causes of patients to seek emergency care in the dental clinic. Depending on the origin of the infection the lesions can be classified as *periapical*, *periodontal* and *pericoronary* abscesses.

CLASSIFICATION

Different classifications have been proposed for periodontal abscesses: *chronic* or *acute*, *single* or *multiple*, *gingival* or *periodontal*, occurring in the supporting periodontal tissues or in the gingiva. A recent proposed classification (Meng 1999) included *gingival abscesses* (in previously healthy sites and caused by impaction of foreign bodies), *periodontal abscesses* (either acute or chronic, in relation to a periodontal pocket), and *pericoronal abscesses* (at incompletely erupted teeth).

The most rational classification is the one based on etiological criteria. Depending on the cause of the acute infectious process, two types of periodontal abscesses may occur:

- *Periodontitis-related abscess*, when the acute infection originates from a biofilm present in a deepened periodontal pocket
- *Non-periodontitis-related abscess*, when the acute infection originates from another local source, such as foreign body impaction or alterations in root integrity.

Periodontitis-related abscess

In a periodontitis patient a periodontal abscess represents a period of active periodontal tissue breakdown and is the result of an extension of the infection into the still intact periodontal tissues. This abscess formation is usually due to the marginal closure of a deep periodontal pocket and lack of proper drainage. Therefore, the existence of deep, tortuous pockets and deep concavities associated with furcation lesions may favor the formation of the acute condition. Once the acute inflammatory process is started, there is a local accumulation of neutrophils, tissue breakdown will occur and pus will be formed. The retention of pus in the pocket may further compromise the drainage and the lesion may rapidly progress into deeper parts of the periodontium. There are different mechanisms behind the formation of a periodontitis-related abscess:

Exacerbation of a chronic lesion
Such abscesses may develop in a deepened periodontal pocket without any obvious external influence, and may occur in: (1) an untreated periodontitis patient, or (2) as a recurrent infection during supportive periodontal therapy.

Post-therapy periodontal abscesses
There are various reasons why an abscess may occur during the course of active therapy:

- *Post-scaling periodontal abscess*. When these lesions occur immediately after scaling or after a routine professional prophylaxis, they are usually related to the presence of small fragments of remaining calculus that obstruct the pocket entrance once the edema in the gingiva has disappeared (Dello Russo 1985,

Carranza 1990). This type of abscess formation can also occur when small fragments of calculus have been forced into the deep, previously non-inflamed portion of the periodontal tissues (Dello Russo 1985).

- *Post-surgery periodontal abscess*. When an abscess occurs immediately following periodontal surgery, it is often the result of an incomplete removal of subgingival calculus or to the presence of foreign bodies in the periodontal tissues, such as sutures, regenerative devices or periodontal pack (Garrett et al. 1997).

- *Post-antibiotic periodontal abscess*. Treatment with systemic antibiotics without subgingival debridement in patients with advanced periodontitis may also cause abscess formation (Helovuo & Paunio 1989, Topoll et al. 1990, Helovuo et al. 1993). In such patients, the microbiota in the subgingival biofilm may be protected from the antibiotic, a super infection may result and massive inflammation occur. Helovou et al. (1993) followed patients with untreated periodontitis who were given broad-spectrum antibiotics (penicillin, erythromycin) for non-oral reasons. They showed that 42% of these patients developed marginal abscesses within 4 weeks of antibiotic therapy.

Non-periodontitis-related abscess

The formation of this type of abscess may also occur in relation to a periodontal pocket, but in such cases there is always an external local factor that explains the acute inflammation. Such factors include:

- Impaction of foreign body in the gingival sulcus or periodontal pocket. It may be related to oral hygiene practices (toothbrush, toothpicks, etc.) (Gillette & Van House 1980, Abrams & Kopczyk 1983), orthodontic devices, food particles, etc.
- Root morphology alterations. In this instance local anatomical factors, such as an invaginated root (Chen et al. 1990), a fissured root (Goose 1981), an external root resorption, root tears (Haney et al. 1992, Ishikawa et al. 1996) or iatrogenic endodontic perforations (Abrams et al. 1992), may be the cause of the abscess formation.

PREVALENCE

The prevalence of periodontal abscesses was studied in emergency dental clinics (Ahl et al. 1986, Galego-Feal et al. 1996), in general dental clinics (Lewis et al. 1990), in periodontitis patients before treatment (Gray et al. 1994), and in periodontitis patients during supportive periodontal therapy (SPT) (Kaldahl et al. 1996, McLeod et al. 1997).

Among all dental conditions in need of emergency treatment, periodontal abscesses represent between 8% and 14% (Ahl et al. 1986, Galego-Feal et al. 1996). Gray et al. (1994) monitored periodontal patients in an army clinic and found that periodontal abscesses had a prevalence of 27.5%. In this population, 13.5% of the patients undergoing active periodontal treatment had experienced abscess formation, while untreated patients showed a higher figure, 59.7%. McLeod et al. (1997) followed 114 patients in SPT and identified 42 patients (27.5%) that had suffered from acute episodes of periodontal abscess.

In a prospective longitudinal treatment study, by Kaldahl et al. (1996), the occurrence of periodontal abscesses during 7 years of periodontal maintenance was also studied. From the 51 patients included, 27 abscesses were detected; 23 of the abscesses occurred at teeth in quadrants treated only by coronal scaling, 3 in areas treated by root planing, and only 1 in areas treated by surgical means; 16 out of the 27 abscess sites had an initial probing pocket depth > 6 mm, while in 8 sites the probing depth was 5-6 mm.

Abscesses often occur in molar sites, and molars represent more than 50% of all cases of abscess formation (Smith & Davies 1986, McLeod et al. 1997, Herrera et al 2000b). The most likely reason for this high prevalence of abscesses in molars could be lesions involving the furcation and the complex root morphology of such teeth.

The occurrence of a periodontal abscess may be important not only because of its relatively high prevalence, but also because of how this acute infection may influence the prognosis of the affected tooth. Since abscesses sometimes develop during SPT in teeth with remaining deep periodontal pockets and teeth with a reduced amount of periodontal support left, the additional periodontal destruction that occurs during the abscess development may call for tooth extraction (Chace & Low 1993, McLeod et al. 1997).

PATHOGENESIS AND HISTOPATHOLOGY

A periodontal abscess contains bacteria, bacterial products, inflammatory cells, tissue breakdown products and serum. Tissue destruction is mainly caused by the inflammatory cells and their extracellular enzymes. The precise pathogenesis of the periodontal abscess is still not known. It is believed that a periodontal abscess is formed by occlusion or trauma to the orifice of the periodontal pocket, resulting in extension of the infection from the pocket into the soft tissues of the pocket wall. An inflammatory infiltrate is formed followed by destruction of the connective tissues, encapsulation of the bacterial mass and pus formation. The lowered tissue resistance and the virulence as well as the number of bacteria present determine the course of the infection. The entry of bacteria

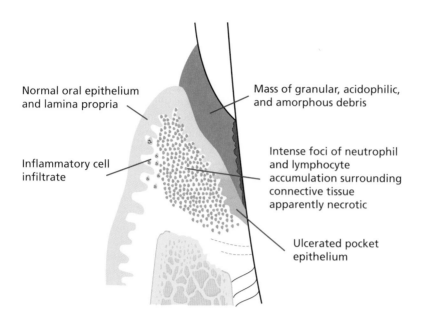

Normal oral epithelium and lamina propria

Inflammatory cell infiltrate

Mass of granular, acidophilic, and amorphous debris

Intense foci of neutrophil and lymphocyte accumulation surrounding connective tissue apparently necrotic

Ulcerated pocket epithelium

Fig. 11-1. Schematic drawing showing the histopathology of a periodontal abscess.

into the soft tissue pocket wall could be the event that initiates the formation of a periodontal abscess.

Histologically, neutrophils are found in the central area of the abscess and close to soft tissue debris. At a later stage, a pyogenic membrane, composed of macrophages and neutrophils, is organized. The rate of tissue destruction within the lesion will depend on the growth of bacteria inside the foci and their virulence, as well as on the local pH. An acidic environment will favor the activity of lysosomal enzymes and promote tissue destruction (DeWitt et al. 1985).

De Witt et al. (1985) studied biopsies sampled from 12 abscesses. The biopsies were taken immediately apical to the center of the abscess and processed for histological examination. They observed that the sites examined had a normal oral epithelium and lamina propria, but an inflammatory cell infiltrate resided lateral to the pocket epithelium. There were foci of neutrophil and lymphocyte accumulations in areas characterized by massive tissue destruction and a mass of granular, acidophilic and amorphous debris present in the pocket (see Fig. 11-1). In seven out of nine biopsies evaluated by electron-microscopy, Gram-negative bacteria were seen invading both the pocket epithelium and the compromised connective tissue.

MICROBIOLOGY

In review articles it was pointed out that purulent oral infections often are poly-microbial, and are caused by endogenous bacteria (Tabaqhali, 1988). However, very few studies have investigated the specific microbiota of periodontal abscesses. Newman & Sims (1979) studied nine abscesses and found that 63.1% of the microbiota was comprised of strict anaerobes. Topoll et al. (1990) analysed 20 abscesses in 10 patients who had taken antibiotics prior to the study. They reported

that 59.5% of the microbiota was made up of strict anaerobes. Herrera et al. (2000b) reported that 45.1% of the bacteria in the abscess material included anaerobes.

The microbiota of the periodontal abscess resembles the microbiota of chronic periodontitis lesions. The microflora found in periodontal abscesses is polymicrobial, dominated by non-motile, Gram-negative, strict anaerobic, rod-shaped species. From this group, *Porphyromonas gingivalis* is probably the most virulent. The occurrence of *P. gingivalis* in periodontal abscesses ranges from 50-100% (Newman & Sims 1979, Van Winkelhoff et al. 1985, Topoll et al. 1990, Hafström et al. 1994, Herrera et al. 2000b). Using a polymerase chain reaction technique, Ashimoto et al. (1998) found *P. gingivalis* in all of the seven cases of abscesses they investigated. Other anaerobic species that can be found include *Prevotella intermedia*, *Prevotella melaninogenica*, *Fusobacterium nucleatum* and *Bacteriodes forsythus*. Spirochetes (*Treponema* species) are also found in most cases (Ashimoto et al. 1998). The majority of the Gram-negative anaerobic species are non-fermentative and display moderate to strong proteolytic activity. Strict anaerobic, Gram-positive bacterial species in periodontal abscesses include *Peptostreptococcus micros*, *Actinomyces* spp. and *Bifidobacterium* spp. Facultative anaerobic Gram-negative bacteria that can be isolated from periodontal abscesses include *Campylobacter* spp., *Capnocytophaga* spp. and *Actinobacillus actinomycetemcomitans* (Hafström et al. 1994).

DIAGNOSIS

The diagnosis of a periodontal abscess should be based on the overall evaluation and interpretation of the patient's chief complaint, together with the clinical

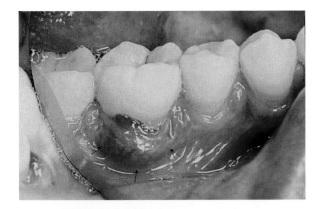

Fig. 11-2. Periodontal abscess (arrows) associated with a lower right first molar. Observe the association between the abscess formation and the furcation lesion in this molar.

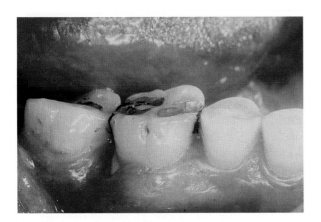

Fig. 11-3. Periodontal abscess associated with a lower second molar. Observe the diffuse swelling affecting all the buccal gingiva of the molar.

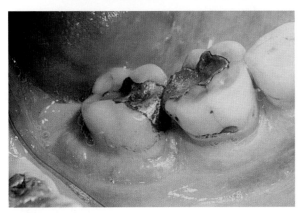

Fig. 11-4. Periodontal abscess associated with the distal surface of a lower right first molar. Observe the spontaneous suppuration expressed through the gingival pocket at the distal surface.

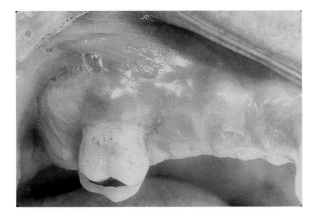

Fig. 11-5. Periodontal abscess associated with an upper right third molar. Observe how this lesion is associated with tooth extrusion and the tooth exhibits an increased mobility.

and radiological signs found during the oral examination.

The most prominent symptom of a periodontal abscess is the presence of an ovoid elevation of the gingiva along the lateral side of the root (Fig. 11-2).

Abscesses located deep in the periodontium may be less easy to identify by the swelling of the soft tissue and may present as diffuse swellings or simply as a red area (Fig. 11-3). Another common finding is suppuration, either from a fistula or, most commonly,

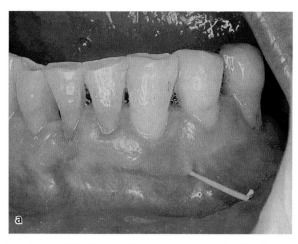 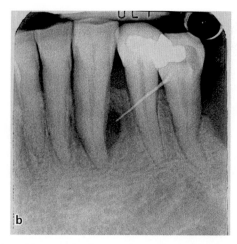

Fig. 11-6. (a) Periodontal abscess associated with a lower left canine. Observe the fistulous tract opening demonstrated with a gutta-percha point. (b) Radiological image of the lower canine from (a). The differential diagnosis with a periapical abscess was done by the positive tooth vitality sign and absence of caries or restoration in the canine, and the presence of a deep periodontal pocket in the lingual aspect of this tooth.

from the pocket (Fig. 11-4). This suppuration may be spontaneous or occur after pressure on the outer surface of the gingiva. The clinical symptoms usually include pain (from light discomfort to severe pain), tenderness of the gingiva, swelling and sensitivity to percussion of the affected tooth. Other related symptoms are tooth elevation and increased tooth mobility (Fig. 11-5).

During the periodontal examination, the abscess is usually found at a site with a deep periodontal pocket. Signs associated with periodontitis such as bleeding on probing, suppuration and sometimes increased tooth mobility are also present (Smith & Davies 1986, Hafström et al. 1994, Herrera et al. 2000b). The radiographic examination may either reveal a normal appearance of the interdental bone, or some bone loss, ranging from a widening of the periodontal ligament space to pronounced bone loss involving most of the affected tooth (Fig. 11-6a,b).

In some patients the occurrence of a periodontal abscess may be associated with elevated body temperature, malaise and regional lymphadenopathy (Smith & Davies 1986, Carranza, 1990, Ibbott et al. 1993, Herrera et al. 2000b). Herrera et al (2000b) provided laboratory data from blood and urine of patients immediately after a periodontal abscess had been identified, and reported that in 30% of the patients there was an elevated number of blood leukocytes. The absolute number of blood neutrophils and monocytes was also enhanced in 20-40% of the patients.

Differential diagnosis

The differential diagnosis of periodontal abscesses should always be made with other abscesses that can occur in the oral cavity. Acute infections, such as periapical abscesses, lateral periapical cysts, vertical root fractures and endo-periodontal abscesses, may have a similar appearance and symptomatology as a periodontal abscess, although with a clearly different etiology. Signs such as lack of pulp vitality, the presence of deep caries lesions, the presence of a sinus tract and findings made in the radiographic examination, will aid in the distinction between abscesses of different etiologies.

Other lesions may appear in the oral cavity with a similar appearance to a periodontal abscess. Parrish et al. (1989) described three cases of osteomyelitis in periodontitis patients, initially diagnosed as periodontal abscess. Also, different tumors may have the appearance of a periodontal abscess. Such tumors include gingival squamous cell carcinoma (Torabinejad & Rick 1980, Kirkham et al. 1985), a metastatic carcinoma from pancreatic origin (Selden et al. 1998) and an eosinophilic granuloma diagnosed by rapid bone destruction after periodontal therapy (Girdler 1991). A pathologic anatomic diagnosis must be made if the abscess fails to respond to conventional therapy (see also Chapter 12).

Treatment

The treatment of the periodontal abscess usually includes two stages: (1) the management of the acute lesion, and (2) the appropriate treatment of the original and/or residual lesion, once the emergency situation has been controlled. For the treatment of the acute lesion, alternatives were proposed, such as: (1) incision and drainage, (2) scaling and root planing, (3) periodontal surgery, (4) the use of different systemically administered antibiotics, and (5) tooth extraction.

Although some authors have recommended a pure mechanical treatment including surgical drainage through the pocket, or scaling and planing of the root surface and compression and debridement of the soft

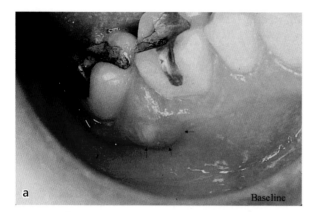
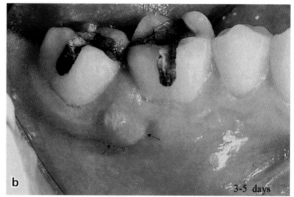
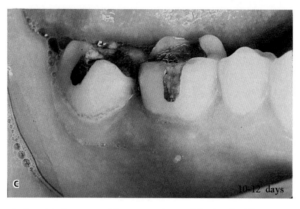

Fig. 11-7. (a) Treatment of a periodontal abscess with systemic antibiotics (azithromycin, 500 mg, 3 days) without any mechanical therapy. Baseline situation. (b) 5 days after antibiotic therapy. (c) 12 days after antibiotic therapy, immediately before the final periodontal instrumentation.

tissue wall (Ahl et al. 1986, Ammons 1996), this purely mechanical treatment may cause irreversible damage to healthy periodontal tissues adjacent to the lesion. Such damage may occur in particular when the swelling is diffuse or is associated with marked tissue tension.

In order to avoid damage to healthy periodontal tissue it is recommended to use systemically administered antibiotics as the only initial treatment in abscesses with marked swelling, tension and pain. In such instances, once the acute condition has receded, mechanical debridement, including root planing, is performed. The effect of treatment of abscesses has been determined in only a few studies. Smith and Davies (1986) studied 62 abscesses in 55 patients. Their proposed treatment included incision, drainage and systemic metronidazole (200 mg, tid, 5 days) and after the acute phase, regular periodontal treatment. Hafström et al. (1994) recommended drainage, irrigation and supragingival debridement, together with systemic tetracycline therapy for 2 weeks. Similar good treatment outcomes were obtained in a recent controlled parallel study in which two systemic antibiotic regimes (amoxicillin/clavulanate, 500+125 mg, tid, 8 days; and azithromycin, 500 mg, once per day, 3 days) were used as the only measure during the phase of initial therapy. This was followed by regular periodontal treatment once the acute phase was resolved

(Herrera et al. 2000c). The study showed that the infectious process in the acute periodontal abscess was controlled by means of systemic antibiotics without concomitant or prior debridement (Fig. 11-7a,b,c). The short-term clinical outcome with the use of both antibiotics regimens was successful. There was a rapid control of the pain levels, significant reduction in the edema, redness and swelling, and further the suppuration was almost entirely eradicated. Periodontal parameters, such as bleeding and periodontal probing depth, were also significantly reduced. Short-term microbiological results demonstrated a reduction of the microbiota in the abscess, as well as the number of selected periodontal pathogens (Herrera et al. 2000c). However, none of the antibiotic therapies were able to entirely resolve the infection. This implies that mechanical debridement, sometimes including surgical means, is an essential measure in the definitive treatment of a periodontal abscess.

Table 11-1 shows a number of different antibiotics that may be used in the treatment of a periodontal abscess. Doses and regimes recommended may differ between different countries. In principle, a high dose of the antibiotic delivered during a short period of time, is recommended. If the patient is recovering properly, the antibiotic regimen may not be extended over a 5-day period.

Table 11-1. Antimicrobial agents that may be used in the treatment of periodontal abscesses

Antimicrobial agent	Effective against	Properties
Penicillin V	Streptococci, some strict anaerobes	Poorly absorbed, affected by β-lactamases, bactericidal
Amoxicillin	Most Gram-positive oral species, many Gram-negative	Well absorbed, affected by β-lactamases but can be protected by clavulanic acid, bactericidal
Cephalexin	Anaerobes streptococci, strict anaerobes, facultative	Well absorbed, affected by β-lactamases, not against meticillin-resistant staphylococci, bactericidal
Ceftibuten	Gram-negative rods broad spectrum against Gram-negative and positive bacteria	Resistent to most β-lactamases, bactericidal, not effective against staphylococci, pseudomonads
Clindamycin	Gram-positive cocci including staphylococci	Bacteriostatic or bactericidal depending on local concentration and susceptibility of the pathogen, drug of choice in case of rapid local spread
Metronidazole	Gram-positive and negative anaerobes	Well absorbed, not effective against facultative bacteria, bactericidal
Azithromycin	Most anaerobes Gram-positive and negative bacteria, many strict anaerobes	Good tissue concentration, bacteriostatic for most pathogens

COMPLICATIONS

Tooth loss

Periodontal abscesses have been suggested as the main cause for tooth extraction during the phase of supportive periodontal therapy (SPT) (Chace & Low 1993). A tooth with a history of repeated abscess formation is considered as a tooth with a questionable prognosis (Becker et al. 1984). In a retrospective study, 45% of teeth with periodontal abscesses in a SPT population were extracted (McLeod et al. 1997). Another retrospective study including 455 teeth with a questionable prognosis, showed that 55 (12%) were lost after a mean of 8.8 years, and that the main reason for tooth extraction was periodontal abscess formation (Chace & Low 1993). Smith & Davies (1986) evaluated 62 teeth with abscesses; 14 (22.6%) teeth were extracted as initial therapy, and 9 (14.5%) after the acute phase. Out of the 22 teeth treated and subsequently monitored, 14 had to be extracted during the following 3 years.

Dissemination of the infection

A number of publications, mainly case reports, have described different systemic infections in different parts of the body, in which the suspected source of infection was a periodontal abscess. Two possibilities have been described: the dissemination of the bacteria inside the tissues during therapy; or bacterial dissemination through the blood stream due to bacteremia from the untreated abscess.

Dento-alveolar abscesses of endodontic origin are more often associated with complications such as bacterial spread than periodontal abscesses. Cellulitis, subcutaneous infection, phlegmone and mediastinitis can result from odontogenic infections but are very uncommon with periodontal abscesses. However, a periodontal abscess can function as a focus for a non-oral infection. A periodontal abscess may be the focus from which bacteria and bacterial products disseminate from the oral cavity to other body sites and may result in a variety of different infectious disorders. Mechanical treatment of a periodontal abscess may result in bacteremia (Flood et al. 1990, Roberts & Sherriff 1990) which, in patients with, for example, endoprosthesis (Van Winkelhoff et al. 1993, Van Waldman et al. 1997) or in immuno-compromised states, can result in non-oral infections.

The lungs may act as a mechanical barrier where periodontal bacteria can be trapped and subsequently may cause disease (Suzuki & Delisle 1984, Kuijper et al. 1992). Occasionally dissemination of periodontal bacteria can result in a brain abscess (Gallaguer et al. 1981). A number of case reports on periodontal pathogens that have been retrieved from brain abscesses are available. *P. micros, F. nucleatum,* black-pigmented anaerobic rods and *Actinomyces* spp. are among the strict anaerobic periodontal species that have been isolated from intra-cranial abscesses (Van Winkelhoff & Slots 1999). Other infections related with periodontal abscesses are: cervical necrotizing fascitis (Chan & McGurk 1997), and cellulites in breast cancer patients (Manian 1997).

REFERENCES

Abrams, H., Cunningham, C. & Lee, S. (1992). Periodontal changes following coronal/root perforation and formocresol pulpotomy. *Journal of Endodontics* **18**, 399-402.

Abrams, H. & Kopczyk, R. (1983). Gingival sequela from a retained piece of dental floss. *Journal of the American Dental Association* **106**, 57-58.

Ahl, D., Hilgeman, J. & Snyder, J. (1986). Periodontal emergencies. *Dental Clinics of North America* **30**, 459-472.

Ammons, W.J. (1996). Lesions in the oral mucous membranes. Acute lesions of the periodontium. In: Wilson, T. & Korman, K., eds. *Fundamentals of Periodontics*. Singapore: Quintessence, pp. 435-440.

Ashimoto, A., Tanaka, T., Ryoke, K. & Chen, C. (1998). PCR detection of periodontal/endodontic pathogens associated with abscess formation. *Journal of Dental Research* **77**, 854.

Becker, W., Berg, L. & Becker, B. (1984). The long-term evaluation of periodontal treatment and maintenance in 95 patients. *International Journal of Periodontics and Restorative Dentistry* **2**, 55-70.

Carranza, F. (1990). *Glickman's Clinical Periodontology*, 7th edn. Philadelphia: W.B. Saunders Company.

Chace, R.J. & Low, S. (1993). Survival characteristics of periodontally-involved teeth: a 40-year study. *Journal of Periodontology* **64**, 701-705.

Chan, C. & McGurk, M. (1997). Cervical necrotising fasciitis – a rare complication of periodontal disease. *British Dental Journal* **183**, 293-296.

Chen, R., Yang, J. & Chao, T. (1990). Invaginated tooth associated with periodontal abscess. *Oral Surgery Oral Medicine Oral Pathology* **69**, 659.

Dello Russo, M. (1985). The post-prophylaxis periodontal abscess: etiology and treatment. *International Journal of Periodontics and Restorative Dentistry* **1**, 29-37.

DeWitt, G., Cobb, C. & Killoy, W. (1985). The acute periodontal abscess: microbial penetration of the tissue wall. *International Journal of Periodontics and Restorative Dentistry* **1**, 39-51.

Flood, T., Samaranayake, L., MacFarlane, T., McLennan, A., MacKenzie, D. & Carmichael, F. (1990). Bacteraemia following incision and drainage of dento-alveolar abscesses. *British Dental Journal* **169**, 51-53.

Galego-Feal, P., García-Quintans, A., Gude-Sampedro, F. & García-García, A. (1996). Tramadol en el tratamiento del dolor de origen dentario en un servicio de urgencias hospitalario. *Emergencias* **8**, 480-484.

Gallaguer, D., Erickson, K. & Hollin, S. (1981). Fatal brain abscess following periodontal therapy: a case report. *Mount Sinai Journal of Medicine* **48**, 158-160.

Garrett, S., Polson, A., Stoller, N., Drisko, C., Caton, J., Harrold, C., Bogle, G., Greenwell, H., Lowenguth, R., Duke, S. & DeRouen, T. (1997). Comparison of a bioabsorbable GTR barrier to a non-absorbable barrier in treating human class II furcation defects. A multi-center parallel design randomized single-blind study. *Journal of Periodontology* **68**, 667-675.

Gillette, W. & Van House, R. (1980). Ill effects of improper oral hygiene procedures. *Journal of the American Dental Association* **101**, 476-481.

Girdler, N. (1991). Eosinophilic granuloma presenting as a chronic lateral periodontal abscess: a lesson in diagnosis? *British Dental Journal* **170**, 250.

Goose, D. (1981). Cracked tooth syndrome. *British Dental Journal* **150**, 224-225.

Gray, J., Flanary, D. & Newell, D. (1994). The prevalence of periodontal abscess. *Journal of Indiana Dental Association* **73**, 18-23.

Hafström, C., Wikström, M., Renvert, S. & Dahlén, G. (1994). Effect of treatment on some periodontopathogens and their antibody levels in periodontal abscesses. *Journal of Periodontology* **65**, 1022-1028.

Haney, J., Leknes, K., Lie, T., Selvig, K. & Wikesjö, U. (1992). Cemental tear related to rapid periodontal breakdown: a case report. *Journal of Periodontology* **63**, 220-224.

Helovuo, H., Hakkarainen, K. & Paunio, K. (1993). Changes in the prevalence of subgingival enteric rods, staphylococci and yeasts after treatment with penicillin and erythromycin. *Oral Microbiology and Immunology* **8**, 75-79.

Helovuo, H. & Paunio, K. (1989). Effects of penicillin and erythromycin on the clinical parameters of the periodontium. *Journal of Periodontology* **60**, 467-472.

Herrera, D., Roldán, S. & Sanz, M. (2000a). The periodontal abscess: a review. *Journal of Clinical Periodontology* **27**, 377-387.

Herrera, D., Roldán, S., O'Connor, A. & Sanz, M. (2000b). The periodontal abscess: I. Clinical and microbiology findings. *Journal of Clinical Periodontology* **27**, 387-394.

Herrera, D., Roldán, S., Gonzalez, I. & Sanz, M. (2000c). The periodontal abscess: II. Short-term clinical and microbiological efficacy of two systemic antibiotics regimes. *Journal of Clinical Periodontology* **27**, 395-404.

Ibbott, C., Kovach, R. & Carlson-Mann, L. (1993). Acute periodontal abscess associated with an immediate implant site in the maintenance phase. *International Journal of Oral and Maxillofacial Implants* **8**, 699-702.

Ishikawa, I., Oda, S., Hayashi, J. & Arakawa, S. (1996). Cervical cemental tears in older patients with adult periodontitis. Case reports. *Journal of Periodontology* **67**, 15-20.

Kaldahl, W., Kalwarf, K., Patil, K., Molvar, M. & Dyer, J. (1996). Long-term evaluation of periodontal therapy: I. Response to four therapeutic modalities. *Journal of Periodontology* **67**, 93-102.

Kawamata, T., Takeshita, M., Ishizukam N. & Hori, T. (2001). Patent forman ovale as a possible risk factor for cryptogenic brain abscess: report of two cases. *Neurosurgery* **49**, 204-206.

Kirkham, D., Hoge, H. & Sadegui, E. (1985). Gingival squamous cell carcinoma appearing as a benign lesion: report of a case. *Journal of the American Dental Association* **111**, 767-768.

Kuijper, E.J., Wiggerts, H.O., Jonker, G.J., Schaal, K.P. & De Gans, J. (1992). Disseminated actinomyces due to *Actinomyces meyeri* and *Actinobacillus actinomycetemcomitans*. *Scandinavian Journal of Infectious Diseases* **24**, 667-672.

Lewis, M., Meechan, C., MacFarlane, T., Lamey, P. & Kay, E. (1990). Presentation and antimicrobial treatment of acute orofacial infections in general dental practice. *British Journal of Oral and Maxillofacial Surgery* **28**, 359-366.

Manian, F. (1997). Cellulitis associated with an oral source of infection in breast cancer patients: report of two cases. *Scandinavian Journal of Infectious Diseases* **29**, 421-422.

Meng, H.X. (1999). Periodontal abscess. *Annals of Periodontology* **4**, 79-82.

McLeod, D., Lainson, P. & Spivey, J. (1997). Tooth loss due to periodontal abscess: a retrospective study. *Journal of Periodontology* **68**, 963-966.

Newman, M. & Sims, T. (1979). The predominant cultivable microbiota of the periodontal abscess. *Journal of Periodontology* **50**, 350-354.

Parrish, L., Kretzschmar, D. & Swan, R. (1989). Osteomyelitis associated with chronic periodontitis: a report of three cases. *Journal of Periodontology* **60**, 716-722.

Roberts, G. & Sherriff, M. (1990). Bacteraemia following incision and drainage of dento-alveolar abscesses. *British Dental Journal* **169**, 149.

Selden, H., Manhoff, D., Hatges, N. & Michel, R. (1998). Metastatic carcinoma to the mandible that mimicked pulpal/periodontal disease. *Journal of Endodontics* **24**, 267-270.

Smith, R. & Davies, R. (1986). Acute lateral periodontal abscesses. *British Dental Journal* **161**, 176-178.

Suzuki, J. & Delisle, A. (1984). Pulmonary actinomycosis of periodontal origin. *Journal of Periodontology* **55**, 581-584.

Tabaqhali, S. (1988). Anaerobic infections in the head and neck region. *Scandinavian Journal of Infectious Diseases* **57**, 24-34.

Topoll, H., Lange, D. & Müller, R. (1990). Multiple periodontal abscesses after systemic antibiotic therapy. *Journal of Clinical Periodontology* **17**, 268-272.

Torabinejad, M. & Rick, G. (1980). Squamous cell carcinoma of the gingiva. *Journal of the American Dental Association*, 870-872.

Van Waldman, B., Mont, M. & Hungerford, D. (1997). Total knee arthroplasty infections associated with dental procedures. *Clinical Orthopaedics and Related Research* **343**, 164-172.

Van Winkelhoff, A.J., Carlee, A. & de Graaff, J. (1985). *Bacteroides endodontalis* and other black-pigmented *Bacteroides* species in odontogenic abscesses. *Infection and Immunity* **49**, 494-497.

Van Winkelhoff, A.J., Overbeek, B.P., Pavicic, M.J.A.M., Van den Bergh, J.P.A., Ernst, J.P.M.G. & De Graaff, J. (1993). Long standing bacteremia by oral *Actinobacillus actinomycetemcomitans* in a patient with a pacemaker. *Clinical and Infectious Diseases* **14**, 216-218.

Van Winkelhoff, A.J. & Slots, J. (1999). *Actinobacillus actinomycetemcomitans* and *Porphyromonas gingivalis in* non-oral infections. *Periodontology 2000* **20**, 122-135.

CHAPTER 12

Non-Plaque Induced Inflammatory Gingival Lesions

PALLE HOLMSTRUP AND DANIEL VAN STEENBERGHE

Gingival diseases of specific bacterial origin

Gingival diseases of viral origin

Gingival diseases of fungal origin

Gingival lesions of genetic origin

Gingival diseases of systemic origin

Traumatic lesions

Gingival inflammation, clinically presenting as gingivitis, is not always due to accumulation of plaque on the tooth surface, and non-plaque induced inflammatory gingival reactions often present characteristic clinical features (Holmstrup 1999). They may occur due to several causes, such as specific bacterial, viral or fungal infection without an associated plaque-related gingival inflammatory reaction. Gingival lesions of genetic origin are seen in hereditary gingival fibromatosis, and several mucocutaneous disorders manifest as gingival inflammation. Typical examples of such disorders are lichen planus, pemphigoid, pemphigus vulgaris and erythema multiforme. Allergic and traumatic lesions are other examples of non-plaque induced gingival inflammation. Dentists, and especially specialists in periodontology, are the key persons in the diagnostic unraveling and treatment of patients affected by such lesions.

This chapter focuses on those non-plaque induced inflammatory gingival lesions of the gingival tissues, which are most relevant, either because they are common or because they are important examples for the understanding of the variety of tissue reactions that take place in the periodontium. For further information the reader is referred to other textbooks (Piette & Reychler 1991, Pindborg 1992, Newman et al. 1993, Porter & Scully 1994a,b). The modifying factors of plaque-related gingivitis such as smoking, sexual hormones and metabolic anomalies (diabetes) are dealt with in Chapter 6 and tumors and cysts are reviewed in Chapter 13.

GINGIVAL DISEASES OF SPECIFIC BACTERIAL ORIGIN

Infective gingivitis and stomatitis may occur on rare occasions in both immunocompromised and non-immunocompromised individuals, when non-plaque related pathogens overwhelm innate host resistance (Rivera-Hidalgo & Stanford 1999). The lesions may be due to bacteria and may not be accompanied by lesions elsewhere in the body. Typical examples of such lesions are due to infections with *Neisseria gonorrhea* (Scully 1995, Siegel 1996), *Treponema pallidum* (Scully 1995, Ramirez-Amador et al. 1996, Siegel 1996, Rivera-Hidalgo & Stanford 1999), *Streptococci, Mycobacterium chelonae* (Pedersen & Reibel 1989) or other organisms (Blake & Trott 1959, Littner et al. 1982). The gingival lesions manifest as fiery red edematous painful ulcerations, as asymptomatic chancres or mucous patches, or as atypical non-ulcerated, highly inflamed gingivitis. Biopsy supplemented by microbiologic examination reveals the background of the lesions.

GINGIVAL DISEASES OF VIRAL ORIGIN

Herpes virus infections

A number of viral infections are known to cause gingivitis (Scully et al. 1998b). The most important are the

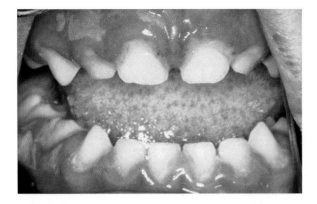

Fig. 12-1. Herpetic gingivostomatitis in a 3-year-old child. Erythematous swelling of attached gingiva with sero-fibrinous exudate along the gingival margin.

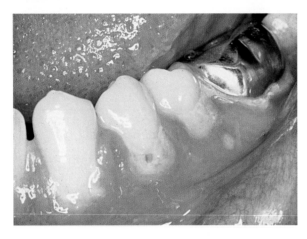

Fig. 12-2. Herpetic gingivostomatitis in a 43-year-old woman. Ulceration along the gingival margin and ruptured vesicle in relation to second lower left premolar. No affection on top of interdental papillae.

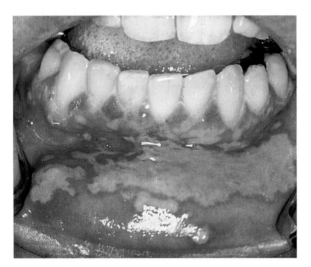

Fig. 12-3. Herpetic gingivostomatitis in a 38-year old woman. Widespread ulceration of lower lip mucosa and gingiva.

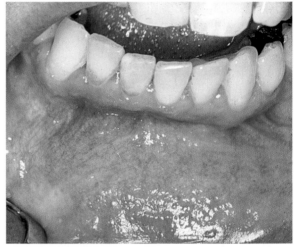

Fig. 12-4. Same patient as shown in Fig. 12-3, 4 weeks later. Healing without loss of tissue or scar formation.

herpes viruses: herpes simplex viruses type 1 and 2 and varicella-zoster virus. These viruses usually enter the human body in childhood and may give rise to oral mucosal disease followed by periods of latency and sometimes reactivation. Herpes simplex virus type 1 (HSV-1) usually causes oral manifestations, whereas herpes simplex virus type 2 (HSV-2) is mainly involved in anogenital infections and only occasionally is involved in oral infection (Scully 1989).

Primary herpetic gingivostomatitis
Herpes simplex infections are among the most com-

mon viral infections. Herpes simplex is a DNA virus with low infectiosity, which after entering the oral mucosal epithelium, penetrates a neural ending and by retrograde transport through the smooth endoplasmatic reticulum (200–300 mm/day) travels to the trigeminal ganglion where it can remain latent for years. The virus has also been isolated in extraneural locations such as the gingiva (Amit et al. 1992). Sometimes herpes simplex viruses may also play a role in recurring erythema multiforme. It is presently unknown whether the virus plays a role in other oral diseases, but herpes simplex virus has been found in

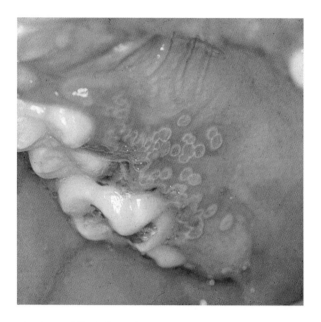

Fig. 12-5. Recurrent intraoral herpes infection. Ruptured vesicles of right palatal gingiva and mucosa.

gingivitis (Ehrlich et al. 1983), acute necrotizing gingivitis (Contreras et al. 1997), and periodontitis (Parra & Slots 1996).

When a baby is infected, sometimes from the parent's recurrent herpes labialis, it is often wrongly diagnosed as "teething". With increased hygiene in the industrialized society, more and more primary infections occur at higher ages, i.e. during adolescence or even adulthood. It is estimated in the US that there are about half a million cases per year (Overall 1982). The primary herpetic infection may run an asymptomatic course in early childhood, but may also give rise to severe gingivostomatitis, which occurs mostly before adolescence (Fig. 12-1). This manifestation includes painful severe gingivitis with redness, ulcerations with serofibrinous exudate and edema accompanied by stomatitis (Figs. 12-2 and 12-3). The incubation period is one week. A characteristic feature is the formation of vesicles, which rupture, coalesce and leave fibrin-coated ulcers (Scully et al. 1991, Miller & Redding 1992). Fever and lymphadenopathy are other classic features. Healing occurs spontaneously without scarring in 10 to 14 days (Fig. 12-4). During this period pain can render eating difficult.

The virus remains latent in the ganglion cell, probably through integration of its DNA in that of the chromosomal DNA (Overall 1982). Reactivation of the virus resulting in recurrent infections occurs in 20-40% of individuals with the primary infection (Greenberg 1996) and usually presents in the form of herpes labialis, but recurrent intraoral herpes infections are also seen. Recurrent infections occur in general more than once per year, usually at the same location as the vermilion border and/or the skin adjacent to it, where neural endings are known to be clustering. A large variety of factors trigger reactivation of latent virus. These are trauma, ultraviolet light exposure, fever, menstruation and others (Scully et al. 1998b).

While recurrences at the vermilion border are well recognized, recurrent intraoral herpes lesions often remain undiagnosed because they are considered

aphtous ulcerations (Lennette & Magoffin 1973), irrespective of the fact that aphtous ulcers do not affect keratinized mucosa. Recurrent intraoral herpes typically presents a less dramatic course than does the primary infection. A characteristic manifestation is a cluster of small painful ulcers in the attached gingiva and hard palate (Yura et al. 1986) (Fig. 12-5). The diagnosis can be made on the basis of the patient history and clinical findings supported by isolation of HSV from lesions. A reliable isolation of virus is best obtained from intact vesicular lesions, for instance in the form of an aspiration of the vesicle fluid with a small syringe. Isolation and growth of herpes viruses are elaborate because of their fragility. The virus must be transferred to a special cell line in the laboratory within 24 hours, or stored at –70°C. The herpes virus is detected within 5 days, and while a positive viral culture can be taken as evidence of viral infection, a negative result does not rule out such an infection. Laboratory diagnosis may also involve examination of a blood sample for increased antibody titer against herpes virus. However, this is most relevant in cases of primary infection, because the antibody titer remains elevated for the rest of the lifetime. The histopathologic features of cytologic smears from the gingival lesions are not specific, but the presence of giant cells and intranuclear inclusion bodies may indicate intra-cellular activity of virus (Burns 1980).

Immunodeficient patients, such as HIV-infected individuals, are at increased risk of acquiring the infection (Holmstrup & Westergaard 1998). In the immunocompromised patient the recurrence of herpes infection, either gingival or elsewhere, may be severe and even life-threatening.

The treatment of herpetic gingivostomatitis includes careful plaque removal to limit bacterial superinfection of the ulcerations, which delays their healing. In severe cases, including patients with immunodeficiency, the systemic use of antiviral drugs such as acyclovir or valacyclovir is recommended (O'Brien & Campoli-Richards 1989, Mindel 1991). Resistance to

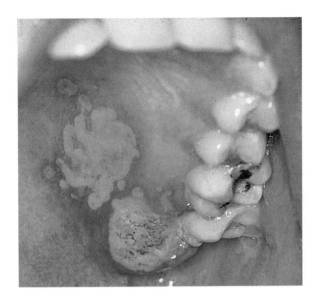

Fig. 12-6. Herpes zoster of left palatal gingiva and mucosa. Irregular fibrin coated ulcerations with severe pain.

acyclovir, especially among immunodeficient patients on long-term therapy, is a growing concern (Westheim et al. 1987) and explain why other antiviral drugs may be relevant.

Herpes zoster

Varicella-zoster virus causes varicella (chicken pox) as the primary self-limiting infection. It occurs mainly in children and later reactivation of the virus in adults causes herpes zoster (shingles). Both manifestations can involve the gingiva (Straus et al. 1988, Scully 1995). Chicken pox is associated with fever, malaise and a skin rash. The intraoral lesions are small ulcers usually on the tongue, palate and gingiva (Miller 1996, Scully et al. 1998b). The virus remains latent in the dorsal root ganglion from where it can be reactivated years after the primary infection (Rentier et al. 1996). Later reactivation results in herpes zoster, with unilateral lesions following the infected nerve (Miller 1996). The reactivation normally affects the thoracic ganglia in elderly or immunocompromised patients. Reactivation of virus from the trigeminal ganglion occurs in 20% of reported cases (Hudson & Vickers 1971). If the second or third branch of the trigeminal nerve is involved, skin lesions may be associated with intraoral lesions, or intraoral lesions may occur alone (Eisenberg 1978), for instance affecting the palatal gingiva (Fig. 12-6). Initial symptoms are pain and paraesthesia, which may be present before lesions occur (Greenberg 1996). The associated pain is usually severe. The lesions, which often involve the gingiva, initiate as vesicles. They soon rupture to leave fibrin-coated ulcers, which often coalesce to irregular forms (Millar & Traulis 1994) (Fig. 12-6). In immunocompromised patients, including HIV-infected individuals, the infection can result in severe tissue destruction with tooth exfoliation and necrosis of alveolar bone and high morbidity (Melbye et al. 1987, Schwartz et al. 1989). The diagnosis is usually obvious due to the unilateral occurrence of lesions associated with severe pain. Healing of the lesions usually takes place in 1-2 weeks.

Treatment consists of soft or liquid diet, rest, atraumatic removal of plaque and diluted chlorhexidine rinses. This may be supplemented by antiviral drug therapy.

GINGIVAL DISEASES OF FUNGAL ORIGIN

Fungal infection of the oral mucosa includes a range of diseases such as aspergillosis, blastomycosis, candidosis, coccidioidomycosis, cryptococcosis, histoplasmosis, mucormycosis and paracoccidioidomycosis infections (Scully et al. 1998b), but some of the infections are very uncommon and not all of them manifest as gingivitis. The present chapter focuses on candidosis and histoplasmosis, both of which may cause gingival infection.

Candidosis

Various *Candida* species are recovered from the mouth of humans including *C. albicans, C. glabrata, C. krusei, C. tropicalis, C. parapsilosis,* and *C. guillermondii* (Cannon et al. 1995). *C. albicans* is by far the most common. It is a normal commensal of the oral cavity but also an opportunistic pathogen. The prevalence of oral carriage of *C. albicans* in healthy adults ranges from 3% to 48% (Scully et al. 1995), the large variation being due to differences in examined populations and the procedures used. The proportion of *C. albicans* in the total oral yeast population can reach about 50-80% (Wright et al. 1985), and by far the most common fungal infection of the oral mucosa is candidosis mainly caused by the organism *C. albicans* (Scully et al 1998b), the proteinase-positive strains of which are associated with disease (Negi et al. 1984, Odds 1985) and invasion of keratinized epithelia such as that of the gingiva. Invasion and increased desquamation is due to the hyaluronidase production. Infection by *C. albicans* usually occurs as a consequence of reduced

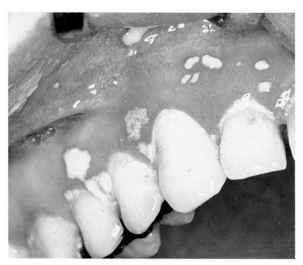

Fig. 12-7. Pseudomembranous candidosis of maxillary gingiva and mucosa in HIV seropositive patient. The lesions can be scraped off, leaving a slightly bleeding surface.

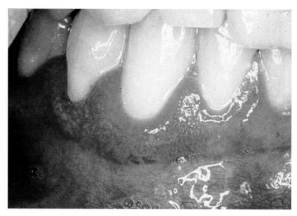

Fig. 12-8. Erythematous candidosis of attached mandibular gingiva of HIV seropositive mucosa. The mucogingival junction is invisible.

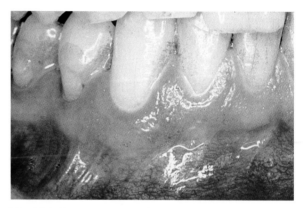

Fig. 12-9. Same patient as shown in Fig. 12-8 after topical antimycotic therapy. The mucogingival junction is visible.

host defense posture (Holmstrup & Johnson 1997), including immunodeficiency (Holmstrup & Samaranayake 1990) (Figs. 12-7 and 12-8), reduced saliva secretion, smoking and treatment with corticosteroids, but may be due to a wide range of predisposing factors. Disturbances in the oral microbial flora, such as after therapy with broad-spectrum antibiotics, may also lead to oral candidosis. The predisposing factors are, however, often difficult to identify. Based on their site, infections may be defined as superficial or systemic. Candidal infection of the oral mucosa is usually a superficial infection, but systemic infections are not uncommon in debilitated patients.

In otherwise healthy individuals, oral candidosis rarely manifests in the gingiva. This is surprising when considering the fact that *C. albicans* is frequently isolated from the subgingival flora of patients with severe periodontitis (Slots et al. 1988). The most common clinical characteristic of gingival candidal infections is redness of the attached gingiva often associated with a granular surface (Fig. 12-10).

Various types of oral mucosal manifestations are pseudomembranous candidosis (also known as thrush in neonates), erythematous candidosis, plaque-type candidosis, and nodular candidosis (Holmstrup & Axéll 1990). Pseudomembranous candidosis shows whitish patches (Fig. 12-7), which can be wiped off the mucosa with an instrument or gauze leaving a slightly bleeding surface. The pseudomembranous type usually has no major symptoms. Erythematous lesions can be found anywhere in the oral mucosa (Fig. 12-10). The intensely red lesions are usually associated with pain, sometimes even severe. The plaque-type of oral candidosis is a whitish plaque, which cannot be removed. There are usually no symptoms and the lesion is clinically indistinguishable from oral leukoplakia. Nodular candidal lesions are infrequent in the gingiva. Slightly elevated nodules of

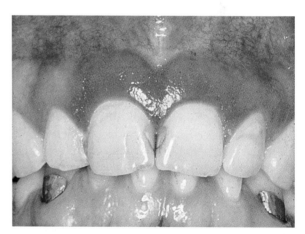

Fig. 12-10. Chronic erythematous candidosis of maxillary attached gingiva of the incisor region.

white or reddish color characterize them (Holmstrup & Axéll 1990).

A diagnosis of candidal infection can be accomplished on the basis of culture, smear and biopsy. A culture on Nickersons medium at room temperature is easily handled in the dental premises. Microscopic examination of smears from suspected lesions is another easy diagnostic procedure, either performed as

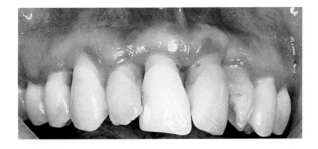

Fig. 12-11. Linear gingival erythema of maxillary gingiva. Red banding along the gingival margin, which does not respond to conventional therapy.

direct examination by phase contrast microscopy or as light microscopic examination of periodic-acid-Schiff-stained or Gram-stained smears. Mycelium forming cells in the form of hyphae or pseudohyphae and blastospores are seen in great numbers among masses of desquamated cells. Since oral carriage of *C. albicans* is common among healthy individuals, positive culture and smear does not necessarily imply candidal infection (Rindum et al. 1994). Quantitative assessment of the mycological findings and the presence of clinical changes compatible with the above types of lesions is necessary to obtain a reliable diagnosis, which can also be obtained on the basis of identification of hyphae or pseudohyphae in biopsies from the lesions.

Topical treatment involves application of antifungals, such as nystatin, amphotericin B or miconazole. Nystatin may be used as an oral suspension. Since it is not resorbed it can be used in pregnant or lactating women. Miconazole exists as an oral gel. It should not be given during pregnancy and it can interact with anticoagulants and phenytoin. The treatment in the severe or generalized forms also involves systemic antifungals such as fluconazole.

Linear gingival erythema

Linear gingival erythema (LGE) is regarded as a gingival manifestation of immunosuppression characterized by a distinct linear erythematous band limited to the free gingiva (Consensus Report 1999) (Fig. 12-11). It is characterized by a disproportion of inflammatory intensity for the amount of plaque present. There is no evidence of pocketing or attachment loss. A further characteristic of this type of lesion is that it does not respond well to improved oral hygiene or to scaling (EC Clearinghouse on Oral Problems 1993). The extent of gingival banding measured by number of affected sites has been shown to depend on tobacco usage (Swango et al. 1991). While 15% of affected sites were originally reported to bleed on probing and 11% exhibited spontaneous bleeding (Winkler et al. 1988), a key feature of linear gingival erythema is now considered to be lack of bleeding on probing (Robinson et al. 1994).

Some studies of various groups of HIV-infected patients have revealed prevalences of gingivitis with band-shaped patterns in 0.5-49% (Klein et al. 1991, Swango et al. 1991, Barr et al. 1992, Laskaris et al. 1992,

Masouredis et al. 1992, Riley et al. 1992, Ceballos-Salobrena et al. 1996, Robinson et al. 1996). These prevalence values reflect some of the problems with nonstandardized diagnosis and selection of study groups. A few studies of unbiased groups of patients have indicated that gingivitis with band-shaped or punctate marginal erythema may be relatively rare in HIV-infected patients, and probably a clinical finding which is no more frequent than in the general population (Drinkard et al. 1991, Friedman et al. 1991).

It is interesting to note that, whereas there was no HIV-related preponderance of red banding, diffuse and punctate erythema was significantly more prevalent in HIV-infected than in non-HIV-infected individuals in a British study (Robinson et al. 1996). Red gingival banding as a clinical feature alone was, therefore, not strongly associated with HIV infection.

There are indications that candidal infection is the background of some cases of gingival inflammation including LGE (Winkler et al. 1988, Robinson et al. 1994), but studies have revealed a microflora comprising both *C. albicans*, and a number of periopathogenic bacteria consistent with those seen in conventional periodontitis, i.e. *Porphyromonas gingivalis*, *Prevotella intermedia*, *Actinobacillus actinomycetemcomitans*, *Fusobacterium nucleatum* and *Campylobacter rectus* (Murray et al. 1988, 1989, 1991). By DNA probe detection, the percentage of positive sites in HIV associated gingivitis as compared with matched gingivitis sites of HIV seronegative patients for *A. actinomycetemcomitans* was 23% and 7% respectively, for *P. gingivalis* 52% and 17%, *P. intermedia* 63% and 29%, and for *C. rectus* 50% and 14% (Murray et al. 1988, 1989, 1991). *C. albicans* has been isolated by culture in about 50% of HIV associated gingivitis sites, in 26% of unaffected sites of HIV seropositive patients and in 3% of healthy sites of HIV seronegative patients. The frequent isolation and the pathogenic role of *C. albicans* may be related to the high levels of the yeasts in saliva and oral mucosa of HIV-infected patients (Tylenda et al. 1989).

An interesting histopathologic study of biopsy specimens from the banding zone has revealed no inflammatory infiltrate but an increased number of blood vessels, which explains the red color of the lesions (Glick et al. 1990). The incomplete inflammatory reaction of the host tissue may be the background of the lacking response to conventional treatment.

A number of diseases present clinical features resembling those of LGE and which, accordingly, do not resolve after improved oral hygiene and debridement.

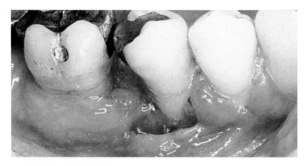

Fig. 12-12. Gingival histoplasmosis with loss of periodontal tissue around second premolar.

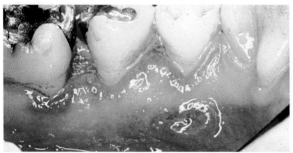

Fig. 12-13. Same patient as shown in Fig. 12-12. Lingual aspect with ulceration in the deeper part of crater-formed lesion.

Examples are oral lichen planus, which is frequently associated with a similar inflammatory red band of the attached gingiva (Holmstrup et al. 1990) and so is sometimes mucous membrane pemphigoid (Pindborg 1992) or erythematous lesions associated with renal insufficiency because of the salivary ammonia production associated with the high levels of urea.

There is little information about treatment based on controlled studies of this type of affection. Conventional therapy plus rinsing with 0.12% chlorhexidine gluconate twice daily has shown significant improvement after 3 months (Grassi et al. 1989). It was mentioned above that LGE in some cases might be related to the presence of *Candida* strains. In accordance with this finding, clinical observations suggest that improvement is frequently dependent on successful eradication of intraoral *Candida* strains, which results in disappearance of the characteristic features (Winkler et al. 1988). Consequently, attempts to identify the presence of fungal infection either by culture or smear is recommendable followed by antimycotic therapy in *Candida*-positive cases.

Histoplasmosis

Histoplasmosis is a granulomatous disease caused by *Histoplasma capsulatum*, a soil saprophyte found mainly in feces from birds and cats. The infection occurs in the north-eastern, south-eastern, mid Atlantic and central states of the US. It is also found in Central and South America, India, East Asia and Australia. Histoplasmosis is the most frequent systemic mycosis in the US. Airborne spores from the mycelial form of the organism mediate it (Rajah & Essa 1993). In the normal host, the course of the infection is subclinical (Anaissie et al. 1986). The clinical manifestations include acute and chronic pulmonary histoplasmosis and a disseminated form, mainly occurring in immunocompromised patients (Cobb et al. 1989). Oral lesions have been seen in 30% of patients with pulmonary histoplasmosis and in 66% of patients with the disseminated form (Weed & Parkhill 1948, Loh et al. 1989). The oral lesions may affect any area of the oral mucosa (Chinn et al. 1995) including the gingiva. They initiate as nodular or papillary and later may become ulcerative with loss of gingival tissue, and painful (Figs. 12-12 and 12-13). They are sometimes granulomatous and the clinical appearance may resemble a malignant tumor (Boutros et al. 1995). The diagnosis is based on clinical appearance and histopathology and/or culture, and the treatment consists of systemic antifungal therapy.

GINGIVAL LESIONS OF GENETIC ORIGIN

Hereditary gingival fibromatosis

Gingival hyperplasia (synonymous with gingival overgrowth, gingival fibromatosis) may occur as a side effect to systemic medications including phenytoin, sodium valproate, cyclosporine and dihydropyridines. These lesions are to some extent plaque-dependent and they are reviewed in Chapter 7. Gingival hyperplasia may also be of genetic origin. Such lesions are known as hereditary gingival fibromatosis (HGF), which is an uncommon condition characterized by diffuse gingival enlargement, sometimes covering major parts of, or the total, tooth surfaces. The lesions develop irrespective of effective plaque removal.

HGF may be an isolated disease entity or part of a syndrome (Gorlin et al. 1990), associated with other clinical manifestations, such as hypertrichosis (Horning et al. 1985, Cuestas-Carneiro & Bornancini 1988),

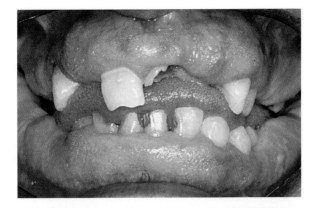

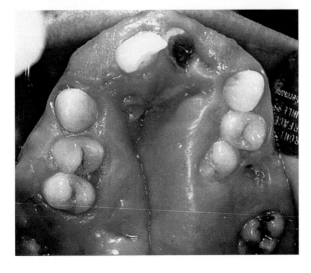

Fig. 12-14. Hereditary gingival fibromatosis. Facial aspect with partial coverage of teeth.

Fig. 12-15. Same patient as shown in Fig.12-15. The maxillary gingival fibromatosis is severe and has resulted in total disfiguration of the dental arch.

mental retardation (Araiche & Brode 1959), epilepsy (Ramon et al. 1967), hearing loss (Hartsfield et al. 1985), growth retardation (Bhowmick et al. 2001) and abnormalities of extremities (Nevin et al. 1971, Skrinjaric & Basic 1989). Most cases are related to an autosomal dominant mode of inheritance, but cases have been described with an autosomal recessive background (Emerson 1965, Jorgensen & Cocker 1974, Singer et al. 1993). The most common syndrome of HGF includes hypertrichosis, epilepsy and mental retardation; the two latter features, however, are not present in all cases (Gorlin et al. 1990).

Typically, HGF presents as large masses of firm, dense, resilient, insensitive fibrous tissue that covers the alveolar ridges and extends over the teeth resulting in extensive pseudopockets. The color may be normal or erythematous if inflamed (Figs. 12-14 and 12-15). Depending on extension of the gingival enlargement, patients complain of functional and esthetic problems. The enlargement may result in protrusion of the lips, and they may chew on a considerable hyperplasia of tissue covering the teeth. HGF is seldom present at birth but may be noted at an early age. If the enlargement is present before tooth eruption, the dense fibrous tissue may interfere with or prevent the eruption (Shafer et al. 1983).

Studies have suggested that an important pathogenic mechanism may be enhanced production of transforming growth factor (TGF-beta 1) reducing the proteolytic activities of HGF fibroblasts, which again favor the accumulation of extracellular matrix (Coletta et al. 1999). Recently a locus for autosomal dominant HGF has been mapped to a region on chromosome 2 (Hart et al. 1998, Xiao et al. 2000), although at least two genetically distinct loci seem to be responsible for this type of HGF (Hart et al. 2000).

The histological features of HGF include moderate hyperplasia of a slightly hyperkeratotic epithelium with extended rete pegs. The underlying stroma is almost entirely made up of dense collagen bundles with only few fibroblasts. Local accumulation of inflammatory cells may be present (Shafer et al. 1983). Histological examination may facilitate the differential diagnosis from other genetically determined gingival enlargements such as Fabry disease, characterized by telangiectasia.

The treatment is surgical removal, often in a series of gingivectomies, but relapses are not uncommon. If the volume of the overgrowth is extensive, a repositioned flap to avoid exposure of connective tissue by gingivectomy may better achieve elimination of pseudopockets.

GINGIVAL DISEASES OF SYSTEMIC ORIGIN

Mucocutaneous disorders

A variety of mucocutaneous disorders present gingival manifestations sometimes in the form of desquamative lesions or ulceration of the gingiva. The most important of these diseases are lichen planus, pemphigoid, pemphigus vulgaris, erythema multiforme and lupus erythematosus.

Lichen planus

Lichen planus is the most common mucocutaneous disease manifesting on the gingiva. The disease may affect skin and oral as well as other mucosal membranes in some patients while others may present either skin or oral mucosal involvement alone. Oral involvement alone is common and concomitant skin lesions in patients with oral lesions have been found in 5-44% of the cases (Andreasen 1968, Axéll & Rundquist 1987). The disease may be associated with severe discomfort and since it has been shown to possess a premalignant potential, although this is still a controversial issue (Holmstrup 1992), it is important to diagnose and treat the patients and to follow them at the regular oral examinations (Holmstrup et al. 1988).

The prevalence of oral lichen planus (OLP) in various populations has been found to be 0.1-4% (Scully et al. 1998a). The disease may afflict patients at any age although it is seldom observed in childhood (Scully et al. 1994).

Skin lesions are characterized by red papules with white striae (Wickham striae) (Fig. 12-16). Itching is a common symptom, and the most frequent locations are the flexor aspects of the arms, the thighs and the neck. In the vast majority of cases the skin lesions disappear spontaneously after a few months, which is in sharp contrast with the oral lesions, which usually remain for years (Thorn et al. 1988).

A variety of clinical appearances is characteristic of OLP. These include:

- papular (Fig. 12-17)
- reticular (Figs. 12-18 and 12-19)
- plaque-like (Fig. 12-20)
- atrophic (Figs. 12-21 to 12-25)
- ulcerative (Figs. 12-22 and 12-27)
- bullous (Fig. 12-29)

Simultaneous presence of more than one type of lesion is common (Thorn et al. 1988). The most characteristic clinical manifestations of the disease and the basis of the clinical diagnosis are white papules (Fig. 12-17) and white striations (Figs. 12-18, 12-19, 12-26 and 12-27), which often form reticular patterns (Thorn et al. 1988). Sometimes atrophic and ulcerative lesions

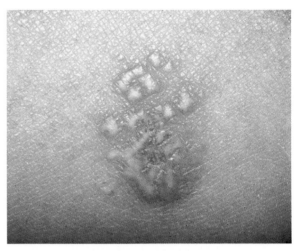

Fig. 12-16. Skin lesions of lichen planus. Red papules with delicate white striations.

are referred to as erosive (Rees 1989). Papular, reticular and plaque-type lesions usually do not give rise to significant symptoms, whereas atrophic and ulcerative lesions are associated with moderate to severe pain, especially in relation to oral hygiene procedures and eating. OLP frequently persists for many years (Thorn et al. 1988). Any area of the oral mucosa may be affected by OLP, but the lesions often change in clinical type and extension over the years. Such changes may imply the development of plaque-type lesions, which are clinically indistinguishable from oral leukoplakia. This may give rise to a diagnostic problem if other lesions more characteristic of OLP have disappeared (Thorn et al. 1988).

A characteristic histopathologic feature in OLP is a subepithelial, band-like accumulation of lymphocytes and macrophages characteristic of a type IV hypersensitivity reaction (Eversole et al. 1994). The epithelium shows hyperortho- or hyperparakeratinization and basal cell disruption with transmigration of lymphocytes into the basal and parabasal cell layers (Eversole 1995). The infiltrating lymphocytes have been identified as CD4+ and CD8+ positive cells (Buechner 1984, Walsh et al. 1990, Eversole et al. 1994). Other characteristic features are Civatte bodies, which are dyskeratotic basal cells. Common immunohistochemical findings of OLP-lesions are fibrin in the basement membrane zone, but deposits of IgM, C3, C4, and C5 may also be found. None of these findings are specific of OLP (Schiødt et al. 1981, Kilpi et al. 1988, Eversole et al. 1994).

The subepithelial inflammatory reaction in OLP lesions is presumably due to a so far unidentified antigen in the junctional zone between epithelium and connective tissue or to components of basal epithelial cells (Holmstrup & Dabelsteen 1979, Walsh et al. 1990, Sugerman et al. 1994). A lichen planus specific antigen in the stratum spinosum of skin lesions has been described (Camisa et al. 1986), but this antigen does not appear to play a significant role in oral lesions since it is rarely identified there. It is still an open

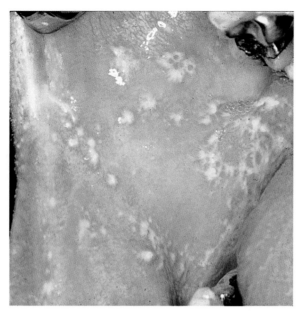

Fig. 12-17. Oral lichen planus. Papular lesion of right buccal mucosa.

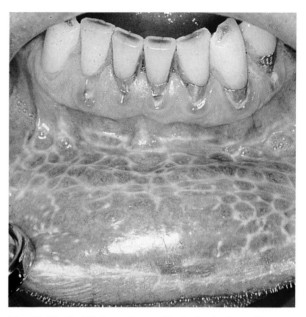

Fig. 12-18. Oral lichen planus. Reticular lesion of lower lip mucosa. The white striations are denoted Wickham striae.

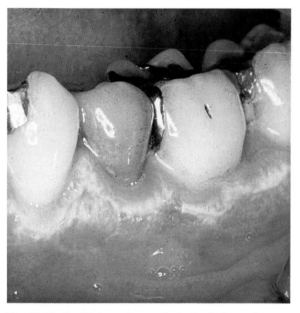

Fig. 12-19. Oral lichen planus. Reticular lesions of gingiva in lower left premolar and molar region.

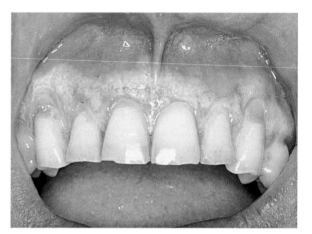

Fig. 12-20. Oral lichen planus. Plaque-type lesion of maxillary gingiva.

question whether OLP is a multivariate group of etiologically diverse diseases with common clinical and histopathological features or a disease entity characterized by a type IV hypersensitivity reaction to an antigen in the basement membrane area. The clinical diagnosis is based on the presence of papular or reticular lesions. The diagnosis may be supported by histopathological findings of hyperkeratosis, degenerative changes of basal cells and subepithelial inflammation dominated by lymphocytes and macrophages (Holmstrup 1999).

The uncertain background of OLP results in several border zone cases of so-called oral lichenoid lesions (OLL) for which a final diagnosis is difficult to establish. The most common OLLs are probably lesions in contact with dental restorations (Holmstrup 1991) (see later in this chapter). Other types of OLL are associated with various types of medications including antimalarials, quinine, quinidine, non-steroidal anti-inflammatory drugs, thiazides, diuretics, gold salts, penicillamine, beta-blockers and others (Scully et al. 1998a). Graft-versus-host reactions are also characterized by a lichenoid appearance (Fujii et al. 1988) and a group of OLL is associated with systemic diseases of which liver disease has been revealed lately (Fortune & Buchanan 1993, Bagan et al. 1994, Carrozzo et al. 1996). This appears to be particularly evident in Southern Europe and Japan where hepatitis C has been found in 20-60% of OLL cases (Bagan et al. 1994, Gandolfo et al. 1994, Nagao et al. 1995).

Several follow-up studies have demonstrated that OLP is associated with increased development of oral cancer, the frequency of cancer development being in the range of 0.5-2% (Holmstrup et al. 1988).

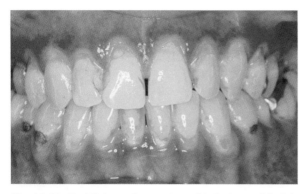

Fig. 12-21. Oral lichen planus. Atrophic lesions of facial maxillary and mandibular gingiva. Such lesions were previously often termed desquamative gingivitis.

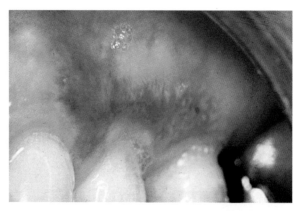

Fig. 12-22. Oral lichen planus. Atrophic and ulcerative lesion of maxillary gingiva. Note that the margin of the gingiva has normal color in upper incisor region, which distinguishes the lesions from plaque induced gingivitis.

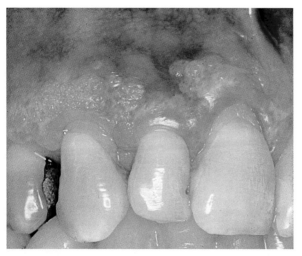

Fig. 12-23. Oral lichen planus. Atrophic and reticular lesion of maxillary gingiva. Several types of lesions are often present simultaneously.

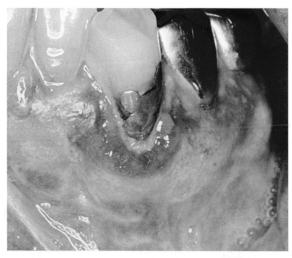

Fig. 12-24. Oral lichen planus. Atrophic and reticular lesion of lower left canine region. Plaque accumulation results in exacerbation of oral lichen planus, and atrophic lesions compromises oral hygiene procedures. This may lead to a vicious circle that the dentist can help in breaking.

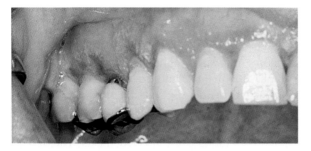

Fig. 12-25. Oral lichen planus. Atrophic and reticular lesion of right maxillary gingiva in a patient using an electric toothbrush, which is traumatic to the marginal gingiva. The physical trauma results in exacerbation of the lesion with atrophic characteristics and pain.

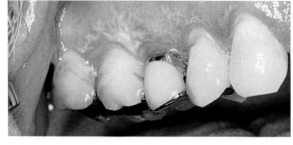

Fig. 12-26. Same patient as shown in Fig. 12-25 after modified toothbrushing procedure with no traumatic action on marginal gingiva.

The most important part of the therapeutic regimen is an atraumatic meticulous plaque control, which results in significant improvement in many patients (Holmstrup et al. 1990) (Figs. 12-25 to 12-28). Individual oral hygiene procedures with the purpose of effective plaque removal without traumatic influence on

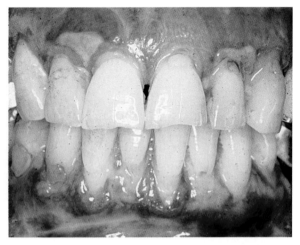

Fig. 12-27. Oral lichen planus. Atrophic and ulcerative/reticular lesions of maxillary and mandibular incisor region. The patient, who is a 48-year-old woman, suffers from severe discomfort from food, beverages and toothbrushing.

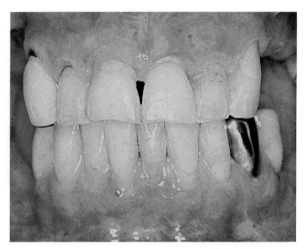

Fig. 12-28. Same patient as shown in Fig. 12-27 after periodontal treatment and extraction of teeth with deep pockets. An individual oral hygiene program, which ensured gentle, meticulous plaque removal has been used by the patient for three months. The atrophic/ulcerative lesions are now healed and no more symptoms left.

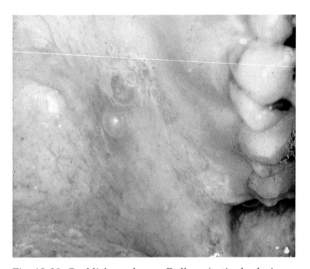

Fig. 12-29. Oral lichen planus. Bullous/reticular lesion of left palatal ucosa.

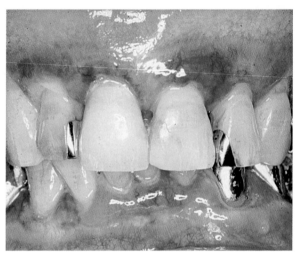

Fig. 12-30. Benign mucous membrane pemphigoid affecting the attached gingiva of both jaws. The lesions are erythematous and resemble atrophic lichen planus lesions. They result in pain associated with oral procedures including eating and oral hygiene.

the gingival tissue should be established for all patients with symptoms. In case of persistent pain, typically associated with atrophic and ulcerative affections, antifungal treatment may be necessary if the affections are hosting yeast, which occurs in 37% of OLP-cases (Krogh et al. 1987). In painful cases, which have not responded to the treatment above, topical corticosteroids, preferably in a paste or an ointment, should be used three times daily for a number of weeks. However, in such cases relapses are very common, which is why intermittent periods of treatment may be needed over an extended period of time.

Pemphigoid
Pemphigoid is a group of disorders in which autoan-

tibodies towards components of the basement membrane result in detachment of the epithelium from the connective tissue. Bullous pemphigoid predominantly affects the skin, but oral mucosal involvement may occur (Brooke 1973, Hodge et al. 1981). If only mucous membranes are affected, the term benign mucous membrane pemphigoid (BMMP) is often used. The term cicatricial pemphigoid is also used to describe subepithelial bullous disease limited to the mouth or eyes and infrequently other mucosal areas. This term is problematic, because usually oral lesions do not result in scarring, whereas this is an important danger for ocular lesions (Scully et al. 1998b). It is now evident that BMMP comprises a group of disease entities characterized by an immune reaction involv-

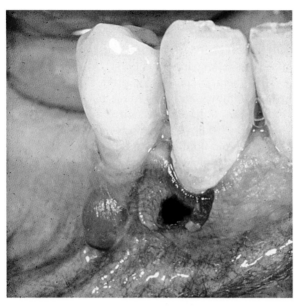

Fig. 12-31. Benign mucous membrane pemphigoid with intact and ruptured gingival bulla.

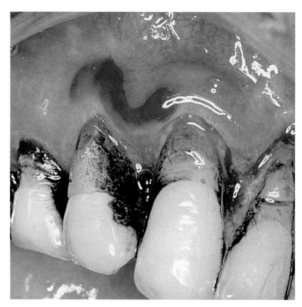

Fig. 12-32. Benign mucous membrane pemphigoid with hemorrhagic gingival bulla. The patient uses chlorhexidine for daily plaque reduction.

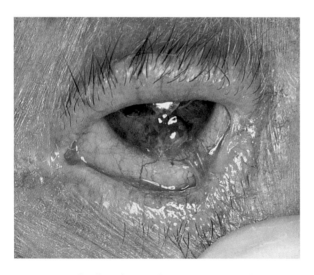

Fig. 12-33. Benign mucous membrane pemphigoid. Eye lesion with scar formation due to coalescence of palpebral and conjunctival mucosa.

ing autoantibodies directed against various basement membrane zone antigens (Scully & Laskaris 1998). These antigens have been identified as hemidesmosome or lamina lucida components (Leonard et al. 1982, 1984, Manton & Scully 1988, Domloge-Hultsch et al. 1992, 1994). In addition, complement-mediated cell destructive processes may be involved in the pathogenesis of the disease (Eversole 1994). The trigger mechanisms behind these reactions, however, have not yet been revealed.

The majority of affected patients are females with a mean age at onset of 50 years or over (Shklar & McCarthy 1971). Oral involvement in BMMP is almost inevitable and usually the oral cavity is the first site of disease activity (Silverman et al. 1986, Gallagher & Shklar 1987). Any area of the oral mucosa may be involved in BMMP, but the main manifestation is desquamative lesions of the gingiva presenting intensely erythematous attached gingival (Laskaris et al. 1982, Silverman et al. 1986, Gallagher & Shklar 1987) (Fig. 12-30). The inflammatory changes, as al-

ways when not caused by plaque, may extend over the entire gingival width and even over the muco-gingival junction. Rubbing of the gingiva may precipitate bulla formation (Dahl & Cook 1979). This is denoted a positive Nicholsky sign and is caused by the destroyed adhesion of the epithelium to the connective tissue. The intact bullae are often clear to yellowish or they may be hemorrhagic (Figs. 12-31 and 12-32). This, again, is due to the separation of epithelium from connective tissue at the junction resulting in exposed vessels inside the bullae. Usually, the bullae rupture rapidly leaving fibrin coated ulcers. Sometimes, tags of loose epithelium can be found due to rupture of bullae. Other mucosal surfaces may be involved in some patients. Ocular lesions are particularly important because scar formation can result in blindness (Williams et al. 1984) (Fig. 12-33).

The separation of epithelium from connective tissue at the basement membrane area is the main diagnostic feature of BMMP. An unspecific inflammatory reaction is a secondary histologic finding. In addition,

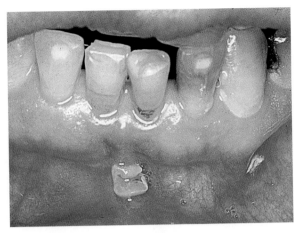

Fig. 12-34. Pemphigus vulgaris. Initial lesion resembling recurrent aphtous stomatitis.

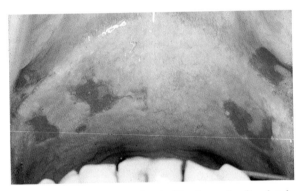

Fig. 12-35. Pemphigus vulgaris. Erosions of soft palatal mucosa. The erosive lesions are due to loss of the superficial part of the epithelium, leaving the connective tissue covered only by the basal cell layers.

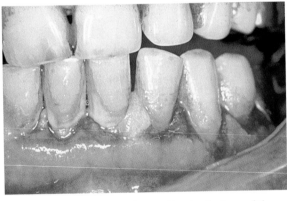

Fig. 12-36. Pemphigus vulgaris. Erosive lesions of the attached gingiva.

immunohistochemical examination can help distinguish BMMP from other vesiculobullous diseases, in particular pemphigus which is life threatening. Deposits of C3, IgG, and sometimes other immunoglobulins as well as fibrin are found at the basement membrane zone in the vast majority of cases (Laskaris & Nicolis 1980, Daniels & Quadra-White 1981, Manton & Scully 1988). It is important to involve peri-lesional tissue in the biopsy because the characteristic features

may be lost within lesional tissue (Ullman 1988). Circulating immunoglobulins are found only occasionally in BMMP by indirect immunofluorescence (Laskaris & Angelopoulos 1981).

The therapy consists of professional atraumatic plaque removal and individual instruction in gentle but careful daily plaque control, eventually supplemented with daily use of chlorhexidine and/or topical corticosteroid application if necessary. As for all the chronic inflammatory oral mucosal diseases, oral hygiene procedures are very important and controlling the infection from plaque bacteria may result in considerable reduction of disease activity and symptoms. However, the disease is chronic in nature and formation of new bullae is inevitable in most patients. Topical corticosteroids, preferably applied as a paste at night, temper the inflammatory reaction.

Pemphigus vulgaris

Pemphigus is a group of autoimmune diseases characterized by formation of intraepithelial bullae in skin and mucous membranes. The group comprises several variants, pemphigus vulgaris (PV) being the most common and most serious form (Barth & Venning 1987).

Individuals of Jewish or Mediterranean background are more often affected by PV than others. This is an indication of a strong genetic background of the disease (Pisanti et al. 1974). The disease may occur at any age, but is typically seen in the middle-aged or elderly. It presents with widespread bulla formation often including large areas of skin, and if left untreated the disease is life threatening. Intraoral onset of the disease with bulla formation is very common and lesions of the oral mucosa including the gingiva are frequently seen. Early lesions may resemble aphtous ulcers (Fig. 12-34), but widespread erosions are common at later stages (Fig. 12-35). Gingival involvement may present as painful desquamative lesions or as erosions or ulcerations, which are remains of ruptured bullae (Fig. 12-36). Such lesions may be indistinguishable from BMMP (Zegarelli & Zegarelli 1977, Sciubba 1996). Since the bulla formation is located in the spinous cell layer, the chance of seeing an intact bulla is even more reduced than in BMMP. Involvement of other mucous membranes is common (Laskaris et al. 1982). The ulcers heal slowly, usually without scar formation, and the disease runs a chronic course with recurring bulla formation (Zegarelli & Zegarelli 1977).

The diagnosis is based on the characteristic histological feature of PV that is intraepithelial bulla formation due to destruction of desmosomes resulting in acantholysis. The bullae contain non-adhering free epithelial cells, denoted Tzank cells, which have lost their intercellular bridges (Coscia-Porrazzi et al. 1985, Nishikawa et al. 1996). Mononuclear cells and neutrophils dominate the associated inflammatory reaction. Immunohistochemistry reveals pericellular epithelial deposits of IgG and C3. Circulating autoantibodies against interepithelial adhesion molecules are detectable in serum samples of most patients, but at the initial stage of intraoral affection antiepithelial antibody may not be elevated (Melbye et al. 1987, Manton & Scully 1988, Lamey et al. 1992, Lever & Schaumburg-Lever 1997). The background of bulla formation in PV is damage to the intercellular adhesion caused by autoantibodies to cadherin-type epithelial cell adhesion molecules (desmoglein 1 and 3) (Nousari & Anhalt 1995, Nishikawa et al. 1996). The mechanism by which these molecules trigger the formation of autoantibodies has not yet been established.

Immediate referral of patients with PV to a dermatologist or internal medicine specialist is important because when recognized late the disease can be fatal, although systemic corticosteroid therapy can presently solve most cases. Supplementary local treatment consists of gentle plaque control and professional cleaning as mentioned for the chronic inflammatory oral mucosal diseases above. Sometimes, additional topical corticosteroid application is needed to control the intraoral disease activity.

Erythema multiforme

Erythema multiforme (EM) is an acute, sometimes recurrent, vesiculobullous disease affecting mucous membranes and skin. A general malaise often precedes the lesions, which involve skin and mucous membranes in various degrees. Two forms of the disease have been described: a minor form with only moderate involvement and a major form, also mentioned as Stevens-Johnson syndrome, with widespread mucous membrane, i.e. oral, ocular and genital, in addition to skin lesions (Lozada-Nur et al. 1989, Assier et al. 1995, Bystryn 1996). This latter multilocular entity has to be differentiated from other disorders such as Reiter and Behçet's syndromes, which also affect the eyes, the oral mucosa and often the genitalia. The pathogenesis of EM remains obscure, but the disease appears to be an immune reaction precipitated by a wide range of factors including herpes simplex virus (Lozada & Silverman 1978, Nesbit & Gobetti 1986, Ruokonen et al. 1988, Miura et al. 1992, Aurelian et al. 1998), mycoplasma pneumoniae (McKellar & Reade 1986, Stutman 1987) and various drugs (Bottiger et al. 1975, Gebel & Hornstein 1984, Kauppinen & Stubb 1984).

EM may occur at any age but most frequently affects young individuals. It may or may not involve the oral mucosa, but oral involvement occurs in as much as 25-60% of cases (Huff et al. 1983) and sometimes is the only involved site. The characteristic oral lesions comprise swollen lips often with extensive crust formation of the vermilion border (Fig. 12-37). The basic lesions, however, are bullae that rupture and leave extensive ulcers usually covered by heavy yellowish fibrinous exudates sometimes described as pseudomembranes (Figs. 12-38 and 12-39). Such lesions may also involve the buccal mucosa and gingiva (Huff et al. 1983, Lozada-Nur et al. 1989, Scully et al. 1991, Barrett et al. 1993). The skin lesions are charac-

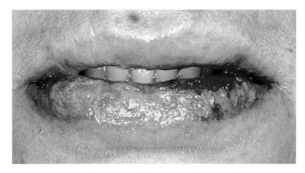

Fig. 12-37. Erythema multiforme with crust formation of the vermilion border of the lower lip.

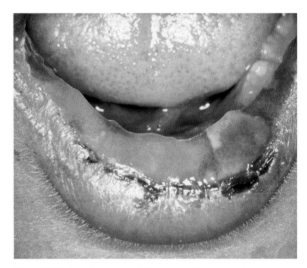

Fig. 12-38. Erythema multiforme with ulceration covered by heavy fibrin exudate.

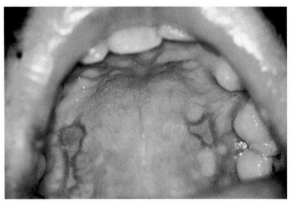

Fig. 12-39. Erythema multiforme with fibrin coated ulceration of palatal mucosa.

teristic due to the iris appearance with a central bulla formation surrounded by a blanched halo within an erythematous zone (Fig. 12-40). Similar intraoral lesions do occur but they are infrequent. The disease is usually self-limiting but recurrences are common. Healing of the lesions may require several weeks (Fabbri & Panconesi 1993).

The histopathology of EM shows intra- or subepi-

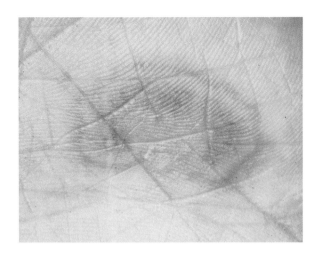

Fig. 12-40. Erythema multiforme. Skin lesion with characteristic iris appearance. Central bulla formation surrounded by a blanched halo within an erythematous zone.

thelial separation of epithelium from connective tissue with non-specific inflammation (Reed 1985). Immunohistochemical findings are non-specific and in most instances the diagnosis relies on the clinical findings.

Although periodontal lesions are not the most frequent intraoral manifestation, they can sometimes pose a differential diagnostic problem. The typical crusty ulcerations of the vermilion border and the heavy fibrin exudates covering intraoral lesions are indicative of erythema multiforme, sometimes therefore denoted erythema multiforme exudativum. The mucosal ulcerations may take weeks to heal and they are painful (Lozada-Nur et al. 1989).

As for any intraoral ulcerations, a gentle plaque control and professional cleaning is mandatory. The treatment often involves systemic corticosteroids, but topical treatment may act in cases with minor lesions.

Lupus erythematosus

Lupus erythematosus (LE) is a group of autoimmune connective tissue disorders in which autoantibodies form to various cellular constituents including nucleus, cytoplasma membrane and others. Women are much more affected than men. The etiology of LE remains unknown, but deposits of antigen-antibody complexes appear to play a role in the tissue damage characteristic of the disease (Schrieber & Maini 1984). LE includes two major forms: discoid LE (DLE) and systemic LE (SLE) which may involve a range of organ systems including kidney, heart, central nervous system, vascular system and bone marrow. The prevalence of LE has been estimated at 0.05% (Condemi 1987).

DLE is a mild chronic form, which involves skin and mucous membranes, sometimes involving the gingiva as well as other parts of the oral mucosa (Schiødt 1984a,b). The typical lesion presents a central atrophic area with small white dots surrounded by irradiating fine white striae with a periphery of telangiectasia (Fig. 12-41). The lesions can be ulcerated or clinically indistinguishable from leukoplakia or atrophic oral lichen planus (Fig. 12-42) (Schiødt 1984b). Sometimes patients present brownish gingival

lesions, which is a side effect of antimalarial drugs prescribed to these patients as part of their treatment (Fig. 12-43). Eight per cent of patients with DLE develop SLE, and ulcerations may be a sign of SLE, which, on the other hand, demonstrates oral lesions in 25-40% of the patients (Schiødt 1984a, Pisetsky 1986, Johnsson et al. 1988). The characteristic bordeaux-colored "butterfly" skin lesions are photosensitive, scaly, erythematous macules located on the bridge of the nose and the cheeks (Standefer & Mattox 1986). The systemic type, which can still be fatal because of nephrological and hematological complications, also has skin lesions on the face but they tend to spread over the entire body.

The diagnosis is based on clinical and histopathological findings. The epithelial changes, characteristic of oral LE lesions, are hyperkeratosis, keratin plugging and variation in epithelial thickness, liquefaction degeneration of basal cells and increased width of the basement membrane. The subepithelial connective tissue harbors inflammation, sometimes resembling OLP but often with a less distinct band-shaped pattern (Schiødt & Pindborg 1984). Immunohistochemical investigation reveals deposits of various immunoglobulins, C3 and fibrin along the basement membrane (Reibel & Schiødt 1986).

Systemic corticosteroid and other anti-inflammatory treatment regimens are required for SLE. Additional topical treatment is sometimes needed for symptomatic intraoral lesions to resolve.

Drug-induced mucocutaneous disorders

A number of drugs show reverse effects in the oral mucosa. Best known in the periodontal field is gingival hyperplasia related to intake of phenytoin, sodium valproate, cyclosporine and dihydropyridines. Because these lesions to some extent are plaque dependent, they are reviewed in Chapter 7. Other types of drugs may give rise to EM as mentioned above.

Several other drugs may be associated with adverse effects that include lesions of the oral mucosa. An example is azathioprine, which is an antimetabolite used for immunosuppression in the treatment of autoimmune and other diseases and to prevent rejec-

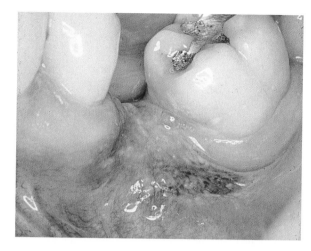

Fig. 12-41. Gingival discoid lupus erythematosus lesion. A central atrophic area with small white dots is surrounded by delicate white striae.

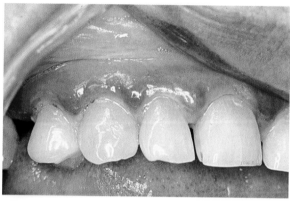

Fig. 12-42. Atrophic gingival discoid lupus erythematosus lesions may resemble plaque-induced gingivitis. Areas of the gingival margin of normal color shows that the lesions are not plaque-induced.

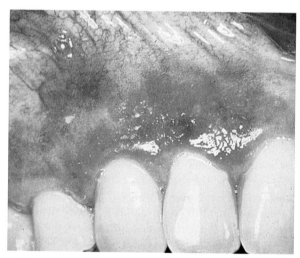

Fig. 12-43. Antimalarial drugs may result in brownish gingival discoloration. This is a patient with discoid lupus erythematosus receiving an antimalarial drug, chloroquine, as part of the treatment regimen.

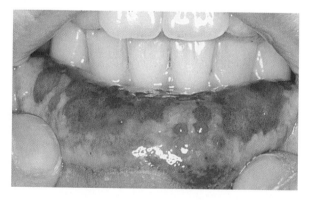

Fig. 12-44. Drug-induced stomatitis sometimes involve the gingiva. This is a gingival lesion with ulceration due to azathioprine, which is an antimetabolite used for immunosuppression.

tion of transplants. Its mode of action is through inhibition of purine base synthesis, resulting in suppression of nucleic acid and protein synthesis, whereby the immune response is inhibited at various stages. Rap-

idly proliferating tissues such as the bone marrow, the hair follicles, the gastrointestinal and the oral mucosa may thereby show side effects, oral ulceration being one such example. These ulcerations may include the gingiva. Other examples of drugs frequently resulting in adverse effects in the form of stomatitis are antineoplastic drugs used in cancer chemotherapy. Methotrexate is a cytostatic drug sometimes used in the treatment of leukemia. Epithelial atrophy, superficial sloughing, intense erythema and ulceration are characteristic findings in the oral mucosa of patients with adverse effects of the chemotherapeutic treatment (Pindborg 1992) (Fig. 12-44). The ulcerative lesions are frequent portals of entry for microorganisms from the mouth, and thereby often sources of serious systemic infection in patients with suppression of the bone marrow and reduced defense systems against infection. Professional plaque removal, mouth rinsing with 0.1% chlorhexidine and prophylactic antibiotic regimen are important in such patients (Sonis 1998, Holmstrup & Glick 2002).

Allergic reactions

Allergic manifestations in the oral mucosa are uncommon. However, several mechanisms may be involved in allergy, which are exaggerated immune reactions. Oral mucosal reactions are type I reactions (immediate type), which is mediated by IgE, or more often they are type IV reactions (delayed type) mediated by T-cells. The rare intraoral occurrence may be due to the fact that much higher concentrations of allergen are required for an allergic reaction to occur in the oral mucosa than in skin and other surfaces (Amlot et al. 1985, Lüders 1987, Holmstrup 1999). This chapter includes allergies to dental restorative materials, toothpastes, mouthwashes and food.

Dental restorative materials

The clinical manifestation of type IV allergy (contact allergy) occurs after a period of 12 to 48 hours following contact with the allergen. The oral mucosal affections have been denoted contact lesions and prior contact with the allergen resulting in sensitization is prerequisite for these reactions to occur (Holmstrup 1991). The oral mucosal reactions to restorative materials include reactions to mercury, nickel, gold, zinc, chromium, palladium and acrylics (Ovrutsky & Ulyanow 1976, Zaun 1977, Bergman et al. 1980, Council on Dental Materials, Instruments and Equipment Workshop 1984, Fisher 1987). The lesions, which may sometimes affect the gingiva, have clinical similarities with oral lichen planus affections, which is why they are denoted OLL (see earlier in this chapter) or oral leukoplakia (Fig. 12-45). They are reddish or whitish, sometimes ulcerated lesions, but one of the crucial diagnostic observations is that the lesions resolve after removal of the offending material. Additional patch testing to identify the exact allergen gives supplementary information, but for dental amalgam it has been shown that there is no obvious correlation between the result of an epicutaneous patch test and the clinical result after removal of the fillings (Skoglund 1994). A

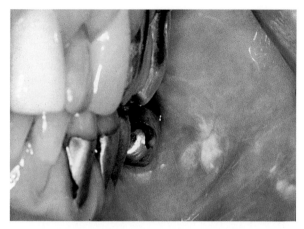

Fig. 12-45. Lichenoid contact lesion of left buccal mucosa due to type IV hypersensitivity to mercury. The lesion is confined to the zone of contact with the amalgam fillings. These lesions usually recover after replacement of the mercury containing fillings with composites or other materials devoid of allergy provoking components.

clinical manifestation confined to the area of contact with the offending restorative material and the result after replacing this material reveals the diagnosis (Holmstrup 1999).

Reactions to oral hygiene products, chewing gum and food

Toothpastes, mouthwashes and chewing gum
Contact allergy rarely occurs after the use of toothpastes (Sainio & Kanerva 1995, Skaare et al. 1997,) and mouthwashes (Sainio & Kanerva 1995). The constituents responsible for the allergic reactions may be flavor additives, for instance carvone and cinnamon (Drake & Maibach 1976) or preservatives (Duffin & Cowan 1985). The flavoring constituents may be used, also, in chewing gum and result in similar forms of gingivostomatitis (Kerr et al. 1971). The clinical manifestations of allergy include a diffuse fiery red edematous gingivitis sometimes with ulcerations or whiten-

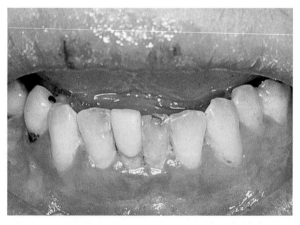

Fig. 12-46. Diffuse gingivitis and cheilitis due to contact allergy to flavor additive in dentifrice.

ing (Fig. 12-46). Similar affections may involve the labial, buccal and tongue mucosa and in addition cheilitis may be seen. The clinical manifestations, which are characteristic, form the basis of the diagnosis, which may be supported by resolving of the lesions after cessation of using the allergen-containing agent (Holmstrup 1999).

Foods

Allergic reactions attributable to food may manifest both as type I and type IV reactions. Type I reaction with severe swelling has been described after intake of food components such as peanuts and pumpkin seed. Birch pollen allergy is associated with some types of oral mucosa allergy, and more than 20% of patients with oral allergy may be hypersensitive to kiwi, peach, apple, chestnut and salami (Yamamoto et al. 1995, Antico 1996, Asero et al. 1996, Liccardi et al. 1996, Rossi et al. 1996, Helbling 1997, Wutrich 1997). Another food allergen resulting in gingivitis or gingivostomatitis is red pepper (Serio et al. 1991, Hedin et al. 1994). Unless it has been demonstrated that the lesions resolve after removal of the allergen, the diagnosis is difficult to establish.

Other gingival manifestations of systemic conditions

Gastro-intestinal diseases

Crohn's disease

Crohn's disease is characterized by chronic granulomatous infiltrates of the wall of the last ileal loops, but any part of the gastro-intestinal tract can be affected.

The oral cavity is part of the gastrointestinal tract. It is thus not surprising that Crohn's disease can occur from the rectum to the lips. The number of reports of lesions involving the periodontium is limited (van Steenberghe et al. 1976), which is probably related to a tradition by many clinicians of using the term aphtous lesions for any ulcerative disease of the oral mucosa. The oral lesions have striking similarity with those of the intestinal tract as revealed by rectoscopy, i.e. irregular long ulcerations with elevated borders with a cobblestone appearance. Usually, the periodontal lesions appear after the diagnosis has been established on the basis of the intestinal affection, but sometimes the oral lesions are the first findings leading to the diagnosis (Fig. 12-47). Exacerbations of the oral lesions appear in parallel with those of the intestine. An increased risk of periodontal destruction has been reported associated with a defective neutrophil function (Lamster et al. 1982).

The term orofacial granulomatosis has been used as a collective diagnosis of Crohn's disease, Melkersson-Rosenthal syndrome and sarcoidosis, because these diseases show the same histopathologic features, i.e. non-caseating, epitheloid cell granulomas in

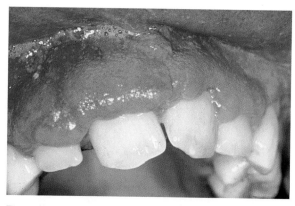

Fig. 12-47. Crohn's disease often presents oral, including gingival, lesions with mucosal hyperplasia. This is a granulomatous gingival hyperplasia of the upper incisor region.

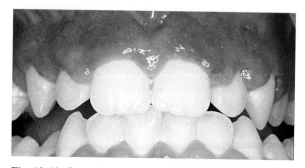

Fig. 12-48. Granulomatous gingival hyperplasia may be due to sarcoidosis, which is one of the orofacial granulomatosis, including also Crohn's disease and Melkersson-Rosenthal syndrome.

the affected tissue; although rarely, all three diseases may present gingival lesions, characterized by swellings (Pindborg 1992), sarcoidosis sometimes being fiery red granular gingival overgrowth (Fig. 12-48). Among 45 cases of oral sarcoidosis, 13% had gingival lesions (Blinder et al. 1997).

The local treatment consists of corticoid paste application daily or twice daily during painful exacerbations and a meticulous oral hygiene to reduce additional inflammation of the oral cavity.

Hematological disorders

Leukemia

Leukemia is a malignant hematological disorder with abnormal proliferation and development of leukocytes and their precursors in blood and bone marrow. It can involve any of the subsets of leukocytes, polymorphonuclear leukocytes, lymphocytes or monocytes. The normal hematopoiesis is suppressed and, in most cases of leukemia, the white blood cells appear in the circulating blood in immature forms. The leukemic cell proliferation at the expense of normal hematopoietic cell lines causes bone marrow failure and depressed blood cell count. As a consequence of the inability to produce sufficient functional white blood cells and platelets, death may result from infec-

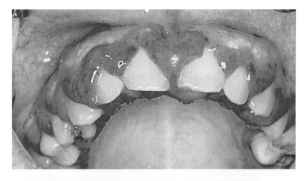

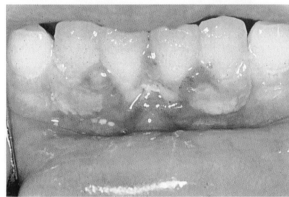

Fig. 12-49. Acute myelogenous leukemia with extensive swelling of the gingiva.

Fig. 12-50. Acute lymphocytic leukemia with gingival ulceration in a child.

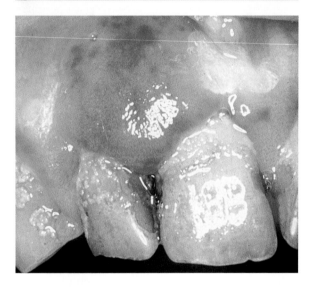

Fig. 12-51. Acute myelogenous leukemia with petecchia and swelling of the gingiva. This patient had several episodes of spontaneous bleeding from the gingiva, which prevented oral hygiene procedures from being undertaken.

tion or bleeding associated with neutropenia and thrombocytopenia.

The classification of leukemia is based on its course, acute or chronic, and origin of cells involved. The basic forms are: acute lymphocytic leukemia (ALL), acute myelogenous leukemia (AML), chronic lymphocytic leukemia (CLL) and chronic myelogenous leukemia (CML). Acute leukemias have an aggressive course resulting in death within 6 months if untreated. They occur rather seldom and patients are usually either under 20 or over 60 years of age. Chronic leukemias, of which the lymphocytic form is the most common, have less pronounced bone marrow failure and a more indolent course usually lasting several years. They occur during adulthood and normally after the age of 40. Whereas the peripheral granulocyte count is markedly elevated in chronic leukemia, it may be elevated, decreased or normal in acute leukemia (McKenna 2000).

Gingival manifestations in leukemia, which include extensive swelling (Fig. 12-49), ulceration (Fig. 12-50), petecchia (Fig. 12-51), and erythema, are much more common in acute than in chronic forms. Sometimes the manifestations lead to the diagnosis of leukemia. Thus, 69% of patients with acute leukemia had oral signs of leukemia on examination and 33% of the patients had gingival swelling (Pindborg 1992). In another study gingival swelling was revealed in 21% of AML patients but in no patients with ALL (Meyer et al. 2000). The latter group, on the other hand, showed both gingival erythema and ulcer in 36%. In leukemic children, only 10-17% appear to possess gingival swelling (Curtis 1971, Michaud et al. 1977). The pronounced gingival swelling seen in leukemic patients is mostly due to plaque-induced inflammation, since a stringent plaque control appears to resolve the swelling (Barrett 1984), but it may be due to the presence of leukemic infiltrates, although this has been reported to be an uncommon feature of leukemic patients (Barrett 1984). Due to secondary thrombocytopenia, gingival bleeding is a common sign in leukemic patients. It has been reported as the initial sign in 17.7% of patients with acute leukemias and in 4.4% of patients with chronic forms (Lynch & Ship 1967).

In general, the periodontal treatment of patients with leukemia is important, and it aims at reducing plaque as a source of bacteremia and damage to the periodontal tissues both during disease and during periods of chemotherapy. In such periods, potentially pathogenic bacteria occur in plaque simultaneous with granulocytopenia in these patients (Peterson et al. 1990). The reduction of periodontal inflammation may also prevent episodes of gingival bleeding. As with many other patients, chemical plaque control in combination with mechanical debridement appears to be most effective and is the preferred method of periodontal therapy in leukemic patients (Holmstrup & Glick 2002). However, the increased tendency to bleeding in many of these patients may necessitate the use of methods alternative to toothbrushing. A study of professional plaque removal preceding mouthrinsing with 0.1% chlorhexidine in patients with AML showed that the additional initial removal of plaque and calculus was more effective in reducing gingival inflammation than mouthrinsing with chlorhexidine alone (Bergman et al. 1992). A one-day antibiotic prophylaxis regimen with a combination of piperacillin and netilmicin was given prior to and after the mechanical debridement.

Periodontal treatment always involves a close cooperation with the medical department or specialist responsible for coordination of the patient's treatment.

TRAUMATIC LESIONS

The background of traumatic lesions of the oral tissues may be factitious, iatrogenic or accidental. Chemical as well as physical and thermal injuries may affect the periodontium (Armitage 1999).

Chemical injury

Surface etching by various chemical products with toxic properties may result in mucosal reactions including reactions of the gingiva. Chlorhexidine-induced mucosal desquamation (Fløtra et al. 1971, Almquist & Luthman 1988) (Fig. 12-52), acetylsalicylic acid burn (Najjar 1977), cocaine burn (Dello Russo & Temple 1982), and slough due to dentifrice detergents are examples of such reactions (Muhler 1970). These lesions are reversible and resolve after quitting the toxic influence. Another chemical injury to the gingival tissue may be caused by incorrect use of caustics

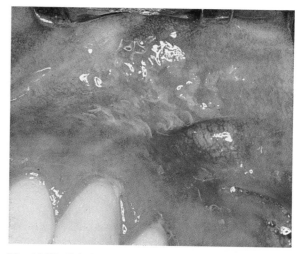

Fig. 12-52. Chlorhexidine-induced mucosal desquamation. This is a reversible type of lesion, which is completely normalized after stopping chlorhexidine use.

by the dentist. Paraformaldehyde used for pulp mummification may give rise to inflammation and necrosis of the gingival tissue if the cavity sealing is insufficient (Di Felice & Lombardi 1998). Usually, the diagnosis is obvious from the clinical findings and the patient history.

Physical injury

Oral hygiene agents and inexpedient procedures can be injurious to the gingival tissues. If the physical traumas are limited, the gingival response is hyperkeratosis, resulting in a white leukoplakia-like, frictional keratosis (Fig. 12-53). In case of more violent trauma the damage varies from superficial gingival laceration to major loss of tissue resulting in gingival recession (Axéll & Koch 1982, Smukler & Landsberg

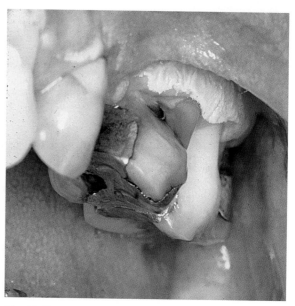

Fig. 12-53. Frictional keratosis due to violent toothbrushing. Note the cervical abrasion of adjacent teeth.

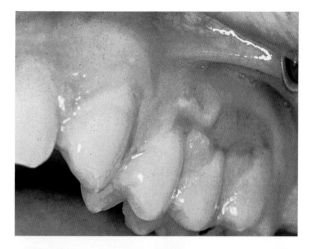

Fig. 12-54. Gingival wounding due to improper tooth-brushing. Note the characteristic horizontal extension of the lesion and the non-inflamed interdental papillae.

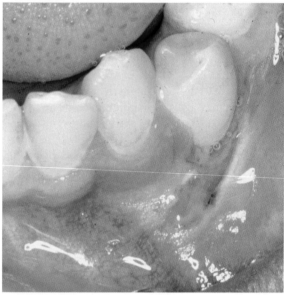

Fig. 12-55. Gingival wounding due to improper tooth-brushing. Note the characteristic horizontal extension of the lesion, which affects the most prominent part of the tooth arch.

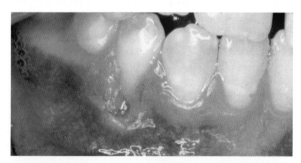

Fig. 12-56. Self-inflicted gingival recession with ulcerated margin due to 7-year-old child's scratching with fingernail.

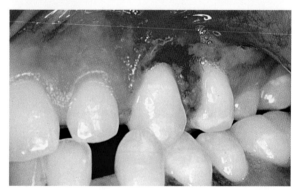

Fig. 12-57. Self-inflicted gingival ulceration with bleeding surface caused by finger scratching.

1984). Abrasivity of dentifrice, great brushing force and horizontal movement of the toothbrush contribute to the gingival injury even in young patients. Characteristic findings in these patients are extremely good oral hygiene, cervical tooth abrasion, and unaffected tops of the interdental papillae in the site of injury (Figs. 12-54 and 12-55). The disease has been termed traumatic ulcerative gingival lesion (Axéll & Koch 1982). Dental flossing may also cause gingival ulceration and inflammation primarily affecting the top of the interdental papillae. The prevalence of such findings is unknown (Gillette & Van House 1980). The diagnosis of physical injuries is based on the clinical findings. An important differential diagnosis is necrotizing gingivitis (Blasberg et al. 1981), see Chapter 10. The latter normally reveals itself as a necrotic gingival margin and interdental papillae, while brushing trauma leads to ulcerations of a few millimeters of the gingival margin.

A type of physical injury to the gingival tissues is self-inflicted. Sometimes the lesions are termed gingivitis artefacta. The lesions often show ulceration of the gingival margin often associated with recession (Fig. 12-56). Such lesions are most common in children and young individuals and two-thirds appear to involve female patients. Picking at or scratching the gingiva with a finger or a fingernail usually produces the lesions, which may be hemorrhagic (Fig. 12-57). Sometimes the lesions are made by instruments (Pattison 1983). The correct diagnosis is often difficult to establish based on clinical findings, and identification of the offending agent may be impossible.

Thermal injury

Extensive thermal burns of the oral mucosa are very rare, but minor burns particularly from hot beverages are seen occasionally. Their predilection by site is the palatal and labial mucosa but any part of the oral mucosa can be involved including the gingiva (Colby et al. 1961). The area involved is painful and erythematous and may slough a coagulated surface. Vesicles may also occur (Laskaris 1994) and sometimes the lesions present as ulceration, petecchia or erosion (Fig. 12-58). Obviously, the history is important for reaching the correct diagnosis. Common causes are hot coffee, pizza and melted cheese, but dental treatments involving improper handling of hot hydrocolloid impression material, hot wax or cautery instruments are other causes (Colby et al. 1961).

Foreign body reactions

Another type of tissue reaction is established through epithelial ulceration that allows entry of foreign material into gingival connective tissue. This can happen

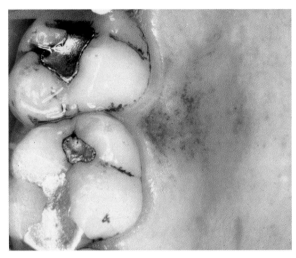

Fig. 12-58. Thermal burn with slight erosion of palatal gingiva due to hot coffee intake.

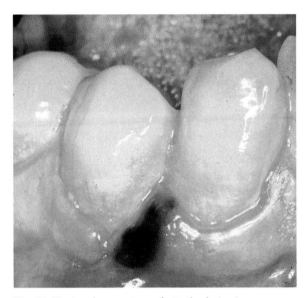

Fig. 12-59. Amalgam tattoo of attached gingiva.

via abrasion or cutting (Gordon & Daley 1997b), a route of tissue injury, which is best exemplified by the amalgam tattoo (Buchner & Hansen 1980) (Fig. 12-59). Gingival inflammation associated with foreign bodies has been termed foreign body gingivitis. A clinical study of this condition has shown that it often presents as a red or combined red/white painful chronic lesion frequently misdiagnosed as lichen planus (Gordon & Daley 1997a). An X-ray microanalysis of foreign body gingivitis showed that most of the identified foreign bodies were of dental material origin, usually abrasives (Gordon & Daley 1997b). Another way of introducing foreign substances into the tissues is self-inflicted injury, for instance due to chewing on sticks or self-induced tattooing (Gazi 1986). It is uncertain whether the inflammatory reaction in such cases is due to a toxic or in some instances an allergic reaction.

References

Almquist, H. & Luthman, J. (1988). Gingival and mucosal reactions after intensive chlorhexidine gel treatment with or without oral hygiene measures. *Scandinavian Journal of Dental Research* **96**, 557-560.

Amit, R., Morag, A., Ravid, Z., Hochman, N., Ehrlich, J. & Zakay-Rones, Z. (1992). Detection of herpes simplex virus in gingival tissue. *Journal of Periodontology* **63**, 502-506.

Amlot, P.L., Urbanek, R., Youlten, L.J., Kemeny, M. & Lessof, M.H. (1985). Type I allergy to egg and milk proteins: comparison of skin prick tests with nasal, buccal and gastric provocation tests. *International Archives of Allergy and Applied Immunology* **77**, 171-173.

Anaissie, E., Kantarjian, H., Jones, P., Barlogie, B., Luna, M., Lopez-Berestein, G. & Bodey, G.P. (1986). *Fusarium*: a newly recognized fungal pathogen in immunosuppressed patients. *Cancer* **57**, 2141-2145.

Andreasen, J.O. (1968). Oral lichen planus. 1. A clinical evaluation of 115 cases. *Oral Surgery Oral Medicine Oral Pathology* **25**, 31-42.

Antico, A. (1996). Oral allergy syndrome induced by chestnut (*Castanea sativa*). *Annals of Allergy, Asthma and Immunology* **76**, 37-40.

Araiche, M. & Brode, H. (1959). A case of fibromatosis gingivae. *Oral Surgery* **12**, 1307-1310.

Armitage, G.C. (1999). Development of a classification system for periodontal diseases and conditions. *Annals of Periodontology* **4**, 1-6.

Asero, R., Massironi, F & Velati, C. (1996). Detection of prognostic factors for oral allergy syndrome in patients with birch pollen hypersensitivity. *Journal of Allergy and Clinical Immunology* **97**, 611-616.

Assier, H., Bastuj-Garin, S., Revuz, J. & Roujeau, J-C. (1995). Erythema multiforme with mucous membrane involvement and Stevens-Johnson syndrome are clinically different disorders with distinct causes. *Archives of Dermatology* **131**, 539-543.

Aurelian, L., Kokuba, H. & Burnett, J.W. (1998). Understanding the pathogenesis of HSV-associated erythema multiforme. *Dermatology* **197**, 219-222.

Axéll, T. & Koch, G. (1982). Traumatic ulcerative gingival lesion. *Journal of Clinical Periodontology* **9**, 178-183.

Axéll, T. & Rundquist, L. (1987). Oral lichen planus – a demographic study. *Community Oral Dentistry and Oral Epidemiology* **15**, 52-56.

Bagan, J.V., Aguirre, J.M., del Olmo, J.A., Milian, A., Penarrocha, M., Rodrigo, J.M. & Cardona, F. (1994). Oral lichen planus and chronic liver disease: a clinical and morphometric study of the oral lesions in relation to transaminase elevation. *Oral Surgery Oral Medicine Oral Pathology* **78**, 337-342.

Barr, C., Lopez, M.R. & Rua-Dobles, A. (1992). Periodontal changes by HIV serostatus in a cohort of homosexual and bisexual men. *Journal of Clinical Periodontology* **19**, 794-801.

Barrett, A.W., Scully, C. & Eveson, J.W. (1993). Erythema multiforme involving gingiva. *Journal of Periodontology* **64**, 910-913.

Barrett, P.A. (1984). Gingival lesions in leukemia: A classification. *Journal of Periodontology* **55**, 585-588.

Barth, J.H. & Venning, V.A. (1987). Pemphigus. *British Journal of Hospital Medicine* **37**, 326, 330-331.

Bergman, M., Bergman, B. & Söremark, R. (1980). Tissue accumulation of nickel released due to electrochemical corrosion of non-previous dental casting alloys. *Journal of Oral Rehabilitation* **7**, 325-330.

Bergman, O.J., Ellegaard, B., Dahl, M. & Ellegaard, J. (1992). Gingival status during chemical plaque control with or without prior mechanical plaque removal in patients with acute myeloid leukemia. *Journal of Clinical Periodontology* **19**, 169-173.

Bhowmick, S.K., Gidvani, V.K. & Rettig, K.R. (2001). Hereditary gingival fibromatosis and growth retardation. *Endocrine Practice* **7**, 383-387.

Blake, G.C. & Trott, J.R. (1959). Acute streptococcal gingivitis. *Dental Practitioner and Dental Record* **10**, 43-45.

Blasberg, B., Jordan-Knox, A. & Conklin, R.J. (1981). Gingival ulceration due to improper toothbrushing. *Journal of the Canadian Dental Association* **47**, 462-464.

Blinder, D., Yahatom, R. & Taicher, S. (1997). Oral manifestations of sarcoidosis. *Oral Surgery Oral Medicine Oral Pathology Oral Radiology and Endodontics* **83**, 458-461.

Bottiger, L.E., Strandberg, I. & Westerholm, B. (1975). Drug induced febrile mucocutaneaous syndrome. *Acta Medica Scandinavica* **198**, 229-233.

Boutros, H.H., Van Winckle, R.B., Evans, G.A. & Wasan, S.M. (1995). Oral histoplasmosis masquerading as an invasive carcinoma. *Journal of Oral Maxillofacial Surgery* **53**, 1110-1114.

Brooke, R.I. (1973). The oral lesions of bullous pemphigoid. *Journal of Oral Medicine* **28**, 36-40.

Buchner, A. & Hansen, L.S. (1980). Amalgam pigmentation (amalgam tattoo) of the oral mucosa. *Oral Surgery Oral Medicine Oral Pathology* **49**, 139-142.

Buechner, S.A. (1984). T cell subsets and macrophages in lichen planus. In situ identification using monoclonal antibodies and histochemical techniques. *Dermatologica* **169**, 325-329.

Burns, J.C. (1980). Diagnostic methods for herpes simplex infection: a review. *Oral Surgery* **50**, 346-349.

Bystryn, J-C. (1996). Erythema multiforme with mucous membrane involvement and Stevens-Johnson syndrome are clinically different disorders. Comment. *Archives of Dermatology* **132**, 711-712.

Camisa, C., Allen, C.M., Bowen, B. & Olsen, R.G. (1986). Indirect immunofluorescence of oral lichen planus. *Journal of Oral Pathology* **15**, 218-220.

Cannon, R.D., Holmes, A.R, Mason, A.B. & Monk, B.C. (1995). Oral candida: Clearance, colonization, or candidiasis? *Journal of Dental Research* **74**, 1152-1161.

Carrozzo, M., Gandolfo, S., Carbone, M., Colombatto, P., Broccoletti, R., Garzino-Demo, P. & Ghizetti, V. (1996). Hepatitis C virus infection in Italian patients with oral lichen planus: a prospective case control study. *Journal of Oral Pathology and Medicine* **25**, 527-533.

Cebaillos-Salobrena, A., Aguirre-Urizar, J.M. & Bagan-Sebastian, J.V. (1996). Oral manifestations associated with human immunodeficiency virus infection in a Spanish population. *Journal of Oral Pathology and Medicine* **25**, 523-526.

Chinn, H., Chernoff, D.N., Migliorati, C.A., Silverman, S. & Green, T.L. (1995). Oral histoplasmosis in HIV-infected patients. *Oral Surgery Oral Medicine Oral Pathology* **79**, 710-714.

Cobb, C.M., Shultz, R.E., Brewer, J.H. & Dunlap, C.L. (1989). Chronic pulmonary histoplasmosis with an oral lesion. *Oral Surgery Oral Medicine Oral Pathology* **67**, 73-76.

Colby, R.A., Kerr, D.A. & Robinson, H.B.G. (1961). *Color Atlas of Oral Pathology*. Philadelphia: JB Lippincott Company, p. 96.

Coletta, R.D., Almeida, O.P., Reynolds, M.A. & Sauk, J.J. (1999). Alteration in expression of MMP-1 and MMP-2 but not TIMP-1 and TIMP-2 in hereditary gingival fibromatosis is mediated by TGF-beta 1 autocrine stimulation. *Journal of Periodontal Research* **34**, 457-463.

Condemi, J.J. (1987). The autoimmune diseases. *Journal of the American Medical Association* **258**, 2920-2929.

Consensus Report (1999). *Ann Periodontol* **4**, 30-31.

Contreras, A., Falkler, W.A., Enwonwu, C.O., Idigbe, E.O., Savage, K.O., Afolabi, M.B., Onwujekwe, D., Rams, T.E. & Slots, J. (1997). Human *Herpesviridae* in acute necrotizing ulcerative gingivitis in children in Nigeria. *Oral Microbiology and Immunology* **12**, 259-265.

Coscia-Porrazzi, L., Maiello, F.M., Ruocco, V. & Pisani, M. (1985).

Cytodiagnosis of oral pemphigus vulgaris. *Journal of Acta Cytologica* **29**, 746-749.

Council on Dental Materials, Instruments and Equipment Workshop (1984). Biocompatibility of metals in dentistry – recommendations for clinical implementation. *Journal of the American Dental Association* **109**, 469-471.

Cuestas-Carneiro, R. & Bornancini, C.A. (1988). Hereditary generalized gingival fibromatosis associated with hypertrichosis: report of five cases in one family. *Journal of Oral Maxillofacial Surgery* **46**, 415-420.

Curtis, A.B. (1971). Childhood leukemias: initial oral manifestations. *Journal of the American Dental Association* **83**, 159-164.

Dahl, M.G. & Cook, L.J. (1979). Lesions induced by trauma in pemphigoid. *British Journal of Dermatology* **101**, 469-473.

Daniels, T.E. & Quadra-White, C. (1981). Direct immunofluorescence in oral mucosal disease: a diagnostic analysis of 130 cases. *Oral Surgery Oral Medicine Oral Pathology* **51**, 38-54.

Dello Russo, N.M. & Temple, H.V. (1982). Cocaine effects on gingiva. *Journal of the American Dental Association* **104**, 13.

Di Felice, R. & Lombardi, T. (1998). Gingival and mandibular bone necrosis caused by a paraformaldehyde-containing paste. *Endodontics & Dental Traumatology* **14**, 196-198.

Domloge-Hultsch, N., Anhalt, G.J., Gammon, W.R., Lazarova, Z., Briggaman, R., Welch, M., Jabs, D.A., Huff, C. & Yancey, K.B. (1994). Antiepiligrin cicatricial pemphigoid. A subepithelial bullous disorder. *Archives of Dermatology* **130**, 1521-1529.

Domloge-Hultsch, N., Gammon, W.R., Briggaman, R.A., Gil, S.G., Carter, W.G. & Yancey, K.B. (1992). Epiligrin, the major human keratinocyte integrin ligand, is a target in both an acquired autoimmune and an inherited subepidermal blistering skin disease. *Journal of Clinical Investigations* **90**, 1628-1633.

Drake, T.E. & Maibach, H.I. (1976). Allergic contact dermatitis and stomatitis caused by cinnamic aldehyde-flavoured toothpaste. *Archives of Dermatology* **112**, 202-203.

Drinkard, C.R., Decker, L., Little, J.W., Rhame, F.S., Balfour, H.H. Jr., Rhodus, N.L., Merry, J.W., Walker, P.O., Miller, C.E., Volberding, P.A. & Melnick, S.L. (1991). Periodontal status of individuals in early stages of human immunodeficiency virus infection. *Community Dentistry and Oral Epidemiology* **19**, 281-285.

Duffin, P. & Cowan, G.C. (1985). An allergic reaction to toothpaste. *Journal of the Irish Dental Association* **32**, 11-12.

EC-Clearinghouse on Oral Problems Related to HIV Infection and WHO Collaborating Centre on Oral Manifestations of the Immunodeficiency Virus. Classification and diagnostic criteria for oral lesions in HIV infection. (1993). *Journal of Oral Pathology and Medicine* **22**, 289-291.

Ehrlich, J., Cohen, G.H. & Hochman, N. (1983). Specific herpes simplex virus antigen in human gingiva. *Journal of Periodontology* **54**, 357-360.

Eisenberg, E. (1978). Intraoral isolated herpes zoster. *Oral Surgery Oral Medicine Oral Pathology* **45**, 214-219.

Emerson, T.G. (1965). Hereditary gingival fibromatosis: a family pedigree of four generations. *Oral Surgery Oral Medicine Oral Pathology* **19**, 1-9.

Eversole, L.R. (1994). Immunopathology of oral mucosal ulcerative, desquamative and bullous diseases. *Oral Surgery Oral Medicine Oral Pathology* **77**, 555-571.

Eversole, L.R. (1995). Oral mucosal diseases. Review of the literature. In: Millard, H.D. & Mason, D.K., eds. *Perspectives on 1993 Second World Workshop on Oral Medicine.* Ann Arbor: University of Michigan, pp. 105-162.

Eversole, L.R., Dam, J., Ficarra, G. & Hwang, C-Y. (1994). Leukocyte adhesion molecules in oral lichen planus: a T cell mediated immunopathologic process. *Oral Microbiology and Immunology* **9**, 376-383.

Fabbri, P. & Panconesi, E. (1993). Erythema multiforme "minus and maius" and drug intake. *Clinics in Dermatology* **11**, 479-489.

Fisher, A.A. (1987). Contact stomatitis. *Clinics in Dermatology* **5**, 709-717.

Fløtra, L., Gjermo, P., Rølla, G. & Wærhaug, J. (1971). Side effects of chlorhexidine mouth washes. *Scandinavian Journal of Dental Research* **79**, 119-125.

Fortune, F. & Buchanan, J.A.G. (1993). Oral lichen planus and coeliac disease. *Lancet* **341**, 1154-1155.

Friedman, R.B., Gunsolley, J., Gentry, A., Dinius, A., Kaplowitz, L. & Settle, J. (1991). Periodontal status of HIV-seropositive and AIDS patients. *Journal of Periodontology* **62**, 623-627.

Fujii, H., Ohashi, M. & Nagura, H. (1988). Immunohistochemical analysis of oral lichen-planus-like eruption in graft-versus-host disease after allogeneic bone marrow transplantation. *American Journal of Clinical Pathology* **89**, 177-186.

Gallagher, G. & Shklar, G. (1987). Oral involvement in mucous membrane pemphigoid. *Clinics in Dermatology* **5**, 18-27.

Gandolfo, S., Carbone, M., Carozzo, M. & Gallo, V. (1994). Oral lichen planus and hepatitis C virus (HCV) infection: is there a relationship? A report of 10 cases. *Journal of Oral Pathology and Medicine* **23**, 119-122.

Gazi, M.I. (1986). Unusual pigmentation of the gingiva. *Oral Surgery Oral Medicine Oral Pathology* **62**, 646-649.

Gebel, K. & Hornstein, O.P. (1984). Drug-induced oral erythema multiforme. Results of a long-term retrospective study. *Dermatologica* **168**, 35-40.

Gillette, W.B. & Van House, R.L. (1980). Ill effects of improper oral hygiene procedure. *Journal of the American Dental Association* **101**, 476-480.

Glick M., Pliskin, M.E., & Weiss, R.C. (1990). The clinical and histologic appearance of HIV-associated gingivitis. *Oral Surgery Oral Medicine Oral Pathology* **69**, 395-398.

Gordon, S.C. & Daley, T.D. (1997a). Foreign body gingivitis: clinical and microscopic features of 61 cases. *Oral Surgery Oral Medicine Oral Pathology* **83**, 562-570.

Gordon, S.C. & Daley, T.D. (1997b). Foreign body gingivitis: identification of the foreign material by energy-dispersive X-ray microanalysis. *Oral Surgery Oral Medicine Oral Pathology* **83**, 571-576.

Gorlin, R.J., Cohen, M.M., & Levis, L.S. (1990). *Syndromes of the head and neck,* 3rd edn. New York: Oxford University Press, pp. 847-855.

Grassi, M., Williams, C.A., Winkler, J.R. & Murray, P.A. (1989). Management of HIV-associated periodontal diseases. In: Robertson, P.B. & Greenspan, J.S., eds. Perspectives on Oral Manifestations of AIDS. *Proceedings of First International Symposium on Oral Manifestations of AIDS.* Littleton: PSG Publishing Company, pp. 119-130.

Greenberg, M.S. (1996). Herpes virus infections. *Dental Clinics of North America* **40**, 359-368.

Hart, T.C., Pallos, D., Bowden, D.W., Bolyard, J., Pettenati, M.J. & Cortelli, J.R. (1998). Genetic linkage of hereditary gingival fibromatosis to chromosome 2p21. *American Journal of Human Genetics* **62**, 876-883.

Hart, T.C., Pallos, D., Bozzo, L., Almeida, O.P., Marazita, M.L., O'Connell, J.R. & Cortelli, J.R. (2000). Evidence of genetic heterogeneity for hereditary gingival fibromatosis. *Journal of Dental Research* **79**, 1758-1764.

Hartsfield, J.K., Bixler, D. & Hazen, R.H. (1985). Gingival fibromatosis with sensoneural hearing loss: an autosomal dominant trait. *American Journal of Medical Genetics* **22**, 623-627.

Hedin, C.A., Karpe, B. & Larsson, Å. (1994). Plasma-cell gingivitis in children and adults. A clinical and histological description. *Swedish Dental Journal* **18**, 117-124.

Helbling, A. (1997). Important cross-reactive allergens. *Schweizerische Medizinische Wochenschrift* **127**, 382-389.

Hodge, L., Marsden, R.A., Black, M.M., Bhogal, B. & Corbett, M.F. (1981). Bullous pemphigoid: The frequency of mucosal involvement and concurrent malignancy related to indirect immunofluorescence findings. *British Journal of Dermatology* **105**, 65-69.

Holmstrup, P. (1991). Reactions of the oral mucosa related to silver amalgam. *Journal of Oral Pathology and Medicine* **20**, 1-7.

Holmstrup, P. (1992). The controversy of a premalignant potential of oral lichen planus is over. *Oral Surgery Oral Medicine Oral Pathology* 73, 704-706.

Holmstrup, P. (1999). Non-plaque induced gingival lesions. *Annals of Periodontology* 4, 20-31.

Holmstrup, P. & Axéll, T. (1990). Classification and clinical manifestations of oral yeast infection. *Acta Odontologica Scandinavica* 48, 57-59.

Holmstrup, P. & Dabelsteen, E. (1979). Changes in carbohydrate expression of lichen planus affected oral epithelial cell membranes. *The Journal of Investigative Dermatology* 73, 364-367.

Holmstrup, P. & Glick, M. (2002). Treatment of periodontal disease in the immunodeficient patient. *Periodontology 2000* 28, 190-205.

Holmstrup, P. & Johnson, N.W. (1997). Chemicals in diagnosis and management of selected mucosal disorders affecting the gingiva. In: Lang, N.P., Karring, T. & Lindhe, J., eds. *Proceedings of the 2nd European Workshop.* Berlin: Quintessence, pp. 366-379.

Holmstrup, P. & Samaranayake, L.P. (1990). Acute and AIDS-related oral candidoses. In: Samaranayake, L.P. & MacFarlane, T.W., eds. *Oral Candidosis.* London: Wright, Butterworth & Co. Ltd, pp. 133-155.

Holmstrup, P., Schiøtz, A.W. & Westergaard, J. (1990). Effect of dental plaque control on gingival lichen planus. *Oral Surgery Oral Medicine Oral Pathology* 69, 585-590.

Holmstrup, P., Thorn, J.J., Rindum, J. & Pindborg, J.J. (1988). Malignant development of lichen-planus-affected oral mucosa. *Journal of Oral Pathology* 17, 219-225.

Holmstrup, P. & Westergaard, J. (1998). HIV infection and periodontal diseases. *Periodontology 2000* 18, 37-46.

Horning, G.M., Fisher, J.G., Barker, F., Killoy, W.J. & Lowe, J.W. (1985). Gingival fibromatosis with hypertrichosis. *Journal of Periodontology* 56, 344-347.

Hudson, C.D. & Vickers, R.A. (1971). Clinicopathologic observations in prodromal herpes zoster of the fifth cranial nerve. *Oral Surgery Oral Medicine Oral Pathology* 31, 494-501.

Huff, J.C., Weston, W.L. & Tonnesen, M.G. (1983). Erythema multiforme: a critical review of characteristics, diagnostic criteria and causes. *Journal of the American Academy of Dermatology* 8, 763-775.

Jonsson, H., Nived, O. & Sturfelt, G. (1988). The effect of age on clinical and serological manifestations in unselected patients with systemic lupus erythematosus. *Journal of Rheumatology* 15, 505-509.

Jorgensen, R.J. & Cocker, M.E. (1974). Variation in the inherence and expression of gingival fibromatosis. *Journal of Periodontology* 45, 472-477.

Kauppinen, K. & Stubb, S. (1984). Drug eruptions: causative agents and clinical types. A series of in-patients during a 10-year period. *Acta Dermatolicica et Venereologica* 64, 320-324.

Kerr, D.A., McClatchey, K.D. & Regezi, J.A. (1971). Allergic gingivostomatitis (due to gum chewing). *Journal of Periodontology* 42, 709-712.

Kilpi, A.M., Rich, A.M., Radden, B.G. & Reade, P.C. (1988). Direct immunofluorescence in the diagnosis of oral mucosal disease. *International Journal of Oral Maxillofacial Surgery* 17, 6-10.

Klein, R.S., Quart, A.M. & Small, C.B. (1991). Periodontal disease in heterosexuals with acquired immuno-deficiency syndrome. *Journal of Periodontology* 62, 535-540.

Krogh, P., Holmstrup, P., Thorn, J.J., Vedtofte, P. & Pindborg, J.J. (1987). Yeast species and biotypes associated with oral leukoplaki and lichen planus. *Oral Surgery Oral Medicine Oral Pathology* 63, 48-54.

Lamey P.J., Rees, T.D., Binnie, W.H., Wright, J.M., Rankin, K.V. & Simpson, N.B. (1992). Oral presentation of pemphigus vulgaris and its response to systemic steroid therapy. *Oral Surgery Oral Medicine Oral Pathology* 74, 54-57.

Lamster, I.B., Rodrick, M.L., Sonis, S.T. & Falchuk, Z.M. (1982). An analysis of peripheral blood and salivary polymorphonuclear leukocyte function, circulating immune complex levels and oral status in patients with inflammatory bowel disease. *Journal of Periodontology* 53, 231-238.

Laskaris, G. (1994). *Color Atlas of Oral Diseases.* Stuttgart: Georg Thieme Verlag, p. 66.

Laskaris, G. & Angelopoulos, A. (1981). Cicatricial pemphigoid: direct and indirect immunofluorescent studies. *Oral Surgery Oral Medicine Oral Pathology* 51, 48-54.

Laskaris, G., Hadjivassiliou, M., Stratigos, J. (1992). Oral signs and symptoms in 160 Greek HIV-infected patients. *Journal of Oral Pathology and Medicine* 21, 120-123.

Laskaris, G. & Nicolis, G. (1980). Immunopathology of oral mucosa in bullous pemphigoid. *Oral Surgery Oral Medicine Oral Pathology* 50, 340-345.

Laskaris, G., Sklavounou, A. & Stratigos, J. (1982). Bullous pemphigoid, cicatricial pemphigoid and pemphigus vulgaris: a comparative clinical survey of 278 cases. *Oral Surgery Oral Medicine Oral Pathology* 54, 656-662.

Lennette, E.H. & Magoffin, R.L. (1973). Virologic and immunologic aspects of major oral ulcerations. *Journal of the American Dental Association* 87, 1055-1073.

Leonard, J.N., Haffenden, G.P., Ring, N.P., McMinn, R.M., Sidgwick, A., Mowbray, J.F., Unsworth, D.J., Holborow, E.J., Blenkinsopp, W.K., Swain, A.F. & Fry, L. (1982). Linear IgA disease in adults. *British Journal of Dermatology* 107, 301-316.

Leonard, J.N., Wright, P., Williams, D.M., Gilkes, J.J., Haffenden, G.P., McMinn, R.M. & Fry, L. (1984). The relationship between linear IgA disease and benign mucous membrane pemphigoid. *British Journal of Dermatology* 110, 307-314.

Lever, W.F. & Schaumburg-Lever, G. (1997). Immunosuppressants and prednisone in pemphigus vulgaris. Therapeutic results obtained in 63 patients between 1961-1978. *Archives of Dermatology* 113, 1236-1241.

Liccardi, G., D'Amato, M. & D'Amato, G. (1996). Oral allergy syndrome after ingestion of salami in a subject with monosentitization to mite allergens. *The Journal of Allergy and Clinical Immunology* 98, 850-852.

Littner, M.M., Dayan, D., Kaffe, I., Begleiter, A., Gorsky, M., Moskana, D. & Buchner, A. (1982). Acute streptococcal gingivostomatitis. Report of five cases and review of the literature. *Oral Surgery Oral Medicine Oral Pathology* 53,144-147.

Loh, F., Yeo, J., Tan, W. & Kumarasinghe, G. (1989). Histoplasmosis presenting as hyperplastic gingival lesion. *Journal of Oral Pathology and Medicine* 18, 533-536.

Lozada, F. & Silverman, S. Jr. (1978). Erythema multiforme. Clinical characteristics and natural history in fifty patients. *Oral Surgery Oral Medicine Oral Pathology* 46, 628-636.

Lozada-Nur, F., Gorsky, M. & Silverman, S. Jr. (1989). Oral erythema multiforme: clinical observations and treatment of 95 patients. *Oral Surgery Oral Medicine Oral Pathology* 67, 36-40.

Lüders, G. (1987). Exogenously induced diseases of the oral mucosa. *Zeitschrift für Hautkrankheiten* 62, 603-606, 611-612.

Lynch, M.A. & Ship, I.I. (1967). Initial oral manifestations of leukemia. *Journal of the American Dental Association* 75, 932-940.

Manton, S.M. & Scully, C. (1988). Mucous membrane pemphigoid – an elusive diagnosis. *Oral Surgery Oral Medicine Oral Pathology* 66, 37-40.

Masouredis, C.M., Katz, M.H., Greenspan, D., Herrera, C., Hollander, H., Greenspan, J.S. & Winkler, J.R. (1992). Prevalence of HIV-associated periodontitis and gingivitis in HIV-infected patients attending an AIDS clinic. *Journal of Acquired Immune Deficiency Syndrome* 5, 479-483.

McKellar, G.M. & Reade, P.C. (1986). Erythema multiforme and mycoplasma pneumoniae infection. Report and discussion of a case presenting with stomatitis. *International Journal of Oral Maxillofacial Surgery* 15, 342-348.

McKenna, S.J. (2000). Leukemia. *Oral Surgery Oral Medicine Oral Pathology Oral Radiology and Endodontics* 89, 137-139.

Melbye, M., Grossman, R.J., Goedert, J.J., Eyster, M.E. & Biggar, R.J. (1987). Risk of AIDS after herpes zoster. *Lancet* 28, 728-731.

Meyer, U., Kleinheinz, J., Handschel, J., Kruse-Losler, B., Weingart, D. & Joos, U. (2000). Oral findings in three different groups of immunocompromised patients. *Journal of Oral Pathology and Medicine* **29**, 153-158.

Michaud, M., Baehner, R.L., Bixler, D. & Kafrawy, A.H. (1977). Oral manifestations of acute leukemia in children. *Journal of the American Dental Association* **95**, 1145-1150.

Millar, E.P. & Traulis, M.J. (1994). Herpes zoster of the trigeminal nerve: the dentist's role in diagnosis and management. *Journal of the Canadian Dental Association* **60**, 450-453.

Miller, C.S. (1996). Viral infections in the immunocompetent patient. *Clinics in Dermatology* **14**, 225-241.

Miller, C.S. & Redding, S.W. (1992). Diagnosis and management of orofacial herpes simplex virus infections. *Dental Clinics of North America* **36**, 879-895.

Mindel, A. (1991). Is it meaningful to treat patients with recurrent herpetic infections? *Scandinavian Journal of Infections* **78**, 27-32.

Miura, S., Smith, C.C., Burnett, J.W. & Aurelian, L. (1992). Detection of viral DNA within skin of healed recurrent herpes simplex infection and erythema multiforme lesions. *Journal of Investigative Dermatology* **98**, 68-72.

Muhler, J.C. (1970). Dentifrices and oral hygiene. In: Bernier, J.L. & Muhler, J.C., eds. *Improving Dental Practice Through Preventive Measures*. St. Louis: C.V. Mosby Co, pp. 133-157.

Murray, P.A., Grassi, M. & Winkler, J.R. (1989). The microbiology of HIV-associated periodontal lesions. *Journal of Clinical Periodontology* **16**, 636-642.

Murray, P.A., Winkler, J.R., Peros, W.J., French, C.K. & Lippke, J.A. (1991). DNA probe detection of periodontal pathogens in HIV-associated periodontal lesions. *Oral Microbiology and Immunology* **6**, 34-40.

Murray, P.A., Winkler, J.R., Sadkowski, L., Kornman, K.S., Steffensen, B., Robertson, P. & Holt, S.C. (1988). The microbiology of HIV-associated gingivitis and periodontitis. In: Robertson, P.B. & Greenspan, J.S., eds. Oral manifestations of AIDS. *Proceedings of First International Sympsosium on Oral Manifestations of AIDS*. Littleton: PSG Publishing Company, pp. 105-118.

Nagao, Y., Sata, M., Tanikawa, K., Itoh, K. & Kameyama, T. (1995). Lichen planus and hepatitis C virus in the northern Kyushu region of Japan. *European Journal of Clinical Investigation* **25**, 910-914.

Najjar, T.A. (1977). Harmful effects of "aspirin compounds". *Oral Surgery Oral Medicine Oral Pathology* **44**, 64-70.

Negi, M., Tsuboi, R., Matsui, T. & Ogawa, H. (1984). Isolation and characterization of proteinase from Candida albicans: substrate specificity. *The Journal of Investigative Dermatology* **83**, 32-36.

Nesbit, S.P. & Gobetti, J.P. (1986). Multiple recurrence of oral erythema multiforme after secondary herpes simplex: Report of case and review of literature. *Journal of the American Dental Association* **112**, 348-352.

Nevin, N.C., Scally, B.G., Kernohan, D.C. & Dodge, J.A. (1971). Hereditary gingival fibromatosis. *Journal of Mental Deficiency Research* **15**, 130-135.

Newman, N.H., Rees, T.D. & Kinane, D.F. (1993). Diseases of the periodontium. Northwood: Science Reviews Limited.

Nishikawa, T., Hashimoto, T., Shimizu, H., Ebihara, T. & Amagai, M. (1996). Pemphigus from immunofluorescence to molecular biology. *Journal of Dermatological Science* **12**, 1-9.

Nousari, H.C. & Anhalt, G.J. (1995). Bullous skin diseases. *Current Opinion on Immunology* **7**, 844-852.

O'Brien, J.J. & Campoli-Richards, D.M. (1989). Acyclovir. An update of its role in antiviral therapy. *Current Therapeutics* **30**, 81-93.

Odds, F.C. (1985). *Candida albicans* proteinase as a virulence factor in the pathogenesis of Candida infections. *Zentralblatt für Bakteriologie und Hygiene, I. Abt. Orig. A* **260**, 539-542.

Overall, J.C. Jr. (1982). Oral herpes simplex: pathogenesis. Clinical and virologic course, approach to treatment. In: Hooks, J.J. & Jordan, G.W., eds. *Viral infections in oral medicine*. New York: Elsevier/North Holland, pp. 53-78.

Ovrutsky, G.D. & Ulyanow, A.D. (1976). Allergy to chromium using steel dental prosthesis. *Stomatologia (Moscow)* **55**, 60-61.

Parra, B. & Slots, J. (1996). Detection of human viruses in periodontal pockets using polymerase chain reaction. *Oral Microbiology and Immunology* **5**, 289-293.

Pattison, G.L. (1983). Self-inflicted gingival injuries: literature review and case report. *Journal of Periodontology* **54**, 299-304.

Pedersen, A. & Reibel, J. (1989). Intraoral infection with *Mycobacterium chelonae. Oral Surgery Oral Medicine Oral Pathology* **67**, 262-265.

Peterson, D.E., Minh, G.E., Reynolds, M.A., Weikel, D.S., Overholser, C.D., DePaola, L.G., Wade, J.C. & Suzuki, J.B. (1990). Effect of granulocytopenia on oral microbial relationships in patients with acute leukemia. *Oral Surgery Oral Medicine Oral Pathology Oral Radiology and Endodontics* **70**, 720-723.

Piette, E. & Reychler, H. (1991) Traité de pathologiques buccale et maxillo-faciale. Bruxelles: De Boeck-Wesmael, p. 1977.

Pindborg, J.J. (1992). Atlas of diseases of the oral mucosa, 5th edn. Copenhagen: Munksgaard, p. 246.

Pisanti, S., Sharav, Y., Kaufman, E. & Posner, L.N. (1974). Pemphigus vulgaris: incidence in Jews of different ethnic groups, according to age, sex and initial lesion. *Oral Surgery Oral Medicine Oral Pathology* **38**, 382-387.

Pisetsky, D.S. (1986). Systemic lupus erythematosus. *Medical Clinics of North America* **70**, 337-353.

Porter, S.R. & Scully, C. (1994a). Periodontal aspects of systemic disease, a classification. In: Lang, N.P. & Karring, T., eds. *Proceedings of the 1st European workshop on periodontology*. London: Quintessence Publishing Co, pp. 375-414.

Porter, S.R. & Scully, C (1994b). Periodontal aspects of systemic disease; therapeutic aspects. In: Lang, N.P. & Karring, T., eds. *Proceedings of the 1st European workshop on periodontology*. London: Quintessence Publishing Co, pp. 415-438.

Rajah, V. & Essa, A. (1993). Histoplasmosis of the oral cavity, oropharynx and larynx. *Journal of Laryngology and Otology* **107**, 58-61.

Ramirez-Amador, V., Madero, J.G., Pedraza, L.E., de la Rosa Garcia, E., Guevara, M.G., Gutierrez, E.R. & Reyes-Teran, G. (1996). Oral secondary syphilis in a patient with human immunodeficiency virus infection. *Oral Surgery Oral Medicine Oral Pathology Oral Radiology & Endodontics* **81**, 652-654.

Ramon, Y., Berman W. & Bubis, J.S. (1967). Gingival fibromatosis combined with cherubism. *Oral Surgery* **24**, 435-448.

Reed, R.J. (1985). Erythema multiforme. A clinical syndrome and a histologic complex. *American Journal of Dermatopathology* **7**,143-152.

Rees, T.D. (1989). Adjunctive therapy. *Proceedings of the World Workshop in Clinical Periodontics*. Chicago: The American Academy of Periodontology, X-1/X-39.

Reibel, J. & Schiødt, M. (1986). Immunohistochemical studies on colloid bodies (Civatte bodies) in oral lesions of discoid lupus erythematosus. *Scandinavian Journal of Dental Research* **94**, 536-544.

Rentier, B., Piette, J., Baudoux, L., Debrus, S., Defechereux, P., Merville, M.P., Sadzot-Delvaux, C. & Schoonbroodt, S. (1996). Lessons to be learned from varicella-zoster virus. *Veterinary Microbiology* **53**, 55-66.

Riley, C., London, J.P. & Burmeister, J,A. (1992). Periodontal health in 200 HIV-positive patients. *Journal of Oral Pathology and Medicine* **21**, 124-127.

Rindum, J.L., Stenderup, A. & Holmstrup, P. (1994). Identification of *Candida albicans* types related to healthy and pathological oral mucosa. *Journal of Oral Pathology and Medicine* **23**, 406-412.

Rivera-Hidalgo, F. & Stanford, T.W. (1999). Oral mucosal lesions caused by infective microorganisms. I. Viruses and bacteria. *Periodontology 2000* **21**,106-124.

Robinson, P.G., Sheiham, A., Challacombe, S.J. & Zakrzewska, J.M. (1996). The periodontal health of homosexual men with HIV infection: a controlled study. *Oral Diseases* **2**, 45-52.

Robinson, P.G., Winkler, J.R., Palmer, G., Westenhouse, J., Hilton, J.F.& Greenspan, J.S. (1994). The diagnosis of periodontal conditions associated with HIV infection. *Journal of Periodontology* **65**, 236-243.

Rossi, R.E., Monasterolo, G., Operti, D. & Corsi, M. (1996). Evaluation of recombinant allergens Bet v 1 and Bet v 2 (profilin) by Pharmacia CAP system in patients with pollen-related allergy to birch and apple. *Allergy* **51**, 940-945.

Ruokonen, H., Malmstrom, M. & Stubb, S. (1988). Factors influencing the recurrence of erythema multiforme. *Proceedings of the Finnish Dental Society* **84**, 167-174.

Sainio, E.L. & Kanerva, L. (1995). Contact allergens in toothpastes and a review of their hypersensitivity. *Contact Dermatitis* **33**, 100-105.

Schiødt, M. (1984a). Oral discoid lupus erythematosus. II. Skin lesions and systemic lupus erythematosus in sixty-six patients with 6-year follow-up. *Oral Surgery Oral Medicine Oral Pathology* **57**, 177-180.

Schiødt, M. (1984b). Oral manifestations of lupus erythematosus. *International Journal of Oral Surgery* **13**, 101-147.

Schiødt, M., Holmstrup, P., Dabelsteen, E. & Ullman, S. (1981). Deposits in immunoglobulins, complement, and fibrinogen in oral lupus erythematosus, lichen planus, and leukoplakia. *Oral Surgery Oral Medicine Oral Pathology* **51**, 603-608.

Schiødt, M. & Pindborg, J.J. (1984). Oral discoid lupus erythematosus. I. The validity of previous histopathologic diagnostic criteria. *Oral Surgery Oral Medicine Oral Pathology* **57**, 46-51.

Schrieber, L. & Maini, R.N. (1984). Circulating immune complexes (CIC) in connective tissue diseases (CTD). *Netherland Journal of Medicine* **27**, 327-339.

Schwartz, O., Pindborg, J.J. & Svenningsen, A. (1989). Tooth exfoliation and necrosis of the alveolar bone following trigeminal herpes zoster in HIV-infected patient. *Danish Dental Journal* **93**, 623-627.

Sciubba, J.J. (1996). Autoimmune aspects of pemphigus vulgaris and mucosal pemphigoid. *Advances in Dental Research* **10**, 52-56.

Scully, C. (1989). Orofacial herpes simplex virus infections: current concepts in the epidemiology, pathogenesis, and treatment, and disorders in which the virus may be implicated. *Oral Surgery Oral Medicine Oral Pathology* **68**, 701-710.

Scully, C. (1995). Infectious diseases: review of the literature. In: Millard, H.D. & Mason, D.R., eds. *Second World Workshop on Oral Medicine*. Ann Arbor: University of Michigan, pp. 7-16.

Scully, C., Almeida, O.P.D. & Welbury, R. (1994). Oral lichen planus in childhood. *British Journal of Dermatology* **130**, 131-133.

Scully, C., Beyli, M., Ferreiro, M.C., Ficarra, G., Gill, Y., Griffiths, M., Holmstrup, P., Mutlu, S., Porter, S. & Wray, D. (1998a). Update on oral lichen planus: etiopathogenesis and management. *Critical Reviews on Oral Biology and Medicine* **9**, 86-122.

Scully, C., El-Kabir, M. & Samaranayake, L. (1995). Candidosis. In: Millard, H.D. & Mason, E.K., eds. *Perspectives on 1993 Second World Workshop on Oral Medicine.* Ann Arbor: University of Michigan, pp. 27-50.

Scully, C., Epstein, J.B., Porter, S.R. & Cox, M.F. (1991). Viruses and chronic diseases of the oral mucosa. *Oral Surgery Oral Medicine Oral Pathology* **72**, 537-544.

Scully, C. & Laskaris, G. (1998). Mucocutaneous disorders. *Periodontology 2000* **18**, 81-94.

Scully, C., Monteil, R. & Sposto, M.R. (1998b). Infectious and tropical diseases affecting the human mouth. *Periodontology 2000* **18**, 47-70.

Serio, F.G., Siegel, M.A. & Slade, B.E. (1991). Plasma cell gingivitis of unusual origin. A case report. *Journal of Periodontolology* **62**, 390-393.

Shafer, W.G., Hine, M.K. & Levy, B.M. (1983). A Textbook of Oral Pathology, 4th edn. Philadelphia: W.B. Saunders, pp. 785-786.

Shklar, G. & McCarthy, P.L. (1971). Oral lesions of mucous membrane pemphigoid. A study of 85 cases. *Archives of Otolaryngology* **93**, 354-364.

Siegel, M.A. (1996). Syphilis and gonorrhea. *Dental Clinics of North America* **40**, 369-383.

Silverman, S. Jr, Gorsky, M., Lozada-Nur, F. & Liu, A. (1986). Oral mucous membrane pemphigoid. A study of sixty-five patients. *Oral Surgery Oral Medicine Oral Pathology* **61**, 233-237.

Singer, S.L., Goldblatt, J., Hallam, L.A. & Winters, J.C. (1993). Hereditary gingival fibromatosis with a recessive mode of inheritance. Case reports. *Austrian Dental Journal* **38**, 427-432.

Skaare, A., Kjaerheim, V., Barkvoll, P. & Rolla, G. (1997). Skin reactions and irritation potential of four commercial toothpastes. *Acta Odontologica Scandinavica* **55**, 133-136.

Skoglund, A. (1994). Value of epicutaneous patch testing in patients with oral mucosal lesions of lichenoid character. *Scandinavian Journal of Dental Research* **102**, 216-222.

Skrinjaric, I. & Basic, M. (1989). Hereditary gingival fibromatosis: report on three families and dermatoglyphic analysis. *Journal of Periodontal Research* **24**, 303-309.

Slots, J., Rams, T.E. & Listgarten, M.A. (1988). Yeasts, enteric rods and pseudomonas in the subgingival flora of severe adult periodontitis. *Oral Microbiology and Immunology* **3**, 47-52.

Smukler, H. & Landsberg, J. (1984). The toothbrush and gingival traumatic injury. *Journal of Periodontology* **55**, 713-719.

Sonis, S.T. (1998). Mucositis as a biological process: a new hypothesis for the development of chemotherapy-induced stomatotoxicity. *Oral Oncology* **34**, 39-43

Standefer, J.A. Jr & Mattox, D.E. (1986). Head and neck manifestations of collagen vascular diseases. *Otolaryngologic Clinic of North America* **19**, 181-210.

Straus, S.E., Ostrove, J.M., Inchauspe, G., Felser, J.M., Freifeld, A., Croen, K.D. & Sawyer, M.H. (1988). NIH Conference. Varicella-zoster virus infections. Biology, natural history, treatment and prevention. *Annals of Internal Medicine* **108**, 221-237.

Stutman, H.R. (1987). Stevens-Johnson syndrome and mycoplasma pneumoniae: Evidence for cutaneous infection. *The Journal of Pediatrics* **111**, 845-847.

Sugerman, P.B., Savage, N.W. & Seymour, G.J. (1994). Phenotype and suppressor activity of T-lymphocyte clones extracted from lesions of oral lichen planus. *British Journal of Dermatology* **131**, 319-324.

Swango, P.A., Kleinman, D.V. & Konzelman, J.L. (1991). HIV and periodontal health. A study of military personnel with HIV. *Journal of the American Dental Association* **122**, 49-54.

Thorn, J.J., Holmstrup, P., Rindum, J. & Pindborg, J.J. (1988). Course of various clinical forms of oral lichen planus. A prospective follow-up study of 611 patients. *Journal of Oral Pathology* **17**, 213-218.

Tylenda, C.A., Larsen, J., Yeh, C-K., Lane, H.E. & Fox, P.C. (1989). High levels of oral yeasts in early HIV-infection. *Journal of Oral Pathology and Medicine* **18**, 520-524.

Ullman, S. (1988). Immunofluorescence and diseases of the skin. *Acta Dermatologica et Venereologica* **140** (suppl.), 1-31.

van Steenberghe, D., Vanherle, G.V., Fossion, E. & Roelens, J. (1976). Crohn's disease of the mouth: report of a case. *Journal of Oral Surgery* **34**, 635-638.

Walsh, L.J., Savage, N.W., Ishii, T. & Seymour, G.J. (1990). Immunopathogenesis of oral lichen planus. *Journal of Oral Pathology and Medicine* **19**, 389-396.

Weed, L.A. & Parkhill, E.M. (1948). The diagnosis of histoplasmosis in ulcerative disease of the mouth and pharynx. *American Journal of Clinical Pathology* **18**, 130-140.

Westheim, A.I., Tenser, R.B. & Marks, J.G. (1987). Acyclovir resistance in a patient with chronic mucocutaneous herpes simplex infections. *Journal of the American Academy of Dermatology* **17**, 875-880.

Williams, D.M., Leonard, J.N., Wright, P., Gilkes, J.J., Haffenden, G.P., McMinn, R.M. & Fry, L. (1984). Benign mucous membrane (cicatricial) pemphigoid revisited: a clinical and immunological reappraisal. *British Dental Journal* **157**, 313-316.

Winkler, J.R., Grassi, M. & Murray, P.A. (1988). Clinical description and etiology of HIV-associated periodontal disease. In: Robertson, P.B. & Greenspan, J.S., eds. Oral Manifestations of AIDS. *Proceedings of First International Symposium on Oral Manifestations of AIDS*. Littleton: PSG Publishing Company, pp. 49-70.

Wright, P.S., Clark, P. & Hardie, J.M. (1985). The prevalence and significance of yeasts in persons wearing complete dentures with soft-lining materials. *Journal of Dental Research* **64**, 122-125.

Wutrich, B. (1997). Oral allergy syndrome to apple after a lover's kiss. *Allergy* **52**, 253-256.

Xiao, S., Wang, X., Qu, B., Yang, M., Liu, G., Bu, L., Wang, Y., Zhu, L., Lei, H., Hu, L., Zhang, X., Liu, J., Zhao, G. & Kong, X. (2000). Refinement of the locus for autosomal dominant hereditary gingival fibromatosis (GINGF) to a 3.8-cM region on 2p21. *Genomics* **68**, 247-252.

Yamamoto, T., Kukuminato, Y., Nui, I., Takada, R., Hirao, M., Kamimura, M., Saitou, H., Asakura, K. & Kataura, A. (1995). Relationship between birch pollen allergy and oral and pha-ryngeal hypersensitivity to fruit. *Journal of Otology Rhinology and Laryngegology of the Society of Japan* **98**, 1086-1091.

Yura, Y., Iga, H., Terashima, K., Yoshida, H., Yanagawa, T., Azuma, M., Hayashi, Y. & Sato, M. (1986). Recurrent intraoral herpes simplex virus infection. *International Journal of Oral Maxillofacial Surgery* **15**, 457-463.

Zaun, H. (1977). Contact allergies related to dental restorative materials and dentures. *Aktuel Dermatol* **3**, 89-93.

Zegarelli, D. & Zegarelli, E. (1977). Intraoral pemphigus vulgaris. *Oral Surgery Oral Medicine Oral Pathology* **44**, 384-393.

CHAPTER 13

Differential Diagnoses: Periodontal Tumors and Cysts

PALLE HOLMSTRUP AND JESPER REIBEL

Reactive processes of periodontal soft tissues

Reactive processes of periodontal hard tissues

Benign neoplasms of periodontal soft tissues

Benign neoplasms of periodontal hard tissues

Malignant neoplasms of periodontal soft tissues

Malignant neoplasms of periodontal hard tissues

Cysts of the periodontium

A common problem in the clinic is differential diagnosis-making between plaque-associated periodontal diseases and other diseases of the periodontal tissues. Tumors and cysts account for a major part of these other diseases. When handling patients who present such differential diagnostic problems, it is important to try explaining the observed features in the simplest way and act accordingly. This includes elimination of such possible causative factors as plaque, inexpedient habits and ill-fitting restorations. In those cases where a simple explanation and appropriate treatment is not satisfactory, it is necessary to proceed with additional possibilities as determined by the clinical and radiographic features. The present descriptions of tumors and cysts comprise a number of characteristic examples and emphasize that the periodontal tissues may be the origin of such lesions. While the descriptions also demonstrate that the reaction of these tissues may differ from reactions observed at other locations, they do not pretend to be a complete account of such lesions related to the periodontal tissues. A distinction is made between a tumor and a neoplasm. Tumor is a clinical term which refers to a process characterized by enlargement which may be a reactive process in response to some kind of irritation. Such processes occasionally show spontaneous regression. Examples of these lesions are pyogenic granuloma and giant cell granuloma. A tumor may also be a true neoplasm, which is a process with autonomous progressive growth that can be either benign or malignant. The malignant process usually grows more rapidly than the benign one and more often gives rise to loosening

of teeth rather than moving them, as is characteristic of some benign processes. The term epulis is sometimes used to designate a tumor originating from the gingiva. Literally, however, it is a non-specific term meaning "on the gum", which is why it is not used in this chapter. Clinical differential diagnostic considerations always rely on the following characteristics of the process in question: surface, color, size, consistency, relation to underlying tissue and radiographic features. It should be emphasized, however, that histopathologic examination is always necessary to establish the correct diagnosis.

REACTIVE PROCESSES OF PERIODONTAL SOFT TISSUES

Fibroma/focal fibrous hyperplasia

Clinical features

True fibromas (i.e. neoplasia) are very rare in the oral cavity (Barker & Lucas 1967). The term fibroma is commonly used, however, to designate a focal fibrous hyperplasia caused by irritation ("irritation fibroma"). Focal fibrous hyperplasia is a common lesion in the oral cavity. It occurs more often in women than in men and it is usually asymptomatic. The majority of these lesions are found in the anterior region (Lee 1968, Kfir et al. 1980).

Focal fibrous hyperplasias may vary in size and

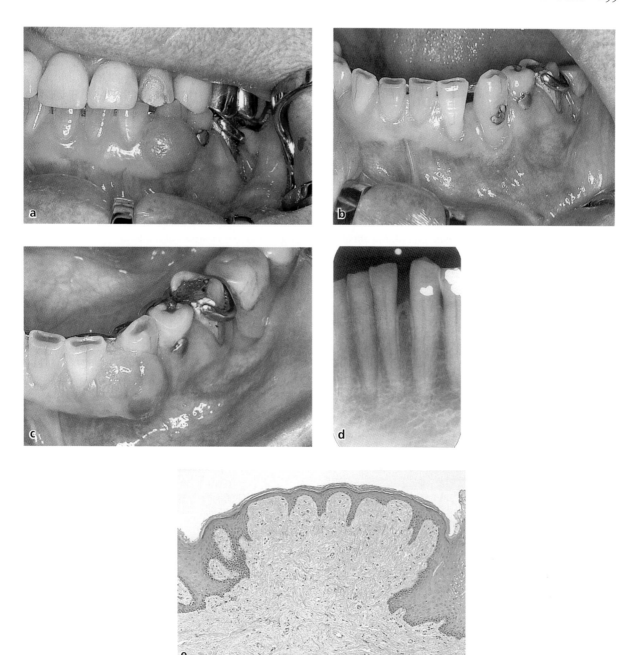

Fig. 13-1. (a) Giant cell fibroma of gingiva between left mandibular lateral incisor and canine of 61-year-old woman. (b) Same patient as (a) after surgical removal and healing. (c) Same patient as (a) and (b). Recurrence of giant cell fibroma 4 years after surgical removal of primary lesion shown in (a). (d) Radiographically, there was no sign of attachment loss associated with the lesion in (c). (e) Photomicrograph of small giant cell fibroma characterized by hyperplastic collageneous tissue with scattered angular cells.

usually present as sessile, well-circumscribed smooth-surfaced nodules. In contrast to pyogenic granuloma and giant cell granuloma, focal fibrous hyperplasia is relatively firm and is similar in color to the adjacent mucosa. Hyperplasias may, however, be whitish due to irritation resulting in hyperkeratosis. Focal fibrous hyperplasia rarely causes erosions in the underlying bone or separation of adjacent teeth from each other.

The so-called giant cell fibroma (Weathers & Callihan 1974), not to be confused with giant cell granuloma, is regarded as a separate entity by many authorities. It occurs frequently in the gingiva (Fig. 13-1a). Clinically, it is indistinguishable from focal fibrous

hyperplasia and it may also be a reactive lesion (Reibel 1982).

Histopathology

Focal fibrous hyperplasia is characterized by cell-poor, hyperplastic collageneous tissue. The covering epithelium may show increased keratinization (hyperkeratinization) due to irritation such as biting. Giant cell fibroma resembles the focal fibrous hyperplasia histologically (Fig. 13-1e) but contains scattered angular and multinucleated cells of a different appearance and nature than the giant cells in giant cell granulomas.

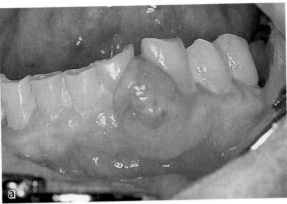
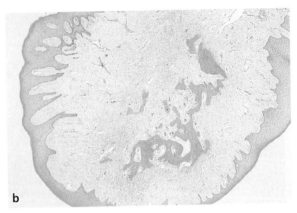

Fig. 13-2. (a) Calcifying fibroblastic granuloma affecting the gingiva between mandibular lateral incisor and canine. (b) Histopathologic features of lesion shown in (a). Note the formation of bone-like tissue.

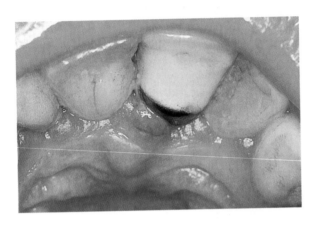

Fig. 13-3. Pyogenic granuloma of marginal gingiva of left maxillary central incisor. The lesion is covered by fibrin.

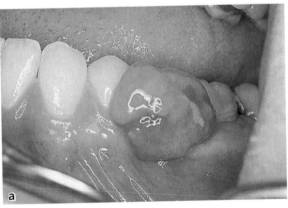
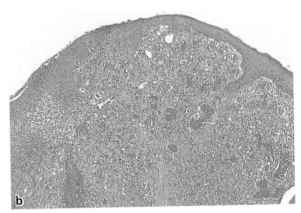

Fig. 13-4. (a) Pyogenic granuloma of gingiva in the left mandibular premolar region. A minor part of the surface is fibrin coated. (b) Histopathologic characteristics of lesion shown in (a). The tissue is highly vascular and part of the surface is ulcerated (left).

Treatment

Focal fibrous hyperplasias are managed by complete surgical excision which sometimes includes the superficial periodontal ligament fibers from where they may originate (Fig. 13-1b-d). Although recurrences occur, they are more infrequent than for pyogenic granulomas, giant cell granulomas and calcifying fibroblastic granulomas.

Calcifying fibroblastic granuloma

Clinical features

This lesion is sometimes referred to as peripheral ossifying fibroma or peripheral fibroma with calcification. It is considered a reactive lesion, although the pathogenesis is uncertain (Lee 1968, Andersen et al. 1973a, Kfir et al. 1980). It occurs exclusively on the gingiva (Fig. 13-2a), predominantly in the second decade. Women are affected more often than men and there is a predilection for the anterior part of the jaws.

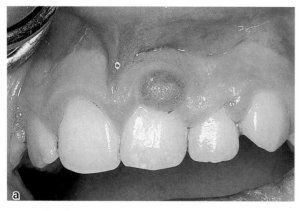 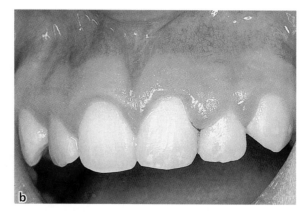

Fig. 13-5. (a) Pregnancy granuloma of gingiva before and after surgical removal and healing (b).

Sometimes they extend between the teeth and involve both the facial and lingual gingiva.

Calcifying fibroblastic granuloma is often reddish and ulcerated (Fig. 13-2a), clinically similar to the pyogenic granuloma, but normal color, non-ulcerated lesions can be seen, resembling focal fibrous hyperplasias.

Histopathology

The lesion is characterized by a fibrous proliferation in which bone- or cementum-like hard tissue is formed (Fig. 13-2b) (Buchner & Hansen 1987a). The surface epithelium is usually ulcerated and highly cell-rich areas are usually found below the ulceration and in areas of hard tissue formation.

Treatment

The treatment is surgical excision but calcifying fibroblastic granuloma has a tendency to recur. It is important to remove any source of irritation such as plaque, calculus and inappropriate restorations.

Pyogenic granuloma

Clinical features

Pyogenic granuloma is more correctly called telangiectatic granuloma, since the lesion is highly vascular and usually is not purulent as the term pyogenic suggests. It is frequently ulcerated and the appearance of the fibrin-coated ulcer may resemble purulence (Fig. 13-3). Pyogenic granuloma may be conceived as an exaggerated reaction to minor trauma without it having been possible to demonstrate a definite infectious organism.

Pyogenic granuloma may occur in all areas of the oral mucosa, but is most frequently found on the marginal gingiva (Figs. 13-3 & 13-4a) (Makek & Sailer 1985). It occurs most often on the vestibular aspect of the anterior part of the jaw with a preference for the maxilla. It may develop rapidly and the size varies considerably. It is reddish (Fig. 13-4a) or bluish, sometimes lobulated, and may be sessile or pedunculated. Bleeding from the ulcerated lesion is common, but

typically it is not painful. Teeth may become separated due to interdental growth of the lesion.

Due to its red color, which may sometimes turn to a cyanotic hue, pyogenic granuloma may be mistaken for giant cell granuloma. The pregnancy tumor (Fig. 13-5a, b) arising from the fourth to the ninth month of pregnancy in women (Daley et al. 1991) is clinically and histologically similar to pyogenic granuloma but often shows regression after parturition.

Histopathology

The lesion is characterized by vascular proliferation that resembles granulation tissue. Numerous vascular spaces and rather solid sheets of endothelial cells may be seen, sometimes organized in lobular aggregates (Fig. 13-4b). The surface epithelium is usually ulcerated and beneath such areas there is heavy acute inflammation. Chronic inflammatory cells are often found deeper in the lesion. The content of erythrocytes in the vascular spaces is responsible for the reddish color of the lesion. The stromal tissue may become fibrotic with time, which is why both clinical and histopathologic features may partly resemble fibrous hyperplasia.

Treatment

The treatment is surgical excision but gingival pyogenic granuloma has a potential for recurrence. It is important to remove any source of irritation such as plaque, calculus and inappropriate restorations.

Peripheral giant cell granuloma

Clinical features

Peripheral giant cell granuloma occurs exclusively on the gingiva or edentulous alveolar ridge. It can be seen in young individuals but occurs in all age groups. It is more frequent in women than in men, and the mandible is more often affected than the maxilla (Andersen et al. 1973b, Katsikeris et al. 1988). It may arise anywhere on the gingival mucosa and sometimes both the facial and lingual gingiva are involved due to extension between the teeth.

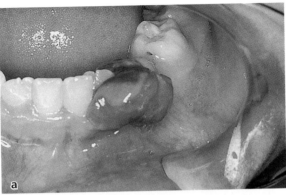
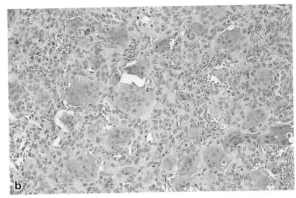

Fig. 13-6. (a) Peripheral giant cell granuloma affecting left mandibular gingiva of 10-year-old boy. Histopathology of the lesion is shown in (b). Note numerous multinuclear giant cells.

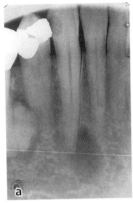
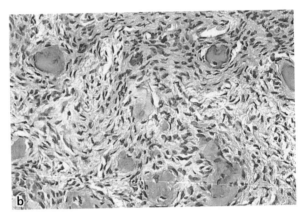

Fig. 13-7. (a) Periapical cemental dysplasia in right mandible. The radiograph demonstrates early osteolytic lesion with well-circumscribed periapical radiolucency of the canine whereas the lesion of the premolar is in a late phase with well circumscribed radiopacity bordered by a distinct radiolucent zone. (b) Photomicrograph of periapical cemental dysplasia in intermediate phase with islands of cementum-like tissue surrounded by cell-rich fibrous tissue.

The lesions are pedunculated or sessile and they are typically red or purple and commonly ulcerated (Fig. 13-6a). Local irritation or trauma appears to be important for these lesions to occur.

Giant cell granuloma has great growth potential and may cause separation of teeth due to the pressure exerted by the growth. Erosion of the underlying bone can be found on radiographs and sometimes it is impossible to determine if the lesion has started centrally (central giant cell granuloma) or if a peripheral growth has extended into the bone. Differentiation from pyogenic granuloma is often difficult.

Histopathology

The lesion is characterized by focal collections of multinucleated osteoclast-like giant cells with a richly cellular and vascular stroma separated by collageneous septa (Fig. 13-6b). Extravasated erythrocytes are typical, often resulting in deposition of hemosiderin pigment. Formation of osteoid can sometimes be noticed. The giant cells probably have their origin from the periodontal ligament (odontoclasts/osteoclasts).

Treatment

The treatment is surgical excision but as with calcifying fibroblastic granuloma and pyogenic granuloma, giant cell granuloma has a tendency to recur (Katsikeris et al. 1988).

REACTIVE PROCESSES OF PERIODONTAL HARD TISSUES

Periapical cemental dysplasia

Clinical features

Periapical cemental dysplasia is sometimes referred to as a type of cementoma, but most authorities agree that it is not a true neoplasm and it does not appear to be developmental in nature (Kramer et al. 1992). It belongs to the group of fibro-osseous cemental lesions (Waldron 1985, van der Waal 1991). The cause of these lesions is unknown but some may be of a reactive nature. Periapical cemental dysplasia affects the apical part of several teeth, which are usually vital. The

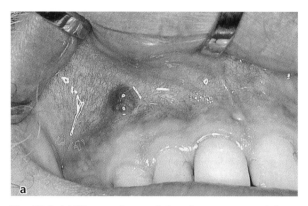 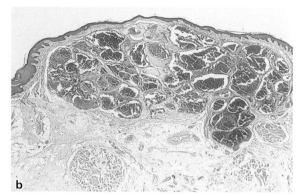

Fig. 13-8. (a) Hemangioma of alveolar mucosa at right maxillary canine. The lobulated blue lesion is a cavernous type of hemangioma as shown in (b).

mandibular incisors are the most commonly affected and the lesions are more frequent in women than in men. They occur most often between the fourth and the fifth decade. There are usually no symptoms.

Radiographical findings depend on the developmental phase of the lesion, varying from well-circumscribed periapical radiolucencies (Fig. 13-7a), an intermediate phase with irregular radiopacities within the radiolucent zones, to a late phase with well-circumscribed periapical radiopacities bordered by distinct radiolucent zones. The significance of the lesion is the differential diagnostic problem in distinguishing it from periapical granuloma and radicular cyst.

Histopathology

The lesion develops from an osteolytic phase in which periapical bone is replaced by cellular fibroblastic tissue through a cementoblastic phase in which a cementum-like tissue is formed within the fibrous tissue (Fig. 13-7b). In the late phase the lesion consists of dense, irregular cementum-like material. The histology resembles that seen in cemento-ossifying fibroma and fibrous dysplasia.

Therapy

Periapical cemental dysplasia is innocuous and needs no surgical treatment as it is usually self-limiting. Radiographic follow-up examination every fifth year may be considered.

Benign neoplasms of periodontal soft tissues

Most of the soft tissue tumors that occur in various sites of the body can be seen in the oral mucosa as well. Examples are neoplasms derived from peripheral nerves (neurilemoma ("schwannoma") and neurofibroma), blood vessels (hemangioma) and smooth muscle (leiomyoma) (Pindborg 1992, Neville et al. 1995). None of them, however, have a special propensity to occur on the gingiva and usually they are clinically indistinguishable from focal fibrous hyperplasias or other non-neoplastic lesions. Exceptions are hemangiomas and nevi, which are described below. Furthermore, squamous papilloma and verruca vulgaris are dealt with in this section.

Hemangioma

Clinical features

Hemangiomas show a predilection for the head and neck region and are rather frequent tumors of the oral mucosa. There is a predilection for women (Neville et al. 1995). Several authors doubt whether hemangiomas are true neoplasms and suggest they be classified as hamartomas or developmental anomalies. Most cases are present at birth or occur shortly thereafter, although some cases develop in adults. Some of them may undergo regression. Hemangiomas present as flat or raised, sometimes lobulated, soft lesions of blue to red color (Fig. 13-8a). They are usually asymptomatic but may bleed when traumatized. Typically, they blanch on pressure and the color returns shortly after releasing the pressure. This is not the case with other bluish lesions such as mucous cysts.

Histopathology

Hemangiomas are divided into capillary and cavernous types (Fig. 13-8b) depending on the size of the vessels. Mixed types are not uncommon. Especially in the capillary type, sheets of proliferating endothelial cells are common. Some hemangiomas resemble pyogenic granulomas but ulceration and an inflammatory component are not typical of hemangiomas.

Treatment

Hemangiomas may give rise to severe bleeding if treated with conventional surgery and cryosurgery may be the treatment of choice where treatment is necessary and possible. Large tumors which are not suitable for surgery may be embolized or injected with agents to induce fibrosis. Episodes of bleeding at eating and toothbrushing are common indications of treatment.

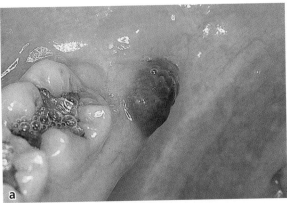

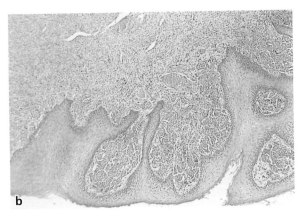

Fig. 13-9. (a) Nevus of lower right mandibular retromolar area. Histopathologic examination showed that the nevus cells were solely located in the subepithelial connective tissue (b), which is why the lesion is an intramucosal nevus. Note melanin formation by the nevus cells.

Nevus

Clinical features

The term "nevus" is used for a variety of lesions of the skin and oral mucosa. Here it will be used synonymously with a pigmented lesion containing nevus cells (brown or nevocellular nevus) or a lesion containing melanocytes in the connective tissue (blue nevus). Nevus cells are derived from the neural crest and are related to melanocytes. Nevus cells are capable of producing melanin pigment, although they do not invariably do so.

Nevi are very common on the skin but rare in the oral mucosa. They usually develop during childhood and they are more common in women than in men. Most intraoral nevi are seen on the palate but the gingiva is not an uncommon location (Buchner & Hansen 1987b). They can present as flat, slightly raised lesions or even as a tumor (Fig. 13-9a). They are usually brown or black or they may show little or no pigmentation. The blue nevus should be differentiated from an amalgam tatoo.

Histopathology

Nevocellular or brown nevus contains nests of nevus cells located along the basal cell layer of the epithelium (junctional activity, junctional nevus), solely in the connective tissue (intramucosal nevus) (Fig. 13-9b), or in both locations (compound nevus). The nevus cells may or may not contain melanin pigment. In blue nevus, dendritic, melanin-producing melanocytes occur in the connective tissue (Neville et al. 1995).

Treatment

Some malignant melanomas of the skin seem to develop from nevi. Especially in adults, nevi with junctional activity should be viewed with caution. In the oral mucosa little is known about malignant transformation of nevi. Excision of oral nevi is generally recommended (Buchner et al. 1990).

Papilloma

Clinical features

The term papilloma covers four or five different types of benign epithelial proliferations: squamous and filiform papilloma, verruca vulgaris, condyloma and focal epithelial hyperplasia (FEH). Malignant transformation is very rare or non-existing and usually there are no symptoms. Human papilloma virus (HPV) is commonly found in these lesions and a causative role of HPV in the development of at least some of these lesions is strongly suggested (Pindborg & Prætorius 1987, Garlick & Taichman 1991). Generally, a relationship between the histomorphology and distinct HPV

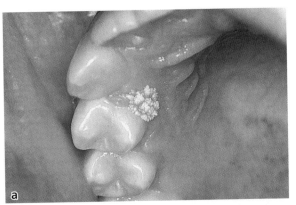

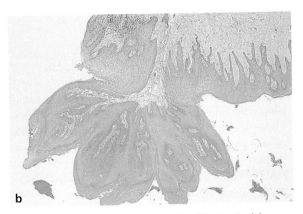

Fig. 13-10. (a) Gingival papilloma of right maxillary first premolar region. (b) Photomicrograph of lesion in (a).

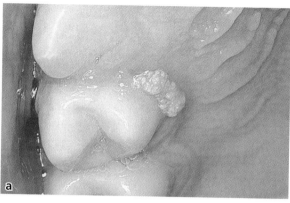
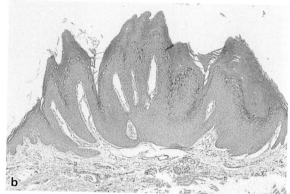

Fig. 13-11. (a) Gingival verruca vulgaris of left maxillary first premolar region. Clinically, it resembles the lesion shown in Fig. 13-10 but histopathologic examination of the surgically removed lesion showed characteristics typical of verruca (b).

types, of which about 70 are known, can be established. Verruca vulgaris is dealt with separately and condyloma and FEH will not be mentioned further here.

Squamous papilloma and filiform papilloma can be distinguished by detailed clinical and histologic features (Prætorius, personal communication). Here, however, they will be dealt with together. They are exophytic, pedunculated or sessile lesions with a reddish/normal or whitish/gray color and a granular/moruloid or filiform/digitated surface (Fig. 13-10a). They are mainly seen in the third to fifth decade, in contrast to verruca vulgaris, which is usually seen in younger age groups. The soft palate is the most common location. It is often difficult to differentiate clinically between verruca vulgaris and squamous and filiform papillomas.

Histopathology
Squamous and filiform papillomas are covered by squamous epithelium with deep crypts in the surface. The epithelium is keratinized or non-keratinized with irregular rete ridges which cover sometimes ramified connective tissue papillae (Fig. 13-10b).

Treatment
Surgical excision, including the base of the lesion, is the treatment of choice. Recurrence is uncommon.

Verruca vulgaris

Clinical features
Verruca vulgaris is common on the skin. In the oral mucosa verrucae are less common and are often seen as a result of autoinoculation in children with warts on the fingers. The majority are located on the lips and in the palate and 10-20% are located on the gingiva (Green et al. 1986, Pindborg & Prætorius 1987). Verruca vulgaris seems to be associated with HPV type 2 and 4.

Clinically the lesions are sessile, exophytic or raised

with a whitish surface with angulated verrucous projections (Fig. 13-11a).

Histopathology
Histologically, they show a papillomatous surface with hyperkeratinization and elongated rete ridges (Fig. 13-11b). Characteristically, the rete ridges bend inward at the margins of the lesion, pointing toward a center below the lesion (Prætorius-Clausen 1972).

Treatment
Some verrucae disappear spontaneously, especially in children. Treatment usually consists of surgical excision. Recurrence occurs in some cases.

Peripheral odontogenic tumors

Clinical features
Odontogenic tumors primarily occur as intraosseous growths but sometimes they present in a peripheral location in the gingiva (Buchner & Sciubba 1987, Pindborg 1992). The following entities may occur as a gingival tumor: ameloblastoma, squamous odontogenic tumor, ameloblastic fibro-odontoma, adenomatoid odontogenic tumor, calcifying odontogenic cyst, calcifying epithelial odontogenic tumor (Fig. 13-12a,b) and odontogenic fibroma. Peripheral odontogenic tumors usually present as non-ulcerated sessile or pendunculated gingival lesions. The clinical features, thus, are nonspecific, resembling focal fibrous hyperplasias or other non-neoplastic lesions (Buchner & Sciubba 1987). Most examples are rather small.

Histopathology
Generally, these lesions show histopathologic features similar to the intraosseous forms of the tumors (Fig. 13-12b).

Treatment
Due to the rather small number of reported cases and the varying behavior of the different odontogenic tumors mentioned above, general guidelines will not be

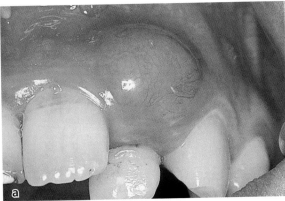

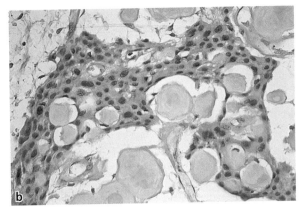

Fig. 13-12. (a) Gingival swelling of left maxillary lateral incisor region. The tumor was surgically removed and the histopathologic examination revealed a calcifying epithelial odontogenic tumor (b).

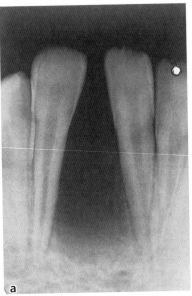

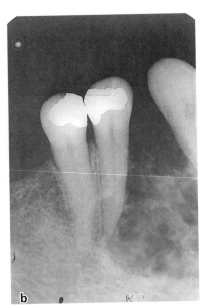

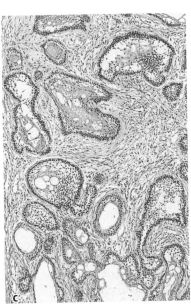

Fig. 13-13. (a) Radiograph shows well-demarcated loss of alveolar bone between displaced mandibular incisors. After surgical removal and histopathologic examination (c) the lesion was diagnosed as an ameloblastoma. (b) Radiograph with irregular radiolucency with scalloped periphery in alveolar bone of mandibular premolar and canine region. The teeth are displaced. Biopsy revealed an ameloblastoma.

given. Apparently an innocuous clinical behavior is characteristic of most reported cases, showing a different biologic behavior than their intraosseous counterparts (Buchner & Sciubba 1987). However, some examples of recurrence have been reported.

It should be mentioned here that odontogenic tumors or hamartomas are frequently detected histologically in the soft tissue in operation specimens from exposure of molars delayed in eruption for no obvious clinical cause (Philipsen et al. 1992). The fate of these lesions, had the surgical exposure not been performed, is unknown.

BENIGN NEOPLASMS OF PERIODONTAL HARD TISSUES

Ameloblastoma

Clinical features

The ameloblastoma is a benign but locally invasive neoplasm derived from odontogenic epithelium (Kramer et al. 1992). It occurs most commonly between 20 and 40 years of age and affects women and men equally. The most common location is the molar regions, with most tumors being localized in the mandible (van der Waal 1991, Reichart et al. 1995). The tumors grow slowly and sometimes reach excessive sizes before symptoms arise. Such symptoms may be expansion of cortical bone and displacement of teeth. The alveolar nerve usually remains undisturbed even in cases of large tumors in the mandible, but roots of

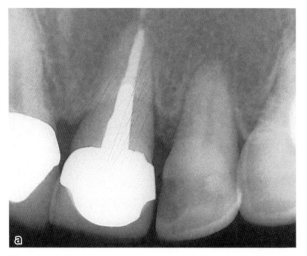 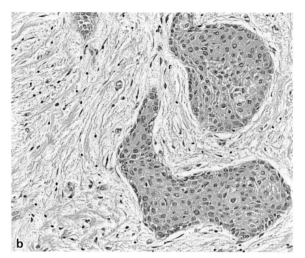

Fig. 13-14. (a) Squamous odontogenic tumor demonstrating substantial diffuse radiolucency of alveolar bone in left maxillary incisor region. The diagnosis was revealed by biopsy showing features presented in (b).

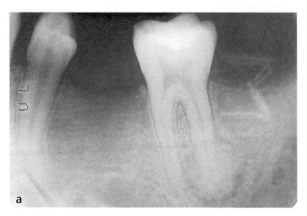 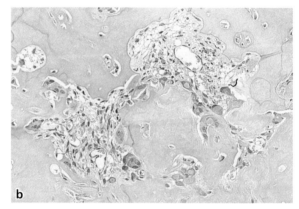

Fig. 13-15. (a) Radiographic presentation of a benign cementoblastoma in a 20-year-old man. The periapical lesion of the mandibular second molar shows an almost circular radiopacity surrounded by a radiolucent margin. Part of the root is resorbed and replaced by lesional tissue. The tumor is composed of cementum-like tissue (b).

adjacent teeth are sometimes resorbed. Intraosseous ameloblastomas rarely demonstrates mucosal involvement in the form of gingival tumor. Radiographically, the ameloblastoma demonstrate unilocular or multilocular radiolucency, which is usually well-circumscribed. The radiographic features may be indistinguishable from jaw cysts but may also resemble loss of bone due to marginal periodontitis (Fig. 13-13a, b).

Histopathology
The general histopathologic features consist of islands and/or strands of odontogenic epithelium in a mature collageneous stroma (Fig. 13-13c). Columnar or cuboidal epithelial cells resembling ameloblasts surround loosely arranged epithelial cells resembling the stellate reticulum of the enamel organ.

Treatment
Conservative and radical surgery are equally common types of treatment, and recurrences are common following both treatment modalities (Reichart et al. 1995). This is probably due to difficulties in removing the proliferating cords of tumor tissue in the marrow spaces at the periphery of the tumor. In general, more radical treatment of maxillary ameloblastomas than of mandibular ones is recommended (Reichart et al. 1995).

Squamous odontogenic tumor

Clinical features
This odontogenic tumor was first described in 1975 (Pullon et al. 1975) and very few examples have been reported. However, as the tumor seems to develop from the periodontal ligament, presumably from the epithelial rests of Malassez, and is most often associated with the lateral root surface of an erupted tooth, it is important to include it here as an example of a periodontal tissue reaction.

Squamous odontogenic tumor has been found in almost all age groups and does not seem to have a predilection for any site or gender. Radiographically, the findings are not specific (Fig. 13-14a). They often show a triangular radiolucent defect between the

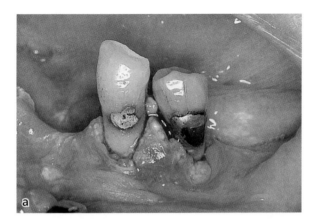
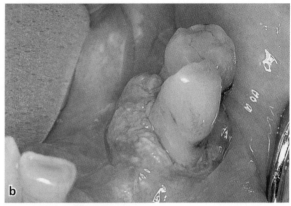
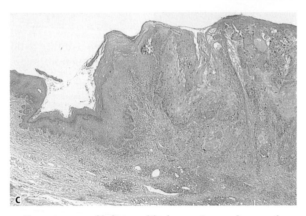

Fig. 13-16. Gingival squamous cell carcinoma of left mandibular canine and premolar region. (a) Facial aspect. (b) Mesial and lingual aspect. (c) Photomicrograph of the lesion showing carcinoma in right half.

roots of two teeth which may suggest vertical bone loss (Neville et al. 1995).

Histopathology
The characteristic findings are islands of squamous epithelium in a mature collageneous stroma (Fig. 13-14b). There are no columnar peripheral cells or stellate reticulum-like cells as in the ameloblastoma.

Treatment
Local excision or enucleation is the most common type of treatment. There seems to be some tendency for recurrence.

Benign cementoblastoma

Clinical features
Benign cementoblastoma is a slow-growing neoplasm forming hard tissue around the apex of a tooth (Kramer et al. 1992). It is most common in the mandibular premolar and molar region, is almost equally common among men and women, and is most often seen in the second decade (Ulmansky et al. 1994). The tumor is slowly growing and may cause swelling and pain.

Radiographically, a periapical radiopacity typically surrounded by a radiolucent margin of uniform width is seen (Fig. 13-15a) (Ulmansky et al. 1994). The tumor may obscure the apex of the involved tooth and root

resorption with fusion of the tumor with the tooth is characteristic. The involved tooth is usually vital.

Histopathology
The tumor is built up of cementum-like tissue with numerous reversal lines, the tissue being attached to the tooth. Between the cementum-like areas the tissue is cellular, and in the periphery it is unmineralized (Fig. 13-15b). A small biopsy of this tumor may be difficult to differentiate from osteosarcoma.

Treatment
Surgical enucleation is the treatment of choice, although this may be difficult due to the relationship between the tumor and the related tooth.

MALIGNANT NEOPLASMS OF PERIODONTAL SOFT TISSUES

Squamous cell carcinoma

Clinical features
In the literature it is rare to see a distinction maintained between gingival cancer and cancer developed on the edentulous alveolar ridge. Thus, many reports deal with cancer of the "gums". In most of these cases men have dominated, and only older people are af-

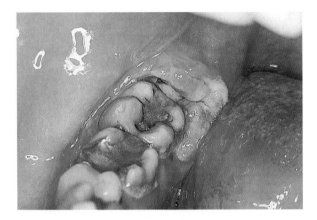

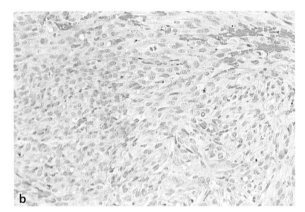

Fig. 13-17. Metastasis from adenocarcinoma of lung. The neoplasm affects lingual gingiva of right mandibular second molar and mucosa covering semi-impacted third molar.

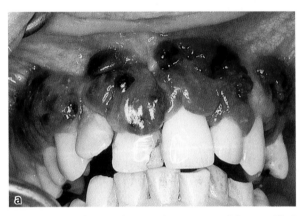

Fig. 13-18. (a) Gingival Kaposi's sarcoma of the maxilla in 33-year-old man with AIDS. (b) Histopathologic features of Kaposi's sarcoma shown in (a).

fected (Pindborg 1980). In England a marked shift in male/female ratio has been observed, since the ratio was 5:1 in 1932-39, but 1:1 by 1960-69 (Easson & Palmer 1976). Most gingival cancers affect the mandible and 60% are located posterior to the premolars. In an American study it has been shown that dentists play an important part in the early recognition of gingival cancer; 60% of these patients are first seen by a dentist (Cady & Catlin 1969). Gingival cancer commonly begins as a nodular lesion (Fig. 13-16a,b) often with ulceration and surrounding leukoplakia. It infiltrates rapidly in depth, frequently extending along the periodontal membrane with osseous involvement and destruction of the supporting bone. Pain and loosening of teeth is common. In the American study, gingival cancer had exceeded 3 cm at admission in 44% of the referred cases and regional lymph-node metastasis on admission was found in 37%.

Histopathology
Squamous cell carcinoma of the gingiva does not differ histologically from squamous cell carcinomas elsewhere in the oral mucosa. Islands and cords of malignant epithelial cells are seen infiltrating underlying tissues (Fig. 13-16c). Varying amounts of horn pearls are formed and usually a strong inflammatory reaction is found in the stroma.

Treatment
Gingival squamous cell carcinomas are usually treated by surgery, irradiation or combinations of these. When irradiation therapy is required, extraction of involved teeth is often necessary before irradiation is instituted if the teeth suffer from severe periodontitis. This is due to an increased risk of osteoradionecrosis after extraction of teeth situated in irradiated bone as the result of permanently reduced vascularization (Beumer et al. 1984).

Metastasis to the gingiva

The majority of metastases to the oral region are intraosseous. The gingiva (including the alveolar mucosa) is most often the seat of soft tissue metastasis in the mouth. In the oral regions, soft tissue metastases from lung cancer (Fig. 13-17) is encountered most frequently in men, while metastases from breast cancer account for most soft tissue metastases in women. About 20% of oral soft tissue metastases were manifested before the primary tumor was diagnosed. Furthermore, in 90% of the cases the clinical manifestation resembled a hyperplastic or reactive lesion (Hirshberg et al. 1993). These observations emphasize the need for a histologic examination of all such tumors.

Histopathology
The histology resembles the tumor of origin. Most cases are carcinomas and sarcomas rarely metastasize to the oral region.

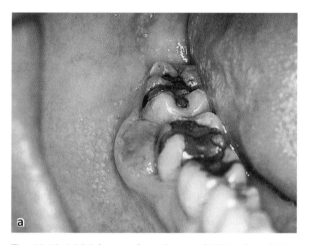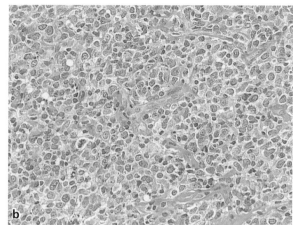

Fig. 13-19. (a) Malignant lymphoma of HIV-infected 36-year-old man. The gingival neoplasm in the right mandibular molar region resembles a pyogenic granuloma, but histopathologic examination revealed a malignant lymphoma shown in (b).

Kaposi's sarcoma

Clinical features

In 1872, Kaposi described what he called "multiple idiopathic hemorrhagic sarcoma", which later came to bear his name. Most of his patients were Jews, especially Ashkenazim. Later it was reported that Kaposi's sarcoma occurred among people living around the Mediterranean.

Then, in the middle of the 1950s, reports came from Sub-Saharan Africa that Kaposi's sarcoma was a prevalent malignant tumor in that area, but oral manifestations of Kaposi's sarcoma in Jews and Africans were rare.

It was later recognized that Kaposi's sarcoma sometimes occurred in individuals who had been treated with immunosuppressive drugs after kidney transplantation.

The latest phase in the occurrence of Kaposi's sarcoma is among individuals suffering from the acquired immunodeficiency syndrome (AIDS). The appearance of a Kaposi's sarcoma is one of the criteria for the development of AIDS in patients infected with human immunodeficiency virus (HIV). In most instances, Kaposi's sarcoma will first manifest as skin lesions followed by oral lesions. In rare cases, oral manifestations may be the first sign of Kaposi's sarcoma. Gingival location is the second most frequently observed after the palate (Pindborg & Reichart 1995).

The typical appearance is that of single or multiple blue, violet or red slightly raised lesions. Ulceration is common and with time the tumors can reach monstrous proportions (Fig. 13-18a).

Histopathology

The typical features are a lesion with bundles of spindle-shaped cells and many thin-walled vascular luminae, often lined by plump endothelial cells (Fig. 13-18b). There are usually a number of mitotic figures of which some are atypical. There is general agreement that the cell of origin of Kaposi's sarcoma is the endothelial cell.

Treatment

There is no curative treatment but palliative treatment includes both cytostatics and irradiation.

Malignant lymphoma

Clinical features

A primary malignant lymphoma is rare in the oral cavity. When it occurs, it is most commonly seen in the palate and gingiva (Takahashi et al. 1989). It presents as a diffuse swelling which is usually ulcerated. The diagnosis may be quite difficult to arrive at as the first manifestations may resemble a non-specific periodontitis, pyogenic granuloma (Fig. 13-19a) or pericoronitis (Maxymiw et al. 1991).

In HIV-infected patients non-Hodgkin's lymphomas occur with increased frequency (Holmstrup & Westergaard 1994). Occasionally, a gingival tumor may be the first manifestation of a non-Hodgkin's lymphoma in an HIV-infected patient (Fig. 13-19a).

Histopathology

Histomorphologic features, immunologic and genetic markers are used to diagnose and classify malignant lymphomas. The lesions contain lymphocytic-appearing cells (Fig. 13-19b); in low-grade tumors the cells are well-differentiated small lymphocytes, whereas high-grade tumors contain less differentiated cells. Common to all lymphomas are infiltrative growth as characteristically seen in all malignant tumors.

Treatment

Depending on the extension and spread of the tumor, surgical removal, irradiation, cytostatics and combinations of these may be the treatment of choice.

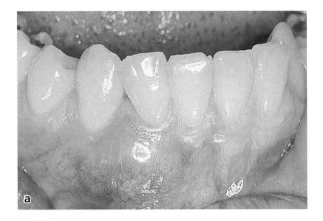

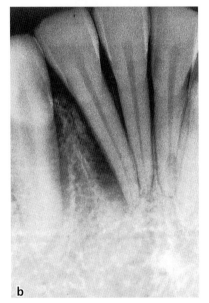

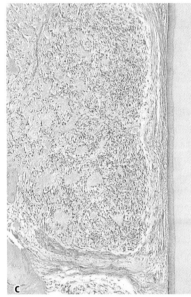

Fig. 13-20. (a) A swelling between the right mandibular canine and lateral incisor was associated with tooth mobility, displacement, and loss of supporting periodontal bone as seen in the radiograph (b). The biopsy showed osteosarcoma (c).

Malignant neoplasms of periodontal hard tissues

Osteosarcoma

Clinical features

Osteosarcoma is the most common primary malignant tumor of bone. About 7% of all osteosarcomas occur in the jaws.

The first symptoms of a jaw osteosarcoma appear when the patients are, on average, about 30 years old, which is a decade older than for osteosarcomas in other bones. The maxilla and mandible are affected with about equal frequency. Men are affected more commonly than women. Symptoms include mobile teeth, swelling (Fig. 13-20a), anesthesia or paresthesia, toothache and nasal obstruction (van der Waal 1991). Radiographically, the neoplasm demonstrates a variety of patterns ranging from radiolucent (Fig. 13-20b) to radiopaque changes. Sometimes the formation of bony trabeculae results in a sunray appearance in a direction perpendicular to the outer surface. A number of jaw osteosarcomas will have, as their first manifestation, a widening of the periodontal membrane (Garrington et al. 1967).

Histopathology

A variety of histologic appearances can be seen (Neville et al. 1995). Some osteosarcomas are primarily osteoblastic, with production of irregular osteoid and bone (Fig. 13-20c). In others, production of cartilage (chondroblastic osteosarcomas) or the presence of fibroblastic cells (fibroblastic osteosarcomas) are the dominant histologic features. Common to all these types are the malignant-appearing cells with pleomorphic nuclei and mitotic figures. The prognosis is not dependent on the histologic subtype.

Treatment

Resection of involved and surrounding bone is the common treatment. Sometimes supplementary chemotherapy and/or radiotherapy are used.

Langerhans cell disease

Clinical features

Langerhans cell disease, formerly named histiocytosis X, is a proliferation of histiocyte-like cells that have

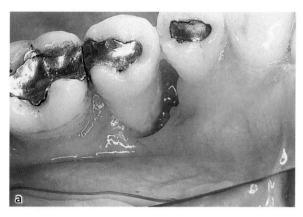
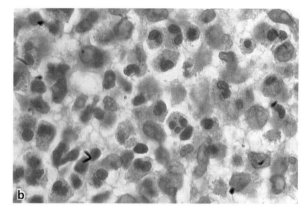

Fig. 13-21. (a) Eosinophilic granuloma of alveolar bone in the mandibular premolar region showed progressive loss of supporting periodontal tissue in a 33-year-old woman. The lesion was biopsied and characteristic features of Langerhans cell disease were revealed (b). Note the numerous eosinophils.

been shown in recent years to be Langerhans cells. Langerhans cells are blood marrow-derived cells normally present in the skin, mucosa, lymph nodes and blood marrow. The disease is difficult to classify as the etiology and pathogenesis are unknown and due to the fact that it is characterized by clinical heterogeneity and an unpredictable course. Some classify this disease, or at least some of its manifestations, as a malignant systemic disorder/neoplastic disease while others classify it as a reactive, proliferative disease. Traditionally, the disease has been divided into three subtypes: a disease with solitary or multiple bone lesions (eosinophilic granuloma), a chronic multi-organ disease associated with considerable morbidity (Hand-Schüller-Christian syndrome) and an acute multi-organ disease occurring mainly in infants and with a common fatal outcome (Letterer-Siwe disease). There are overlapping clinical features between these subtypes.

Manifestations in the jaws are seen in 10-20% of all cases. Swelling, tenderness, pain and loosening of teeth (Fig. 13-21a) are frequent symptoms. The jaw lesions often appear as punched-out radiolucencies but ill-defined radiolucencies are also seen, sometimes mimicking periodontal disease (Neville et al. 1995, van der Waal 1991).

Histopathology

The lesions are characterized by a diffuse infiltration of rather large mononuclear cells representing Langerhans cells with varying numbers of eosinophilic granulocytes and other inflammatory cells (Fig. 13-21b). Identification of Langerhans cells by electron microscopy or immunohistochemical methods is sometimes used to confirm the diagnosis.

Treatment

The prognosis for patients with jaw lesions in the absence of visceral involvement is generally good. Such lesions are usually treated surgically, sometimes with supplementary radiotherapy. Recurrence and progression of the disease can be seen. Chronic and acute disease with multiorgan involvement is usually treated with chemotherapeutic agents and the prognosis is generally moderate or poor.

CYSTS OF THE PERIODONTIUM

The origin of jaw cysts is either developmental or inflammatory and the background of the frequent occurrence of these cysts is the abundance of epithelial remnants residing within the jaws (Shear 1992, 1994).

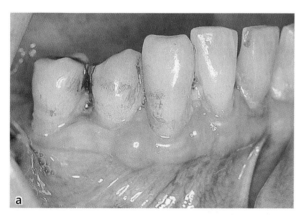
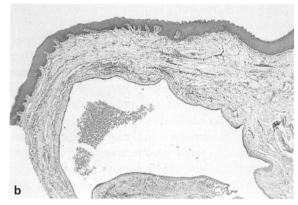

Fig. 13-22. (a) Gingival cyst between right mandibular first premolar and canine. (b) Characteristic histopathologic features of a cyst lined by a thin non-keratinized squamous epithelium.

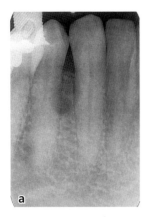
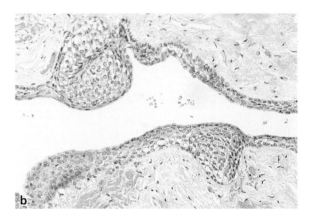

Fig. 13-23. (a) Radiographic manifestation of lateral periodontal cyst between right mandibular first premolar and canine. The cyst was surgically removed, and the tissue histologically examined. (b) Characteristic histopathologic features of a non-keratinized lining epithelium with focal thickenings.

The epithelial remnants most frequently forming the background of cysts of the periodontal tissues are of odontogenic origin.

Gingival cyst

Clinical features

Gingival cysts are of developmental origin. Whereas the frequency of gingival cysts is high in newborns, they are rarely seen after 3 months of age because most of the gingival cysts in newborns undergo involution and disappear or rupture through the surface epithelium and exfoliate (Shear 1992). Such cysts are frequently referred to as Epstein's pearls or Bohn's nodules, but there is some confusion about the terminology. Studies have revealed gingival cysts of infants in 76% and 85%, the majority occurring in the maxilla. Gingival cysts in infants arise from remnants of the dental lamina.

Gingival cysts in adults are uncommon. They are most often found in patients aged more than 40 (Nxumalo & Shear 1992). Some cases are diagnosed clinically, but others are recognized histologically in biopsies from the gingiva. They may occur with or without bone involvement in the form of a superficial erosion and they may give rise to gingival swelling (Fig. 13-22a), although they are most often unnoticed. The gingival cyst in adults has a predilection for occurrence in the mandibular canine and premolar region, which are also predilection sites for the lateral periodontal cyst. This is why there is some confusion about the relationship between the two types of cysts, a confusion which is further complicated by the fact that many cysts in the lateral periodontal position are in fact keratocysts, while others are of inflammatory origin, for instance associated with accessory root canals of necrotic teeth (Shear 1992). Clinically recognizable gingival cysts are most frequent in the mandible. A gingival cyst may arise from (1) odontogenic epithelial cell nests, (2) degenerative, cystic changes in proliferating epithelial ridges from the gingival surface epithelium, (3) traumatic implantation of surface epithelium into the connective tissue, or (4) junctional epithelium, which in turn is derived from the reduced enamel epithelium. Shear (1992) has been impressed by the many similarities between the gingival cyst in adults and the lateral periodontal cyst. He proposed that the gingival cyst in adults is derived from junctional epithelium after eruption of the tooth, whereas the lateral periodontal cyst is formed from the reduced enamel epithelium by dilation of the follicle before eruption of the tooth.

Histopathology

The gingival cysts in infants are usually small, with a diameter of 2-3 mm. They are lined by a stratified squamous epithelium with a parakeratotic surface and flat basal cells. The cyst lumen is filled with keratin (Shear 1992).

The gingival cyst of adults (Fig. 13-22b) is lined with a thin, non-keratinized squamous epithelium sometimes exhibiting focal thickenings of the epithelial lining as can also be seen in the lateral periodontal cyst (Nxumalo & Shear 1992).

Treatment

There is no reason to treat gingival cysts in infants.

Gingival cysts of adults are treated by local surgical excision and usually there is no tendency to recur.

Lateral periodontal cyst

Clinical features

The lateral periodontal cysts are rare developmental cysts most often occurring in adults, predominantly localized to the canine and premolar region and most often affecting the mandible as mentioned also for the gingival cyst (Shear 1992). Lateral periodontal cysts occur in the lateral periodontal position and the diagnosis implies that an inflammatory background is excluded, as is a collateral keratocyst. The cyst may present as a gingival swelling but it is usually symptomless. It is usually observed by routine radiography and sometimes it has features in common with mar-

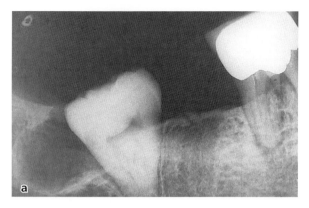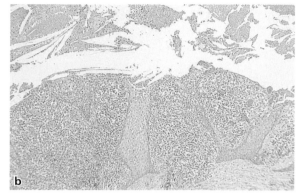

Fig. 13-24. (a) Radiography of inflammatory paradental cyst associated with partially erupted mandibular third molar. The cyst is lined by irregular non-keratinized squamous epithelium (b). Severe inflammation is seen in the connective tissue wall.

ginal periodontitis. The radiograph shows a round or oval radiolucency often less than 1 cm in diameter and usually with a margin of radiopacity. It is situated somewhere between the cervical margin and the apex of the tooth (Fig. 13-23a). The cyst probably arises initially as a dentigerous cyst developing by expansion of the tooth follicle along the lateral surface of the crown (Altini & Shear 1992).

Histopathology

The cyst is lined by a thin, non-keratinized stratified squamous epithelium, sometimes with focal epithelial thickenings (Fig. 13-23b) (Shear & Pindborg 1975). Inflammatory cells are only manifest in the case of secondary infection.

Treatment

The treatment is surgical enucleation with careful handling of the root surfaces and vascular supply of the associated tooth. Clinicians are advised to follow the cases for a number of years as some variants of the cysts may have a tendency to recur.

Inflammatory paradental cyst

Clinical features

The inflammatory paradental cyst has previously been described as the collateral inflammatory cyst, the inflammatory lateral periodontal cyst, the paradental cyst, and the mandibular infected buccal cyst (Vedtofte & Prætorius 1989). The site of predilection for this cyst is the mandibular molar area, most frequently the third molar, and the associated tooth is vital. Bilateral occurrence has been reported and similar cysts have been described in the globulomaxillary region between lateral incisors and canines (Vedtofte & Holmstrup 1989). The cyst develops most frequently in children and young adults, equally often in women and men. The cysts are often infected and pain, swelling and discharge of pus from the periodontal pocket are common due to communication with the periodontal pocket. Frequently, the cysts are diagnosed as periodontitis or pericoronitis (Vedtofte & Prætorius 1989). Radiographically, the inflammatory paradental cyst presents a well-defined radiolucency in a position predominantly distal to the involved tooth (Fig. 13-24a). A buccal superimposition may give an impression of a periapical lesion. The cyst may cause displacement of the tooth distal to the cyst. The cyst is frequently diagnosed shortly after tooth eruption and it is probably initiated by pericoronitis at the time of tooth eruption, the most likely origin of the cyst epithelium being the epithelial cell rests of Malassez and the reduced enamel epithelium (Craig 1976, Vedtofte & Prætorius 1989).

Histopathology

The cyst is lined with a thick non-keratinized stratified squamous epithelium, and the underlying connective tissue is infiltrated by inflammatory cells (Fig. 13-24b). The histology is non-specific.

Treatment

It has been demonstrated that the tooth associated with the cyst can in almost all cases be preserved. Cystectomy is the treatment, and usually the surgical treatment is followed by regeneration of bone and a periodontal sulcus of 2-3 mm (Vedtofte & Prætorius 1989).

Odontogenic keratocyst

Clinical features

Keratocysts may occur at any age and they are most frequent in males. The cysts are most often seen in the mandibular third molar region but may occur anywhere in the jaws including the alveolar bone. Radiographically, they may be small, round or ovoid, radiolucent areas with a smooth periphery or they may have scalloped margins or even be multilocular (Fig. 13-25a) (Shear 1992). It has been reported that a keratocyst-like lesion can be seen in the gingival soft tissues as well (Fardal & Johannesen 1994, Chehade et al. 1994).

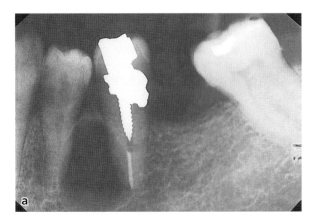

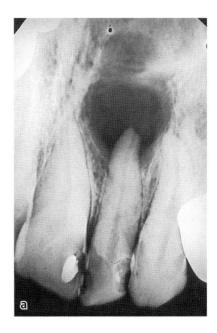

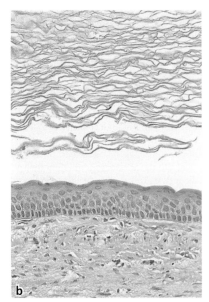

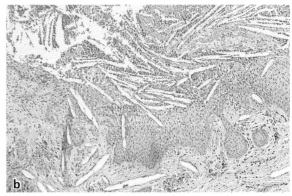

Fig. 13-25. (a) Keratocyst shows well demarcated ovoid radiolucency between right mandibular premolars. (b) The cyst is lined by keratinized squamous epithelium piling up in the cyst lumen (top). Note palisading of nuclei in the basal cell layer of the epithelium.

Fig. 13-26. (a) The radicular cyst shows a radiolucency surrounding the apex of a maxillary lateral incisor. (b) The radicular cyst is lined by an irregular non-keratinized stratified epithelium. Note cholesterol clefts in cyst lumen and connective tissue wall.

Histopathology

The cyst lining is a thin connective tissue capsule covered by an ortho- or parakeratinized stratified squamous epithelium with cuboidal or columnar basal cells (Fig. 13-25b). Inflammatory cells are not present unless the cyst is secondarily infected.

Treatment

Surgical intervention results in cure in most cases, but in contrast to other jaw cysts, the keratocysts show a propensity for recurrence (Forssell et al. 1988) even after what appears to be total removal. This is especially true for the parakeratinized cysts. Large cysts may be initially treated with marsupialization, i.e. opening of the cyst cavity into the mouth. This procedure usually leads to progressive reduction in the size of cysts in the jaws.

Radicular cyst

Clinical features

The radicular cyst is the most common cyst of the jaws, accounting for about 60% of jaw cysts (Shear 1992). The background of these cysts is a non-vital tooth with periapical granuloma in which rests of Malassez are stimulated to proliferate and finally form a cyst cavity which grows, probably due to accumulation of fluid within the cavity. Radiographically, the cysts show a well-circumscribed round or oval radiolucency related to the apical part of the root (Fig. 13-26a). The diameter varies from a few millimeters to a few centimeters.

Histopathology

The cyst cavity is lined by a non-keratinized stratified squamous epithelium of varying thickness and with irregular ridges proliferating into the underlying connective tissue (Fig. 13-26b). Sometimes mucous cells form part of the cyst lining, presumably due to metaplasia of the epithelium. There is usually a heavy inflammatory reaction in the underlying connective tissue, the inflammatory cells usually penetrating the epithelium and entering the cyst cavity. Numerous cholesterol clefts may be seen. As with the inflammatory paradental cyst, the histology is non-specific.

Treatment

Radicular cysts need surgical removal, possibly preceded by marsupialization if the cyst cavity is very large. Endodontic treatment or revision of previous endodontic treatment of the tooth involved is important.

References

Altini, M. & Shear, M. (1992). The lateral periodontal cyst: an update. *Journal of Oral Pathology & Medicine* **21**, 245-250.

Andersen, L., Fejerskov, O. & Philipsen, H.P. (1973a). Calcifying fibroblastic granuloma. *Journal of Oral Surgery* **31**, 196-200.

Andersen, L., Fejerskov, O. & Philipsen, H.P. (1973b). Oral giant cell granulomas. A clinical and histologic study of 129 new cases. *Acta Pathologica Microbiologica Scandinavica Section A* **81**, 606-616.

Barker, D.S. & Lucas, R.B. (1967). Localized fibrous overgrowths of the oral mucosa. *British Journal of Oral Surgery* **5**, 86-92.

Beumer, J., Harrison, R., Sanders, B. & Kurrasch, M. (1984). Osteoradionecrosis: predisposing factors and outcomes of therapy. *Head & Neck Surgery* **6**, 819-827.

Buchner, A. & Hansen, L.S. (1987a). The histomorphologic spectrum of peripheral ossifying fibroma. *Oral Surgery, Oral Medicine, Oral Pathology* **63**, 452-461.

Buchner, A. & Hansen, L.S. (1987b). Pigmented nevi of the oral mucosa: A clinicopathologic study of 36 new cases and review of 155 cases from the literature. Part I. A clinicopathologic study of 36 new cases. *Oral Surgery, Oral Medicine, Oral Pathology* **63**, 566-572.

Buchner, A., Leider, A.S., Merrell, P.W. & Carpenter, W.M. (1990). Melanocytic nevi of the oral mucosa: a clinicopathologic study of 130 cases from northern California. *Journal of Oral Pathology & Medicine* **19**, 197-201.

Buchner, A. & Sciubba, J.J. (1987). Peripheral epithelial odontogenic tumors: A review. *Oral Surgery, Oral Medicine, Oral Pathology* **63**, 688-697.

Cady, B. & Catlin, D. (1969). Epidermoid carcinoma of the gum. A 20-year survey. *Cancer* **23**, 551-569.

Chehade, A., Daley, T.D., Wysocki, G.P. & Miller, A.S. (1994). Peripheral odontogenic keratocyst. *Oral Surgery, Oral Medicine, Oral Pathology* **77**, 494-497.

Craig, G.T. (1976). The paradental cyst. A specific inflammatory odontogenic cyst. *British Dental Journal* **141**, 9-14.

Daley, T.D., Nartey, N.O. & Wysocki, G.P. (1991). Pregnancy tumor: an analysis. *Oral Surgery, Oral Medicine, Oral Pathology* **72**, 196-199.

Easson, E.C. & Palmer, M.K. (1976). Prognostic factors in oral cancer. *Clinical Oncology* **2**, 191-202.

Fardal, Ø. & Johannessen, A.C. (1994). Rare case of keratin-producing multiple gingival cysts. *Oral Surgery, Oral Medicine, Oral Pathology* **77**, 498-500.

Forssell, K., Forssell, H. & Kahnberg, K-E. (1988). Recurrence of keratocysts. A long-term follow-up study. *International Journal of Oral & Maxillofacial Surgery* **17**, 25-28.

Garlick, J.A. & Taichman, L.B. (1991). Human papillomavirus infection of the oral mucosa. *American Journal of Dermatopathology* **13**, 386-395.

Garrington, G.E., Scofield, H.H., Cornyn, J. & Hooker, S.P. (1967). Osteosarcoma of the jaws. Analysis of 56 cases. *Cancer* **20**, 377-391.

Green, T.L., Eversole, L.R. & Leider, A.S. (1986). Oral and labial verruca vulgaris: clinical, histologic and immunohistochemical evaluation. *Oral Surgery, Oral Medicine, Oral Pathology* **62**, 410-416.

Hirshberg, A., Leibovich, P. & Buchner, A. (1993). Metastases to the oral mucosa: analysis of 157 new cases. *Journal of Oral Pathology & Medicine* **22**, 385-390.

Holmstrup, P. & Westergaard, J. (1994). Periodontal diseases in HIV-infected patients. *Journal of Clinical Periodontology* **21**, 270-280.

Katsikeris, N., Kakarantza-Angelopoulou, E. & Angelopoulos, A.P. (1988). Peripheral giant cell granuloma. Clinicopathologic study of 224 new cases and review of 956 reported cases. *International Journal of Oral & Maxillofacial Surgery* **17**, 94-99.

Kfir, Y., Buchner, A. & Hansen, L.S. (1980). Reactive lesions of the gingiva. A clinicopathological study of 741 cases. *Journal of Periodontology* **51**, 655-661.

Kramer, I.R.H., Pindborg, J.J. & Shear, M. (1992). The WHO histological typing of odontogenic tumours. A commentary on the second edition. *Cancer* **70**, 2988-2994.

Lee, K.W. (1968). The fibrous epulis and related lesions. (Granuloma pyogenicum, "Pregnancy tumour", fibro-epithelial polyp and calcifying fibroblastic granuloma.) A clinicopathological study. *Periodontics* **6**, 277-292.

Makek, M.S. & Sailer, H.F. (1985). Endothelial pseudotumor (so-called pyogenic granuloma) – a report on 140 cases. *Schweizerische monatsscrift für Zahnmedizin* **95**, 248-260.

Maxymiw, W.G., Wood, R.E. & Lee, L. (1991). Primary, multifocal non-Hodgkin's lymphoma of the jaws presenting as periodontal disease in a renal transplant patient. *International Journal of Oral & Maxillofacial Surgery* **20**, 69-70.

Neville, B.W., Damm, D.D., Allen, C.M. & Bouquot, J.E. (1995). *Oral & maxillofacial pathology.* Philadelphia: Saunders.

Nxumalo, T.N. & Shear, M. (1992). Gingival cysts in adults. *Journal of Oral Pathology & Medicine* **21**, 309-313.

Philipsen, H.P., Thosaporn, W., Reichart, P. & Grundt, G. (1992). Odontogenic lesions in opercula of permanent molars delayed in eruption. *Journal of Oral Pathology & Medicine* **21**, 38-41.

Pindborg, J.J. (1980). *Oral cancer and precancer.* Copenhagen: Munksgaard.

Pindborg, J.J. (1992). *Atlas of diseases of the oral mucosa*, 5th edn. Copenhagen: Munksgaard.

Pindborg, J.J. & Prætorius, F. (1987). Oral human papillomavirus infections. *Tandlaegebladet* **91**, 404-409.

Pindborg, J.J. & Reichart, P.A. (1995). *Atlas of diseases of the oral cavity in HIV-infection.* 1st edn. Copenhagen: Munksgaard.

Prætorius-Clausen, F. (1972). Rare oral viral disorders. Review. *Oral Surgery, Oral Medicine, Oral Pathology* **34**, 604-618.

Pullon, P.A., Shafer, W.G., Elzay, R.P., Kerr, D.A. & Corio, R.L. (1975). Squamous odontogenic tumor. Report of six cases of a previously undescribed lesion. *Oral Surgery, Oral Medicine, Oral Pathology* **40**, 616-630.

Reibel, J. (1982). Oral fibrous hyperplasias containing stellate and multinucleated cells. *Scandinavian Journal of Dental Research* **90**, 217-226.

Reichart, P.A., Philipsen, H.P. & Sonner, S. (1995). Ameloblastoma: Biological profile of 3677 cases. *Oral Oncology, European Journal of Cancer* **31B**, 86-99.

Shear, M. (1992). *Cysts of the oral regions*, 3rd edn. Oxford: Wright.

Shear, M. (1994). Developmental odontogenic cysts. An update. *Journal of Oral Pathology & Medicine* **23**, 1-11.

Shear, M. & Pindborg, J.J. (1975). Microscopic features of the lateral periodontal cyst. *Scandinavian Journal of Dental Research* **83**, 103-110.

Takahashi, H., Tsuda, N., Tezuka, F. & Okabe, H. (1989). Primary extranodal non-Hodgkin's lymphoma of the oral region. *Journal of Oral Pathology & Medicine* **18**, 84-91.

Ulmansky, M., Hjørting-Hansen, E., Prætorius, F. & Haque, M.F. (1994). Benign cementoblastoma. A review and five new cases. *Oral Surgery, Oral Medicine, Oral Pathology* **77**, 48-55.

Vedtofte, P. & Holmstrup, P. (1989). Inflammatory paradental cysts in the globulomaxillary region. *Journal of Oral Pathology & Medicine* **18**, 125-127.

Vedtofte, P. & Prætorius, F. (1989). The inflammatory paradental cyst. *Oral Surgery, Oral Medicine, Oral Pathology* **68**, 182-188.

Waal, I. van der (1991). *Diseases of the jaws. Diagnosis and treatment.* Copenhagen: Munksgaard.

Waldron, C.A. (1985). Fibro-osseous lesions of the jaws. *Journal of Oral & Maxillofacial Surgery* **43**, 249-262.

Weathers, D.R. & Callihan, M.D. (1974). Giant-cell fibroma. *Oral Surgery, Oral Medicine, Oral Pathology* **37**, 374-384.

CHAPTER 14

Endodontics and Periodontics

GUNNAR BERGENHOLTZ AND GUNNAR HASSELGREN

Influence of pathologic conditions in the pulp on the periodontium

Manifestations of acute endodontic lesions in the marginal periodontium

Impact of endodontic treatment measures on the periodontium

Influence of external root resorptions

Influence of periodontal disease on the condition of the pulp

Influence of periodontal treatment measures on the pulp

Endodontic considerations in root resection of multirooted teeth in periodontal therapy

Differential diagnostic considerations

Treatment strategies for combined endodontic and periodontal lesions

---

The fact that the periodontium is anatomically interrelated with the dental pulp by virtue of apical foramina and lateral canals creates pathways for exchange of noxious agents between the two tissue compartments when either or both of the tissues are diseased. Resorptive processes involving the root surface, and treatment measures aimed at managing periodontal disease enhance this potential as the accompanying exposure of dentinal tubules establishes yet another passage across the body of the tooth structure. Consequently, under certain clinical conditions discussed in this chapter, disease in one of the tissue compartments may result in pathological conditions in the other.

Not only may interactions occur between the periodontium and the pulp to induce or even aggravate an existing lesion, they may also present the clinician with the challenge of deciding the direct cause of an inflammatory condition in the periodontium. Hence, inflammatory symptoms often seen as typical of periodontal disease including deep periodontal pockets with or without swelling and suppuration of the marginal gingivae, increased tooth mobility and angular bony defects may also represent symptoms of a pathological condition present in the root canal system of the affected tooth.

The differential diagnosis between an endodontic lesion (the term endodontic lesion is used to denote an inflammatory process in the periodontal tissues resulting from noxious agents present in the root canal system of the tooth, usually a root canal infection) and a periodontal lesion (the term periodontal lesion is used to denote an inflammatory process in the periodontal tissues resulting from accumulation of dental plaque on the external tooth surfaces) can often be established without much difficulty, since endodontic lesions most often induce symptoms in the apical periodontium, while symptoms of periodontal disease usually are confined to the marginal periodontium. However, the character of the clinical symptoms may occasionally be confusing and cause the misinterpretation of their etiology. What appears to be a periodontal lesion may actually be symptoms of an endodontic disorder and *vice versa*. The establishment of a correct diagnosis may also be complicated when both a periodontal and an endodontic lesion affect the same tooth simultaneously and may present as a single lesion. This condition has been termed "true endodontic-periodontal lesion" and implies that the lesion either is the result of, or the cause of, the other, or the lesion may just represent two separate processes, an endodontic and a periodontal, which have developed independently.

Proper diagnosis of the various disorders affecting the periodontium and the pulp is important to exclude unnecessary and even detrimental treatment. The clinician should therefore be well acquainted with the pathogenesis as well as with available diagnostic measures aimed at identifying disease conditions of these tissues. For this purpose, possible interrelationships between disease processes of the dental pulp and the periodontium are described in this chapter. Emphasis is placed upon diagnosis and treatment.

Since, in addition, root fractures and iatrogenic root perforations may be associated with inflammatory lesions of a similar nature in the periodontium as those of pulpal and periodontal disease, the clinical features of these complications are addressed as well. The mechanisms and the clinical management of different forms of external root surface resorptions have also been included in this chapter.

INFLUENCE OF PATHOLOGIC CONDITIONS IN THE PULP ON THE PERIODONTIUM

Impact of disease conditions in the vital pulp

Disease processes of the dental pulp frequently involve inflammatory changes. Caries, restorative procedures and traumatic injuries are the most common causes. In fact, any loss of hard tissue integrity, exposing dentin or the pulp directly, may allow bacteria and bacterial elements present in the oral environment to adversely affect the normal condition of the pulp. The resulting inflammatory lesion will then be directed towards the source of irritation and be confined for as long as the inflammatory defense does not collapse and convert into a destructive breakdown of the pulpal tissue. Consequently, inflammatory alterations in the vital pulp will not sustain distinct lesions in the adjoining periodontium. Yet, occasionally, disruption of the apical lamina dura or widening of the periodontal ligament space may be seen in the periodontium. Even a minor periapical radiolucency may be present in spite of the fact that vital pulp functions prevail (Langeland 1987). In such instances, typical clinical signs of pulpitis, including spontaneous pain, thermal sensitivity or tenderness to percussion, may or may not be present.

If the pulp survives the acute phase of the inflammatory response, repair and scarring of the tissue frequently develop. Reparative dentin (synonymous with irregular secondary dentin, irritation dentin, tertiary dentin) within areas of the previous lesion, fibrosis and dystrophic mineralizations represent typical sequelae to pulpal repair (Fig. 14-1). Such tissue changes do not *per se* warrant further concern except that they may interfere with the nervous and vascular supply of the tissue, which in turn may jeopardize its continued vital function upon an iterated insult.

Conclusion
From a diagnostic point of view it is important to realize that as long as the pulp maintains vital functions, although inflamed or scarred, it is unlikely to produce irritants that are sufficient to cause pronounced marginal breakdown of the periodontium. Consequently no benefit will be gained from pulp

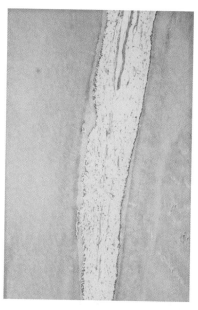

Fig. 14-1. Histologic section showing emerging hard tissue repair (reparative dentin) along the root canal wall of a monkey tooth exposed to scaling and root planing 30 days earlier. Specimen is from an experimental study by Bergenholtz & Lindhe (1978).

extirpation (pulpectomy) as an adjunct or alternative to the treatment of teeth for periodontal disease.

Impact of pulpal necrosis

Contrary to disease conditions in the vital pulp, pulp necrosis is frequently associated with inflammatory involvement of the periodontal tissue. The location of these lesions is most often at the apex of the tooth (Fig. 14-2). They may also occur at any site where lateral canals exit into the periodontium (Fig. 14-3, see also below).

While sterile necrotic pulps are unable to sustain overt inflammation in the periodontal tissue (Bergenholtz 1974, Sundqvist 1976, Möller et al. 1981), animal experiments (Kakehashi et al. 1965, Fabricius et al. 1982) and clinical studies (Bergenholtz 1974, Sundqvist 1976) have convincingly demonstrated the infectious nature of these processes. In this respect pulpal disease shares an identical etiology with periodontal disease. In fact, the two disease entities show many characteristics in common in terms of their microbiologic (Kerekes & Olsen 1990, Sundqvist 1990, 1994) and immunologic/histopathologic features (Bergenholtz et al. 1983, Stashenko et al. 1998, Marton & Kiss 2000). Similar to periodontal disease, potential pathogens most often associated with endodontic infections are found in the anaerobic segment of the flora with *Fusobacterium, Prevotella, Porphyromonas, Peptostreptococcus, Eubacterium, Capnocytophaga*, and *Lactobacillus* belonging to the genera most frequently isolated by culture (Sundqvist 1990, 1994, Baumgartner & Falkler 1991, Wasfy et al. 1992). Also spirochetes (Thilo et al. 1986, Molven et al. 1991, Dahle et al. 1996)

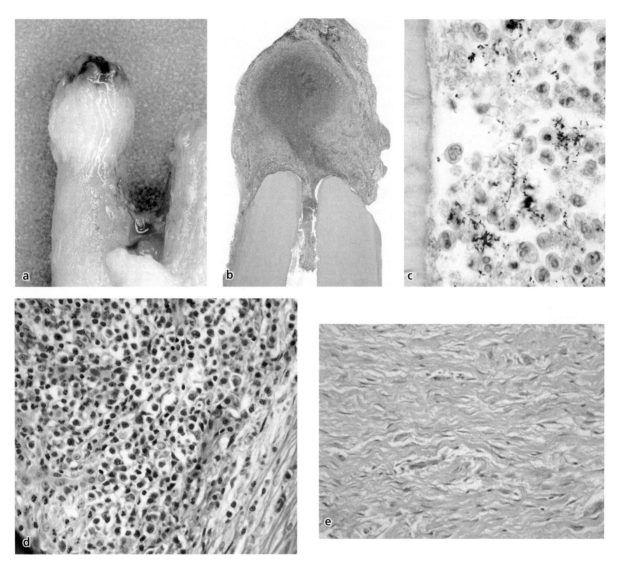

Fig. 14-2. Series of images demonstrating features of apical inflammatory lesions caused by a root canal infection. A lesion at the tip of an extracted palatal root of an upper molar (a). The longitudinally cut tissue section through the root tip shows an overview (b). The outer collagen rich connective tissue confines the soft tissue lesion and attaches it to the root surface. High magnification of a bacterial front–host tissue interface inside a root canal, where bacterial organisms (stained blue) are being battled by polymorphonuclear leukocytes (c). A typical mixed inflammatory cell response is common at the center of a lesion (d). In the most peripheral portion the connective tissue of an established lesion is rich in collagen and devoid of inflammatory cells (e). Figs 14-2 (a-c) and (e) have been kindly provided by Dr Domenico Ricucci. Microphotograph in (d) is from a lesion in a monkey (unpublished study by Bergenholtz & Wikesjö).

and fungi (Waltimo et al. 1997) may reside in infected root canals. It should be noted that the composition of the microbiota in necrotic pulps is not as complex as the one in deep periodontal pockets associated with periodontal disease and usually comprises a limited number of bacterial species of which one or two may predominate.

The host tissue response to the infection will take the form of either an acute abscess (Fig. 14-4) or a chronic inflammatory response (Fig. 14-2). Which of the forms occurs is largely dependent on the quality and quantity of the bacteria present in the root canal and the capacity of the host defense to confine and neutralize the bacterial elements that are released from the root canal system into the periodontium. Following the initial expansion, which involves de-

struction of the periodontal ligament and the adjacent alveolar bone, a balanced host-parasite relationship is usually established (Yu & Stashenko 1987, Stashenko & Yu 1989, Nair 1997, Stashenko et al 1998). The inflammatory process may then remain unchanged in size for years, although cyst transformation occasionally occurs that can result in substantial destruction of the alveolar bone.

Histologically, the established lesion is characterized by a richly vascularized granulation tissue, which, to a varying degree, is infiltrated by inflammatory cells. Neutrophilic granulocytes play a most important role in confining the infection to the pulpal space (Fig. 14-2c) (Stashenko et al. 1995) and constitute a cellular front line that may establish itself even inside the apical portion of the canal (Nair 1987). The remain-

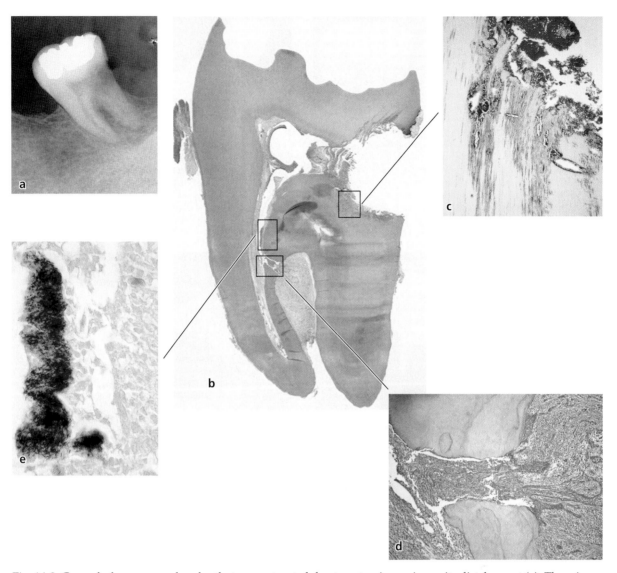

Fig. 14-3. Case of a lower second molar that was extracted due to extensive caries on its distal aspect (a). There is an apical radiolucency associated with the distal root tip. Histologic sections demonstrate different features (b-e). In the overview the coronal pulp tissue shows evidence of severe breakdown (b). Vital pulp tissue seems to remain in the mesial root while it is necrotic in the distal root (not shown). Stainings for bacteria reveal invasion of carious dentin (c) and deep into the pulp tissue of the mesial root (e). A lateral canal is clearly visible and connects the pulpal space with the periodontium in the furcal region, where an inflammatory lesion has developed (d). Note the proliferating epithelium adjacent to the exit of this canal into the periodontium (d). There was no increased pocket probing depth associated with this tooth. Courtesy of Dr Domenico Ricucci.

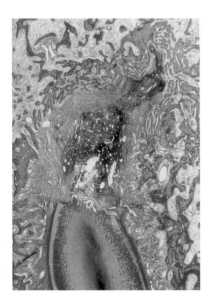

Fig, 14-4. Microphotograph showing an experimentally induced periapical inflammatory lesion in a monkey. Section is through a maxillary incisor with adjacent alveolar bone. The inflammatory response shows evidence of spreading. Note also the resorption of the root tip. From Syed et al. 1982.

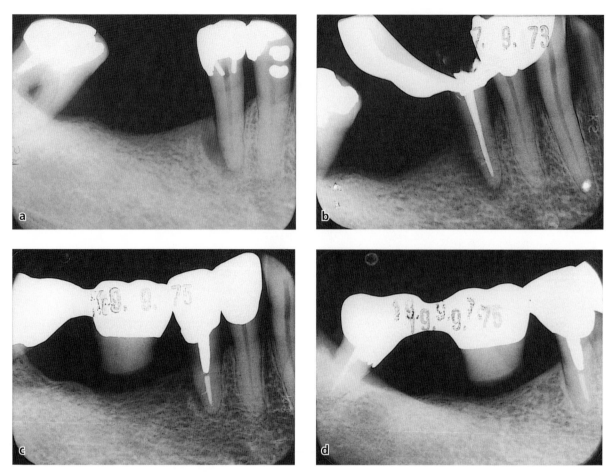

Fig. 14-5. (a) Radiolucent area along the distal root surface of tooth #45 combined with a horizontal marginal bone destruction. (b) The pulp was non-vital and the tooth was endodontically treated. After prosthetic therapy (c), the 2-year follow-up radiograph in (d) shows bone fill in the previous angular bony defect, whereas the marginal bone remains at the same level. On careful examination one can see that a lateral canal communicating with the lateral bone defect was filled.

der of the lesion will be composed of a mixed cellular response (Fig 14-2d) typical of a longstanding infectious process where various immunocompetent cells (dendritic cells, macrophages, T and B-cells) are prevalent (Torabinejad & Kettering 1985, Babal et al. 1987, Okiji et al. 1994, Stashenko et al 1998, Marton & Kiss 2000). With increasing distances from the root canal apertures, the established lesion harbors a decreasing number of inflammatory cells and an increasing amount of fibro-vascular elements representing attempts to repair. More peripherally there is a much stronger expression of fibroblastic activity and formation of new vessels and in the most peripheral portions of the lesion, a collagen-rich connective tissue normally separates it from the surrounding bone tissue (Fig. 14-2a,e).

Some, but far from all, lesions contain proliferating epithelial cells (Nair 1997). The origin of these epithelial strands is thought to be the epithelial rests of Malassez. In the lesion, they appear to take a random course, but sometimes they also attach to the root surface (Fig 14-3d). Their contribution to periodontal pocket formations, upon an endodontic lesion, developing in close proximity to the epithelial sulcus of the marginal periodontium, remains obscure.

In its established form, the lesion is clearly localized and constitutes an immunologically active protection zone of importance to preventing the dissemination of intracanal pathogens into the surrounding periodontal tissue (Stashenko 1990). While most often effective in this respect (Byström et al. 1987, Haapasalo et al. 1987, Nair 1987, Molven et al. 1991), bacteria may occasionally overcome the host defense and be present in the periapical tissue environment. This is particularly true on purulent lesions. It is also well known that *Actinomyces* related species, especially *Actinomyces israeli* and *Propionibacterium propionicum* may produce bacterial masses or nests within the lesion site (Happonen 1986).

Conclusion

Inflammatory processes in the periodontium associated with necrotic dental pulps have, similar to periodontal disease, an infectious etiology. The essential difference between the two disease entities is their respective source of infection. While periodontal disease is maintained by bacterial accumulation in the dento-gingival region, endodontic lesions are directed towards infectious elements released from the pulpal space. Rarely will established endodontic lesions in-

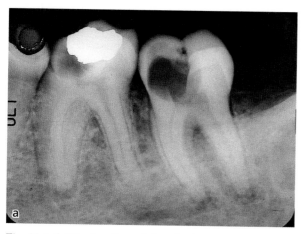
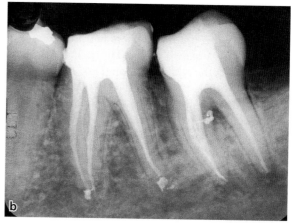

Fig. 14-6. (a) Destruction of alveolar bone is observed in the furcal region of the second lower left molar. (b) Upon endodontic treatment a lateral became filled suggesting that the furcal lesion had an endodontic origin. Courtesy of Dr Pierre Machtou.

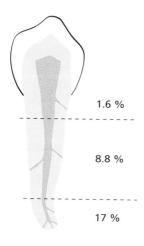

1.6 %

8.8 %

17 %

Fig. 14-7. Frequency of accessory canals at different levels of the root. The data are average values obtained from De Deus (1975). Observations were made after the teeth had been rendered transparent and the root-canal system filled with China ink. The figures for the coronal portion of the root include those of the bi- and trifurcations.

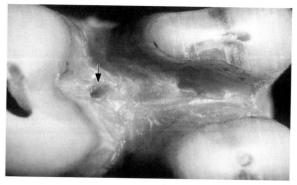

Fig. 14-8. Photograph of the furcation area of an extracted maxillary molar with cut roots demonstrating the opening of an accessory canal (arrow). Scanning electron microscopic observations indicate that the frequency of such furcation foramina is great (Burch & Hulen 1974, Koenigs et al. 1974), whereas the number of openings at the pulpal floor is small (Perlich et al. 1981). This suggests that furcation foramina at the external surface of the root do not necessarily represent patent communications with the pulpal chamber. Courtesy of Dr Robert C. Bowers.

volve the marginal periodontium, unless they are developing close to the bone margin. A potential pathway for infectious elements in root canal in such instances may be lateral canals.

Manifestations of endodontic lesions in the marginal periodontium from lateral canals

Endodontic lesions, where bacterial elements reach the periodontium by way of lateral canals, may, except for lateral aspects of roots (Fig. 14-5), appear in furcation areas of two and three-rooted teeth (Fig. 14-3). If there is an existing periodontal lesion, the two soft tissue lesions may merge and in the radiograph appear as one lesion (Fig. 14-5a). Although, clinically, one may be able to bring a probe through both lesions, it

is important from a therapeutic point of view to understand that the coronal part is directed towards an infection in the marginal periodontium, and the apical part to an infection emanating from the root canal system. This means that in order to obtain healing, elimination of both the sources of infection is required (see further below).

Lateral canals normally harbor connective tissue and vessels, which connect the circulatory system of the pulp with that of the periodontal ligament. Such anastomoses are formed during the early phases of tooth development. During the completion of root formation, several anastomoses become blocked and reduced in width by continuous deposition of dentin and root cementum. This may explain why endodontic lesions are rarely seen in furcal areas of the adult dentition, while in primary and young permanent molars such lesions often are the first sign of an infected pulp necrosis. Patent communications of varying sizes (10-250 μm), numbers and locations in the root, however, may remain and bring about endodontic lesions in the adult dentition (Figs. 14-3, 14-6).

Lateral canals can be observed in all groups of teeth. The majority are found in the apical portion of the root. In the middle and cervical root portions, the prevalence is small. In a study of 1140 extracted human teeth from adult subjects, De Deus (1975) reported lateral canals in 27%. These canals were distributed at various levels of the root as depicted in Fig. 14-7.

The frequency of lateral canals in the furcation area of two and three-rooted teeth has been determined in numerous studies of extracted human teeth (Fig. 14-8). A variety of techniques have been employed, which may explain the divergent results obtained. While some studies found furcation canals in between 20% and 60% of examined teeth (Lowman et al. 1973, Vertucci & Williams 1974, Gutmann 1978), others have failed to demonstrate the presence of such canals at furcation sites (Pineda & Kuttler 1972, Hession 1977). Radiographically, it is seldom possible to identify lateral canals unless they have been filled with a contrasting root-filling material following endodontic therapy (Figs. 14-5, 14-6). A lateral position of a radiolucency associated with a tooth with a necrotic and infected pulp may also indicate the presence of a lateral canal (Fig. 14-5a).

The clinical significance of lateral canals for the dissemination of infectious elements from an infected pulp to the periodontium is not well established. In fact, there is no documentation as to how often such lesions occur. It is conceivable that the wider the lateral canal, the greater is the likelihood for a lateral lesion to develop. Although clinical observations demonstrate their occurrence (Figs. 14-3, 14-5 and 14-6), the rate at which endodontic lesions appear in the marginal periodontium seems to be low.

In this context, it should be recognized that there is little evidence suggesting that infectious products from a necrotic pulp can affect the periodontal tissue through intact walls of dentin and cementum. Even if the width of the dentinal tubules is large enough to allow passage of both bacteria and their components, an intact outer layer of cementum evidently acts as an effective barrier against such penetration. Once cementum has been damaged, for example by root resorption, inflammatory periodontal lesions may be sustained by an active root canal infection (see below, Fig. 14-26).

Conclusion

Inflammatory lesions may develop from a root canal infection at the lateral aspects of the root and in furcation regions of two and multirooted teeth. In these instances, the lesions may be induced and maintained by bacterial products, which reach the periodontium through lateral canals. These types of lesions appear to be rare and do not seem to emerge at a rate that corresponds to the frequency with which lateral canals occur in teeth.

MANIFESTATIONS OF ACUTE ENDODONTIC LESIONS IN THE MARGINAL PERIODONTIUM

Inflammatory lesions in the periodontal tissue, induced and maintained by root canal infection, often have a limited extension around the apex of the tooth (Fig. 14-2) or at the orifice of a lateral canal (Fig. 14-3).

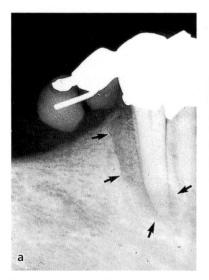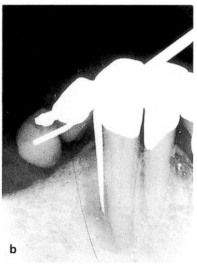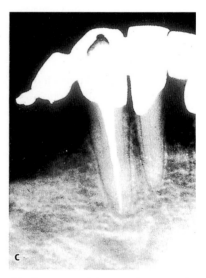

Fig. 14-9. Angular bone defect is observed along the distal root surface of a mandibular canine (a). Apical-marginal communication was confirmed by periodontal probing (b). Endodontic treatment resulted in complete reestablishment of the periodontal structures, demonstrating that the periodontal defect in this case was the result of endodontic infection only. Courtesy of Dr Ralph Milthon.

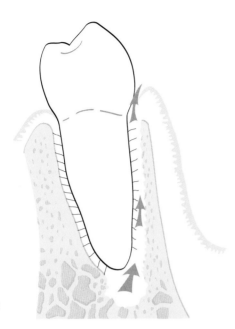 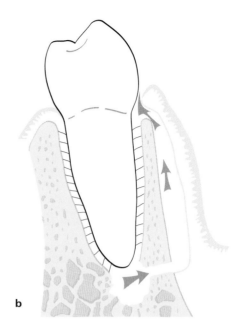

a   b

Fig. 14-10. Schematic illustration demonstrating possible pathways for drainage of a periapical abscess into the gingival sulcus/pocket. (a) periodontal ligament fistulation. (b) extraosseous fistulation.

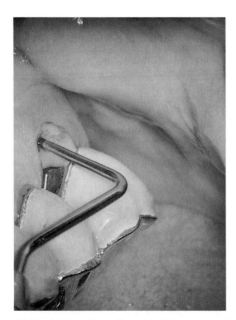

Fig. 14-11. Drainage of pus from probing a periodontal ligament fistulation of an endodontic lesion associated with an upper molar.

In conjunction with the initial expansion of an endodontic lesion, the periodontal tissue support can be lost to the extent that an apical-marginal communication emerges, in particular when there is already a substantial loss of periodontal tissue support due to periodontal disease (Fig. 14-5). Following the exacerbation of an established lesion, the subsequent abscess formation may cause the destruction of the supporting tissue structures along the entire root length (Fig. 14-9). This may occur even in a tooth with a normal height of the attachment apparatus.

The emergence of these processes may or may not be associated with clinical signs of acute inflammation including throbbing pain, tenderness to percussion and apical palpation, increased tooth mobility and swelling of the marginal gingiva. Note that the same symptoms are typical of a periodontal abscess due to either periodontal disease, root fracture, root resorption or iatrogenic root perforation (see also Fig. 14-27).

In general, drainage of endodontic abscesses into the sulcus/pocket follows one of two routes (Fig. 14-10):

1. The suppurative process may cause a sinus tract along the periodontal ligament space (periodontal ligament fistulation; Fig. 14-10a). This usually results in only a narrow opening of the fistula into the gingival sulcus/pocket and may not be detected unless careful probing of the sulcus is carried out at multiple sites. *Such a fistula may readily be probed down to the apex of the tooth (Fig. 14-9b), where no increased probing depth otherwise exists around the tooth.* In multirooted teeth a periodontal ligament fistulation can drain off into the furcation area (Fig. 14-11). The resulting lesion may then resemble a "through and through" furcation defect from periodontal disease (Fig. 14-12).

2. A periapical abscess can also perforate the cortical bone close to the apex and elevate the soft tissue including the periosteum from the bone surface, and drain into the gingival sulcus/pocket (Fig. 14-10b). This type of drainage will result in a wide opening of the fistula into the sulcus/pocket (extraosseous fistulation), and is most often seen at the buccal aspect of the tooth. Since this type of fistula is not associated with loss of bone tissue at the inner walls of the alveolus, a periodontal probe cannot penetrate into the periodontal ligament space.

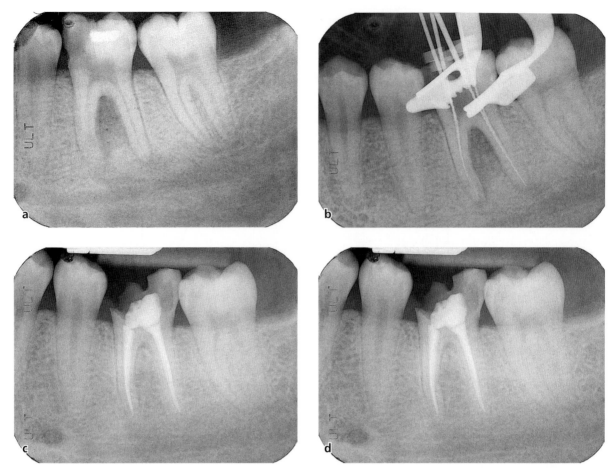

Fig. 14-12. A large radiolucent area is seen in the furcation region of the lower left first molar (tooth #36) mimicking what potentially could be a through and through furcation involvement (a). There is, however, a distinct caries lesion and the pulp is necrotic. Upon endodontic therapy (b,c) the 18-month follow-up radiograph demonstrates complete bone fill in the region (d). Courtesy of Dr Kevin Martin.

It is important to realize that the lesions described are strictly of endodontic origin. Therefore, following conventional endodontic therapy, directed to eliminate the root canal infection, both types of marginal communications should, following proper treatment, heal rapidly without a persistent periodontal defect (Figs. 14-5, 14-12 and 14-13). Thus, there is generally no need for adjunctive periodontal therapy. The endodontic treatment of the involved tooth should be performed without delay to prevent repeated exacerbations and the establishment of a permanent apical-marginal communication.

Conclusion

Acute manifestations of root canal infections can result in rapid and extensive destruction of the attachment apparatus. Abscesses may drain off in different directions of which (1) a sinus tract along the periodontal ligament space and (2) an extraosseous fistulation into the gingival sulcus/pocket warrant particular attention from a differential diagnostic point of view. Following proper endodontic therapy, these lesions should be expected to heal without a persistent periodontal defect.

IMPACT OF ENDODONTIC TREATMENT MEASURES ON THE PERIODONTIUM

When breakdown of periodontal tissue is associated with a root-filled tooth, endodontic etiology should be taken into account, particularly if the root filling is of poor quality. From unfilled spaces in the root canal, sustaining bacterial growth, infectious products may emerge into the periodontium along the very same pathways as in an untreated tooth with infected pulp. Clinical observations suggest that such infections may contribute to increased probing depth (Jansson et al. 1993) and results of clinical follow-ups have shown retarded or impaired periodontal tissue healing subsequent to periodontal therapy of endodontically treated teeth with periapical pathology (Ehnevid et al. 1993a,b). From these observations, it follows that endodontic retreatment may be considered as an adjunct to periodontal therapy whenever a root canal filling is defective and/or displays signs of periapical inflammation. Root-filled teeth in general, however, do not seem to be associated with an impaired periodontal status (Miyashita et al. 1998).

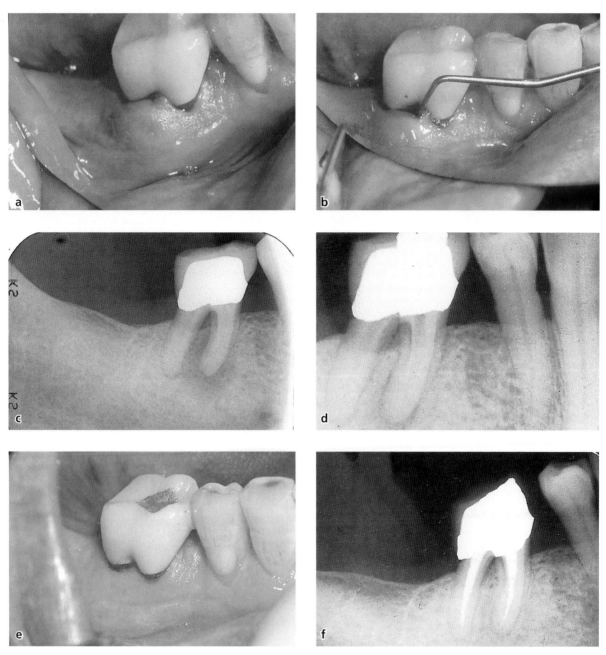

Fig. 14-13. Facial swelling associated with tooth #46 as a result of a periapical abscess (a). Patient had experienced pain and tenderness in the area for 1 week. Periodontal probing disclosed a deep facial pocket along the mesial root (b). Radiographically, the lesion circumscribed the mesial root with marginal extension in the furcation (c). It was not possible to determine the condition of the pulp by conventional pulp-vitality tests. Test cavity preparation revealed a necrotic pulp that was endodontically treated including intracanal dressing with calcium hydroxide. Obvious reduction in lesion size was observed 3 months after treatment (d). Gingival lesion resolved leaving no abnormal probing depth (e), although radiographically a small bone defect remained in the furcation area (d, f) Endodontic treatment was completed by filling the root canals with gutta-percha. Twelve months after root filling complete resolution of the bone defect had occurred (f). Diagnosis and treatment of this case was carried out by one of the authors (G.B.) in collaboration with Dr David Simpson.

Periodontal inflammatory lesions may also result from mechanical as well as chemical irritation initiated by root canal treatment. However, medicaments for canal irrigation and disinfection as well as materials for filling used in modern endodontics are comparatively well tolerated by the connective tissue of the periodontium, even if, during treatment, they are forced into the periodontal ligament. On the other hand, strong antiseptic drugs used for root canal disinfection and pulp devitalization cause severe damage if they leak into the periodontal tissue (Fig. 14-14a,b).

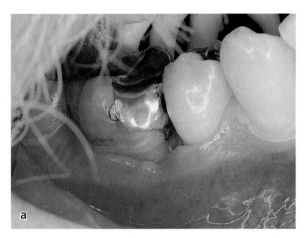
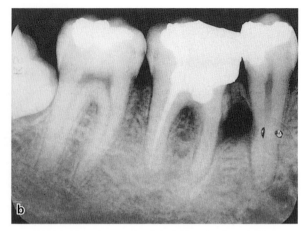

Fig. 14-14. (a) Clinical photograph showing a periodontal defect at the mesial aspect of tooth #46. The pulp of the tooth had been subjected to a treatment with paraformaldehyde applied in order to cause its devitalization. Leakage of the agent along a defect temporary restoration had obviously occurred as indicated by the loss of proximal bone and presence of a bone sequestrum (b).

Root perforations

During endodontic treatment, and in conjunction with preparation of root canals for the insertion of posts, instrumentation can accidentally cause perforation of the root and wounding of the periodontal ligament (Alhadainy 1994). Perforations can be made through the lateral walls of the root or through the pulpal floor in multirooted teeth. At the site of perforation, the subsequent inflammatory reaction can result in the formation of a periodontal pocket, if the perforation is located close to the gingival margin (Lantz & Persson 1967, Strömberg et al. 1972, Petersson et al. 1985). Other complications include exacerbation of a preexisting periodontal lesion and development of clinical symptoms, similar to those of a periodontal abscess, e.g. acute pain, swelling, drainage of pus from the pocket, increased tooth mobility and further loss of fibrous attachment (Fig. 14-15).

Early detection of the complication is crucial to provide reasonable conditions for successful treatment. Diagnosis may be based on the occurrence of sudden pain and bleeding during preparation of root canals coronal to the working length. Such signs are likely to be less distinct if the perforation occurs during a procedure conducted under local anesthesia. In such cases bleeding may not invariably be provoked. For example, when post preparations are carried out by means of a machine-driven instrument, a smear layer is formed that may clog up the blood vessels. Thus, in many instances no bleeding will be noticed until the following visit, when granulation tissue is formed and has proliferated into the root canal space from the site of perforation. These granulations sometimes bleed profusely on attempts to remove them, which in turn may jeopardize adequate placement of an internal perforation seal. For this reason treatment of a root perforation should be initiated once discovered.

The series of radiographs in Fig. 14-16 demonstrates the successful outcome of a treatment of a

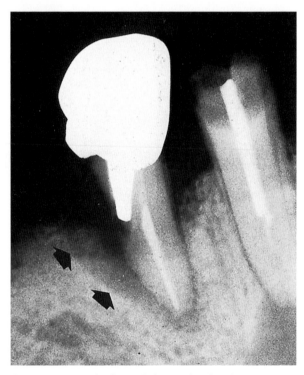

Fig. 14-15. Angular bone defect at the distal root surface of a mandibular premolar (arrows). The root is perforated. Conceivably, this occurred in conjunction with preparation of the root canal for a post and core. Clinical symptoms included drainage of pus from the pocket and increased tooth mobility. The tooth was extracted.

perforation made in the furcation of a mandibular molar. Healing of the lesion in the periodontium depends largely on whether bacterial infection can be excluded from the wound site by a tight seal of the perforation (Beavers et al. 1986). If the perforation is close to the sulcus area, or conducted through the floor of a multirooted tooth, the inflammatory response may induce the proliferation of sulcular epithelium to form a deepened periodontal pocket (Petersson et al. 1985).

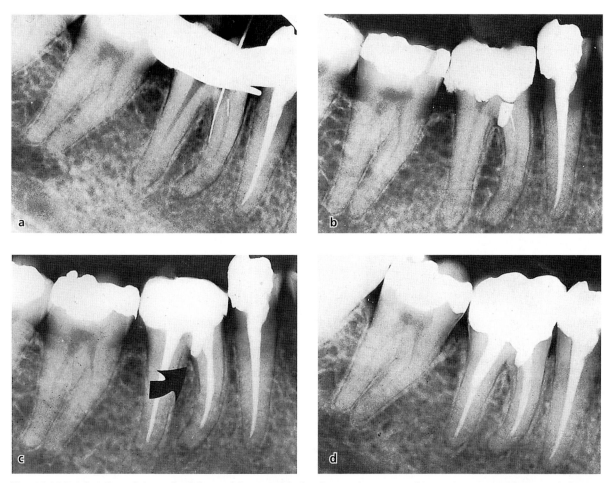

Fig. 14-16. Perforation of the pulpal floor of the mandibular first molar occurred in conjunction with a search for root canal openings (a). The perforation was immediately sealed with gutta-percha (b). One month after treatment a slight radiolucency appeared at the perforation site (arrow) in the periodontium (c). After an observation period of 2 years, normal periodontal conditions were re-established both clinically and radiographically (d). Courtesy of Dr Gunnar Heden.

Repair of root perforations is unpredictable and a questionable prognosis of treatment should be anticipated (Petersson et al. 1985). Major reasons are that perforations frequently are difficult to access for a proper seal. Furthermore, the perforation is often made at an oblique angle in the lateral wall of the root and the artificial canal may then have an oval-shaped orifice into the periodontium. Obturation of such defects with gutta-percha, for example, can result in a poor seal and a risk of subsequent bacterial irritation of the periodontal tissue.

Over the years a large number of therapeutic agents and methods have been proposed for the management of root perforations (Alhadainy 1994). Materials suggested for sealing include amalgam, zinc oxide and eugenol cements, calciumhydroxide-containing pastes both chemically cured and light cured and plaster of Paris. More recently, mineral trioxide aggregate (MTA) has come into vogue by virtue of promising clinical results (Arens & Torabinejad 1996, Schwartz et al. 1999) and by observation in animal experiments of cementum depositions against the material (Torabinejad et al. 1997, Holland et al. 2001).

For mid-root and cervical perforations, non-surgi-

cal approaches including placement of an internal seal are preferable to surgical procedures as the latter often results in pocket formation and furcation involvement. Furthermore, surgical approaches are not always feasible because of the inherent difficulty in accessing many perforation sites. In such cases, as a last resort, extraction followed by repair and re-implantation of the tooth has been attempted. In multi-rooted teeth, hemisection and extraction of one or two roots may be the treatment of choice.

Conclusion

Inflammatory lesions in the marginal periodontium as manifested by increased probing depth, suppuration, increased tooth mobility and loss of fibrous attachment may result from an undetected or unsuccessfully treated root perforation. If an iatrogenic root perforation occurs during instrumentation of root canals, filling of the artificial canal to the periodontium should be carried out immediately. Outcome of treatment depends on how well the wound site can be sealed and protected from infection. The closer the perforation is to the marginal gingiva, the greater the

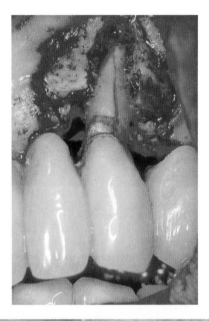

Fig. 14-17. Vertical root fracture of a maxillary root-filled upper canine included as abutment in a prosthetic reconstruction. Due to the inflammatory breakdown, alveolar bone facial to the root surface is absent.

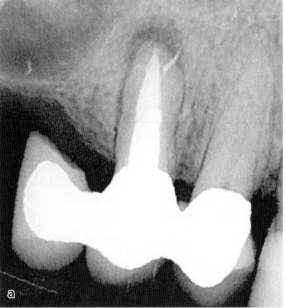
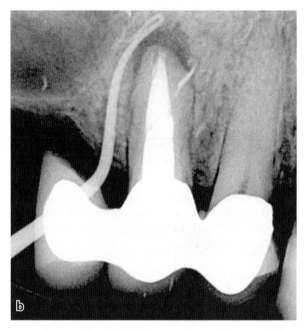

Fig. 14-18. Periapical radiolucency associated with an upper second premolar (a) which turned out to be caused by a longitudinal root fracture. There was a buccal deep pocket probing depth. (b) A gutta-percha point has been inserted in a fistulous tract. The widely prepared root canal and the cantilever most likely contributed to the risk for fracture in this case. Courtesy of Dr Tomas Kvist.

likelihood of proliferation of sulcular epithelium to the perforation site.

Vertical root fracture

Clinical symptoms that are typical for endodontic and periodontal lesions may also appear at teeth with vertical root fractures. A vertical root fracture is defined as a fracture of the root that is longitudinally oriented at a more or less oblique angle towards the long axis of the tooth (Fig. 14-17). It can traverse the root in different directions mesially/distally or facially/lingually and may or may not involve the pulpal chamber. A vertical root fracture can extend the

entire length of a tooth and involve the gingival sulcus/pocket area but may also be incomplete and confined to either the coronal or apical ends. Furthermore, it should be noted that even though vertical root fractures usually involve opposite sides of the root, occasionally only one aspect of the root is involved.

As a result of bacterial growth in the fracture space, the adjacent periodontal ligament will become the seat of an inflammatory lesion, which causes breakdown of connective tissue fibers and alveolar bone (Fig. 14-17). Breakdown can manifest itself radiographically in a number of different ways (Figs. 14-18, 14-19c, 14-20). Thus, the radiographic defect may be similar to those found at endodontic and periodontal lesions. In other situations the appearance may be atypical of

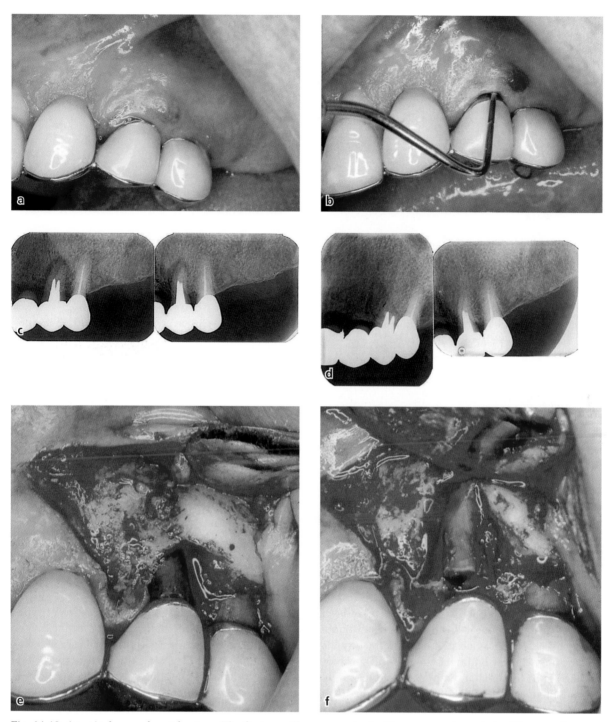

Fig. 14-19. A typical case of root fracture. The first maxillary premolar had been asymptomatic for 20 years after completion of endodontic treatment and bridge work. Patient sought treatment because of suddenly occurring pain, tenderness and facial swelling (a). A deep periodontal pocket can be probed at the buccal aspect of the tooth (b), while other sites showed no abnormal probing depths. Radiographs (c) revealed a radiolucent area along the mesial aspect of the tooth. A set of radiographs taken 6 months earlier at a recall session (d) showed no such lesion. The elevation of a mucoperiosteal flap (e) revealed substantial loss of marginal bone at the buccal aspect of the root and a fracture in a mesiodistal direction could be confirmed. Following removal of bone, the root was separated from the crown (f) and extracted.

these disorders. A widening of the periodontal ligament space along one or both of the lateral root surfaces may indicate the presence of a root fracture. A thin halo-like apical radiolucency is another example of a radiographic lesion suggestive of a vertical root fracture (Pitts & Natkin 1983, Testori et al. 1993, Tamse et al. 1999a).

Clinical symptoms associated with vertical root fractures show a varying character. Occasionally, there may be pronounced pain symptoms and abscess formation – symptoms similar to those occurring with

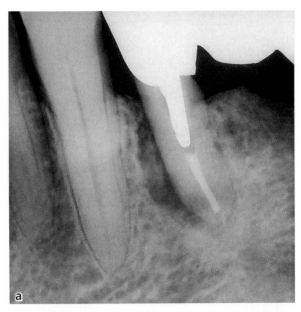

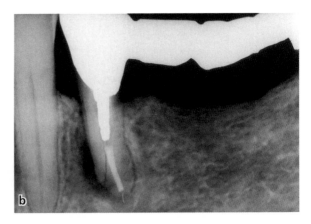

Fig. 14-20. Mandibular premolar included in a 4-unit bridge showing a bone lesion at the mesial aspect. In one of the projections there is no evidence of fracture (a) while in another radiograph, taken with a slight shift of angulation, a fracture line is clearly visible (b). Courtesy of Dr K-G. Olsson.

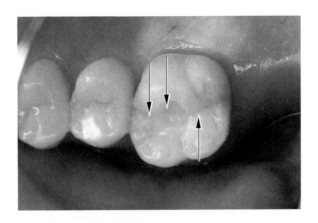

Fig. 14-21. Unrestored, cracked left maxillary first molar causing symptoms of pulpitis. The patient, a 47-year-old male, had complained of pain in the TMJ-region. Following the preparation of a test cavity a clear split line was observed at the bottom of the cavity, confirming the cause of the pain symptoms. Courtesy of Dr H. Suda.

periodontal or endodontic abscesses. In other instances, a narrow, local deepening of a periodontal pocket (Fig. 14-19), associated with the fracture, may be the only clinical finding. Other clinical symptoms occurring in conjunction with root fractures are tenderness to mastication, fistulous tract, mild pain and dull discomfort. The diagnosis of a vertical root fracture is often difficult because the fracture is usually not readily detectable by clinical inspection unless there is a clear separation of the root fragments. By radiographic examination the central X-ray beam has to be parallel to the fracture plane to give a radiographic appearance (Fig. 14-20). The suspicion of a vertical root fracture is often inferred from a pocket probing depth in an aberrant position, for example at a buccal or lingual aspect of a tooth in a dentition which otherwise is free from symptoms of periodontal disease (Fig 14-18). Another strong indication is the sudden appearance of clinical symptoms and/or radiographic lesion on a root-filled tooth that has remained asymptomatic and without lesion for many years (Fig. 14-19a-d).

A number of diagnostic procedures can be undertaken to confirm the diagnosis. Application of various dye solutions, e.g. methylene blue or iodine tincture, on to the crown and the root surface can sometimes be indicative. As the dye enters the fracture space, it will show up as a distinct line against the surrounding tooth substance. Indirect illumination of the root, using fiber-optic light, can also be of value. The fiber-optic probe should then be placed at various positions on the crown or the root, whereby the fracture line may clearly present itself. The surgical microscope or an endoscope, providing both enlargement and directed light, are other valuable tools to detect a fracture.

In premolars and molars the diagnosis may be supported from observation of varying pain sensations elicited by loading facial and lingual cusps. The procedure includes asking the patient to bite down on a Burlew disc or a specially designed plastic stick (FracFinder). Separate loading of either buccal or lingual cusps eliciting pain sensation from one, but not the other, loaded portion indicates the potential of a fracture. Often the diagnosis of a vertical root fracture has to be confirmed by surgical exposure of the root for direct visual examination (Fig. 14-19e,f; Walton et al. 1984).

Data on prevalence of vertical root fractures are scarce in the literature. While the prevalence appears to be low, vertical root fractures probably occur more often than clinicians are able to diagnose (Tamse et al. 1999b). There seems to be an overrepresentation of endodontically treated teeth compared to teeth with vital pulps (Fig. 14-21), with molars and premolars more often affected than incisors and canines (Meister et al. 1980, Testori et al. 1993). In longitudinal clinical follow-up studies of patients treated with fixed prostheses, vertical root fractures were frequent in root-filled teeth with posts and, in particular, among those teeth serving as terminal abutments in cantilever bridges (Randow et al. 1986).

It is of clinical interest to note that root fracture of endodontically treated teeth may occur and/or be diagnosed several years after the completion of endodontic therapy and final restoration of the tooth (Fig. 14-19). In a study comprising 32 vertical root fractures, the average time between the completion of endodontic treatment and diagnosis of fracture was 3.25 years, with a range varying between 3 days and 14 years (Meister et al. 1980). In another study comprising 36 teeth, symptoms of root fracture developed on average more than 10 years after completion of treatment (Testori et al. 1993).

Although the subject of considerable study, the etiology of vertical root fractures is not well established. In some situations the cause is undoubtedly iatrogenic from pin and post placements, root canal filling procedures, and seating of intracoronal restorations. Results of experimental studies suggest that loss of tooth structure from caries, trauma and restorative procedure weakens teeth and makes them susceptible to fracture from mastication forces (Reeh et al. 1989, Sedgley & Messer 1992). The reason vertical root fractures appear to be associated with endodontically treated teeth may be that the access opening preparation as well as overzealous root canal preparation results in substantial loss of fracture resistance. It has also been speculated that, along with loss of vital pulp tissue, mechanoreceptive functions are lost concomitantly, allowing larger loads to be placed during mastication than the patient would normally tolerate (Löwenstein & Rathkamp 1955, Randow & Glantz 1986). Suggestions that endodontically treated teeth with time become brittle due to changes in the biomechanical properties of dentin and, thus, less resistant to mastication forces have not been substantiated in careful analyses (Sedgley & Messer 1992).

Also, clinically intact teeth with no or minimal restorations may be subjected to vertical root fracture (Fig. 14-21). Traumatic occlusal forces may induce fracture, and mandibular molars appear to be especially at risk (Yang et al. 1995, Chan et al. 1999). Subsequent to these fractures typical pulpitis symptoms may be initiated followed by breakdown of the pulp and abscess formation, if the fracture involves the pulp tissue directly.

Vertical root fractures that involve the gingival sulcus/pocket area usually have a hopeless prognosis due to continuous bacterial invasion of the fracture space from the oral environment. While there are reports on successful management of fractured teeth by reattaching the fragments with a bonding resin after extraction and re-implantation, fractured teeth are normally candidates for extraction. In multirooted teeth a treatment alternative is hemisection and extraction of the fractured root.

Conclusion

Symptoms and signs associated with vertical root fractures show a varying character and may be difficult to distinguish from those associated with periodontal and endodontic lesions. A variety of diagnostic procedures should be considered. Except for the leads obtained from anamnestic findings and pocket probing depths in buccal or lingual positions or both, clinical examination should include measures to make fracture lines visible: application of dye solutions, the use of fiberoptic light, inspection in the surgical microscope or endoscope and by a surgical flap. Pain on selective loading of cusps may be an indication of root fracture. A vertical root fracture should be anticipated in root-filled teeth, which, after a long history of being asymptomatic and without signs of endodontic infection, suddenly present with tenderness, pain symptoms and radiographic bone destruction (Fig. 14-20). Roots with vertical root fracture usually have a hopeless prognosis and should be extracted.

INFLUENCE OF EXTERNAL ROOT RESORPTIONS

External resorption of roots normally progresses without clinical symptoms and without causing periodontal defects that can be mistaken for endodontic or periodontal disease. However, in their advanced stages they may interfere with the gingival sulcus and cause the development of a periodontal abscess (Fig. 14-22). Since such lesions may be associated with both increased pocket probing depths and drainage of pus upon probing, this section of the chapter addresses various forms of external root resorptions, their mechanisms, clinical features and management.

Mechanisms of hard tissue resorption

The hard tissues of the body consist of two major components, mineral and matrix. The ratio of these two components varies between bone, cementum and dentin, but the same tools – acids and enzymes – are used by nature to monitor the degradation of these tissues. Bone is normally remodeled to adapt to func-

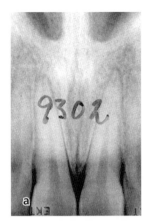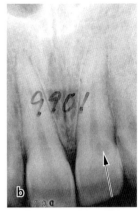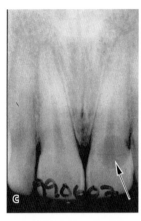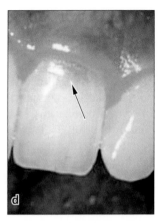

Fig. 14-22. Series of radiographs taken at different time periods showing the appearance of an external root resorption in a young adult patient (a-c). At the age of 15 years there is no sign of resorption (a). Six years later a small radiolucency is seen (arrow) (b). In just 6 months the lesion had expanded considerably (arrow) (c) and appeared clinically as a pink area (arrow) (d). Courtesy Dr Anders Molander.

tional changes, but as far as dental hard tissues in permanent teeth are concerned resorption should be seen as an expression of a pathological process. Bone as well as cementum and dentin and also enamel, when applicable, are resorbed by clast cells (Hammarström & Lindskog 1992). Osteoclasts are large, multi-nucleated, motile cells emanating from hematopoietic precursor cells in the bone marrow (Marks 1983, Vaes 1988, Pierce et al. 1991). Mononucleated cells are also involved when dental hard tissue is resorbed (Wedenberg & Lindskog 1985, Lindskog et al. 1987, Sasaki et al. 1990).

Under normal conditions, hard tissues are protected from resorption by their surface layers of blast cells. It appears that as long as these layers are intact, resorption cannot occur. It is known that hormonal regulation of bone resorption is mediated by osteoblasts (Chambers 1988). Stimulation by parathyroid hormone will make osteoblasts contract to expose the bone surface for the osteoclasts (Jones & Boyde 1976, Rodan & Martin 1981). However, parathyroid hormone exerts no influence on cementoblasts (Lindskog et al. 1987). This may explain why bone and not teeth are remodeled to adapt to functional changes.

A denuded hard tissue surface attracts resorbing cells. It has been suggested that the removal of the organic matrix of bone will make it possible for phagocytic cells to recognize the mineral component (Chambers 1981). Thus it appears that the blast cell layer on hard tissues forms a protective barrier that has to be broken down to trigger osteoclastic activity. Under clinical conditions various forms of damage can affect the blast cell layer, e.g. trauma or excessive scaling and root planing in periodontal therapy (Andreasen 1981). Subsequent to the injury, mobile osteoclasts come and seal themselves to the exposed hard tissue surface and excrete acids into the extracellular environment under their ruffled border to demineralize the tissue. This event further creates the necessary acid environment essential for the function of lysosomal enzymes with

low pH optima, to degrade the tissue matrix (Vaes 1968).

Conclusion

Two mechanisms are involved in resorption of a hard tissue:

1. a trigger mechanism
2. a reason for the resorption to continue.

The trigger mechanism in root resorption is a root surface detached from its protective blast cell layer. Detachment may follow any damage to the cementoblastic cell layer. For the resorption to continue, a stimulus is required, e.g. an infection or a continuous mechanical force such as the one in orthodontic treatment. Consequently, the treatment of root resorption should be directed towards the cause for the continuance of the resorption, e.g. removal of infected material in a root canal, or the halt of an orthodontic tooth movement.

Clinical manifestations of external root resorptions

Root resorptions *per se* do not cause painful symptoms. Unless a resorptive process is located coronally and is undermining the enamel, giving it a pinkish appearance (Fig. 14-22d), the only way to detect and diagnose a dental resorption is by means of radiography (Fig. 14-22a-c). If only one radiograph is taken it is usually not possible to exactly define a radiolucent area found inside the confines of a root. It may be a resorptive process inside the root canal, or a radiolucent resorptive defect located buccally or lingually and superimposed on the image of the root. It may also just be an artifact. Therefore, one should always take more than one radiograph and use different angulations to observe whether the radiolucent area belongs to the root or not.

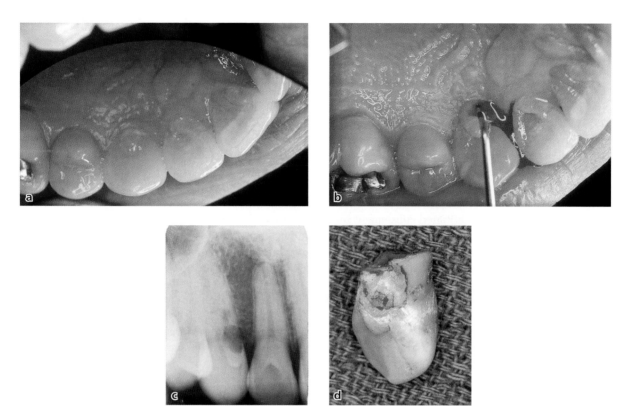

Fig. 14-23. Painful condition associated with a peripheral inflammatory root resorption (PIRR). The 30-year-old male patient had experienced pain and tenderness of the right maxilla for several weeks (a). Clinically, all teeth were sensible to pulp testing. Periodontal probing revealed pus drainage from the lingual aspect of tooth #13 (b). An angulated radiograph revealed the presence of a resorptive defect (c). The tooth was deemed beyond recovery and was extracted. An extensive resorptive defect had undermined the clinical crown (d).

Root resorptions always start at a surface and are termed external if emanating from the root surface and internal if initiated in the root canal wall. If the radiolucent area is situated within the confines of the root, at least two angulations or tomography are useful to determine whether it is related to the root canal or the root surface. If the outline of the root canal space is clearly visible within the radiolucency, as in Figs. 14-22c and 14-23, this is a strong case for an external origin. Due to its relatively rare occurrence internal resorptions will not be further discussed in this chapter.

The initial stage of a resorptive process usually passes undetected as radiographs can only demonstrate a resorptive cavity after a certain size has been reached (Fig. 14-23a-c; Andreasen et al. 1987). The location of the lesion is also important for the detection. A facial or lingual root resorption cavity is more difficult to visualize radiographically than a proximal cavity. Be aware that in the cervical region it may be difficult to differentiate radiographically between cavities caused by caries and those caused by resorption. Resorptive processes and caries develop by different mechanisms, which is useful for distinguishing these lesions. Bacterial acids, which demineralize dentin, create carious defects, but the organic part will remain and render the cavity soft on exploration. A simultaneous removal of the mineral phase and the organic matrix of the hard tissue forms the resorptive defect. This results in a cavity floor, which is hard on probing.

Different forms of external root resorption

There are different forms of external root resorption. The underlying mechanism is understood for some of these, whereas other forms still remain unexplained. In some instances external root resorptions appear to be genetically linked, as they run in families. There are also instances when only the enamel of an unerupted tooth is being resorbed. Furthermore, external resorptions can be caused by precipitation of oxalate crystals in the hard tissues of patients as a result of increased concentration of oxalates in the blood due to kidney failure (Moskow 1989).

Andreasen (1981) has proposed a classification of those external root resorptions that have a known mechanism:

- Surface resorption
- Replacement resorption associated with ankylosis
- Inflammatory resorption associated with inflammation in the periradicular tissues adjacent to the resorption site.

Subforms are:
- Peripheral inflammatory root resorption (PIRR)
- External inflammatory root resorption (EIRR)

Surface resorption

This type of resorption is common, self-limiting and reversible (Harding 1878). In a microscopic study of human teeth in individuals varying in age from 16 to 58, only 10% of the teeth showed neither active resorption nor signs of healed resorption (Henry & Weinman 1951). Resorptions were noted twice as often in older than in young subjects. Other studies have demonstrated up to 88% of teeth with active or, in most instances, healed resorptions (Hötz 1967). Reports on surface resorptions are sparse as most are self-limiting and spontaneously repaired upon injury.

A surface resorption is initiated subsequent to injury of the cementoblastic cell layer. Osteoclasts are attracted by substances from the damaged tissue on the denuded root surface and resorb the hard tissue for as long as activating factors are released at the site of injury, usually for a few days (Hammarström & Lindskog 1992). The resorptive process stops following the disappearance of the osteoclasts and the defect will become populated with hard tissue repairing cells leading to cementum repair (Lindskog et al. 1983a,b, 1987).

These resorptions may be caused by a localized injury in conjunction with external trauma (Andreasen 1981) and by trauma from occlusion. Resorption may also result from excessive orthodontic forces. The mechanism of the latter kind of resorption is thought to be a function of the hyaline zone that is formed subsequent to the orthodontic compression of the periodontal ligament. Along with the resorption of the hyaline layer, clast cells will resorb the root surface for as long as the orthodontic force is in place. Major loss of dental hard tissue giving root foreshortening may occur from this kind of iatrogenic injury.

Conclusion

The large majority of teeth show signs of active or healed surface resorptions or both. It is conceivable that minor traumata caused by unintentional biting on hard objects, bruxism, high fillings, etc., cause localized damage to the periodontal ligament and trigger the initiation of this type of resorption. The process is self-limiting and self-healing – no active treatment is required. During orthodontic treatment caution should be exercised in monitoring the forces to minimize the risk of foreshortening of roots.

Replacement resorption

This type of resorptive process results in a replacement of the dental hard tissues by bone, hence the name (Andreasen 1981). When a surface resorption stops, cells from the periodontal ligament will proliferate and populate the resorbed area (Lindskog et al. 1983a,b, 1987). If the resorption is large it will take some time for the PDL cells to cover the entire surface. Cells from the nearby bone tissue may then arrive first and establish themselves on the resorbed surface (An-

dreasen & Kristersson 1981, Gottlow et al. 1986). Bone is thus being formed directly upon the dental hard tissue. This results in a fusion between bone and tooth which is known as ankylosis.

Replacement resorption and ankylosis are often used as synonyms. While replacement resorption describes the active process during which the tooth is resorbed and replaced by bony tissue, ankylosis is the Greek word for immobile. It describes the situation of a tooth lacking normal mobility due to the fusion between tooth and bone. This fusion can be permanent or transient and appears to depend on the size of the resorbed area. If the ankylotic area is small, the bone on the tooth surface can resorb and be replaced with reparative cementum (Andreasen & Skougaard 1972, Andreasen & Kristersson 1981, Andersson et al. 1985, Hammarström et al. 1986). If the ankylotic area is large, a sufficient amount of bone will be formed on the root surface to make the fusion between bone and tooth permanent (Andreasen 1981, Andreasen & Kristersson 1981, Hammarström et al. 1986). It has been shown that long-term rigid splinting following external trauma results in a higher incidence of dentoalveolar ankylosis than with a short-term, less rigid fixation. The latter allows for some movement during the splinting period and probably prevents ankylosis (Andreasen 1975).

Clinically, ankylosis is diagnosed by absent tooth mobility and by a percussion tone that is higher than in a normal tooth (Andreasen 1975, Andersson et al. 1985). Radiographically, a local disappearance of the periodontal ligament contour may show an initial stage of fusion. However, even in non-ankylosed teeth it is not always possible to observe the entire contour of the periodontal ligament. Percussion and tooth mobility testing appear therefore more sensitive diagnostic tools than radiography in the early stages of replacement resorption (Andersson et al. 1985). When dentoalveolar ankylosis occurs at a young age, the tooth will not erupt but will follow the growth pattern of the bone resulting in so-called infra-occlusion (Andreasen & Hjörting-Hansen 1966, Kürol 1984, Malmgren et al. 1984).

The formation of bone on a dentin surface is not necessarily a pathological process, but one to be regarded as a form of repair. The bone has accepted the dental hard tissue as a part of itself and the tooth becomes involved in the normal skeletal turnover (Löe & Waerhaug 1961, Hammarström et al 1986). The turnover phase is fast in the growing child, but slower in the adult individual. Hence, the rate of bone replacement follows this pattern. However, the detailed mechanism of the resorptive process is not clearly understood.

Conclusion

Ankylosis is a prerequisite for replacement resorption. It may be seen as a form for repair of root surface

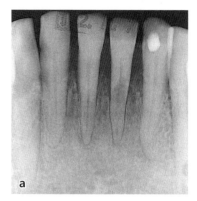

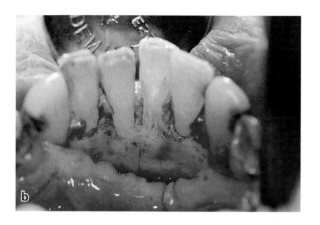

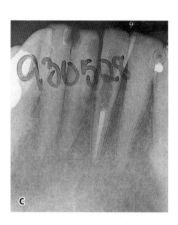

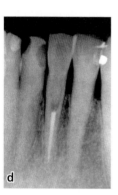

Fig. 14-24. Radiograph from a 78-year-old lady who presented herself to the clinic after an episode of severe pain and with a lingual periodontal abscess (a). The medical history was unremarkable. Radiograph revealed external root resorption on the lingual aspect of both the central incisors (a). The patient was initially managed by antibiotic treatment. Upon flap elevation and accessing the resorbing area and removing the granulation tissue an exposure to a necrotic pulp of tooth #31 was noted (b). Endodontic treatment was carried out during the surgery procedure (c). Tooth #41 was left without any further treatment and the case was followed clinically and radiographically. No recurrence of resorption did occur on either tooth and the patient has remained comfortable. Radiograph at the last follow-up 8 years after treatment (d). Note that there is no obvious progression of the resorptive process associated with tooth #41.

resorptions, which from a clinical standpoint is not desirable. No treatment for this condition is available.

External inflammatory resorption

The term external inflammatory resorption suggests the presence of an inflammatory lesion in the periodontal tissues adjacent to a resorptive process (Andreasen 1985). There are two main forms – peripheral inflammatory root resorption (PIRR) and external inflammatory root resorption (EIRR). Both forms are triggered by a destruction of the cementoblasts and the cementoid. In PIRR the factors activating osteoclasts are thought to be provided by an inflammatory lesion in the adjacent periodontal tissues (Andreasen 1985, Gold & Hasselgren 1992). EIRR, on the other

hand, receives its stimulus from an infected necrotic pulp (Andreasen 1985, Andreasen & Andreasen 1992).

Peripheral inflammatory root resorption (PIRR)

The outstanding feature of this type of resorption is its cervical location and invasive nature (Heithersay 1999a). It has therefore been termed invasive cervical root resorption. However, in the adult, the periodontal tissue may have receded apical to the cervical area. Therefore, other names have been used for this lesion such as subosseous resorption (Antrim et al. 1982) and (the complete opposite) supraosseous extra-canal invasive resorption (Frank & Bakland 1987). The different names reflect the confusion that has surrounded this type of resorptive lesion. Since the resorptive process extends into the dentin peripherally towards the pulp, and the clast activating factors seem to emanate from a periodontal inflammatory lesion, a name which reflects the etiology of this phenomenon, peripheral inflammatory root resorption (PIRR), was proposed (Gold & Hasselgren 1992).

The clinical features of PIRR include granulation tissue formation that bleeds freely on probing. Occasionally, a periodontal abscess may develop due to marginal infection, which may mimic a periodontal or endodontic condition (Fig. 14-23). When the lesion is located more apically or proximally, probing is usually difficult. Radiographically the lesion may only be seen after a certain size has been reached (Fig 14-22). Sometimes the appearance is mottled due to formation of hard tissue within the resorptive defect (Seward 1963). The outline of the root canal can often be seen within the radiolucent area (Fig. 14-22c). The presence of a profuse bleeding upon probing and granulation tissue in combination with a hard cavity bottom confirm the diagnosis. Electric pulp test and cold tests are usually positive, but will not distinguish this condition from caries or internal resorption, which are the two major differential diagnostic options (Frank & Bakland 1987).

The mechanism for this form of resorption is far from completely understood. Predisposing factors seem to be orthodontic treatment, trauma and intracoronal bleaching, while periodontal therapy took a low incidence among 222 examined cases (Heithersay 1999b). The reason for the low incidence following periodontal treatment could be that even upon excessive scaling and root planing, the damaged area of the root surface usually becomes covered by junctional epithelium. Yet, it appears that in the presence of a periodontal inflammatory lesion the onset of a resorptive process is triggered and that its continuance has an infectious cause (Brosjö et al. 1990, Gold & Hasselgren 1992).

Unmineralized, newly formed tissue in cementum (Gottlieb 1942), in osteoid (Chambers et al. 1985), and in predentin (Stenvik & Mjör 1970) has been observed to be resistant to resorption. This seems to explain the pattern of progression this form of resorption normally takes as it avoids invasion of the pulp and expands laterally instead. Yet, this peripheral extension can markedly undermine the tooth structure (Fig. 14-23). If there is a non-vital pulp and thus no resorption inhibition in the form of odontoblast supported predentin, PIRR will go straight to the pulpal space (Fig. 14-24). In root-filled teeth, which have been subjected to intracoronal bleaching, tissue toxic bleaching agents such as hydrogen peroxide have been found to be capable of penetrating through dentin and cementum (Fuss et al. 1989). If this occurs under clinical conditions, damage will be inflicted upon the periodontal ligament cells and cause resorption (Harrington & Natkin 1979, Montgomery 1984). Subsequently, bacteria may colonize the chemically emptied dentinal tubules and maintain inflammation and the resorptive process (Cvek & Lindvall 1985).

The most common form of treatment for PIRR is surgical exposure of the area, including removal of the granulation tissue. A base material is subsequently placed followed by a permanent filling and suturing of the flap. Other treatment forms include repositioning of the flap apical to the filling or orthodontic extrusion of the tooth (Gold & Hasselgren 1992). Recently, it has been suggested that guided tissue regeneration can be used, after surgical removal of the granulation tissue, to promote ingrowth of periodontal ligament cells into the resorbed area (Rankow & Krasner 1996). This kind of resorption may also be approached from within the tooth structure. Usually pulpectomy is required. To aid in removal of the resorbing tissue the use of 90% aqueous solution of trichloracetic acid has been proposed (Heithersay 1999c).

External inflammatory root resorption (EIRR)

This type of resorption is usually a complication that follows a dental trauma. It begins as a surface resorption due to damage of the periodontal ligament and the root surface in conjunction with the traumatic injury. The stimulus for EIRR is infectious products released into the adjacent tissues by way of the dentinal tubules exposed by the resorption (Bergenholtz 1974, Andreasen 1985, Andreasen & Andreasen 1992). The bacterial components will then maintain an inflammatory process in the adjacent periodontal tissues that in turn will trigger the continuance of the resorption. The osteoclastic resorption, basically aimed at eliminating the irritants, will thus move in the direction of the infected pulp tissue. As dentin is being further resorbed, more infectious and inflammatory byproducts are released into the surrounding area, thus perpetuating the inflammatory reaction and the resorptive process (Andreasen 1985).

The earliest stages are usually hard to detect as the resorptive cavity needs to reach a certain size to become radiographically visible. The first radiographic signs of resorption following trauma cannot usually be seen for several weeks (Andreasen et al. 1987). Treatment will be directed towards the cause of the resorption, that is, the root canal infection (Cvek 1993). In this context the use of calcium hydroxide has been advocated (Cvek 1993) as it is a useful antibacterial intracanal medicament (Byström et al. 1985). Calcium hydroxide also aids the cleaning of the canal by its soft tissue dissolving capability (Hasselgren et al. 1987), thus eliminating sources for bacterial nutrition. However, the positive effect of any medicament appears to be secondary to the elimination of root canal infection. Hence, clinical follow-ups suggest no difference in outcome between teeth treated long-term with calcium hydroxide and teeth subjected to instrumentation and filling with gutta-percha (Cvek 1973).

Conclusion

Peripheral inflammatory root resorption (PIRR) and external inflammatory root resorption (EIRR) are two

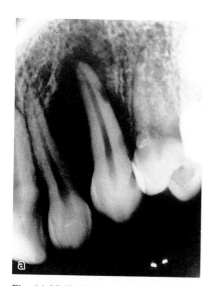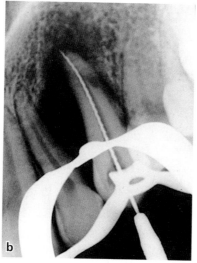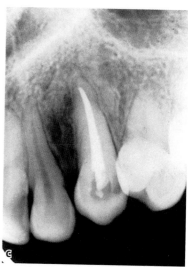

Fig. 14-25. Radiographs from a 27-year-old woman, showing the left maxillary canine which had been autotransplanted into a surgically prepared socket 2 months earlier. External inflammatory root resorption (EIRR) is visible on the distal aspect of the root (a). Endodontic treatment was initiated (b) and following the preparation of the canal, calcium hydroxide was placed as a long-term dressing. Radiograph following root filling (c) shows that the external resorption cavity is more rounded and a periodontal contour can be seen between the root and bone which has grown into the prepared socket.

forms of progressing external root resorption associated with inflammation in the periodontal tissues. The mechanism of EIRR is thought to be the release of bacterial elements from an infected pulp devitalized in conjunction with trauma. By focusing the treatment on the endodontic infection the resorption can usually be stopped as this takes away the reason for the continuance of the resorption (Fig. 14-25). In the subsequent healing phase there is risk of ankylosis. The greater the resorbed area, the greater is the risk for this complication (Andreasen & Kristersson 1981, Gottlow et al. 1986).

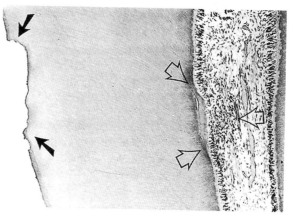

Fig. 14-26. Histologic section of a monkey tooth exposed to experimental periodontal tissue breakdown. Beneath resorptive defects in the external root surface a slight infiltrate of inflammatory cells and a small rim of reparative dentin are observed in the pulp. From Bergenholtz & Lindhe (1978).

INFLUENCE OF PERIODONTAL DISEASE ON THE CONDITION OF THE PULP

The formation of bacterial plaque on detached root surfaces following periodontal disease has the potential to induce pathologic changes in the pulp along the very same pathways as an endodontic infection can affect the periodontium in the opposite direction. Thus, bacterial products and substances released by the inflammatory process in the periodontium may gain access to the pulp via exposed lateral canals and apical foramina, as well as dentinal tubules.

A clearcut relationship between progressive periodontal disease and pulpal involvement, however, does not invariably exist. In fact, while inflammatory alterations as well as localized necrosis of pulp tissue have been observed adjacent to lateral canals in teeth exposed by periodontal disease (Seltzer et al. 1963a, Rubach & Mitchell 1965), a number of clinical studies

have failed to confirm a direct correlation between periodontal disease and pulp tissue changes (Mazur & Massler 1964, Czarnecki & Schilder 1979, Torabinejad & Kiger 1985). In a study in monkeys, Bergenholtz & Lindhe (1978) observed the nature and frequency of tissue changes in the pulp of teeth following an experimentally induced breakdown of the attachment apparatus. They found that the majority of the root specimens examined (70%) exhibited no pathologic pulp tissue changes, despite the fact that approximately 30-40% of the periodontal attachment was lost. The remaining roots (30%) displayed only small inflammatory cell infiltrates and/or formations of reparative dentin in areas of the pulp subjacent to root areas exposed through the periodontal tissue destruction.

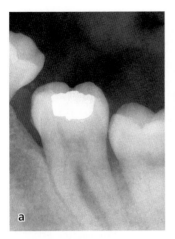
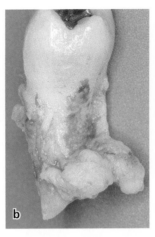
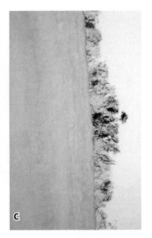
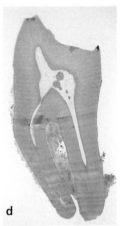

Fig. 14-27. Case of a lower second molar with severe periodontal tissue breakdown and furcation involvement (a) that was extracted and subjected to histologic examination. Upon extraction substantial amounts of calculus is seen on the distal root surface (b). While there was bacterial accumulation on the cementum layer (c), the pulp tissue has remained functional and without inflammatory involvement (d). Courtesy of Dr Domenico Ricucci.

These tissue changes were frequently associated with root surface resorption (Fig. 14-26), suggesting that dentinal tubules have to be uncovered before irritation can be transmitted. This observation further suggests that the presence of an intact cementum layer is important for the protection of the pulp from injurious elements produced by the plaque microbiota (Fig. 14-27). Consequently, the lack of correlation found in clinical observations between periodontal disease and pulp tissue alterations may simply depend on the fact that few open pathways exist in many periodontally involved teeth. Furthermore, once the dentin/pulp complex has been exposed to a bacterial challenge, repair and healing will often be instituted, leaving the remaining tissue relatively unaffected (Warfvinge & Bergenholtz 1986, Bergenholtz 2000).

In the study by Bergenholtz & Lindhe (1978), destructive periodontal disease was produced experimentally during a comparatively short period (5-7 months), while in humans a similar degree of destruction of periodontal tissue normally requires several years. It has been reported that the pulp of teeth with long-standing periodontal disease develops fibrosis and various forms of mineralizations (Fig. 14-1; Bender & Seltzer 1972, Lantelme et al. 1976). The number of blood vessels and nerve fibers can also be reduced. It seems reasonable that tissue changes of this nature represent the accumulated response of the pulp to the relatively weak, but repeatedly occurring, insults of the tissue via exposed dentinal tubules and lateral canals.

Conclusion

It seems that periodontal disease rarely jeopardizes the vital functions of the pulp. In teeth with moderate breakdown of the attachment apparatus, the pulp usually remains in proper function. Breakdown of the pulp presumably does not occur until the periodontal disease process has reached a terminal state, i.e. when bacterial plaque involves the main apical foramina

(Langeland et al. 1974). Apparently, as long as the blood supply through the apical foramen remains intact, the pulp is capable of withstanding injurious elements released by the lesion in the periodontium.

INFLUENCE OF PERIODONTAL TREATMENT MEASURES ON THE PULP

Scaling and root planing

Scaling and root planing are indispensable procedures in the treatment of periodontal disease. However, not only will bacterial deposits be removed from the root surface but so also may cementum and superficial parts of dentin. Therefore, by this instrumentation, dentinal tubules will be exposed and normally left unprotected to the oral environment. Subsequent microbial colonization of the exposed root dentin may result in bacterial invasion of the dentinal tubules (Adriaens et al. 1988). As a consequence, inflammatory lesions may develop in the pulp (Bergenholtz & Lindhe 1978). Yet, the vitality of the pulp is not normally put at risk (Bergenholtz & Lindhe 1978, Nilvéus & Selvig 1983, Hattler & Listgarten 1984), even though root dentin hypersensitivity frequently develops following such measures, presenting an uncomfortable and difficult problem to manage (see below).

During the maintenance phase of periodontal therapy, scaling and planing of roots are frequently repeated procedures. At each recall session, the root surfaces are debrided and some dentin is removed. This therapy can result not only in weakening of the tooth structure but also in extensive reparative dentin formation in the pulp (Fig. 14-28). Whether such repair processes impair pulp functions on a long-term basis is not well studied. In a patient material subjected to

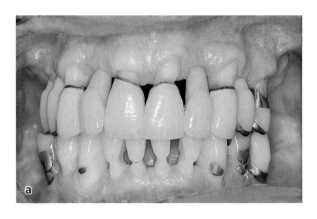

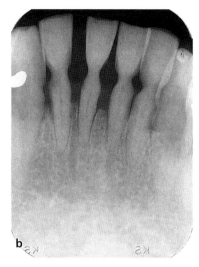

Fig. 14-28. Clinical photograph of a patient, who has been in the maintenance phase after treatment for periodontal disease (a). While there are excellent gingival conditions and no pocket probing depths, there is substantial loss of cervical root dentin. One of the lower incisors later fractured off, but without a pulpal exposure due to accumulation reparative dentin in the coronal portion of the pulp chamber (b). Courtesy of Dr Sture Nyman.

maintenance therapy for over 4-13 years, pulp tissue necrosis was a rare finding (3%), and, when occurring, it was attributed to caries and progression of periodontal disease rather than to the periodontal treatment *per se* (Bergenholtz & Nyman 1984). On rare occasions deep periodontal scaling may expose lateral canals that in turn can induce severe painful symptoms of pulpitis.

Conclusion
Results of clinical observations and animal experiments support the view that scaling and root planing procedures normally do not threaten the vitality of the pulp. Adjacent to instrumented root surfaces localized inflammatory alterations may on occasion emerge, but in most instances these will be followed by repair processes. (Figs. 14-1, 14-28b).

Root dentin hypersensitivity

Patients subjected to scaling and root planing in periodontal therapy may after the instrumentation procedure experience increased sensitivity of the treated teeth to evaporative, tactile, thermal and osmotic stimuli (Fischer et al. 1991, Kontturi-Närhi 1993, Chabanski et al. 1996). Usually, the symptoms, when occurring, develop and peak during the first week to subside or disappear within the subsequent weeks and are, although uncomfortable, most often a temporary and sustainable complication. However, occasionally the condition may become a chronic pain problem and may persist for months or years. Patients appear to be especially at risk after periodontal surgery. In a comprehensive questionnaire survey, severe painful symptoms were reported to prevail in 26% of the subjects 6 months to 5 years after the completion of treatment, while 16% treated non-surgically had pain symptoms (Kontturi-Närhi 1993). In a clinical trial

comprising 35 patients, Tammaro et al (2000) observed that, while a majority of patients subjected to non-surgical periodontal instrumentation developed sensitive teeth, only a few teeth in a small number of the patients developed highly sensitive root surfaces.

The main initial symptom is sharp pain of rapid onset that disappears once the stimulus is removed. In more severe, long-standing cases, shorter or longer periods of lingering, dull or aching pain symptoms may be provoked. Even a minimal contact of a toothbrush with the root dentin surface may result in intense pain – a condition not only uncomfortable but one likely to hinder proper oral hygiene measures.

The pain condition is termed dentin hypersensitivity (Holland et al. 1997). But the ailment has also been given many other names such as sensitive dentin, cervical dentinal sensitivity and root sensitivity, which reflect the confusion that still exists regarding its etiologic background (Orchardson et al. 1994). The fact that root surfaces become sensitive to a variety of externally derived stimuli after periodontal instrumentation is not surprising as dentinal tubules become uncovered to the oral environment and subject to hydrodynamic forces. Hence, a variety of pain-evoking stimuli including evaporative, tactile, thermal and osmotic stimuli may elicit sudden fluid shifts in the exposed tubules thereby inducing a painful sensation according to the hydrodynamic theory of dentin sensitivity (Brännström 1966, Pashley 1996). This mechanism alone can certainly explain the sensitivity patients experience immediately after the instrumentation procedure and during a short period afterwards, while it does not make clear why the symptoms increase over time and why the pain condition may prevail in certain patients and in certain teeth.

The increase in pain intensity may have one or both of the following two explanations. Firstly, the smear layer formed on the root surface by the scaling proce-

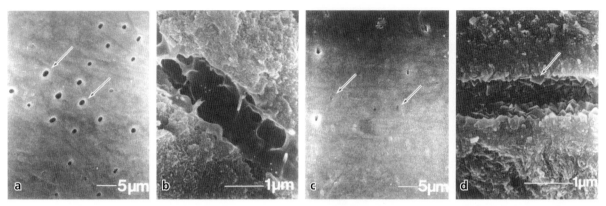

Fig. 14-29. Scanning electron microscopic images of specimens of hypersensitive (a, b) and non-sensitive root dentin areas of human teeth (c, d). In (a) there are numerous wide tubular apertures. These tubules show no evidence of hard tissue depositions after being fractured open (b). Most tubules are occluded (c) and below the surface rhombohedral crystals of from 0.1-0.3 μm are present (d). The images are kindly provided by Dr Masahiro Yoshiyama and published with permission of the *Journal of Dental Research*.

dure will be dissolved within a few days (Kerns et al. 1991). This in turn will increase the hydraulic conductance of the involved dentinal tubules (Pashley 1996) and thus decrease the peripheral resistance to fluid flow across dentin. Thereby pain sensations are more readily evoked. Secondly, open dentinal tubules serve as pathways for diffusive transport of bacterial elements in the oral cavity to the pulp, which is likely to cause a localized inflammatory pulpal response (Bergenholtz & Lindhe 1975, 1978). Indeed, experiments in dogs have shown that pulpal inflammation greatly enhances the sensitivity of responding nerve fibers (Närhi et al. 1994). A large number of intradental A-delta fibers, normally inactive, are now able to respond upon stimulation (Närhi et al. 1996). It has furthermore been shown that the receptive field of individual fibers gets wider (Närhi et al. 1996). In addition, shallow oral exposures of root dentin in the rat are accompanied by sprouting of new terminal branches from pulpal axons in areas subjacent to the root surface injury (Taylor et al. 1988). Sprouting of nerves is a temporary event and will subside if inflammation disappears – a feature consistent with their involvement in root dentin hypersensitivity (Byers & Närhi 1999). In other words, an essential component of the increasing root sensitivity that patients experience after an instrumentation procedure in periodontal therapy is likely to be related to a peripheral sensitization of pulpal nociceptors due to release of inflammatory mediators.

The fact that root dentin hypersensitivity often disappears a few weeks after the scaling procedure is best explained by the development of a natural occlusion of the exposed dentinal tubules by mineral deposits (Fig. 14-29; Yoshiyama et al. 1989, 1990). The hydrodynamic mechanism for dentinal pain will thereby be inactivated. Furthermore, the potential for an inward diffusion of bacterial elements to the pulp will be substantially reduced. The observations of few if any open tubules in non-sensitive radicular dentin (Hiatt & Johansen 1972, Absi et al. 1987, Yoshiyama et al.

1989, Cuenin et al. 1991, Oyama & Matsumoto 1991, Kontturi-Närhi 1993), while hypersensitive root areas show large numbers of tubular apertures on their surfaces (Absi et al. 1987, Yoshiyama et al. 1989, Cuenin et al. 1991, Oyama & Matsumoto 1991, Kontturi-Närhi 1993), support this view.

The fact that only certain individuals become seriously affected may be related to local factors in the oral cavity, as well as to the level of the subjects' pain perception. Certain dietary factors, in particular fruit juices, yoghurt and wines, have been implicated in the pathogenesis of dentin hypersensitivity (Addy et al. 1987). By their acidity and ability to etch dentin, natural occlusions of dentinal tubules by mineralizations may thus be dissolved or prevented from forming. It needs also to be recognized that pain is not only an expression of injury and noxious stimuli, but also a psychobiological phenomenon having both a physiological and psychological basis for its perception and reaction to it. Indeed, a variety of emotional elements may influence the subjective interpretation of pain (Eli 1992), and anxiety, fear and depression are factors that are known to affect pain perception and the subject's ability to identify coping methods (McGrath 1994).

A further factor that is potentially involved in the symptomatology associated with root dentin hypersensitivity is the enhancement of the responsiveness of the central nervous system. Indeed it has been shown that neuroplastic changes in the central nociceptive pathways, including expanded receptive fields and heightened excitability, may occur following peripheral injury and inflammation (see review by Sessle 2000). Such changes may be maintained even if peripheral sensitization phenomena are bypassed and seem to become more prominent in long-lasting pain conditions (Sessle 2000).

In cases of severe root dentin hypersensitivity, active treatment is urgent. However, the methods presently available provide an unpredictable remedy and only temporary relief is at best attained (Orchardson et al. 1994, Ikola 2001). Since tubular patency seems to play a crucial role in the pathogenesis of root dentin hypersensitivity, most procedures hitherto attempted are logically aimed to induce a block of their peripheral ends by an astringent or coagulating effect. Examples of agents commonly employed for both self-applied and dentist-applied treatments are strontium chloride, sodium monofluorophosphate, sodium fluoride, calcium hypophosphate, calcium hydroxide, potassium nitrate, potassium oxalates, glutaraldehyde, stannous fluoride, cavity varnishes, and dentin-bonding agents (for reviews see Gangarosa 1994, Zappa 1994, Ikola 2001). Why these methods fail to provide an effective clinical treatment result may have several explanations. One is likely to be technical in nature in that it is often difficult to attain a completely dry dentin surface during the application procedure due to continuous release of gingival fluid from the sulcus, which is not easily restrained by compressed air or other methods. Consequently, upon application of an astringent agent, protein from this exudate might primarily be brought to coagulation rather than the tubular content. The precipitate is then easily removed upon subsequent tooth cleaning measures. Most agents furthermore may only cause a superficial block that may be dissolved over the course of time. Also topical applications do not address the pain mechanisms associated with either peripheral or central sensitization of nociceptors. Agents able to decrease the excitability of intradental nerves have therefore been proposed based on the assumption that potassium ions released from formulations containing potassium salts (e.g. chlorides, nitrates, citrate and oxalates) diffuse along the dentinal tubules to inactivate intradental nerve activity (Markowitz & Kim 1992, Orchardson & Peacock 1994). Recent experiments employing electrophysiological recordings in dogs, however, have shown that the effect of topical application is weak and becomes abolished after irrigation (Ikola 2001). A review of clinical trials employing potassium-containing preparations in gels, mouthwashes and toothpastes revealed inconsistent results (Orchardson & Gillam 2000). While several early studies reported significant reductions in sensitivity to tactile and air stimuli, properly controlled studies have shown that a significant placebo effect operates (Orchardson & Gillam 2000), which also applies to clinical trials employing agents aimed to block the dentinal tubules (Yates et al. 1998).

Any treatment approach to root dentin hypersensitivity should be preceded by a careful analysis of conditions that may be the cause of, or contribute to, the symptoms. Cracked teeth including cusp fractures, fractured or leaky restorations, caries, as well as a variety of other exposures of dentin to the oral environment, may cause pain sensations to the same stimuli which cause root dentin hypersensitivity. An area of exposed dentin may be more sensitive if there is irritation of the pulp from other areas of the tooth, for example from a leaky restoration (Närhi et al. 1994) and enhanced treatment effect on root dentin hypersensitivity has actually been obtained if restorations were replaced concomitantly (Hovgaard et al. 1991). Particular care should be taken to eliminate traumatic occlusion. Furthermore, dietary advice should be given to patients who admit excessive consumption of citrus fruits, apples or any other food or drinks that are acidic by nature.

Plaque control is an important integral part of the prevention and treatment of root dentin hypersensitivity. It has been observed clinically that, with time, teeth in patients with excellent oral hygiene habits develop hard, smooth and insensitive root surfaces. Electron microscopic examination of the dentin of such root surfaces has revealed that mineral deposits obliterate the tubular openings (Hiatt & Johansen 1972). However, when severe symptoms of root hypersensitivity have emerged it is difficult to motivate the patient to maintain the degree of plaque control that is necessary to allow for a natural occlusion of the dentinal tubules. In such situations an agent may be beneficial which has a reasonable capacity to block the tubular openings, at least temporarily, so that proper oral hygiene measures can be reinforced. In severe cases, where no remedy is achieved with any advice or treatment approach, pulpectomy and root filling may be the last resort.

Conclusion

Root dentin hypersentivity frequently develops as an uncomfortable and sometimes difficult ailment to treat, subsequent to scaling and root planing procedures in periodontal therapy. Although the exact mechanism is not well established, the condition is clearly related to open dentinal tubules that allow hydrodynamic mechanisms to elicit painful sensations upon external stimuli. Treatment planning should consider contributory etiologic factors including overconsumption of acidic food items. Root dentin hypersensitivity should also be checked against other conditions that can cause similar symptoms, e.g. cracked teeth (Fig. 14-21). A large number of therapeutic techniques are available that seek to block the tubular openings. Most of these agents induce at least a temporary block so that proper oral hygiene measures can be reinforced for a natural occlusion of the dentinal tubules.

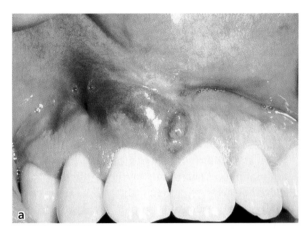
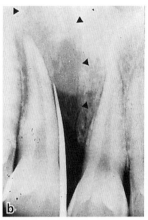
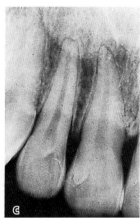

Fig. 14-30. Gingival swelling at the buccal aspect of tooth #11 (a). Radiographic appearance of the area. Note the advanced destruction of alveolar bone along the mesial aspect of the root (arrowheads) (b). Healing of the area 7 months following periodontal treatment (c). Courtesy of Dr Harald Rylander.

ENDODONTIC CONSIDERATIONS IN ROOT RESECTION OF MULTIROOTED TEETH IN PERIODONTAL THERAPY

Treatment of periodontally diseased, multirooted teeth may involve separation and extraction of one or two roots (see Chapter 29). As a rule, endodontic treatment of the root to be retained should be performed prior to surgery. Information will thus be gained regarding the effect of the endodontic treatment before alternative roots are extracted. This rule should be followed for teeth with both vital and nonvital pulps. The root canals of molars are sometimes difficult to prepare, in particular when the tooth has been exposed to longstanding periodontal disease. Such teeth may harbor mineralizations (pulp stones, dystrophic calcifications, reparative dentin formations) that make proper endodontic treatment precarious. In multirooted teeth with advanced periodontal destruction, it is not always possible to decide before surgery which root(s) can be preserved. As an alternate to permanent filling of all root canals in such teeth, pulpectomy may be performed and the canals may be temporarily filled with calcium hydroxide. Each of the canal orifices is then sealed with a temporary, bacteria tight cement. Root separation can thus be performed without bacterial contamination of the root canals. Permanent root filling of the root(s) retained is performed after surgery.

DIFFERENTIAL DIAGNOSTIC CONSIDERATIONS

It is clear from the previous text that during treatment of periodontal disease one is not infrequently presented with the dilemma of accurately assessing the contribution of an endodontic infection to deep peri-odontal pockets. In this chapter, several examples of lesions in the periodontium have been presented which are not associated with periodontal disease. Two cases are described below showing clinical and radiographic symptoms similar to those of an acute endodontic condition. The cases demonstrate that diagnostic entities such as location, form and extension of radiolucencies, clinical symptoms of pain or swelling, and increased probing depths are not always accurate diagnostic criteria for differentiating a periodontal lesion from an endodontic disorder.

The clinical photograph in Fig. 14-30 shows swelling of the marginal gingiva on the buccal aspect of tooth #11. The swelling had for a few days been preceded by severe throbbing pain. Radiographic examination (Fig. 14-30a) disclosed the presence of an angular bony defect that involved the apical portions of the tooth. In this case the pulp demonstrated vital signs upon testing, indicating that the pathologic condition was not of endodontic origin. Pocket debridement was combined with irrigation with 0.2% chlorhexidine digluconate solution and systemic administration of an antibiotic. The lesion healed rapidly. Seven months after treatment new bone had formed around the apex and along the mesial root surface (Fig. 14-30c). This case demonstrates that the periodontal destruction observed was caused by periodontal disease.

Fig. 14-31 illustrates another case of differential diagnostic interest. A radiograph taken of the front tooth region of the mandible demonstrates bone loss associated with the apex of tooth #31 in addition to a generalized horizontal loss of alveolar bone (Fig. 14-31a). The form and extension of the apical radiolucency around tooth #31 are similar to those resulting from an endodontic lesion. Clinically, a deep periodontal pocket could be probed along the distobuccal root surface. The patient had been on a recall program after treatment for periodontal disease and had previously shown excellent gingival conditions. Sensibility tests indicated that the pulp was vital. Therefore, endodontic treatment was not performed. Following

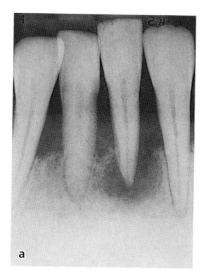
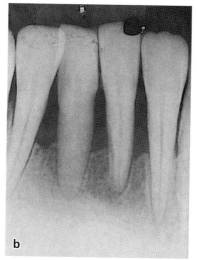
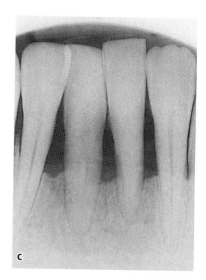
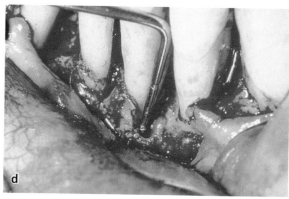

Fig. 14-31. Advanced destructions of alveolar bone including an angular bone defect simulating an endodontic periapical lesion around tooth #31 (a). The pulp responded vital on testing and the tooth was therefore not subjected to endodontic therapy but only to periodontal treatment. On raising a flap (d) the lesion was at the buccal aspect and obviously had not destroyed the neuro-vascular supply of the pulp as evidenced by the healing of the lesion in 6 months (b) and deposition of hard tissue in the pulp, which became obvious 2 years after therapy (c). Courtesy of Dr Ingvar Magnusson.

elevation of a mucoperiosteal flap, an angular bone defect was found at the buccal aspect of the root but without involving the root tip. The wound area was debrided along with scaling of the root surface. Rapid bone fill followed after surgery (Fig. 14-31b) and the pulp maintained its vitality, although later the root canal became obliterated by hard tissue repair, most likely as a consequence of the surgical procedure (Fig 14-31c). The mechanism behind the apically positioned radiolucency in Fig 14-31a is explained by superimposition of the buccal loss of alveolar bone on the root tip of tooth #31, which went beyond its most apical level (Fig. 14-32).

These two cases demonstrate that neither clinical symptoms nor radiographic findings invariably lead to a correct diagnosis. The only significant observation for the differential diagnosis was pulp vitality. Pulp vitality means that the pulp chamber is occupied by connective tissue supplied by nerves and blood vessels. Sensory nerve function is normally present. Vital pulp tissue may or may not be subjected to inflammatory and degenerative tissue changes. In most situations its vitality must be determined by indirect

means and such measures are based on the assumption that a vital pulp is able to respond to sensory stimuli such as mechanical, thermal and electric stimulation. This means that the *sensibility* of the pulp is tested rather than the *vitality* of the tissue. There is ample documentation to support the concept that a tooth which responds to sensory stimuli has vital functions. Conversely, if a tooth does not respond to sensory stimuli, the pulp may be non-vital. It must be recognized that both false positive and false negative readings occur (Seltzer et al. 1963b, Mumford 1964, Peters et al. 1994). Therefore, a combination of different test methods should always be used to ensure a correct diagnosis. Pulpal sensibility can be examined by thermal stimulation with the use of ethyl chloride, carbon dioxide snow, ice, or heated gutta-percha sticks and by the use of electric stimulation with a pulp tester.

Conclusion

It is important to remember that the recognition of pulp vitality is essential for a differential diagnosis and for the selection of primary measures for treat-

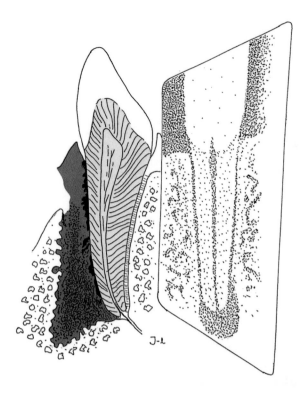

Fig. 14-32. The drawing attempts to picture a potential mechanism for the radiographic radiolucency in Fig 14-31a. Due to the periodontal infection a substantial amount of the supporting tissue was broken down. Yet the neuro-vascular supply of the pulp was not engaged. The appearance of an apical lesion is explained by the superimposition of the alveolar bone destruction at the buccal aspect of the tooth. Courtesy of Dr Mats Joatell.

ment of inflammatory lesions in the marginal and apical periodontium. Deep restorations, dental trauma, endodontic treatment, previous pulp capping, etc., are factors to consider when assessing the need for endodontic treatment as a part of the overall periodontal therapy. Location, form and extension of radiolucencies, as well as clinical symptoms of pain, tenderness, abscess formation, increased probing depth, etc., may not always distinguish a periodontal lesion from an endodontic lesion.

Table 14-1. Treatment strategies

Cause	Condition of the pulp	Treatment
Endodontic	Non-vital	Endodontic
Periodontal	Vital	Periodontal
Endodontic/ periodontal	Non-vital	Endodontic – first observe the result of this therapy and institute periodontal therapy later if necessary

TREATMENT STRATEGIES FOR COMBINED ENDODONTIC AND PERIODONTAL LESIONS

Occasionally, endodontic and periodontal lesions may affect one and the same tooth. Lesions may be totally separated from each other and present no extraordinary therapeutic consideration. In a few other situations there is no obvious demarcation between the two lesions, which both radiographically and clinically appear as one lesion (see Figs. 14-5 and 14-12b,c). This type of combined lesion defect may be identified by probing along the root to the apical region of the tooth.

Treatment of combined endodontic and periodontal lesions does not differ from the treatment given when the two disorders occur separately. The part of the lesion sustained by the root canal infection can usually be expected to resolve after proper endodontic treatment (Figs. 14-5b, 14-12d-f). The part of the lesion caused by the plaque infection may also heal follow-

ing periodontal therapy, although little or no regeneration of the attachment apparatus can be expected (see Chapter 28). This suggests that the larger the part of the lesion caused by the root canal infection, the more favorable the prognosis is for regeneration of the attachment apparatus. It is important to realize that it is clinically not possible to determine the extent to which one or the other of the two disorders (endodontic or periodontal) has affected the supporting tissues. Therefore, the treatment strategy must be first to focus on the pulpal infection and to perform debridement and disinfection of the root canal system. The second phase includes a period of observation whereby the extent of periodontal healing resulting from the endodontic treatment is followed. Reduced probing depth can usually be expected within a couple of weeks while bone regeneration may require several months before it can be radiographically detected. Thus, periodontal therapy including deep scaling with and without periodontal surgery should be postponed until the result of the endodontic treatment can be properly evaluated (Figs. 14-5, 14-12).

Conclusion

It should be understood that periodontal disease may be responsible for the entire loss of the supporting apparatus around a tooth (see Fig. 14-30) and may in addition be the cause of the breakdown of the pulpal tissue. In such cases endodontic treatment will not contribute to periodontal healing and the problem will have to be solved by a periodontal treatment approach (Fig. 14-30). When there is doubt as to whether a lesion in the periodontium is of endodontic or periodontal origin, or both, the treatment strategy listed in Table 14-1 may be followed.

REFERENCES

Absi, E.G., Addy, M. & Adams, D. (1987). Dentine hypersensitivity. A study of the patency of dentinal tubules in sensitive and non-sensitive cervical dentin. *Journal of Clinical Periodontology* **14**, 280-284.

Addy, M., Absi, E.G. & Adams, D. (1987). Dentine hypersensitivity. The effects *in vitro* of acids and dietary substances on root-planed and burred dentine. *Journal of Periodontology* **14**, 274-279.

Adriaens, P.A., De Boever, J.A. & Loesche, W.J. (1988). Bacterial invasion in root cementum and radicular dentin of periodontally diseased teeth in humans. *Journal of Periodontology* **59**, 222-230.

Alhadainy, H.A. (1994). Root perforations. A review of literature. *Oral Surgery* **78**, 368-374.

Andersson, L., Blomlöf, L., Lindskog, S., Feiglin, B. & Hammarström, L. (1984). Tooth ankylosis. Clinical, radiographic and histological assessments. *International Journal of Oral Surgery* **13**, 423-431.

Andersson, L., Lindskog, S., Blomlöf, L., Hedström, K-G. & Hammarström, L. (1985). Effect of masticatory stimulation on dentoalveolar ankylosis after experimental tooth replantation. *Endodontics and Dental Traumatology* **1**, 13-16.

Andreasen, J.O. (1975). Periodontal healing after replantation of traumatically avulsed human teeth. Assessment by mobility testing and radiography. *Acta Odontologica Scandinavica* **33**, 325-335.

Andreasen, J. O. (1981). Relationship between surface and inflammatory resorption and changes in the pulp after replantation of permanent incisors in monkeys. *Journal of Endodontics* **7**, 294-301.

Andreasen, J.O. (1985). External root resorptions: its implication in dental traumatology, paedodontics, periodontics, orthodontics and endodontics. *International Journal of Endodontics* **8**, 109-118.

Andreasen, J.O. & Andreasen, F.M. (1992). Root resorption following traumatic dental injuries. *Proceedings of the Finnish Dental Society* **88**, Suppl. 1, 95-114.

Andreasen, J.O. & Hjörting-Hansen, E. (1966). Replantation of teeth. I. Radiographic and clinical study of human teeth replanted after accidental loss. *Acta Odontologica Scandinavica* **24**, 263-286.

Andreasen, J.O. & Kristerson, L. (1981). Evaluation of different types of autotransplanted connective tissues as potential periodontal ligament substitutes. *International Journal of Oral Surgery* **10**, 189-201.

Andreasen, F.M., Sewerin, I., Mandel, U. & Andreasen, J.O. (1987). Radiographic assessment of simulated root resorption cavities. *Endodontics and Dental Traumatology* **3**, 21-27.

Andreasen, J.O. & Skougaard, M. (1972). Reversibility of surgically induced dental ankylosis in rats. *International Journal of Oral Surgery* **1**, 98-102.

Antrim, D.D., Hicks, M.L. & Altaras, D.E. (1982). Treatment of subosseous resorption: a case report. *Journal of Endodontics* **8**, 567-569.

Arens, D.E. & Torabinejad, M. (1996). Repair of furcal perforations with mineral trioxide aggregate: two case reports. *Oral Surgery* **82**, 84-88.

Babal, P., Soler, P., Brozman, M., Jakubovsky, J., Beyly, M. & Basset, F. (1987). *In situ* characterization of cells in periapical granuloma by monoclonal antibodies. *Oral Surgery* **64**, 348-352.

Baumgartner, J.C. & Falkler, W.A. (1991). Bacteria in the apical 5 mm of infected root canals. *Journal of Endodontics* **17**, 380-383.

Beavers, R.A., Bergenholtz, G. & Cox, C.F. (1986). Periodontal wound healing following intentional root perforations in permanent teeth of *Macaca mulatta*. *International Journal of Endodontics* **19**, 36-44.

Bender, I.B. & Seltzer, S. (1972). The effect of periodontal disease on the pulp. *Oral Surgery* **33**, 458-474.

Bergenholtz, G. (1974). Micro-organisms from necrotic pulp of traumatized teeth. *Odontologisk Revy* **25**, 347-358.

Bergenholtz, G. (2000). Evidence for bacterial causation of adverse pulpal responses in resin-based dental restorations. *Critical Reviews in Oral Biology and Medicine* **11**, 467-480.

Bergenholtz, G., Lekholm, U., Liljenberg, B. & Lindhe, J. (1983). Morphometric analysis of chronic inflammatory periapical lesions in root filled teeth. *Oral Surgery* **55**, 295-301.

Bergenholtz, G. & Lindhe, J. (1975). Effect of soluble plaque factors on inflammatory reactions in the dental pulp. *Scandinavian Journal of Dental Research* **83**, 153-158.

Bergenholtz, G. & Lindhe J. (1978). Effect of experimentally induced marginal periodontitis and periodontal scaling on the dental pulp. *Journal of Clinical Periodontology* **5**, 59-73.

Bergenholtz, G. & Nyman, S. (1984). Endodontic complications following periodontal and prosthetic treatment of patients with advanced periodontal disease. *Journal of Periodontology* **55**, 63-68.

Bissada, N.F. (1994). Symptomatology and clinical features of hypersensitive teeth. *Archives of Oral Biology* **39**, Suppl., 31S-32S.

Brännström, M. (1966). Sensitivity of dentine. *Oral Surgery* **21**, 517-526.

Brosjö, M., Andersson, K., Berg, J.O. & Lindskog, S. (1990). An experimental model for cervical resorption in monkeys. *Endodontics and Dental Traumatology* **6**, 118-120.

Burch, J.G. & Hulen, S. (1974). A study of the presence of accessory foramina and the topography of molar furcations. *Oral Surgery* **38**, 451-455.

Byers, M.R. & Närhi, M.V.O. (1999). Dental injury models: Experimental tools for understanding neuroinflammatory interactions and polymodal nociceptor functions. *Critical Reviews in Oral Biology and Medicine* **10**, 4-39.

Byström, A., Claesson, R. & Sundqvist, G. (1985). The antibacterial effect of camphorated phenol, paramonochlorphenol, and calcium hydroxide in the treatment of infected root canals. *Endodontics and Dental Traumatology* **1**, 170-175.

Byström, A., Happonen, R-P., Sjögren, U. & Sundqvist, G. (1987). Healing of periapical lesions of pulpless teeth after endodontic treatment with controlled asepsis. *Endodontics and Dental Traumatology* **3**, 58-63.

Chabanski, M.B, Gillam, D.G. & Newman, H.N. (1996). Prevalence of cervical dentine sensitivity in a population of patients referred to a specialist Periodontology Department. *Journal of Clinical Periodontology* **23**, 989-992.

Chambers, T.J. (1981). Phagocytic recognition of bone by macrophages. *Journal of Pathology* **135**, 1-7.

Chambers, T.J. (1988). Resorption of bone. In: Davidovitch, Z., ed. *Biological mechanisms of tooth eruption and root resorption.* Birmingham, AL: Ebsco Media, pp. 93-100.

Chambers, T.J., Darby, J.A. & Fuller, K. (1985). Mammalian collagenase predisposes bone surface to osteoclastic resorption. *Cell Tissue Research* **241**, 671-675.

Chan, C.P., Lin, C.P., Tseng, S.C. & Jeng, J.H. (1999). Vertical root fracture in endodontically versus nonendodontically treated teeth: a survey of 315 cases in Chinese patients. *Oral Surgery* **87**, 504-507.

Cuenin, M.F., Scheidt, M.J., ONeal, R.B., Strong, S.L., Pashley, D.H., Horner, J.A. & Van Dyke, T.E. (1991). An *in vivo* study of dentin sensitivity: The relation of dentin sensitivity and the patency of dentin tubules. *Journal of Periodontology* **62**, 668-673.

Cvek, M. (1973). Treatment of non-vital permanent incisors with calcium hydroxide. II. Effect on external root resorption in luxated teeth compared with effect of root filling with guttapercha. *Odontologisk Revy* **25**, 343-354.

Cvek, M. (1993) Endodontic management of traumatized teeth. In: Andreasen, J.O., & Andreasen, F.M., ed. *Textbook and color atlas of traumatic injuries to the teeth.* Copenhagen: Munksgaard.

Cvek, M. & Lindvall, A.M. (1985). External root resorption following bleaching of pulpless teeth with hydrogen peroxide. *Endodontics and Dental Traumatology* **1**, 56-60.

Czarnecki, R.T. & Schilder, H. (1979). A histological evaluation of the human pulp in teeth with varying degrees of periodontal disease. *Journal of Endodontics* **5**, 242-253.

Dahle, U.R., Tronstad, L. & Olsen, I. (1996). Characterization of new periodontal and endodontic isolates of spirochetes. *European Journal of Oral Sciences* **104**, 41-47.

DeDeus, Q.D. (1975). Frequency, location, and direction of the lateral secondary and accessory canals. *Journal of Endodontics* **1**, 361-366.

Ehnevid, H., Jansson, L.E., Lindskog, S.F. & Blomlöf, L.B. (1993a). Periodontal healing in relation to radiographic attachment and endodontic infection. *Journal of Periodontology* **64**, 1199-1204.

Ehnevid, H., Jansson, L., Lindskog, S. & Blomlöf, L. (1993b). Periodontal healing in teeth with periapical lesions. A clinical retrospective study. *Journal of Clinical Periodontology* **20**, 254-258.

Eli, I. (1992). Oral psychophysiology. Stress, pain, and behavior in dental care. Boca Raton: CRC Press, pp. 41-58.

Fabricius, L., Dahlén, G., Holm, S.E. & Möller, Å.J.R. (1982). Influence of combinations of oral bacteria on periapical tissues of monkeys. *Scandinavian Journal of Dental Research* **90**, 200-206.

Fischer, C., Wennberg, A., Fischer, R.G. & Attström, R. (1991). Clinical evaluation of pulp and dentine sensitivity after supragingival and subgingival scaling. *Endodontics and Dental Traumatology* **7**, 259-263.

Frank, A.L. & Bakland, L.K. (1987). Nonendodontic therapy for

supraosseous extracanal invasive resorption. *Journal of Endodontics* **13**, 348-355.

Fuss, Z., Szjakis, S. & Tagger, M. (1989). Tubular permeability to calcium hydroxide and to bleaching agents. *Journal of Endodontics* **15**, 3362-3364.

Gangarosa Sr, L.P. (1994). Current strategies of dentist-applied treatment in the management of hypersensitive dentine. *Archives of Oral Biology* **39**, Suppl., 101S-106S.

Gold, S. & Hasselgren, G. (1992). Peripheral inflammatory root resorption; a review of the literature with some case reports. *Journal of Clinical Periodontology* **19**, 523-534.

Gottlieb, B. (1942). Biology of the cementum. *Journal of Periodontology* **13**, 13-17.

Gottlow, J., Nyman, S., Lindhe, J., Karring T. & Wennström, J. (1986). New attachment formation in the human periodontium by guided tissue regeneration: Case reports. *Journal of Clinical Periodontology* **13**, 604-616.

Gutmann, J.L. (1978). Prevalence, location and patency of accessory canals in the furcation region of permanent molars. *Journal of Periodontology* **49**, 21-26.

Haapasalo, M., Ranta, K. & Ranta, H. (1987). Mixed anaerobic periapical infection with sinus tract. *Endodontics and Dental Traumatology* **3**, 83-85.

Hammarström, L.E. & Lindskog, S. (1992). Factors regulating and modifying dental root resorption. *Proceedings of the Finnish Dental Society* **88**, Suppl. 1, 115-123.

Hammarström, L.E., Pierce, A., Blomlöf, L., Feiglin, B. & Lindskog, S. (1986). Tooth avulsion and replantation - a review. *Endodontics and Dental Traumatology* **2**, 1-8.

Happonen, R-P. (1986). *Immunocytochemical diagnosis of cervicofacial actinomycosis with special emphasis on periapical inflammatory lesions.* Thesis. University of Turku, Finland.

Harding, G.H. (1878). The process of absorption in bone and tooth structure. *British Journal of Dental Science* **21**, 308-315.

Harrington, G.W. & Natkin, E. (1979). External resorption associated with bleaching of the pulpless teeth. *Journal of Endodontics* **5**, 344-348.

Hasselgren, G., Cvek, M. & Olsson, B. (1987). Effects of calcium hydroxide and sodium hypochlorite on the dissolution of necrotic porcine muscle tissue. *Journal of Endodontics* **14**, 125-127.

Hattler, A.B. & Listgarten, M.A. (1984). Pulpal response to root planing in a rat model. *Journal of Endodontics* **10**, 471-476.

Heithersay, G.S. (1999a). Clinical, radiologic, and histopathologic features of invasive cervical resorption. *Quintessence International* **30**, 27-37.

Heithersay, G.S. (1999b). Invasive cervical resorption: An analysis of potential predisposing factors. *Quintessence International* **30**, 83-95.

Heithersay, G.S. (1999c). Treatment of invasive cervical resorption: An analysis of results using topical application of trichloracetic acid, curettage and restoration. *Quintessence International* **30**, 96-110.

Henry, J.L. & Weinmann, J.P. (1951). The pattern of resorption and repair of human cementum. *Journal of the American Dental Association* **42**, 270-290.

Hession, R.W. (1977). Endodontic morphology. II. A radiographic analysis. *Oral Surgery* **44**, 610-620.

Hiatt, W.H & Johansen, E. (1972). Root preparation. I. Obturation of dentinal tubules in treatment of root hypersensitivity. *Journal of Periodontology* **43**, 373-380.

Holland, G.R., Närhi, M., Addy, M., Gangarosa, L. & Orchardson R. (1997). Guidelines for the design and conduct of clinical trials on dentine hypersensitivity. *Journal of Clinical Periodontology* **24**, 808-813.

Holland, R., Filho, A.O.J., de Souza, V., Nery, M.J., Bernabé, P.F.E. & Dezan Junior, E. (2001). Mineral trioxide aggregate repair of lateral root perforations. *Journal of Endodontics* **4**, 281-284.

Hovgaard, O., Larsen, M.J. & Fejerskov, O. (1991). Tooth hypersensitivity in relation to quality of restorations. *Journal of Dental Research* **70** (Spec issue), IADR abstract 1667.

Hötz, R. (1967). Wurzel resorptionen an bleibenden Zähnen. *Fortschritte der Kieferorthopädie* **28**, 217-224.

Ikola, S. (2001). *Dentin hypersensitivity and its treatment methods.* Thesis. Institute of Dentistry, University of Turku, Finland.

Jansson, L., Ehnevid, H., Lindskog, S. & Blomlöf, L. (1993). Relationship between periapical and periodontal status. A clinical retrospective study. *Journal of Clinical Periodontology* **20**, 117-123.

Jones, S.J. & Boyde, A. (1976). Experimental study of changes in osteoblastic shape induced by calcitonin and parathyroid extract in an organ culture system. *Cell Tissue Research* **169**, 449-465.

Kakehashi, S., Stanley, H.R. & Fitzgerald, R.J. (1965). The effects of surgical exposures of dental pulps in germ-free and conventional laboratory rats. *Oral Surgery* **20**, 340-349.

Kerekes, K. & Olsen, I. (1990). Similarities in the microfloras of root canals and deep periodontal pockets. *Endodontics and Dental Traumatology* **6**, 1-5.

Kerns, D.G., Scheidt, M.J., Pashley, D.H., Horner, J.A., Strong, S.L. & Van Dyke, T.E. (1991). Dentinal tubule occlusion and root hypersensitivity. *Journal of Periodontology* **62**, 421-428.

Koenigs, J.F., Brilliant, J.D. & Foreman, D.W. (1974). Preliminary scanning electron microscope investigations of accessory foramina in the furcation areas of human molar teeth. *Oral Surgery* **38**, 773-782.

Kontturi-Närhi, V. (1993). *Dentin hypersensitivity. Factors related to the occurrence of pain symptoms.* Academic Dissertation, University of Kuopio, Finland.

Kürol, J. (1984). Infraocclusion of primary molars. An epidemiological, familial, longitudinal, clinical and histological study. *Swedish Dental Journal*, Supplement.

Langeland, K. (1987). Tissue response to dental caries. *Endodontics and Dental Traumatology* **3**, 149-171.

Langeland, K., Rodrigues, H. & Dowden, W. (1974). Periodontal disease, bacteria and pulpal histopathology. *Oral Surgery* **37**, 257-270.

Lantelme, R.L., Handelman, S.L. & Herbison, R.J. (1976). Dentin formation in periodontally diseased teeth. *Journal of Dental Research* **55**, 48-51.

Lantz, B. & Persson, P. (1967). Periodontal tissue reactions after root perforations in dogs teeth: a histologic study. *Odontologisk Tidskrift* **75**, 209-236.

Lindskog, S., Blomlöf, L. & Hammarström, L. (1983a). Mitosis and microorganisms in the periodontal membrane after storage in milk or saliva. *Scandinavian Journal of Dental Research* **91**, 456-472.

Lindskog, S., Blomlöf, L. & Hammarström, L. (1983b). Repair of periodontal tissues *in vivo* and *in vitro*. *Journal of Periodontology* **10**, 188-205.

Lindskog, S., Blomlöf, L. & Hammarström, L. (1987). Comparative effects of parathyroid hormone on osteoblasts and cementoblasts. *Journal of Clinical Periodontology* **14**, 386-389.

Löe, H. & Waerhaug, J. (1961). Experimental replantation of teeth in dogs and monkeys. *Archives of Oral Biology* **3**, 176-184.

Löwenstein, N.R., & Rathkamp, R. (1955). A study on the pressoreceptive sensibility of the tooth. *Journal of Dental Research* **34**, 287-294.

Lowman, J.V., Burke, R.S. & Pelleu, G.B. (1973). Patent accessory canals: Incidence in molar furcation region. *Oral Surgery* **36**, 580-584.

Malmgren, B., Cvek, M., Lundberg, M. & Frykholm, A. (1984). Surgical treatment of ankylosed and infrapositioned reimplanted incisors in adolescents. *Scandinavian Journal of Dental Research* **92**, 391-399.

Markowitz, K. & Kim, S. (1992) The role of selected cations in the desensitization of intradental nerves. *Proceedings of the Finnish Dental Society* **88** (Suppl. I), 39-54.

Marks, S.C. Jr. (1983). The origin of the osteoclast: Evidence, clinical implications and investigative challenges of an extraskeletal source. *Journal of Oral Pathology* **12**, 226-256.

Marton, I.J. & Kiss, C. (2000). Protective and destructive immune reactions in apical periodontitis. *Oral Microbiology and Immunology* **15**, 139-150.

Mazur, B. & Massler, M. (1964). Influence of periodontal disease on the dental pulp. *Oral Surgery* **17**, 592-603.

Meister, F., Lommel, T.J. & Gerstein, H. (1980). Diagnosis and possible causes of vertical root fractures. *Oral Surgery* **49**, 243-253.

McGrath, P.A. (1994). Psychological aspects of pain perception. *Archives of Oral Biology* **39** (suppl.), 55S-62S.

Miyashita, H., Bergenholtz, G. & Wennström, J. (1998). Impact of endodontic conditions on marginal bone loss. *Journal of Periodontology* **69**, 158-164.

Möller, Å.J.R., Fabricius, L., Dahlén, G., Öhman, A.E. & Heyden, G. (1981). Influence on periapical tissues of indigenous oral bacteria and necrotic pulp tissue in monkeys. *Scandinavian Journal of Dental Research* **89**, 475-484.

Molven, O., Olsen, I. & Kerekes, K. (1991). Scanning electron microscopy of bacteria in the apical part of root canals in permanent teeth with periapical lesions. *Endodontics and Dental Traumatology* **7**, 226-229.

Montgomery, S. (1984). External cervical resorption after bleaching a pulpless tooth. *Oral Surgery* **57**, 203-206.

Moskow, B.M. (1989). Periodontal manifestations of hyperoxaluria and oxalosis. *Journal of Periodontology* **60**, 271-278.

Mumford, J.M. (1964). Evaluation of gutta percha and ethyl chloride in pulp testing. *British Dental Journal* **116**, 338-342.

Nair, P.N.R. (1987). Light and electron microscopic studies of root canal flora and periapical lesions. *Journal of Endodontics* **13**, 29-39.

Nair, P.N.R. (1997). Apical periodontitis a dynamic encounter between root canal infection and host response. *Periodontology 2000* **13**, 121-148.

Närhi, M., Yamamoto, H., Ngassapa, D. & Hirvonen, T. (1994). The neurophysiological basis and the role of the inflammatory reactions in dentine hypersensitivity. *Archives of Oral Biology* **39**, Suppl., 23S-30S.

Närhi, M., Yamamoto, H. & Ngassapa, D. (1996). *Function of intradental nociceptors in normal and inflamed teeth. Proceedings of the International Conference on Dentin/Pulp Complex* 1995. Berlin: Quintessence, pp. 136-140.

Nilvéus, R. & Selvig, K.A. (1983). Pulpal reactions to the application of citric acid to root-planed dentin in beagles. *Journal of Periodontal Research* **18**, 420-428.

Okiji, T., Kawashima, N., Kosaka, T., Kobayashi, C. & Suda, H. (1994). Distribution of Ia antigen-expressing nonlymphoid cells in various stages of induced periapical lesions in rat molars. *Journal of Endodontics* **20**, 27-31.

Orchardson, R. & Gillam, D.G. (2000). The efficacy of potassium salts as agents for treating dentin hypersensitivity. *Journal of Orofacial Pain* **14**, 9-19.

Orchardson, R., Gangarosa Sr, L.P., Holland, G.R., Pashley, D.H., Trowbridge, H.O., Ashley, F.P., Kleinberg, I. & Zappa, U. (1994). Consensus report. Dentine hypersensitivity into the 21st century. *Archives of Oral Biology* **39**, Suppl., 113S-119S.

Orchardson, R., & Peacock, J.M. (1994). Factors affecting nerve excitability and conduction as a basis for desensitizing dentine. *Archives of Oral Biology* **39**, Suppl., 81S-86S.

Oyama, T. & Matsumoto, K. (1991). A clinical and morphological study of cervical hypersensitivity. *Journal of Endodontics* **17**, 500-502.

Pashley, D.H. (1996). Dynamics of the pulpo-dentin complex. *Critical Reviews in Oral Biology & Medicine* **7**, 104-133.

Perlich, MA., Reader, A. & Foreman, D.W. (1981). A scanning electron microscopic investigation of accessory foramens on the pulpal floor of human molars. *Journal of Endodontics* **7**, 402-406.

Peters, D.D., Baumgartner, J.C. & Lorton L. (1994). Adult pulpal diagnosis. I. Evaluation of the positive and negative responses to cold and electrical pulp tests. *Journal of Endodontics* **20**, 506-511.

Petersson, K., Hasselgren, G. & Tronstad, L. (1985). Endodontic treatment of experimental root perforations in dog teeth. *Endodontics and Dental Traumatology* **1**, 22-28.

Pierce, A.M., Lindskog, S. & Hammarström, L.E. (1991). Osteoclasts: structure and function. *Electron Microscopical Revue* **4**, 1-5.

Pineda, F. & Kuttler, Y. (1972). Mesiodistal and buccolingual roentgenographic investigation of 7,275 root canals. *Oral Surgery* **33**, 101-110.

Pitts, D.L. & Natkin, E. (1983). Diagnosis and treatment of vertical root fractures. *Journal of Endodontics* **9**, 338-346.

Randow, K. & Glantz, P.-O. (1986). On cantilever loading of vital and non-vital teeth. An experimental clinical study. *Acta Odontologica Scandinavica* **44**, 271-277.

Randow, K., Glantz, P.O. & Zöger, B. (1986). Technical failures and some related clinical complications in extensive fixed prosthodontics. An epidemiological study of long-term clinical quality. *Acta Odontologica Scandinavica* **44**, 241-255.

Rankow, H.J. & Krasner, P.R. (1996). Endodontic applications of guided tissue regeneration in endodontic surgery. *Journal of Endodontics* **22**, 34-43.

Reeh, E.S., Messer, H.H. & Douglas, W.H. (1989). Reduction in tooth stiffness as a result of endodontic and restorative procedures. *Journal of Endodontics* **15**, 512-516.

Rodan, G.A. & Martin, T.J. (1981). Role of osteoblasts in hormonal control of bone resorption. A hypothesis. *Calcified Tissue Research* **33**, 349-355.

Rubach, W.C. & Mitchell, D.F. (1965). Periodontal disease, accessory canals and pulp pathosis. *Journal of Periodontology* **36**, 34-38.

Sasaki, T., Shimizu, T., Watanabe, C. & Hiyoshi, Y. (1990). Cellular roles in physiological root resorption of deciduous teeth in the cat. *Journal of Dental Research* **69**, 67-74.

Schwartz, R.S., Mauger, M., Clement, D.J. & Walker, W.A. 3rd (1999). Mineral trioxide aggregate: a new material for endodontics. *Journal of American Dental Association* **130**, 967-975.

Sedgley, C.M. & Messer, H.H. (1992). Are endodontically treated teeth more brittle? *Journal of Endodontics* **18**, 332-335.

Seltzer, S., Bender, I.B. & Ziontz, M. (1963a). The interrelationship of pulp and periodontal disease. *Oral Surgery* **16**, 1474-1490.

Seltzer, S., Bender, I.B. & Ziontz, M. (1963b). The dynamics of pulp inflammation: correlations between diagnostic data and actual histologic findings in the pulp. *Oral Surgery* **16**, 1846-1871.

Sessle, B.J. (2000). Acute and chronic craniofacial pain: Brainstem mechanism of nociceptive transmission and neuroplasticity, and their clinical correlates. *Critical Reviews in Oral Medicine and Biololgy* **11**, 962-981.

Seward, G.R. (1963). Periodontal disease and resorption of teeth. *British Dental Journal* **34**, 443-449.

Stashenko, P. (1990). Role of immune cytokines in the pathogenesis of periapical lesions. *Endodontics and Dental Traumatology* **6**, 89-96.

Stashenko, P., Teles, R. & D'Souza, R. (1998). Periapical inflammatory responses and their modulation. *Critical Reviews in Oral Biology and Medicine* **9**, 498-521

Stashenko, P., Wang, C.Y., Riley, E., Wu, Y., Ostroff, G. & Niederman, R. (1995). Reduction of infection-stimulated periapical bone resorption by the biological response modifier PGG Glucan. *Journal of Dental Research* **74**, 323-330.

Stashenko, P. & Yu, S.M. (1989). T-helper and T suppressor cell reversal during the development of induced rat periapical lesions. *Journal of Dental Research* **68**, 830-834.

Stenvik, A. & Mjör, I.A. (1970). Pulp and dentin reactions to experimental tooth intrusion. *American Journal of Orthodontics* **57**, 370-385.

Strömberg, T., Hasselgren, G., Bergstedt, H. (1972). Endodontic treatment of traumatic root perforations in man. *Swedish Dental Journal* **65**, 457-466.

Sundqvist, G. (1976). *Bacteriologic studies of necrotic dental pulps.* Umeå University Odontological Dissertation #7.

Sundqvist, G. (1990). Endodontic microbiology. In: Spångberg,

L.S.W., ed. *Experimental endodontology.* Boca Raton, FL: CRC Press, pp. 131-153.

Sundqvist, G. (1994). Taxonomy, etiology, and pathogenecity of the root canal flora. *Oral Surgery* **78**, 552-530.

Syed, S.A., Bergenholtz, G., Cox, C.F. & Loesche, W.J. (1982). Microbiological and histopathological correlation of induced periapical lesions in monkeys. *Journal of Dental Research* 61, IADR Abstract 251.

Tammaro, S., Wennström, J. & Bergenholtz, G. (2000). Root dentin sensitivity following non-surgical periodontal treatment. *Journal of Clinical Periodontology* **27**, 690-697.

Tamse, A., Fuss, Z., Lustig, J., Ganor, Y. & Kaffe, I. (1999a). Radiographic features of vertically fractured, endodontically treated maxillary premolars. *Oral Surgery* **88**, 348-352.

Tamse, A., Fuss, Z., Lustig, J & Kaplavi, J. (1999b). An evaluation of endodontically treated vertically fractured teeth. *Journal of Endodontics* **25**, 506-508.

Taylor, P.E., Byers, M.R. & Redd, P.E. (1988). Sprouting of CGRP nerve fibers in response to dentin injury in rat molars. *Brain Research* **461**, 371-376.

Ten Cate, A.R. (1972). The epithelial cell rests of Malassez and the genesis of the dental cyst. *Oral Surgery* **34**, 956-964.

Testori, T., Badino, M. & Castagnola, M. (1993). Vertical root fractures in endodontically treated teeth. *Journal of Endodontics* **19**, 87-90.

Thilo, B.E., Baehni, P. & Holz, J. (1986). Dark-field observation of the bacterial distribution in root canals following pulp necrosis. *Journal of Endodontics* **12**, 202-205.

Torabinejad, M. & Kettering, J.D. (1985). Identification and relative concentration of B and T lymphocytes in human chronic periapical lesions. *Journal of Endodontics* **11**, 122-125.

Torabinejad, M. & Kiger, R.D. (1985). A histologic evaluation of dental pulp tissue of a patient with periodontal disease. *Oral Surgery* **59**, 198-200.

Torabinejad, M., Pitt Ford, T.R., McKendry, D.J., Abedi, H.R., Miller, D.A. & Kariyawasan, S.P. (1997). Histologic assessment of mineral trioxide aggregate as a root-end filling material in monkeys. *Journal of Endodontics* **23**, 225-228.

Waltimo, T.M., Siren, E.K., Torkko, H.L., Olsen, I. & Haapasalo, M.P. (1997). Fungi in therapy-resistant apical periodontitis. *International Endodontic Journal* **30**, 96-101.

Walton, R.E., Michelich, R.J. & Smith, G.N. (1984). The histopathogenesis of vertical root fractures. *Journal of Endodontics* **10**, 48-56.

Warfvinge, J. & Bergenholtz, G. (1986). Healing capacity of human and monkey dental pulps following experimentally induced pulpitis. *Endodontics and Dental Traumatology* **2**, 256-262.

Wasfy, M.O., McMahon, K.T., Minah, G.E. & Falker Jr., W.A. (1992). Microbiological evaluation of periapical infections in Egypt. *Oral Microbiology and Immunology* **7**, 100-105.

Wedenberg, C. & Lindskog, S. (1985). Experimental internal resorption in monkey teeth. *Endodontics and Dental Traumatology* **1**, 221-227.

Vaes, G. (1968). On the mechanism of bone resorption: the action of parathyroid hormone on the excretion and synthesis of lysosomal enzymes and the extracellular release of acid by bone cells. *Journal of Cell Biology* **39**, 676-697.

Vaes, G. (1988). Cellular biology and biochemical mechanism of bone resorption. *Clinical Orthopedics* **23**, 239-271.

Vertucci, F.J. & Williams, R.G. (1974). Furcation canals in the human mandibular first molar. *Oral Surgery* **38**, 308-314.

Yang, S.F., Rivera, E.M. & Walton, R.E. (1995). Vertical root fracture in nonendodontically treated teeth. *Journal of Endodontics* **21**, 337-339.

Yates, R., Owens, R., Jackson, R., Newcombe, R.G. & Addy, M. (1998). A split mouth placebo-controlled study to determine the effect of amorphous calcium phosphate in the treatment of dentine hypersensitivity. *Journal of Clinical Periodontology* **25**, 687-692.

Yoshiyama, M., Masada, A., Uchida, A. & Ishida, H. (1989).

Scanning electron microscopic characterization of sensitive vs. insensitive human radicular dentin. *Journal of Dental Research* **68**, 1498-1502.

Yoshiyama, M., Noiri, Y., Ozaki, K., Uchida, A., Ishikawa, Y. & Ishida, H. (1990). Transmission electron microscopic characterization of hypersensitive human radicular dentin. *Journal of Dental Research* **69**, 1293-1297.

Yu, S.M. & Stashenko, P. (1987). Identification of inflammatory cells in developing rat periapical lesions. *Journal of Endodontics* **13**, 535-540.

Zappa, U. (1994). Self-applied treatments in the management of dentine hypersensitivity. *Archives of Oral Biology* **39**, Suppl., 107S-112S.

CHAPTER 15

Trauma from Occlusion

JAN LINDHE, STURE NYMAN AND INGVAR ERICSSON

DEFINITION AND TERMINOLOGY

Trauma from occlusion is a term used to describe pathologic alterations or adaptive changes which develop in the periodontium as a result of undue force produced by the masticatory muscles. *Trauma from occlusion* is only one of many terms that have been used to describe such alterations in the periodontium. Other terms often used are: *traumatizing occlusion, occlusal trauma, traumatogenic occlusion, periodontal traumatism, overload,* etc. In addition to producing damage in the periodontal tissues, excessive occlusal force may also cause injury in, for example, the temporomandibular joint, the masticatory muscles, the pulp tissue. This chapter deals exclusively with the effects of *trauma from occlusion* on the periodontal tissues.

Trauma from occlusion was defined by Stillman (1917) as "a condition where injury results to the supporting structures of the teeth by the act of bringing the jaws into a closed position". WHO in 1978 defined *trauma from occlusion* as "damage in the periodontium caused by stress on the teeth produced directly or indirectly by teeth of the opposing jaw". In "Glossary of Periodontic Terms" (American Academy of Periodontology 1986), *Occlusal Trauma* was defined as "An injury to the attachment apparatus as a result of excessive occlusal force".

Traumatizing forces may act on an individual tooth or on groups of teeth in premature contact relationship; may occur in conjunction with parafunctions such as clenching and bruxism, in conjunction with loss or migration of premolar and molar teeth with an accompanying, gradually developing spread of the anterior teeth of the maxilla, etc.

In the literature, the tissue injury associated with *trauma from occlusion* is often divided into *primary* and *secondary*. The *primary* form includes a tissue reaction (damage), which is elicited around a tooth with normal height of the periodontium, while the *secondary* form is related to situations in which occlusal forces cause injury in a periodontium of reduced height. The distinction between a *primary* and a *secondary* form of injury – *primary* and *secondary occlusal trauma* – serves no meaningful purpose, since the alterations which occur in the periodontium as a consequence of trauma from occlusion are similar and independent of the height of the target tissue, i.e. the periodontium. It is, however, important to understand that symptoms of *trauma from occlusion* may develop only in situations when the magnitude of the load elicited by occlusion is so high that the periodontium around the exposed tooth cannot properly withstand and distribute the resulting force with unaltered position and stability of the tooth involved. This means that in cases of severely reduced height of the periodontium even comparatively small forces may produce traumatic lesions or adaptive changes in the periodontium.

TRAUMA FROM OCCLUSION AND PLAQUE-ASSOCIATED PERIODONTAL DISEASE

Ever since Karolyi (1901) postulated that an interaction may exist between "*trauma from occlusion*" and "*alveolar pyrrohea*" different opinions have been presented in the literature regarding the validity of this claim. Already in the 1930s Box (1935) and Stones (1938) reported experiments in sheep and monkeys, the result of which seemed to indicate that "trauma from occlusion is an etiologic factor in the production of that variety of periodontal disease in which there is

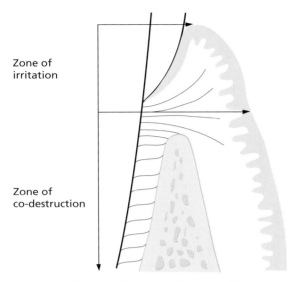

Fig. 15-1. Schematic drawing of the zone of irritation and the zone of co-destruction according to Glickman.

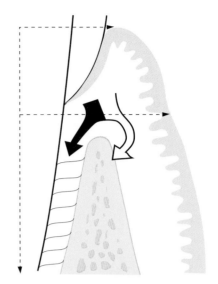

Fig. 15-2. The inflammatory lesion in the zone of irritation can, in teeth not subjected to trauma, propagate into the alveolar bone (open arrow), while in teeth also subjected to trauma from occlusion, the inflammatory infiltrate spreads directly into periodontal ligament (filled arrow).

vertical pocket formation associated with one or a varying number of teeth" (Stones 1938). The experiments by Box and Stones, however, have been criticized because they lacked proper controls and because the experimental design of the studies did not justify the conclusions drawn.

The interaction between *trauma from occlusion* and plaque-associated periodontal disease in humans was in the period 1955-70 frequently discussed in connection with "report of a case", "in my opinion statements", etc. Even if such anecdotal data may have some value in clinical dentistry, it is obvious that conclusions drawn from research findings are much more pertinent. The research-based conclusions are not always indisputable but they invite the reader to a critique which anecdotal data do not. In this chapter, therefore, the presentation will be limited to findings collected from research endeavors involving: (1) human autopsy material, (2) clinical trials and (3) animal experiments.

Analysis of human autopsy material

Results reported from carefully performed research efforts involving examinations of human autopsy material have been difficult to interpret. In the specimens examined (1) the histopathology of the lesions in the periodontium have been described, as well as (2) the presence and apical extension of microbial deposits at adjacent root surfaces, (3) the mobility of the teeth involved and (4) "the occlusion" of the sites under scrutiny. It is obvious that assessments made in specimens from cadavers have a limited to questionable value when "cause-effect" relationships between occlusion, plaque and periodontal lesions are to be de-

scribed. It is not surprising, therefore, that *conclusions* drawn from this type of research can be controversial. This can best be illustrated if "Glickman's concept" is compared with "Waerhaug's concept" of what autopsy studies have revealed regarding trauma from occlusion and periodontal disease.

Glickman's concept

Glickman (1965, 1967) claimed that the pathway of the spread of a plaque-associated gingival lesion can be changed if forces of an abnormal magnitude are acting on teeth harboring subgingival plaque. This would imply that the character of the progressive tissue destruction of the periodontium at a "traumatized tooth" will be different from that characterizing a "non-traumatized" tooth. Instead of an even destruction of the periodontium and alveolar bone (suprabony pockets and horizontal bone loss), which according to Glickman occurs at sites with uncomplicated plaque-associated lesions, sites which are also exposed to abnormal occlusal force will develop angular bony defects and infrabony pockets.

Since the concept of Glickman regarding the effect of *trauma from occlusion* on the spread of the plaque-associated lesion is often cited, a more detailed presentation of his theory seems pertinent:

The periodontal structures can be divided into two zones:

1. the *zone of irritation* and
2. the *zone of co-destruction* (Fig. 15-1).

The *zone of irritation* includes the marginal and interdental gingiva. The soft tissue of this zone is bordered by hard tissue (the tooth) only on one side and is not affected by forces of occlusion. This means that gingi-

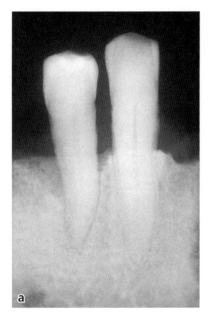

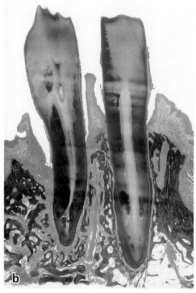

Fig. 15-3. A radiograph of a mandibular premolar-canine region. Note the angular bony defect at the distal aspect of the premolar. (b) Histologic mesiodistal section of the specimen illustrated in (a). Note the infrabony pocket at the distal aspect of the premolar. From Glickman & Smulow (1965).

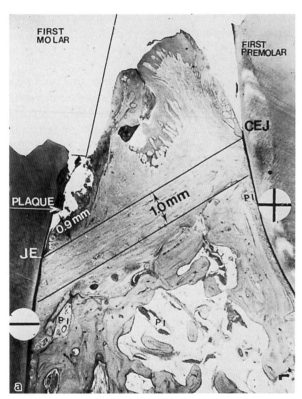

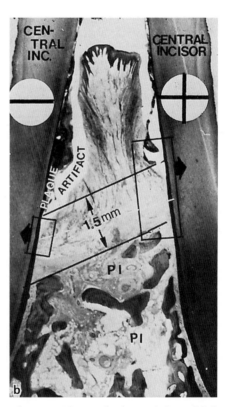

Figs. 15-4a,b. Microphotographs illustrating two interproximal areas with angular bony defects. "-" denotes a tooth not subjected and "+" denotes a tooth subjected to trauma from occlusion. In categories "-" and "+" the distance between the apical cells of the junctional epithelium and the supporting alveolar bone is about 1-1.5 mm, and the distance between the apical extension of plaque and the apical cells of the junctional epithelium about 1 mm. Since the apical cells of the junctional epithelium and the subgingival plaque are located at different levels on the two adjacent teeth, the outline of the bone crest becomes oblique. A radiograph from such a site would disclose the presence of an angular bony defect at a nontraumatized ("-") tooth.

val inflammation cannot be induced by *trauma from occlusion* but is the result of irritation from microbial plaque. The plaque-associated lesion at a "non-traumatized" tooth propagates in apical direction by first involving the alveolar bone and only later the periodontal ligament area. The progression of this lesion results in an even (horizontal) bone destruction.

The zone of *co-destruction* includes the periodontal ligament, the root cementum and the alveolar bone and is coronally demarcated by the transseptal (interdental) and the dentoalveolar collagen fiber bundles (Fig. 15-1). The tissue in this zone may become the seat of a lesion caused by *trauma from occlusion*.

The fiber bundles which separate the zone of co-destruction from the zone of irritation can be affected from two different directions:

1. from the inflammatory lesion maintained by plaque in the *zone of irritation*
2. from trauma-induced changes in the *zone of co-destruction*.

Through this exposure from two different directions the fiber bundles may become dissolved and/or oriented in a direction parallel to the root surface. The spread of an inflammatory lesion from the *zone of irritation* directly down into the periodontal ligament (i.e. not via the interdental bone) may hereby be facilitated (Fig. 15-2). This alteration of the "normal" pathway of spread of the plaque-associated inflammatory lesion results in the development of angular bony defects. Glickman (1967) in a review paper stated that *trauma from occlusion* is an etiologic factor (co-destructive factor) of importance in situations where angular bony defects combined with infrabony pockets are found at one or several teeth (Fig. 15-3).

Waerhaug's concept

Waerhaug (1979) examined autopsy specimens (Fig. 15-4) similar to Glickman's, but measured in addition the distance between the subgingival plaque and (1) the periphery of the associated inflammatory cell infiltrate in the gingiva and (2) the surface of the adjacent alveolar bone. He concluded from his analysis that angular bony defects and infrabony pockets occur equally often at periodontal sites of teeth which are not affected by trauma from occlusion as in traumatized teeth. In other words, he refuted the hypothesis that *trauma from occlusion* played a role in the spread of a gingival lesion into the "zone of co-destruction". The loss of connective attachment and the resorption of bone around teeth are, according to Waerhaug, exclusively the result of inflammatory lesions associated with subgingival plaque. Waerhaug concluded that angular bony defects and infrabony pockets occur when the subgingival plaque of one tooth has reached a more apical level than the microbiota on the neighboring tooth, and when the volume of the alveolar bone surrounding the roots is comparatively large. Waerhaug's observations support findings presented by Prichard (1965) and Manson (1976) which imply that the pattern of loss of supporting structures is the result of an interplay between the form and volume of the alveolar bone and the apical extension of the microbial plaque on the adjacent root surfaces.

It is obvious, as stated above, that examinations of autopsy material have a limited value when "cause-effect" relationships with respect to trauma and progressive periodontitis are to be determined. As a consequence, the conclusions drawn from this field of research have not been generally accepted. A number of authors tend to accept Glickman's conclusions that trauma from occlusion is an aggravating factor in periodontal disease (e.g. Macapanpan & Weinmann

1954, Posselt & Emslie 1959, Glickman & Smulow 1962, 1965) while others accept Waerhaug's concept, i.e. that there is no relationship between occlusal trauma and the degree of periodontal tissue breakdown (e.g. Lovdahl et al. 1959, Belting & Gupta 1961, Baer et al. 1963, Waerhaug 1979).

Clinical trials

In addition to the presence of angular bony defects and infrabony pockets, *increased tooth mobility* is frequently listed as an important sign of occlusal trauma. For details regarding tooth mobility, see Chapter 30 "Occlusal Therapy". Conflicting data have been reported also regarding the periodontal conditions of mobile teeth. In one clinical study by Rosling et al. (1976) patients with advanced periodontal disease associated with multiple angular bony defects and mobile teeth were exposed to antimicrobial therapy (i.e. subgingival scaling after flap elevation). Healing was evaluated by probing attachment level measurements and radiographic monitoring. The authors reported that "the infrabony pocket located at hypermobile teeth exhibited the same degree of healing as those adjacent to firm teeth".

In another study, however, Fleszar et al. (1980) reported on the influence of tooth mobility on healing following periodontal therapy including both root debridement and occlusal adjustment. They concluded that "pockets of clinically mobile teeth do not respond as well to periodontal treatment as do those of firm teeth exhibiting the same disease severity".

A third study (Pihlstrom et al. 1986) studied the association between *trauma from occlusion* and periodontitis by assessing a series of clinical and radiographic features at maxillary first molars. Parameters included in this study were: probing depth, probing attachment level, tooth mobility, wear facets, plaque and calculus, bone height, widened periodontal space, etc. Pihlstrom and his associates concluded from their measurements and examinations that teeth with increased mobility and widened periodontal ligament space had, in fact, deeper pockets, more attachment loss and less bone support than teeth without these symptoms.

Burgett et al. (1992) studied the effect of occlusal adjustment in the treatment of periodontitis. Fifty subjects with periodontitis were examined at baseline and subsequently treated for their periodontal condition with root debridement ± flap surgery. Twenty-two out of the 50 patients, in addition, received comprehensive occlusal therapy. Reexaminations performed 2 years later disclosed that probing attachment gain was on the average about 0.5 mm larger in patients who received the combined treatment, i.e. scaling and occlusal adjustment, than in patients in whom the occlusal adjustment was not included.

The findings by Fleszar, Pihlstrom and Burgett and co-workers lend some support to the concept that

Tipping movement

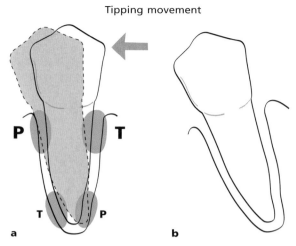

a   b

Bodily movement

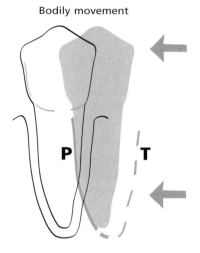

Figs. 15-5. If the crown of a tooth is exposed to excessive, horizontally directed forces (arrow), pressure (P) and tension (T) zones will develop within the marginal and apical parts of the periodontium (a). The supraalveolar connective tissue remains unaffected by force application. Within the pressure and tension zones tissue alterations take place which eventually allow the tooth to tilt in the direction of the force. When the tooth has escaped the trauma, complete regeneration of the periodontal tissues takes place (b). There is no apical downgrowth of the dentogingival epithelium.

Fig. 15-6. When a tooth is exposed to forces which produce "bodily tooth movement", e.g. in orthodontic therapy, the pressure (P) and tension (T) zones, depending on the direction of the force, are extended over the entire tooth surface. The supraalveolar connective tissue is not affected in conjunction either with tipping or with bodily movements of teeth. Forces of this kind, therefore, will not induce inflammatory reactions in the gingiva. No apical downgrowth of the dentogingival epithelium occurs.

trauma from occlusion (and increased tooth mobility) may have a detrimental effect on the periodontium. Neiderud et al. (1992), however, in a beagle dog study demonstrated that tissue alterations which occur at mobile teeth with clinically healthy gingivae (and normal height of the tissue attachment) may reduce the resistance offered by the periodontal tissues to probing. In other words, if the probing depth at two otherwise similar teeth – one non-mobile and one hypermobile – is recorded, the tip of the probe will penetrate 0.5 mm deeper at the mobile than at the non-mobile tooth. This finding must be taken into consideration when the above clinical data are interpreted.

Since neither analysis of autopsy material nor data from clinical trials can be used to properly determine the role *trauma from occlusion* may play in periodontal pathology, it is necessary to describe the contributions made by means of animal research in this particular field. Results from such experiments, describing the reactions of the normal and subsequently the diseased periodontium to occlusal forces, are presented below.

Animal experiments

Orthodontic type trauma

The reaction of the periodontal tissues to traumatic forces initiated by occlusion has been studied principally in animal experiments. In early experiments the reaction of the normal periodontium was studied following the application of forces which were inflicted

on teeth in one direction only. Biopsies including tooth and periodontium were harvested after varying experimental time intervals and prepared for histologic examinations. Analysis of the tissue sections (Häupl & Psansky 1938, Reitan 1951, Mühlemann & Herzog 1961, Ewen & Stahl 1962, Waerhaug & Hansen 1966, Karring et al. 1982) revealed the following: when a tooth is exposed to unilateral forces of a magnitude, frequency or duration that its periodontal tissues are unable to withstand and distribute while maintaining the stability of the tooth, certain well-defined reactions develop in the periodontal ligament, eventually resulting in an adaptation of the periodontal structures to the altered functional demand. If the crown of a tooth is affected by such horizontally directed forces, the tooth tends to tilt (tip) in the direction of the force (Fig. 15-5). This tilting force results in the development of *pressure* and *tension zones* within the marginal and apical parts of the periodontium. The tissue reactions which develop in the *pressure zone* are characterized by increased vascularization, increased vascular permeability, vascular thrombosis, and disorganization of cells and collagen fiber bundles. If the magnitude of forces is within certain limits, allowing the maintenance of the vitality of the periodontal ligament cells, bone-resorbing osteoclasts soon appear on the bone surface of the alveolus in the *pressure zone*. A process of bone resorption is initiated. This phenomenon is called *"direct bone resorption"*.

If the force applied is of higher magnitude, the result may be necrosis of the periodontal ligament tissue in the *pressure zone*, i.e. decomposition of cells,

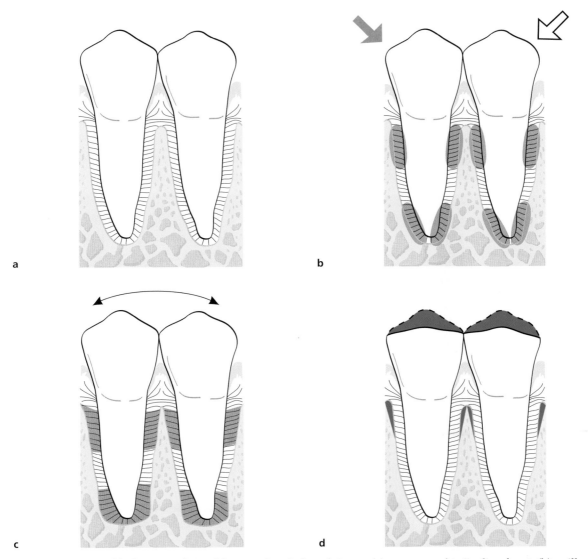

Fig. 15-7. Two mandibular premolars with normal periodontal tissues (a) are exposed to jiggling forces (b) as illustrated by the two arrows. The combined tension and pressure zones (encircled areas) are characterized by signs of acute inflammation including collagen resorption, bone resorption and cementum resorption. As a result of bone resorption the periodontal ligament space gradually increases in size on both sides of the teeth as well as in the periapical region. When the effect of the force applied has been compensated for by the increased width of the periodontal ligament space (c), the ligament tissue shows no sign of inflammation. The supraalveolar connective tissue is not affected by the jiggling forces and there is no apical downgrowth of the dentogingival epithelium. After occlusal adjustment the width of the periodontal ligament becomes normalized (d) and the teeth are stabilized.

vessels, matrix and fibers (*hyalinization*). "Direct bone resorption" therefore cannot occur. Instead, osteoclasts appear in marrow spaces within the adjacent bone tissue where the stress concentration is lower than in the periodontal ligament and a process of undermining or "*indirect bone resorption*" is initiated. Through this reaction the surrounding bone is resorbed until there is a breakthrough to the hyalinized tissue within the *pressure zone*. This breakthrough results in a reduction of the stress in this area, and cells from the neighboring bone or adjacent areas of the periodontal ligament can proliferate into the *pressure zone* and replace the previously hyalinized tissue, thereby reestablishing prerequisites for "direct bone resorption". Irrespective of whether the bone resorp-

tion is of a direct or an indirect nature the tooth moves (tilts) further in the direction of the force.

Concomitant with the tissue alterations in the *pressure zone*, apposition of bone occurs in the *tension zone* in order to maintain the normal width of the periodontal ligament in this area. Because of the tissue reactions in the *pressure* and *tension* zones the tooth becomes, temporarily, hypermobile. When the tooth has moved (tilted) to a position where the effect of the forces is nullified, healing of the periodontal tissues takes place in both the *pressure* and the *tension zones* and the tooth becomes stable in its new position. In orthodontic tilting (tipping) movements, neither gingival inflammation nor loss of connective tissue attachment will occur in a healthy periodontium and – as long as the tooth is not moved through the envelope of the alveo-

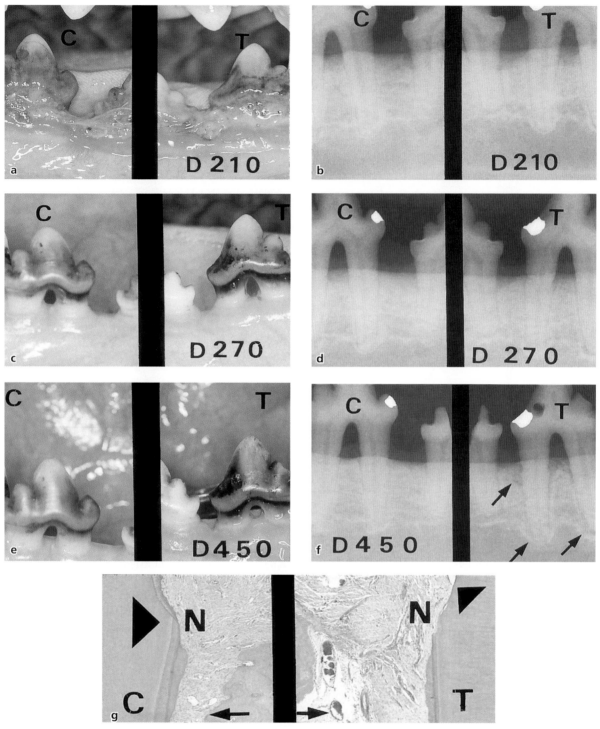

Fig. 15-8. Dogs were allowed to accumulate plaque and calculus in the mandibular premolar regions over a 210-day period (a). When around 40-50% of the periodontal tissue support had been lost (b) the animals were treated by scaling, root planing and pocket elimination. During surgery, a notch was prepared in the root at the level of the bone crest. The dogs were subsequently placed on a plaque control program and 2 months later (Day 270) all experimental teeth (the lower fourth premolars; 4P and P4) were surrounded by a healthy periodontium with reduced height (c and d). The mandibular **left** fourth premolar (T) was exposed to jiggling forces (e). As a consequence, a widened periodontal ligament and increased tooth mobility resulted (f). This increase in tooth mobility and the development of widened periodontal ligament space did not, however, result in apical downgrowth of the dentogingival epithelium (g). Arrowheads indicates the apical extension of the junctional epithelium which coincides with the apical border of the notch (N), prepared in the root surface prior to jiggling. C= control tooth. T= test tooth.

lar process – there is no apical migration of the dentogingival epithelium. In other words, since the supraalveolar connective tissue is only bordered by hard tissue (the tooth) on one side (in the direction of the force), this structure remains unaffected by this type of force.

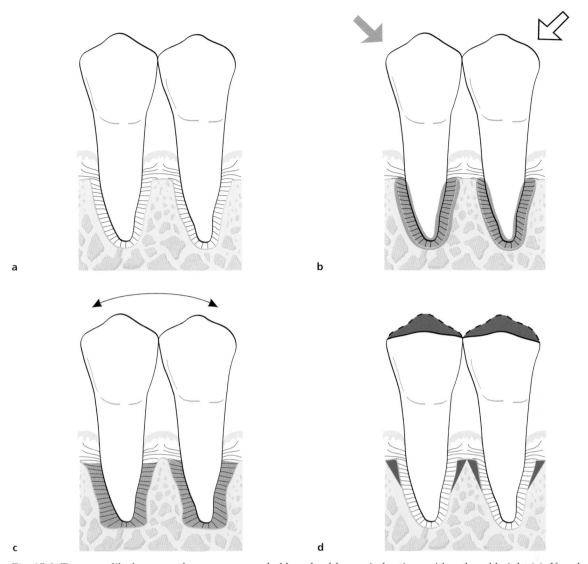

Fig. 15-9. Two mandibular premolars are surrounded by a healthy periodontium with reduced height (a). If such premolars are subjected to traumatizing forces of the jiggling type (b) a series of alterations occurs in the periodontal ligament tissue. These alterations result in a widened periodontal ligament space (c) and in an increased tooth mobility but do not lead to further loss of connective tissue attachment. After occlusal adjustment (d) the width of the periodontal ligament is normalized and the teeth stabilized.

These tissue reactions do not differ fundamentally from those which occur as a consequence of *bodily tooth movement* in orthodontic therapy (Reitan 1951). The main difference is that the *pressure* and *tension zones*, depending on the direction of the force, are more extended in an apical-coronal direction along the root surface than in conjunction with tipping movement (Fig. 15-6). Neither in conjunction with tipping nor in conjunction with bodily movements of the tooth is the supraalveolar connective tissue affected by the *force*. Unilateral forces directed to the crown of teeth, therefore, will not induce inflammatory reactions in the gingiva or cause loss of connective tissue attachment.

Studies (Steiner et al. 1981, Wennström et al. 1987) have demonstrated, however, that orthodontic forces producing bodily (or tipping) movement of teeth may result in gingival recession and loss of connective tissue attachment. This breakdown of the attachment apparatus occurred at sites with gingivitis when, in addition, the tooth was moved through the envelope of the alveolar process. At such sites a bone dehiscence becomes established and, if the covering soft tissue is thin (in the direction of the movement of the tooth), recession (attachment loss) may occur.

Criticism has been directed, however, at experiments in which only unilateral trauma is exerted on teeth (Wentz et al. 1958). It has been suggested that in humans, unlike in the animal experiments described above, the occlusal forces act alternately in one and then in the opposite direction. Such forces have been termed *jiggling forces*.

Jiggling-type trauma

Healthy periodontium with normal height
Experiments have been reported in which traumatic forces were exerted on the crowns of the teeth, alternately in buccal and lingual or mesial and distal direc-

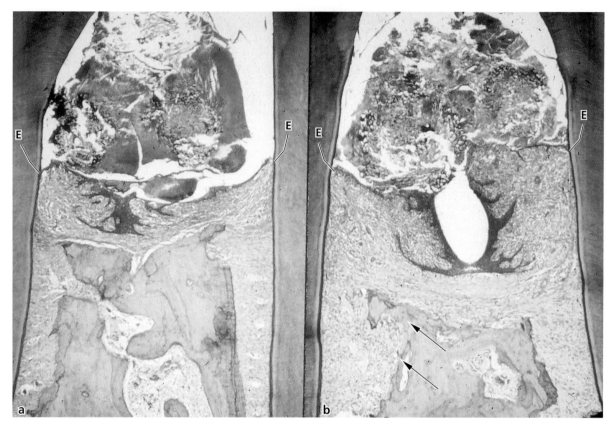

Fig. 15-10. A composite photomicrograph illustrating the interdental space between two pairs of teeth. The teeth have been subjected to experimental, ligature-induced periodontitis and in (b) also to repetitive mechanical injury. In (b), there is considerable loss of alveolar bone and an angular widening of the periodontal ligament space (arrows). However, the apical downgrowth of the dentogingival epithelium in the two areas (a) and(b) is similar. E indicates the apical level of the dentogingival epithelium. Courtesy of Dr. Meitner.

tions, and in which the teeth were not allowed to move away from the force (e.g. Wentz et al. 1958, Glickman & Smulow 1968, Svanberg & Lindhe 1973, Meitner 1975, Ericsson & Lindhe 1982). In conjunction with *"jiggling-type trauma"* no clearcut *pressure* and *tension zones* can be identified but rather there is a combination of pressure and tension on both sides of the jiggled tooth (Fig. 15-7).

The tissue reactions in the periodontal ligament provoked by the combined *pressure* and *tension* forces were found to be similar, however, to those reported for the pressure zone at orthodontically moved teeth, with the one difference that the periodontal ligament space at jiggling gradually increased in width on both sides of the tooth. During the phase when the periodontal space gradually increased in width (1) inflammatory changes were present in the ligament tissue, (2) active bone resorption occurred, and (3) the tooth displayed signs of gradually increasing (*progressive*) mobility. When the effect of the forces applied had been compensated for by the increased width of the periodontal ligament space, the ligament tissue showed no signs of increased vascularity or exudation. The tooth was hypermobile but the mobility was no longer *progressive* in character. Distinction should thus be made between *progressive* and *increased* tooth mobility.

In *"jiggling-type trauma"* experiments, performed on animals with a normal periodontium, the supraalveolar connective tissue was not influenced by the occlusal forces, the reason being that this tissue compartment is bordered by hard tissue on one side only. This means that a gingiva which was noninflamed at the start of the experiment remained noninflamed, but also that an overt inflammatory lesion residing in the supraalveolar connective tissue was not aggravated by the jiggling forces.

Healthy periodontium with reduced height

Progressive periodontal disease is characterized by gingival inflammation and a gradually developing loss of connective tissue attachment and alveolar bone. Treatment of periodontal disease, i.e. removal of plaque and calculus and elimination of pathologically deepened pockets, will result in the reestablishment of a healthy periodontium but with reduced height. The question is whether a healthy periodontium with reduced height has a capacity similar to that of the normal periodontium to adapt to traumatizing occlusal forces (secondary occlusal trauma).

This problem has also been examined in animal experiments (Ericsson & Lindhe 1977). Destructive periodontal disease was initiated in dogs by allowing the animals to accumulate plaque and calculus for a

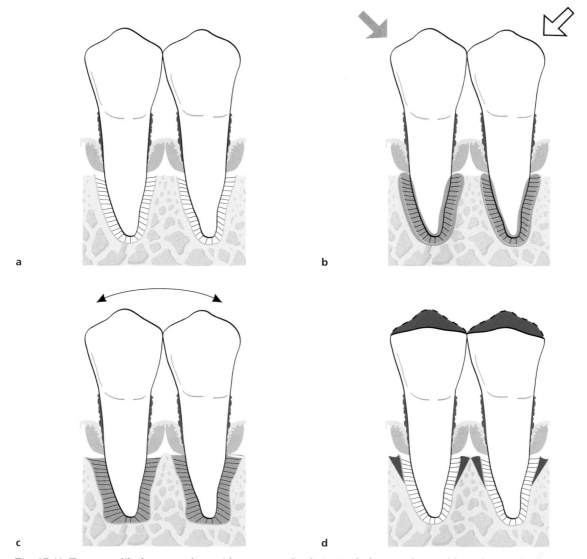

Fig. 15-11. Two mandibular premolars with supra- and subgingival plaque, advanced bone loss and periodontal pockets of a suprabony character (a). Note the connective tissue infiltrate (shadowed areas) and the noninflamed connective tissue between the alveolar bone and the apical portion of the infiltrate. If these teeth are subjected to traumatizing forces of the jiggling type (b), pathologic and adaptive alterations occur within the periodontal ligament space. These tissue alterations, which include bone resorption, result in a widened periodontal ligament space and increased tooth mobility but no further loss of connective tissue attachment (c). Occlusal adjustment results in a reduction of the width of the periodontal ligament (d) and in less mobile teeth.

period of 6 months (Fig. 15-8). When around 50% of the periodontal tissue support had been lost (Fig. 15-8a,b), the progressive disease was subjected to treatment by scaling, root planing and pocket elimination (Fig. 15-8c). During a subsequent 8-month period, the animals were enrolled in a careful plaque control program. During this period certain premolars were exposed to traumatizing jiggling forces. The periodontal tissues in the combined *pressure* and *tension zones* reacted to the forces by vascular proliferation, exudation and thrombosis, as well as by bone resorption. In radiographs, widened periodontal ligaments (Fig. 15-8d) could be found around the traumatized teeth, which at clinical examination displayed signs of *progressive* tooth mobility. The gradual increase in the width of the periodontal ligament and the resulting progressive increase in tooth mobility

took place during a period of several weeks but eventually terminated. The active bone resorption ceased and the markedly widened periodontal ligament tissue regained its normal composition; healing had occurred (Fig. 15-8e). The teeth were hypermobile but surrounded by periodontal structures which had adapted to the altered functional demands.

During the entire experimental period the supraalveolar connective tissue remained unaffected by the jiggling forces. There was no further loss of connective tissue attachment and no further downgrowth of dentogingival epithelium (Fig. 15-8e). The results from this study clearly reveal that within certain limits a healthy periodontium with reduced height has a capacity similar to that of a periodontium with normal height to adapt to altered functional demands (Fig. 15-9).

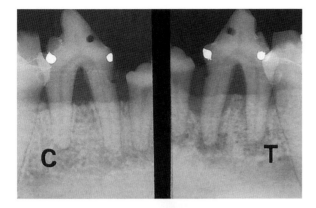

Fig. 15-12. Radiographic appearance of one test tooth (T) and one control tooth (C) at the termination of an experiment in which periodontitis was induced by ligature placement and plaque accumulation and in which trauma of the jiggling type was induced. Note angular bone loss particularly around the mesial root of the mandibular premolar (T) and the absence of such a defect at the mandibular premolar (C). From Lindhe & Svanberg (1974).

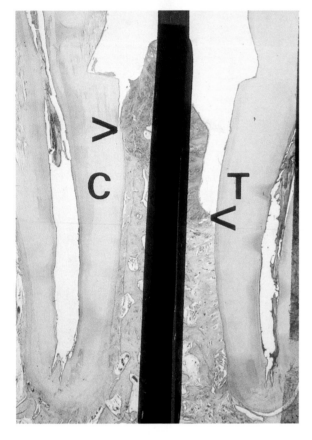

Fig. 15-13. Microphotographs from one control (C) and one test (T) tooth after 240 days of experimental periodontal tissue breakdown and 180 days of trauma from occlusion of the jiggling type (T). The arrowheads denote the apical position of the dentogingival epithelium. The attachment loss is more pronounced in T than in C. From Lindhe & Svanberg (1974).

Plaque-associated periodontal disease

Experiments carried out on humans and animals have demonstrated that *trauma from occlusion* cannot induce pathologic alterations in the supraalveolar connective tissue, i.e. cannot produce inflammatory lesions in a normal gingiva or aggravate a gingival lesion associated with plaque and cannot induce loss of connective tissue attachment. The question remains if abnormal occlusal forces can influence the spread of the plaque-associated lesion and enhance the rate of tissue destruction in periodontal disease. This has been studied in animal experiments (Lindhe & Svanberg 1974, Meitner 1975, Nyman et al. 1978, Ericsson & Lindhe 1982, Polson & Zander 1983). In these experiments progressive and destructive periodontal disease was first initiated in dogs or monkeys by allowing the animals to accumulate plaque and calculus. Teeth thus involved in a progressive periodontal disease process were also subjected to trauma from occlusion.

"Traumatizing" jiggling forces (Lindhe & Svanberg 1974) were exerted on premolars and were found to induce certain tissue reactions in the combined *pressure/tension zones*. The periodontal ligament tissue in these zones, within a few days of the onset of the jiggling forces, displayed signs of inflammation, had increased numbers of vessels, showed increased vascular permeability and exudation, thrombosis, as well as retention of neutrophils and macrophages. On the adjacent bone surfaces there were a large number of osteoclasts. Since the teeth could not orthodontically move away from the jiggling forces, the periodontal ligament of both sides of the tooth gradually increased in width, the teeth became hypermobile (*progressive tooth mobility*) and angular bony defects could be detected in the radiographs. The forces were eventually nullified by the increased width of the periodontal ligament.

If the forces applied were of a magnitude to which

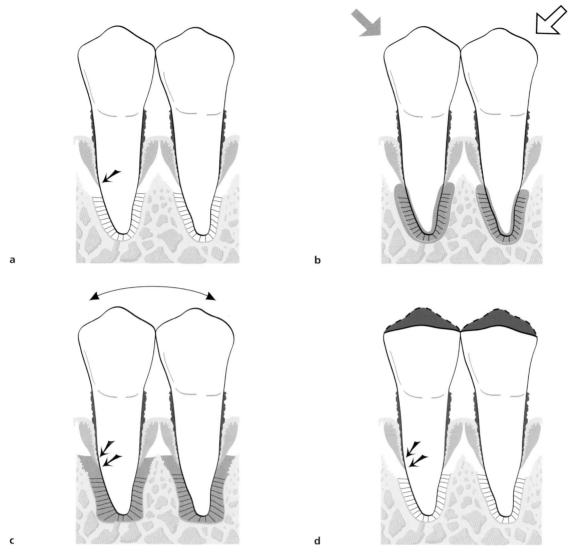

Fig. 15-14. Illustration of a tooth where subgingival plaque has mediated the development of an infiltrated soft tissue (shadowed area) and an infrabony pocket (a). When trauma from occlusion of the jiggling type is inflicted (arrows) on the crown of this tooth (b), the associated pathologic alterations occur within a zone of the periodontium which is also occupied by the inflammatory cell infiltrate (shadowed area). In this situation the increasing tooth mobility may also be associated with an enhanced loss of connective tissue attachment and further downgrowth of dentogingival epithelium; compare arrows in (c) and (d). Occlusal adjustment will result in a narrowing of the periodontal ligament, less tooth mobility, but no improvement of the attachment level (d) (Lindhe & Ericsson 1982).

the periodontal structures could adapt, the *progressive* increase of the tooth mobility terminated within a few weeks. The active bone resorption ceased but the angular bone destruction persisted as well as the increased tooth mobility. The periodontal ligament had an increased width but a normal tissue composition. Histologic examination of biopsies revealed that this adaptation had occurred with no greater apical proliferation of the dentogingival epithelium than was caused by the plaque-associated lesion (Fig. 15-10a,b; Meitner 1975). This means that occlusal forces which allow adaptive alterations to develop in the *pressure/tension* zones of the periodontal ligament will not aggravate a plaque-associated periodontal disease (Fig. 15-11).

If, however, the magnitude and direction of the jiggling forces were such that during the course of the study (6 months) the tissues in the *pressure/tension* zones could not become adapted, the injury in the *zones of co-destruction* had a more permanent character. The periodontal ligament in the *pressure/tension* zones displayed for several months signs of inflammation (vascular proliferation, exudation, thrombosis, retention of neutrophils and macrophages, collagen destruction). Osteoclasts residing on the walls of the alveolus maintained the bone-resorptive process, which resulted in a gradual widening of the periodontal ligament in the *pressure/tension* zones (Fig. 15-12). As a consequence, the resulting angular bone destruction was continuous and the mobility of the teeth remained progressive. The plaque-associated lesion in the "zone of irritation" and the inflammatory lesion in the "zone of co-destruction" merged; the dentogingival epithelium proliferated in an apical direc-

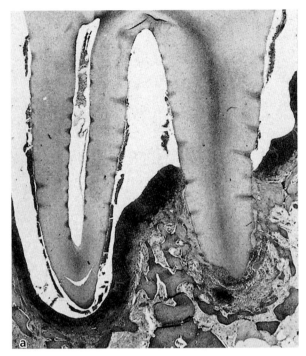
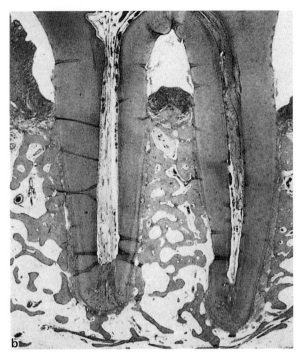

Fig. 15-15. (a) Periodontal conditions around a tooth which has been exposed to trauma from occlusion (of the jiggling type) for 300 days in combination with plaque-associated experimental periodontitis. (b), Condition of a control tooth from the same dog in which experimental periodontitis but no jiggling trauma had been in operation. Note the difference between (a) and (b) regarding the degree of bone destruction and loss of connective tissue attachment. Note also in (a) the location of the subgingival plaque at the apex of the root. From Ericsson & Lindhe (1982).

tion and periodontal disease was aggravated (Figs. 15-13 & 15-14; Lindhe & Svanberg 1974).

Similar findings were reported from another experiment in the dog (Ericsson & Lindhe 1982) in which the effect was assessed of a *prolonged* period of jiggling force application on the rate of progression of plaque-associated, marginal periodontitis. Thus, in dogs with continuing periodontal disease, certain teeth were exposed to jiggling forces during a period of 10 months. Control teeth were not jiggled. Fig. 15-15a illustrates the marked periodontal tissue breakdown around a tooth which for several months was exposed to plaque infection combined with jiggling trauma and Fig. 15-15b illustrates a control tooth which was exposed to plaque infection only.

On the other hand, more short-term experiments in the monkey (Polson & Zander 1983), evaluating the effect of *trauma from occlusion* on teeth involved in an ongoing process of periodontitis, failed to support the findings by Lindhe & Svanberg (1974) and Ericsson & Lindhe (1982). Polson & Zander (1983) observed that trauma superimposed on periodontal lesions associated with angular bony defects (1) caused increased loss of alveolar bone but (2) failed to produce additional loss of connective tissue attachment.

CONCLUSIONS

Experiments carried out in humans as well as animals, have produced convincing evidence that neither unilateral forces nor jiggling forces, applied to teeth with a healthy periodontium, result in pocket formation or in loss of connective tissue attachment. *Trauma from occlusion cannot induce periodontal tissue breakdown.* Trauma from occlusion does, however, result in resorption of alveolar bone leading to an increased tooth mobility which can be of a transient or permanent character. This bone resorption with resulting increased tooth mobility should be regarded as a physiologic adaptation of the periodontal ligament and surrounding alveolar bone to the traumatizing forces, i.e. to altered functional demands.

In teeth with progressive, plaque-associated periodontal disease, trauma from occlusion may, however, under certain conditions enhance the rate of progression of the disease, i.e. act as a co-factor in the destructive process. From a clinical point of view, this knowledge strengthens the demand for proper treatment of plaque associated with periodontal disease. This treatment will arrest the destruction of the periodontal tissues even if the occlusal trauma persists. A treatment directed towards the trauma alone, however, i.e. occlusal adjustment or splinting, may reduce the mobility of the traumatized teeth and result in some regrowth of bone, but it will not arrest the rate of further breakdown of the supporting apparatus caused by plaque. (For a detailed discussion of treatment of teeth exhibiting increased mobility, see Chapter 30.)

REFERENCES

Baer, P., Kakehashi, S., Littleton, N.W., White, C.L. & Lieberman, J.E. (1963). Alveolar bone loss and occlusal wear. *Periodontics* **1**, 91.

Belting, C.M. & Gupta, O.P. (1961). The influence of psychiatric disturbances on the severity of periodontal disease. *Journal of Periodontology* **32**, 219-226.

Box, H.K. (1935). Experimental traumatogenic occlusion in sheep. *Oral Health* **25**, 9-25.

Burgett, F., Ramfjord, S., Nissle, R., Morrison, E., Charbeneau, T. & Caffesse, R. (1992). A randomized trial of occlusal adjustment in the treatment of periodontitis patients. *Journal of Clinical Periodontology* **19**, 381-387.

Ericsson, I. & Lindhe, J. (1977). Lack of effect of trauma from occlusion on the recurrence of experimental periodontitis. *Journal of Clinical Periodontology* **4**, 115-127.

Ericsson, I. & Lindhe, J. (1982). The effect of longstanding jiggling on experimental marginal periodontitis in the beagle dog. *Journal of Clinical Periodontology* **9**, 497-503.

Ewen, S.J. & Stahl. S.S. (1962). The response of the periodontium to chronic gingival irritation and long-term tilting forces in adult dogs. *Oral Surgery, Oral Medicine, Oral Pathology* **15**, 1426-1433.

Fleszar, T.J., Knowles, J.W., Morrison, E.C., Burgett, F.G., Nissle, R.R. & Ramfjord, S.P. (1980). Tooth mobility and periodontal therapy. *Journal of Clinical Periodontology* **7**, 495-505.

Glickman, I. (1965). Clinical significance of trauma from occlusion. *Journal of the American Dental Association* **70**, 607-618.

Glickman, I. (1967). Occlusion and periodontium. *Journal of Dental Research* **46**, Supplement 1, 53.

Glickman, I. & Smulow, J.B. (1962). Alterations in the pathway of gingival inflammation into the underlying tissues induced by excessive occlusal forces. *Journal of Periodontology* **33**, 7-13.

Glickman, I. & Smulow, J.B. (1965). Effect of excessive occlusal forces upon the pathway of gingival inflammation in humans. *Journal of Periodontology* **36**, 141-147.

Glickman, I. & Smulow, J.B. (1968). Adaptive alteration in the periodontium of the Rhesus monkey in chronic trauma from occlusion. *Journal of Periodontology* **39**, 101-105.

Häupl, K. & Psansky, R. (1938). Histologische Untersuchungen der Wirdungsweise der in der Funktions-Kiefer-Orthopedie verwendeten Apparate. *Deutsche Zahn-, Mund- und Kieferheilkunde* **5**, 214.

Karolyi, M. (1901). Beobachtungen über Pyorrhea alveolaris. *Osterreichisch-Ungarische Viertel Jahresschrift für Zahnheilkunde* **17**, 279.

Karring, T., Nyman, S., Thilander, B. & Magnusson, I. (1982). Bone regeneration in orthodontically produced alveolar bone dehiscences. *Journal of Periodontal Research* **17**, 309-315.

Lindhe, J. & Ericsson, I. (1982). The effect of elimination of jiggling forces on periodontally exposed teeth in the dog. *Journal of Periodontology* **53**, 562-567.

Lindhe, J. & Svanberg, G. (1974). Influences of trauma from occlusion on progression of experimental periodontitis in the Beagle dog. *Journal of Clinical Periodontology* **1**, 3-14.

Lovdahl, A., Schei, O., Waerhaug, J. & Arno, A. (1959). Tooth mobility and alveolar bone resorption as a function of occlusal stress and oral hygiene. *Acta Odontologica Scandinavica* **17**, 61-77.

Macapanpan, L.C. & Weinmann, J.P. (1954). The influence of injury to the periodontal membrane on the spread of gingival inflammation. *Journal of Dental Research* **33**, 263-272.

Manson, J.D. (1976). Bone morphology and bone loss in periodontal disease. *Journal of Clinical Periodontology* **3**, 14-22.

Meitner, S.W. (1975). *Co-destructive factors of marginal periodontitis and repetitive Mechanical injury.* Thesis. Rochester, USA: Eastman Dental Center and The University of Rochester, USA.

Mühlemann, H.R. & Herzog, H. (1961). Tooth mobility and microscopic tissue changes reproduced by experimental occlusal trauma. *Helvetica Odontologia Acta* **5**, 33-39.

Neiderud, A-M., Ericsson, I. & Lindhe, J. (1992). Probing pocket depth at mobile/nonmobile teeth. *Journal of Clinical Periodontology* **19**, 754-759.

Nyman, S., Lindhe, J. & Ericsson, I. (1978). The effect of progressive tooth mobility on destructive periodontitis in the dog. *Journal of Clinical Periodontology* **7**, 351-360.

Pihlstrom, B.L., Anderson, K.A., Aeppli, D. & Schaffer, E.M. (1986). Association between signs of trauma from occlusion and periodontitis. *Journal of Periodontology* **57**, 1-6.

Polson, A. & Zander, H. (1983). Effect of periodontal trauma upon infrabony pockets. *Journal of Periodontology* **54**, 586-591.

Posselt, U. & Emslie, R.D. (1959). Occlusal disharmonies and their effect on periodontal diseases. *International Dental Journal* **9**, 367-381.

Prichard, J.F. (1965). *Advanced periodontal disease.* Philadelphia: W.B. Saunders.

Reitan, K. (1951). The initial tissue reaction incident to orthodontic tooth movement as related to the influence of function. *Acta Odontologica Scandinavica* **10**, Supplement 6.

Rosling, B., Nyman, S. & Lindhe, J. (1976). The effect of systematic plaque control on bone regeneration in infrabony pockets. *Journal of Clinical Periodontology* **3**, 38-53.

Steiner, G.G., Pearson, J.K. & Ainamo, J. (1981). Changes of the marginal periodontium as a result of labial tooth movement in monkeys. *Journal of Periodontology* **56**, 314-320.

Stillman, P.R. (1917). The management of pyorrhea. *Dental Cosmos* **59**, 405.

Stones, H.H. (1938). An experimental investigation into the association of traumatic occlusion with periodontal disease. *Proceedings of the Royal Society of Medicine* **31**, 479-495.

Svanberg, G. & Lindhe, J. (1973). Experimental tooth hypermobility in the dog. A methodological study. *Odontologisk Revy* **24**, 269-282.

Waerhaug, J. (1979). The infrabony pocket and its relationship to trauma from occlusion and subgingival plaque. *Journal of Periodontology* **50**, 355-365.

Waerhaug, J. & Hansen, E.R. (1966). Periodontal changes incident to prolonged occlusal overload in monkeys. *Acta Odontologica Scandinavica* **24**, 91-105.

Wennström, J., Lindhe, J., Sinclair, F. & Thilander, B. (1987). Some periodontal tissue resections to orthodontic tooth movement in monkeys. *Journal of Clinical Periodontology* **14**, 121-129.

Wentz, F.M., Jarabak, J. & Orban, B. (1958). Experimental occlusal trauma imitating cuspal interferences. *Journal of Periodontology* **29**, 117-127.

CHAPTER 16

Periodontitis as a Risk for Systemic Disease

RAY C. WILLIAMS AND DAVID PAQUETTE

Early 1900 beliefs

The concept of risk

  Understanding the concept of risk

Periodontitis as a risk for:

  Coronary heart disease
  Pregnancy complications
  Diabetic complications
  Respiratory infections

Summary

Throughout the history of mankind, there has been the belief that diseases and maladies which affect the mouth, such as periodontal disease, can have an effect on the rest of the body. Over the centuries, writings from the ancient Egyptians, Hebrews, Assyrians, Greeks and Romans to name a few, have all noted the importance of the mouth in overall health and well-being. Thus, one could say that the concept linking periodontitis and systemic disease can be traced back to the beginning of recorded history and medicine (O'Reilly & Claffey 2000).

This chapter examines the emerging new evidence collected since the early 1990s implicating periodontal infection as a risk factor for several systemic conditions such as coronary heart disease, preterm low birthweight infants, diabetes and pulmonary disease. But first, it is helpful for the student of dentistry to understand the historical perspective under which this relationship emerged. The concept of "focal infection" which emerged around 1900 (but died out in the 1940s) has resurfaced and stimulated much debate and research to elucidate and understand the true nature of the role of periodontitis as a risk for systemic disease.

EARLY 1900 BELIEFS THAT ORAL INFECTION CAUSED SYSTEMIC DISEASE

At the beginning of the twentieth century, medicine and dentistry were searching for reasons to explain why people became afflicted with a wide range of systemic diseases. Medicine at that time had very little insight into what caused diseases such as arthritis, pneumonia and pancreatitis, to name a few. Then, through the writings and lectures of principally two individuals, W. D. Miller and William Hunter, the concept that oral bacteria and infection were the likely cause of most of a person's systemic illnesses suddenly became very popular (O'Reilly & Claffey 2000). For the next 40 years physicians and dentists would embrace the idea that infections, especially those originating in the mouth, caused most of man's suffering and illness. This era, which came to be known as the "era of focal infection", can be attributed primarily to a microbiologist in Philadelphia, Willoughby D. Miller and a London physician, William Hunter (O'Reilly & Claffey 2000).

Willoughby Miller was a highly regarded Professor at the University of Pennsylvania School of Dental Medicine around the turn of the nineteenth century. Miller had earlier trained in microbiology with Robert Koch, a scientific pioneer in microbiology and the father of the modern "germ theory" of disease. While under the tutelage of Robert Koch, Miller too became intensely interested in the role of "germs" or bacteria in causing diseases. Miller returned to the US following his trainings convinced that the bacteria residing in the mouth could cause or be attributed to most systemic diseases in patients. In a paper published in 1891, entitled "The human mouth as a focus of infection", Miller argued that the oral flora caused ostitis, osteomyelitis, septicemia, pyemia, disturbances of the alimentary tract, noma, dyptheria, tuberculosis, syphilis and thrush (Miller 1891). Clearly from this one publication, one can appreciate just how extensively the mouth and oral infection were blamed for causing systemic disease (O'Reilly & Claffey 2000).

While attending one of Miller's lectures at the International Congress of Hygiene, William Hunter, a physician from the London Fever Hospital, noted that he and Miller were in strong agreement about the systemic impact of oral infections or oral sepsis. Shortly after, Hunter was invited to speak at the opening of the Strathcona Medical Building at McGill University in Montreal in 1910. In his address to the audience, he blamed poor dentistry and the resulting oral sepsis for causing most of mankind's morbidity. Hunter remarked that the crowns, bridges and partial dentures he saw in his patients in London were built on teeth surrounded by a "mass of sepsis". Indeed this oral sepsis could explain why most individuals developed chronic diseases (Hunter 1900, O'Reilly & Claffey, 2000). It is likely that Hunter was referring to the untreated periodontal disease, caries and defective restorations in his patients at the London Fever Hospital (Fig. 16-1). But whatever Hunter thought he observed in the mouths of his sick patients, his speech at McGill University and his subsequent publication on the role of sepsis and antisepsis in medicine (Hunter 1910) ushered in an era of blaming periodontal disease, caries and poor oral hygiene as the primary cause of systemic illness. The term "oral sepsis" used by Hunter was replaced with the term "focal infection" in 1911 (Billings 1912). "Focal infection" implied that there was a nidus of infection somewhere in the body, such as periodontitis, which via the bloodstream could affect distant sites and organs. Throughout the 1920s and 1930s, dentists and physicians believed that the bacteria on the teeth and the resultant infectious diseases such as caries, gingivitis and periodontitis that followed, were a "focus of infection" that led to a wide variety of systemic problems. It became popular during this period to extract teeth as a means of ridding the body of oral bacteria and preventing and/or treating diseases affecting the joints, as well as diseases of the heart, liver, kidneys and pancreas (Cecil & Angevine 1938, O'Reilly & Claffey 2000).

However, by 1940, medicine and dentistry were realizing that there was much more to explain a patient's general systemic condition than bacteria in his or her mouth. Dentists and physicians realized that (1) extracting a person's teeth did not necessarily make the person better or make their disease go away, (2) people with very healthy mouths and no obvious oral infection developed systemic disease, and (3) people who had no teeth and thus no apparent oral infection still developed systemic diseases (Galloway 1931, Cecil & Angevine 1938).

By 1950 it was apparent to medicine and dentistry that oral infections such as dental caries, gingivitis and periodontitis could not explain why individuals developed a wide range of systemic diseases. Medicine was, by this time, making great strides in discovering

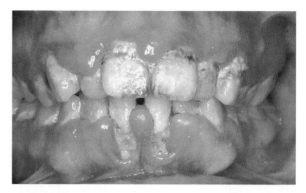

Fig. 16-1. Poor oral conditions including large plaque accumulation, caries, gingivitis and periodontitis were popularly blamed for causing systemic diseases in the early 1900s.

the true etiologies of many diseases, and dentistry was making great strides in the prevention as well as the treatment of caries and periodontal disease. And so the era of "focal infection" as a primary cause of systemic diseases finally came to an end (O'Reilly & Claffey 2000).

Throughout the second half of the twentieth century, several researchers and clinicians continued to ask the question whether oral infection (and inflammation) might in some way contribute to a person's overall health, but the reasons given were mostly speculative. Clinicians continued to propose that bacteria and bacterial products within the periodontal pocket, which reached the bloodstream from the mouth, could surely in some way be harmful to the body as a whole (Thoden van Velzen et al. 1984). However, it was not until the last decade of the twentieth century that dentistry and medicine again began to examine the relationship of oral infection as a risk for systemic disease. The student of dentistry thus needs to appreciate the intense focus on oral infection as a "possible" cause of many systemic diseases from 1900-1950, then the era of retreat from the focal infection theories of disease causation from 1950 to around 1989, and now the careful new look at periodontitis as a possible risk for systemic disease using discreet scientific levels of evidence.

THE CONCEPT OF RISK

Since around 1989 dentistry has again turned its attention to examining a possible relationship of oral infection in contributing to an individual's risk for systemic disease. The student should note that dentistry has come a long way in how we study such a relationship. In the first half of the twentieth century, the evidence was primarily anecdotal and based on testimony and statements from dentists and physicians. There was no scientific evidence. At present, however, a group of highly trained epidemiologists, basic scientists and clinical scientists are using modern scientific method-

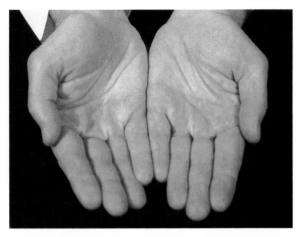

Fig. 16-2. In a patient having 28 teeth and with advanced periodontitis of all teeth, the subgingival surface area of infection could be roughly similar to the surface area represented by the two hands.

ology, to carefully and, hopefully, accurately examine the relationship of periodontitis to systemic disease.

In 1989, Kimmo Matilla and his co-workers in Finland conducted a case-control study on patients who had experienced an acute myocardial infarction, and they compared these patients to control subjects selected from the community. A dental examination was performed on all of the patients and subjects studied and a dental index computed. The dental index used by Matilla was the sum of scores from the number of carious lesions, missing teeth and periapical lesions, and probing depth measures to indicate periodontitis and the presence or absence of pericoronitis. Matilla and his group reported a highly significant association between poor dental health, as measured by the dental index, and acute myocardial infarction. The association was independent of other risk factors for heart attack such as age, total cholesterol, high density lipoprotein (HDL) triglycerides, C peptide, hypertension, diabetes and smoking (Matilla et al. 1989).

Matilla's provocative findings generated a great deal of interest in the scientific community. Medicine and dentistry were actively studying the concept of "risk" and were seeking "risk factors" that might help explain why certain individuals were more susceptible to disease or why certain individuals responded better than others to treatment of disease. Might it be possible that periodontitis and dental infection did in fact confer risk on a person for an acute myocardial infarction? In looking back, it appears that Matilla's findings came at a critical time in dentistry and the study of "risk".

Dental scientists first turned their attention to understanding the "biologic plausibility" of how periodontitis might confer risk for systemic disease. Offenbacher, Page, Loesche, Genco, Beck and their colleagues, to name a few scientists, noted that periodontitis and the anaerobic subgingival infection associated with periodontitis certainly had the potential, via the bloodstream, to reach and affect distant sites and

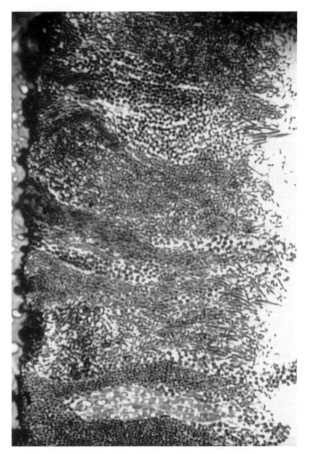

Fig. 16-3. A highly organized biofilm within a periodontal pocket consisting primarily of Gram-negative anaerobic bacteria.

organs. Periodontal investigators noted that a patient who had, for example, 28 teeth with pocket depths of 6-7 mm and bone loss, had a large overall surface area of infection and inflammation (Waite & Bradley 1965). In patients with moderate periodontitis, the surface area could be the size of the palm of the hand or larger (Fig. 16-2). In addition, the subgingival bacteria in deep periodontal pockets exists in a highly organized biofilm (Fig. 16-3). Subgingival biofilms would represent a large and continuing bacterial load and would be a constant source of lipopolysaccharide (LPS) as well as Gram-negative bacteria to the bloodstream. Proinflammatory cytokines such as TNF-α, 1L-1β, IFN-γ and PGE$_2$ can reach high concentrations in the tissues of the periodontium. The periodontium can then serve as a renewing reservoir for spillover of these mediators into the circulation. Thus, periodontal pockets containing a Gram-negative biofilm and periodontitis-affected tissues would have the striking potential to flood the circulation with bacteria, bacterial products such as LPS and inflammatory cytokines, all of which could reach all parts of the body and possibly affect distant sites and organs (Loesche 1994, Beck et al. 1996, 1998, Offenbacher 1996, Page 1998a, Genco et al. 1999).

Recognizing that it was indeed possible to comprehend how periodontitis could contribute to systemic disease (the "biologic plausibility" of such an idea), the dental profession then turned its attention to examining existing epidemiological data to see if a relationship between periodontitis and systemic disease could be extracted from these existing data sets. Over the years, several large epidemiological studies had been conducted on the health status of various populations. Examples of these studies are the National Health and Nutrition Examination Surveys I, II and III (NHANES I, II, III) and the Veterans Administration Normative Aging Study. When these epidemiological studies were conducted there was no actual study of the relationship of periodontitis to systemic health and disease. Further, the measures of dental disease and periodontitis in these studies were diverse. For example, one study noted periodontitis "present" if a pocket depth was greater than 5 mm while another study noted periodontitis was "present" if a pocket depth was greater than 4 mm. Another study simply asked the individual whether or not she/he had periodontitis. Thus the clinical measures of periodontitis in these epidemiological data sets are diverse at best and almost non-existent at worst. Still, by just examining these large epidemiology data sets of human subjects, dental researchers have found compelling evidence that periodontitis may be a risk for certain systemic conditions (Loesche 1994, Beck et al. 1996, 1998, Offenbacher 1996, Garcia et al. 2001).

UNDERSTANDING THE CONCEPT OF RISK

If periodontitis is in fact a risk for systemic disease then it is important for the student and the dental profession as a whole to understand how "risk" is studied and evaluated. We need to understand what is meant by "risk factor", "risk indicator", "risk marker" and "background characteristic" (Beck 1994).

In studying risk, the main question is what exactly is a "risk factor". Risk factor implies that the factor in question is part of the cause of the disease. Risk factor is customarily defined as an exposure that increases the probability that disease will occur. In contrast, a risk indicator is a suspected risk factor that is correctly identified through cross-sectional case control study designs but there are not yet longitudinal cohort study data available. Risk markers denote those characteristics that have the ability to predict individuals at high risk for disease, but are not a likely part of the causal chain. Finally, background characteristics are those risk markers that may be strongly predictive of disease, but at present are not changeable (Table 16-1) (Beck 1994, Offenbacher 1996).

Using the above distinctions, medicine continues to focus on identifying exposures that may help explain why certain individuals develop disease. Through these efforts it is hoped that in identifying risk factors one can (1) more accurately identify the cause(s) of a disease, (2) predict which patients are at high risk for

Table 16-1. Definitions of terms commonly used to study and to describe "risk"

Risk factor	An exposure that increases the probability that disease will occur
Risk indicator	A suspected risk factor that is correctly identified through cross-sectional study designs but there are not yet longitudinal study data
Risk marker	A characteristic or factor that has the ability to predict individuals at high risk for disease, but is not likely to be part of the causal chain
Background characteristic	A risk marker or predictor that may be strongly predictive of disease but at present is not changeable

disease or disease progression, (3) aid in the diagnosis of a disease or condition, and (4) provide clues on how to better prevent the disease or condition (Lilienfeld 1967, Beck 1994).

Beck and co-workers, as well as other epidemiologists, teach us that it is not easy to determine whether a suspected risk factor is actually part of the cause of a disease. This can only be done through experimentation, i.e. the randomized controlled trial, and conducting such human experiments is usually neither ethical nor possible. For example, to establish smoking as causative in heart disease in a clinical trial one would have to ask one group of subjects to smoke heavily over several years while control subjects did not smoke, and then examine the evidence of heart disease in the two groups. Thus, criteria were established some years ago by Sir Bradford Hill and later refined by Lilienfeld to help epidemiologists decide whether the evidence from observational studies will support interpreting a possible "risk factor" as causal. It is helpful to understand these criteria, because all of the evidence collected on periodontitis as a risk for systemic disease may be categorized under these criteria (Table 16-2) (Lilienfeld 1967, Beck 1994, Offenbacher 1996, Beck et al. 1998):

1. *Consistency of association*: A risk factor is more likely to be causal if most, if not all, studies dealing with the relationship produce similar positive results. This is especially true if the studies involve different populations, methods or time periods.
2. *Strength of associations*: A valid study is one that is free from error. The stronger the association, the less likely the association is entirely due to error that might distort the results. The strength of association is usually quantified with an odds-ratio in case control studies and a risk ratio in cohort studies.
3. *Correct time sequence*: The potential risk factor must precede the occurrence of the disease. The inability of cross-sectional studies to determine whether the factor occurred before the onset of disease is a major problem in determining causality and thus whether it is a true risk factor.

Table 16-2. Criteria for considering a possible risk factor for a disease as important in causing the disease

Consistency of associations	A factor is more likely to be causal if all studies dealing with the relationship produce similar results. This is especially true if the studies involve different populations, methods or time periods.
Strength of associations	A valid study is one that is free from error. The stronger the association, the less likely that the association is entirely due to error that might distort the results.
Correct time sequence	The potential factor must precede the occurrence of the disease.
Specificity of associations	If a given factor is related to other diseases, its association with the disease is less likely to be interpreted as causal. While a specific association may be more likely to be causal, lack of specificity cannot justify rejecting causality, because many diseases have multiple causes.
Degree of exposure (dose-response effect)	If a factor is of causal importance, then the risk of developing the disease should be related to the degree of exposure to the factor.
Biologic plausibility	The association must make sense in light of current knowledge.
Support from experimental evidence	Experimental reproduction of the disease should occur frequently in animals (humans when possible) exposed to the risk factor. Randomized controlled trials testing interventions to prevent disease occurrence are strong evidence.

4. *Specificity of associations*: If a given factor is related to other diseases, its association with the disease is less likely to be interpreted as causal. While a specific association may be more likely to be causal, lack of specificity cannot justify rejecting causality because many diseases have multiple causes; a single factor may produce a number of different diseases; and a single factor may be a vehicle for other factors.
5. *Degree of exposure*: If a risk factor is of causal importance, then the risk of developing the disease should be related to the degree of exposure to the risk factor. Accordingly, persons with higher levels of exposure should be at higher risk for the condition as compared to those persons with lower levels of exposure.
6. *Biologic plausibility*: The association of the risk factor must make sense in light of current knowledge of the biology or pathogenesis of the disease.
7. *Support from experimental evidence*: Experimental reproduction of the disease should occur frequently in animals exposed to the risk factor. Randomized controlled human trials which test the effect of intervention to prevent disease occurrence are also strong evidence of a causal relationship.

With the above criteria in mind, periodontal investigators began to examine the large epidemiological data sets which were available to ask the question: is there a relationship between existence and severity of periodontal disease and specific systemic diseases? Much of the research so far using the existing data sets has examined a relationship between periodontitis and coronary heart disease. These findings are summarized in the next section.

PERIODONTITIS AS A RISK FOR CORONARY HEART DISEASE

To date, a number of investigators have reported that an association between periodontitis and coronary heart disease/atherosclerosis may exist (Matilla et al. 1995, Beck et al. 1996, 1998, Garcia & Vokonas 1996, Genco et al. 1997, Loesche et al. 1998, Mendez et al. 1998, Morrison et al. 1999, Valtonen et al. 1999, Wu et al. 2000a,b).

Atherosclerosis is a progressive disease process in which large to medium-sized muscular and large elastic arteries become occluded with fibro-lipid lesions (atheromas). Approximately 50% of the deaths in most industrialized countries are attributable to the complications of atherosclerosis, with coronary thrombosis and acute myocardial infarction representing about half of these (Beck et al. 1996). Beck and his colleagues note that atherosclerosis and periodontitis appear to have a number of characteristics in common (Beck et al. 1996). For example, both diseases are more likely to occur in persons who are older, male, of lower educational status, who smoke, are hypertensive, who are stressed and are socially isolated. Beck and Offenbacher suggest that these common characteristics may indicate that periodontal disease and heart disease share a similar etiologic pathway (Beck 1994, Beck et al. 1998, Beck & Offenbacher 1998).

One of the initial compelling reasons for considering periodontitis as a risk factor for cardiovascular disease relates to the strong body of emerging evidence on infections or inflammatory etiologies for atherosclerosis and coronary heart disease. A summary of the evidence is as follows (Beck et al. 1998):

• Prior flu-like symptoms are more common in cases of myocardial infarction than in controls studied at the same time.
• High levels of cytomegalovirus antibodies were associated with elevated carotid intimal-medial wall thickness 18 years later.
• Prior infection with cytomegalovirus is a strong independent risk factor for restenosis after coronary atherectomy.
• Dental infections are more common in cases of cerebral infarction compared to control subjects matched for age and gender.

Table 16-3. Strength and consistency of associations between oral conditions and atherosclerosis/coronary heart disease (CHD). From Beck et al. 1998 with permission.

Study	Design	Association	Measure
Mattila et al. 1989/Finland	Case-control	Total dental index and heart attack	OR = 1.3
Mattila et al. 1993/Finland	Case-control	Total dental index and atheromatosis	OR = 1.4
Mattila et al. 1995/Finland	Follow-up	Total dental index and new events	HR = 1.2
DeStefano et al. 1993/USA	Cohort	PI, OHI, and admits and death due to CHD	RR = 1.2
Beck et al. 1996/Boston	Cohort	PD, bone levels, and new CHD, fatal CHD & stroke	OR = 1.5, 1.9, 2.8
Genco et al. 1997/USA	Cohort	Bone loss and new CHD	OR = 2.7
Joshipura et al. 1996/USA	Cohort	Tooth loss in men with periodontal disease and CHD	RR = 1.7

PI = plaque index; OHI = oral hygiene instruction; PD = probing depth.

Table 16-4. Specificity of associations between oral conditions and atherosclerosis/coronary heart disease (CHD). From Beck et al. 1998 with permission.

Study	Association	Measure	Adjusted
Mattila et al. 1989/Finland	Total dental index and heart attack	OR = 1.3	Yes
Mattila et al. 1993/Finland	Total dental index and atheromatosis	OR = 1.4	Yes
Mattila et al. 1995/Finland	Total dental index and new events	HR = 1.2	Yes
DeStefano et al. 1993/USA	PI, OHI, and admits and death due to CHD	RR = 1.2	Yes
Beck et al. 1996/Boston	PD, bone levels, and new CHD, fatal CHD and stroke	OR = 1.5, 1.9, 2.8	Yes
Genco et al. 1997/USA	Bone loss and new CHD	OR = 2.7	Yes
Joshipura et al. 1996/USA	Tooth loss in men with periodontal disease and CHD	RR = 1.7	Yes

Table 16-5. Time sequence for associations between oral conditions and atherosclerosis/coronary heart disease (CHD). From Beck et al. 1998 with permission.

Study	Association	Sequence
Mattila et al. 1995/Finland	Total dental index and new events	Oral condition prior to 7-year follow-up of patients with myocardial infarction
DeStefano et al. 1993/USA	PI, OHI, and admits and death due to CHD	Oral status prior to 14-year follow-up; assumed to be w/o CHD at baseline
Beck et al. 1996/Boston	PD, bone levels, and new CHD, fatal CHD and stroke	PD and bone loss prior to 18-year follow-up of men w/o CHD
Genco et al. 1997/USA	Bone loss and new CHD	Bone loss prior to 10-year follow-up
Joshipura et al. 1996/USA	Tooth loss in men with periodontal disease and CHD	Men reporting signs and symptoms of CHD excluded from follow-up analysis

- The gingival index is significantly correlated with fibrinogen and white cell counts in periodontal patients and controls, adjusted for age, smoking and socio-economic status.
- Plasma levels of cholesterol, low density lipoprotein cholesterol and triglycerides were significantly higher in 46 periodontitis patients aged 50-60 compared to age and gender-matched controls. In addition, successful periodontal therapy was more likely in persons with lower lipid values (Beck et al. 1998).

As noted earlier, in order to evaluate the data contained in large existing data sets which may link periodontitis to systemic disease, investigators used the criteria for studying risk outlined by Lilienfeld (1967). What follows is a summary of evidence gathered to date from these epidemiological studies and the data are presented in Tables 16-3, 16-4 and 16-5.

Consistency, strength and specificity of associations

Matilla and co-workers conducted two separate case-control studies totaling 100 patients with acute myocardial infarction and 102 controls selected from the community. In Matilla's original 1989 report, subjects with evidence of oral infection were 30% more likely to present with myocardial infarction relative to subjects without oral infections (Matilla et al. 1989, Matilla 1989).

In a second case control report, Matilla and co-workers noted associations between dental infections and the degree of atherosclerosis. This study examined the same subjects as the first report but pertained to information obtained with diagnostic coronary angiography. Accordingly, the left main coronary artery, the a, b, and c portions of the right coronary artery, the circumflex artery, and the left anterior descending artery were assessed diagnostically and graded for a degree of occlusion on a 5-point scale. Again, the total dental index score was used as a general score for dental caries, endodontics and periodontal infections. In a multivariate analysis, significant associations were found between dental infections, age and triglycerides and severe coronary atheromatosis. These associations remained significant even after adjusting for other known risk factors like total cholesterol, HDL, smoking, hypertension, socio-economic status and body mass index. The authors postulated that bacterial infections have profound effects on endothelial cells, monocyte-macrophages, thrombocytes and blood coagulation and lipid metabolism, and concluded that dental infections are the only factor outside the scope of the classic coronary risk factors which have shown an independent association with the severity of adult coronary atherosclerosis in their multivariate assessment (Matilla et al. 1993, Beck et al. 1998). Continuing to monitor for myocardial infarction among the cases in these first case control reports, Matilla et al. (1995) presented Cox proportional hazard models further implicating dental infection as a significant risk factor for new cardiovascular events.

DeStefano and co-workers assessed the association between periodontal disease and coronary heart disease within the National Health and Nutrition Examination Survey I (NHANES I), which followed subjects for 14 years. This cohort study examined several potentially confounding variables including age, gender, race, education, marital status, systolic blood pressure, total cholesterol levels, body mass index, diabetes, physical activity, alcohol consumption, poverty and cigarette smoking. These investigators reported that among the 9760 subjects examined longitudinally, those with periodontitis had a 25% increased risk of coronary heart disease relative to those with minimal periodontal disease, adjusted for the co-variables mentioned above (DeStefano et al. 1993). Interestingly, males younger than 50 years old with periodontitis

were 72% more likely to develop coronary heart disease compared to their periodontally healthy counterparts.

Using data obtained in the Normative Aging Study, Beck and co-workers evaluated 921 men aged 21-80 years who were free of coronary heart disease at baseline. Over an 18-year follow-up period, 207 men developed coronary heart disease, 59 died of coronary heart disease and 40 had strokes. Odds ratios adjusted for age and established cardiovascular risk factors were 1.5, 1.9 and 2.8 for periodontal bone loss and total coronary heart disease, fatal coronary heart disease and stroke respectively (Bell et al. 1966, Kapur et al. 1972, Beck et al. 1996, Garcia & Vokonas 1996). These data indicated that persons with radiographic evidence of periodontitis were 0.5 to 2.8 times more likely to develop coronary heart disease or suffer from a vascular event.

In a larger six-year cohort study, Joshipura and co-workers followed 44 119 men in the health professions who reported no coronary heart disease symptoms at baseline, no notable dietary histories and no missing information on age or number of teeth. All information was obtained via mailed questionnaires. Joshipura and her group found that the association between self-reported history of periodontal disease and incidence of heart disease was not significant after adjusting for other risk factors such as age, body mass, exercise, smoking habits, alcohol consumption, family history of myocardial infarction before age 60 and intake of vitamin E (relative risk = 1.04). It should be noted that most of the studies showing a positive association between periodontal disease and coronary heart disease have highlighted the importance of the extent of periodontal disease burden in the relationship. Since the subjects in this study dichotomously responded to a question about periodontal disease (yes/no) it is not possible to quantify the extent of the periodontal disease present in these participants. In addition, misclassification from self-reported periodontal disease seems very likely. The study did however demonstrate that men with tooth loss and periodontal disease were 70% more likely to exhibit coronary heart disease (Joshipura et al. 1996).

Genco and co-workers investigated the association between periodontal infection and risk of cardiovascular disease in 1372 Native Americans of the Gila River Indian Community, a group with a high prevalence of diabetes mellitus. At baseline, alveolar bone level was measured and cardiovascular status was monitored for up to 10 years. Among all age groups, alveolar bone level was predictive of coronary heart disease, but did not remain significant in a multivariate analysis. In contrast, for persons younger than 60 years of age, alveolar bone level was predictive of coronary heart disease, with an odds ratio of 2.68 (Genco et al. 1997).

A recent report of another examination of the NHANES I data did not find an association between periodontal disease and subsequent heart disease.

Hujoel and co-workers evaluated the same population cohort as DeStefano and colleagues but for a longer 21-year follow-up. The Hujoel et al. study extensively adjusted for possible confounding factors, and this may account for the lack of any detected significant relationship after adjustment. It is also likely that significant misclassification occurred in the periodontal status over time, with those classified as having no periodontal disease at baseline developing periodontal disease over the 21 years of study. Lastly, misclassification of those having periodontal disease at baseline may have occurred over time as a result of treatment and extractions (Hujoel et al. 2000).

Table 16-3 summarizes the strength and consistency of associations for oral conditions as risk factors for coronary heart disease. It is interesting to note the consistency of the associations across studies that used different study designs and a variety of measures for both the exposure and outcome.

Specificity of the associations between periodontitis and coronary heart disease

The specificity of the associations between oral conditions and heart disease are summarized in Table 16-4. The associations in these studies have been adjusted for established risk factors for atherosclerosis and coronary heart disease, indicating that the associations found are not confounded by those factors. The student should remember that the criterion of specificity suggests that the condition being studied such as periodontitis is more likely to be a risk factor if it is specifically related to a single disease and not multiple diseases. Data relating periodontitis as a risk for preterm low birthweight infants, diabetes and other systemic conditions suggest that periodontitis does not fully meet the criterion of specificity. However, it is the combined weight of the evidence that is most important. It is of course possible for an exposure to be a risk factor for multiple conditions. Cigarette smoking is one such example (Beck et al. 1998).

Correct time sequence

Table 16-5 presents data which examine the time sequence for an association between oral conditions and atherosclerosis/coronary heart disease. Because the reviewed case control studies conducted by Matilla and co-workers (1989, 1993) selected subjects on the basis of diagnosed coronary heart disease, they lack information on whether periodontitis preceded the cardiovascular diagnosis. The Matilla et al. (1995) study is a follow-up of patients who were hospitalized with myocardial infarction; therefore the disease was present prior to oral status measurement. The DeStefano et al. study is a cohort study so it is assumed that any NHANES I subjects who had heart disease at baseline were not included in the analysis. The Beck

and co-workers study enrolled only participants who were systemically healthy, so oral disease present at baseline did not precede the development of the cardiovascular outcome. The outcome variable in the Genco et al. study was new cardiovascular disease. The outcome variable in the Joshipura et al. study was new coronary heart disease. Thus there are at least a few studies that meet the time sequence criterion for establishing periodontitis as a risk for coronary heart disease (Beck et al. 1998, Garcia et al. 2001).

Degree of exposure

The degree of exposure of the suspected risk factor is considered important in establishing causation because increasing dose levels of the purported risk factor or exposure should lead to increasing probabilities for the disease.

Figs. 16-4, 16-5 and 16-6 are taken from Beck and co-workers' reports (Beck et al. 1996, 1998). One can note that with increasing periodontitis severity as measured with bone loss there is a higher cumulative frequency of occurrence of coronary heart disease. Levels of alveolar bone loss and cumulative incidence of total coronary heart disease and fatal coronary heart disease indicated a biologic gradient between severity of exposure and occurrence of disease.

Figs. 16-7 and 16-8 are new analyses from Beck and co-workers' research (Beck et al. 1996, 1998) that looked more closely at the amount of exposure to periodontal infection. Fig. 16-7 presents the number of sites with > 20% bone loss adjusted for age in an attempt to describe whether the extent of the infection was related to total coronary heart disease. The line represents the values predicted from the logistic regression model, assuming a linear dose-response relationship between increasing numbers of sites with greater than 20% bone loss and total coronary heart disease, adjusting for age. The model is significant with a P value of 0.02 and shows that the predicted odds ratios run from 1.04 for 1 or 2 sites up to 2.5 for 11 to 20 sites with bone loss greater than 20%.

Fig. 16-8 presents the same information, except that the relationship between the number of sites of bone loss and total coronary heart disease was adjusted for all relevant risk factors. Both figures provide support for a dose-response gradient between extent of periodontal bone loss and coronary heart disease independent of other known risk factors.

Arbes et al. (1999) recently evaluated the association between periodontal disease and coronary heart disease in the third National Health and Nutrition Examination Survey (NHANES III) and found that the odds for a history of heart attack increased with the severity of periodontal disease. With the highest severity of periodontal disease, the odds ratio was 3.8 (95% confidence interval; 1.5-9.7) as compared to no periodontal disease after adjustment for age, gender, race, poverty, smoking, diabetes, high blood pressure,

Cumulative incidence of CHD, %

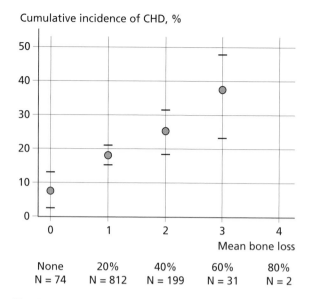

Fig. 16-4. Age-adjusted level of bone loss and cumulative incidence of coronary heart disease.

Cumulative incidence of fatal CHD, %

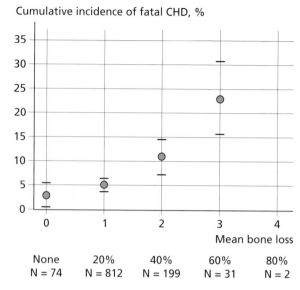

Fig. 16-5. Age-adjusted level of bone loss and cumulative incidence of fatal coronary heart disease.

Cumulative incidence of stroke, %

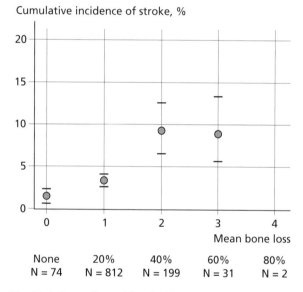

Fig. 16-6. Age-adjusted level of bone loss and cumulative incidence of stroke.

body mass index and serum cholesterol. This cross-sectional study adds additional evidence for an association seen in the Beck et al. (1996) study, and shows a dose response with high levels of periodontal disease associated with higher prevalence of reported heart attack.

Biological plausibility

It has been particularly helpful in the ongoing study of risk to try to understand the "biologic plausibility" or scientific logic that would explain a link between periodontitis and atherosclerosis/coronary heart disease. As noted earlier, for many years infection has been suspected as a risk factor for atherosclerosis and coronary heart disease (Thorn et al. 1992, Loesche 1994, Danesh et al. 1997). Other suspected etiologic

infectious agents in atherogenesis include cytomegalovirus, herpes virus, *H. pylori* and *C. pneumoniae*. The inflammatory response to these infections, and the large body of evidence on inflammatory pathways in atherogenesis, certainly provide reasons to believe that the inflammation resulting from periodontal infection and periodontitis may contribute to coronary heart disease (Beck et al. 1998, Ross 1999).

Several investigators have suggested that there is marked variability in individual host responses to bacterial challenge with periodontitis (Offenbacher 1996, Beck et al. 1998, Page 1998a,b). Such variability has been attributed to individual differences in T cell and monocyte functions, with such differences in part having a genetic basis. Some individuals may respond to a microbial or lipopolysaccharide (LPS) challenge with an abnormally high inflammatory response, as reflected in the release of high levels of pro-inflammatory mediators such as PGE_2, IL-1β, and TNF-α. In laboratory tests, peripheral blood monocytes from these hyperinflammatory monocyte phenotype patients secrete three-fold to ten-fold greater amounts of these mediators in response to LPS than those from normal monocyte phenotype individuals. Such observations have led to the hypothesis that the variation in inflammatory responses may be a direct consequence of at least two factors: those genes that regulate the T cell-monocyte response, and the host-microbial environment, which can trigger and modulate the response (Offenbacher 1996, Beck et al. 1998, Page 1998a,b).

Beck, Offenbacher and colleagues propose that the natural histories of both periodontitis and coronary heart disease/atherosclerosis may in fact be related to a common hyper-reactive inflammatory phenotype or response. They further list several pathogenic characteristics shared by the two diseases (Beck & Offenbacher 1998, Beck et al. 1998, Offenbacher et al. 1999):

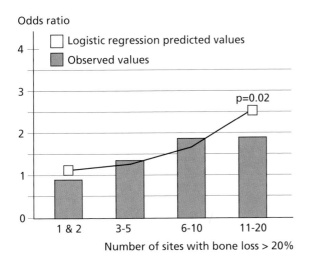

Fig. 16-7. Odds ratios and 95% confidence intervals for number of sites with > 20% bone loss and total coronary heart disease adjusted for age.

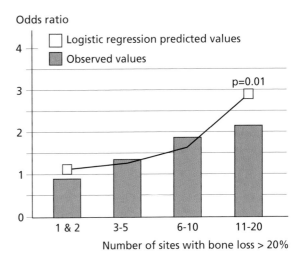

Fig. 16-8. Odds ratios and 95% confidence intervals for number of sites with > 20% bone loss and total coronary heart disease adjusted for age and other relevant risk factors.

1. Cells of the monocytic lineage and the attendant cytokines play a critical role in initiating and propagating both atheroma formation and periodontitis.
2. The hyper-inflammatory phenotype appears to be under both genetic and environmental influence. Monocytic hyper-responsiveness to LPS has been genetically mapped tentatively to the area of HLA-DR3/3 or -DQ which is the region where increased susceptibility to Type 1 diabetes mellitus has been proposed to reside. Furthermore, dietary-induced elevation of serum low-density lipoprotein has been shown to upregulate monocytic responses to LPS, thereby providing a behavorial or environmental influence on the macrophage phenotype. Known risk factors for coronary heart disease such as dietary fat intake may therefore enhance monocyte secretion of inflammatory and tissue destructive cytokines, and via this common mechanism, may contribute to the severity of the expression of coronary heart disease and periodontal disease.
3. Periodontal infections may directly contribute to the pathogenesis of atherosclerosis and thromboembolic events by providing repeated systemic challenges with LPS and inflammatory cytokines.

There is also evidence that some of the bacteria found in dental plaque may have a direct effect on atherosclerosis and thromboembolic events. Herzberg and co-workers have reported that the oral Gram-positive bacterium *S. sanguis* and the Gram-negative periodontal pathogen *P. gingivalis* have been shown to induce platelet aggregation and activation through the expression of collagen-like platelet aggregation-associated proteins. The aggregated platelets may then play a role in atheroma formation and thromboembolic events (Herzberg et al. 1983, Herzberg & Meyer 1996, 1998).

A recent study by Haraszthy et al. identified periodontal pathogens in human carotid atheromas

(Haraszthy et al. 2000). Fifty carotid atheromas obtained at endarterectomy were analyzed for the presence of bacterial 16-S rDNA by PCR using synthetic oligonucleotide probes specific for the periodontal pathogens *A.a.*, *B. forsythus*, *P. gingivalis* and *P. intermedia*. Thirty per cent of the specimens were positive for *B. forsythus*, 26% positive for *P. gingivalis*, 18% positive for *A. a.* and 14% positive for *P. intermedia*. *Chlamydia pneumoniae* DNA was detected in 18% of the atheromas. These and other studies suggest that periodontal pathogens may be present in atherosclerotic plaques, where, like other infectious organisms, they may play a role in atherogenesis (Genco et al. 1999).

Experimental evidence

There is ongoing research to see if well-controlled prospective studies in animal models and in human subjects can confirm or extend the evidence for a role for periodontitis as a risk for systemic disease. Beck and co-workers (1998) have studied the effects of *P. gingivalis* infection and high-fat diets in atheroma formation in mice. Using a knock-out mouse model genetically susceptible to cardiovascular disease (heterozygotic APOE), animals were given a high-fat or low-fat diet. Small steel coil chambers were implanted subcutaneously and the rejection of the chambers after inoculation with *P. gingivalis* HG405 was examined. The animals were first immunized with a dose of heat-killed *P. gingivalis* and 21 days later challenged with live *P. gingivalis*. The sloughing of the chamber would represent an intense inflammatory reaction to the infectious agent. Initial findings suggest that a high-fat diet in the susceptible mouse strain was associated with a tendency to exhibit increased risk of serious inflammation. This initial study at least links dietary fat intake in a susceptible mouse to an inflammatory response to a periodontal pathogen, *P. gingi-*

valis. Geva et al. (2000) in this group have reported that infection of mice with a more virulent *P. gingivalis* strain leads to increased atheroma size and calcification with the amount of calcification increasing with the length of exposure. In no instance was calcification found in mice not exposed to *P. gingivalis*. Further, significantly greater amounts of bone morphogenic protein-2 (BMP-2) were found in the atheromas of the *P. gingivalis* challenged mice (Chung et al. 2002). These data indicate that infection with a virulent strain of *P. gingivalis* can promote atheroma formation and arterial calcification via up-regulation of BMPs in a mouse model.

When one looks at the collective evidence gathered so far, it seems clear that, at least from historical epidemiological data, there is a compelling link between periodontitis and coronary heart disease. There are also emerging data which strongly suggest that periodontitis may be a risk for pregnancy complications such as preterm low birthweight infants.

PERIODONTITIS AS A RISK FOR PREGNANCY COMPLICATIONS

Beginning around 1996, with a landmark report by Offenbacher and colleagues (Offenbacher et al. 1996), there has been an increasing interest and much research into whether periodontitis may be a possible risk factor for preterm low birthweight infants.

Preterm infants who are born with low birthweights represent a major social and economic public health problem, even in industrialized nations. Although there has been an overall decline in infant mortality in the US over the past 40 years, preterm low birthweight remains a significant cause of perinatal mortality and morbidity. Accordingly, a 47% decrease in the infant mortality rate to a level of 13.1 per 1000 live births occurred between 1965 and 1980, but the mortality rate and the incidence of preterm delivery have not significantly changed since the early 1990s (Offenbacher et al. 1996, 1998, Champagne et al. 2000).

Preterm low birthweight deliveries represent approximately 10% of annual births in industrialized nations and account for two-thirds of overall infant mortality. Approximately one-third of these births are elective while two-thirds are spontaneous preterm births. About a half of the spontaneous preterm births are due to premature rupture of membranes and the other half are due to preterm labor. For the spontaneous preterm births, 10-15% occur before 32 weeks gestation, result in very low birthweight (<1500 g) and often cause long-term disability, such as chronic respiratory diseases and cerebral palsy (Offenbacher et al. 1996, 1998, Champagne et al. 2000).

Among the known risk factors for preterm low birthweight deliveries are young maternal age (<18 years) drug, alcohol and tobacco use, maternal stress, genetic background, and genitourinary tract infec-

tions. Although 25-50% of preterm low birthweight deliveries occur without any known etiology, there is increasing evidence that infection may play a significant role in preterm delivery (Hill 1998, Goldenberg et al. 2000, Sobel 2000, Williams et al. 2000).

One of the more important acute exposures that have been implicated in preterm birth is an acute maternal genitourinary tract infection at some point during the pregnancy. Bacterial vaginosis (BV) is a Gram-negative, predominantly anaerobic infection of the vagina, usually diagnosed from clinical signs and symptoms. It is associated with a decrease in the normal lactobacillus-dominated flora and an increase in anaerobes and facultative species including *Gardnerella vaginalis*, *Mobiluncus curtsii*, *Prevotella bivia* and *Bacteroides ureolyticus*. Bacterial vaginosis is a relatively common condition that occurs in about 10% of all pregnancies. It may ascend from the vagina to the cervix and even result in inflammation of the maternal-fetal membranes (chorioamnionitis). Extending beyond the membranes, the organisms may appear in the amniotic fluid compartment that is shared with the fetal lungs and/or may involve placental tissues and result in exposure to the fetus via the bloodstream. Despite the observed epidemiological linkage of bacterial vaginosis with preterm birth, the results from randomized clinical trials to determine the effects of treating bacterial vaginosis with systemic antibiotics on incident preterm birth are equivocal (Goldenberg et al. 2000). Still, there are compelling data linking maternal infection and the subsequent inflammation to preterm birth. It appears that inflammation of the uterus and membranes represents a common effector mechanism that results in preterm birth, and thus, either clinical infection or subclinical infection is a likely stimulus for increased inflammation.

In the early 1990s, Offenbacher and his group hypothesized that oral infections, such as periodontitis, could represent a significant source of both infection and inflammation during pregnancy. Offenbacher noted that periodontal disease is a Gram-negative anaerobic infection with the potential to cause Gram-negative bacteremias in persons with periodontal disease. He hypothesized that periodontal infections, which serve as reservoirs for Gram-negative anaerobic organisms, lipopolysaccharide (LPS, endotoxin) and inflammatory mediators including PGE_2 and TNF-α, may be a potential threat to the fetal-placental unit (Collins et al. 1994a,b).

As a first step in testing this hypothesis, Offenbacher and colleagues conducted a series of experiments in the pregnant hamster animal model. It had been noted earlier by Lanning et al. (1983) that pregnant hamsters challenged with *E. coli* LPS had malformation of fetuses, spontaneous abortions and low fetal weight. The work by Lanning and co-workers clearly demonstrated that infections in pregnant animals could elicit many pregnancy complications including spontaneous abortion, preterm labor, low birthweight, fetal growth restriction and skeletal abnormalities. It was not clear however if these findings from *E. coli* endotoxin would be similar if endotoxin from oral anaerobes was studied. First of all, LPS from Gram-negative enteric organisms differs in structure and biological activity from oral LPS. Thus, Offenbacher needed to demonstrate that LPS from oral organisms had similar effects on fetal outcomes when administered to pregnant animals. Secondly, the oral cavity represents a distant site of infection. Although pneumonia has been a recognized example of a distant site of infection triggering maternal obstetric complications, it was important to demonstrate that distant, non-disseminating infections with oral pathogens could elicit pregnancy complications in animal models. Thirdly, oral infections are chronic in nature. Increased obstetric risk is generally associated with acute infections that occur during pregnancy. Thus, in concept, maternal adaptation to a chronic infectious challenge was assumed to afford protection to the fetus, even during acute flare-ups that may occur during pregnancy.

Offenbacher's landmark hamster studies (Collins et al. 1994a,b) demonstrated that chronic exposure to oral pathogens like *P. gingivalis* in a chamber model (Genco & Arko 1994) does not in fact afford protection, but actually enhances the feto-placental toxicity of exposure during pregnancy. Thus during pregnancy the mother does not become "tolerant" of infectious challenge from oral organisms. Offenbacher also wanted to demonstrate that the low-grade infections with low numbers of oral pathogens were not of sufficient magnitude to induce maternal malaise or fever. He noted however a measurable local increase of PGE_2 and TNF-α in chamber fluid with *P. gingivalis* infection as well as a 15-18% decrease in fetal weight. Further, the magnitude of the PGE_2 and TNF-α response was inversely related to the weight of the fetuses, mimicking the intra-amniotic changes seen in humans with preterm low birthweight. LPS dosing experiments demonstrated that higher levels of LPS could induce fever and weight loss in pregnant animals and resulted in more severe pregnancy outcomes including spontaneous abortions and malformations. These more noteworthy outcomes were not seen in the low challenge-oral infection models, but rather resulted in a consistent decrease in fetal weight. Previous sensitization or exposures to these pathogens prior to pregnancy enhanced the severity of the fetal growth restriction when a secondary exposure occurred during pregnancy.

Offenbacher and colleagues then went on to study infection and pregnancy in the hamster by experimentally inducing periodontal disease in the animal model (Collins et al. 1994b). Four groups of animals were fed either control chow or plaque-promoting chow for an 8-week period to induce experimental periodontitis prior to mating. Two additional groups of animals (i.e. one control chow and one plaque-promoting chow) received exogenous *P. gingivalis* via oral gavage. Animals fed the plaque-promoting diet begin-

ning 8 weeks prior to mating developed periodontitis. These animals also had litters with a mean fetal weight of 1.25 ± 0.07 g that was 81% of the weight of the control groups. Animals receiving both plaque-promoting diet and *P. gingivalis* gavage also had significantly smaller fetuses. The mean fetal weight for this group was 1.20 ± 0.19 g which represented a significant 22.5% reduction in fetal weight compared to controls. Exogenous *P. gingivalis* challenge by gastric gavage did not appear to promote either more severe periodontal disease or more severe fetal growth restriction. This experiment indicated that experimentally induced periodontitis in the hamster could also alter fetal weight in the hamster.

Other factors appear also to be involved in the findings of low fetal weight in the hamster study. There was a statistically significant elevation of intra-amniotic fluid levels of both PGE_2 and TNF-α. This finding suggests that periodontal infection can result in a change in the fetal environment. It is possible that both PGE_2 and TNF-α are produced by the periodontium and appear in the systemic circulation to eventually cross the chorioamniotic barrier and finally appear in the fluid. It is more likely, however, that blood-borne bacterial products such as endotoxin target the chonoamniotic plexus to trigger local PGE_2 and TNF-α synthesis. These animal studies by Offenbacher and colleagues provided important proof-of-concept experiments and raised the possibility that distant, low grade oral infections might also trigger inflammation of the human maternal-fetal unit in a manner analogous to that seen with reproductive tract infections (Collins et al. 1994a,b).

In a subsequent landmark study, Offenbacher and colleagues conducted a case-control study on 124 pregnant or postpartum women (Offenbacher et al. 1996). Preterm low birthweight cases were defined as a mother whose infant had a birthweight of less than 2500 g and also had one or more of the following: gestational age < 37 weeks, preterm labor or preterm premature rupture of membranes. Controls were all mothers whose infant had a normal birthweight. Assessments included a broad range of known obstetric risk factors such as tobacco usage, drug use and alcohol consumption, level of prenatal care, parity, genitourinary tract infections and weight gain during pregnancy. Each subject received a full-mouth periodontal examination to determine clinical attachment levels. Mothers of preterm low birthweight cases and first birth PLBW cases had significantly more advanced periodontal disease as measured with attachment loss than the respective mothers of normal birthweight controls. Multivariate logistic regression models, controlling for other known risk factors and covariates, demonstrated that periodontitis was a statistically significant risk factor for preterm low birthweight, with adjusted odds ratios of 7.9 and 7.5 for all PLBW cases and primiparous PLBW cases respectively. This research by Offenbacher and colleagues was the first to demonstrate an association between periodontal infection and adverse pregnancy outcomes in humans (Offenbacher et al. 1996).

Jeffcoat and Hauth have recently confirmed this association in a larger case-control study. Gathering data on 1313 mothers, Jeffcoat and Hauth reported that maternal periodontitis was an independent risk factor for preterm birth. With increasing severity of periodontal disease as an exposure, there was an increased risk for preterm birth with odds ratios ranging from 4.45 to 7.07 for moderate to severe periodontitis, adjusting for age, race, smoking and parity (Jeffcoat et al. 2001a,b).

Offenbacher's group at the University of North Carolina has been conducting a large prospective molecular epidemiological study designed to examine the role of maternal periodontal infections on abnormal pregnancy outcomes. The principal goal of the study is to determine whether the presence of maternal periodontal disease represents a significant independent risk factor for preterm birth and low birthweight in the context of other established risk factors. Maternal periodontal disease was assessed at baseline (prior to 26 weeks gestation) and at postpartum to examine for periodontal disease progression during pregnancy. This group measured periodontal disease as an exposure in three ways: (1) clinical signs – by assessment of disease extent and severity (Carlos et al. 1986), (2) inflammatory response – by concentrations of inflammatory mediators (PGE$_2$ and IL-1β) within the gingival crevicular fluid (GCF), and (3) microbial burden – by determining levels of periodontal pathogens. Serum antibody responses to specific oral organisms were also measured. Extensive maternal obstetric data were collected including medical, social and clinical OB histories. The presence of bacterial vaginosis as a potential covariate or confounder was assessed by clinical exam, history and quantitative examination of the composition of the vaginal flora by wet mount, Gram stain and whole chromasomal DNA macroarray for specific indicator vaginal and cervical organisms. Neonatal exposures and outcomes were determined including fetal cord blood measures of antibody to oral organisms and levels of inflammatory mediators. Data have to date been collected in over 1200 mothers.

The findings from this large prospective cohort study very nicely confirm and extend the case-control observations that Offenbacher reported earlier. At baseline, periodontal disease independently enhances the risk of preterm birth, e.g. for moderate-severe disease adjusted odds ratio = 3.0 for GA< 37 weeks and odds ratio of 7.9 adjusting for race, age, socio-economic status, smoking, parity, bacterial vaginosis and chorioamnionitis (Lieff et al. 2000). In addition, periodontal disease increased the relative risk for fetal growth restriction (decreased weight for gestational age, adjusting for parity, race and baby sex) as well as pregnancy-induced hypertension, preeclampsia and neonatal death.

Of particular interest in this ongoing study is the finding that not only does the presence of periodontal disease early in pregnancy appear to confer risk, but also if periodontal disease becomes more severe during pregnancy, this periodontitis worsening independently enhances the risk of preterm birth. When periodontal disease is present both at baseline and also progressing during pregnancy the odds ratio for preterm birth is 10.9 adjusting for age, race, previous preterm births, parity, smoking and social status (Lieff et al. 2000). Clinical diagnosis of vaginosis or subclinical vaginosis chorioamnionitis did not confound the relationship between periodontal disease and preterm birth. Complementing these recent epidemiologic findings, Madianos et al. (2002) have presented initial findings of fetal immunoglobulin (IgM) specific for periodontal pathogens. Although they detected IgM specific to *P. gingivalis* and *B. forsythus*, among others, in fetal cord blood samples from both low and normal birthweight infants, these preliminary data at least confirm that the fetus can be challenged by maternal periodontal bacteria and can mount an independent host response.

PERIODONTITIS AS A RISK FOR DIABETIC COMPLICATIONS

Similar to cardiovascular disease, diabetes mellitus is a common, multifactorial disease process involving genetic, environmental and behavioral risk factors. Affecting up to 5% of the general population and over 124 million persons worldwide (King et al. 1998), this chronic condition is marked by defects in glucose metabolism that produce hyperglycemia in patients. Diabetes mellitus is broadly classified under two major types (American Diabetes Association Expert Committee on the Diagnosis and Classification of Diabetes Mellitus 1997). In patients with Type 1 diabetes, (formerly called insulin-dependent diabetes mellitus), the defect occurs at the level of the pancreatic beta cells that are destroyed. Consequently Type 1 diabetics produce insufficient levels of the hormone insulin for homeostasis. In contrast, patients with Type 2 diabetes (formerly called non-insulin-dependent diabetes mellitus), exhibit the defect at the level of the insulin molecule or receptor. Cells in Type 2 diabetics cannot respond or are resistant to insulin stimulation. Diabetes mellitus is usually diagnosed via laboratory fasting blood glucose levels that are greater than 126 mg/dL. Additionally, casual or non-fasting blood glucose values are elevated above 200 mg/dL. Thirdly, diabetic patients exhibit abnormal glucose tolerance tests (i.e. blood glucose levels greater than 140 mg/dL at 2 hours following a 100 g glucose load). Elevated glycated hemoglobin levels (HbAl and HbA1c) comprise a fourth laboratory parameter and one that provides a 30 to 90-day record of the patient's glycemic status. Classic signs and symptoms of diabetes include polyuria, polydipsia, polyphagia, pruritis, weakness and fatigue. End-stage diabetes mellitus is characterized by problems with several organ systems including micro and macro-vascular disease (atherosclerosis), retinopathy, nephropathy, neuropathy and indeed periodontal disease.

Although environmental exposures, viral infection, autoimmunity and insulin resistance are currently considered to play principal roles in the etiology of diabetes mellitus (Yoon 1990, Atkinson & Maclaren 1990), pathogenesis of the disease and end-organ damage relies heavily on the formation and accumulation of advanced glycation end products (AGEs) (Brownlee 1994). Accordingly, the chronic hyperglycemia in diabetes results in the non-enzymatic and irreversible glycation of body proteins. These AGEs, in turn, bind to specific receptors for advanced glycation end products (RAGEs) on monocytes, macrophages and endothelial cells, and alter intracellular signaling (transduction) pathways (Esposito et al. 1992, Kirstein et al. 1992). With AGE-RAGE binding, monocytes and macrophages are stimulated to proliferate, up-regulate pro-inflammatory cytokines and produce oxygen free radicals (Vlassara et al. 1988, Yan et al. 1994, Yui et al. 1994). While oxygen free radicals directly damage host tissues, pro-inflammatory cytokines like IL-1, IL-6 and TNF-α exacerbate this damage via a cascade of catabolic events and the recruitment of other immune cells (T and B lymphocytes). Patients with diabetes exhibit elevated levels of AGEs in tissues including those of the periodontium (Brownlee 1994, Schmidt et al. 1998). Diabetics also present with elevated serum and gingival crevicular fluid levels of pro-inflammatory cytokines (Nishimura et al. 1998, Salvi et al. 1998). Furthermore, monocytes isolated from diabetics and stimulated with LPS secrete higher concentrations of pro-inflammatory cytokines and prostaglandins (Salvi et al. 1998). Chronic hyperglycemia, the accumulation of AGEs and the hyper-inflammatory response may promote vascular injury and altered wound healing via increased collagen cross-linking and friability, thickening of basement membranes and altered tissue turnover rates (Weringer & Arquilla 1981, Lien et al. 1984, Salmela et al. 1989, Cagliero et al. 1991). Lastly, diabetic patients exhibit impairments in neutrophil chemotaxis, adherence and phagocytosis, (Bagdade et al. 1978, Manoucherhr-Pour et al. 1981, Kjersem et al. 1988) and thus are at high risk for infections like periodontitis.

Numerous epidemiologic surveys demonstrate an increased prevalence of periodontitis among patients with uncontrolled or poorly controlled diabetes mellitus. For example, Cianciola et al. (1982) reported that 13.6% and 39% of Type 1 diabetics, 13-18 and 19-32 years of age respectively, had periodontal disease. In contrast, none of the non-diabetic sibling controls and 2.5% of the non-diabetic, unrelated controls exhibited clinical evidence of periodontitis. In a classic study, Thorstensson and Hugoson (1993) examined the severity of periodontitis in patients with diabetes mellitus and compared severity of periodontitis with the

duration a patient had been diagnosed with diabetes. In looking at three age cohorts, 40-49 years, 50-59 years and 60-69 years, the 40-49 years age group diabetics had more periodontal pockets $\geq$ 6 mm and more extensive alveolar bone loss than non-diabetics. In this same age group, there were also more subjects with severe periodontal disease experience among the diabetics than among the non-diabetics. In noting that the younger age diabetics had more periodontitis than the older age diabetics, these authors reported that early onset of diabetes is a much greater risk factor for periodontal bone loss than mere disease duration. Safkan-Seppala & Ainamo (1992) conducted a cross-sectional study of 71 Type 1 diabetics diagnosed with the condition for an average of 16.5 years. Diabetics identified with poor glycemic control demonstrated significantly more clinical attachment loss and radiographic alveolar bone resorption as compared to well-controlled diabetics with the same level of plaque control. Two longitudinal cohort studies monitoring Type 1 diabetics for 5 and 2 years respectively documented significantly more periodontitis progression among diabetics overall and among those poorly controlled (Sappala et al. 1993, Firatli 1997). Investigators from the State University of New York at Buffalo have published a number of landmark papers documenting the periodontal status of Pima Indians, a population with a high prevalence of Type 2 diabetes mellitus. Shlossman et al. (1990) first documented the periodontal status of 3219 subjects from this unique population. Diagnosing Type 2 diabetes with glucose tolerance tests, the investigators found a higher prevalence of clinical and radiographic periodontitis for diabetics versus non-diabetics independent of age. This investigative group next focused on a cross-sectional analysis of 1342 dental subjects (Emrich et al. 1991). A logistic regression analysis indicated that Type 2 diabetics were 2.8 times more likely to exhibit clinical attachment loss and 3.4 times more likely to exhibit radiographic alveolar bone loss indicative of periodontitis relative to non-diabetic controls. In a larger study of 2273 Pima subjects, 60% of Type 2 diabetics were affected with periodontitis versus 36% of non-diabetic controls (Nelson et al. 1990). When a cohort of 701 subjects with little or no evidence of periodontitis at baseline were followed for approximately 3 years, diabetics were 2.6 times more likely to present with incident alveolar bone resorption as compared to non-diabetics. Taylor et al. (1998a,b) similarly reported higher odds ratios of 4.2 and 11.4 for the risk of progressive periodontitis among diabetic Pima Indians in general and poorly controlled diabetics (i.e. with glycated hemoglobin levels > 9%) respectively.

The studies cited above reiterate diabetes as a modifier or risk factor for periodontitis. Recently, new data have emerged indicating that the presence of periodontitis or periodontal infection can increase the risk for diabetic complications, principally poor glycemic control. Taylor et al. (1996) first tested this hypothesis using longitudinal data on 88 Pima subjects. Severe periodontitis at baseline as defined clinically or radiographically was significantly associated with poor glycemic control (glycated hemoglobin > 9%). Other significant covariates in the regression modeling included subject age, smoking, and baseline severity and duration of Type 2 diabetes. Given these findings the next logical question is whether periodontal treatment can improve glycemic control. Several investigators have sought to answer this question using periodontal mechanical treatment as the intervention (Seppala & Ainamo 1994, Aldridge et al. 1995, Smith et al. 1996, Christgau et al. 1998, Stewart et al. 2001). These studies in general have failed to detect an improvement in glycated hemoglobin level with scaling and root planing alone. Grossi et al. (1997) reported more compelling findings from an intervention trial featuring 113 Pima Indians with Type 2 diabetes and periodontitis who received both mechanical and antimicrobial treatment. At baseline, participants were treated with scaling and root planing plus one of five antimicrobial regimens: (1) water (placebo) rinse and peroral doxycycline (100 mg q.d. for 2 weeks), (2) 0.12% chlorhexidine rinse and peroral doxycycline, (3) povidone-iodine rinse and peroral doxycycline, (4) 0.12% chlorhexidine rinse and peroral placebo, or (5) povidone-iodine rinse and peroral placebo. Subjects were evaluated using clinical, microbiological and laboratory parameters prior to therapy and at 3 and 6 months. All treatment groups on average demonstrated clinical and microbiological improvements; however, those groups treated with adjunctive peroral tetracycline exhibited significant and greater reductions in pocket depth and subgingival detection rates for *P. gingivalis* as compared to the groups receiving peroral placebo. Most strikingly, diabetic subjects receiving mechanical therapy plus peroral tetracycline demonstrated significant, 10% reductions in their glycated hemoglobin levels. Two small, uncontrolled cohort studies with nine Type 1 diabetic-periodontitis patients each similarly reported improvements in glycemic control with combination mechanical-antimicrobial therapy (Williams & Mahan 1960, Miller et al. 1992). These limited lines of evidence suggest that untreated periodontal infections may increase a diabetic patient's risk for poorer glycemic control and subsequent systemic complications.

PERIODONTITIS AS A RISK FOR RESPIRATORY INFECTIONS

There is lastly emerging evidence that in certain at risk populations, periodontitis and poor oral health may be associated with several respiratory conditions. Respiratory diseases contribute considerably to morbidity and mortality in human populations. Lower respiratory infections were ranked as the third most common cause of death worldwide in 1990, and chronic obstructive pulmonary disease was ranked sixth (Scannapieco 1999).

Bacterial pneumonia is either community-acquired or hospital-acquired (nosocomial). Community-acquired pneumonia is usually caused by bacteria that reside on the oropharyngeal mucosa, such as *Streptococcus pneumonia* and *Haemophilus influenza*. Alternatively, hospital-acquired pneumonia is often caused by bacteria within the hospital or health care environment, such as Gram-negative bacilli, *Pseudomonas aeruginosa* and *Staphylococcus aureus* (Scannapieco 1999). As many as 250 000 to 300 000 hospital-acquired respiratory infections occur in the US each year with an estimated mortality rate of about 30%. Pneumonia also contributes to a significant number of other deaths by acting as a complicating or secondary factor with other diseases or conditions.

Chronic obstructive pulmonary disease (COPD) is another common severe respiratory disease characterized by chronic obstruction to airflow with excess production of sputum resulting from chronic bronchitis and/or emphysema. Chronic bronchitis is the result of irritation to the bronchial airway causing an expansion of the propagation of mucus-secreting cells within the airway epithelium. These cells secrete excessive tracheobronchial mucus sufficient to cause cough with expectoration for at least 3 months of the year over two consecutive years. Emphysema is the distention of the air spaces distal to the terminal bronchiole with destruction of the alveolar septa (Scannapieco 1999).

Beginning in 1992 with a report by Scannapieco's group at SUNY-Buffalo (Scannapieco et al. 1992), several investigators have hypothesized that oral and/or periodontal infection may increase the risk for bacterial pneumonia or COPD.

It seems quite plausible from all the evidence reviewed in this chapter that the oral cavity may also have a critical role in respiratory infections. For example, oral bacteria from the periodontal pocket can be aspirated into the lung to cause aspiration pneumonia. The teeth may also serve as a reservoir for respiratory pathogen colonization and subsequent nosocomial pneumonia. Typical respiratory pathogens have been shown to colonize the dental plaque of hospitalized intensive care and nursing home patients. Once established in the mouth, these pathogens may be aspirated into the lung to cause infection. Also, periodontal disease-associated enzymes in saliva may modify mucosal surfaces to promote adhesion and colonization by respiratory pathogens, which are then aspirated into the lungs. These same enzymes may also destroy salivary pellicles on pathogenic bacteria to hinder their clearance from the mucosal surface. Lastly, cytokines originating from periodontal tissues may alter respiratory epithelium to promote infection by respiratory pathogens (Scannapieco 1999).

At present, cross-sectional epidemiologic studies from Frank Scannapieco's group in Buffalo and Catherine Hayes's group in Boston are pointing to a sig-

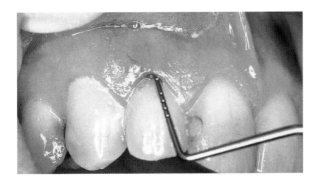

Fig. 16-9. Mean probing depth measurements of 4-5 mm have been customarily used in epidemiology studies to designate a subject as being healthy or having periodontitis.

nificant association between poor oral health such as periodontitis and pulmonary conditions. In a recent report examining data from the third National Health and Nutrition Examination Survey (NHANES III), Scannapieco and Ho reported that patients with a history of chronic obstructive pulmonary disease had significantly more periodontal attachment loss (1.48 ± 1.35 mm) than subjects without COPD (1.17 ± 1.09 mm) p = 0.0001 (Scannapieco & Ho 2001).

SUMMARY

This chapter has examined the evidence, gathered by many investigators since the early 1990s, which suggests that periodontitis may be a risk for certain systemic conditions such as cardiovascular disease, preterm low-birthweight infants, diabetes mellitus and pulmonary disease. Collectively, the findings gathered for the most part from large epidemiological data sets, are very compelling. It would certainly appear that at the least, in a diverse group of study subjects, periodontitis is strongly associated with systemic conditions. But there is much yet to be done to elucidate and understand the exact nature of the relationship of periodontitis to a person's overall risk for systemic disease.

The student of dentistry will note that in this chapter the measures of periodontal disease used in the epidemiological data sets were "all over the board". Most of the studies tried to relate some type of clinical sign of periodontitis such as pocket depth, attachment loss or bone loss on radiographs to a systemic condition (Fig. 16-9). Two studies used self-reported disease and asked the subject if he/she had periodontitis with a yes/no answer. And as was noted in this chapter, while one study might distinguish between health and periodontitis if pocket depths were < 4mm (health) or ≥ 4 mm (periodontitis), another study might use 5 mm to distinguish between health and periodontitis. Thus in one study subjects having pocket depths of ≥ 4 mm would be diagnosed with periodontitis while in another study that subject would have been called healthy. Further, "self-reported" periodontal disease with a yes/no answer is likely to have considerable error such that those data may be of limited use. Still, collectively, the epidemiol-

ogical data point to a strong and noteworthy relationship between periodontitis and systemic conditions. In April 2001, an AAP-NIDCR Conference was held in Bethesda, MD, which focused on "The periodontitis-systemic connection". One of the major points made at this conference focused on the need for future studies to go far beyond trying to link clinical signs of periodontitis (such as pocket depth) with systemic complications (Fig. 16-10). Scientists and clinicians at this conference noted that it is the anaerobic infection in periodontal pockets and the host inflammatory response to the infection that then leads to the clinical signs of periodontitis (Fig. 16-11). However, it is probably more relevant to examine the relationship of anaerobic infection and the inflammatory response in the periodontal tissues to systemic disease (Fig. 16-12) than to focus on clinical signs of periodontitis as has been done in the epidemiological studies to date. Thus, research workers in the future need to explore how infection and inflammation in the periodontal pocket may better explain the role of periodontitis as a risk for systemic disease.

Lastly, students of dentistry will ask, "if you treat periodontitis, do you prevent the onset or reduce the severity of systemic complications?" It is clear that dentistry must now focus on intervention studies to determine whether treating periodontitis will have a beneficial effect on systemic diseases. This is not an easy task and some studies will take considerable time before we know the answer. However, there are exciting initial data which examine intervention and the impact of periodontal treatment on preterm low birthweight infants. In a preliminary study, Lamster and his colleagues reported that periodontal intervention decreased the risk of preterm low birthweight infants. In a study of 195 young women at the School of Pregnant and Parenting Teens in Central Harlem, the overall prevalence of preterm low birthweight was 14.6%. PLBW occurred in 18.8% of the women who did not receive periodontal intervention but in only 6.7% of the women who received periodontal therapy (Mitchell-Lewis et al. 2000). Lopez and co-workers, in a noteworthy abstract, have recently reported that periodontal therapy significantly reduces the risk of preterm low birthweight in a study of 351 pregnant women. The total incidence of PLBW in this cohort of subjects was 6.26%. In women treated for periodontitis, the incidence of PLBW was only 1.84% while this

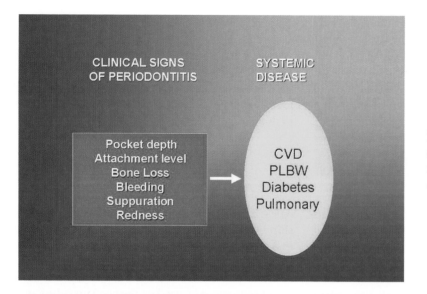

Fig. 16-10. Most studies to date have used a clinical sign of periodontitis such as probing depth to relate periodontitis to systemic complications.

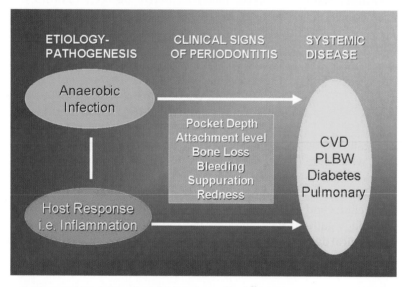

Fig. 16-11. In addition to clinical measures of disease severity, the anaerobic bacterial burden and the inflammatory response must be taken into account in linking periodontitis to systemic disease.

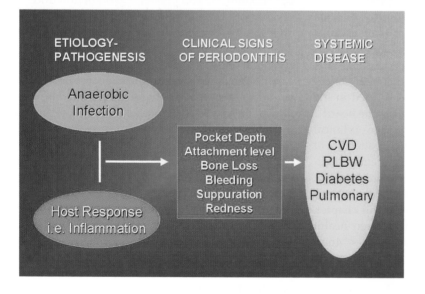

Fig. 16-12. Studying the anaerobic bacterial burden and the inflammatory response may be more critical than measures of pocket depth in finding a relationship between periodontitis and systemic complications.

incidence was 10.11% in untreated women. Lopez concluded that periodontitis was an independent risk factor for PLBW and that periodontal treatment significantly reduced the risk of PLBW. These two studies are compelling findings indeed and suggest that at least for preterm low birthweight babies, reducing

periodontal infection and disease can be very beneficial. There are also studies being designed to look at the effect of intervention on cardiovascular disease. Our group, along with colleagues at Boston University, SUNY-Buffalo, University of Maryland and Oregon Health Science University, have initiated plans for the "Periodontal Intervention and Vascular Events" (PAVE) pilot trial. This proposed multicenter study hopes to ultimately design and conduct a large clinical trial of periodontal therapy in patients at risk for cardiovascular events.

Dentistry has come a long way since 1900 when Willoughby Miller and William Hunter proclaimed that oral disease caused most systemic disease. A hundred years later we are developing a scientifically-based understanding of how in fact periodontitis may be a risk for certain systemic diseases. As these more recent observations are confirmed and clarified, dentistry will have a new responsibility in caring for patients who may develop or who have periodontitis. It is no longer just teeth that are at risk.

REFERENCES

Aldridge, J.P., Lester, V., Watts, T.L.P., Collins, A., Viberti, G. & Wilson, R.F. (1995). Single-blind studies of the effects of improved periodontal health on metabolic control in Type 1 diabetes mellitus. *Journal of Clinical Periodontology* 22, 271-275.

American Diabetes Association Expert Committee on the Diagnosis and Classification of Diabetes Mellitus (1997). Committee Report. *Diabetes Care* 20,1183-1197.

Arbes, S.J., Slade, G.D., & Beck, J.D. (1999). Association between extent of periodontal attachment loss and self-reported history of heart attack: An analysis of NHANES III data. *Journal of Dental Research* 78,1777-1782.

Atkinson, M.A. & Maclaren, N.K. (1990). What causes diabetes? *Scientific American* 164, 95-123.

Bagdade, J.D., Stewart, M. & Walters, E. (1978). Impaired granulocyte adherence. A reversible defect in host defense in patients with poorly controlled diabetes. *Diabetes* 27, 677-681.

Beck, J.D. (1994). Methods of assessing risk for periodontitis and developing multifactional models. *Journal of Periodontology* 65, 316-323.

Beck, J.D., Garcia, R., Heiss, G., Vokonas, P. & Offenbacher, S. (1996). Periodontal disease and cardiovascular disease. *Journal of Periodontology* 67, 1123-1137.

Beck, J.D. & Offenbacher, S. (1998). Oral health and systemic disease: periodontitis and cardiovascular disease. *Journal of Dental Education* 62, 859-870.

Beck, J.D., Offenbacher, S., Williams, R.C., Gibbs, P. & Garcia, K. (1998). Periodontitis: a risk factor for coronary heart disease? *Annals of Periodontology* 3, 127-141.

Beck, J.D., Slade, G. & Offenbacher, S. (2000). Oral disease, cardiovascular disease and systemic inflammation. *Periodontology 2000* 23, 110-120.

Bell, B., Rose, C.L. & Damon, A. (1966). The Veterans Administration longitudinal study of health and aging. *Gerontologist* 6, 179-184.

Billings, F. (1912). Chronic focal infections and their etiologic relations to arthritis and nephritis. *Archive Internal Medicine* 9, 484-498.

Brownlee, M. (1994). Glycation and diabetic complications. *Diabetes* 43, 836-841.

Cagliero, E., Roth, T., Roy, S. & Lorenzi, M. (1991). Characteristics and mechanisms of high-glucose-induced overexpression of basement membrane components in cultured human endothelial cells. *Diabetes* 40, 102-110.

Carlos, J., Wolfe, M. & Kingman, A. (1986). The extent and severity index: a simple method for use in epidemiologic studies of periodontal disease. *Journal of Clinical Periodontology* 13, 500-506.

Cecil, R.L. & Angevine, D.M. (1938). Clinical and experimental observations on focal infection with an analysis of 200 cases of rheumatoid arthritis. *Annals Internal Medicine* 12, 577-584.

Champagne, C.M.E., Madianos, P.N., Lieff, S., Murtha, A.P., Beck, J.D. & Offenbacher, S. (2000). Periodontal medicine: emerging concepts in pregnancy outcomes. *Journal of the International Academy of Periodontology* 2, 9-13.

Christgau, M., Pallitzsch, K.D., Schmalz, G., Kreiner, U. & Frenzel, S. (1998). Healing response to non-surgical periodontal therapy in patients with diabetes mellitus: Clinical, microbiological, and immunologic results. *Journal of Clinical Periodontology* 25, 112-124.

Chung, H.J., Champagne, C.E., Southerland, J.H., Geva S., Liu, Y., Paquette, D.W., Madianos, P.N., Beck, J.D. & Offenbacher, S. (2002). Effects of *P. gingivalis* infection on atheroma formation in ApO-E (+/-) mice. *Journal of Dental Research* 79, 59 (Abstract).

Cianciola, L.J., Park, B.H., Bruck, E., Mosovich, L. & Genco, R.J. (1982). Prevalence of periodontal disease in insulin-dependent diabetes mellitus (juvenile diabetes). *Journal of the American Dental Association* 104, 653-660.

Collins, J.G., Smith, M.A., Arnold, R.R. & Offenbacher, S. (1994a). Effects of *E. coli* and *P. gingivalis* lipopolysaccharide on pregnancy outcome in the golden hamster. *Infection and Immunity* 62, 4652-4655.

Collins, J.G., Windley, H.W., Arnold, R.R. & Offenbacher, S. (1994b). Effects of a *Porphyromonas gingivalis* infection on inflammatory mediator response and pregnancy outcomes in hamsters. *Infection and Immunity* 62, 4356-4361.

Danesh, J., Collins, R. & Peto, R. (1997). Chronic infections and coronary heart disease: is there a link? *Lancet* 350, 430-436.

Davenport, E.S., Williams, C.E., Sterne, J.A., Sivapathasundram, V., Fearne, J.M. & Curtis, M.A. (1998). The East London study of maternal chronic periodontal disease and preterm low birthweight infants: study design and prevalence data. *Annals of Periodontology* 3, 213-221.

DeStefano, F., Anda, R.F., Kahn, H.S., Williamson, D.F. & Russell, C.M. (1993). Dental disease and risk of coronary heart disease and mortality. *British Medical Journal* 306, 688-691.

Ebersole, K.L., Machen, R.L., Steffen, M.J. & Willman, D.E. (1997). Systemic acute-phase reactants, C-reactive protein and haptoglobin in adult periodontitis. *Clinical Experimental Immunology* 107, 347-352.

Emrich, L.J., Shlossman, M. & Genco, R.J. (1991). Periodontal disease in non-insulin dependent diabetes mellitus. *Journal of Periodontology* 62, 123-131.

Esposito, C., Gerlach, H., Brett, J., Stern, D. & Vlassara, H. (1992). Endothelial receptor-mediated binding of glucose-modified albumin is associated with increased monolayer permeability and modulation of cell surface coagulant properties. *Journal of Experimental Medicine* 170, 1388-1407.

Firatli, E. (1997). The relationship between clinical periodontal status and insulin-dependent diabetes mellitus. Results after 5 years. *Journal of Periodontology* 68, 136-140.

Fourrier, F., Duvivier, B., Boutigny, H., Roussel-Delvallez, M. & Chopin, C. (1998). Colonization of dental plaque: a source of nosocomial infections in intensive care unit patients. *Critical Care Medicine* 26(2), 301-308.

Galloway, C.E. (1931). Focal infection. *American Journal of Surgery* 14, 643-645.

Garcia, R. & Vokonas, P. (1996). Periodontal disease and all-cause mortality in the VA dental longitudinal study. *Journal of Dental Research* 75, 48 (abstract 246).

Garcia, R.I., Henshaw, M.M. & Krall, E.A. (2001). Relationship between periodontal disease and systemic health. *Periodontology 2000* **24**, 21-36.

Garcia, R.I., Krall, E.A. & Vokonas, P.S. (1998). Periodontal disease and mortality from all causes in the VA dental longitudinal study. *Annals of Periodontology* **3**, 339-349.

Genco, C.A. & Arko, R.J. (1994). Animal chamber models for study of host-parasite interactions. *Methods in Enzymology* **235**, 120-140.

Genco, R., Chadda, S. & Grossi, S. (1997). Periodontal disease is a predictor of cardiovascular disease in a Native American population. *Journal of Dental Research* **76**, 408 (abstract 3158).

Genco, R.J., Wu, T.J., Grossi, S.G., Fulkner, K., Zambon, J.J. & Trevesan, M. (1999). Periodontal microflora related to the risk for myocardial infarction. A case control study. *Journal of Dental Research* **78**, 457 (abstract 2811).

Geva, S., Liu, Y., Champagne, C., Southerland, J.H., Madianos, P.N. & Offenbacher, S. (2000). *Porphyromonas gingivalis* enhances atherosclerotic plaque calcification in Apo E (+/-) mice. *Journal of Dental Research* **79**, 599 (abstract 2980).

Gibbs, R.S., Romero, R., Hillier, S.L., Eschenbach, D.A. & Sweet, R.L. (1992). A review of premature birth and subclinical infections. *American Journal of Obstetrics and Gynecology* **166**, 1515-1528.

Goldenberg, R., Hauth, J.C. & Andrews, W.W. (2000). Intrauterine infection and preterm delivery. *New England Journal of Medicine* **3432**, 1500-1507.

Grau, A.J., Buggle, F., Ziegler, C. & Schwarz, W. (1997). Association between acute cerebrovascular eschemia and chronic recurrent infection. *Stroke* **28**, 1724-1729.

Grossi, S.G., Skrepcinski, F.B., DeCaro, T., Robertson, D.C., Ho, A.W., Dunford, R.G. & Genco, R.J. (1997). Treatment of periodontal disease in diabetics reduces glycated hemoglobin. *Journal of Periodontology* **68**, 713-719.

Haraszthy, V.I., Zambon, J.J., Trevisan, M., Zeid, M. & Genco, R.J. (2000). Identification of periodontal pathogens in atheromatous plaques. *Journal of Periodontology* **71**, 1554-1560.

Hayes, C., Sparrow, D., Cohen, M., Vokonas, P. & Garcia, R. (1998). Periodontal disease and pulmonary function: The VA longitudinal study. *Annals of Periodontology* **3**, 257-261.

Herzberg, M.C., Brintzenhofe, K.L. & Clawson, C.C. (1983). Aggregation of human platelets and adhesion of *Streptococus sanguis*. *Infection and Immunity* **39**, 1457-1469.

Herzberg, M.C. & Meyer, M.W. (1996). Effects of oral flora on platelets: possible consequences in cardiovascular disease. *Journal of Periodontology* **67**, 1138-1142.

Herzberg, M.E. & Meyer, M.W. (1998). Dental plaque, platelets and cardiovascular diseases. *Annals of Periodontology* **3**, 152-160.

Hill, G.B. (1998). Preterm birth: associations with genital and possibly oral microflora. *Annals of Periodontology* **3**, 222-232.

Hujoel, P.P., Drangsholt, M., Spiekerman, C. & Derouen, T.A. (2000). Periodontal disease and coronary heart disease risk. *Journal of the American Medical Association* **284**, 1406-1410.

Hunter, W. (1900). Oral sepsis as a cause of disease. *British Medical Journal* **1**, 215-216.

Hunter, W. (1910). The role of sepsis and antisepsis in medicine. *Lancet* **1**, 79-86.

Jeffcoat, M.K., Geurs, N., Reddy, M.S., Cliver, S.O., Goldenberg, R.L. & Hauth, J.C. (2001a). Periodontal infection and preterm birth. *JADA* **132**, 875-880.

Jeffcoat, M.K., Geurs, N.C., Reddy, M.S., Cliver, S., Goldenberg, R. & Hauth, J. (2001b). Periodontal infections and preterm birth: results of a prospective study. *Journal of Dental Research* **80**, 956 (abstract 1222).

Joshipura, K.J., Rimm, E.B., Douglass, C.W., Trichopoulos, D., Ascherio, A. & Willett, W.C. (1996). Poor oral health and coronary heart disease. *Journal of Dental Research* **75**, 1631-1636.

Kapur, K., Glass, R., Loftus, E., Alman, J. & Fuller, R. (1972). The Veterans Administration longitudinal study of oral health and disease. *Aging and Human Development* **3**, 125-137.

King, H., Aubert, R.E. & Herman, W.H. (1998). Global burden of diabetes 1995-2025; prevalence, numerical estimates and projections. *Diabetes Care* **21**, 1414-1431.

Kirstein, M., Aston, C., Hintz, R. & Vlassara, H. (1992). Receptor-specific induction of insulin-like growth factor 1 in human monocytes by advanced glycosylation end product-modified proteins. *Journal of Clinical Investigation* **90**, 439-446.

Kjersem, H., Hilsted, J., Madsbad, S., Wandall, J.H., Johnsen, K.S. & Borregaard, N. (1988). Polymorphonuclear leucocyte dysfunction during short-term metabolic changes from normo- to hyperglycemia in type 1 (insulin dependent) diabetic patients. *Infection* **16**, 215-221.

Lanning, J.C., Kilbelink, D.R. & Chen, L.T. (1983). Teratogenic effects of endotoxin in the golden hamster. *Teratogenesis, Carcinogenesis, & Mutagenesis* **3**, 145-149.

Lieff, S., Jared, H., McKaig, R., Herbert, W., Murtha, A., Moss, K., Worley, M., Smith, F., Block, M., Brown, P., Beck, J. & Offenbacher, S. (2000). Periodontitis and preterm low birthweight risk in pregnant women. *Journal of Dental Research* **79**, 608 (abstract 3713).

Lien, Y.H., Stern, R., Fu, J.C.C. & Siegel, R.C. (1984). Inhibition of collagen fibril formation *in vitro* and subsequent cross-linking by glucose. *Science* **225**, 1489-1491.

Lilienfeld, A. (1967). *Foundations of Epidemiology*. New York: Oxford University Press.

Loesche, W.J. (1994). Periodontal disease as a risk factor for heart disease. *Compendium of Continuing Education in Dentistry* **15**, 976-991.

Loesche, W.J., Schook, A., Terpenning, M.S., Chen, Y-M., Dominguez, L. & Grossman, N. (1998). Assessing the relationship between dental disease and coronary heart disease in elderly US veterans. *Journal of the American Dental Association* **129**, 301-311.

Lopez, H.J., Smith, P. & Guitierrez, J. (2001). Periodontal therapy reduces the risk of preterm low birthweight. *Journal of Dental Research* **80**, abstract 1223.

Madianos, P.N., Lieff, S., Murtha, A.P., Boggess, K.A., Auten, R.L., Beck, J.D. & Offenbacher, S. (2002). Maternal periodontitis and prematurity: Part II – maternal infection and fetal exposure. *Annals of Periodontology* (in press).

Manoucherhr-Pour, M., Spagnuolo, P.J., HM, Bissada, N.F. (1981). Impaired neutrophil chemotaxis in diabetic patients with severe periodontitis. *Journal of Dental Research* **60**, 729-730.

Matilla, K.J. (1989). Viral and bacterial infections in patients with acute myocardial infarction. *Journal of Internal Medicine* **225**, 293-296.

Matilla, K., Nieminen, M., Valtonen, V., Rasi, V., Kesaniemi, Y., Syrjala, S., Jungul, P., Isoluoma, M., Hietaniemi, K., Jokinen, M. & Huttunen, J. (1989). Association between dental health and acute myocardial infarction. *British Medical Journal* **298**, 779-782.

Matilla, K.J., Valle, M.S., Nieminen, M.S., Valtonen, V.V. & Hietaniemi, K.L. (1993). Dental infections and coronary atherosclerosis. *Atherosclerosis* **103**, 205-211.

Matilla, K.J., Valtonen, V.V., Nieminen, M. & Huttunen, J.K. (1995). Dental infection and the risk of new coronary events: prospective study of patients with documented coronary artery disease. *Clinical Infectious Disease* **20**, 588-592.

McDonald, H.M., O'Loughlin, J.A., Jolley, P., Vigneswaren, P. & McDonald, P.J. (1991). Vaginal infections and preterm labor. *British Journal of Obstetrics and Gynecology* **98**, 427-435.

Mendez, M.V., Scott, T., LaMonte, W., Vokonas, P., Menzoian, J.O. & Garcia, R. (1998). An association between periodontal disease and peripheral vascular disease. *American Journal of Surgery* **176**, 153-157.

Miller, L.S., Manwell, M.A., Newbold, D., Redding, M.E., Rasheed, A., Blodgett, J. & Kornman K.S. (1992). The relationship between reduction in periodontal inflammation and diabetes control: A report of 9 cases. *Journal of Clinical Periodontology* **63**, 843-848.

Miller, W.D. (1891). The human mouth as a focus of infection. *Dental Cosmos* **33**, 689-713.

Mitchell-Lewis, D.A., Papapanou, P.N., Engebretson, S., Grbic, J., Herrera-Abreu, M., Celenti, R., Chen, J.C. & Lamster, I.B. (2000). Periodontal intervention decreases the risk of preterm low birthweight. *Journal of Dental Research* **79**, abstract 3712.

Mojon, P., Budtz-Jorgensen, E., Michel, J. & Limebach, H. (1997). Oral health and history of respiratory tract infection in frail institutionalized elders. *Gerodontology* **14**, 9-16.

Morrison, H.I., Ellison, L.F. & Taylor, G.W. (1999). Periodontal disease and risk of fatal coronary heart and cerebrovascular diseases. *Journal of Cardiovascular Risk* **6**, 7-11.

Nelson, R.G., Shlossman, M., Budding, L.M., Pettitt, D.J., Saad, M.F., Genco, R.J. & Knowler, W.C. (1990). Periodontal disease and NIDDM in Pima Indians. *Diabetes Care* **13**, 836-840.

Nishimura, F., Takahashi, K., Kurihara, M., Takashiba, S. & Murayama, Y. (1998). Periodontal disease as a complication of diabetes mellitus. *Annals of Periodontology* **3**, 20-29.

Offenbacher, S. (1996). Periodontal diseases: pathogenesis. *Annals of Periodontology* **1**, 821-878.

Offenbacher, S., Jared, H.L., O'Reilly, P.G., Wells, S.R., Salvi, G.E., Lawrence, H.P., Socransky, S.S. & Beck, J.D. (1998). Potential pathogenic mechanisms of periodontitis-associated pregnancy complication. *Annals of Periodontology* **3**, 233-250.

Offenbacher, S., Katz, V., Fertik, G., Collins, J., Boyd, D., Maynor, G., McKaig, R & Beck, J. (1996). Periodontal infection as a possible risk factor for preterm low birthweight. *Journal of Periodontology* **67**, 1103-1113.

Offenbacher, S., Lieff, S., Boggess, K., Murtha, A., Madianos, P., Champagne, C., McKaig, R., Jared, H., Mauriello, S., Auten, R., Herbert, W. & Beck, J. (2002). Maternal periodontitis and prematurity: Part I – obstetric outcome of prematurity and growth restriction. *Annals of Periodontology* (in press).

Offenbacher, S., Madianos, P.N., Champagne, C.M., Southerland, J., Paquette, D.W., Williams, R.C., Slade, G. & Beck, J. (1999). Periodontitis-atherosclerosis syndrome: An expanded model of pathogenesis. *Journal of Periodontal Research* **34**, 346-352.

O'Reilly, P.G. & Claffey, W.M. (2000). A history of oral sepsis as a cause of disease. *Periodontology 2000* **23**, 13-18.

Page, R.C. (1998a). The pathobiology of periodontal diseases may affect systemic diseases: inversion of a paradigm. *Annals of Periodontology* **3**, 108-120.

Page, R.C. (1998b) Periodontal diseases: a new paradigm. *Journal of Dental Education* **62**, 812-821.

Ross, R. (1999). Mechanisms of disease: atherosclerosis – an inflammatory disease. *New England Journal of Medicine* **340**, 115-126.

Russell, S.L., Boylan, R.J., Kaslick, R.S., Scannapieco, F.A. & Katz, R.V. (1999). Respiratory pathogen colonization of the dental plaque of institutionalized elders. *Special Care in Dentistry* **19**, 1-7.

Safkan-Seppala, B. & Ainamo, J. (1992). Periodontal conditions in insulin-dependent diabetes mellitus. *Journal of Clinical Periodontology* **19**, 24-29.

Salmela, P.I., Oikarinen, A., Pirtiaho, H., Knip, M., Niemi, M. & Ryhänen, L. (1989). Increased non-enzymatic glycosylation and reduced solubility of skin collagen in insulin-dependent diabetic patients. *Diabetes Research* **11**, 115-120.

Salvi, G.E., Beck, J.D. & Offenbacher, S. (1998). PGE2, IL-1 beta, and TNF-alpha responses in diabetics as modifiers of periodontal disease expression. *Annals of Periodontology* **3**, 40-50.

Scannapieco, F.A. (1999). Role of oral bacteria in respiratory infection. *Journal of Periodontology* **70**, 793-802.

Scannapieco, F.A. & Ho, A.W. (2001). Potential associations between chronic respiratory disease and periodontal disease: Analysis of National Health and Nutrition Examination Survey III. *Journal of Periodontology* **72**, 50-56.

Scannapieco, F.A., Papandonatos, G.D. & Dunford, R.G. (1998). Associations between oral conditions and respiratory disease in a national sample survey population. *Annals of Periodontology* **3**, 251-256.

Scannapieco, F.A., Stewart, E.M. & Mylotte, J.M. (1992). Coloni-

zation of dental plaque by respiratory pathogens in medical intensive care patients. *Critical Care Medicine* **20**, 740-745.

Schmidt, A.M., Weidman, E., Lalla, E., Yan, S.D., Hori, O., Cao, R., Brett, J.G. & Lamster, I.B. (1996). Advanced glycation endproducts (AGEs) induce oxidant stress in the gingiva: a potential mechanism underlying accelerated periodontal disease associated with diabetes. *Journal of Periodontal Research* **31**, 508-515.

Seppälä, B. & Ainamo, J. (1994). A site-by-site follow-up study on the effect of controlled versus poorly controlled insulin-dependent diabetes mellitus. *Journal of Clinical Periodontology* **21**, 161-165.

Seppälä, B., Seppälä, M. & Ainamo, J. (1993). A longitudinal study on insulin-dependent diabetes mellitus and periodontal disease. *Journal of Clinical Periodontology* **20**, 161-165.

Seppälä, B., Shlossman, M., Knowler, W.C., Pettit, D.J. & Genco, R.J. (1990). Type 2 diabetes mellitus and periodontal disease. *Journal of American Dental Association* **121**, 532-536.

Shlossman, M., Knowler, W.C., Pettit, D.J. & Genco, R.J. (1990). Type 2 diabetes mellitus and periodontal disease. *Journal of the American Dental Association* **121**, 532-536.

Slavkin, H.C. & Baum, B.J. (2000). Relationship of dental and oral pathology to systemic illness. *Journal of the American Medical Association* **284**, 1215-1217.

Smith, G.T., Greenbaum, C.J., Johnson, B.D. & Persson, G.R. (1996). Short-term responses to periodontal therapy in insulin-dependent diabetic patients. *Journal of Periodontology* **67**, 794-802.

Sobel, J.D. (2000). Bacterial vaginosis. *Annual Reviews of Medicine* **51**, 349-356.

Stewart, J.E., Wager, K.A., Friedlander, A.H. & Zadeh, H.H. (2001). The effect of periodontal treatment on glycemic control in patients with type 2 diabetes mellitus. *Journal of Clinical Periodontology* **28**, 306-310.

Taylor, G.W., Burt, B.A., Becker, M.P., Genco, R.J., Shlossman, M., Knowler, W.C. & Pettit, D.J. (1996). Severe periodontitis and risk for poor glycemic control in patients with non-insulin-dependent diabetes mellitus. *Journal of Periodontology* **67**(10 Suppl), 1085-1093.

Taylor, G.W., Burt, B.A., Becker, M.P., Genco, R.J., Shlossman, M., Knowler, W.E. & Pettit, D.J. (1998a). Non-insulin dependent diabetes mellitus and alveolar bone loss progression over 2 years. *Journal of Periodontology* **69**, 76-83.

Taylor, G.W., Burt, B.A., Becker, M.P., Genco, R.J. & Schlossman, M. (1998b). Glycemic control and alveolar bone loss progression in type 2 diabetics. *Annals of Periodontology* **3**, 30-39.

Thoden van Velzen, T., Abraham-Inpijin, L. & Moore, W.R. (1984). Plaque and systemic disease: reappraisal of the focal concept. *Journal of Clinical Periodontology* **11**, 209-220.

Thorn, D.H., Grayson, J.T., Siscovick, D.S., Wang, S., Weiss, N.S. & Daling, J.R. (1992). Association of prior infection with *Chlamydia pneumoniae* and angiographically demonstrated coronary artery disease. *Journal of the American Medical Association* **268**, 68-72.

Thorstensson, H. & Hugoson, A. (1993). Periodontal disease experience in adult long-duration insulin-dependent diabetics. *Journal of Clinical Periodontology* **20**, 352-358.

Valtonen, V.V. (1999). Role of infections in atherosclerosis. *American Heart Journal* **138**, 5431-5433.

Vlassara, H., Brownlee, M., Manogue, K.R., Dinarello, C.A. & Pasagian, A. (1988). Cachectin/TNF and IL-1 induced by glucose-modified proteins: role in normal tissue remodeling. *Science* **240**(4858), 1546-1548.

Waite, D.E. & Bradley, R.E. (1965). Oral infections. *Journal of American Dental Association* **71**, 587-592.

Weringer, E.J. & Arquilla, E.R. (1981). Wound healing in normal and diabetic Chinese hamsters. *Diabetologia* **21**, 394-401.

Williams, C.E., Davenport, E.S., Sterne, J.A., Sivapathasundaram, V., Fearne, J.M. & Curtis, M.A. (2000). Mechanisms of risk in preterm low birthweight infants. *Periodontology 2000* **23**, 142-150.

Williams, R. & Mahan, C. (1960). Periodontal disease and diabetes in young adults. *JAMA* **172**, 776-778.

Wu, T., Trevisan, M., Genco, R., Falkner, K., Dorn, J. & Sempos, C. (2000a). An examination of the relation between periodontal health status and cardiovascular risk factors: serum total and HDL cholesterol, C-reactive protein and plasma fibrinogen. *American Journal of Epidemiology* **151**, 273-282.

Wu, T., Trevisan, M., Genco, R.J., Dorn, J.P., Falkner, K.L. & Sempos, C.T. (2000b). Periodontal disease and risk of cerebrovascular disease. The first national health and nutrition examination survey and its follow-up study. *Archives of Internal Medicine* **160**, 2749-2755.

Yan, S.D., Schmidt, A.M., Anderson, G.M., Zhang, J., Brett, J.,

Zou, Y.S., Pinsky, D. & Stern, D. (1994). Enhanced cellular oxidant stress by the interaction of advanced glycation end products with their receptors/binding proteins. *Journal of Biological Chemistry* **269**, 9889-9897.

Yoon, J.W. (1990). The role of viruses and environmental factors in the induction of diabetes. *Current Topics in Microbiology and Immunology* **164**, 95-123.

Yui, S., Sasaki, T., Araki, N., Horiuchi, S. & Yamazaki, M. (1994). Induction of macrophage growth by advanced glycation end products of the Maillard reaction. *Journal of Immunology* **152**, 1943-1949.

CHAPTER 17

Genetics in Relation to Periodontitis

BRUNO G. LOOS AND UBELE VAN DER VELDEN

INTRODUCTION AND DEFINITIONS

Periodontitis is a multifactorial disease for which several risk and susceptibility factors are proposed in the natural history of periodontitis (Page et al. 1997). A *risk factor* for periodontitis is a factor (environmental, behavioral or biologic) confirmed by temporal sequence, usually in longitudinal studies. The presence of a risk factor directly increases the probability of a disease occurring, and the absence of a risk factor reduces this possibility (Norderyd 1998). Risk factors are part of the causal chain, or expose the host to the causal chain. Risk factors are by definition modifiable. Good examples of risk factors in relation to periodontitis are plaque and smoking. In cross-sectional or case-control studies a *risk indicator* may be observed, therefore when such a factor is not (yet) identified in longitudinal studies, the term *putative* risk factor is used.

In contrast to modifiable risk factors, non-modifiable determinants or background factors, like age, gender and genotype (genetic make-up) are recognized as *susceptibility factors*. *Putative* susceptibility factors are determinants, only confirmed in cross-sectional or case-control studies.

In this chapter the terms *severity factor* and *putative severity factor* will also be used. These terms are employed when factors are studied in patients only, and no control subjects without periodontitis are included in these investigations. For example, if a given genotype is more frequently observed in patients with severe periodontitis than in patients with the moderate form of the disease (cross-sectional study), one can regard that genotype as a putative severity factor. If a putative severity factor is confirmed in a longitudinal patient population study, it becomes a severity factor. Such a severity factor may or may not turn out to be a susceptibility factor as well.

The area of research related to the role of genetic factors in periodontitis frequently uses specific patient populations. During the years, however, the nomenclature of the diagnosis of the various forms of periodontitis has changed. In this chapter the diagnosis of the form of periodontitis as mentioned in the original research papers is used as much as possible. These include early onset periodontitis (currently aggressive periodontitis) subdivided into prepubertal periodontitis, juvenile periodontitis and rapidly progressive periodontitis. The latter diagnosis is frequently a synonym for post juvenile periodontitis and generalized juvenile periodontitis. Adult periodontitis is currently referred to as chronic periodontitis.

The definitions above are important in studies of the etiology and pathogenesis of periodontitis, of which genetics forms an important aspect.

Evidence for the role of genetics in periodontitis

Heritability of aggressive periodontitis (early onset periodontitis)

It was recognized a long time ago that frequently siblings of patients with juvenile periodontitis (JP) also suffer from periodontitis. This was mainly based on case reports of one or a few families ascertained on the basis of one subject (the proband) with JP. In an American study on 77 siblings of 39 probands with localized (L) or generalized (G) JP, it was shown that almost 50% of the siblings also suffered from JP (Boughman et al. 1992). In 11 families a co-occurrence of LJP and GJP was present. As an epidemiological survey in the US showed that the prevalence of JP varies between 0.16 and 2.49% (Löe & Brown 1991), the high prevalence of JP in these families suggests a genetic background for the disease. The largest JP family study included 227 probands with aggressive periodontitis (Marazita et al. 1994). There were 26 GJP individuals whose earlier records were consistent with LJP, i.e. demonstrating progression from the localized to a more generalized form.

Furthermore, there were 16 families with co-occurrence of LJP and GJP, confirming the findings of Boughman et al. (1992). Out of the 227 probands, 104 had at least one first-degree relative clinically examined. Now it was possible to carry out a segregation analysis on 100 families (four families each had two probands). Segregation analysis is a formal method of studying families with a disease to assess the likelihood that the condition is inherited as a genetic trait. The family members included 527 subjects: 60 with LJP, 72 with GJP, 254 unaffected subjects and 141 subjects with an unknown periodontal condition. The group of unaffected subjects included edentulous subjects, subjects with adult periodontitis and periodontally healthy subjects. The majority of the families were of African-American origin. The authors concluded that the most likely mode of inheritance was autosomal dominant in both African-American and Caucasian kindreds, with 70% penetrance in African-Americans and 73% in Caucasians.

Heritability of chronic periodontitis (adult periodontitis)

Very few investigations exist with regard to family studies of probands with chronic (adult) periodontitis or younger subjects with minor periodontitis. Van der Velden et al. (1993) studied the effect of sibling relationship on the periodontal condition in a group of young Indonesians deprived of regular dental care. The study population included 23 family units consisting of three or more siblings. In all, 78 subjects aged 15-25 years were studied. The mean interproximal amount of loss of attachment in this population was 0.29 mm. The individual mean ranged from 0 to 1.27 mm. In 33% of the subjects, ≥ 1 sites with a probing depth of 5 mm or more in conjunction with 2 mm loss of attachment were present. The results of the analysis showed a significant siblingship effect for plaque, calculus, loss of attachment, spirochetes on the tongue and in the pocket, P. gingivalis on the gingiva and in the saliva and P. intermedia in the saliva. However, the microbiological parameters which showed a significant siblingship effect were not significantly correlated with attachment loss (Van der Velden et al. 1993). These findings suggest that also in less severe forms of periodontitis there may be a genetic background for the disease.

In order to study familial aspects of chronic (adult) periodontitis in a Dutch population, 24 families were selected at the Academic Center for Dentistry Amsterdam (Petit et al. 1994), each consisting of a proband with chronic (adult) periodontitis, a spouse and 1-3 children. The mean age of the probands was 39 years, with a range from 30 to 50 years. In total, 49 children were investigated with an age range of 3 months to 15 years. The results showed that none of the children under the age of 5 years was affected by periodontitis, whereas in the group of 5-15 years, 21% had at least one pocket ≥ 5 mm in conjunction with loss of attachment. In the group of 10-15 years this was 45%. In contrast, in an epidemiological study carried out in the city of Amsterdam, it was shown that the prevalence of pockets ≥ 5 mm in conjunction with loss of attachment in 15-year-old adolescents is about 5% (Van der Velden et al. 1989). Therefore, collectively, these results suggest that periodontitis also aggregates in families.

The twin model

The twin model is probably the most powerful method by which to study genetic aspects of periodontal diseases. Monozygous (MZ) twins arise from a single fertilized ovum and are therefore genetically identical and of the same sex. Dizygous (DZ) twins arise from the fertilization of two separate ova and share, on average, one half of their descendent genes in the same way as siblings do. In twin studies the terms concordance and disconcordance are often used. This means the degree of similarity or dissimilarity between twins in respect of one or more particular characteristics. Any discordance in disease between MZ twins must be due to environmental factors. Any discordance between DZ twins could arise from environmental and/or genetic variance. For a condition that is predominantly environmental in origin, the concordance rates of MZ and DZ twins would be expected to be similar. However, if a disease has a genetic background, concordance rates would be greater in MZ twins compared to DZ twins. Even more powerful is the addition of monozygous twins who

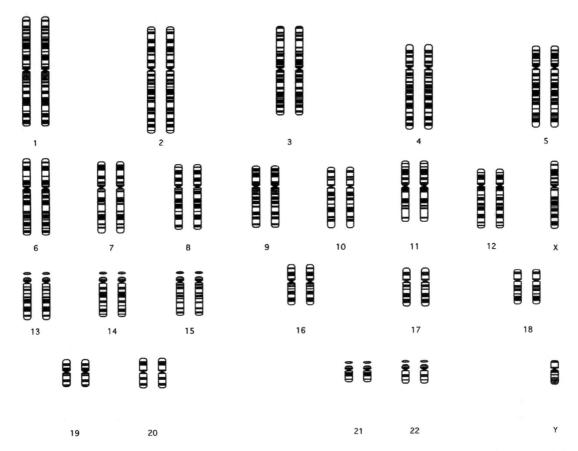

Fig. 17-1. Schematic drawing of 23 pairs of chromosomes (the diploid human genome). 22 pairs of autosomal chromosomes and 1 pair of sex chromosomes are present. In this case the genome of a male is shown (one X and one Y chromosome). In the case of a female, two X chromosomes would have been present. G-banding generates a characteristic lateral series of bands in each member of the chromosome set. Adapted from Hart et al. (2000a).

were separated at birth and reared apart (MZA), since in that case the effects of shared genes can be examined without the confounding effects of a common family environment.

The largest twin study included 4908 twin pairs of which, on the basis of questionnaire data, 349 (116 MZ and 233 DZ) pairs reported a history of periodontal disease in one or both pair members (Corey et al. 1993). The mean age of the MZ twins was 33 years and of the DZ twins 35 years. The concordance rates ranged from 0.23 to 0.38 for MZ twins and 0.08 to 0.16 for DZ twins. Michalowicz and co-workers evaluated the periodontal condition (attachment loss, pocket depth, gingival index and plaque index) of 110 adult twins with a mean age of 40 years ranging from 16 to 70 years (Michalowicz et al. 1991). This study included 63 MZ twin pairs reared together, 33 like-sexed DZ twin pairs reared together and 14 MZA twin pairs. Their results showed that the correlations of reared together MZ twins are consistently greater than those of DZ twins. Heritability estimates from the MZA twins were 0.38 for attachment loss, 0.46 for plaque, 0.69 for pocket depth and 0.82 for the gingival index. These values were, for the twins reared together, 0.48, 0.38, 0.51 and 0.40 respectively. These results indicate that between 38 and 82% of the population variance for these measures may be attributed to genetic fac-

tors. In a recent study on 117 adult pair twins (Michalowicz et al. 2000), the analysis included the evaluation of the environmental factors like smoking and utilization of dental services. The study included 64 MZ twin pairs (mean age 41 years) and 53 DZ pair twins (mean age 42 years). The results showed that chronic (adult) periodontitis was estimated to have approximately 50% heritability, which was unaltered following adjustments for behavioral variables including smoking. In contrast, while MZ twins were also more similar than DZ twins for gingivitis scores, there was no evidence of heritability for gingivitis after behavioral covariates such as utilization of dental care and smoking were incorporated in the analysis.

Another study on 169 adult twins with early periodontitis (Michalowicz et al. 1999) looked at whether host genetic factors influence the presence of *A. actinomycetemcomitans*, *P. gingivalis*, *P. intermedia*, *F. nucleatum* and *P. corrodens*. The study included 21 MZ twins and 17 DZ twins reared apart as well as 83 MZ twins and 48 DZ twins reared together. The MZ twins ranged in age from 16 to 80 years with a mean of 44 years, the DZ twins ranged in age from 22 to 67 years with a mean of 48 years. The subject-based prevalences of the bacteria in the twin groups were: *P. gingivalis* 11%, *A. actinomycetemcomitans* 22%, *P. inter-*

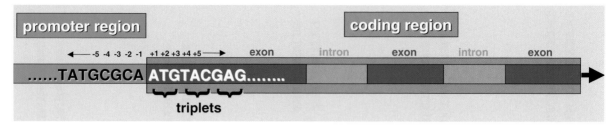

Fig. 17-2. Schematic representation of a gene. The gene consists of a promoter and a coding region. Within the coding region, intermittent areas of non-coding DNA exist (intron). Exons contain triplets of nucleotides (codons) that code for a specific amino acid. The number and length of exons and introns within the coding region is variable per gene.

media 19%, *E. corrodens* 0.34% and *F. nucleatum* 40%. Interestingly, for all species examined the concordance rates were not significantly different between MZ and DZ twin groups. These findings were apparent despite similar smoking histories, self-reported oral hygiene practices and antibiotic use. Furthermore, MZ twins reared together were no more similar than MZ reared apart twins with respect to any bacterial species examined.

Therefore it can be concluded that the basis for familial aggregation of periodontitis appears not bacterial/environmental/behavioural in nature; rather, genetics seem to form the basis for the familial aggregation of periodontitis.

Human genes and polymorphisms

Each normal human being has 23 pairs of *chromosomes* (the *diploid* human genome), 22 pairs of *autosomal* chromosomes and 1 pair of *sex* chromosomes (XX for females and XY for males) (Fig. 17-1). From each pair, one chromosome is inherited from the father and one from the mother. Chromosomes show differences in size and have characteristic lateral series of bands (G-banding); therefore each chromosome can be identified by its characteristic size and banding pattern. Each chromosome contains a single, very long *duplex* of deoxyribonucleic acid (DNA). DNA consists of chemically linked sequences of *nucleotides*; these are the "building blocks" of the DNA and always contain a nitrogenous base. Four nitrogenous bases exist: adenine (A), guanine (G), cytosine (C) and thymine (T). The bases are linked to a sugar (2-deoxyribose), where a phosphate group is also added. The *haploid* human genome (i.e. one copy of 22 autosomal chromosomes and one sex chromosome) consists of 3.3×10^9 nucleotides (also written as 3.3×10^9 base pairs (bp)).

In the chromosomes, DNA is arranged in a double helix model: two polynucleotide chains in the duplex are associated together by hydrogen bonding between the nitrogenous bases. These reactions are described as *base pairing* and they are complementary: G pairs only with C, and A pairs only with T. Therefore, if one

chain of DNA is sequenced, the complementary chain of the duplex can be deduced.

DNA contains the genetic code and a given specific sequence of nucleotides encodes for the sequence of amino acids that constitutes the corresponding protein (Fig. 17-2). The genetic code is read in groups of three nucleotides; each trinucleotide sequence (triplet) is called a *codon*. Written in the conventional direction from left to right, the nucleotide sequence of the DNA strand that codes for a protein has a starting point and an end point. In this way on the DNA strand, a gene can be deciphered. A gene consists of two parts (Fig. 17-2): (1) a *coding region*, i.e. a reading frame starting at nucleotide position +1, containing a multitude of triplets that codes for a sequence of amino acids to form a protein; and (2) a *promoter* region, i.e. a sequence of nucleotides upstream (left) of the coding region starting with nucleotide position –1 read from right to left, that is not organized in a series of triplets but contains stretches of nucleotides that are essential for the regulation of the *transcription* of the coding region. Within the coding region intermittent areas of non-coding DNA exist; these regions are called *introns*. The true coding areas within the coding region are called *exons* (Fig. 17-2). From the recent results of the human genome project, it is estimated that about 30 000–40 000 human genes exist.

Variant forms of a gene that can occupy a specific chromosal site *(locus)* are called *alleles*. For example, hemoglobin is a complex molecule consisting of two α-type and two β-type chains. The gene for the β chain may have in some instances a mutation, causing sickle cell anemia. In this case, the *rare* β^s sickle allele, responsible for sickle cell anemia, is a variant of the *normal* β^A allele for the β gene. Two or more alleles for a given locus may exist in nature throughout evolution, but may develop any time. A *polymorphic* locus is one whose alleles are such that the most common, *normal* variant (*N*-allele) among them occurs with < 99 % frequency in the population. Thus, if a locus is for example *bi-allelic*, the rarer allele (designated *R*-allele) must occur with a frequency > 1% in the population. This way, when different alleles of a given gene co-exist in the human population, we speak about *genetic polymorphisms*.

Polymorphisms arise as a result of mutation. All organisms suffer from certain numbers of spontane-

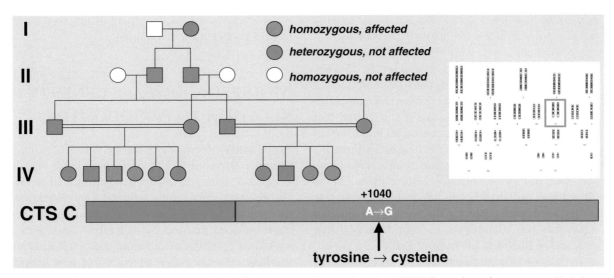

Fig. 17-3. A functional recessive mutation in the gene encoding cathepsin C (CTS C gene) on chromosome 11, is inherited in generation IV from a common ancestral grandmother in generation I (Hart et al. 2000a). O = male, □ = female, single horizontal line between O and □ is marriage between unrelated spouses, double horizontal lines between O and □ is marriage with a related family member. Vertical lines represent children from a marriage. Subjects with the CTS C *R*-allele are indicated.

ous mutations as the result of normal cellular operation or random interactions with the environment. An alteration that changes only a single base pair is called a point mutation. Not all such mutations are repaired and they can therefore be inherited and transmitted for generations. The most common class of point mutations is the *transition*, comprising the substitution of one nucleotide with another. The variation at the site harboring such changes has recently been termed a "single nucleotide polymorphism" (SNP) (Schork et al. 2000).

The SNP may have no effects or may have some important biological effects. For example, if a transition has taken place within the coding region of a gene, it may result in an amino acid substitution and therefore an altered protein, perhaps with an altered function. Or, when such mutations have taken place in the promoter region of the gene, it may or may not result in altered gene regulation. The altered regulation due to the mutation in the promoter region may give rise to reduced or inhibited gene expression or, alternatively, result in overexpression of the gene, perhaps with biological consequences. SNPs occur the most over any other type of polymorphism; the frequency of SNPs across the human genome is estimated at every 0.3-1 kilobases (Kb) (Schork et al. 2000).

Other types of genetic polymorphisms result from *insertions* or *deletions* (Schork et al. 2000). The simple form of this polymorphism is where a single nucleotide pair may be deleted or may be inserted with the same potential effects as described above for the transition. The most common type of insertion/deletion polymorphism is the existence of variable numbers of repeated bases or nucleotide patterns in a genetic region. Repeated base patterns can consist of several hundreds of basepairs, known as a variable number of tandem repeats (VNTRs or *mini-satellites*). Also very common are *micro-satellites*, which consist of two,

three or four nucleotides repeats, a variable number of times; micro-satellites are also referred to as *simple tandem repeats* (STRs). Such repeats are considered highly polymorphic and often result in many alleles or gene variants due to the existence of many different repeat sizes within the population. The STRs may occur every 3-10 Kb genome wide (Schork et al. 2000).

Genetic polymorphisms are highly useful in population genetic studies. After genotyping of individuals and assessing genotype frequencies among groups of interest, one can also calculate the frequency of the *N*-allele and the *R*-allele among the groups or populations under study. Each of the alleles and each of the resulting genotypes have a particular frequency in the population. It is important to realize that populations with different genotype frequencies may have comparable or equal allele frequencies. Furthermore, frequencies of genotypes and alleles may differ between a diseased group and a healthy group. Subsequently, when a given allele is identified to be associated with disease (as susceptibility and/or as severity factor), functional studies can be started to investigate the possible role of that gene in the etiology and pathogenesis of the disease.

GENETICS IN RELATION TO DISEASE IN GENERAL

Most human diseases have a complex pathogenesis. For example, it is widely known that for heart diseases, hypertension, cancer and Alzheimer's disease, interactions between genetic and environmental factors determine disease expression. The genes that are identified to be involved in complex multifactorial diseases are called *modifying disease genes* (Hart 1996, Hart et al. 2000b). They contrast with *major disease genes*, which, when a given aberrant allelic form is present, are responsible for disease expression according to Mendel's laws (Hart 1996, Hart et al. 2000b), for example, the fatal inherited disease cystic fibrosis. This disease is caused by a recessive mutation in the cystic fibrosis transmembrane conductance regulator (CFTR) gene. This gene encodes for a protein that functions as a plasma membrane chloride channel in epithelial tissues, in particular in lung epithelium. If a person is *homozygous* for the rare disease allele (*R*-allele), then he/she will develop cystic fibrosis. On the other hand, individuals will not develop the disease if they are homozygous for the normal (*N*) allele or when they are *heterozygous*, i.e. they have both the *dominant N*-allele and the *recessive R*-allele.

To date, genetic studies in relation to periodontitis have revealed only one major disease gene (see the next section) that follows the principles of Mendel. Most forms of periodontitis are likely to be associated with multiple modifying genes, i.e. the disease is said to be *polygenic*. Analogous to other complex diseases, it is estimated that for periodontitis between 10 and 20 genes may be involved. However, it is important to realize that the number and type of modifying disease genes for the same disease may not be equal for different ethnic populations and may also be influenced by environmental factors.

A MAJOR DISEASE GENE ASSOCIATED WITH PERIODONTITIS

Through an internal marriage event in a family of Jordanian descent, Hart and co-workers have identified and localized a gene on chromosome 11 that is responsible for a severe form of prepubertal periodontitis (Hart et al. 2000a). Starting with four affected children from generation IV of two families, a disease causing *R*-allele of the cathepsin C (CTS C) gene was discovered (Fig. 17-3). Cathepsin C is a proteinase which is found in neutrophils and lymphocytes as well as epithelial cells. Affected children, but not their brothers and sisters, were homozygous for an A to G transition polymorphism at gene position +1040. This resulted in a substitution of the amino acid tyrosine by a cysteine. This polymorphism was shown to be functional as there was a decreased cathepsin C activity (Hart et al. 2000a).

Interestingly, other mutations in the CTS C gene have been identified and have been linked to the Papillon-Lefèvre syndrome, a disease which is also associated with a severe form of prepubertal periodontitis (Hart et al. 1999, Toomes et al. 1999). Therefore, certain functional CTS C gene mutations need to be considered causative for prepubertal periodontitis and Papillon-Lefèvre syndrome. However, the mechanism by which an altered function of cathepsin C plays a role in the pathogenesis of the prepubertal form of periodontitis is unknown.

MODIFYING DISEASE GENES IN RELATION TO PERIODONTITIS

Periodontitis develops in a limited subset of humans (Chapter 2). About 10-15% of the population will develop severe forms of destructive periodontal disease. The disease is importantly influenced by the microorganisms in the subgingival lesion, by acquired systemic diseases that reduce or hamper optimal host resistance, and by environmental factors. Plaque and smoking are such well-accepted risk factors. In addition, modifying disease genes contribute to susceptibility and severity of periodontitis. For these modifying disease genes Mendelian principles do not apply (Hart 1996, Hart et al. 2000b), because it is thought that both carriers (heterozygotes) as well as homozygous subjects for a given modifying disease gene, may not necessary develop the disease if no other risk factors are simultaneously present.

Currently very little is known about which genes may be involved in periodontitis as modifying disease genes. However, as the immune system is thought to play a crucial role in the pathogenesis of periodontitis, researchers have concentrated on the identification of genetic polymorphisms in several aspects of the host immunity. In particular, genetic variation in the genes of immune mediators, such as cytokines, has been used as a potential target for susceptibility factors in relation to periodontitis.

The text below reviews progress in the search for genetic polymorphisms that are associated with destructive periodontal disease.

CYTOKINE GENE POLYMORPHISMS

There are several arguments why the genes encoding for interleukin-1 (IL-1) and tumor necrosis factor-α (TNF-α) seem good candidates for genetic studies in relation to periodontitis (Cox & Duff 1996, Kornman et al. 1997, Verweij 1999, Craandijk et al. 2002):

1. There is evidence to suggest that IL-1 and TNF-α play important roles in the pathogenesis of periodontitis. IL-1α and IL-1β and TNF-α are potent immunologic mediators with proinflammatory properties. Moreover, IL-1 and TNF-α have the capacity to increase bone resorption and can regulate fibroblast cell proliferation, both from gingival and periodontal ligament origin. IL-1 and TNF-α levels are increased in the gingival crevicular fluid in periodontitis and these cytokines are found in

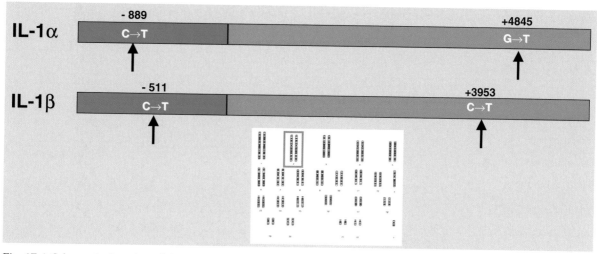

Fig. 17-4. Schematic drawing of the genes for IL-1α and IL-1β located on chromosome 2. Genetic polymorphisms are indicated.

higher levels in the inflamed periodontal tissues compared to healthy periodontal tissues.

2. Genetically determined, interindividual differences have been observed for the IL-1 and TNF-α production by peripheral blood mononuclear cells or oral leukocytes, isolated from individuals with and without periodontitis. It is conceivable that these differences in IL-1 and TNF-α production and secretion play a role as susceptibility and/or severity factors.

3. Some IL-1 and TNF-α alleles have been suggested as potential genetic markers for disease. For example, IL-1 polymorphisms have been associated with inflammatory bowel disease, Sjögren syndrome and psoriasis. TNF-α gene polymorphisms have been associated with (chronic) inflammatory and infectious disease processes, including leishmaniasis, alopecia areata, meningococcal disease, leprosy and cerebral malaria.

IL-1 gene polymorphisms

The genes encoding IL-1α and IL1-β are located in close proximity in the IL-1 gene cluster on chromosome 2 (Fig. 17-4). The first study that reported polymorphisms for the IL-1 genes in relation to periodontitis was presented by Kornman et al. (1997). The combined presence of the R-allele of the IL-1α gene at nucleotide position –889 (IL-1α^{-889T}) and the R-allele of IL-1β gene at nucleotide position +3953 (IL-1β^{+3953T}) was associated with *severity* of periodontitis in non-smoking Caucasian patients. The combined carriage rate of the R-alleles IL-1α^{-889T} and IL-1β^{+3953T} is designated the *IL-1 composite genotype* (Kornman et al. 1997). Other investigators have reported similar findings (Table 17-1), also in cross-sectional studies (McDevitt et al. 2000, Papapanou et al. 2001). It is important to note that the above studies were carried out in Caucasians (Table 17-1). Therefore, the IL-1 composite geno-

type can be considered a putative severity factor for periodontitis in Caucasians.

After these encouraging results, several studies have investigated genetic polymorphisms in the IL-1α and IL-1β genes in relation to *susceptibility* for periodontitis mostly in Caucasian populations (Table 17-1). Diehl and co-workers suggest that aggressive periodontitis is a complex but oligogenic condition, with polymorphisms in the IL-1 gene cluster as (putative) susceptibility factors (Diehl et al. 1999). However, Hodge et al. (2001) failed to show an association between the IL-1 composite genotype and GJP. Lack of association with IL-1 composite genotype was also reported for chronic (adult) periodontitis patients in two case control studies (Laine et al. 2001, Papapanou et al. 2001). It has also been reported that patients with the IL-1 composite genotype more often harbored putative periodontal pathogens and had increased counts of these pathogens (Socransky et al. 2000). Interestingly, Laine et al. (2001) reported increased frequency of the R-alleles of the IL-1α, Il-1β and IL-1 receptor antagonist genes in non-smoking patients in whom *P. gingivalis* and *A. actinomycetemcomitans* could not be detected. These latter results suggest that IL-1 gene polymorphisms play a role in the absence of other (putative) risk factors. Similar studies in Chinese and African-Americans have not resulted in significant findings, because the IL-1 composite genotype was hardly or not at all present in these ethnic populations (Armitage et al. 2000, Walker et al. 2000).

Several longitudinal studies on IL-1 polymorphisms have been performed (Table 17-1); from these studies it may be possible to assess whether a given genotype can be considered a true susceptibility and/or severity factor. For example, it was reported among periodontitis patients in maintenance over 5 to 14 years, that the IL-1 composite genotype increased the risk of tooth loss by 2.7 times (McGuire & Nunn 1999). The IL-1 composite genotype in combination with heavy smoking increased the risk of tooth loss by

Table 17-1. Summary of studies investigating the IL-1 composite genotype (Kornman et al. 1997) in relation to periodontitis

A. Cross-sectional studies

Study[1]	n patients	n controls	putative susceptibility	putative severity
Kornman et al. 1997[2]	99		not tested	+
Gore et al. 1998	32	32	–	not tested
Walker et al. 2000[3]	37	37	–	not tested
Armitage et al. 2000[4]	300		–[5]	–
McDevitt et al. 2000[6]	90		not tested	+
Hodge et al. 2001[7]	56	56	–	not tested
Papapanou et al. 2001	132	73	–	+
Laine et al. 2001	105	53	–	not tested

B. Longitudinal studies

Study[1]	n patients	susceptibility	severity
McGuire & Nunn 1999	42	not tested	+
Ehmke et al. 1999	33	not tested	–
De Sanctis & Zucchelli 2000	40	not tested	+
Cattabriga et al. 2001	60	not tested	–
Cullinan et al. 2001	295	trend	+[8]

+ or – indicates whether or not the IL-1 composite genotype can be considered a (putative) susceptibility and/or (putative) severity factor.
[1] All studies included Caucasians only, unless otherwise specified
[2] Non-smokers only
[3] African-Americans with localized juvenile periodontitis (LJP)
[4] Chinese
[5] Formally not possible to test as there is no control group; however the genotype was virtually non-existent in this population, therefore it can be deduced that the composite genotype is not a putative susceptibility factor
[6] A private practice study population
[7] Early onset periodontitis (EOP)
[8] For non-smokers > 50 years and for smokers testing positive for *P. gingivalis*

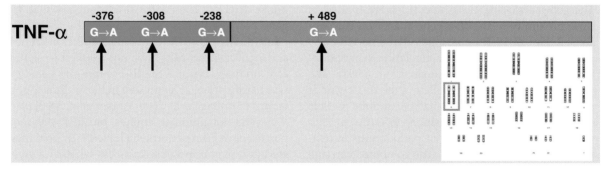

Fig. 17-5. Schematic drawing of the TNF-α gene located on chromosome 6. Genetic polymorphisms are indicated.

7.7 times (McGuire & Nunn 1999). Cullinan et al. (2001) presented a study in which 295 gingivitis and moderate periodontitis subjects were followed for 5 years and the IL-1 composite genotype was determined. Among non-smoking subjects > 50 years who were IL-1 composite genotype positive, deeper probing depths were observed than in IL-1 composite genotype negative. Furthermore, a significant interac-

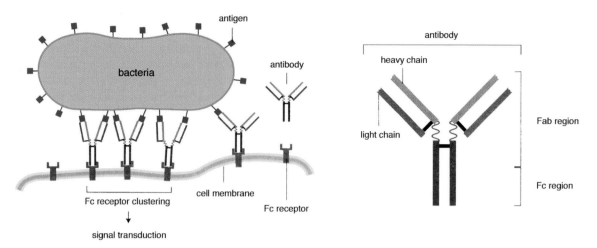

Fig. 17-6. Antibodies (immunoglobulins (Ig)) have a Fab-region (antigen binding, hypervariable region) and an Fc-region (constant for each of the Ig classes). For example, the antibodies recognize antigens on a microorganism through the Fab-region. Subsequently Fc regions bind to Fc-receptors on immune cells and this process may activate the cell. A cluster of activated receptors will initiate signal transduction and dependent on the type of immune effector cell, may induce for example phagocytosis (Van der Pol & Van de Winkel 1998a,b).

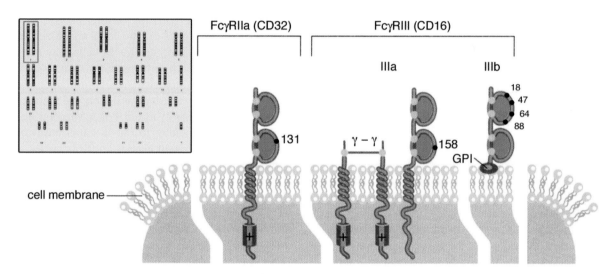

Fig. 17-7. Schematic drawing of three of the human Fc receptors for IgG. They have an extracellular part, a transmembrane region and a cytoplasmic tail (except FcγRIIIb, which is anchored in the outer leaflet of the cell membrane via a glycosyl-phosphatidyl-inositol (GPI) molecule). The extracellular part of leukocyte FcγR class II and III consists of two immunoglobulin-like domains. The + sign in the intracellular signaling motifs (cylinder) indicates the capacity of signaling to the cytoplasmic environment of the cell. The FcγRIIa-mediated effector functions can be established through the intracellular signaling motif (cylinder) within the cytoplasmic tail of the molecule. The FcγRIIIa is associated with a γ-chain homodimer, which serves as signaling subunit. The FcγRIIIb-mediated effector functions are transmitted through the GPI. The functional genetic polymorphisms are depicted as black dots (•) in the extracellular Ig-like domains. For the FcγRIIa at amino acid position 131, arginine (R) or histidine (H) is present. For the FcγRIIIa at amino acid position 158, valine (V) or phenylalanine (F) is present. The FcγRIIIb polymorphism is caused by four amino acid substitutions at positions 18, 47, 64 and 88 and results in glycosylation differences, affecting receptor affinity. The CD indication in parentheses indicates the numbering within the cluster of differentiation system of immunological markers (Van der Pol & Van de Winkel 1998a,b).

tion was found between IL-1 composite genotype positive and age, smoking and presence of *P. gingivalis*, which suggests that the IL-1 composite genotype is a contributory but non-essential susceptibility factor.

In summary, for the global population, IL-1 gene polymorphisms cannot be regarded as a susceptibility or severity factor for periodontitis. However, in Caucasian patients with chronic periodontitis, the IL-1 composite genotype may behave as a severity factor, in particular in non-smoking subjects.

TNF-α gene polymorphisms

The TNF-α gene is located on chromosome 6 within the major histocompatibility complex (MHC) gene cluster. Several studies have investigated genetic polymorphisms in the TNF-α gene as putative susceptibility and severity factors in relation to periodontitis. The genetic polymorphisms are mainly G to A transitions (Fig. 17-5). Craandijk et al. (2002) found that the frequencies of R-alleles (an A) at nucleotide positions –376, –308, –238 and +489 of the TNF-α gene in 90 patients were no different from those in 264 reference controls.

TNF-α gene polymorphisms in relation to aggressive periodontitis were also investigated, but the TNF-α^{-308} R-allele was found not to be associated with aggressive periodontitis (Shapira et al. 2001). Also, another gene marker in the TNF-α gene was investigated in relation to susceptibility for aggressive periodontitis. This concerned a marker based on a variable number of microsatellite repeats; again no indication was found for an association with GJP (Kinane et al. 1999).

Investigations into severity of periodontitis in relation to any of the TNF-α gene R-alleles also did not reveal a positive association. The carriage of a R-allele at nucleotide positions –308 and –238 revealed no differences in the % of teeth with ≥ 50% bone loss (Craandijk et al. 2002). Moreover, the carriage rates of the R-alleles at nucleotide positions –376, –308, –238, and +489 were no different among patients with moderate or severe periodontitis. Lack of association of TNF-α genetic polymorphisms with periodontitis severity was also reported by others (Kornman et al. 1997, Galbraith et al. 1998).

Based on the literature to date on TNF-α genetics in relation to periodontitis, there is no indication that any of the reported gene variations are related to the susceptibility or severity of periodontitis.

IL-10 gene polymorphisms

IL-10 is located on chromosome 1, in a cluster with closely related interleukin genes, including IL-19, IL-20 and IL-24. IL-10 plays a role in the regulation of pro-inflammatory cytokines such as IL-1 and TNF-α. Functional disturbance in IL-10 due to genetic polymorphisms could be detrimental to host tissues and could be linked to periodontal disease susceptibility. IL-10 gene polymorphisms have been investigated in relation to aggressive periodontitis; 79 Caucasian patients from West Scotland with GJP were included and matched with a control population (Kinane et al. 1999). Two microsatellite markers located in the promoter region of the gene were used; these were previously implicated in systemic lupus erythematosus (Kinane et al. 1999). However, no significant differences in frequencies of various IL-10 alleles in comparison to periodontally healthy controls were ob-

served. Also, in Japanese patients either with GJP (n = 18) or with adult periodontitis (n = 34), as well as 52 controls, polymorphisms in the promoter region of the IL-10 gene were analyzed (Yamazaki et al. 2001). No significant differences for the carriage rates of the various IL-10 alleles were seen between patients and controls. The carriage rates of the studied alleles in the IL-10 promoter region were different in Japanese from those of Caucasian heritage (Yamazaki et al. 2001), again emphasizing that allele frequencies in relation to disease for one ethnic group may not be extrapolated to another population.

FcγR GENE POLYMORPHISMS

Leukocytes exhibit receptors (R) for the constant region (Fc) of immunoglobulin (Ig) molecules. In the case of IgG, these receptors are termed FcγR. The FcγRs are found on leukocytes from both the myeloid and lymphoid lineages. The FcγR links the humoral part of the host defense with the cellular aspects of the immune system (Fig. 17-6). Thus, IgG opsonized antigens, particles, microorganisms or cells may trigger cellular effects, including phagocytosis, antibody dependent cellular cytotoxicity (ADCC), antigen presentation, cytokine release, degranulation and regulation of antibody synthesis (Van der Pol & Van de Winkel 1998a). The FcγR belong to the Ig superfamily and exist, like Ig, in different classes and subclasses. The genes for the FcγR are found on the long arm (q) of chromosome 1, and encode for three main classes of FcR: FcγRI, FcγRII and FcγRIII. Several subclasses exist, like FcγRIa and b, FcγRIIa, b and c, and FcγRIIIa and b (Van der Pol & Van de Winkel 1998a).

The FcγRIIa is the most widely distributed of the IgG receptor molecules. It is expressed on all granulocytes, on antigen presenting cells (APC), platelets, endothelial cells and a subset of T cells (Van der Pol & Van de Winkel 1998a). It has been shown that structural and functional differences in FcγRIIa are due to genetic polymorphisms. The G to A transition polymorphism in the FcγRIIa gene at nucleotide position +392 results in the substitution of histidine (H) for arginine (R) at amino acid position 131 of the receptor molecule (Fig. 17-7). Subjects homozygous for the FcγRIIa^{H131} allele (N-allele) bind IgG2 immune complexes efficiently, while individuals homozygous for the FcγRIIa^{R131} allele (R-allele) are deficient for this interaction (Warmerdam et al. 1991). Because IgG2 is generally elevated in patients with LJP, it has been speculated that the FcγRIIa R-allele may be associated with susceptibility for aggressive periodontitis: patients with the FcγRIIa^{R131} allele could be more susceptible for periodontitis due to a diminished capacity to phagocytose IgG2 opsonized *A. actinomycetemcomitans* (Wilson & Kalmar 1996). However, this hypothesis may have to be rejected since Loos et al. (2003) recently found that the N-allele carriage rate

(FcγRII[H131]) is higher in aggressive periodontitis subjects than in controls. Moreover, periodontitis patients (aggressive and chronic periodontitis) homozygous for the N-allele (H/H131 genotype) have more periodontal bone loss than the other patients carrying one or two R-alleles. Also, both the Japanese studies (Kobayashi et al. 1997, 2001) and two studies with Caucasian subjects (Colombo et al. 1998, Meisel et al. 2001), have not been able to substantiate the hypothesis by Wilson & Kalmar (1996).

The FcγRIIIa and IIIb are expressed on a limited number of immune cell types (Van der Pol & Van de Winkel 1998a). FcγRIIIa is found on monocytes and macrophages, natural killer (NK) cells and a subset of T cells. The G to T transition polymorphism in the FcγRIIIa gene at the nucleotide position +559, results in the substitution of valine (V) for phenylalanine (F) at amino acid position 158 (Fig. 17-7). Individuals who are homozygous for the FcγRIIIa[V158] allele (N-allele) have a higher affinity for IgG1 and IgG3 than subjects homozygous for the R-allele (FcγRIIIa[F158]). Moreover, subjects carrying the N-allele can bind IgG4 while the persons with the R-allele are unable to do so (Van der Pol & Van de Winkel 1998a). The FcγRIIIa N-allele (V158) is proposed as a putative susceptibility factor for periodontitis, in particular for aggressive periodontitis in a group of Dutch patients (Loos et al. 2003). Also, Meisel et al. (2001), in a German population, studied FcγRIIIa polymorphisms in relation to periodontitis severity; they observed more severe periodontal bone destruction in homozygous FcγRIIIa N-allele patients (V/V158). In a Japanese population it was found that the FcγRIIIa R-allele (F158) was overrepresented in patients with periodontal disease recurrence (Sugita et al. 1999). In contrast, a recent Japanese study showed that the FcγRIIIa N-allele was overrepresented in patients with severe periodontitis versus subjects with the moderate form (Kobayashi et al. 2001). Again, it is apparent that comparisons between the different studies are difficult as the prevalences of FcγR genotypes are different among subjects of different ethnic background (Van der Pol & Van de Winkel 1998a).

The FcγRIIIb is the most abundantly expressed IgG receptor on neutrophils, and also in the FcγRIIIb gene a bi-allelic polymorphism exists (Van der Pol & Van de Winkel 1998a). The FcγRIIIb-neutrophil antigen (NA) 1 or NA2 polymorphism is caused by four amino acid substitutions in the Fc binding region with different glycosylation patterns (Fig. 17-7). The FcγRIIIb[NA2] allele is considered the R-allele, while the NA1 allele is the N-allele. The NA2 type receptor binds less efficiently with IgG1 and IgG3 immune complexes (Van der Pol & Van de Winkel 1998a). In Japanese patients, the FcγRIIIb R-allele (NA2) was associated with early onset periodontitis (Kobayashi et al. 2000) and was found more often in adult patients with disease recurrence (Kobayashi et al. 1997). Also the combined carriage of both the R-allele of the FcγRIIIb gene and the R-allele of the FcγRIIIa gene was more frequently detected in Japanese aggressive periodontitis patients over healthy Japanese controls (Kobayashi et al. 2000).

The possibility that genes encoding for Fcγ receptors are associated with the susceptibility and severity of several forms of periodontitis in different ethnic groups seems promising. Further research is needed in larger groups of subjects from different global populations to confirm the current observations. Furthermore, functional studies among subjects with different FcγR genotypes need to be undertaken to investigate the corresponding phenotypes and unravel the role of the Fcγ receptors in the pathogenesis of periodontitis.

CONCLUSIONS AND FUTURE DEVELOPMENTS

An important problem related to research in the heredity of periodontitis is that, whatever the cause of the disease, the symptoms are the same: deepening of the periodontal pocket, loss of attachment and bone loss. In the majority of cases, the development of periodontitis in an individual depends probably on the collective presence of a number of environmental risk factors in conjunction with a number of susceptibility factors at a given time point during life. The more susceptibility factors an individual has inherited, the greater the genetic predisposition and the higher the chance for early development of periodontitis. If an individual has inherited a major disease gene this will also result in early development of periodontitis. Since children of patients with chronic periodontitis show a relatively high prevalence of minor periodontitis, it is likely that some forms of early periodontitis share a common pathogenic pathway with that of adult periodontitis.

With the increasing knowledge of major and modifying disease genes it is conceivable that a number of genetic tests will be developed. These tests could be used to diagnose the degree of genetic predisposition at an early age when periodontitis has not yet developed, e.g. children of parents suffering from periodontitis. Depending on the degree of predisposition of a child the appropriate preventive measures can be taken. However, the use of genetic tests only makes sense if enough major and modifying disease genes have been identified. In addition, before a genetic test can be used, data of the test for the various ethnic groups/races should be available.

REFERENCES

Armitage, G.C., Wu, Y., Wang, H-Y., Sorrell, J., di Giovine, F.S. & Duff, G.W. (2000). Low prevalence of a periodontitis-associated interleukin-1 composite genotype in individuals of Chinese heritage. *Journal of Periodontology* **71**, 164-171.

Boughman, J.A., Astemborski, J.A. & Suzuki, J.B. (1992). Phenotypic assessment of early onset periodontitis in sibships. *Journal of Clinical Periodontology* **19**, 233-239.

Cattabriga, M., Rotundo, R., Muzzi, L., Nieri, M., Verrocchi, G., Cairo, F. & Pini Prato, G. (2001). Retrospective evaluation of the influence of the interleukin-1 genotype on radiographic bone levels in treated periodontal patients over 10 years. *Journal of Periodontology* **72**, 767-773.

Colombo, A.P., Eftimiadi, C., Haffajee, A.D., Cugini, M.A. & Socransky, S.S. (1998). Serum IgG2 level, Gm(23) allotype and FcγRIIa and FcγRIIIb receptors in refractory periodontal disease. *Journal of Clinical Periodontology* **25**, 465-474.

Corey, L.A., Nance, W.E., Hofstede, P. & Schenkein, H.A. (1993). Self-reported periodontal disease in a Virginia twin population. *Journal of Periodontology* **64**, 1205-1208.

Cox, A. & Duff, G.W. (1996). Cytokines as genetic modifying factors in immune and inflammatory diseases. *Journal of Pediatric Endocrinology and Metabolism* **9** suppl. 1, 129-132.

Craandijk, J., Van Krugten, M.V., Verweij, C.L., Van der Velden, U. & Loos, B.G. (2002). Tumor necrosis factor-α gene polymorphisms in relation to periodontitis. *Journal of Clinical Periodontology* **29**, 28-34.

Cullinan, M.P., Westerman, B., Hamlet, S.M., Palmer, J.E., Faddy, M.J., Lang, N.P. & Seymour, G.J. (2001). A longitudinal study of interleukin-1 gene polymorphisms and periodontal disease in a general adult population. *Journal of Clinical Periodontology* **28**, 1137-1144.

De Sanctis, M. & Zucchelli, G. (2000). Interleukin-1 gene polymorphisms and long-term stability following guided tissue regeneration. *Journal of Periodontology* **71**, 606-613.

Diehl, S.R., Wang, Y., Brooks, C.N., Burmeister, J.A., Califano, J.V., Wang, S. & Schenkein, H.A. (1999). Linkage disequilibrium of interleukin-1 genetic polymorphisms with early-onset periodontitis. *Journal of Periodontology* **70**, 418-430.

Ehmke, B., Kreb, W., Karch, H., Grimm, T., Klaiber, B. & Flemmig, T.F. (1999). Interleukin-1 haplotype and periodontal disease progression following therapy. *Journal of Clinical Periodontology* **26**, 810-813.

Galbraith, G.M.P., Steed, R.B., Sanders, J.J. & Pandey, J.P. (1998). Tumor necrosis factor alpha production by oral leukocytes: influence of tumor necrosis factor genotype. *Journal of Periodontology* **69**, 428-433.

Gore, E.A., Sanders, J.J., Pandey, J.P., Palesch, Y. & Galbraith, G.M. (1998). Interleukin-1beta+3953 allele 2: association with disease status in adult periodontitis. *Journal of Clinical Periodontology* **25**, 781-785.

Hart, T.C. (1996). Genetic risk factors for early-onset periodontitis. *Journal of Periodontology* **67**, 355-366.

Hart, T.C., Hart, P.S., Bowden, D.W., Michalec, M.D., Callison, S.A., Walker, S.J., Zhang, Y. & Firatli, E. (1999). Mutations of the cathepsin C gene are responsible for Papillon-Lefèvre syndrome. *Journal of Medical Genetics* **36**, 881-887.

Hart, T.C., Hart, P.S., Michalec, M.D., Zhang, Y., Marazita, M.L., Cooper, M., Yassin, O.M., Nusier, M. & Walker, S. (2000a). Localisation of a gene for prepubertal periodontitis to chromosome 11q14 and identification of a cathepsin C gene mutation. *Journal of Medical Genetics* **37**, 95-101.

Hart, T.C., Marazita, M.L. & Wright, J.T. (2000b). The impact of molecular genetics on oral health paradigms. *Critical Reviews in Oral Biology and Medicine* **11**, 26-56.

Hodge, P.J., Riggio, M.P. & Kinane, D.F. (2001). Failure to detect an association with IL1 genotypes in European Caucasians with generalised early onset periodontitis. *Journal of Clinical Periodontology* **28**, 430-436.

Kinane, D.F., Hodge, P.J., Eskdale, J., Ellis, R. & Gallagher, G. (1999). Analysis of genetic polymorphisms at the interleukin-10 and tumour necrosis factor loci in early-onset periodontitis. *Journal of Periodontal Research* **34**, 379-386.

Kobayashi, T., Westerdaal, N.A.C., Miyazaki, A., van der Pol, W-L., Suzuki, T., Yoshie, H., van de Winkel, J.G.J. & Hara, K. (1997). Relevance of immunoglobulin G Fc receptor polymorphism to recurrence of adult periodontitis in Japanese patients. *Infection and Immunity* **65**, 3556-3560.

Kobayashi, T., Sugita, N., van der Pol, W-L., Nunokawa, Y., Westerdaal, N.A.C., Yamamoto, K., van de Winkel, J.G.J. & Yoshie, H. (2000). The Fcγ receptor genotype as a risk factor for generalized early-onset periodontitis in Japanese patients. *Journal of Periodontology* **71**, 1425-1432.

Kobayashi, T., Yamamoto, K., Sugita, N., van der Pol, W-L., Yasudo, K., Kaneko, S., van de Winkel, J.G.J. & Yoshie, H. (2001). The Fcγ receptor genotype as a severity factor for chronic periodontitis in Japanese patients. *Journal of Periodontology* **72**, 1324-1331.

Kornman, K.S., Crane, A., Wang, H-Y., di Giovine, F.S., Newman, M.G., Pirk, F.W., Wilson Jr., T.G., Higginbottom, F.L. & Duff, G. (1997). The interleukin 1 genotype as a severity factor in adult periodontal disease. *Journal of Clinical Periodontology* **24**, 72-77.

Laine, M.L., Farre, M.A., Gonzalez, G., van Dijk, L.J., Ham, A.J., Winkel, E.G., Crusius, J.B., Vandenbroucke, J.P., van Winkelhoff, A.J. & Pena, A.S. (2001). Polymorphisms of the interleukin-1 gene family, oral microbial pathogens, and smoking in adult periodontitis. *Journal of Dental Research* **80**, 1695-1699.

Löe, H. & Brown, L.J. (1991). Early onset periodontitis in the United States of America. *Journal of Periodontology* **62**, 608-616.

Loos, B.G., Leppers-van de Straat, F.G.J., van de Winkel, J.G.J. & van der Velden, U. (2003). Fcγ receptor gene polymorphisms in relation to periodontitis. *Journal of Clinical Periodontology* (in press).

Marazita, M.L., Burmeister, J.A., Gunsolly, J.C., Koertge, T.E., Lake, K. & Schenkein, H.A. (1994). Evidence for autosomal dominant inheritance and race-specific heterogeneity in early-onset periodontitis. *Journal of Periodontology* **65**, 623-630.

McDevitt, M.J., Wang, H-Y., Knobelman, C., Newman, M.G., di Giovine, F.S., Timms, J., Duff, G.W. & Kornman, K.S. (2000). Interleukin-1 genetic association with periodontitis in clinical practice. *Journal of Periodontology* **71**, 156-163.

McGuire, M.K. & Nunn, M.E. (1999). Prognosis versus actual outcome. IV. The effectiveness of clinical parameters and the IL-1 genotype in accurately predicting prognoses and tooth survival. *Journal of Periodontology* **70**, 49-56.

Meisel, P., Carlsson, L.E., Sawaf, H., Fanghaenel, J., Greinacher, A. & Kocher, T. (2001). Polymorphisms of Fcγ-receptors RIIa, RIIIa, and RIIIb in patients with adult periodontal diseases. *Genes and Immunity* **2**, 258-262.

Michalowicz, B.S., Aeppli, D., Virag, J.G., Klump, D.G., Hinrichs, J.E., Segal, N.L., Bouchard, T.J. & Philstrom, B.L. (1991). Periodontal findings in adult twins. *Journal of Periodontology* **62**, 293-299.

Michalowicz, B.S., Wolff, L.F., Klump, D., Hinrichs, J.E., Aeppli, D.M., Bouchard, T.J.J. & Pihlstrom, B.L. (1999). Periodontal bacteria in adult twins. *Journal of Periodontology* **70**, 263-273.

Michalowicz, B.S., Diehl, S.R., Gunsolley, J.C., Sparks, B.S., Brooks, C.N., Koertge, T.E., Califano, J.V., Burmeister, J.A. & Schenkein, H.A. (2000). Evidence of a substantial genetic basis for risk of adult periodontitis. *Journal of Periodontology* **71**, 1699-1707.

Norderyd, O. (1998). Risk for periodontal disease in a Swedish adult population. Cross-sectional and longitudinal studies over two decades. *Swedish Dental Journal Supplement* **132**, 1-67.

Page, R.C., Offenbacher, S., Schroeder, H.E., Seymour, G.J. & Kornman, K.S. (1997). Advances in the pathogenesis of periodontitis: Summary of developments, clinical implications and future directions. *Periodontology 2000* **14**, 216-248.

Papapanou, P.N., Neiderud, A.M., Sandros, J. & Dahlen, G. (2001). Interleukin-1 gene polymorphism and periodontal status. A case-control study. *Journal of Clinical Periodontology* **28**, 389-396.

Petit, M.D.A., van Steenbergen, T.J.M., Timmerman, M.F., de Graaff, J. & van der Velden, U. (1994) Prevalence of periodontitis and suspected periodontal pathogens in families of adult periodontitis patients. *Journal of Clinical Periodontology* **21**, 76-85.

Schork, N.J., Fallin, D. & Lanchbury, S. (2000). Single nucleotide polymorphisms and the future of genetic epidemiology. *Clinical Genetics* **58**, 250-264.

Shapira, L., Stabholz, A., Rieckmann, P. & Kruse, N. (2001). Genetic polymorphism of the tumor necrosis factor (TNF)-alpha promoter region in families with localized early-onset periodontitis. *Journal of Periodontal Research* **36**, 183-186.

Socransky, S.S., Haffajee, A.D., Smith, C. & Duff, G.W. (2000). Microbiological parameters associated with IL-1 gene polymorphisms in periodontitis patients. *Journal of Clinical Periodontology* **27**, 810-818.

Sugita, N., Yamamoto, K., Kobayashi, T., van der Pol, W-L., Horigome, T., Yoshie, H., van de Winkel, J.G.J. & Hara, K. (1999). Relevance of FcγRIIIa-158V-F polymorphism to recurrence of adult periodontitis in Japanese patients. *Clinical and Experimental Immunology* **117**, 350-354.

Toomes, C., James, J., Wood, A.J., Wu, C.L., McCormick, D., Lench, N., Hewitt, C., Moynihan, L., Roberts, E., Woods, C.G., Markham, A., Wong, M., Widmer, R., Ghaffar, K.A., Pemberton, M., Hussein, I.R., Temtamy, S.A., Davies, R., Read, A.P., Sloan, P., Dixon, M.J. & Thakker, N.S. (1999). Loss-of-function mutations in the cathepsin C gene result in periodontal disease and palmoplantar keratosis. *Nature Genetics* **23**, 421-424.

Van der Pol, W-L. & Van de Winkel, J.G.J. (1998a). IgG receptor polymorphisms: risk factors for disease. *Immunogenetics* **48**, 222-232.

Van der Pol, W-L. & Van de Winkel, J.G.J. (1998b). Immunologie in de medische praktijk. X. IgG-receptoren: structuur, functie en immunotherapie. *Nederlands Tijdschrift voor Geneeskunde* **142**, 335-340.

Van der Velden, U., Abbas, F., Van Steenbergen, T.J.M., De Zoete, O.J., Hesse, M., De Ruyter, C., De Laat, V.H.M. & De Graaff, J. (1989). Prevalence of periodontal breakdown in adolescents and presence of Actinobacillus actinomycetemcomitans in subjects with attachment loss. *Journal of Periodontology* **60**, 640-610.

Van der Velden, U., Abbas, F., Armand, S., de Graaff, J., Timmerman, M.F., van der Weijden, G.A., van Winkelhoff, A.J. & Winkel, E.G. (1993). The effect of sibling relationship on the periodontal condition. *Journal of Clinical Periodontology* **20**, 683-690.

Verweij, C.L. (1999). Tumour necrosis factor gene polymorphisms as severity markers in rheumatoid arthritis. *Annals of Rheumatoid Disease* **58** (Suppl. 1), I20-I26.

Walker, S.J., Van Dyke, T.E., Rich, S., Kornman, K.S., di Giovine, F.S. & Hart, T.C. (2000). Genetic polymorphisms of the IL-1alpha and IL-1beta genes in African-American LJP patients and an African-American control population. *Journal of Periodontology* **71**, 723-728.

Warmerdam, P.A.M., van de Winkel, J.G.J., Vlug, A., Westerdaal, N.A.C. & Capel, P.J.A. (1991). A single amino acid in the second Ig-like domain of the human Fcγreceptor II is critical for human IgG2 binding. *Journal of Immunology* **147**, 1338-1343.

Wilson, M.E. & Kalmar, J.R. (1996). FcγRIIa (CD32): A potential marker defining susceptibility to localized juvenile periodontitis. *Journal of Periodontology* **67**, 323-331.

Yamazaki, K., Tabeta, K., Nakajima, T., Ohsawa, Y., Ueki, K., Itoh, H. & Yoshie, H. (2001). Interleukin-10 gene promoter polymorphism in Japanese patients with adult and early-onset periodontitis. *Journal of Clinical Periodontology* **28**, 828-832.

CLINICAL CONCEPTS

Chapter 18

Examination of Patients with Periodontal Disease

Sture Nyman and Jan Lindhe

SYMPTOMS OF PERIODONTAL DISEASE

Clinically, both aggressive and chronic forms of periodontal disease are characterized by color and texture alterations of the gingiva, e.g. redness and swelling, as well as an increased tendency to bleeding on probing in the gingival sulcus/pocket area. In addition, the periodontal tissues may exhibit a reduced resistance to probing (increased depth of the clinical pocket) and/or tissue recession (Figs. 18-1a-c). More advanced stages of the disease are also frequently associated with increased tooth mobility as well as drifting and crowding of teeth.

In the radiograph, periodontal disease may be recognized by moderate to advanced loss of alveolar bone (Fig. 18-2). If bone loss has progressed at a similar rate in a certain part of the dentition, the crestal contour of the remaining bone in the radiograph is even: "horizontal" bone loss. Angular bony defects are the result of bone loss which has developed at different rates around different teeth/tooth surfaces: "vertical" bone loss.

In the histological section, periodontal disease is characterized by the presence of an inflammatory cell infiltrate (ICT; Fig. 18-3) within a 1-2 mm wide zone of the gingival connective tissue adjacent to the biofilm on the tooth. Within the infiltrated area there is a pronounced loss of collagen. In more advanced forms of periodontal disease, marked loss of connective tissue attachment to the root and apical downgrowth of dentogingival epithelium along the root are important findings.

Results from clinical and animal research have demonstrated that aggressive and chronic forms of periodontal disease

1. affect different parts of the dentition to a varying degree
2. are often progressive in character and, if left untreated, may result in tooth loss
3. can be arrested following proper therapy.

In order to arrive at a meaningful treatment plan, the various periodontal lesions must be recognized and their involvement in various parts of the dentition identified.

Thus, examination of a patient with respect to periodontal disease must not only identify sites in the dentition with inflammatory alterations but also the extent of tissue breakdown in such sites. The examination should therefore include all parts of the dentition and describe the periodontal conditions at all buccal, lingual and approximal tooth surfaces. Since periodontal disease includes inflammatory alterations of the gingiva and a progressive loss of periodontal ligament and alveolar bone, the comprehensive examination must include measures describing such pathologic alterations.

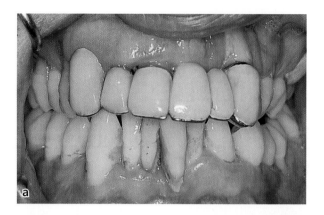

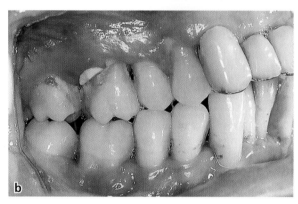
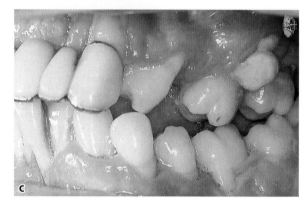

Fig. 18-1. (a-c) Clinical status of a patient suffering from advanced periodontal disease. Note the presence of different signs of periodontal disease such as texture alterations of the gingiva, gingival recessions (in the region of teeth 23, 24, 31, 33, 36 and 41), crowding of teeth (the mandibular front teeth), pus formation (tooth 14) and drifting of the premolars and molars.

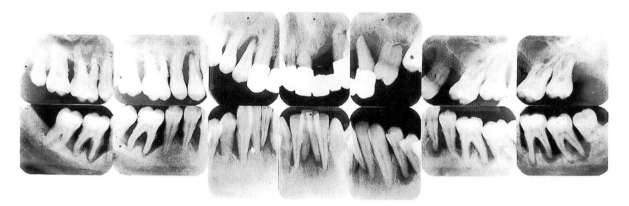

Fig. 18-2. Radiographic status of the patient described in Fig. 18-1a-c.

Fig. 18-4a-c illustrates the clinical status of a 55-year-old male with periodontal disease. The examination procedures used to assess the location and extension of periodontal disease will be demonstrated by using this case as an example.

THE GINGIVA

Clinical signs of gingival inflammation include changes in color and texture of the soft marginal tissue and an increased tendency for bleeding on probing.

Various index systems have been developed to de-scribe gingivitis in epidemiologic and clinical research. In the individual patient, refined and qualitative distinctions between various forms of gingivitis, i.e. initial, early and established gingival lesions (Page & Schroeder 1976), serve no meaningful purpose since the correct diagnosis of the gingival lesion can be made only in the histologic section. Since, however, the symptom "bleeding on probing" to the bottom of the gingival sulcus/pocket is associated with the presence of an inflammatory cell infiltrate in this area, the occurrence of such bleeding is an important indicator of disease. The identification of the apical extent of the gingival lesion is made in conjunction with *pocket depth measurements*. In sites where "shallow" pockets

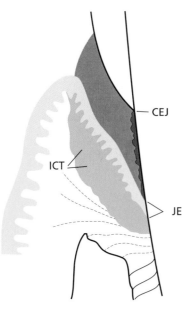

Fig. 18-3. Schematic drawing illustrating the histologic features of periodontal disease. Note the infiltrated connective tissue area (ICT).

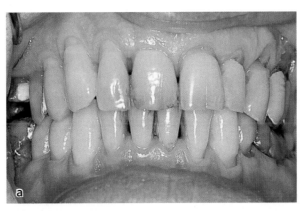

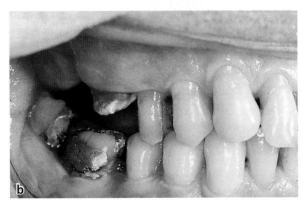

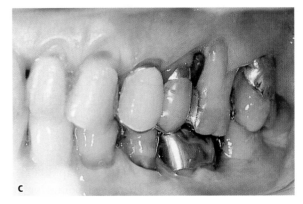

Fig. 18-4. (a-c) Clinical status of a 55-year-old male with periodontal disease.

are present, inflammatory lesions residing in the overt portion of the gingiva are distinguished by probing in the superficial marginal tissue. When the infiltrate resides in sites with deepened pockets and attachment loss, the inflammatory lesion in the apical part of the pocket must be identified by probing to the bottom of the deepened pocket.

Bleeding on probing: a blunt periodontal probe is inserted to the "bottom" of the gingival pocket and is moved gently along the tooth (root) surface (Fig. 18-5).

If bleeding is provoked by this instrumentation, the site examined is considered inflamed.

Fig. 18-6 illustrates the chart used to identify gingival sites which at the initial examination of the 55-year-old patient referred to above were found to bleed on probing. Each tooth in the chart is represented by a square and each tooth surface by a triangle. The upper triangle represents the palatal/lingual gingival unit, the bottom triangle the buccal unit and the remaining fields the two approximal gingival units. A cross is inserted in the fields of the chart which corre-

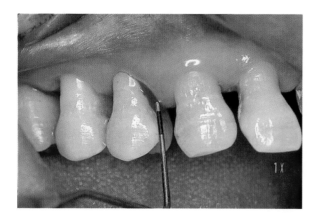

Fig. 18-5. Pocket probing used to identify gingival inflammation. A site is considered inflamed if bleeding is provoked by gentle probing to the bottom of the pocket.

Sites with gingivitis

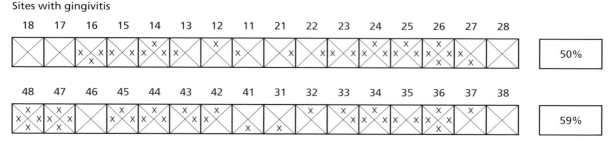

Fig. 18-6. The gingivitis chart of the patient seen in Fig. 18-4.

spond to the inflamed gingival units. The mean gingivitis score is given as a percentage figure. In the present patient (Fig. 18-4a-c), 27 out of a total number of 52 gingival units in the maxilla bled on probing. The gingivitis score for the maxillary dentition is thus 50%. The corresponding score for the mandibular dentition is 59%. This method of charting not only serves as a means of documenting areas of health and disease in the dentition but similar charting during the course of therapy will disclose sites which turn healthy or remain inflamed.

THE PERIODONTAL LIGAMENT – THE ROOT CEMENTUM

In order to evaluate the amount of tissue lost in periodontal disease and also to identify the apical extension of the inflammatory lesion, the following parameters should be recorded:

1. pocket depth (probing depth)
2. attachment level (probing attachment level)
3. furcation involvement
4. tooth mobility

Assessment of pocket depth

The pocket (-probing-) depth, i.e. the distance from the gingival margin to the bottom of the gingival pocket, is measured by means of a graduated probe (Fig. 18-7).

The pocket depth should be assessed at each surface of all teeth in the dentition. In the periodontal chart (Fig. 18-10) it may be sufficient to identify only the deepest value recorded at each tooth surface. Pocket depth values of < 4 mm may be excluded from the chart since such pockets can be regarded as falling within normal variations.

Results from pocket depth measurements will only in rare situations (when the gingival margin coincides with the cemento-enamel junction) give proper information regarding the extent of loss of probing attachment. For example, an inflammatory edema may cause a swelling of the free gingiva resulting in a coronal displacement of the gingival margin without a concomitant migration of the dentogingival epithelium to a level apical to the cemento-enamel junction. In such a situation a pocket depth exceeding 3-4 mm represents a "pseudopocket". In other situations, an obvious loss of attachment may have occurred without a concomitant increase of the pocket depth. A situation of this kind is shown in Fig. 18-7 at the buccal aspect of teeth 21 and 22 (two-digit systems; FDI 1970) where recessions of the gingiva can be seen.

Assessment of attachment level

Attachment levels may be assessed by means of a graduated probe and expressed as the distance in mm from the cemento-enamel junction to the bottom of the probeable gingival pocket. The longest distance for each tooth surface is recorded and may be included in the periodontal chart.

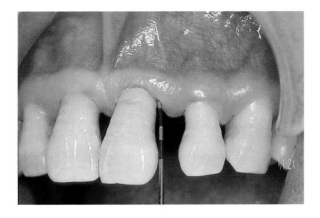

Fig. 18-7. Measurement of probing depth. Note the gingival recession at the buccal aspect of teeth 21 and 22.

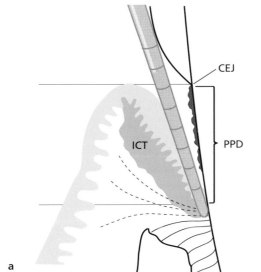

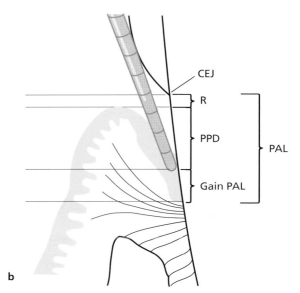

Fig. 18-8. (a) In the presence of an inflammatory cell infiltrate (ICT) in the gingiva, the probe penetrates apically to the bottom of the histologic pocket. (b) Following successful therapy the swelling is reduced (R = recession) and the cell infiltrate is replaced by collagen. The probe fails to reach the apical part of the dentogingival epithelium. CEJ = cemento-enamel junction. PPD = probing pocket depth. PAL = probing attachment level, R = recession. Gain PAL = recorded-false-gain of attachment ("clinical attachment").

Errors inherent in periodontal probing

The distances recorded in a periodontal examination using a periodontal probe have generally been assumed to represent a fairly accurate estimate of the pocket depth or attachment level at a given site. In other words, the tip of the probe has been assumed to identify the level of the most apical cells of the dentogingival epithelium. Results from research published in the 1970s have demonstrated, however, that this is seldom the case (Saglie et al. 1975, Listgarten et al. 1976, Armitage et al. 1977, Ezis & Burgett 1978, Spray et al. 1978, Robinson & Vitek 1979, van der Velden 1979, Magnusson & Listgarten 1980, Polson et al. 1980). Listgarten (1980) listed a variety of factors which influence the result of a measurement made with a periodontal probe. These factors include (1) the thickness of the probe used, (2) malposition of the probe due to anatomic features such as the contour of the tooth surface, (3) the pressure applied on the instrument during probing, and (4) the degree of inflam-

matory cell infiltration in the soft tissue and accompanying loss of collagen. Listgarten suggested that "a distinction should be made between the histological and the clinical pocket depth to differentiate between the depth of the actual anatomic defect and the measurement recorded by the probe".

Measurement errors depending on factors such as the thickness of the probe, the contour of the tooth surface and improper angulation of the probe can be reduced or avoided by the selection of a proper instrument and careful management of the examination procedure. More difficult to avoid, however, are errors resulting from variations in probing force and the extent of inflammatory alterations of the periodontal tissues. As a rule, the greater the probing force, the deeper the penetration of the probe into the tissue. In this context it should be realized that in investigations designed to disclose the force used by different clinicians, the probing force was found to range from 3 to 130 g (Gabathuler & Hassell 1971, Hassell et al. 1973), and also to differ by as much as 2:1 for the same dentist

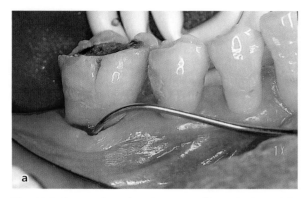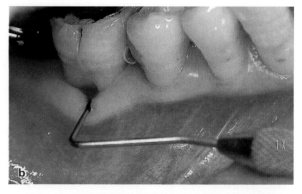

Fig. 18-9. A periodontal probe inserted into the buccal furcation area of a mandibular molar. A furcation involvement of degree 2 was found.

Periodontal chart						Diagnosis		
						Gingivitis	Parodontitis levis	Parodontitis gravis et complicata
Tooth	Pocket depth M	B	D	L	Furcation involvement	Tooth mobility		
18								
17	4	4	4		3			
16	4		6			1		
15	5		6	4				
14	4		4					
13	4		6	6				
12								
11			6	5				
21	6		7	4				
22	4		8	5				
23	6							
24		4	7			1		
25	6		4		m,b,d 2			
26	4	4	8	8	3			
27								
28								
	8	8	4	4	b 2	2		
48	6	14	8	4	3	1		
47								
46	4		6	4				
45			6	4				
44			4					
43	6							
42			4					
41			4					
31			4					
32	6							
33			4			1		
34	5		6	6				
35	10		8		b 2			
36	6	4	10	6	b 2			
37								
38								

Fig. 18-10. Periodontal chart including the data obtained from the examination of the patient presented in Fig. 18-4.

from one examination to another. In order to exclude measurement errors related to the effect of variations in probing force, so-called pressure sensitive probes have been developed. Such probes will enable the examiner to probe with a predetermined force (van der Velden & de Vries 1978, Vitek et al. 1979, Polson et al. 1980). However, over and underestimation of the "true" pocket depth or attachment level may also

occur when this type of probing device is employed (Armitage et al. 1977, Robinson & Vitek 1979, Polson et al. 1980). Thus, when the connective tissue subjacent to the pocket epithelium is infiltrated by inflammatory cells, the periodontal probe will most certainly penetrate beyond the apical termination of the dentogingival epithelium. This results in an overestimation of the "true" depth of the pocket. Conversely, when the inflammatory infiltrate decreases in size following successful periodontal treatment, and a concomitant deposition of new collagen takes place within the previously inflamed tissue area, the dentogingival tissue will become more resistant to penetration by the probe. The probe may now fail to reach the apical termination of the epithelium. This results in an underestimation of the "true" pocket depth or attachment level. The magnitude of the difference between the probing measurement and the histologic "true" pocket depth (Gain PAL; Fig. 18-8b) may range from fractions of a millimeter to several millimeters (Listgarten 1980).

From this discussion it should be understood that reduction of pocket depth following periodontal treatment and/or gain of attachment, assessed by periodontal probing, are not necessarily signs of formation of a new connective tissue attachment in the bottom of the previous pocket. Rather, such a change may merely represent a resolution of the inflammatory process and may thus occur without an accompanying attachment gain (Fig. 18-8). In this context it should be realized that the terms "pocket depth" and "gain and loss of attachment" in modern literature have often been changed to the more exact terms "probing depth" and "gain and loss of clinical attachment" or "probing pocket depth" and "probing attachment level".

Current knowledge of the histopathology of periodontal lesions and healing of such lesions has thus resulted in an altered concept regarding the validity of periodontal probing. However, despite difficulties in interpreting the proper significance of pocket depth and attachment level measurements, such determinations still give the clinician a useful estimate of the degree of disease involvement, and particularly so

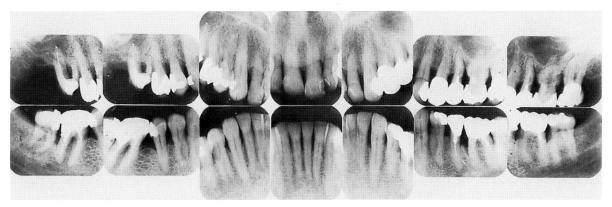

Fig. 18-11. Radiographic status of the patient presented in Fig. 18-4.

when the information obtained is related to other findings of the examination procedure such as "bleeding on probing", and alveolar bone height alterations.

Assessment of furcation involvement

In the progression of periodontal disease around multi-rooted teeth, the destructive process may involve the supporting structures of the furcation area (Fig. 18-9). Elaborate therapeutic techniques must often be used to treat such *furcation involvements* properly. Therefore, the precise identification of the presence and extension of periodontal tissue breakdown within the furcation area is of importance for proper diagnosis and treatment planning.

Furcation involvements may be classified into:

Degree 1: Horizontal loss of supporting tissues not exceeding ⅓ of the width of the tooth.

Degree 2: Horizontal loss of supporting tissues exceeding ⅓ of the width of the tooth, but not encompassing the total width of the furcation area.

Degree 3: Horizontal "through-and-through" destruction of the supporting tissues in the furcation.

The degree of furcation involvement is presented in the periodontal chart (Fig. 18-10) together with a description of which tooth surface the involvement has been identified on (e.g. tooth 26: m, b, d 2; tooth 48: b 2; tooth 36: b 2). A detailed discussion regarding diagnosis of furcation involvements and treatment of furcation-involved teeth is presented in Chapter 28.

Assessment of tooth mobility

The continuous loss of the supporting tissues in progressive periodontal disease may result in increased tooth mobility. Increased tooth mobility may be classified in the following way:

Degree 1: Movability of the crown of the tooth 0.2-1 mm in horizontal direction

Degree 2: Movability of the crown of the tooth exceeding 1 mm in horizontal direction

Degree 3: Movability of the crown of the tooth in vertical direction as well.

It must be understood that plaque-associated periodontal disease is not the only cause of increased tooth mobility. For instance, overloading of teeth and trauma may result in tooth hypermobility. Increased tooth mobility can frequently also be observed in conjunction with periapical lesions, immediately following periodontal surgery, etc. From a therapeutic point of view it is important, therefore, to assess not only the degree of increased tooth mobility but also the cause of the observed hypermobility (see Chapters 15 and 27).

All data collected in conjunction with measurements of pocket (-probing-) depth as well as from the assessments of furcation involvement and tooth mobility are included in the periodontal chart (Fig. 18-10). The various teeth in this chart are denoted according to the two-digit system adopted by FDI in 1970.

THE ALVEOLAR BONE

Radiographic analysis

The height of the alveolar bone and the outline of the bone crest are examined in the radiographs in Fig. 18-11. The radiographs provide information of the height and configuration of the interproximal alveolar bone. Covering structures (bone tissue, teeth) often make it difficult to identify properly the outline of the buccal and lingual alveolar bone crest. The analysis of the radiographs must therefore be combined with a detailed evaluation of the pocket depth and attachment level data in order to arrive at a correct estimate concerning "horizontal" and "vertical" bone loss.

Following active treatment, patients must be enrolled in a follow-up and maintenance care program aimed at preventing recurrence of periodontal disease. This program includes regular reexaminations to study the periodontal conditions. Such reexamina-

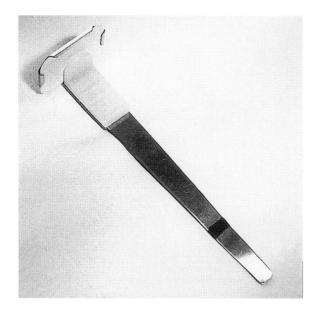

Fig. 18-12. The Eggen device for obtaining "standardized" radiographs.

tions often require repeated radiographic analysis of teeth and jaws at given time intervals. To enable meaningful comparative analysis, a radiographic technique should be used which produces periodic reproducible roentgenograms. A technique of this kind has been described by, for example, Eggen (1969) (Fig. 18-12).

Sounding

In order to arrive at a correct diagnosis with respect to the alveolar bone level, the presence of angular bony defects and interdental osseous craters etc., an additional method, called "sounding", may be used. Following local anesthesia the periodontal probe is inserted into the pocket. The tip of the probe is forced through the supraalveolar connective tissue to make contact with the bone and the distance from the cemento-enamel junction to the bone level is assessed in mm.

DIAGNOSIS OF PERIODONTAL LESIONS

The information regarding the condition of the various periodontal structures (the gingiva, the periodontal ligament, the root cementum and the alveolar bone) which has been obtained through the comprehensive examination presented above should form the basis for a proper assessment of the periodontal condition (Fig. 18-13). It is advantageous to give each tooth in the dentition an individual "diagnosis". Four different "diagnoses" may be used:

Gingivitis

This diagnosis is used when one or several gingival units around a particular tooth are found to bleed on probing. Probing pocket depth and probing attachment level measurements and the radiographic analysis *must fail* to indicate loss of supporting tissues. "Pseudopockets" may be present.

Diagnosis of the periodontal lesion		
Diagnosis	**Criteria**	
	Periodontal charting	*Miscellaneous*
	Radiographic analysis	
Gingivitis	No loss of supporting tissues (pseudopockets)	Bleeding on probing
Periodontitis levis	Horizontal loss of supporting tissues ≤ $\frac{1}{3}$ of the root length	Bleeding on probing
Periodontitis gravis	Horizontal loss of supporting tissues > $\frac{1}{3}$ of the root length	Bleeding on probing
Supplementary diagnosis		
... et complicata	Angular bony defects: interdental craters infrabony pockets Furcation involvement 2, 3	

Fig. 18-13. The conditions of the periodontal tissues around each individual tooth in the dentition are described using different criteria (periodontal charting, radiographic analysis) and diagnosis.

Tooth	Symptom	Diagnosis	Tooth	Symptom	Diagnosis
			48	furcation involvement (2)	gravis et complicata
			47	furcation involvement (3)	gravis et complicata
16	furcation involvement (3)	gravis et complicata			
15	"horizontal" loss of supporting tissues > 1/3 of the root length	gravis	45	"horizontal" loss of supporting tissues > 1/3 of the root length	gravis
14	"horizontal" loss of supporting tissues > 1/3 of the root length	gravis	44	"horizontal" loss of supporting tissues < 1/3 of the root length	levis
13	"horizontal" loss of supporting tissues < 1/3 of the root length	levis	43	"horizontal" loss of supporting tissues < 1/3 of the root length	levis
12	angular bony defect (bottom of the defect located on "gravis level")	gravis et complicata	42	"horizontal" loss of supporting tissues < 1/3 of the root length	levis
11	"horizontal" loss of supporting tissues < 1/3 of the root length	levis	41	"horizontal" loss of supporting tissues > 1/3 of the root length	gravis
21	"horizontal" loss of supporting tissues > 1/3 of the root length	gravis	31	"horizontal" loss of supporting tissues > 1/3 of the root length	gravis
22	"horizontal" loss of supporting tissues > 1/3 of the root length	gravis	32	"horizontal" loss of supporting tissues < 1/3 of the root length	levis
23	"horizontal" loss of supporting tissues < 1/3 of the root length	levis	33	"horizontal" loss of supporting tissues < 1/3 of the root length	levis
24	"horizontal" loss of supporting tissues < 1/3 of the root length	levis	34	"horizontal" loss of supporting tissues < 1/3 of the root length	levis
25	angular bony defect (bottom of the defect located on "gravis level"	gravis et complicata	35	"horizontal" loss of supporting tissues > 1/3 of the root length	gravis
26	furcation involvement (2)	gravis et complicata	36	angular bony defect (bottom of the defect located on "gravis level") furcation involvement (2)	levis et complicata
27	furcation involvement (3)	gravis et complicata	37	angular bony defect (bottom of the defect located on "gravis level") furcation involvement (2)	levis et complicata

Periodontitis levis (overt periodontitis)

The pocket depth and attachment level measurements and radiographic analysis indicate an even ("horizontal") loss of supporting tissues not exceeding one third of the length of the root. Inflammation must be present, i.e. "bleeding on probing" will occur when the site is probed to the "bottom of the pocket".

Periodontitis gravis (advanced periodontitis)

Pocket depth and attachment level measurements and the radiographic analysis indicate an even ("horizontal") loss of supporting tissues exceeding one third of the length of the root. "Bleeding on probing" to the "bottom of the pocket" must be present.

A supplementary diagnosis *periodontitis complicata* is used

1. when an angular bony defect (infrabony pocket, interdental osseous crater) is present adjacent to a tooth, and
2. for a multi-rooted tooth in which furcation involvements of degree 2 or 3 have been identified.

A chart of diagnosis is shown in Fig. 18-14. This particular chart refers to the patient whose clinical status is shown in Fig. 18-4a-c, periodontal chart in Fig. 18-10 and radiographic status in Fig. 18-11. The various teeth have received the diagnoses described in Fig. 18-14.

Periodontal diagnosis

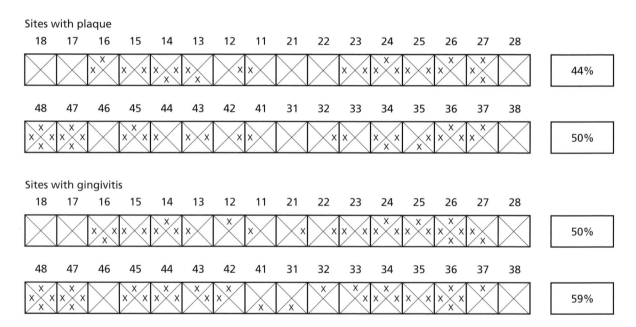

	18	17	16	15	14	13	12	11	21	22	23	24	25	26	27	28
Gingivitis	▓	▓														▓
Periodontitis levis	▓	▓				×		×			×	×				▓
Periodontitis gravis	▓	▓	×	×	×		×		×	×				×	×	×	▓
... et complicata	▓	▓	×											×	×	×	▓

	48	47	46	45	44	43	42	41	31	32	33	34	35	36	37	38
Gingivitis			▓													▓
Periodontitis levis			▓		×	×	×			×	×	×		×	×	▓
Periodontitis gravis	×	×	▓	×			×	×				×			▓
... et complicata	×	×	▓											×	×	▓

Fig. 18-14. Chart of diagnosis describing the patient in Fig. 18-4.

Sites with plaque

| 18 | 17 | 16 | 15 | 14 | 13 | 12 | 11 | 21 | 22 | 23 | 24 | 25 | 26 | 27 | 28 |

44%

| 48 | 47 | 46 | 45 | 44 | 43 | 42 | 41 | 31 | 32 | 33 | 34 | 35 | 36 | 37 | 38 |

50%

Sites with gingivitis

| 18 | 17 | 16 | 15 | 14 | 13 | 12 | 11 | 21 | 22 | 23 | 24 | 25 | 26 | 27 | 28 |

50%

| 48 | 47 | 46 | 45 | 44 | 43 | 42 | 41 | 31 | 32 | 33 | 34 | 35 | 36 | 37 | 38 |

59%

Fig. 18-15. The plaque and gingivitis chart of the patient presented in Fig. 18-4.

Oral hygiene status

In conjunction with examination of the periodontal tissues, the patient's oral hygiene must also be evaluated. Absence or presence of plaque on each tooth surface in the dentition is recorded. The bacterial deposits may be stained with a disclosing solution to facilitate their detection. The presence of plaque is marked in appropriate fields in the plaque chart shown in Fig. 18-15. The mean plaque score for the dentition is given as a percentage value in correspondence with the system used for gingivitis.

Alterations with respect to the presence of plaque and gingival inflammation are illustrated in a simple way by the repeated use of the combined plaque and gingivitis chart (Fig. 18-15) during the course of treatment.

In addition to the assessment of plaque, retention factors for plaque, such as supra and subgingival calculus and defective margins of dental restorations, should also be identified and included in the periodontal chart.

Conclusion

The methods described above for the examination of patients with respect to periodontal disease provide a thorough analysis of the presence, extent and severity of the disease in the dentition. The correct diagnosis for each individual tooth should form the basis for the treatment planning of the individual case.

REFERENCES

Armitage, G.C., Svanberg, G.K. & Löe, H. (1977). Microscopic evaluation of clinical measurements of connective tissue attachment level. *Journal of Clinical Periodontology* **4**, 173-190.

Eggen, S. (1969). Standardisered intraoral röntgenteknik. *Sveriges Tandläkareförbunds Tidning* **17**, 867-872.

Ezis, I. & Burgett, F. (1978). Probing related to attachment levels on recently erupted teeth. *Journal of Dental Research* **57**, Spec Issue A 307, Abstract No. 932.

Gabathuler, H. & Hassell, T. (1971). A pressure sensitive periodontal probe. *Helvetica Odontologica Acta* **15**, 114-117.

Hassell, T.M., Germann, M.A. & Saxer, V.P. (1973). Periodontal probing: investigator discrepancies and correlations between probing force and recorded depth. *Helvetica Odontologica Acta* **17**, 38-42.

Listgarten, M.A. (1980). Periodontal probing: What does it mean? *Journal of Clinical Periodontology* **7**, 165-176.

Listgarten, M.A., Mao, R. & Robinson, P.J. (1976). Periodontal probing and the relationship of the probe tip to periodontal tissues. *Journal of Periodontology* **47**, 511-513.

Magnusson, I. & Listgarten, M.A. (1980). Histological evaluation of probing depth following periodontal treatment. *Journal of Clinical Periodontology* **7**, 26-31.

Page, R.C. & Schroeder, H.E. (1976). Pathogenesis of chronic inflammatory periodontal disease. A summary of current work. *Laboratory Investigations* **33**, 235-249.

Polson, A.M., Caton, J.G., Yeaple, R.N. & Zander, H.A. (1980). Histological determination of probe tip penetration into gingival sulcus of humans using an electronic pressure-sensitive probe. *Journal of Clinical Periodontology* **7**, 479-488.

Robinson, P.J. & Vitek, R.M. (1979). The relationship between gingival inflammation and resistance to probe penetration. *Journal of Periodontal Research* **14**, 239-243.

Saglie, R., Johansen, J.R. & Flötra, L. (1975). The zone of completely and partially destructed periodontal fibers in pathological pockets. *Journal of Clinical Periodontology* **2**, 198-202.

Spray, J.R., Garnick, J.J., Doles, L.R. & Klawitter, J.J. (1978). Microscopic demonstration of the position of periodontal probes. *Journal of Periodontology* **49**, 148-152.

van der Velden, U. (1979). Probing force and the relationship of the probe tip to the periodontal tissues. *Journal of Clinical Periodontology* **6**, 106-114.

van der Velden, U. & de Vries, J.H. (1978). Introduction of a new periodontal probe: The pressure probe. *Journal of Clinical Periodontology* **5**, 188-197.

Vitek, R.M., Robinson, P.J. & Lautenschlager, E.P. (1979). Development of a force-controlled periodontal instrument. *Journal of Periodontal Research* **14**, 93-94.

CHAPTER 19

Treatment Planning

JAN LINDHE, STURE NYMAN AND NIKLAUS P. LANG

Screening for periodontal disease

Diagnosis

Treatment planning
  Initial treatment plan
  Case presentation

Initial (cause-related) therapy

Re-evaluation
  Planning of additional therapy

Additional (corrective) therapy

Supportive periodontal therapy

Case reports

Caries and periodontal diseases are opportunistic infections associated with biofilm formation on the surfaces of teeth. Factors such as bacterial specificity and pathogenicity as well as the disposition of the individual for disease, e.g. local and general resistance, may influence the onset, the rate of progression and clinical character of the plaque-associated dental disorders. Findings from animal experiments and longitudinal studies in humans, however, have demonstrated that treatment, including the elimination or the control of the plaque infection and the introduction of careful plaque control measures, in most, if not all, cases results in dental and periodontal health. Even if health cannot always be achieved and maintained, the arrest of disease progression following treatment must be the goal of modern dental care.

The treatment of patients affected by caries and periodontal disease, including symptoms of associated pathologic conditions such as pulpitis, periapical periodontitis, marginal abscess, tooth migration, etc., may from a didactic point of view be divided into three different stages: initial, cause-related therapy, additional therapeutic measures (corrective phase) and supportive periodontal therapy (or maintenance therapy).

Treatment goals
In every patient with periodontitis, a treatment strategy which includes the elimination of the opportunistic infection must be defined and followed. This treatment strategy must also define the clinical outcome parameters to be reached. Such clinical parameters include:

1. Reduction or resolution of gingivitis (bleeding on probing; BoP)
2. Reduction in probing pocket depth (PPD)
3. Elimination of open furcations in multirooted teeth
4. Individually satisfactory esthetics and function.

Based on data obtained from longitudinal clinical studies, which included surgical as well as non-surgical approaches of therapy, the treatment goals may be further specified:

1. < 10 % of sites BoP+
2. No sites with PPD > 5 mm, but preferably ≤ 4 mm
3. No furcation involvement of degree II or III.

In this context it must also be emphasized that risk factors for periodontitis that can be controlled must be addressed as well. The two main risk factors for chronic periodontitis are *improper plaque control* and *smoking*. Hence the treatment plan must include measures to improve the patient's plaque control performance. In addition, efforts must be made to stimulate a smoker to enroll in smoking cessation programs.

Initial, cause-related therapy
The objective of this treatment is the removal or control of the various biofilms.

Additional therapeutic measures
This includes traditional therapeutic measures such as periodontal surgery, endodontic therapy, restorative and prosthetic treatment. The volume of corrective therapy required and the selection of means for the restorative and prosthetic therapy can be determined only when the level of success of the causative therapy

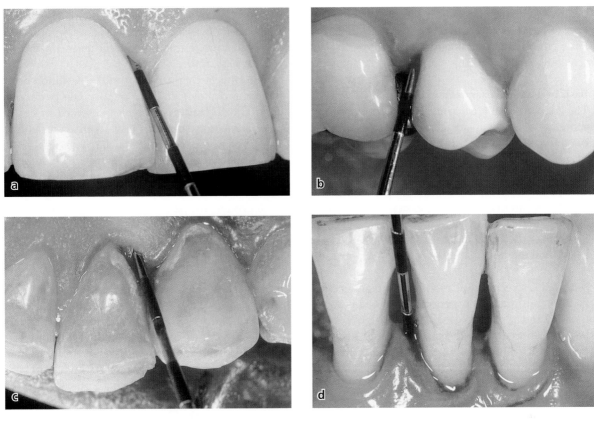

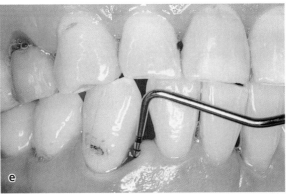

Fig. 19-1a-e. Clinical illustration of the basic periodontal examination scores. (a) BPE score 0. (b) BPE score 1. (c) BPE score 2. (d) BPE score 3. (e) BPE score 4.

can be properly evaluated. The patient's ability to cooperate in the overall therapy must determine the content of the corrective treatment. If this ability is failing or lacking, it may at times not be worth initiating treatment procedures which only in the fully cooperative patient will permanently improve oral esthetics and function. The validity of this statement can be exemplified by the results of studies aimed at assessing the relative value of different types of surgical methods in the treatment of periodontal disease. Thus, a number of clinical trials (Lindhe & Nyman 1975, Nyman et al. 1975, 1977, Rosling et al. 1976a,b, Nyman & Lindhe 1979) have demonstrated that gingivectomy and flap procedures performed in patients with proper plaque control levels often result in gain of alveolar bone and clinical attachment, while surgery in plaque-contaminated dentitions may cause additional destruction of the periodontium.

Supportive periodontal therapy (SPT)

The aim of this treatment is the prevention of disease recurrence. For each individual patient a recall system must be designed which includes (1) self-performed but professionally monitored plaque control programs, (2) scaling and root planing measures, (3) fluoride application, etc. In addition, this treatment involves the regular control of fillings and other restorations made during the corrective phase of therapy.

SCREENING FOR PERIODONTAL DISEASE

A patient seeking dental care is usually screened for the presence of carious lesions by means of clinical probing and bitewing radiographs. Likewise it is imperative that such a patient is screened for the presence of periodontitis using a basic procedure termed basic periodontal examination (BPE) (or periodontal screening record (PSR)).

Basic periodontal examination (BPE)

The goal of the BPE is to screen the periodontal condition of a new patient and to facilitate treatment planning. BPE scoring will allow the therapist to identify:

1. A patient with reasonably healthy periodontal conditions, but in need of long term preventive measures
2. A patient with periodontitis and in need of periodontal therapy.

In the BPE screening each tooth or implant is evaluated. A thin graduated periodontal probe is recommended and applied to at least two sites (mesio-buccal and disto-buccal) of the teeth or implants. Each dentate sextant within the dentition is given a BPE score, whereby the *highest* individual site score is used.

BPE scoring system

Score 0 = PPD ≤ 3 mm, BoP negative, no calculus or overhanging fillings (Fig. 19-1a)

Score 1 = PPD ≤ 3 mm, BoP positive, but no calculus or overhanging fillings (Fig. 19-1b)

Score 2 = PPD ≤ 3 mm, BoP positive, presence of supra and/or subgingival calculus and/or overhanging fillings (Fig. 19-1c)

Score 3 = PPD > 3 mm but ≤ 5 mm, BoP positive (Fig. 19-1d)

Score 4 = PPD > 5 mm (Fig. 19-1e).

If an examiner identifies one single site with a PPD > 5 mm within a sextant, the sextant will receive a score of 4, and no further assessment needs to be made in this particular sextant. Patients with sextants scored 0, 1 or 2 belong to the relatively healthy category. A patient that exhibits a sextant scoring 3 or 4 must undergo a more comprehensive periodontal examination (for details see Chapter 18).

The aim of the present text is to explain the overall objectives of the treatment planning for patients with BPE scores of 3 and 4 and who therefore have undergone a comprehensive diagnostic process.

DIAGNOSIS

The basis for the treatment planning described in this chapter is established by the clinical data collected from the examination of the patient presented in Chapter 18. This particular patient (U.N., male, 55 years of age) was examined with respect to his periodontal conditions, i.e. gingival sites displaying signs of *bleeding on probing* were identified, *pocket depths* and *furcation involvements* were measured and graded, *tooth mobility* was assessed and the radiographs were analyzed to determine the *height* and *outline* of the *alveolar bone crest*.

The clinical characteristics of the dentition of this patient are shown in Fig. 19-2a-c. The periodontal chart and the radiographs are presented in Fig. 19-3a,b. Based on the findings, each tooth in the dentition was given a proper periodontal diagnosis (Fig. 19-3b). In addition to the examination of the periodontal condition, detailed assessments of primary and recurrent caries were made for all tooth surfaces in the dentition. Furthermore, the patient was also examined with respect to endodontic problems, occlusal problems, temporomandibular joint dysfunction etc.

The present patient had secondary caries lesions adjacent to several restorations, particularly in the molar regions (Fig. 19-2b), and root caries in the distal surface of 25 and mesial surface of 26 (Fig. 19-3a). It should be observed that in a patient with a large number of caries lesions an additional number of examination procedures, e.g. assessments of secretion rate and buffering capacity of the saliva, number of lactobacilli and *Streptococcus mutans* etc., will facilitate the selection of proper therapeutic measures. In addition, a periapical lesion was observed in 47 and several defective root fillings were identified (Fig. 19-3a).

TREATMENT PLANNING

Initial treatment plan

Not until a detailed diagnosis of all pathologic conditions has been made, have proper prerequisites been established for an appropriate tentative treatment plan. At this early stage in the management of a patient, it is in most instances impossible to make definite decisions regarding all aspects of the corrective therapy, because:

1. *The degree of success of the initial treatment remains unknown*: the result of the initial cause-related treatment of an individual case forms the basis for the selection of means for additional therapy. The degree of disease elimination that can be reached depends on the outcome of subgingival scaling and root planing, but also on the patient's ability to adopt adequate dietary habits and to exercise proper plaque control techniques.
2. *The patient's "subjective" need for treatment is not known*: when the dentist has completed the examination of the patient and an inventory has been made regarding, for example, periodontal disease, caries, pulpal disease and temporomandibular joint disease, the observations are presented – "the case presentation" – for the patient. During the case presentation session it is important to find out if the patient's subjective need for dental therapy coin-

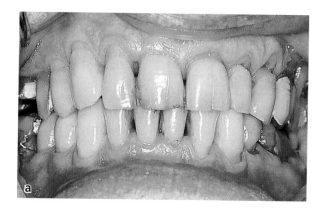

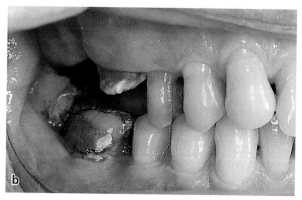

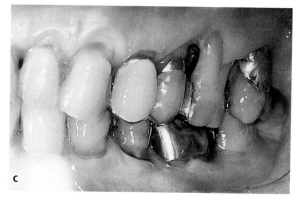

Fig. 19-2a-c. Clinical status of a 55-year-old male patient (U.N.) with periodontitis.

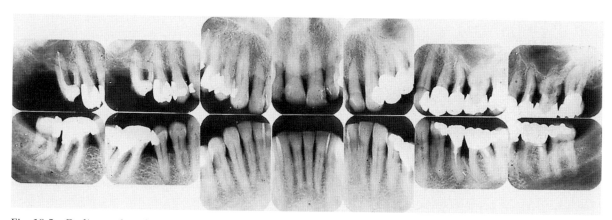

Fig. 19-3a. Radiographs relating to patient U.N. described in Fig. 19-2.

cides with the dentist's professional appreciation of the kind and volume of therapy that is required. It is important that the dentist understands that the main objective of dental therapy, besides *elimination of pain, is to satisfy the patient's demands regarding esthetics and chewing function (comfort)*, demands which certainly vary considerably from one individual to another.

3. *The result of certain parts of the treatment cannot be predicted*: in patients exhibiting advanced forms of caries and periodontal disease it is often impossible to anticipate if all teeth which are present at the initial examination can be successfully treated, or to predict the result of certain parts of the intended therapy. In other words, critical and difficult parts of the treatment must be performed first, and the outcome of this treatment must be evaluated before

all aspects of the definitive corrective treatment can be properly anticipated and described.

Single tooth risk assessment

Based on the result of the comprehensive examination (including assessments of periodontitis, caries and the endodontal status) and the resulting diagnosis, as well as considering the patient's needs regarding esthetics and function, a pre-therapeutic risk assessment is made for all teeth (roots) present.

Three major questions are addressed:

1. Which tooth/root has a *good* prognosis?
2. Which tooth/root is *"irrational-to-treat"*?
3. Which tooth/root has a *questionable* prognosis?

Tooth	Pocket depth M B D L	Furcation involvement	Tooth mobility	Gingivitis	Parodontitis levis	Parodontitis gravis et complicata

Periodontal chart — **Diagnosis**

Tooth	M	B	D	L	Furcation involvement	Tooth mobility	Gingivitis	Parodontitis levis	Parodontitis gravis et complicata
18̶									
17̶	4	4	4		3		X	X	
16	4		6			1	X		
15	5		6	4			X		
14	4		4					X	
13	4		6	6			X	X	
12									X
11			6	5			X		
21	6		7	4			X	X	
22	4		8	5					X
23	6								X
24		4	7			1	X	X	
25	6		4		m,b,d 2		X	X	
26	4	4	8	8	3		X	X	
27									
28̶							X	X	
	8	8	4	4	b 2	2	X	X	
48	6	14	8	4	3	1			
47							X		
46̶	4		6	4					X
45			6	4					X
44			4						X
43	6						X		
42			4				X		
41			4						X
31			4						X
32	6								X
33			4			1	X		
34	5		6	6			X		X
35	10		8		b, l 2		X		X
36	6	4	10	6	b 2				
37									
38̶									

Fig. 19-3b. Periodontal chart relating to patient U.N. (Fig. 19-2).

Teeth with a *good* prognosis will require a relatively simple therapy and may be regarded as secure abutments for function.

Teeth which are considered "irrational-to-treat" should be extracted during initial, cause-related therapy. Such teeth may be identified on the basis of the following criteria:

Periodontal
- Recurrent periodontal abscesses
- Periodontic-endodontic lesions
- Attachment loss to the apex

Endodontal
- Root perforation in the apical half of the root
- Periapical pathology in the presence of obturating post and core

Dental
- Long fracture of the root
- Oblique fracture in the middle third of the root
- Caries lesions that extend into the root canal

Functional
- Third molars without antagonists and with periodontitis/caries

Teeth with a *questionable* prognosis are in need of comprehensive therapy and must be brought into the category of teeth that have a *good* prognosis. Such teeth may be identified on the basis of the following critera:

Periodontal
- Furcation involvement
- Angular bone defects
- "Horizontal" bone loss involving > two-thirds of the root

Endodontal
- Incomplete root canal therapy
- Periapical pathology
- Presence of voluminous posts/screws

Dental
- Extensive root caries

Case presentation

The "Case presentation" is an essential component of the initial treatment and must include a description for the patient of different therapeutic goals. At the case presentation for Mr. U.N. the following treatment plan was described:

- The teeth in the dentition from 15 to 24 and from 45 to 35 probably will not present the dentist with any major therapeutic challenges. For the remaining teeth in the dentition, however, the treatment may involve several complicated or unpredictable measures.

Based on the pre-therapeutic risk assessment (Fig. 19-4), the following scenario was presented to the patient:

- 48 *and* 47 extraction: cannot be treated due to the advanced loss of supporting tissue at the buccal aspect of the teeth in combination with deep furcation involvements and periapical periodontitis as far as 47 is concerned (Fig. 19-3).
- 16 extraction: even if it is possible, from a therapeutic point of view, to preserve the palatal root, the maintenance of this root does not improve esthetics or chewing comfort; the tooth has no antagonist after extraction of 47 (Fig. 19-3).
- 25 *and* 27 extraction: 25 cannot be treated due to advanced root caries in combination with advanced loss of periodontal tissue support at the distal aspect of the tooth; 27 has a periodontal pocket communicating with periapical lesions in combination with furcation involvement of degree 3 (Fig. 19-3).
- 26, 36 *and* 37 present a number of therapeutic problems:
  26 shows signs of deep and extended root caries

	16	15	14	13	12	11	21	22	23	24	25	26	27
Good prognosis		+	+	+	+	+	+	+	+	+			
Questionable prognosis												+	
Irrational-to-treat	+										+		+

	48	47		45	44	43	42	41	31	32	33	34	35	36	37
Good prognosis				+	+	+	+	+	+	+	+	+	+		
Questionable prognosis														+	+
Irrational-to-treat	+	+													

Fig. 19-4. Outcome of the pre-therapeutic risk assessment made for patient U.N. described in Fig. 19-2.

in the mesiobuccal root in combination with furcation involvement of degree 2 m,b,d (Figs. 19-2c & 19-3). Note the unfavorable root- and root canal anatomy of the buccal roots; predictable endodontic treatment? The palatal root of 26 can, however, be maintained.

In 36 there is a deep angular bony defect at the mesial aspect and furcation involvements of degree 2 at both the buccal and lingual surface; 37 has a deep infrabony pocket at the distal surface (10 mm, see the periodontal chart) and furcation involvement of degree 2 b. The distal root of 36 or the mesial root of 37 (or both) are available for treatment.

Two different *alternatives for treatment* were presented to the patient:

• *Alternative 1*. Extraction of 25 and all molars and the maintenance of a dentition comprising 15-24 and 45-35. This alternative may be adequate with respect to "chewing comfort" but may be questionable from an esthetic point of view.
• *Alternative 2*. Extraction of the molars in the right side of the maxilla and mandible (16, 48, 47) and also of 25 and 27; root separation of 26 with the maintenance of the palatal root to be used as abutment for a 3-unit bridge to replace the extracted 25; root separation of one of the molars 36 or 37 with the maintenance of one root to be used as abutment for a 3-unit bridge to obtain occlusal contact with the maxillary bridge.

It should be observed that *alternative 2* involves a considerably larger volume of therapy than *alternative 1*. In a situation like this, expected benefits inherent in a certain treatment versus obvious disadvantages should always be explained to and discussed with the patient. His/her attitude to the alternatives presented must guide the dentist in the design of a proper plan for the overall treatment. In the present case the patient preferred the treatment described as *alternative 2*.

INITIAL (CAUSE-RELATED) THERAPY

The treatment was initiated and included the following measures to eliminate or control the plaque infection:

1. *Instruction* in oral hygiene measures with subsequent check-ups and reinstruction.
2. *Scaling and root planing* in combination with removal of retention factors for plaque.
3. *Excavation and restoration* of carious lesions.
4. *Endodontic treatment* 26 (palatal root) and 37 (mesial root). Endodontic treatment was carried out at an early stage to allow a proper evaluation of healing before the restorative treatment was initiated.
5. *Extraction* of 16, 48, 47. Temporary prosthetic replacement (for esthetic and functional reasons) of teeth which, during this initial phase of the treatment, have to be extracted should preferably be made in the form of removable partial dentures. The use of a removable prosthesis allows the dentist to eventually choose between a removable partial denture and a fixed bridge as permanent prosthetic therapy. If, on the other hand, the temporary prosthetic reconstruction is made in the form of a fixed bridge, the permanent prosthetic therapy must inevitably include fixed bridgework. Such an alternative may, however, during the course of treatment appear to be contraindicated. In the present case a temporary prosthesis was not made.

RE-EVALUATION

The initial phase of therapy is terminated with a thorough analysis of the results obtained with respect to the elimination or degree of control of the dental infections. This implies that a re-evaluation of the patient's caries activity must be performed as well as new assessments of gingival conditions, pocket depths, tooth mobility, etc. The result of this re-evaluation forms the basis for the selection, if necessary, of additional or corrective measures which are to be performed in the phase of definitive treatment.

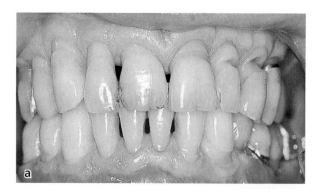

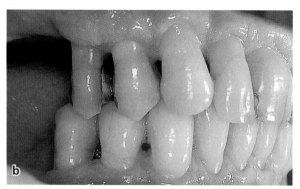
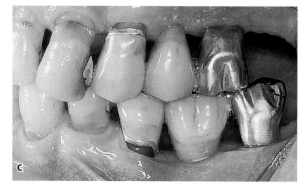

Fig. 19-5a-c. Clinical status of patient U.N. after periodontal and restorative treatment. Compare with Fig. 19-2.

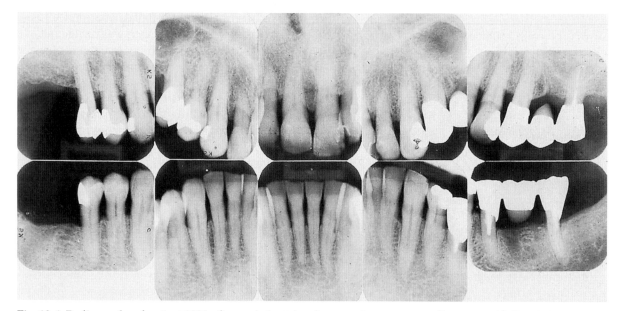

Fig. 19-6. Radiographs of patient U.N. after periodontal and restorative treatment. Compare with Fig. 19-3a.

Planning of additional therapy (definitive treatment plan)

If the results from the re-evaluation, made 1-2 months after the termination of the initial treatment phase, show that caries and periodontal disease have been brought under control, the additional treatment may be carried out in the following sequence:

1. *Extraction* of teeth that cannot be maintained. If such extractions include teeth which must be replaced for esthetic or functional reasons, a tempo-

rary removable partial denture or a temporary fixed bridge must be inserted.
2. *Additional endodontic treatment*
3. *Periodontal surgery*: The type and extent of surgical treatment should be based on probing depth, and "bleeding on probing" measurements should be made at re-evaluation. Periodontal surgery is often limited to those areas of the dentition where the inflammatory lesions were not resolved by scaling and root planing and in areas where furcation involvements persist.
4. *Installation of dental implants*: In regions of the dentition where tooth abutments are missing, implant

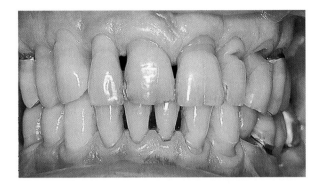

Fig. 19-7. Clinical status of patient U.N. 11 years after active treatment.

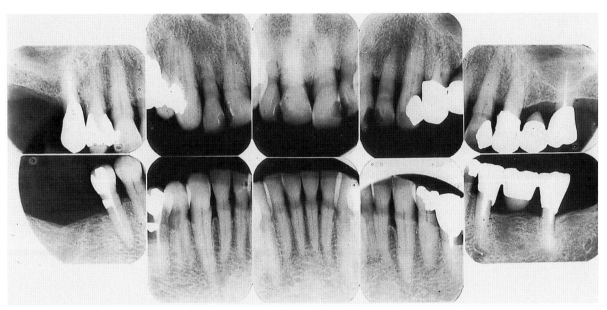

Fig. 19-8. Radiographs of patient U.N. obtained 11 years after treatment.

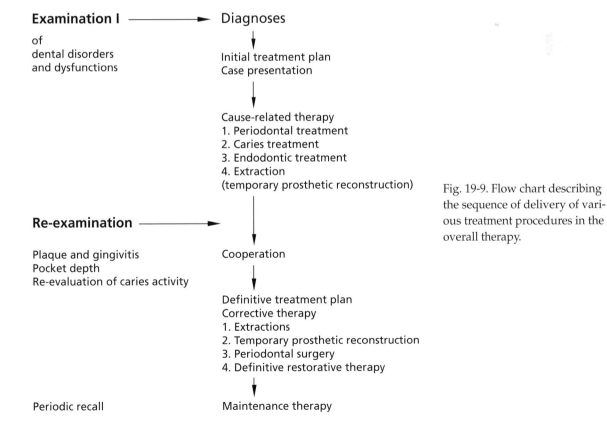

Examination I ⟶ Diagnoses

of
dental disorders
and dysfunctions

Initial treatment plan
Case presentation

Cause-related therapy
1. Periodontal treatment
2. Caries treatment
3. Endodontic treatment
4. Extraction
(temporary prosthetic reconstruction)

Fig. 19-9. Flow chart describing the sequence of delivery of various treatment procedures in the overall therapy.

Re-examination ⟶

Plaque and gingivitis
Pocket depth
Re-evaluation of caries activity

Cooperation

Definitive treatment plan
Corrective therapy
1. Extractions
2. Temporary prosthetic reconstruction
3. Periodontal surgery
4. Definitive restorative therapy

Periodic recall

Maintenance therapy

therapy for esthetic and functional reasons may be considered. It is essential to realize that implant therapy must be initiated first when dental infections are under control, i.e. after successful periodontal therapy.

5. *Definitive restorative and prosthetic treatment* including permanent restorative therapy (crown and bridge, removable partial dentures, etc.).

Additional (corrective) therapy

The present patient exhibited, after initial therapy, low plaque and gingivitis scores (5-10%) and no active carious lesions. The corrective treatment therefore included the following components:

1. *Periodontal surgery* at sites which bled on probing and with probing depths > 4 mm.
2. *Root separation* 37 and extraction of the distal root. *Root separation* 26 and extraction of the buccal roots.
3. *Extraction* 36, 25 and 27.
4. Preparation and installation of *fixed bridges* 24, 25, 26 (palatal root) and 35, 36, 37 (mesial root).

The result of the overall treatment is shown in Figs. 19-5a-c & 19-6.

Supportive periodontal therapy

Following completion of initial, *cause-related and additional therapy* the patient must be enrolled in a recall system which aims to prevent the recurrence of disease. The time interval between the recall appointments must be related to the ability of the patient to maintain a proper oral hygiene standard. Findings reported from several long-term clinical trials have suggested that a maintenance program based on recall appointments once every 3 months is, for most patients, effective in preventing disease recurrence. *It is important to emphasize, however, that the recall program must be designed to meet the individual patient's need. Some patients must be recalled every month, while other patients may have to be checked only once a year.*

At the various recall visits the following procedures should be carried out:

1. Evaluation of the oral hygiene standard
2. Scaling and polishing of the teeth (if indicated).

At least once a year a comprehensive examination should be performed including assessments of (1) caries, (2) gingivitis, (3) pathologically deepened pockets, (4) furcation involvements, (5) tooth mobility and (6) alterations of the alveolar bone level.

The patient (Mr. U.N.) used in this chapter to describe the guiding principles of treatment planning was, during the first 6 months after the active treatment, recalled once every 2 months, during the next 6 months once every 3 months, and subsequently only once every 6 months. The clinical and radiographic status 11 years after active treatment is shown in Figs. 19-7 & 19-8. In the course of this 11-year period there were no signs of recurrence of caries or periodontal disease. The buccal cusp of the crown of 15 was fractured approximately 5 years after active therapy and the tooth was restored with a gold crown with a porcelain facing.

The large variety of treatment problems that different patients present may obviously require that deviations are made from the sequence of treatment steps (initial cause-related therapy, corrective therapy, etc.) discussed above. Such deviations may be accepted as long as the fundamental principles regarding the overall therapy are understood (Fig. 19-9: flow chart).

Three patients will be presented below together with a brief description of their specific dental problems and the treatment delivered in order to demonstrate the rationale behind such variations in the sequence of therapy.

Case reports

Patient K.A. (female, 29 years old)

Initial examination
The periodontal status (pocket depths, furcation involvements, tooth mobility, radiographs and diagnoses) from the initial examination of patient K.A. is shown in Fig. 19-10a,b. The data obtained from this examination disclosed the presence of an advanced destruction of the supporting tissues in most parts of the dentition and the presence of a large number of angular bony defects. The teeth 14, 12, 11, 21, 22, 23, 24, 25, 43, 42, 41, 31, 32, 33, 37 exhibited increased mobility. The plaque and gingivitis scores were 75 and 70%, respectively.

Treatment planning
In the planning of the treatment of this case, it seemed reasonable to anticipate the extraction of some teeth in this severely compromised dentition, namely 14, 11, 21 and 31 (see radiograph: Fig. 19-10a). The extraction of these teeth, however, calls for extensive prosthetic therapy. Should additional teeth be scheduled for extraction in order to facilitate or make the outcome of prosthetic therapy more predictable? The neighboring teeth of 11, 21, 31, also exhibited advanced loss of supporting structures and showed signs of increased mobility. It could be questioned, therefore, if these teeth (i.e. 12, 22, 41, 32) could serve as proper abutments for a fixed bridge. The extraction of tooth 31 would most likely enforce the additional extraction of

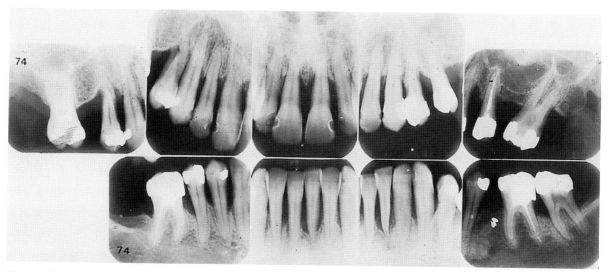

Fig. 19-10a. Case K.A. (29-year-old female patient). Radiographs prior to therapy.

the remaining three mandibular incisors, and consequently a therapy could be anticipated which included the preparation and installation of a fixed bridge extending from tooth 44 to tooth 34. Extraction of 11 and 21 would motivate the extraction of 12, 22, 14 and 24 as well, and call for a bridge construction that extended from tooth 16 to 25 or 26. The prerequisites for a proper prognosis for the prosthetic therapy described above are (1) optimal self-performed oral hygiene, (2) proper healing of the periodontal tissues following cause-related and corrective therapy, and (3) a carefully monitored maintenance care program. If these prerequisites can be met, it may, on the other hand, be possible to avoid all anticipated tooth extractions in this patient and the prosthetic therapy avoided. As stated above most of the teeth had increased mobility. This mobility, however, did not disturb the chewing comfort of this patient. The tooth mobility *per se*, therefore, was not regarded as an indication for splinting.

Conclusions: In a case of this character extensive efforts should be made to properly treat inflammatory periodontal disease in the entire dentition *before* decisions are made to extract one or several teeth. Decisions regarding tooth extraction should, if possible, not be made until after healing following periodontal surgery.

Treatment

Subsequent to initial examination, the patient was given a detailed "case presentation" and information regarding alternative goals of and prerequisites for the overall treatment. This information included a description of the role of dental plaque in the etiology of periodontal disease and the significance of optimal plaque control for a successful outcome of therapy. A treatment program was subsequently planned which aimed at maintaining all teeth, thereby avoiding extensive prosthetic therapy. The overall treatment was performed in the following sequence:

Periodontal chart

Tooth	Pocket depth M	B	D	L	Furcation involvement	Tooth mobility	Gingivitis	Parodontitis levis	Parodontitis gravis et complicata
18̶									
17̶									
16					b 1				X
15̶									
14	8	8	7		m, d 1	2		X	X
13		5	5						X
12	8	5				1			X
11	8	5	5			2		X	X
21	8	7	6			2		X	X
22	6	6	5			1			X
23		4	5			1			X
24	6	8	4		m, d 1	1		X	X
25		5							X
26									
27		6			b, d 1				X
28̶									
48̶									
47̶									
46	5	5			b 1				X
45		7						X	X
44	8	8	4					X	X
43	8	6	6			1		X	X
42	6	5				1			X
41	4					1			X
31	6	6	6			2		X	X
32	4	5				1			X
33	8	7	5			1		X	X
34								X	X
35̶									
36		5			b 1				X
37	7	7	6		b 1	1			X
38̶									

Fig. 19-10b. Periodontal chart relating to case K.A. (Fig. 19-10a).

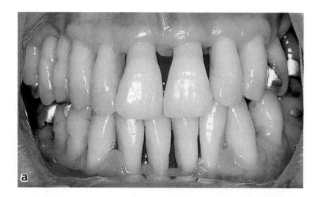

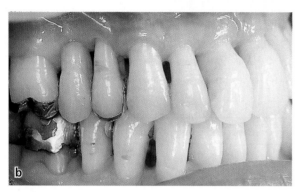
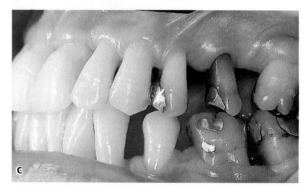

Fig. 19-11a-c. Case K.A. Clinical status 5 years after initial treatment.

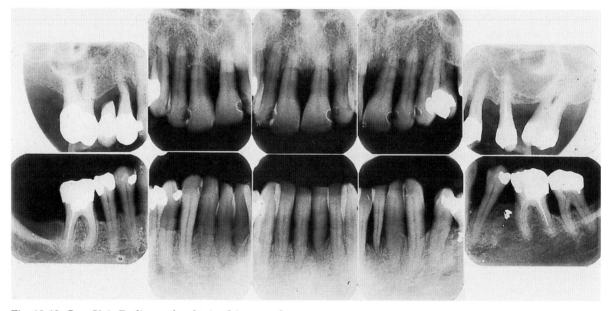

Fig. 19-12. Case K.A. Radiographs obtained 8 years after treatment.

Initial therapy

Oral hyiene instruction and plaque control evaluation. Scaling and root planing. Adjustment of improper amalgam restorations.

Additional therapy (following evaluation at re-examination)

Periodontal surgery involving careful removal of subgingival soft and hard deposits and root planing. All teeth in the dentition could be maintained and the furcation involvements in the premolar and molar areas could be treated successfully with furcation

plasty (see Chapter 29). After healing, a fixed bridge (16, 15, 14) was fabricated and inserted on esthetic indications.

Supportive therapy

During the first 6 months after completion of the initial and corrective therapy, the patient was recalled for maintenance care every 3 weeks. This interval between the recall appointments was then gradually extended to 3 months.

Periodontal chart				
Tooth	Pocket depth M B D L	Furcation involvement	Tooth mobility	
18				
17				
16				
15				
14				
13				
12			1	
11				
21			1	
22			1	
23				
24				
25				
26				
27				
28				
48				
47				
46				
45				
44				
43				
42			1	
41			1	
31			2	
32			1	
33				
34				
35				
36				
37				
38				

Fig. 19-13. Case K.A. Periodontal chart from recordings made 8 years after treatment. (Fig. 19-12).

Concluding remarks

The result of the treatment is shown in Fig. 19-11a-c (clinical status 5 years after initial treatment), Fig. 19-12 (radiographs 8 years after treatment) and Fig. 19-13 (periodontal chart 8 years after treatment).

There was no recurrence of destructive periodontal disease during the period of maintenance.

The planning of the overall treatment and the sequence of the different treatment procedures used in this case were selected for presentation in order to illustrate the following principle: *In patients exhibiting a generalized advanced breakdown of the periodontal tissues, but with an intact number of teeth, considerable efforts should be made to maintain all teeth.* Extraction of one single tooth in such a dentition will frequently also call for the extraction of several others for "prosthetic reasons". The end result of such an approach thus includes an extensive, prosthetic rehabilitation which, if the treatment planning had been properly done, would have been entirely unneccessary.

Patient B.H. (female, 40 years old)

Initial examination

The periodontal status (pocket depths, furcation involvements, tooth mobility, radiographs) from the initial examination is shown in Fig. 19-14a,b. The data obtained from this examination disclosed essentially shallow pockets in most parts of the dentition except for isolated areas (the region 11-24) where some sites exhibited probing depths varying between 4 and 7 mm. It should be observed that, particularly in the maxillary front region, pronounced gingival recessions prevailed. This means that even the moderate probing depth values obtained reflected advanced loss of the supporting tissues. This was further confirmed by the severe loss of alveolar bone (see radiographs: Fig. 19-14) in this region where, in addition, some of the teeth exhibited increased mobility (tooth 11: degree 2 in combination with elongation; tooth 23: degree 3 and tooth 24: degree 2). In the posterior tooth regions there was a loss of periodontal tissues varying between $1/3$ and $1/2$ of the length of the roots. In the mandibular front tooth region the destruction was severe, particularly around tooth 31. This tooth was found to be non-vital and exhibited a mobility of degree 2. The plaque and gingivitis scores were 25 and 30%, respectively.

Treatment

In discussing with the patient different treatment alternatives, it was first suggested that tooth 23 was to be extracted. Not more than 2-3 mm of the apical portion of the root was still invested in supporting bone. The tooth exhibited a degree 3 mobility in conjunction with premature occlusal contact in the intercuspal position and on laterotrusive movement of the mandible. The question arose, however, what consquences extraction of tooth 23 would have for the overall therapy. For instance: the neighboring teeth (22 with advanced periodontal destruction at the distal aspect, and 24 with severe loss of supporting tissue including increased mobility) could not be considered proper abutment teeth for a 3-unit bridge replacing tooth 23. The demand for proper abutment teeth would therefore require a further extension of the bridge to include teeth 21 and 25 (following extraction also of 24). This extension of the bridge implies, however, that tooth 11 will be the first nonsplinted neighboring tooth. Considering the small amount of periodontium which persisted around this tooth, it may from a prosthetic point of view be reasonable to extract 11 as well, and to extend the bridge to tooth 13, since tooth 12 may also be considered improper as the terminal abutment.

From this discussion, it is apparent that extraction of one single tooth (23) in this dentition will lead to extraction of a number of additional teeth to exclude their incorporation in the permanent reconstruction. The result is, thus, an extensive bridge therapy which can be avoided if only the critical tooth (23) can be

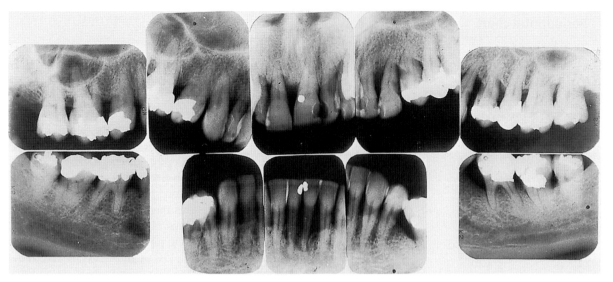

Fig. 19-14a. Case B.H. (40-year-old female patient). Radiographs from the initial examination.

Periodontal chart					
Tooth	Pocket depth M B D L		Furcation involvement	Tooth mobility	
18					
17	4				
16	4	4			
15					
14	4				
13	4				
12					
11	6	4		2	
21	4				
22	4				
23	5	6 5		3	
24	4	7		2	
25					
26	5		d 1		
27	6 4				
28					
48					
47					
46	4				
45	4	4			
44					
43					
42					
41					
31				2	
32					
33	4				
34	4				
35					
36	4		b 1		
37	4		b 1		
38					

Fig. 19-14b. Periodontal chart relating to case B.H. (Fig. 19-14a).

maintained. Therefore it was decided to treat all teeth and postpone the decision of tooth extractions until the result of the periodontal treatment could be properly evaluated.

Initial (cause-related) therapy
Oral hygiene instruction and plaque control evaluation. Scaling and root planing. Occlusal adjustment of 11, 23 and 24. Correction of improper amalgam restorations.

Additional therapy (following re-evaluation)
Periodontal surgery in the region of 11-24. Extraction of 28 and 48 (semi-impacted molars). Endodontic treatment of 31.

Six months following this part of the corrective treatment, a new evaluation disclosed that no pathologically deepened pockets were present and that the mobility had decreased in all initially hypermobile teeth (11: from degree 2 to 1; 23: from degree 3 to 2; 24: from degree 2 to 0; 31 from degree 2 to 1). All teeth could, thus, be maintained and there were no indications for additional tooth extractions. The treatment was completed with a crown restoration in tooth 25.

Supportive therapy
During the first year after completion of the corrective therapy, the patient was enrolled in a maintenance care program with recall appointments once every 3 months and thereafter once every 6 months.

The result of the treatment (12 years after) is shown in Fig. 19-15a-c (clinical status) and Fig. 19-16 (radiographs). No further loss of supporting tissues had occurred during this observation period.

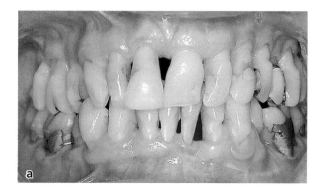

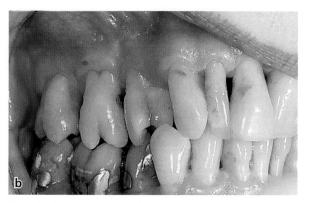

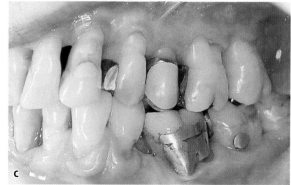

Fig. 19-15a-c. Case B.H. Clinical status 12 years after treatment.

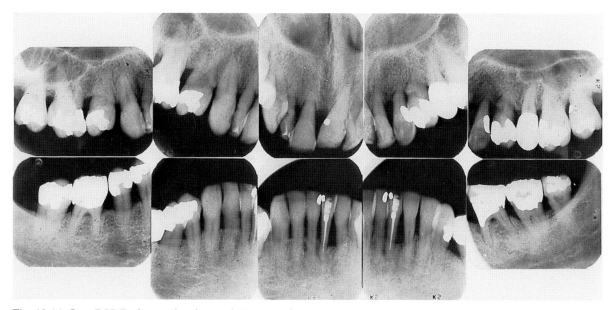

Fig. 19-16. Case B.H. Radiographs obtained 12 years after active therapy. Note that no loss of alveolar bone has occurred during the 12 years of maintenance. Compare with Fig. 19-14.

Patient P.O.S. (male, 30 years old)

Initial examination
The clinical status of this patient is illustrated in Fig. 19-17a-c and the periodontal status (pocket depths, furcation involvements, tooth mobility, radiographs and diagnoses) from the initial examination in Fig. 19-18. The dentition was characterized by severe destruction of the supporting apparatus, including advanced loss of the interradicular periodontal tissues in all molars and the two first maxillary premolars.

Most teeth were markedly mobile, particularly the incisors in both jaws. The plaque and gingivitis scores were close to 100%.

Treatment planning
A thorough analysis of the periodontal conditions in this patient revealed that certain teeth could no longer be treated and maintained but had to be extracted. Hence, it was decided to extract teeth 14 and 24 (furcation involvement of degree 2 from both mesial and distal aspects) and 12, 11, 21, 22 (loss of the supporting

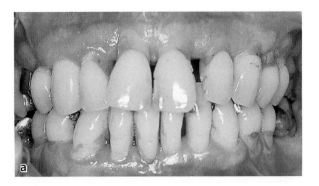

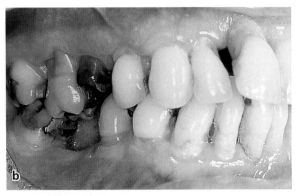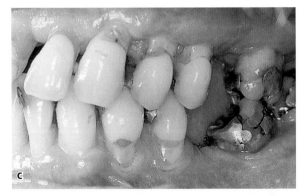

Fig. 19-17a-c. Case P.O.S. (30-year-old male patient). Clinical status prior to surgery.

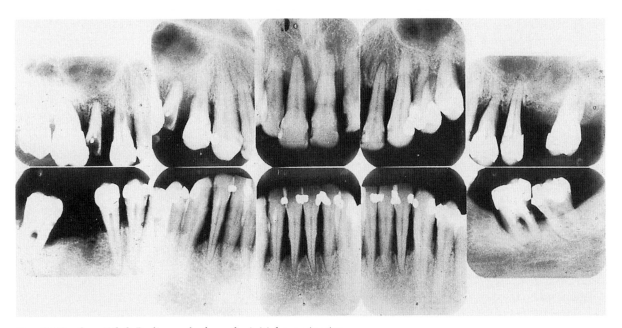

Fig. 19-18a. Case P.O.S. Radiographs from the initial examination.

tissues to a level close to or beyond the apices in combination with a mobility of degree 3). In the mandible, 42, 41, 31, 32 and 37 could not be maintained. The overall treatment of this patient, therefore, had to include prosthetic replacement of a number of teeth.

Alternative 1
Mandible: In the planning phase, it was anticipated that the prosthetic rehabilitation of the mandibular dentition should not involve any technical difficulties since 33 and 43 as well as 34, 35 and 44, 45 were

available for periodontal therapy and, hence, could be used as abutment teeth for a cross-arch fixed bridge. It did not seem reasonable to maintain the furcation-involved 47 and 38. Hence these teeth were scheduled for extraction. In this context it should be understood that if 47 and 38 were to be maintained, the treatment would have included not only endodontic measures but also root separation and periodontal surgery, production of posts and cores, and the incorporation of the preserved roots as abutments in the cross-arch bridge construction.

Periodontal chart						Diagnosis
Tooth	Pocket depth M B D L			Furcation involvement	Tooth mobility	Gingivitis / Parodontitis levis / Parodontitis gravis et complicata
18						
17	9	8 6		m, d 2	1	X X
16	8	8		m, b, d 2	2	X X
15	8	7 4			1	X
14	8 4	8 5		m, d 2	2	X X
13	6	5 4			1	X
12	8 4	7 8			3	X X
11	10 8	10			3	X X
21	7	10 8			3	X
22	8 5	7 5			3	X
23	8	10 6			2	X X
24	9	10 7		m, d 2	2	X X
25	8 6	8 7			2	X
26						
27	10 8	8 4		m, d 2, d 1	2	X X
28						
48						
47	10 5	8 7		3	1	X X
46						
45	8	7 5				X
44	8	8 7			1	X
43	7	8 5			1	X X
42	7 4	7 7			3	X X
41	7 4	7 7			3	X X
31	7 4	7 7			3	X
32	7 4	7 7			3	X
33	8	5 6			1	X
34	10	6 7			1	X X
35	5	4				X
36						
37	10 7	8 7		3	2	X X
38	6 8	9 8		b, 1 2	2	X X

Fig. 19-18b. Periodontal chart relating to case P.O.S. (Fig. 19-18a).

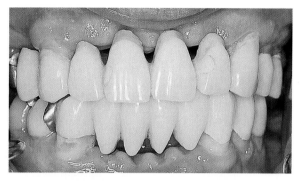

Fig. 19-19. Case P.O.S. Clinical status of the front tooth region at completion of the initial, cause-related treatment.

removable, partial denture was not considered appropriate since the various abutment teeth for such a denture displayed a markedly increased mobility. For the same reason, it was considered inappropriate to *temporarily* replace the extracted teeth by means of a provisional, removable partial denture. The provisional prosthesis had to be fabricated in the form of a fixed bridge in order to enable proper stabilization (splinting) of the hypermobile 13, 23 and 25 prior to periodontal surgery. In the present case the temporary bridge did not include tooth 15 and the maxillary molars. Tooth 15 was to be left uncovered in order to facilitate endodontic therapy and the preparation and insertion of a post and core. In addition, the maxillary molars had to be accessible for periodontal therapy including endodontic treatment and root separation. In order to facilitate the surgical procedures and also to avoid the risk of a further increase of the tooth mobility, the extraction of 14, 12, 11, 21 and 22 and the insertion of the temporary bridge had to be carried out prior to the start of the surgical phase of treatment.

Alternative 2
The alternative treatment to the one outlined above is a complete denture in the maxilla and a removable partial denture in the mandible with the use of 45, 44, 43 and 33, 34, 35 as abutment teeth.

Treatment
The clinical and radiographical symptoms of the advanced disease as well as the therapeutic alternatives were thoroughly discussed with the patient. This dis-

Maxilla: The maxillary dentition presented more difficult therapeutic problems. If the patient was to be restored with a fixed bridge, it was considered pertinent to maintain the two maxillary canines (teeth 13 and 23) and at least one tooth in the premolar (molar) regions on both sides of the jaw (15 and 25) and one or more roots of 17, 16 and 27. *Definitive* prosthetic treatment of the maxillary dentition by means of a

	17	16	15	14	13	12	11	21	22	23	24	25	27
Good prognosis					+								
Questionable prognosis	+		+							+		+	+
Irrational-to-treat		+		+		+	+	+	+		+		

	47		45	44	43	42	41	31	32	33	34	35	37	38
Good prognosis			+	+						+		+		
Questionable prognosis					+						+			
Irrational-to-treat	+					+	+	+	+				+	+

Fig. 19-18c. Pre-therapeutic risk assessment made for patient P.O.S. described in Figs. 19-17 and 19-19a,b.

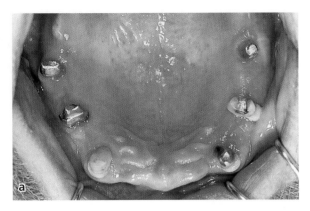
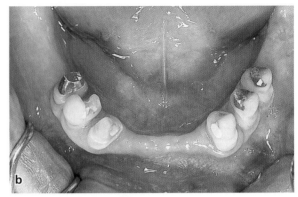

Fig. 19-20a-b. Case P.O.S. The abutment teeth used for a maxillary (a) and a mandibular (b) bridge.

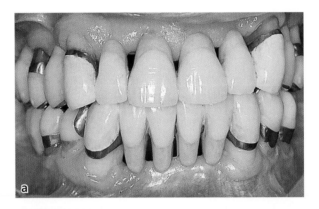

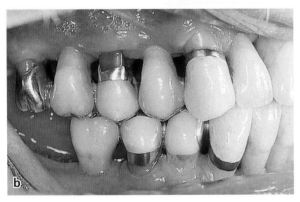
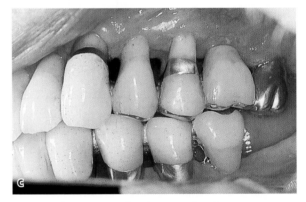

Fig. 19-21a-c. Case P.O.S. Clinical photographs illustrating the result of treatment after 8 years of maintenance.

cussion included a detailed explanation of the role of optimal plaque control for the long-term good prognosis. The treatment was performed according to *alternative 1* and in the following sequence:

Initial (cause-related) therapy
Instruction regarding oral hygiene measures. Scaling and root planing. Evaluation of the ability of the patient to maintain a high standard of oral hygiene.

Extraction of 14, 12, 11, 21, 22. Temporary acrylic bridge 14, 13, 12, 11, 21, 22, 23, 24, 25; (24 was temporarily maintained in order to ensure proper stability of the temporary bridge).

Extraction of 47, 42, 41, 31, 32, 37, 38. Temporary acrylic bridge 44, 43, 42, 41, 31, 32, 33, 34, 35; (45: because the tooth was non-vital it was not incorpo-

rated in the temporary bridge to facilitate endodontic treatment). Endodontic treatment 15, 45. The clinical status at the completion of the initial treatment is seen in Fig. 14-19.

Additional therapy
Periodontal surgery around the teeth which at the re-evaluation after initial therapy still exhibited pathologically deepened pockets which bled on probing. The palatal roots of 17 and 27 were maintained and the buccal roots were extracted following separation.

Extraction of 16 and 24. Following healing after surgery, posts and cores were inserted in 17, 15, 27 and 45 (Fig. 19-20a,b) and permanent fixed bridges were designed and fabricated with the following outline:

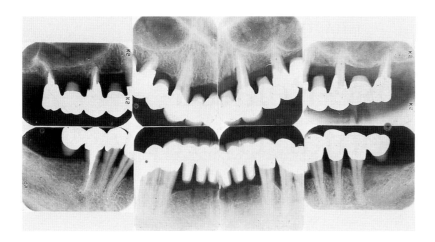

Fig. 19-22. Case P.O.S. Radiographs obtained 8 years after completion of active therapy. Note that no further loss of alveolar bone has occurred during the 8 years of maintenance.

Maxilla: 17 (palatal root), 16, 15, 14, 13, 12, 11, 21, 22, 23, 24, 25, 26, 27 (palatal root).

Mandible: 46, 45, 44, 43, 42, 41, 31, 32, 33, 34, 35, 36.

Supportive therapy
After completion of active treatment this patient was enrolled in a maintenance care program including recall appointments once every 3 months. Clinical photographs (Fig. 19-21a-c) and radiographs (Fig. 19-22) illustrate the result of the treatment at the 8-year control. No further loss of supporting tissues occurred during the maintenance period.

REFERENCES

Lindhe, J. & Nyman, S. (1975). The effect of plaque control and surgical pocket elimination on the establishment and maintenance of periodontal health. A longitudinal study of periodontal therapy in cases of advanced disease. *Journal of Clinical Periodontology* **2**, 67-79.

Nyman, S. & Lindhe, J. (1979). A longitudinal study of combined periodontal and prosthetic treatment of patients with advanced periodontal disease. *Journal of Periodontology* **50**, 163-169.

Nyman, S., Lindhe, J. & Rosling, B. (1977). Periodontal surgery in plaque-infected dentitions. *Journal of Clinical Periodontology* **4**, 240-249.

Nyman, S., Rosling, B. & Lindhe, J. (1975). Effect of professional tooth cleaning on healing after periodontal surgery. *Journal of Clinical Periodontology* **2**, 80-86.

Rosling, B., Nyman, S. & Lindhe, J. (1976a). The effect of systematic plaque control on bone regeneration in infrabony pockets. *Journal of Clinical Periodontology* **3**, 38-53.

Rosling, B., Nyman, S., Lindhe, J. & Jern, B. (1976b). The healing potential of the periodontal tissues following different techniques of periodontal surgery in plaque-free dentitions. A 2-year clinical study. *Journal of Clinical Periodontology* **3**, 233-250.

Chapter 20

Cause-Related Periodontal Therapy

Harald Rylander and Jan Lindhe

Objectives of initial, cause-related periodontal therapy

Means of initial, cause-related periodontal therapy
  Scaling and root planing
  Removal of plaque-retention factors

Healing after initial, cause-related therapy
  Clinical measurements
  Structural measurements

Evaluation of the effect of the initial, cause-related therapy

---

The overall treatment of patients with caries and periodontal disease, including associated pathologic conditions (e.g. pulpal and periapical lesions, tooth migration, tooth loss) can be divided into three different but frequently overlapping phases (see Chapter 19):

The phase of initial, cause-related therapy is aimed at bringing caries and gingivitis under control and at arresting the further progression of periodontal tissue destruction.

The phase of additional therapy is aimed at restoring function and esthetics.

The phase of supportive therapy is aimed at preventing recurrence of caries and periodontal disease.

OBJECTIVES OF INITIAL, CAUSE-RELATED PERIODONTAL THERAPY

The measures used in initial, cause-related periodontal therapy aim at the elimination – and the prevention of their recurrence – of supra and subgingivally located bacterial deposits from the tooth surfaces. This is accomplished by:

- motivating the patient to understand and combat dental disease (*patient information*)
- giving the patient *instruction* on how to properly clean his/her teeth (*self-performed plaque control methods*), see Chapter 21
- *scaling and root planing*

- *removal* of additional *retention factors* for plaque such as overhanging margins of restorations, ill-fitting crowns, etc.

MEANS OF INITIAL, CAUSE-RELATED PERIODONTAL THERAPY

Scaling and root planing

Definitions

Scaling is a procedure which aims at the removal of plaque and calculus from the tooth surface. Depending on the location of the deposits, scaling is performed by supragingival and/or subgingival instrumentation. *Root planing* denotes a technique of instrumentation by which the "softened" cementum is removed and the root surface is made "hard" and "smooth". Subgingival scaling and root planing can be performed as either *closed* or *open* procedures and often under local anesthesia. The *closed* procedure implies subgingival instrumentation without intentional displacement of the gingiva. The root surface is, thus, not accessible for direct visual inspection. The *open* procedure calls for exposure of the affected root surface by measures which displace the gingival tissue. The gingiva is thus incised and reflected or resected to facilitate access and visibility in the field of operation.

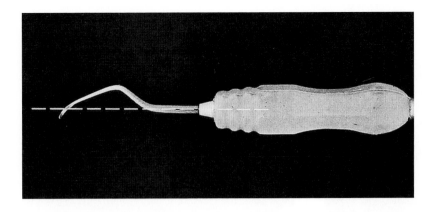

Fig. 20-1. A double-ended hand instrument with col-grip. The cutting edges of the blades are centered over the long axis of the handle.

Instruments and instrumentation

Instruments used for scaling and root planing are classified as:

1. Hand instruments
2. Ultrasonic and sonic instruments
3. Rotating instruments
4. Reciprocating instruments
5. Laser instruments

Hand instruments
A hand instrument is composed of three parts: The *working part* (the blade), the *shank* and the *handle*. The cutting edges of the blade are centered over the long axis of the handle in order to give the instrument proper balance (Fig. 20-1). The blade is often made of *carbon steel, stainless steel* or *tungsten carbide*.

Curettes (Fig. 20-2): Curettes are instruments used for both scaling and root planing. The working part of the curette is the spoon-shaped blade which has two curved cutting edges. The two edges are united by the rounded toe. The curettes are usually made "double-ended" with mirror-turned blades. The length and angulation of the shank as well as the dimensions of the blade differ between different brands of the instrument (Fig. 20-3).

Sickles (Fig. 20-4): The sickle is manufactured with either a curved or a straight blade which has a triangular cross section and two cutting edges. The "facial" surface between the two cutting edges is flat in lateral direction but may be curved in the direction of its long axis. The "facial" surface converges with the two lateral surfaces of the blade. The sickles are mainly used for supragingival debridement or scaling in shallow pockets.

Hoes (Fig. 20-5): The hoe has only one cutting edge. The blade is turned at a 100° angle to the shank with the cutting edge beveled at a 45° angle. The blade can be positioned at four different inclinations in relation to the shank: facial, lingual, distal and mesial. The hoe is mainly used for supragingival scaling but is an excellent instrument to use for root planing during periodontal surgery.

Instrumentation
Supragingival scaling: The debridement of the dentition of a patient with periodontal disease often starts with supragingival scaling. Supragingival calculus and gross overhangs of restorations are removed (Fig. 20-6). This initial phase of the debridement can be performed with the use of hand instruments or ultrasonic instruments (see below). When hand instrumentation is preferred for the initial debridement, a curette or a sickle is often used to simply split off calculus from its attachment to the enamel and/or the exposed part of the root. Following hand instrumentation the clinical crowns should be polished using rubber cups and first pumice and subsequently more fine-grained (grainsize of 2-3μm) polishing pastes. In many cases the *supragingival scaling* effort can be completed in one session. This will allow the patient, without further delay, to implement the new and "improved" self-performed plaque control program.

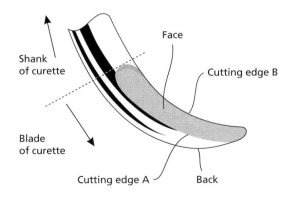

Fig. 20-2. Schematic illustration of the design of the blade of a curette.

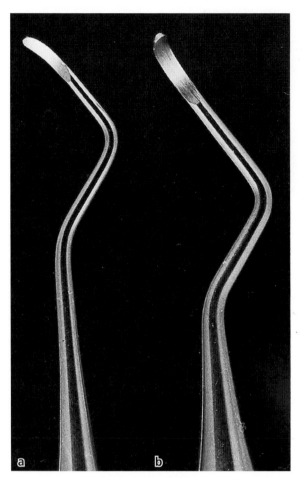
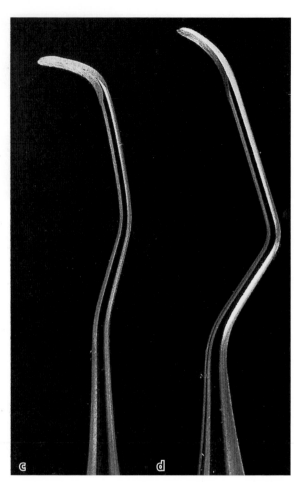

Fig. 20-3. Curettes with different lengths and angulations of the shank. (a) and (b) are curettes used for supragingival and (c) and (d) curettes for subgingival instrumentation. Increased angulation of the shank (b and d) of the curettes permits proper instrumentation in posterior tooth regions.

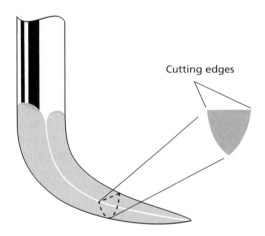

Fig. 20-4. Schematic illustration of the cross section of the blade of a sickle. Note the positions of the cutting edges.

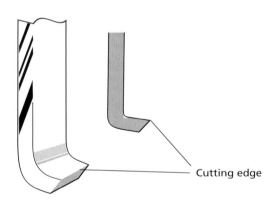

Fig. 20-5. The cross section of a hoe. Note the position of the cutting edge.

Subgingival scaling and root planning: Performed with hand instruments, these treatment procedures aim at removing not only soft and hard deposits from the root surface but also small amounts of tooth substance. Root cementum and also root dentine are removed in the shape of small chips which carry the deposits and which during the cutting operation are curled up at the front side (in the cutting direction) of the blade of the instrument. This method of instrumentation is denoted "orthogonal cutting", which implies the removal of tooth substance by means of an edge which to a varying extent penetrates the hard substance of the root. The result of the cutting opera-

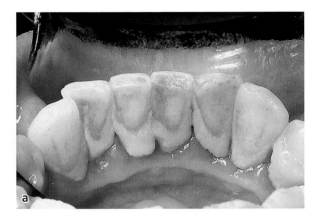
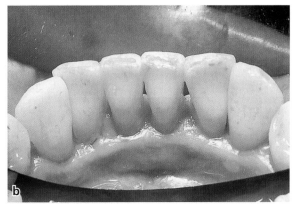
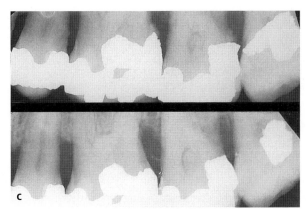

Fig. 20-6. (a) Photograph illustrating the lingual aspect of the mandibular front tooth region with supragingival plaque and calculus. (b) The same tooth region 3 weeks after supragingival scaling and institution of proper oral hygiene. (c) Radiographs of left maxilla before and after removal of calculus and amalgam overhangs.

tion is dependent on the material and geometry of the edge, the sharpness of the edge and the forces used during instrumentation (Lindhe 1964). Even if subgingival scaling and root planing often are regarded as two separate procedures with different objectives (see definition), in clinical work they cannot always be separated from each other.

Subgingival instrumentation aims at resolving the inflammation in the gingiva and arresting the progressive destruction of the attachment apparatus by removing the biofilm present in the gingival pocket. Coupled with an effective supragingival plaque control program, therefore, subgingival debridement is the most important measure in the treatment of periodontitis. As a matter of fact, in many patients who adopt proper self-performed plaque control habits, subgingival instrumentation results in gingival health (Fig. 20-7).

Prior to the start of subgingival instrumentation, the presence and extent of gingivitis and breakdown of the supporting apparatus in all parts of the dentition must have been properly assessed (see Chapter 18). Depending on the severity of the case, and the skill of the operator, the number of teeth that may be included in each treatment session of subgingival scaling and root planing may vary. As a general rule, in a patient with moderate/severe periodontitis, each session should not involve treatment of more than one quadrant.

The subgingival instrumentation should preferably be performed under local anesthesia. The root surface of the diseased site is first explored with a probe to identify (1) the probing depth, (2) the anatomy of the root surface (irregularities, root furrows, open furcation, etc.), and (3) the location of the calcified deposits.

When all root surfaces selected for treatment in a given session have been examined, the order in which the various sites are to be instrumented is determined. The curette is inserted into the first pocket. The instrument is held in a so-called *modified pen grasp* and with *finger rest* – fourth finger rest or third finger rest – with the face of the blade parallel to and in light contact with the root surface (Fig. 20-8). It is important that all root surface instrumentation is performed with a proper finger rest. This implies that one finger – the third or the fourth – must act as a fulcrum for the movement of the blade of the instrument. A proper finger rest should (1) provide a stable fulcrum, (2) permit optimal angulation of the blade, and (3) enable the use of wrist-forearm motion. In addition, to optimize instrumentation and to avoid undue tissue damage, the finger rest must be secured as close as possible to the particular root surface selected for treatment.

After the base of the periodontal pocket has been identified with the distal edge of the blade, the instrument is turned into a proper "cutting" position (Fig. 20-9). The grasp of the instrument is tightened, the

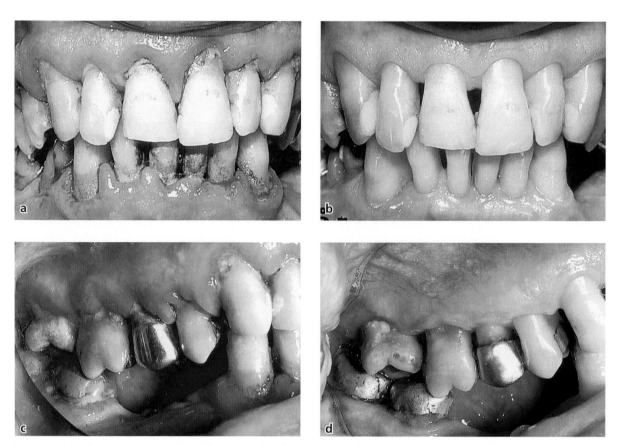

Fig. 20-7a-d. Photographs illustrating the effect of scaling, root planing and proper self-performed plaque control on the gingival tissues. Note gingival recession and the stippled outer surface of the gingiva after treatment (b,d) compared to the status before treatment (a,c).

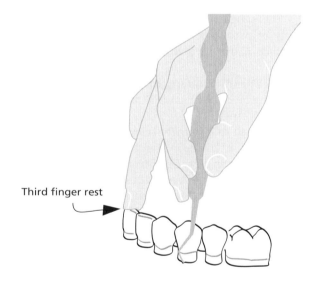

Third finger rest

Fig. 20-8. Schematic illustration demonstrating the proper "third finger rest" using a modified pen grasp in the molar region in the left mandible.

force between the cutting edge and the root surface is increased, and the blade is moved in a firm stroke (working stroke) in coronal direction. Due to the structural and chemical composition of root cementum and dentine, the cutting operation *should always be initiated at the bottom of the pocket and be guided in coronal direction*. In this movement the edge is moved into the root surface, and root substance with attached calculus is removed. The working stroke is followed by a finishing stroke which will produce a smooth root surface. Working and finishing strokes must be made in differ-

ent directions to cover all aspects of the root surface (crosswise, back and forth) but, as stated above, the strokes should always start from an apical position and be guided in coronal direction. After the *working* and *finishing strokes* have been made, the probe is inserted in the pocket again and the surface of the root surface assessed anew. The root surface is considered properly treated when the operator, using a periodontal probe, finds the surface "smooth" and "hard".

The importance of removing "diseased" cementum during root planing was questioned by several

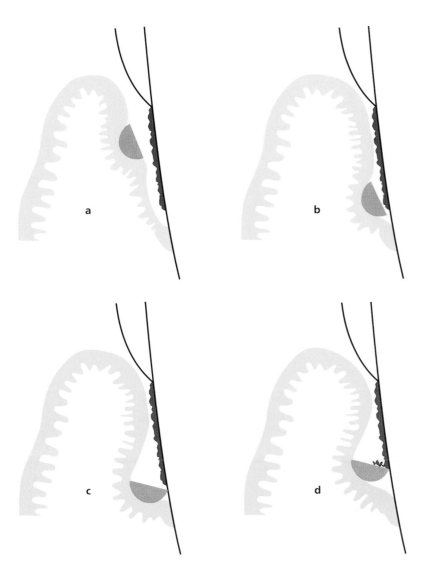

Fig. 20-9. (a) The curette is inserted into the periodontal pocket. Note the close-to-zero degree angulation of the face of the curette against the root surface to facilitate the accessibility of the pocket. (b) The bottom of the periodontal pocket is identified with the distal edge of the blade of the curette. (c) The curette is turned to a proper cutting position for scaling. (d) The blade is moved along the root surface in a scaling stroke to remove calculus.

authors. Nyman et al. (1986, 1988) monitored the outcome of surgical periodontal therapy at sites where the teeth were exposed to either extensive root instrumentation to remove all of the cementum and some dentin, or gentle removal of plaque to leave most of the root cementum. The authors found that in patients with proper self-performed plaque control, both procedures allowed for excellent soft tissue healing. This observation was confirmed by Oberholzer et al. (1996) who concluded – from a clinical study – that the establishment of a smooth and hard root surface was not a critical factor in periodontal therapy. This means that "overinstrumentation" also during non-surgical therapy may cause more harm than good.

In this context it must also be realized that the complete removal of subgingival plaque and calculus in a "non-surgical" procedure is difficult if not impossible. Waerhaug (1978) first assessed the pocket depth of periodontally involved teeth that were subsequently exposed to comprehensive scaling and root planing. Following the completion of this treatment, which was carried out by a skilled periodontist, the teeth were extracted and the root surfaces examined under the microscope. It was concluded that at sites with a pocket depth of > 5 mm, subgingival scaling

and root planing in most cases (about 90%) left deposits of plaque and calculus behind. A similar conclusion was reached by, for example, Rabbani et al. (1981) and Magnusson et al. (1984), and also by Sherman et al. (1990) who in a clinical study demonstrated that "closed" subgingival instrumentation was a procedure which consistently failed to eliminate all deposits of calculus. In their study, periodontally involved teeth were first exposed to subgingival scaling and root planing. Following the completion of this treatment, soft tissue flaps were elevated to expose the root surfaces. The authors observed that small remnants of calculus had been left behind in several locations.

The studies quoted above imply that residual plaque and calculus may remain even after careful and repeated subgingival instrumentation. It is therefore the responsibility of the clinician to monitor treatment outcome. If a site fails to heal properly, i.e.bleeding on probing persists, and if the clinical attachment level in deep pocket sites is not improved, additional therapy such as access flap surgery must be considered. The reason for this is that findings by, for example, Eaton et al. (1985) and Caffesse et al. (1986) have shown that scaling during access therapy may improve the efficacy of root instrumentation.

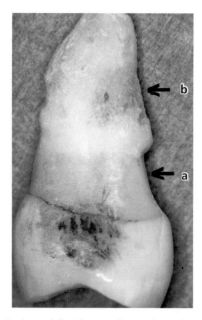

Fig. 20-10. A tooth has been subjected to subgingival scaling and root planing and extensive tooth substance has been removed due to repeated intense instrumentation (arrow a). However, the periodontal pocket was not properly diagnosed and calculus has been left (arrow b).

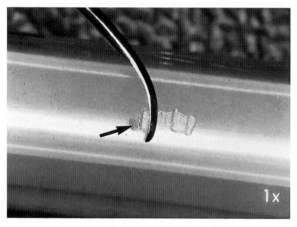

Fig. 20-11. The sharpness of a curette is tested on a plastic stick. A chip (arrow) is easily produced by a sharp instrument.

Fig. 20-10 shows a tooth that has been subjected to repeated scaling and root planing. The clinician did not, however, reach the bottom of the periodontal pocket, plaque and calculus were left behind, the periodontitis lesion progressed and the tooth eventually had to be extracted.

Factors important for the outcome of subgingival instrumentation
Root anatomy: The surface of a single-rooted tooth is often easier to reach by subgingival instrumentation than the furcation complex of multirooted teeth. However, concavities and tooth furrows exist in booth single and multirooted teeth. Such root irregularities may contain small deposits of plaque and calculus which are difficult to reach. In such sites ultrasonic instruments with specially designed tips may facilitate local therapy (Kocher & Plagmann 1997). The technical problems inherent in subgingival instrumentation increase with increasing probing depth. Specially designed instruments with a long shank (Fig. 20-3) may be used in deep pockets.

Skill of the operator: The outcome of the subgingival instrumentation is "operator sensitive". Thus, the technical skill of the dentist/dental hygienist influences the result of this procedure. Brayer et al. (1989) demonstrated that experienced dentists were more efficient in subgingival debridment than more inexperienced operators. The difference between the two categories of therapists was most pronounced in the treatment of deeper (> 6 mm) pocket sites. Also, in surgical therapy the technical skill of the operator remains important for the outcome of the root debridement part of the treatment.

Time allowed: The time allowed for the instrumentation will also influence the treatment result. In a study by Badersten et al. (1981) it was demonstrated that as much as 6-8 minutes were required for a comprehensive subgingival treatment of one single tooth when hand instruments were used. When ultrasonic instruments were used 4-6 minutes were required.

Instrument sharpening
The hand instruments must have proper cutting edges

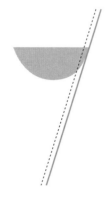

Fig. 20-12. Schematic drawing illustrating the sharpening of a curette. The original geometry of the cutting edge must be maintained during the sharpening procedure.

in order to make subgingival instrumentation a precise and efficient procedure. A curette with a *blunt cutting edge* must be *pressed* against the root surface with a larger force than is required when a sharp instrument is used. Scaling with instruments with blunt cutting edges often results in an incomplete removal of calculus but in the establishment of a "smoothened" root surface. Remaining calculus on such a "smoothened" root surface is difficult to detect with a periodontal probe. The cutting edge of the hand instrument, therefore, must be controlled repeatedly during scaling. This can be done by planing a plastic stick (Fig. 20-11).

The sharpening of hand instruments can be performed by the use of either "rotating" (cylindrical or cone-shaped) or "plain" stones (India or Arkansas stones). Curettes and sickles are sharpened by grinding the lateral surfaces and/or the face of the blade. It is important that the original geometry of the instrument is not changed by the sharpening procedure (Fig. 20-12).

Ultrasonic and sonic instruments
For many years ultrasonic scalers (e.g. Cavitron®, Amdent®, Odontoson®) have been used for the removal of plaque, calculus and stain. Scaling with ultrasonic instruments often results in the establishment of an uneven root surface. It has been suggested, therefore, that ultrasonic scaling should be supplemented with hand instrumentation to establish a smooth root surface (Björn & Lindhe 1962). Clinical studies have evaluated the effect of scaling using ultrasonic or hand instruments (Torafson et al. 1979, Badersten et al. 1981). The authors found that debridement of 4-7 mm pockets with ultrasonic instrumentation was as successful for healing diseased periodontal sites as was scaling with hand instruments (curettes). It has also been questioned whether indeed a *smooth* root surface after treatment is important for successful healing (Rosenberg & Ash 1974). Waerhaug (1956) found that a junctional epithelium readapted and a normal "epithelial cuff" also formed to uneven root surfaces. Properly used, therefore, ultrasonic instrumentation must be regarded as a valuable substitute for conventional scaling with hand instruments and may even be the best instrument for scaling at furcation areas (Leon & Vogel 1987).

Recently a new type of instrument for tooth debridement was introduced – *the sonic scaler* (e.g. Titan-S®, Micro-Mega Air Scaler®). This instrument is air-driven and produces vibrations in the sonic range (2300-6300 cycles per second). In an *in vitro* study (Lie & Leknes 1985) and in clinical studies (Loos et al. 1987, Baehni et al. 1992) it was shown that the sonic scaler was as effective for calculus removal as the ultrasonic instrument and, besides, the sonic scaler caused less root surface roughness than the ultrasonic device.

The removal of plaque and calculus by ultrasonic and sonic instrumentation is accomplished by (1) the vibration of the tip of the instrument, and (2) the

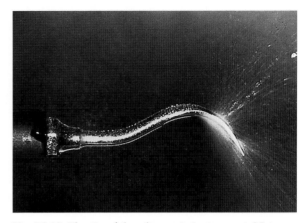

Fig. 20-13. The tip of the ultrasonic instrument. Note the spraying and cavitation of the fluid used for cooling.

spraying and cavitation effect of the fluid coolant. The vibrations (amplitude ranging from 0.006-0.1 mm) in the ultrasonic instruments are produced by a metal core which can change its dimension in an electromagnetic field with an operating frequency between 25 000 and 42 000 cycles per second. In the sonic instruments, the vibrations are generated mechanically. During the generation of the ultrasonic vibrations heat is produced, which is why the tip during instrumentation always has to be irrigated with a coolant.

Before use, the ultrasonic instrument must be adjusted regarding the power (tuning) and cooling according to the manual (Fig. 20-13). The tip should be applied to the tooth surface with very light pressure and be moved back and forth over the surface in sweeping movements and in such a way that its pattern of vibration is orientated parallel to the tooth surface. This will prevent damage to the root. A periodontal probe should always be used to check the root surface characteristics after instrumentation.

A novel, diamond-coated, *sonic scaler insert* was introduced by Kocher & Plagmann (1997) The authors claimed that this type of insert facilitated scaling and root planing in furcation areas.

Rotating instruments
Root furrows, furcation areas and root surfaces in deep, narrow, infrabony pockets are difficult to properly debride with the use of hand instruments. At such sites, therefore, rotating instruments such as fine-grained diamonds (or sonic scalers with diamond-

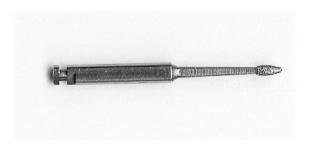

Fig. 20-14. A fine-grained diamond for mechanical debridement. Magnification × 1.5.

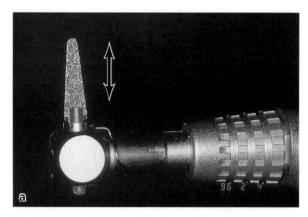
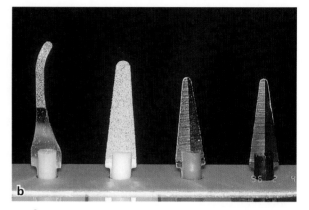

Fig. 20-15. (a) A diamond tip inserted in a handpiece (The Profin® Directional System). Arrows indicate the directions of the movement. (b) A set of tips (Lamineer®) of different design.

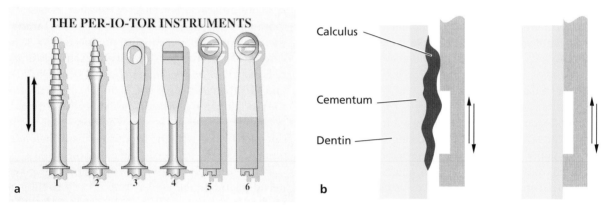

Fig. 20-16. (a) A collection of the PER-IO-TOR® instrument tips for scaling and root planing. (b) A schematic illustration of the effect of the PER-IO-TOR® instrument on the root surface with deposits (left). When the root cementum is clean and planed, no more cementum can be removed because of the design of the instrument (right).

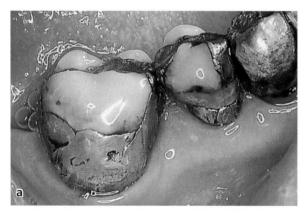
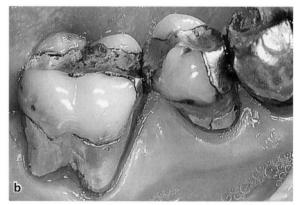

Fig. 20-17. Amalgam restorations before (a) and after (b) the adjustment of the overhangs. The buccal restoration in tooth 46 is prepared in order to reduce the degree of furcation involvement.

coated inserts, see above) can be used (Fig. 20-14). Care should be taken, however, to avoid excessive removal of tooth substance with such cutting procedures.

Reciprocating instruments
The Profin® Directional System offers a specially designed handpiece (a second generation of the so called Eva® system which was introduced in 1969) with a 1.2

mm reciprocating motion of the working tips set in self-steering or fixed mode (Fig. 20-15). A recommended engine speed of 10 000-15 000 rpm will give 20 000-30 000 tip strokes per minute. Specially designed working tips have been developed for the Profin Directional System (Axelsson 1993). The PER-IO-TOR® instruments will optimize cleaning and planing of rough root cementum surfaces and prevent further removal of root cementum once the surface is clean and smooth (Fig. 20-16). Mengel et al. (1994) evaluated the PER-IO-TOR® instruments in an *in vitro* study. They stated that the PER-IO-TOR® instruments have similar planing properties as manual hand instruments, but cause minimal removal of tooth structures.

Laser instruments

Laser instruments have been used in dentistry for cavity preparation since 1964 and for root debridement in combination with periodontal surgery. In a recent clinical study by Schwarz et al. (2001), the Er:YAG (erbium-doped:yttrium, aluminium and garnet laser) was used for "closed" subgingival scaling and root planing. The laser treatment was compared to conventional instrumentation with curettes. The authors concluded that the laser method gave better results in terms of pocket reduction at sites with deep pockets. Further studies are needed, however, to evaluate the laser instrument and the long-term outcome of this kind of treatment.

Removal of plaque-retention factors

In an epidemiological study, Björn et al. (1969, 1970) observed that ill-fitting artificial crowns and fillings were associated with a reduced height of the periodontal bone level. Jeffcoat & Howell (1980) reported that marginal bone loss was more pronounced around teeth with overhanging amalgam restorations than around teeth without restorations. Rodriguez-Ferrer et al. (1980) concluded that "the presence of a subgingival overhanging defective margin may be the only important clinically significant feature of an amalgam restoration related to the pathogenesis of chronic inflammatory periodontal disease". It is not the overhang of the restoration *per se*, however, which causes or maintains periodontal disease. Waerhaug (1960) pointed out that the more advanced gingival inflammation observed in sites with ill-fitting restorations was the result of extensive plaque accumulation and not of mechanical or chemical irritation caused by the filling material. Thus, overhangs of restorations must be removed to (1) facilitate the removal of plaque and calculus, and (2) to establish an anatomy of the tooth surface which facilitates self-performed tooth cleaning.

Overhanging margins of dental restorations can be removed using a flame-shaped diamond stone mounted on a handpiece for rotator movements, or a flat diamond stone mounted on a handpiece for horizontal reciprocal movements (Eva-system®, Profin® Directional System) (Fig. 20-15). The overhang is removed and the restoration is given a proper form and a smooth surface. The triangular or V-shaped tips (Lamineer®) are appropriately tailored for use in narrow interproximal spaces and can reach 2-3 mm sub-

gingivally for the reshaping and polishing of restorations (Fig. 20-15b).

The adjustment of an improperly designed filling or artificial crown is often a difficult and time-consuming procedure. It is sometimes more convenient to remove the improper filling (crown) and insert a new one with a proper marginal fit. Fig. 20-17 illustrates the effect on the periodontal tissues of the adjustment of an amalgam overhang.

HEALING AFTER INITIAL, CAUSE-RELATED THERAPY

Clinical measurements

The potential of subgingival instrumentation to eliminate inflammation and arrest progression of periodontal disease was studied in a number of early clinical trials, e.g. Lövdal et al. (1961), Suomi et al. (1971), Axelsson & Lindhe (1978, 1981), Hirschfeld & Wasserman (1978), Morrison et al. (1980), Badersten et al. (1984).

Lövdal et al. (1961) examined around 1500 individuals in Norway regarding their oral hygiene status, gingival conditions, alveolar bone loss and tooth loss. The patients were subsequently, on an individual basis, given careful oral hygiene instruction, including

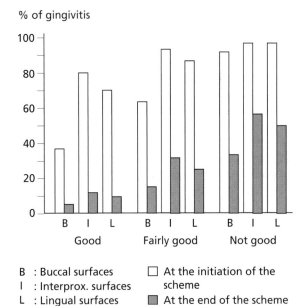

Fig. 20-18. The patients were divided into three groups after the initial examination according to their oral hygiene, "good", "fairly good", "not good". During a 5-year period the patients were subjected to scaling and root planing measures two to four times per year. In all three categories of patients there was a remarkable improvement of gingival conditions after 5 years of repeated plaque control measures. Data from Lövdal et al. 1961.

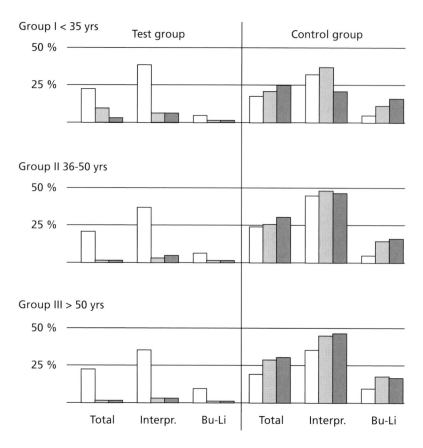

Fig. 20-19. Histogram showing the frequency distribution of inflamed gingival units in the test and control groups at the baseline (open bars) and re-examinations after 3 and 6 years (hatched and black bars respectively). The individual mean (total) figures describe unaltered gingival conditions in the control groups but marked improvements in the test groups during the trial. Data from Axelsson & Lindhe 1981.

detailed information in the proper use of toothbrush, toothpick, dental floss, etc. In addition, their teeth were subjected to meticulous supra and subgingival scaling and root planing. The oral hygiene instruction as well as the scaling and root planing measures were repeated two to four times per year over a 5-year period, at the end of which the patients were re-examined. The authors reported (Fig. 20-18) that "the combined effect of subgingival scaling and controlled oral hygiene definitely reduced the incidence of gingivitis and tooth loss". The improvement was remarkable also in patients whose home-care habits did not improve during the 5 years of trial. Similar findings were reported by Suomi et al. (1971) from a study comprising about 350 subjects in California. A test group of patients received, during a 3-year period, oral hygiene instruction and scaling three to four times per year, while a control group during the same period received restorative oriented dental care. At the end of the 3 years the test group patients had significantly less gingivitis and less attachment loss than the controls.

Axelsson & Lindhe (1978, 1981) compared the effect of a prophylactic program including (1) oral hygiene control and (2) scaling and root planing repeated once every 2-3 months over a 6-year period with the effect of traditional dental therapy, i.e. a therapy which was directed towards the symptoms of dental disorders rather than towards the elimination of the etiological factors. It was observed that in the patients of the control groups there was only a minor improvement in oral hygiene, while in the test groups at the re-examinations after 3 and 6 years, the mean plaque scores were consistently low (< 20%). In the control groups

there was no improvement of the gingival conditions (Fig. 20-19), while in the test groups the gingivitis scores had approached 0 values (meaning gingival health) at the re-examinations. Fig. 20-20 gives the attachment level alterations that occurred between 1972 and 1978. It can be seen that, while in the patients of the control groups there was a substantial further loss of attachment, in the test patients there was no further breakdown of the attachment apparatus.

Hirschfeld & Wasserman (1978) presented a long-term survey of tooth loss in 600 patients treated for periodontal disease. The patients were re-examined at an average of 23 years after the active treatment, which included primarily subgingival scaling, and root planing followed by careful maintenance therapy. The authors observed that "during the post-treatment period 300 patients had lost no teeth from periodontal disease", and "199 had lost 1-3 teeth". This means that periodontal therapy directed towards the elimination of the subgingival infection using a non-surgical approach can be effective in preventing tooth loss in most patients and also in those with advanced periodontal disease.

Morrison et al. (1980) studied the short-term effect of non-surgical treatment in 90 subjects with moderately advanced periodontal disease. Following an initial examination the patients were given oral hygiene instruction and the pockets were treated by subgingival scaling and root planing. Re-examination performed 4 weeks after active therapy revealed that (1) the patients had improved their oral hygiene, (2) the gingivitis scores had decreased, and (3) the initial depth of the periodontal pockets was substantially

Attachment level alteration 1972-1975-1978

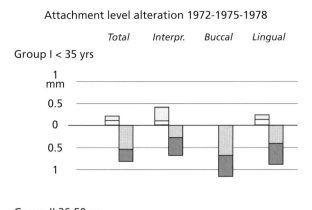

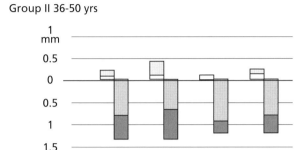

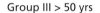

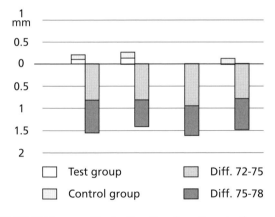

Fig. 20-20. Histogram illustrating the alterations in the clinical attachment levels between the baseline (1972) and re-examinations (1975, 1978) in various test and control groups. The attachment level remained unaltered in the test groups but was reduced in all the control groups (below the O-line). The average attachment loss per year in control groups was: I: 0.13 mm, II: 0.23mm, III: 0.26 mm. Data from Axelsson & Lindhe 1981.

reduced (Fig. 20-21). The authors concluded that already, 1 month following cause-related periodontal therapy, the clinical severity of periodontal disease was markedly reduced.

Badersten et al. (1984) studied the effect of subgingival scaling and root planing in 16 patients with moderate-advanced periodontitis. The patients received oral hygiene instruction and all single-rooted teeth were exposed to meticulous subgingival debridement using either handscalers or an ultrasonic device. Re-examination carried out after 2 years

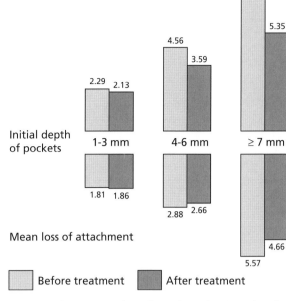

Fig. 20-21. Histogram describing the reduction of probing depth 4 weeks after active therapy comprising scaling and root planing. Data from Morrison et al. 1980.

Table 20-1. The mean probing reduction and probing attachment gain/loss (mm) that can be expected following scaling and root planing in non-molar sites

Initial probing depth	Probing pocket depth reduction	Probing attachment change
< 3	0.5	–0.5 (loss)
3-6	1.0-1.5	–0.5-+0.5
7-> 10	2.5-5.0	+0.5-+2.0

showed that this treatment had resulted in the establishment of healthy gingival conditions (only about 10% of the gingival sites bled on probing) and in a marked reduction in the overall probing depth (Fig. 20-22; Badersten 1984). The authors concluded that careful subgingival scaling and root planing was an effective means to eliminate gingivitis and reduce the probing depth even at sites with initially very deep (> 9 mm) periodontal pockets. Similar observations have also been reported in later clinical studies (for review see Cobb 1996).

It may be concluded that in patients who adopt proper oral hygiene measures:

- Healing after non-surgical therapy seems to be complete after about 3-6 months
- The number of sites that bleed on probing will be markedly reduced
- More gingival recession and gain of probing attach-

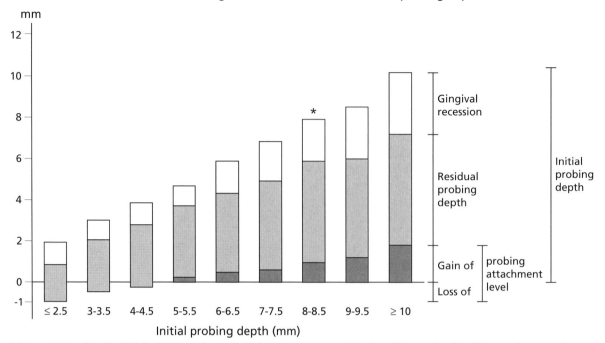

Dimensional changes for sites with different initial probing depths

* Interpretation: For sites initially 8-8.5 mm deep, gingival recession amounted to about 2mm, gain of probing attachment to 1 mm and residual probing depth to 5 mm.

Fig. 20-22. Histogram illustrating clinical results after non-surgical periodontal therapy. Data from Badersten et al. 1981, 1984.

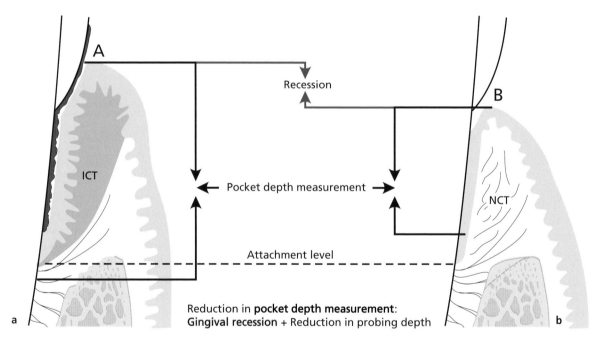

Fig. 20-23. A schematic illustration of a gingival unit (a) before and (b) after periodontal therapy. Probing depth measurements (blue lines) before (a) and after (b) therapy. The dotted line indicates the "histologic" attachment level. Recession = green line. Location of the gingival margin before therapy (A) and after therapy (B). ICT = infiltrated connective tissue, NCT = non-infiltrated connective tissue.

ment will be obtained in initially deeper than more shallow pocket sites. See Fig. 20-22 and Table 20-1.

• In sites with initial probing depths of 6-9 mm, the residual probing depth will be 4-5 mm, and the amount of gingival recession about 2 mm.

• In sites with initial pockets of < 3 mm, a probing attachment loss of 0.5 mm will occur.

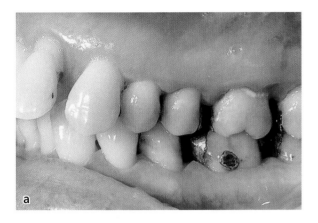

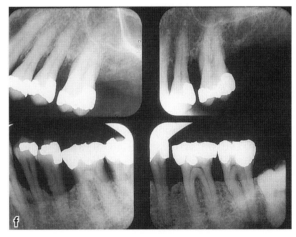

Before	23	24	25	26	27
Mesial	7	5	8	9	7
Buccal			4	6	5
Distal	4	6	0	7	9
Palatal	5	4	4	6	7
	33	34	35	36	37
Mesial	6	8	9	7	6
Buccal			7		
Distal	7	7	10	6	7
Palatal	5	7	8	5	5

b

After	23	24	25	26	27
Mesial	4			4	#
Buccal					#
Distal		4	4		#
Palatal					#
	33	34	35	36	37
Mesial		5	4	4	4
Buccal			5		
Distal		4	5		
Palatal		4	5		

d

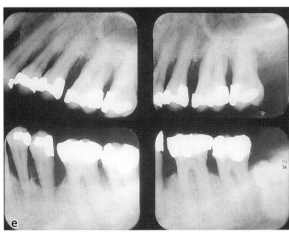

e

f

Fig. 20-24. Photographs illustrating the buccal surfaces of premolars and molars before (a) and 1 year after cause-related periodontal therapy (c). Note the recession of the gingival margin following therapy. The reduction of probing depths and absence of bleeding on probing from the bottom of the pockets after treatment indicate resolution of gingivitis (b,d). A comparison between the radiographs obtained before (e) and after (f) scaling and root planing demonstrates that treatment has also changed the outline of the alveolar bone crest.

Structural measurements

The schematic illustration in Fig. 20-23 demonstrates the difference between an *untreated* and a *treated and healed* periodontal unit as it can be seen in a histologic section.

The untreated unit (Fig. 20-23a) is characterized by the presence of an ulcerated pocket epithelium harboring inflammatory cells. A biofilm is present be-

tween the pocket epithelium and the tooth/root surface. Lateral to the pocket epithelium, a well-defined area (ICT) is located. The ICT contains a large number of vessels, numerous inflammatory cells but only small amounts of collagen. When such a diseased periodontal unit is probed, the instrument penetrates the tissue to a level apical to the pocket epithelium.

The treated and healed periodontal unit (Fig. 20-23b) is characterized by the presence of a thin junc-

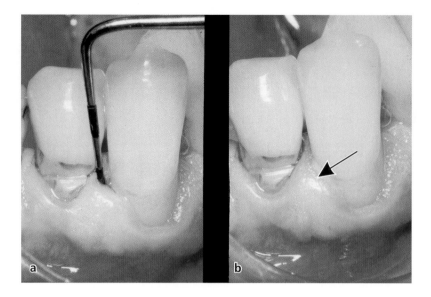

Fig. 20-25. Tooth no. 44 and 43 after cause-related therapy. (a) probing of a 6 mm pocket distal 33 and (b) illustrating bleeding and suppuration after probing (arrow).

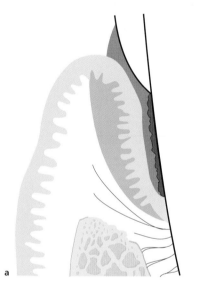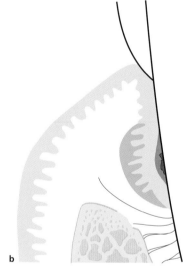

Fig. 20-26. Schematic drawing illustrating a gingival unit before (a) and after (b) cause-related therapy. Clinical signs such as reduced plaque and gingivitis scores and reduced probing depth values as a result of recession indicate healing after the cause-related therapy. Remaining plaque and calculus in the apical part of the root surface of the pocket area (b) may, however, maintain the inflammatory lesion (shadowed area) in the apical part of the pocket. Probing to the bottom of the pocket will result in bleeding.

tional epithelium closely adapted to the tooth/root surface. The connective tissue lateral to the junctional epithelium contains only few inflammatory cells, but has a high content of collagen. In an infrabony defect some new bone and periodontal ligament tissue may have been formed as a result of treatment. When such a healed unit is probed, the instrument will not reach the "before treatment" position but the tip of the probe will stop at a more coronal location. This difference between "before" and "after" treatment probing is regarded *as gain of probing attachment*. The reduced probing depth that is observed after successful treatment is the result of some gingival recession and some gain of probing attachment.

EVALUATION OF THE EFFECT OF THE INITIAL, CAUSE-RELATED THERAPY

The outcome of cause-related therapy must be prop-

erly determined. The clinical examination after this treatment must include data describing (1) resolution of gingivitis, (2) reduction of probing pocket depth and if possible changes in probing attachment levels, (3) reduced tooth mobility, and (4) improvement of the self-performed plaque control.

The finding made at the clinical re-evaluation will form the basis for the selection of measures to be included in the phase of additional treatment. It is usually possible at re-evaluation to classify a patient into one of the following categories:

1. A patient with a proper oral hygiene standard, no gingival or minute inflammation (few sites which bleed on probing), few sites with deepened pockets and several sites which exhibit gain in probing attachment. In such a patient, no further periodontal treatment may be indicated. (Fig. 20-24). The patient should be enrolled in a maintenance program (Supporting Periodontal Therapy, SPT).
2. A patient who has a proper standard of self-performed plaque control, but in whom a number of gingival sites still bleed on probing (Fig. 20-25), and

in whom a significant reduction of the probing depth at such sites has not been achieved. In such a patient, the additional treatment may include surgical means in order to gain access to root surfaces for a more comprehensive debridement (Fig. 20-26).

3. A patient who, despite repeated instruction in self-performed plaque control, has a poor standard of oral hygiene. This patient evidently lacks motivation or ability to exercise proper home care and should not be regarded as a candidate for periodontal surgery. The patient must be made aware of the fact that even though the professional part of the initial therapy has been performed to perfection, reinfection of the periodontal pockets may sooner or later result in recurrence of destructive periodontal disease.

REFERENCES

Axelsson, P. (1993). New ideas and advancing technology in prevention and non-surgical treatment of periodontal disease. *International Dental Journal* **43**(3), 223-238.

Axelsson, P. & Lindhe, J. (1978). Effect of controlled oral hygiene procedures on caries and periodontal disease in adults. *Journal of Clinical Periodontology* **5**, 133-151.

Axelsson, P. & Lindhe, J. (1981). The significance of maintenance care in the treatment of periodontal disease. *Journal of Clinical Periodontology* **8**, 281-294.

Badersten, A., Nilvéus, R. & Egelberg, J. (1981). Effect of nonsurgical periodontal therapy. I. Moderately advanced periodontitis. *Journal of Clinical Periodontology* **8**, 57-72.

Badersten, A., Nilvéus, R. & Egelberg, J. (1984). Effect of nonsurgical periodontal therapy. II. Severely advanced periodontitis. *Journal of Clinical Periodontology* **11**, 63-76.

Baehni, P., Thilo, B., Chapuis, B. & Pernet, D. (1992). Effects of ultrasonic and sonic scalers on dental plaque microflora *in vitro* and *in vivo*. *Journal of Clinical Periodontology* **19**, 455-459.

Bergenholz, G. & Lindhe, J. (1978). Effect of experimentally induced marginal periodontitis and periodontal scaling on the dental pulp. *Journal of Clinical Periodontology* **5**, 59-73.

Björn, A-L., Björn, H. & Grkovic, B. (1969). Marginal fit of restorations and its relation to periodontal bone level. Part I: Metal fillings. *Odontologisk Revy* **20**, 311-322.

Björn, A-L., Björn, H. & Grkovic, B. (1970). Marginal fit of restorations and its relation to periodontal bone level. Part II: Crowns. *Odontologisk Revy* **21**, 337-346.

Björn, H. & Lindhe, J. (1962). The influence of periodontal instruments on the tooth surface. A methodological study. *Odontologisk Revy* **13**, 355-369.

Brayer, W.K., Mellonig, J.T., Dunlap, R.M., Marinak, K.W. & Carson, R.W. (1989). Scaling and root planing effectiveness: the effect of root surface access and operator experience. *Journal of Periodontology* **60**, 67-72.

Caffesse, R.G., Sweemey, P.L. & Smith, B.A. (1986). Scaling and root planing with and without periodontal flap surgery. *Journal of Clinical Periodontology* **13**, 205-210.

Cobb, C.M. (1996). Non-surgical pocket therapy; mechanical. *Annals of Periodontology* **1**, 443-490.

Eaton, K.A., Kieser, J.B. & Davies, R.M. (1985). The removal of root surface deposits. *Journal of Clinical Periodontology* **12**, 141-152.

Hirschfeld, L. & Wasserman, B. (1978). A longterm survey of tooth loss in 600 treated periodontal patients. *Journal of Periodontology* **5**, 225-237.

Jeffcoat, M.K. & Howell, T.H. (1980). Alveolar bone destruction due to overhanging amalgam in periodontal disease. *Journal of Periodontology* **51**, 599-602.

Kocher, T. & Plagmann, H-C. (1997). The diamond-coated sonic scaler tip. Part I. Oscillation pattern of different sonic scaler inserts. *International Journal of Periodontics and Restorative dentistry* **17**, 393-399.

Leon, E.L. & Vogel, R.I. (1987). A comparison of the effectiveness of hand scaling and ultrasonic debridement in furcations as evaluated by differential dark-field microscopy. *Journal of Periodontology* **58**, 86-94.

Lie, T. & Leknes, K.N. (1985). Evaluation of the effect on root surfaces of air turbine scalers and ultrasonic instrumentation. *Journal of Periodontology* **56**, 522-531.

Lindhe, J. (1964). Orthogonal cutting of dentine. *Odontologisk Revy* **15**, suppl. 8.

Loos, B., Kieger, R. & Egelberg, J. (1987). An evaluation of basic periodontal therapy using sonic and ultrasonic scalers. *Journal of Clinical Periodontology* **14**, 29-33.

Lövdal, A., Arno, A., Schei, O. & Waerhaug, J. (1961). Combined effect of subgingival scaling and controlled oral hygiene on the incidence of gingivitis. *Acta Odontologica Scandinavica* **19**, 537-555.

Magnusson, I., Lindhe, J., Yoneyama, T. & Liljenberg, B. (1984). Recolonization of subgingival microbiota following scaling in deep pockets. *Journal of Clinical Periodontology* **11**, 193-207.

Mengel, R., Buns, C., Stelzel, M. & Flores-de-Jacoby, L. (1994). An in vitro study of oscillating instruments for root planing. *Journal of Clinical Periodontology* **21**(8), 513-518.

Morrison, E.C., Ramfjord, S.P. & Hill, R.W. (1980). Short-term effects of initial, non-surgical periodontal treatment (hygiene phase). *Journal of Clinical Periodontology* **7**, 199-211.

Nyman, S., Sarhed, G. Ericsson, I., Gottlow, J. & Karring, T. (1986). The role of "diseased" root cementum for healing following treatment of periodontal disease. *Journal of Clinical periodontology* **13**, 496-503.

Nyman, S., Westfelt, E., Sarhed & Karring, T. (1988). Role of "diseased" root cementum in healing following treatment of periodontal disease. A clinical study. *Journal of Clinical periodontology* **15**, 464-468.

Oberholzer, R. & Rateischak, K.H., (1996). Root planing or root smoothing. *Journal of Clinical Periodontology* **23**, 326-330.

Rabbani, G.M., Ash, M.M. & Caffese, R.G. (1981). The effectiveness of subgingival scaling and root planing in calculus removal. *Journal of Periodontology* **52**, 119-123.

Rodriguez-Ferrer, H.J., Strahan, J.D. & Newman, H.N. (1980). Effect on gingival health of removing overhanging margins of interproximal subgingival amalgam restorations. *Journal of Clinical Periodontology* **7**, 457-462.

Rosenberg, R.M. & Ash, N.N. Jr. (1974). The effect of root roughness on plaque accumulation and gingival inflammation. *Journal of Periodontology* **45**, 146-150.

Rosling, B., Nyman, S. & Lindhe, J. (1976). The effect of systematic plaque control on bone regeneration in infrabony pockets. *Journal of Clinical Periodontology* **3**, 38-53.

Schwarz, F., Sculean, T., Georg, T. & Reich, E. (2001). Periodontal treatment with an Er:Yag Laser compared to scaling and root planing. A controlled clinical study. *Journal of Periodontology* **72**, 361-367.

Sherman, P.R., Hutchens, L.H., Jewson, L.G., Moriarty, J.M., Greco, G.W. & Mc Fall, W.T. (1990). The effectiveness of subgingival scaling and root planing. I. Clinical detection of residual calculus. *Journal of Periodontology* **61**, 3-8.

Suomi, J.D., Greene, J.C., Vermillion, J.R., Doyle, J., Chang, J.J. &

Leatherwood, E.C. (1971). The effect of controlled oral hygiene procedures on the progression of periodontal disease in adults: results after third and final year. *Journal of Periodontology* **42**, 152-60.

Torafson, T., Kiger, R., Selvig, K.A. & Egelberg, J. (1979). Clinical improvement of gingival conditions following ultrasonic versus hand instrumentation of periodontal pockets. *Journal of Clinical Periodontology* **6**, 165-176.

Waerhaug, J. (1956). Effect of rough surfaces upon gingival tissue. *Journal of Dental Research* **35**, 323-325.

Waerhaug, J. (1960). Histologic considerations which govern where the margin of restorations should be located in relation to the gingiva. *Dental Clinics of North America* 167-176.

Waerhaug, J. (1978). Healing of the dento-epithelial junction following subgingival plaque control. As observed on extracted teeth. *Journal of Periodontology* **49**, 119-134.

CHAPTER 21

Mechanical Supragingival Plaque Control

JOSÉ J. ECHEVERRÍA AND MARIANO SANZ

IMPORTANCE OF SUPRAGINGIVAL PLAQUE REMOVAL

The role of plaque in the etiology of gingivitis and periodontitis is well established and has been thoroughly discussed in other chapters in this book. The pivotal study of Löe et al (1965) clearly demonstrated that gingival inflammation consistently follows the build-up of plaque, and that conversely, removal of plaque can reverse this process. This finding not only demonstrated the central role of supragingival plaque in the development of gingivitis, but also that mechanical removal of plaque by oral hygiene practices can reverse these inflammatory changes.

Dental plaque is a biofilm that is not easily removed from the surface of teeth. The biofilms consist of complex communities of bacterial species that reside on tooth surfaces or soft tissues. It has been estimated that between 400 and 1000 species may, at some time, colonize oral biofilms. In these microbial communities, there are observable associations between specific bacteria due in part to synergistic or antagonistic relationships and in part to the nature of the available surfaces for colonization or nutrient availability. Supragingival plaque is exposed to saliva and to the natural self-cleansing mechanisms existing in the oral cavity. However, although such mechanisms may eliminate food debris they do not adequately remove dental plaque. Therefore, the regular use of oral hygiene practices is a requisite for proper supragingival plaque elimination. These practices require not only

the appropriate motivation and instruction of the patient but also the adequate tools.

Although oral hygiene measures can prevent the presence of gingivitis, different studies have shown that regular, non-supervised self-administered oral hygiene alone cannot be considered an effective system of periodontal treatment in the absence of a cause-related periodontal therapy (Loos et al. 1988, Lindhe et al. 1989). However, excellent long-term personal oral hygiene can modify both the quantity and composition of subgingival plaque, without further loss of attachment (Dahlén et al. 1992). Studies on the long-term outcome of periodontal treatment have demonstrated that maintenance of a high status of oral cleanliness prevents or reduces the progression of periodontitis (Axelsson & Lindhe 1978, 1981, Axelsson et al. 1991, Kaldahl et al. 1993). Only minimal loss of periodontal attachment was recorded over the years in these studies in which oral cleanliness was ensured by bi-monthly or tri-monthly debridement and re-instruction of the patients in proper oral hygiene. Accordingly, periodontal diseases can be delayed or even prevented through adequate oral hygiene practices and a periodontal maintenance program. In fact, as part of the healing phase of periodontal surgery, the control of bacterial plaque has a direct beneficial impact on healing and prevention of tissue inflammation (Sanz & Herrera 1998) and on the expected clinical outcomes, especially in cases of periodontal regenerative procedures (Cortellini et al. 1993). Without an adequate level of oral hygiene, periodontal health tends to deteriorate, and further loss of attachment may occur (Lindhe & Nyman 1984). Moreover, adequate and sustained personal oral hygiene is the best

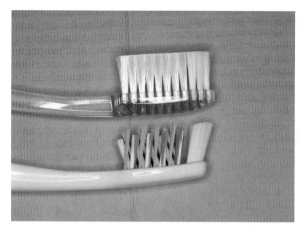

Fig. 21-1. Traditional (top) and novel (bottom) design of manual toothbrushes. The latter shows multiple tufts of bristles angled in different directions.

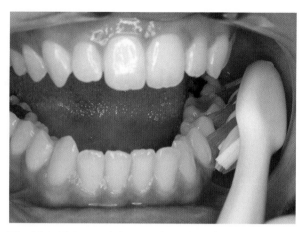

Fig. 21-2. This novel design of toothbrush allows bristles to be easily angled in the direction of approximal tooth surfaces. In this particular case, the Stillman method of toothbrushing is being used.

guarantee of periodontal health. Its impact on periodontal stability could be even superior to that of the frequency of maintenance visits (Westfeld et al. 1983)

SELF-PERFORMED PLAQUE CONTROL

Procedures for control of supragingival plaque are as old as recorded history. Hippocrates (460-377 BC) included in his writings commentaries on the importance of removing deposits from the tooth surfaces. Currently, the use of a toothbrush and fluoridated toothpastes is almost universal. The use of interdental cleaning devices, mouthrinses and other oral hygiene aids is less well documented, but available evidence tends to suggest that only a small percentage of the population use such additional measures on a regular basis (Bakdash 1995). There is an increasing public awareness of the value of good oral health practices. This fact is proven by a recorded increase in both public spending on oral hygiene products (over $3.2 billion a year in the US) and industry spending on consumer related advertising (over $272 million a year in the US) (Bakdash 1995).

Brushing

Although different cleaning devices have been used in different cultures (toothbrushes, chewing sticks, chewing sponges, etc.) the conventional toothbrush is the instrument most frequently used to remove dental plaque. The efficacy of brushing with regard to plaque removal is dictated by three main factors: (1) the design of the brush, (2) the skill of the individual using the brush, and (3) the frequency and duration of use (Frandsen 1986). If tooth brushing is performed using a properly designed brush with an effective technique and for a sufficient duration of time, plaque control

can be achieved on a long-term basis. Unfortunately, it appears that most individuals use a simple horizontal brushing action and the brushing time remains markedly shorter than the one recommended by professionals (2 minutes twice per day) (Cancro & Fischman 1995). Therefore, most individuals carry out ineffective oral hygiene practices.

Toothbrush
At the European Workshop on Mechanical Plaque Control, it was agreed that the features of an ideal manual toothbrush should include (Egelberg & Claffey 1998):

1. Handle size appropriate to user age and dexterity
2. Head size appropriate to the size of the patient's mouth
3. Use of end-rounded nylon or polyester filaments not larger than 0.009 inches in diameter
4. Use of soft bristle configurations as defined by the acceptable international industry standards (ISO)
5. Bristle patterns which enhance plaque removal in the approximal spaces and along the gum line.

There are numerous manual toothbrushes available on the market. However, there is still insufficient evidence that one specific toothbrush design is superior to another (Jepsen 1998). In recent years, industry has introduced novel toothbrush designs with the aim of improving plaque removal in approximal areas (Colgate Total®, Crest Complete®, Jordan Exact®, Oral-B Cross Action®, Reach Advanced Design®, etc.). These designs are based on the premise that the majority of the subjects in any population use a simple horizontal brushing action and regular flat-headed brush, which is ineffective to reach the approximal surfaces in the dentition. Therefore, the design of the brush head has been changed and multiple tufts of bristles angled in different directions are now used (Fig. 21-1). Thus, when the head is located horizontal to the tooth surface, there are bristles angled in the direction of the

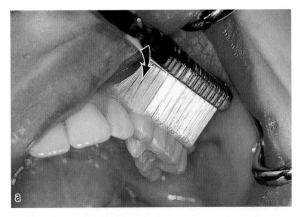

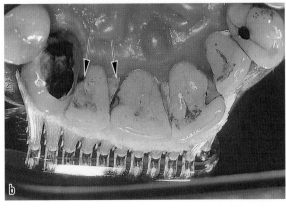

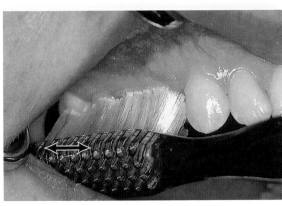

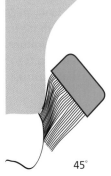

Fig. 21-3. (a) The Charters' method of toothbrushing. The head of the toothbrush is placed in the left maxilla. Note the angulation of the bristles against the buccal tooth surfaces. The bristles are forced into the interproximal areas. (b) The palatal aspect of the incisor region in the maxilla illustrating the penetration of the bristles through the interproximal spaces (arrows).

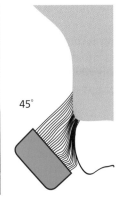

Fig. 21-4. The Bass method of toothbrushing. The head of the toothbrush is in this illustration placed against the buccal surfaces of the posterior teeth of the right maxilla. Note the angulation of the bristles against the tooth and the direction (arrows) of the motion.

approximal tooth surfaces (Fig. 21-2). Toothbrushes with this design may facilitate more plaque removal in such difficult to reach areas when compared with flat-headed brushes (Sharma et al. 1992, 2000, Singh & Deasy 1993, Cronin et al. 2000). The clinical relevance of these enhanced toothbrush designs in plaque removal remains to be proved.

Double and triple-headed toothbrushes have been proposed in order to reach more easily lingual surfaces, especially in molar areas, which are normally the tooth sufaces hardest to reach with a regular toothbrush. Although some studies have indicated that the use of such multiheaded toothbrushes may improve plaque control in lingual areas (Agerholm 1991, Yankell et al. 1996), their use is not widespread. Several studies have also investigated differences in plaque removal between brushes with different handle design. In such studies brushes with long and

contoured handles removed more plaque than brushes with traditional handles. Another point of interest is the stiffness and density of toothbrush bristles. When brushes with hard, soft, multitufted and space-tufted bristles were compared, no significant clinical differences were found with respect to plaque removal. It is worth considering that most of these toothbrush studies are short-term, often involving highly motivated participants such as dental students, who do not represent the general population. Therefore, there is no clear scientific evidence suggesting that one specific toothbrush design is superior in removing plaque; thus, the best toothbrush continues to be the one properly used (Cancro & Fischman 1995, Jepsen 1998).

Methods of toothbrushing

The ideal brushing technique is the one that allows the

complete plaque removal in the least possible time, without causing any lesion to the tissues (Hansen & Gjermo 1971). A variety of toothbrushing methods or techniques have been described in the literature. These methods can be classified into different categories with respect to the pattern of motion that the brush performs:

Horizontal brushing (scrub): is the most widespread technique and despite the efforts of the dental profession to instruct patients to adopt other more convenient brushing techniques, most individuals use such a technique since it is the simplest. The head of the brush is positioned at a 90° angle to the tooth surface and then movement is applied horizontally. The occlusal, lingual and palatal surfaces of the teeth are brushed with the mouth open and the vestibular surfaces are cleaned with the mouth closed.

Vertical brushing (Leonard technique): is similar to the horizontal brushing technique, but the movement is applied in vertical direction using an up-down motion.

Vibratory technique (Stillman technique): the head of the brush is positioned in an oblique direction toward the apex, with the bristles placed partly in the gingival margin and partly on the tooth surface. Light pressure together with a vibratory movement is then applied to the handle, without moving the brush from its original position.

Roll technique (modified Stillman technique): the brush is positioned in a similar manner to the Stillman technique, but after applying a small vibratory pressure, the head of the brush rotates progressively in an occlusal direction.

Charters technique: the head of the brush is positioned in an oblique direction to the tooth surface, with the bristles directed towards the oclusal surface. The brush is then moved back and forth with a rotatory motion. This method is particularly effective in cases with receded interdental papillae, since with this particular situation the brush bristles can penetrate the interdental space (Fig. 21-3).

Bass technique: the head of the brush is positioned in an oblique direction towards the apex, in order to introduce the bristles into the gingival sulcus. The brush is then moved in an anterior-posterior direction using short strokes. This brushing technique is particularly useful in removing plaque not only at the gingival margin, but also subgingivally. A few studies have been carried out on teeth affected with periodontal disease and scheduled for extraction, where the gingival margin was marked with a groove and the depth of subgingival cleaning was measured. These studies showed that using this brushing method the cleaning efficiency could reach a depth of about 0.5 mm subgingivally (Fig. 21-4).

Modified Bass technique: the brush is positioned similarly to the Bass technique, but after applying the small movement in anterior-posterior direction, the head of the brush is rotated applying a movement in occlusal direction. It is a combination of the Bass and the modified Stillman techniques.

Different studies comparing the plaque-removing efficacy of different toothbrushing methods have shown small or no differences. In addition, all methods have been found to be inefficient in removing plaque from approximal tooth surfaces. As early as 1986, Frandsen commented on this issue: "improvement in oral hygiene is not as dependent upon the development of better brushing methods as upon improved performance by the persons using any one of the accepted methods".

Although each of these toothbrushing methods can be effective regarding plaque removal, their implementation must be made according to patient needs. For example, since the Bass method has been associated with gingival recession (O'Leary 1980), it would be hardly indicated in individuals with energetic toothbrushing habits having a thin gingival biotype. On the other hand, since no toothbrushing method has been found to be clearly superior to another, there is no reason to introduce a particular toothbrushing technique in each new periodontal patient. In most cases, small changes in the patient's own method of toothbrushing will suffice, always bearing in mind that more important than the selection of a certain method of toothbrushing is the willingness on the part of the patients to effectively clean their teeth.

Frequency and effectiveness of toothbrushing

How often and how much plaque has to be removed in order to prevent gingivitis and loss of attachment has not been determined. In cross-sectional studies, when the self-reported frequency of tooth cleaning has been related to caries and periodontal disease, the results have been equivocal, suggesting that disease is more related to quality of cleaning than to its frequency (Bjertness 1991). The minimum frequency needed to prevent the development of gingivitis has also been investigated. In one study, dental students and young dental faculty with healthy periodontal condition were assigned to study groups with different cleaning frequencies over periods of 4-6 weeks. The results showed that brushing plus interdental cleaning once daily and also even every second day prevented the development of gingivitis (Lang et al. 1973). Since the majority of individuals, including periodontal patients, are usually not able to remove dental plaque completely as a result of daily brushing, the results from this and other similar studies have limited clinical relevance. From a practical standpoint, it is generally accepted that toothbrushing should be performed at least once a day, particularly in patients showing gingival inflammation, because in such cases the condition of the soft tissues favours plaque accumulation (Ramberg et al. 1994). Thus, in spite of the lack of scientific basis, a general recommendation to brush the teeth twice daily is generally accepted. There are also other reasons that move individuals to

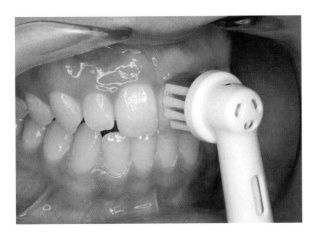

Fig. 21-5. Some electric tootbrushes have better plaque removal efficacy than conventional toothbrushes, especially in approximal tooth surfaces. Here, the electric toothbrush is used according to the scrub (horizontal) method.

clean their teeth more often, e.g. showing whiter teeth and oral freshness. In summary, dental professionals should suggest adequate toothbrushing frequency according to each particular case, always bearing in mind that the quality of the procedure is, by far, more important than its frequency.

Similarly, although numerous studies have monitored the actual time of toothbrushing in controlled clinical settings, what actually occurs in real life may vary. Saxer et al. (1998) demonstrated that regular patients usually believe they spend more time than they actually do. The best estimate of actual mean toothbrushing time for adults seems to range between 30 and 60 seconds.

Toothbrush wear and replacement

The extent of toothbrush wear, such as the amount and degree of splaying and matting, may eventually decrease cleaning efficacy of the brush. Kreifeldt et al (1980) showed that new brushes were more efficient in removing dental plaque than old brushes and, therefore, a recommendation was made that the toothbrush should be replaced when it starts to show signs of matting, regardless of how long it has been in use. However, other studies have shown that the wear status of a toothbrush may not be critical in ensuring optimal plaque control (Daly et al. 1996, Sforza et al. 2000).

Electric toothbrushes

Electric toothbrushes were introduced to the market more than 50 years ago. They were considered an alternative to manual toothbrushes, generally for special categories of individuals such as handicapped patients or just subjects with poor manual dexterity. At the World Workshop in Periodontics in 1966, it was agreed that in subjects not highly motivated to oral health care, as well as in those having difficulty in mastering a suitable handbrush, "the use of an electric brush with its standard movements may result in more frequent and better cleansing of the teeth". However, since then, many modifications of both design and technology of electric toothbrushes have been made. In contrast with old electric toothbrushes, using a combination of horizontal and vertical movements, the new ones apply rotary and oscillating movements

(Fig. 21-5) with bristles moving at high frequencies (Van der Weijden et al. 1998). In several studies, this new generation of electric brushes has proven to have better plaque removal efficacy and gingival inflammation control than conventional brushes, mostly in the approximal tooth surfaces (Egelberg & Claffey 1998). This superiority was clearly demonstrated in a study carried out on extracted teeth (Rapley & Killoy 1994). In the group using a manual toothbrush, 30.6% of the approximal surfaces were plaque-free compared with 53.2% in the group using an electric toothbrush (p < 0.0001). In general, however, the electric toothbrush should not be considered a substitute for a specific interdental cleaning method, such as flossing, but may offer some advantages in terms of an overall approach to oral hygiene, considering that most people do not use any system of interdental cleaning, even in well-developed countries (Johnson & McInnes 1994).

Another interesting aspect of electric toothbrushes is that they are potentially faster than manual toothbrushes at cleaning tooth surfaces. Several studies have focused specifically on the relationship between toothbrushing duration and plaque-removing efficacy (Van der Weijden et al. 1993, 1996). These studies have clearly shown that a manual toothbrush removes less plaque than an electric toothbrush given the same brushing time. It is also worth considering the motivational impulse of most people when they purchase an electric toothbrush. This motivation often disappears after the novelty effect has worn off, and although consumers may find the use of electric toothbrushes initially appealing (Ash 1963), their interest may decrease over time, thus returning to the traditional system of toothbrushing (Baab & Johnson 1989).

In summary, electric toothbrushes can be particularly beneficial in poorly motivated patients, in periodontal patients whose maintenance care shows poor plaque control or in patients demonstrating poor manual dexterity or being physically or mentally handicapped, since in these circumstances they may reduce plaque levels in a significant way.

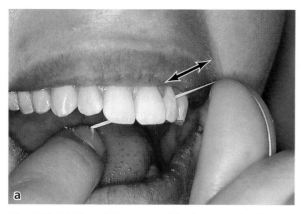
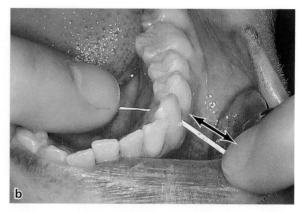

Fig. 21-6. (a) Dental floss is used for interproximal cleaning. The floss is carefully guided through the contact point between teeth 22 and 23. When contact has been established between the floss and the distal/mesial tooth surface, the floss is moved, by minute sawing movements, against the surface for cleaning. (b) The dental floss is guided through the interdental contact point between teeth 34 and 33 by the two *index* fingers.

Interdental cleaning

There is confusion in the literature with respect to the definitions of approximal, interproximal, interdental and proximal sites. Commonly used indices are not suitable for assessing interdental plaque (directly under the contact area), and thereby limit interpretation of interdental plaque removal. The European Workshop on Mechanical Plaque Control in 1999 proposed the following definitions: *Approximal* (proximal) areas are the visible spaces between teeth that are not under the contact area. In health these areas are small, although may increase after periodontal attachment loss. The terms *interproximal* and *interdental* may be used interchangeably and refer to the area under and related to the contact point. The fundamental importance of effective and regular plaque removal with respect to the maintenance of gingival health raises the issue of interdental cleaning and its role in the primary prevention of gingivitis and periodontitis. In patients susceptible to periodontal diseases, the proper removal of plaque in the approximal spaces is of particular importance, since in these areas plaque deposition not only appears earlier but is also more prevalent. However, toothbrushing alone cannot effectively control interproximal plaque, and adjunctive methods of cleaning are required to remove the plaque from these hard-to-reach sites (Lang et al. 1977, Hugoson & Koch 1979). As mentioned previously, a better plaque removal ability in these approximal areas has been demonstrated with electric toothbrushes; however, these devices cannot be considered a substitute for a specific interdental cleaning method, particularly in subjects susceptible to periodontal disease.

Interdental cleaning is important not just to reduce the incidence of gingivitis and caries, but also to improve the overall level of oral hygiene. However, interdental cleaning is not regularly practiced by the majority of the general population, even in the most advanced societies. In spite of this fact, and even considering the high prevalence of gingivitis, the pro-

gression to periodontitis is restricted to a small segment of the population (10-15%). Therefore, the role of interdental cleaning in the primary prevention of periodontitis is still open to discussion. On the other hand, patients treated for periodontitis are more prone to clean interdentally as part on an ongoing supportive therapy.

A number of interdental cleaning methods have been used for this purpose, ranging from floss to the more recently introduced electrically powered cleaning aids. Flossing is the most universally applicable method, since it may be used effectively in nearly all clinical situations. However, not all interdental cleaning devices suit all patients or all types of dentitions. Factors such as the contour and consistency of gingival tissues, the size of the interproximal embrasure, tooth position and alignment and the ability and motivation of the patient should be taken into consideration when recommending an interdental cleaning method. The size of the interdental space to be cleaned is one of the most important determinants regarding the device to be selected. In subjects with normal gingival contours and embrasures, dental floss or tape should be recommended. As recession becomes more pronounced, flossing becomes progressively less effective, mostly when root contours are concave. Then an alternative method (either woodsticks or interdental brushes) should be recommended. A review on interdental cleaning methods (Warren & Chater 1996) has concluded that all conventional devices are effective, but each method should be suited not only to a particular patient but also to a particular situation in the mouth.

Dental floss and tape

Of all the methods for removing interproximal plaque, flossing is the most universal (Fig. 21-6). Clinical studies clearly show that, when toothbrushing is used together with flossing, more plaque is removed from the proximal surfaces than by toothbrushing alone (Reitman et al. 1980, Kinane et al. 1992). Dental floss

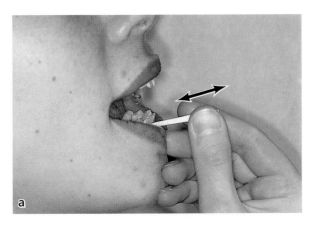
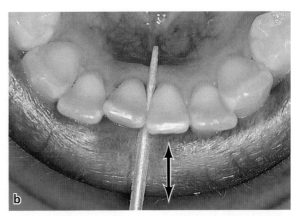
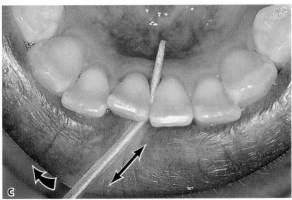
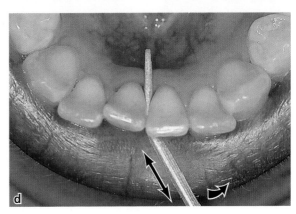

Fig. 21-7. (a) A triangular toothpick is used for interproximal toothcleaning. The toothpick is secured in its position with "finger rest" on the cheek for stabilization of movements. (b) The toothpick is properly inserted in an interproximal site in the mandibular front tooth region. (c,d.) By changing the direction of insertion of the toothpick, the two proximal tooth surfaces are properly cleaned.

and tape – a type of broader dental floss – are most useful where the interdental papillae completely fill the embrasure space. When properly used, flossing effectively removes up to 80% of proximal plaque. Even subgingival plaque can be removed, since dental floss can be introduced 2-3.5 mm below the tip of the papilla (Waerhaug 1981). Several types of floss (waxed, unwaxed) are available; however no clear differences in their effectiveness were demonstrated when comparisons were made. Recently, powered flossing devices have been introduced. In comparison with manual flossing no differences have been found in terms of plaque and gingivitis reduction, although patients preferred flossing with the automated device (Gordon et al. 1996).

The most important factor that influences daily flossing is ease of use. For some individuals it is not easy to perform, especially in posterior areas, since it requires manual dexterity, is time-consuming, there is a risk of frequent shredding when passing through the contact point and there is risk of tissue damage if improperly used. On the other hand, although it is clear that flossing, when properly used, removes plaque in a very efficient manner, there is no evidence that flossing in adult patients with preserved interproximal periodontal tissues should be routinely indicated (Burt & Eklund 1999). Finally, when interproximal spaces are open due to previous loss of

attachment, dental plaque is best removed using other interdental devices.

Toothpicks

Toothpicks are an excellent substitute to dental floss for interproximal open spaces (Bergenholtz et al. 1980). Toothpicks may also be used in primary prevention, since they are easy to use, even in cases of poor manual dexterity, including posterior areas. Probably this is the main reason why toothpicks are more used than dental floss, especially in Scandinavia. However, when used in healthy dentition, they may depress the gingival margin by up to 2 mm, and in long-term use this may cause a permanent loss of the papilla and opening of the embrasure, which may have important esthetic implications in the anterior dentition.

Toothpicks are usually made of soft wood and have a triangular shape, since the rectangular ones do not fit properly in the interdental space at lingual sites (Mandel 1990). These cleaning devices should be clearly recommended in patients with open interdental spaces as secondary prevention for periodontal diseases (Fig. 21-7).

Interproximal brushes

Introduced as an alternative to toothpicks, interproximal brushes are also effective in the removal of plaque from the proximal tooth surfaces (Bergenholtz &

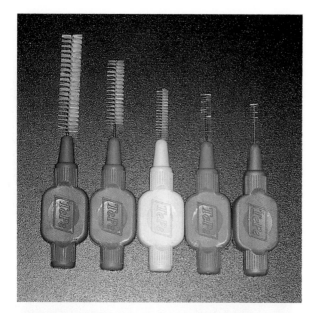

Fig. 21-8. Interproximal brushes of five different sizes.

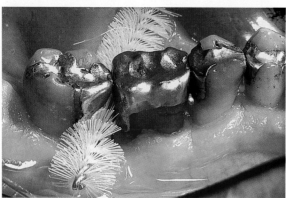

Fig. 21-9. An interproximal brush has been inserted in a wide interdental space between teeth 46 and 47. Lingual view.

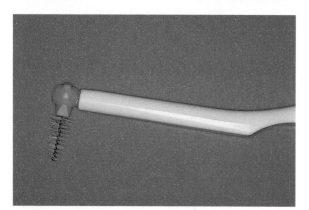

Fig. 21-10. A small interproximal brush inserted in a custom-made handle.

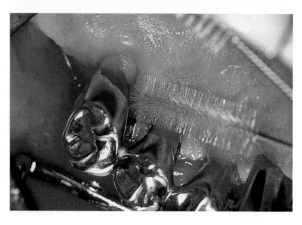

Fig. 21-11. A large interproximal brush inserted in the furcation area of the hemirooted tooth 16.

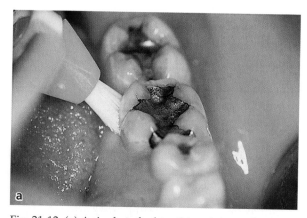
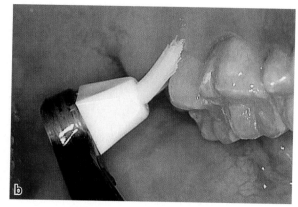

Fig. 21-12. (a) A single-tufted toothbrush is used in tooth regions where cleaning by the use of an ordinary toothbrush is difficult to master. The lingual surfaces of mandibular molars are cleaned. (b) The palatal and distal surfaces of maxillary molars are cleaned by means of a single-tufted toothbrush.

Olsson 1984). Interproximal brushes are manufactured in different sizes and forms (Fig. 21-8) and should be selected to fit, as closely as possible, to the individual interdental space (Fig. 21-9). Small interproximal brushes can be inserted into handles (Fig. 21-10), which may facilitate the cleaning of interproximal areas in the posterior parts of the dentition. The interproximal brush is also the aid of choice when exposed root surfaces have concavities or grooves. In "through and through" furcation defects, the interproximal brush is also the most suitable cleaning device (Fig. 21-11) and can also be used as a carrier of antimicrobial agents, e.g. chlorhexidine. Like toothpicks, interproximal brushes are easy to use, although they may have some drawbacks, including the fact that different types may be needed to fit different open interproximal spaces and when not adequately used, they may elicit dentin hypersensitivity.

Single-tufted brush
A single-tufted brush can be recommended in regions of the dentition not easily reached with other oral hygiene devices, e.g. furcation areas, distal surfaces of the most posterior molars and oral or lingual tooth surfaces with an irregular gingival margin (Fig. 21-12).

Adjunctive aids

Dental irrigation devices
Powered dental irrigation devices are designed to eliminate plaque and soft debris through the mechanical action of a jet stream of water. Dental irrigation with water using a pulsating irrigation device has been shown to reduce adjunctive gingivitis when used to supplement mechanical plaque control (Hugoson 1978, Cutler et al. 2000). Irrigation devices may be used with water or with antimicrobial agents (Lang & Raber 1982); however, results from many studies show that the added effect of the antimicrobials is very limited. Although the use of these devices has shown a limited effect on plaque, gingivitis and periodontitis

when used as an adjunctive to traditional mechanical plaque control, some patients report that their use facilitates the removal of food debris in posterior areas, especially in cases of fixed bridges or orthodontic appliances, when the proper use of interdental cleaning devices is difficult.

Tongue scrapers
The dorsum of the tongue harbors a great number of microorganisms. These bacteria may serve as a source of bacterial dissemination to other parts of the oral cavity, e.g. the tooth surfaces. Therefore, tongue brushing has been advocated as part of daily home oral hygiene together with toothbrushing and flossing, since this might reduce a potential reservoir of microorganisms contributing to plaque formation (Christen & Swanson 1978). However, results of studies on tongue brushing as an adjunct to toothbrushing in order to reduce plaque formation are inconclusive (Badersten et al. 1975).

The bacterial accumulations on the dorsum of the tongue may also be the source of bad breath. In individuals with healthy periodontal conditions, bacterial accumulations in the dorsum of the tongue are the

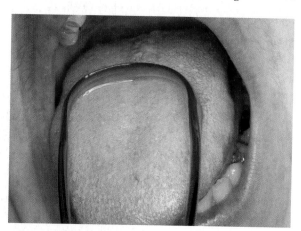

Fig. 21-13. Tongue scrapers facilitate the removal of bacterial accumulations in the dorsum of the tongue, which are a major cause of halitosis.

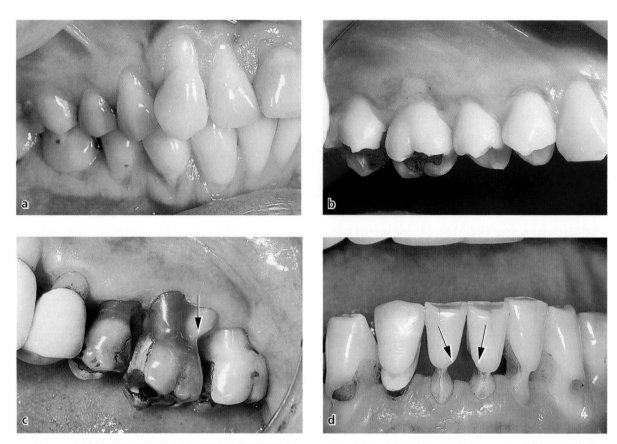

Fig. 21-14. (a) Soft-tissue damage as a result of extensive toothbrushing. Note gingival recession on the buccal gingival surface of tooth 13. (b) Note multiple ulcerations of the buccal gingival margin in the right maxilla. (c,d) Hard-tissue damage (arrows) has resulted after extensive use of interdental brushes.

most important source of the volatile sulfide gases responsible for malodor (van Steenberghe & Rosenberg 1996). Therefore, tongue brushing and the use of tongue scrapers (Fig. 21-13) should be recommended in the management of patients suffering from halitosis (Spielman et al. 1996), often in combination with the use of mouthwashes containing antibacterial agents (Löesche 1999). Tongue brushing has also been advocated as a component of the so called "full mouth disinfection" approach in the treatment of periodontitis, with the aim of reducing possible reservoirs of pathogenic bacteria (Quirynen et al. 2000).

Dentifrices

A dentifrice is usually used in combination with toothbrushing with the purpose of facilitating plaque removal and applying agents to the tooth surfaces for therapeutic or preventive reasons. The addition of abrasives facilitates plaque and stain removal without producing gingival recession/tooth abrasion or altering the remaining components of the dentifrice (Wulknitz 1997). Fluoride is usually omnipresent in commercially available toothpastes. The first successfully formulated fluoride containing dentifrice was reported more than 50 years ago. However, although the fluoride salt form is beneficial in the prevention of caries, it has not routinely exhibited efficacy in controlling gingival inflammation. For this reason, dentifrices have also included in their formulations substances claiming antibacterial, anticalculus and desensitizing properties.

With a few exceptions, chemical agents with antibacterial properties have not been formulated successfully in dentifrices. Chorhexidine, although very effective when used as a mouthrinse, has demonstrated limited efficacy when formulated in dentifrices. Due to its highly cationic formulation, detergents and flavoring agents usually inactivate it. Even when the formulation has shown clinical efficacy, its side effects limit the use of chlorhexidine to specific indications and for short periods of time (Sanz et al. 1994). Triclosan is another antibacterial agent that interferes with plaque growth (Gaffar et al. 1994). As an additional property, triclosan has shown anti-inflammatory effects on gingival tissues (Gaffar et al. 1995). Triclosan can be effectively formulated into a dentifrice, either in combination with a co-polymer or with zinc citrate (Lindhe et al. 1993, Saxton et al. 1993). Results from 6-month clinical studies report a beneficial effect on plaque formation and gingivitis when compared with subjects using a regular fluoridated dentifrice. However, these differences have generally been of limited magnitude. Additionally, the daily use of a triclosan/co-polymer dentifrice may have some effect on the progression of periodontitis (Rosling et al. 1997).

Dentifrices with claims of reducing supragingival calculus formation are also available. The anticalculus formulation usually includes pyrophosphates able to inhibit the nucleation and crystal growth of calcium phosphate minerals. In this way the mineralization of plaque is delayed and it becomes more susceptible to mechanical removal. Calculus reductions from these specially formulated dentifrices when compared to control dentifrices vary between 15% and 50%. Anti-calculus dentifrices do not affect subgingival calculus, since agents applied supragingivally generally do not penetrate subgingivally (Lobene 1986, Sanz & Herrera 1998).

Effects and sequelae of the incorrect use of mechanical plaque removal devices

Since a variety of mechanical and chemical products are used in the self-control of supragingival plaque, the possibility exists that some deleterious effects may appear as a consequence of these oral hygiene practices (Echeverría 1998).

Toothbrushing can cause damage both to soft and hard tissues (Fig. 21-14). Trauma to soft tissues results in gingival erosion and gingival recession. Trauma to hard tissues leads to cervical abrasion of the tooth surface. These lesions have been associated with toothbrush stiffness, the method of brushing and the brushing frequency.

Cervical tooth abrasion has a multifactorial etiology, but in most cases it is the consequence of toothbrushing due to an excessive pressure of the brush and an excessive number of toothbrushing episodes/time. Both situations are probably linked to personality traits (*compulsive brushers*). Tooth wear has also been associated with toothbrush characteristics, especially related to the finishing and hardness of the bristles (Fishman 1997). Abrasives in toothpastes may also play a minor role in the development of tooth abrasion (Axelsson et al. 1997).

In many instances, *tooth abrasion* is found in combination with *gingival recession*. Whereas gingival recession is associated with different etiologic/risk factors, e.g. periodontal inflammation, smoking, gingival biotype or repeated periodontal instrumentation, inadequate toothbrushing is probably the most significant one (Björn et al. 1981). Inadequate toothbrushing that leads to gingival recession has been related to the brushing method (e.g. Bass system), the direction, frequency and magnitude of brushing and also to the characteristics of the toothbrush, such as the end, hardness and material of the bristles. When manual and electric toothbrushes have been compared in terms of their damaging potential, it seems that the latter tend to better preserve both the dental and the gingival tissues (Wilson et al. 1993).

The use of dental floss, interproximal brushes and toothpicks may also induce soft tissue damage. However, in most cases this damage is limited to acute lesions, such as lacerations and gingival erosions (Gillette & Van House 1980).

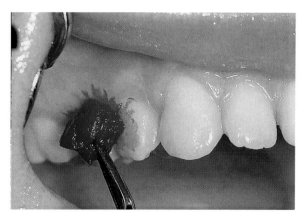

Fig. 21-15. Wafers containing disclosing solutions are often used to identify plaque.

Some substances in toothpastes may induce local or systemic side effects. Chlorhexidine in toothpastes may foster tooth staining (Yates et al. 1993). Pyrophosphates, flavorings and detergents, specially sodium lauryl sulfate, which are present in most commercially available toothpastes, have been implicated as causative factors in certain oral hypersensitive reactions, like aphthous ulcers, stomatitis and cheilitis (Sainio & Kenerva 1995, DeLattre 1999), burning sensation (Kowitz et al 1990) and oral mucosal desquamation (Herlofson & Barkvoll 1996). In these cases, the dental professional should be ready to identify this condition and advise the patient to discontinue the use of the suspected dentifrice.

Importance of instruction and motivation in mechanical plaque control

Mechanical plaque control demands active participation of the individual subject, and therefore the establishment of proper oral home-care habits is a process that to a great extent involves and depends on behavioral changes. When implementing behavioral changes, dental professionals should try to ensure that the patient recognizes his/her oral health status and the role of his/her personal oral hygiene procedures in the prevention of caries and periodontal diseases and they should encourage the patient to take responsibility for his/her own oral health.

Oral hygiene programs, therefore, should include components such as self-assessment, self-examination, self-monitoring and self-instruction. With this purpose, several devices and chemical agents have been used in order to make dental plaque more evident to the patient.

Disclosing agents: Since dental plaque is white, sometimes it cannot easily be identified, particularly if it is not thick enough and/or the observer is not well trained. A disclosing agent is a chemical compound such as erythrosine (Fig. 21-15), fuchsin or a fluorescein-containing dye that stains dental plaque and

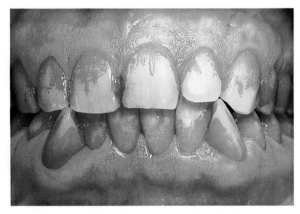

Fig. 21-16. Disclosing agents are used to disclose the presence of dental plaque. Note remaining dental plaque on the buccal tooth surfaces after staining.

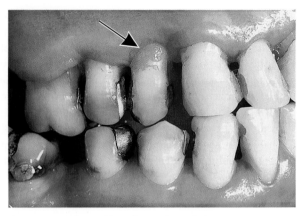

Fig. 21-18. After self-performed toothcleaning, remaining plaque can be identified by the patient following rinsing with a disclosing solution (arrow).

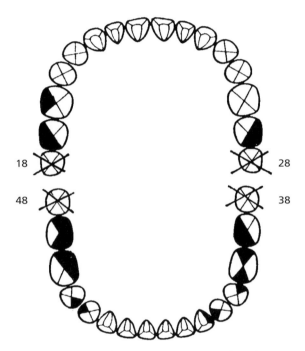

Fig. 21-17. A chart illustrating the teeth and tooth surfaces in the maxilla and mandible. The distribution of tooth surfaces with dental plaque (shadowed areas) is identified. In this case the plaque score is 17%.

thus makes it fully evident to the patient, either with a regular or ultraviolet light. When applied immediately before toothbrushing, the patient can identify the amount of plaque built after the last toothbrushing episode, thus receiving an immediate feedback about his/her cleaning performance. This procedure is useful during the early phase of plaque control. Later on, the disclosing agent should be applied after toothbrushing, which allows the patient to identify those areas needing additional cleaning efforts.

However, knowledge of the role of plaque and the disclosing of plaque in the patient's mouth is usually not enough to establish good oral hygiene habits. Other factors might influence the individual to modify or determine his or her behavior. These factors may be

more or less beyond the control of the dental personnel (such as social and personal factors, environmental setting and past dental experiences) or may lie within the control of dental personnel (such as conditions of treatment, instruction and education of the patient). However, all of them should be considered in the design of an individualized oral hygiene program. The effect of various oral hygiene instruction programs, administered individually or in groups, has been evaluated in a number of clinical studies. These studies have evaluated whether instruction given during one visit only is similar to step-by-step instruction provided during several visits, or whether the use of pamphlets or video-tapes is superior to self-instruction manuals and to personal instruction given by a hygienist or a dentist. Different types and amounts of feedback to the patients using disclosed plaque scores and phase contract demonstrations have also been investigated. These studies have usually reported similar improvements in plaque and gingivitis scores, irrespective of the mode of instruction. However, these results should be interpreted with caution since the subjects participating in these studies were examined at regular intervals, and therefore it is difficult to separate the influx of repeated examinations from the effect of the instructions (Renvert & Glavind 1998).

Rylander and Lindhe (1997) have recommended that oral hygiene instruction be given during a series of visits allowing the possibility of giving the patient immediate feedback and reinforcing the patient in his/her home care activities. The protocol below is based on the one used in several clinical trials by Lindhe & Nyman (1975), Rosling et al. (1976) and Lindhe et al. (1982), where the role of plaque control in preventing and arresting periodontal diseases was clearly proven.

First session

1. Apply a plaque-disclosing solution to the teeth and with aid of a hand mirror, demonstrate to the patient all sites with plaque (Fig. 21-16). The plaque

score should be recorded using a plaque control record (Fig. 21-17).

2. Ask the patient to clean the teeth using his/her traditional technique. With the aid of a hand mirror, demonstrate the results of the toothbrushing to the patient, again identifying all sites with plaque (Fig. 21-18).

3. Without changing the technique, ask the patient to clean the surfaces with plaque. Depending on the plaque remaining after this second toothbrushing, the dentist/dental hygienist should either improve the technique or introduce an alternative system of toothbrushing. In order not to overload the patient with too much information during the first session, the use of adjunctive devices for interproximal brushing can be introduced or improved in the second session.

Second session

1. A few days after the previous session, the disclosing solution is again applied. The results, in terms of plaque deposits, are identified in the mouth, recorded in the plaque control record, and discussed with the patient.

2. The patient is then invited to clean the teeth, according to the directions previously given in the first session, until all staining is removed. In many cases, toothbrushing instructions will need to be reinforced. If necessary, the use of interproximal cleaning aids can now be introduced or improved.

Third and following sessions

1. One or two weeks later the same procedure used in the second session is repeated. However, the efficacy of self-performed plaque control should be evaluated and presented to the patient at each appointment. This repeated instruction, supervision and evaluation aims to reinforce the necessary behavioral changes.

The long-term result of oral hygiene instruction is dependent on these behavioral changes. Therefore patients may fail to comply with given instructions for many reasons, ranging from unwillingness to perform oral self-care, poor understanding, lack of motivation, poor dental health beliefs and unfavourable dental health values, to stressful life events or low socio-economic status. Although the use of behavior modification techniques may offer an advantage over traditional instruction techniques, there is limited research in this area to clarify the relationship between health beliefs and compliance.

In conclusion

- Oral hygiene instruction should be tailored to each individual patient on the bases of his/her personal needs and other factors
- The patient should be involved in the instructional process
- An individualized maintenance program should follow the basic oral hygiene instruction.

References

Agerholm, D.M. (1991). A clinical trial to evaluate plaque removal with a double-headed toothbrush. *British Dental Journal* **170**, 411-413.

Ash, M.M. (1963). A review of the problems and results of studies on manual and power toothbrushes. *Journal of Periodontology* **34**, 375-379.

Axelsson, P. & Lindhe, J. (1978). Effect of controlled oral hygiene procedures on caries and periodontal disease in adults. *Journal of Clinical Periodontology* **5**, 133-151

Axelsson P. & Lindhe, J. (1981). The significance of maintenance care in the treatment of periodontal disease. *Journal of Clinical Periodontology* **8**, 281-294.

Axelsson, P., Lindhe, J. & Nystrom B (1991). On the prevention of caries and periodontal disease, result of a 15 year longitudinal study in adults. *Journal of Clinical Periodontology* **18**, 182-198.

Axelsson, P., Kocher, T. & Vivien, N. (1997). Adverse effects of toothpastes on teeth, gingiva and bucal mucosa. In: Lang, N.P., Karring, T. & Lindhe, J. eds. *Proceedings of the 2nd European Workshop on Periodontology. Chemicals in Periodontics.* London: Quintessence, pp. 259-261.

Baab, D.A. & Johnson, R.H. (1989). The effect of a new electric toothbrush on supra-gingival plaque and gingivitis. *Journal of Periodontology* **60**, 336-341.

Badersten, A., Egelberg, J., Jonsson, G. & Kroneng, M. (1975). Effect of tongue brushing on formation of dental plaque. *Journal of Periodontology* **46**, 625-627.

Bakdash, B. (1995). Current patterns of oral hygiene product use and practices *Periodontology 2000* **8**, 11-14.

Bergenholtz, A., Bjorne, A., Glanzt P-O. & Vikström, B. (1980). The plaque-removing ability of some common interdental aids. An intra-individual study. *Journal of Clinical Periodontology* **1**, 160-165.

Bergenholtz, A. & Olsson, A. (1984). Efficacy of plaque-removal using interdental brushes and waxed dental floss. *Scandinavian Journal of Dental Research* **92**, 198-203.

Bjertness, E. (1991). The importance of bucal hygiene on variation in dental caries in adults. *Acta Odontologica Scandinavica* **49**, 97-102.

Björn, A.L., Andersson, U. & Olsson, A. (1981). Gingival recession in 15-year-old pupils. *Swedish Dental Journal* **5**, 141-146.

Burt, B.A. & Eklund, S.A. (1999). Prevention of periodontal diseases. In: Burt, B.A. & Eklund, S.A., eds. *Dentistry, Dental Practice and the Community*, Philadelphia: W.B. Saunders Company, pp. 358-370.

Cancro, L.P. & Fischman, S.L. (1995). The expected effect on bucal health of dental plaque control through mechanical removal. *Periodontology 2000* **8**, 60-74.

Christen, A. G. & Swanson, B.Z. Jr. (1978). Oral hygiene: a history of tongue scraping and brushing. *Journal of the American Dental Association* **96**, 215-219.

Cortellini, P., Pini Prato, G. & Tonetti, M. (1993). Periodontal regeneration of human intrabony defects. IV. Determinants of healing response. *Journal of Periodontology* **64**, 934-940.

Cronin, M.J., Demblilng, W.Z., Low, M.W., Jacobs, D.M. & Weber, D.A. (2000). A comparative clinical investigation of a novel toothbrush designed to enhance plaque removal efficacy. *American Journal of Dentistry* **13** (spec. issue), 21-26.

Cutler, C.W., Stanford, T.W., Abraham, C, Cederberg, R.A., Boardman, T.J. & Ross, C. (2000). Clinical benefits of bucal irrigation for periodontitis are related to reduction of pro-inflammatory cytokine levels and plaque. *Journal of Clinical Periodontology* **27**, 134-143.

Dahlén, G., Lindhe, J., Sato, K., Hanamura, H. & Okamoto, H. (1992). The effect of supragingival plaque control on the subgingival microbiota in subjects with periodontal disease. *Journal of Clinical Periodontology* **19**, 802-809.

Daly, C. G., Chapple C.C. & Cameron, A.C. (1996). Effect of toothbrush wear on plaque control. *Journal of Clinical Periodontology* **23**, 45-49.

DeLattre, V.F. (1999). Factors contributing to adverse soft tissue reactions due to the use of tartar control toothpastes: report of a case and literature review. *Journal of Periodontology* **70**, 803-807.

Echeverría, J.J. (1998). Managing the use of bucal hygiene aids to prevent damage: Effects and sequelae of the incorrect use of mechanical plaque removal devices. In: Lang, N.P., Attström, R. & Löe, H., eds. *Proceedings of the European Workshop on Mechanical Plaque Control.* London: Quintessence, pp. 268-278.

Egelberg, J. & Claffey, N. (1998). Role of mechanical dental plaque removal in prevention and therapy of caries and periodontal diseases. Consensus Report of Group B. In: Lang, N.P., Attström, R. & Löe, H., eds. *Proceedings of the European Workshop on Mechanical Plaque Control.* London: Quintessence, pp. 169-172.

Fishman, S.L. (1997). The history of oral hygiene products: How far have we come in 6000 years? *Periodontology 2000* **15**, 7-14.

Frandsen, A. (1986). Mechanical oral hygiene practices. In: Löe, H. & Kleinman, D.V., eds. *Dental Plaque Control Measures and Oral Hygiene Practices.* Oxford-Washington DC: IRL Press, pp. 93-116.

Gaffar, A., Afflito, J. & Nabi, N. (1994). Recent advances in plaque, gingivitis, tartar and caries prevention technology. *International Dental Journal* **44** (suppl. 1), 63-70.

Gaffar, A., Scherl, D., Afflito, J. & Coleman, E.J. (1995). The effect of triclosan on mediators of gingival inflammation. *Journal of Clinical Periodontology* **22**, 480-484.

Gillette, W.B. & Van House, R.L. (1980). The effects of improper oral hygiene procedures. *Journal of the American Dental Association* **101**, 476-481.

Gordon, J.M., Frascella, J.A. & Reardon, R.C. (1996). A clinical study of the safety and efficacy of a novel electric interdental cleaning device. *Journal of Clinical Dentistry* **7**, 70-73.

Hansen, F. & Gjermo, P. (1971). The plaque-removal effect of four toothbrushing methods. *Scandinavian Journal of Dental Research* **79**, 502-506.

Herlofson, B.B. & Barkvoll, P. (1996). Oral mucosal desquamation of pre- and post-menopausal women. A comparison of response to sodium lauryl sulphate in toothpastes. *Journal of Clinical Periodontology* **23**, 567-571.

Hugoson, A. (1978). Effect of the Water-Pik® device on plaque accumulation and development of gingivitis. *Journal of Clinical Periodontology* **5**, 95-104.

Hugoson, A. & Koch, G. (1979). Oral health in 1000 individuals aged 3-70 years in the Community of Jönköping, Sweden. *Swedish Dental Journal* **3**, 69-87.

Jepsen, S. (1998). The role of manual toothbrushes in effective plaque control: advantages and limitations. In: Lang, N.P., Attström, R. & Löe, H., eds. *Proceedings of the European Workshop on Mechanical Plaque Control.* London: Quintessence, pp. 121-137.

Johnson, B. D. & McInnes, C. (1994). Clinical evaluation of the efficacy and safety of a new sonic toothbrush. *Journal of Periodontology* **65**, 692-697.

Kaldahl, W.W., Kalkwarf, K.L. & Patil, K.D. (1993). A review of longitudinal studies that compared periodontal therapies. *Journal of Periodontology* **64**, 243-253.

Kinane, D. F., Jenkins, W.M. & Paterson, A.J. (1992). Comparative efficacy of the standard flossing procedure and a new floss applicator in reducing interproximal bleeding. *Journal of Periodontology* **63**, 757-760.

Kowitz, G., Jacobson, J., Meng, Z. & Lucatorto, F. (1990). The effects of tartar-control toothpaste on the oral soft tissues. *Oral Surgery, Oral Medicine and Oral Pathology* **70**, 529-536.

Kreifeldt, J., Hill, P. & Calisti, L. (1980). A systematic study of the plaque-removing efficiency of worn tooth-brushes. *Journal of Dental Research* **59**, 2047-2055.

Lang, N.P., Cumming, B.R. & Löe, H. (1973). Toothbrushing frequency as it relates to plaque development and gingival health. *Journal of Periodontology* **44**, 396-405.

Lang, N.P., Cummings, B.R. & Löe, H.A. (1977). Oral hygiene and gingival helath in Danish dental students and faculty. *Community Dentistry and Oral Epidemiology* **5**, 237-242.

Lang, N.P. & Räber, K. (1982). Use of oral irrigators as vehicle for the application of antimicrobial agents in chemical plaque control. *Journal of Clinical Periodontology* **8**, 177-188.

Lindhe, J. & Nyman, S. (1975). The effect of plaque control and surgical pocket elimination on the establishment and maintenance of periodontal health. A longitudinal study of periodontal therapy in cases of advanced disease. *Journal of Clinical Periodontology* **2**, 67-69.

Lindhe, J & Nyman, S. (1984). Long-term maintenance of patients treated for advanced periodontal disease. *Journal of Clinical Periodontology* **11**, 504-514.

Lindhe, J., Okamoto H., Yoneyama, T., Haffajee, A. & Socransky, S.S. (1989). Longitudinal changes in periodontal disease in untreated subjects. *Journal of Clinical Periodontology* **16**, 662-670.

Lindhe, J., Rosling, B., Socransky, S.S. & Volpe, A.R. (1993). The effect of a triclosan-containing dentifrice on established plaque and gingivitis. *Journal of Clinical Periodontology* **20**, 327-334.

Lindhe, J., Westfeld, E., Nyman, S., Socransky, S.S., Heijl, L. & Bratthall, G. (1982). Healing following surgical/non-surgical treatment of periodontal disease. *Journal of Clinical Periodontology* **9**, 115-128.

Lobene, R.R. (1986). A clinical study of the anticalculus effect of a dentifrice containing soluble pyrophosphate and sodium fluoride. *Clinical Preventive Dentistry* **8**, 5-7.

Löe, H., Theilade, E. & Jensen, S.B. (1965). Experimental gingivitis in man. *Journal of Periodontology* **36**, 177-187.

Löesche, W. (1999). The effects of antimicrobial mouthrinses on oral malodor and their status relative to US Food and Drug Administration regulations. *Quintessence International* **30**, 311-318.

Loos, B., Claffey, N. & Crigger, M. (1988). Effects of oral hygiene measures on clinical and microbiological parameters of periodontal disease. *Journal of Clinical Periodontology* **15**, 211-216.

Mandel, I.D. (1990). Why pick on teeth? *Journal of the American Dental Association* **121**, 129-132.

O'Leary, T.J. (1980). Plaque control. In: Shanley, D., ed. *Efficacy of Treatment Procedures in Periodontology.* Chicago: Quintessence, pp. 41-52.

Quirynen, M., Mongardini, C., De Soete, M., Pauwels, M., Coucke, W., Van Eldere, J. & Van Steenberghe, D (2000). The role of chlorhexidine in the one-stage full-mouth disinfection treatment of patients with advanced adult periodontitis. *Journal of Clinical Periodontology* **27**, 578-589.

Ramberg, P., Lindhe, J. & Eneroth, L. (1994). The influence of gingival inflammation on de novo plaque formation. *Journal of Clinical Periodontology* **21**, 51-56.

Rapley, J.W. & Killoy, W.J. (1994). Subgingival and interproximal plaque removal using a counter-rotational electric toothbrush and a manual toothbrush. *Quintessence International* **25**, 39-42.

Reitman, W.R., Whiteley, R.T. & Robertson, P.B. (1980). Proximal surface cleaning by dental floss. *Clinical Preventive Dentistry* **2**, 7-10.

Renvert, S. & Glavind, L. (1998). Individualized instruction and compliance in oral hygiene practices: recommendations and means of delivery. In: Lang, N.P., Attström, R. & Löe, H., eds.

Proceedings of the European Workshop on Mechanical Plaque Control. London: Quintessence, pp. 300-309.

Rosling, B., Nyman, S. & Lindhe, J. (1976). The effect of systematic plaque control on bone regeneration in infrabony pockets. *Journal of Clinical Periodontology* **3**, 38-53.

Rosling, B., Wannfors, B., Volpe, A.R., Furuichi, Y., Ramberg, P. & Lindhe, J. (1997). The use of a triclosan/copolymer dentifrice may retard the progression of periodontitis. *Journal of Clinical Periodontology* **24**, 873-880.

Rylander, H. & Lindhe, J. (1997). Cause-related periodontal therapy. In: Lindhe, J., Karring, T & Lang N.P., eds. *Clinical Periodontology and Implant Dentistry*. Copenhagen: Munksgaard, pp. 438-447.

Sainio, E.L. & Kanerva, L. (1995). Contact allergens in toothpastes and a review of their hypersensitivity. *Contact Dermatitis* **33**, 100-105.

Sanz, M. & Herrera, D. (1998). Role of oral hygiene during the healing phase of periodontal therapy. In: Lang, N.P., Attström, R. & Löe, H., eds. *Proceedings of the European Workshop on Mechanical Plaque Control*. London: Quintessence, pp. 248-267.

Sanz, M., Vallcorba, N., Fábregues, S., Müller, I. & Herkströter, F. (1994). The effect of a dentifrice containing chlorhexidine and zinc on plaque, gingivitis, calculus and tooth staining. *Journal of Clinical Periodontology* **21**, 431-437.

Saxer U.P., Barbakow, J. & Yankell, S.L. (1998). New studies on estimated and actual toothbrushing times and dentifrice use. *Journal of Clinical Dentistry* **9**, 49-51.

Saxton, C.A., Huntington, E. & Cummings, D. (1993). The effect of dentifrices containing triclosan on the development of gingivitis in a 21-day experimental gingivitis study. *International Dental Journal* **43** (suppl. 1), 423-429.

Sforza, N. M., Rimondini, L., di Menna, F. & Camorali C. (2000). Plaque removal by worn toothbrush. *Journal of Clinical Periodontology* **27**, 212-216.

Sharma, N., Galustians, J., Rustogi, K.N., Volpe, A., Korn, L.R. & Petrone, D. (1992). Comparative plaque removal efficacy of three toothbrushes in two independent clinical studies. *The Journal of Clinical Dentistry* **3** (suppl. C), 13-20.

Sharma, N., Qaqish, J.G., Galustians, J., King, D.W., Low, M.W., Jacobs, D.M. & Weber, D.A. (2000). An advanced toothbrush with improved plaque removal efficacy. *American Journal of Dentistry* **13** (spec. issue), 15-20.

Singh, S.M. & Deasy, M.J. (1993). Clinical plaque removal performance of two manual toothbrushes. *The Journal of Clinical Dentistry* **4** (suppl. D), 13-16.

Spielman, A.I., Bivona, P. & Rifkin, B.R. (1996). Halitosis. A common oral problem. *New York State Dental Journal* **62**, 36-42.

Stillman, P.R. (1932). A philosophy of treatment of periodontal disease. *Dental Digest* **38**, 315-322.

Van der Weijden, G.A., Timmerman, M.F., Danser, M.M. & Van der Velden, U. (1998). The role of electric toothbrushes: advantages and limitations. In: Lang, N.P., Attström, R. & Löe, H., eds. *Proceedings of the European Workshop on Mechanical Plaque Control*. Berlin: Quintessence, pp. 138-155.

Van der Weijden, G.A., Timmerman, M.F., Nijboer, A. & Van der Velden, U. (1993). A comparative study of electric toothbrushes for the effectiveness of plaque removal in relation to toothbrushing duration. *Journal of Clinical Periodontology* **20**, 476-481.

Van der Weijden, G.A., Timmerman, M.F., Snoek, I., Reijerse, E. & Van der Velden, U. (1996). Toothbrushing duration and plaque removal efficacy of electric toothbrushes. *American Journal of Dentistry* **9**, 31-36.

van Steenberghe, D. & Rosenberg, M. (1996). *Bad Breath: A multidisciplinary approach,* 1st edn. Leuven: Leuven University Press.

Waerhaug, J. (1981). Healing of the dento-epithelial junction following the use of dental floss. *Journal of Clinical Periodontology* **8**, 144-150.

Warren, P.R. & Charter, B.V. (1996). An overview of established interdental cleaning methods. *Journal of Clinical Dentistry* **7** (Spec. No. 3), 65-69.

Westfeld, E., Nyman, S., Socransky, S. & Lindhe, J. (1983). Significance of frequency of professional tooth cleaning for healing following periodontal surgery. *Journal of Clinical Periodontology* **10**, 148-156.

Wilson, S., Levine, D., Dequincey, G. & Killoy, W.J. (1993). Effects of two toothbrushes on plaque, gingivitis, gingival abrasion and recession: a 1-year longitudinal study. *Compendium of Dental Education in Dentistry* **16** (suppl. 1), 569-579.

Winkler, S., Garg, A.K., Mekayarajjananonth, T., Bakaeen, L.G. & Khan, E. (1999). Depressed taste and smell in geriatric patients. *Journal of the American Dental Association* **130**, 1759-1765.

Wulknitz, P. (1997). Cleaning power and abrasivity of European toothpastes. *Advances in Dental Research* **11**, 576-579.

Yankell, S.L., Emling, R. C. & Pérez, B. (1996). A six-month clinical evaluation of the Dentrust toothbrush. *Journal of Clinical Dentistry* **7**, 106-109.

Yates, R., Jenkins, S., Newcombe, R., Wade, W., Moran, J. & Addy, M. (1993). A 6-month home usage trial of a 1% chlorhexidine toothpaste (1). Effects on plaque, gingivitis, calculus and toothstaining. *Journal of Clinical Periodontology* **20**, 130-138.

CHAPTER 22

The Use of Antiseptics in Periodontal Therapy

MARTIN ADDY

The concept of chemical supragingival plaque control
   Vehicles for the delivery of chemical agents

Chemical plaque control agents

Chlorhexidine

Clinical uses of chlorhexidine

Evaluation of chemical agents and products

Clinical trial design considerations

THE CONCEPT OF CHEMICAL SUPRAGINGIVAL PLAQUE CONTROL

Epidemiological studies revealed a peculiarly high correlation between supragingival plaque levels and chronic gingivitis (Ash et al. 1964), and clinical research (Löe et al. 1965) led to the proof that plaque was the primary etiological factor in gingival inflammation. Subgingival plaque, derived from supragingival plaque, is also intimately associated with the advancing lesions of chronic periodontal diseases. On the basis that plaque-induced gingivitis always precedes the occurrence and re-occurrence of periodontitis (Lindhe 1986, Löe 1986), the mainstay of primary and secondary prevention of periodontal diseases is the control of supragingival plaque (for reviews see World Workshop on Periodontics 1996a, Hancock 1996). Periodontal diseases appear to occur when a pathogenic microbial plaque acts on a susceptible host (for reviews see Haffajee & Socransky 1994, Moore & Moore 1994, Johnson 1994). What constitutes a pathogenic plaque is much researched and certain microorganisms have been identified as true or putative pathogens, but much remains unknown (for reviews see Zambon 1996, World Workshop on Periodontics 1996b). Susceptibility to periodontal disease is less well understood and, at this time, certainly difficult to predict and quantify although risk factors have been identified (for reviews see Johnson 1994, Porter & Scully 1994). The relationship of plaque levels to pathogenicity and susceptibility are also poorly un-

derstood and therefore, for any one individual, what constitutes a satisfactory level of oral hygiene cannot be stated. This aside, there is evidence which demonstrates that the improving oral hygiene and gingival health, over several decades, noted in developed countries (Hugoson et al. 1998a), has been associated with a decreasing incidence of periodontal disease (Hugoson et al. 1998b). Additionally, long-term follow-up of treated periodontal disease patients has shown that success is dependent on maintaining plaque levels compatible with gingival health (Axelsson & Lindhe 1981a,b). Supragingival plaque control is thus fundamental to the prevention and management of periodontal diseases and, with appropriate advice and instruction from professionals, is primarily the responsibility of the individual (for review see Axelsson 1994).

It could be argued that the heavy reliance on mechanical methods to prevent what are microbially associated diseases is outdated. Very few hygiene practices against microorganisms used by humans on themselves, in the home, at the workplace or in the environment rely on mechanical methods alone and some methods are only chemical. The contrary argument must be that the prevention of periodontitis, through the control of gingivitis, would require the discovery of a safe and effective agent. Also, such a preventive agent would have to be applied from an early age to a large proportion of all populations, many of whom would have low or no susceptibility to periodontal disease (Baelum et al. 1986, for review see Papapanou 1994).

These discussions aside, chemical preventive agents, aimed at the microbial plaque, have been a feature of periodontal disease management for almost a century (for reviews see Fischman 1992, 1997). The consensus appears to be that the use of preventive agents should be as adjuncts and not replacements for the more conventional and accepted effective mechanical methods and only then when these appear partially or totally ineffective alone.

Mechanical tooth cleaning through toothbrushing with toothpaste is arguably the most common and potentially effective form of oral hygiene practiced by peoples in developed countries (for reviews see Frandsen 1986, Jepsen 1998); although, *per capita* in the world, wood sticks are probably more commonly used. Interdental cleaning is a secondary adjunct and would seem particularly important in individuals who, through the presence of disease, can be retrospectively assessed as susceptible (for reviews see Hancock 1996, World Workshop on Periodontics 1996a, Kinane 1998). Unfortunately, it is a fact of life that a significant proportion of all individuals fail to practice a high enough standard of plaque removal such that gingivitis is highly prevalent and from an early age (Lavstedt et al. 1982, Addy et al. 1986). This, presumably, arises either or both from a failure to comply with the recommendation to regularly clean teeth or lack of dexterity with tooth cleaning habits (Frandsen 1986). Certainly, many individuals remove only around half of the plaque from their teeth even when brushing for 2 minutes (de la Rosa 1979). Presumably this occurs because certain tooth surfaces receive little or no attention during the brushing cycle (Rugg-Gunn & MacGregor 1978, MacGregor & Rugg-Gunn 1979). The adjunctive use of chemicals would therefore appear a way of overcoming deficiencies in mechanical tooth cleaning habits as practiced by many individuals. This chapter will consider the past and present status and success of chemical supragingival plaque control to the prevention of gingivitis and thereby periodontitis. Since chemical agents are usually considered as adjuncts, some aspects of mechanical plaque control will be considered.

Supragingival plaque control

The formation of plaque on a tooth surface is a dynamic and ordered process, commencing with the attachment of primary plaque forming bacteria. The attachment of these organisms appears essential for initiating the sequence of attachment of other organisms such that, with time, the mass and complexity of the plaque increases (see Chapter 3). Left undisturbed, supragingival plaque reaches a quantitative and qualitative level of bacterial complexity that is incompatible with gingival health, and gingitivis ensues. Even though, as yet, the microbiology of gingivitis is poorly understood, the sequencing of plaque formation highlights how interventions may prevent the development of gingivitis. Thus, any method of plaque control which prevents plaque achieving the critical point where gingival health deteriorates, will stop gingivitis. Unfortunately, the lack of knowledge of bacterial specificity for gingivitis does not allow targeting of the control of particular organisms except for perhaps the primary plaque formers. Plaque inhibition has, therefore, targeted plaque formation at particular points – bacterial attachment, bacterial proliferation and plaque maturation – and these will be discussed in more detail in the later section "Approaches to chemical supragingival plaque control".

The mainstay of supragingival plaque control has been regular plaque removal using mechanical methods which, in developed countries, means the toothbrush, manual or electric, and in less well developed countries the use of wood or chewing sticks (for review see Frandsen 1986, Hancock 1996). These devices primarily access smooth surface plaque and not interdental deposits. Interdental cleaning devices include wood sticks, floss, tape, interdental brushes and, more recently, electric interdental devices (for review see Egelberg & Claffey 1998, Kinane 1998). Regular mechanical tooth cleaning is directed towards maintaining a level of plaque, quantitatively and/or qualitatively, which is compatible with gingival health, and not rendering the tooth surface bacteria free. Theoretically, mechanical cleaning of teeth could prevent caries but workshops have concluded that tooth brushing *per se* and interdental cleaning as performed by the individual do not prevent caries (for review see Frandsen 1986). Clearly, but outside the scope of this chapter, the toothbrush and other mechanical devices do provide a vehicle whereby anticaries agents, such as fluoride, can be delivered to the tooth surface. Under the conditions of clinical experimentation, tooth cleaning performed once every two days was shown to prevent gingivitis (Lang et al. 1973, Kelner et al. 1974, McNabb et al. 1992). However, the professional recommendation has been to brush twice per day, for which there is evidence of a benefit to gingival health over less frequent cleaning with no additional benefit for more frequent brushing (for review see Frandsen 1986). The duration of brushing is somewhat controversial given that most surveys or studies reveal average brushing time of 60 s or less (Rugg-Gunn & MacGregor 1978, MacGregor & Rugg-Gunn 1979). However, it is worth noting that one study showed less than 50% plaque removal after 2 minutes brushing (de la Rosa 1979). This perhaps highlights that many individuals spend little or no time during the brushing cycle at some tooth surfaces, notably lingually (Rugg-Gunn & MacGregor 1978, MacGregor & Rugg-Gunn 1979).

Oral hygiene, oral hygiene instruction and the effect of supragingival plaque control alone on subgingival plaque and therefore periodontal disease are the subject of other chapters. Nevertheless, some further comments on mechanical tooth cleaning are pertinent in this chapter, particularly in respect of comparative efficacy of devices. The manual toothbrush as known today – man-made filaments in a plastic head – was invented as recently as the 1920s. Evidence for such devices dates back to China approximately 1000 years ago, re-emerging in the 1800s in Europe, but too expensive for common usage (for reviews see Fischman 1992, 1997). Numerous changes in manual toothbrush design have occurred, particularly recently, and similarly numerous claims have been made for the efficacy of individual designs. Despite this, researchers, workshop reports and consensus views have repeatedly concluded that there is no best design of manual toothbrush nor an optimal method of tooth cleaning, the major variable being the person using the brush (for reviews see Frandsen 1986, Jepsen 1998). Limited evidence is available comparing the modern toothbrush with chewing sticks but what is available suggests similar efficacy (Norton & Addy 1989), perhaps not surprisingly if indeed the user is the important factor. Interdental cleaning is considered important particularly for those individuals who are known to be susceptible to or have periodontal disease (for reviews see Egelberg & Claffey 1998, Kinane 1998,). Here again, there is little evidence supporting one interdental cleaning method over another, leaving patients and professionals to hold subjectively related preferences (for review see Kinane 1998). Electric toothbrushes of the counter rotation type found prominence for a short time in the 1960s and 1970s but were unreliable and proven of no greater efficacy over manual brushes, except for handicapped individuals (for reviews see Frandsen 1986). More recently, ranges of new electric brushes have appeared with a variety of head, tuft and filament actions. For these, consensus reports conclude that there is evidence for greater efficacy over manual brushes particularly when professional advice in their use is provided (for reviews see Hancock 1996, World Workshop on Periodontics 1996a, Egelberg & Claffey 1998, van der Weijden et al. 1998). There is, at this time, no evidence for concern over potential harmful effects to hard and soft tissues because the force applied to electric brushes tends to be less than with manual brushes (for review see van der Weijden et al. 1998). Finally, there is no evidence that any one electric toothbrush design is superior and, again, the user appears the major variable.

Chemical supragingival plaque control

History of oral hygiene products

The terminology "oral hygiene products" is recent but there is evidence dating back at least 6000 years that formulations and recipes existed to benefit oral and dental health (for reviews see Fischman 1992, 1997). This includes the written Ebers Papyrus 1500 BC containing recipes for tooth powders and mouthrinses dating back to 4000 BC. A considerable number of formulations can be attributed to the writer and scientist Hippocrates (circa 480 BC). By today's standards the early formulations appear strange if not disgusting but they were not always without logic. Thus, bodies or body parts of animals perceived to have good or continuously erupting teeth were used in the belief that they would impart health and strength to the teeth of the user. Hippocrates, for example, recommended the head of one hare and three whole mice, after taking out the intestines of two, mixing the powder derived from burning the animals with greasy wool, honey, anise seeds, myrrh and white wine. This early toothpaste was to be rubbed on the teeth frequently.

Mouthrinses similarly contained ingredients which would have had some salivary flow stimulating effect, breath odor masking and antimicrobial actions, albeit not necessarily formulated with all these activities in mind. Alcohol-based mouthrinses were particularly popular with the Romans and included white wine and beer. Urine, as a mouthrinse, appeared to be popular with many peoples and over many centuries. There even appeared differences in opinion, with the Cantabri and other peoples of Spain preferring stale urine, whereas Fauchard (1690-1761) in France recommended fresh urine. The Arab nations were purported to prefer children's urine and the Romans to prefer Arab urine. Anecdotal reports suggest the use of urine as a mouthrinse to this very day with individuals rinsing with their own urine. There could, indeed, be benefits to oral health from rinsing with urine by virtue of the urea content; however this has never been evaluated, and given today's Guidelines for Good Clinical Practice, it is unlikely that study protocols would receive ethical approval.

Throughout the centuries, most tooth powders, toothpastes and mouthrinses appear to have been formulated for cosmetic reasons including tooth cleaning and breath freshening rather than the control of dental and periodontal diseases. Many formulations contain very abrasive ingredients and/or acidic substances. However, ingredients with antimicrobial properties were used, perhaps not intentionally, and included arsenic and herbal materials. Herbal extracts are, perhaps, increasingly being used in toothpastes and mouthrinses, although there are little data to support efficacy for gingivitis and none for caries. Many agents prescribed well into the twentieth century, usually as rinses, had the potential to cause local damage to tissues, if not systemic toxicity, including aromatic sulfuric acid, mercuric perchloride, carbolic acid and formaldehyde (Dilling & Hallam 1936).

Perhaps the biggest change to toothpastes came with the chemo-parasitic theory of tooth decay of W. D. Miller in 1890. The theory that organic acids were produced by oral bacteria acting on fermentable carbohydrates in contact with enamel led to both the introduction of agents into toothpaste, which might influence this process, and the production of alkaline products. Shortly after, and at the beginning of the twentieth century, various potassium and sodium salts were added to toothpaste as a therapy for periodontal disease. The first half of the twentieth century saw numerous claims for toothpastes for oral health benefits, including tooth decay and periodontal disease. For example, with the early recognition that periodontal diseases were associated with microorganisms, emetin hydrochloride was added to toothpaste to treat possible amoebic infections. Perhaps with the exception of the well-known essential oil mouthrinse marketed at the end of the nineteenth century, the addition of antimicrobial and/or antiseptic agents to toothpastes and mouthrinses is a relatively recent practice by manufacturers. During the nineteenth and twentieth centuries, toothpastes also became less abrasive. Interestingly, the importance of a level of abrasivity in toothpastes to the prevention of extrinsic dental stain became apparent when one manufacturer marketed a non-abrasive liquid dentifrice. The unsightly brown tooth staining that developed in many users resulted in the early removal of this product from the marketplace. More recently also, standards organizations, notably the British Standards Institute and the International Standards Organization, have laid down standards for toothpastes (BS 5136: 1981, ISO 11609: 1995) and a standard for mouthrinses is under development. Such standards are concerned with safety rather than efficacy. Throughout the ages, and until relatively recently, scientific evaluations of agents and formulations for gum health were not performed and claims for efficacy appear based on anecdotal reports at best. Indeed, given the nature of many ingredients and the recipes recommended in the past for oral hygiene benefits, it is unlikely that efficacy will ever be tested. In the 6000 years history of oral hygiene products, scientific evaluation must be seen as an extremely recent event – an observation which can, of course, be applied to almost all aspects of chemo-prevention and chemo-therapy of human diseases. Indeed, perhaps the first ever, double-blind, randomized cross-over design clinical trial in dentistry was just over 40 years ago (Cooke & Armitage 1960).

Rationale for chemical supragingival plaque control

The epidemiological data and clinical research (Ash et al. 1964, Löe et al. 1965) directly associating plaque with gingivitis perhaps, unfortunately, led to a rather simplistic view that regular tooth cleaning would prevent gingivitis and thereby periodontal disease. Theoretically correct, this concept did not appear to consider the multiplicity of factors which influence the ability of individuals to clean their teeth sufficiently well to prevent disease, not the least of which are those factors which affect individual compliance with advice and dexterity in performing such tasks. The need for research into those psychosocial factors which might influence attitude to and performance in oral hygiene, was stated in a workshop report on plaque control and oral hygiene practices (Frandsen 1986) but appears not to have been heeded to this day. Moreover, and as described in other chapters, epidemiological

data suggest that not all individuals are particularly susceptible to periodontal disease. The most severe disease is accounted for by a relatively small proportion of any population and then by only a proportion of sites in their dentition (Baelum et al. 1986). Even accepting that a considerable proportion of middle-aged adults will have one or more sites in the dentition with moderate periodontal disease, this will be of the chronic adult type and a minimal threat to the longevity of their dentition (Papapanou 1994). This requires that prevention, through improved oral hygiene practices, will be grossly overprescribed.

Given our knowledge concerning the microbiological specificity of periodontal disease and, more particularly, host susceptibility to the disease, it is at present difficult, if not impossible, to predict probable future disease in the, as yet unaffected, host. At present, host susceptibility is described retrospectively in the already diseased individual but, even here, an explanation for their susceptibility, except for a few risk factors, cannot be made. These risk factors include smoking, diabetes and polymorph defects and possible stress (for review see Johnson 1994, Porter & Scully 1994). Genetic markers for periodontal disease have been identified but, at present, appear to be applied retrospectively rather than prospectively (Kornman et al. 1997) and the value to early onset disease has been questioned (Hodge et al. 2001).

One definition of periodontal disease is chronic gingivitis with loss of attachment. This is a particularly useful definition since not only does it describe the pathogenic processes occurring but also alludes to the approach to prevent, treat or prevent re-occurrence of the disease. Therefore prevention through supragingival plaque control still remains the mainstay of controlling gingivitis and therefore the occurrence or re-occurrence of periodontitis (for review see Addy & Adriaens 1998). As alluded to, the importance of oral hygiene to outcome and long-term success of therapy for periodontal disease is hampered by the often ineffectiveness of mechanical cleaning to specific sites using a toothbrush and the limited or lack of use of interdental cleaning by many individuals (for reviews see Axelsson 1994). Despite the encouraging improvements in oral hygiene, gingivitis and, to some extent, periodontitis in developed countries, gingival inflammation is still highly prevalent (for reviews see Baehni & Bourgeois 1998). Taken with the microbial etiology of both gingivitis and periodontitis, this supports the concept of employing agents to control plaque which require minimal compliance and skill in their use. This is the concept that underlies chemical supragingival plaque control, but as with oral hygiene instruction in mechanical methods, it will have to be vastly overprescribed if periodontal disease prevention is to be achieved in susceptible individuals. Chemical supragingival plaque control has thus been the subject of extensive research using scientific methodologies for approximately 40 years. The question to be addressed here is whether a chemical or chemicals

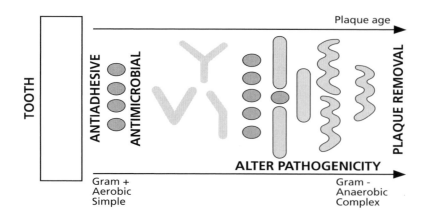

Fig. 22-1. Bacterial succession plaque formation. There is increasing mass and bacterial complexity as plaque bacteria attach and proliferate. Ideal sites of action for chemicals which might influence plaque accumulation are shown. Acknowledgement to Dr William Wade for permission to publish this diagram.

have been discovered and proven efficacious in, firstly, the prevention of gingivitis and, secondly, periodontitis.

Conclusions

- Gingivitis and periodontitis are highly prevalent diseases and prevention of occurrence or re-occurrence is dependent on supragingival plaque control.
- Tooth cleaning is largely influenced by the compliance and dexterity of the individual and little by design features of oral hygiene appliances and aids.
- The concept of chemical plaque control may be justified as a means of overcoming inadequacies of mechanical cleaning.
- Gingivitis is highly prevalent and from a young age in all populations, but the proportion of individuals susceptible to tooth loss through periodontal disease is small.
- Prediction of susceptibility to periodontal disease from an early age is at present impossible.
- Mechanical and/or chemical supragingival plaque control measures for prevention of periodontitis will have to be greatly overprescribed.

Approaches to chemical supragingival plaque control

The well-ordered and dynamic process of plaque formation as described previously and in other chapters, can be summarized in Fig. 22-1. It is apparent that this process can be interrupted, interfered with, reversed or modified at several points and before the plaque mass and/or complexity reaches a level whereby gingival health deteriorates. Mechanical cleaning aims to regularly remove sufficient microorganisms to leave a "healthy plaque" present, which cannot induce gingival inflammation. Chemical agents, on the other hand, could influence plaque quantitatively and qualitatively via a number of processes and these are summarized in Fig. 22-1. The action of the chemicals could fit into four categories:

1. Antiadhesive
2. Antimicrobial
3. Plaque removal
4. Antipathogenic

Antiadhesive agents

Antiadhesive agents would act at the pellicle surface to prevent the initial attachment of the primary plaque forming bacteria. Such antiadhesive agents would probably have to be totally preventive in their effects, acting most effectively on an initially clean tooth surface. Antiadhesive agents do exist and are used in industry, domestically and in the environment. Such chemicals prevent the attachment and development of a variety of biofilms and are usually described as antifouling agents. Unfortunately the chemicals found in such applications are either too toxic for oral use or ineffective against dental bacteria plaques. Nevertheless, the concept of antiadhesives continues to attract research interest (Moran et al. 1995, for review see Wade & Slayne 1997). To date, effective formulations or products with antiadhesive properties are not available to the general public, although the amine alcohol, delmopinol, which appears to interfere with bacterial matrix formation and therefore fits somewhere between the concepts of antiadhesion and plaque removal, has been shown effective against plaque and gingivitis (Collaert et al. 1992, Claydon et al. 1996). Were antiadhesive agents to be discovered, a secondary benefit to extrinsic stain prevention of teeth may be expected (Addy et al. 1995a).

Antimicrobial agents

The bacterial nature of dental plaque, not surprisingly, attracted interest in prevention of plaque formation through the use of antimicrobial agents. Antimicrobial agents could inhibit plaque formation through one of two mechanisms alone or combined. The first would be the inhibition of bacterial proliferation and would be directed, as with antiadhesive agents, at the primary plaque forming bacteria. Antimicrobial agents therefore could exert their effects either at the pellicle coated tooth surface before the primary plaque formers attach or after attachment but before division of these bacteria. This plaque inhibitory effect would be bacteriostatic in type, with the result that the lack of bacterial proliferation would not allow attachment of subsequent bacterial types on to the primary plaque forming bacteria. The second effect could be bacteriocidal whereby the antimicrobial agent destroys all of the microorganisms either attaching or already attached to the tooth surface. Many antimicrobial agents exist which could produce this effect; however, as will be discussed, to be effective in inhibiting plaque, the bacteriocidal effect would have to be absolute or persistent. If not, other bacteria within the oral environment would colonize the tooth surface immediately following the loss of the bacteriocidal effect and the biofilm would be re-established. For the most part biofilms in themselves are fairly resistant to total bacteriocidal effects of antimicrobial agents and, thus far, there does not appear to have been any agent discovered which effectively would sterilize the tooth surface after each application. If such an agent were found it could, of course, have potentially dangerous implications for the oral cavity since it would almost certainly destroy most of the commensal bacteria which normal colonize the oral cavity. This would open up the potential for exogenous microorganisms, with dangerous pathogenic potential, colonizing the oral cavity. In the event, it is probable that antimicrobial agents exert both a bacteriocidal effect followed by a bacteriostatic action of variable duration. The bactertiocidal effect will occur when the antimicrobial agent is at high concentration within the oral cavity and usually this will represent the time when the formulation is actually within the oral cavity. The bacteriocidal effect would be expected to be lost very soon after expectoration.

As will be discussed in respect of chlorhexidine, it is almost certainly the persistence of the bacteriostatic action of antimicrobial agents which accounts for their plaque inhibitory activity. Calculations by Stralfors (1961) indicated that plaque inhibition through a bacteriocidal effect would require the immediate killing of 99.9% of the oral bacteria to effect a plaque inhibitory action of significant duration. Antimicrobial agents for plaque inhibition, to date, are the only agents that have found common usage in oral hygiene products. The efficacy of these agents and products varies at the extremes (for reviews see Addy 1986, Kornman 1986, Mandel 1988, Addy et al. 1994, Addy & Renton-Harper 1996a, Rolla et al. 1997).

Plaque removal agents
The idea of employing a chemical agent which would act in an identical manner to a toothbrush and remove bacteria from the tooth surface, is an attractive proposition. Such an agent, contained in a mouthrinse, would be expected to reach all tooth surfaces and thereby be totally effective. For this reason, the idea of chemical plaque removal agents has attracted the terminology of "the chemical toothbrush". As with antiadhesives, there are potentially agents, such as the hypochlorites, which might be expected to remove bacterial deposits and are commonly employed within the domestic environment. Again, such chemi-

cals would be potentially toxic were they to be applied within the oral cavity. Perhaps the nearest success was with enzymes directed at both the pellicle, e.g. proteases, or the bacterial matrices, e.g. dextranase and mutanase (for review see Kornman 1986). Again, as will be discussed, these enzymes, albeit potentially effective, lacked substantivity within the oral cavity.

Antipathogenic agents
It is theoretically possible that an agent could have an effect on plaque microorganisms, which might inhibit the expression of their pathogenicity without necessarily destroying the microorganisms. In some respects antimicrobial agents, which exert a bacteriostatic effect, achieve such results. At present the understanding of the pathogenesis of gingivitis is so poor that this approach has received no attention. Were our knowledge on the microbial etiology of gingivitis to improve, clearly there exists the possibility of an alternative, but related, approach: the introduction into the oral cavity of organisms which have been modified to remove their pathogenic potential to the gingival tissues. This is not a new concept and was an approach experimented with to replace pathogenic staphylococci within the nasal cavities of surgeons with the idea of reducing the potential for wound infection caused by the operator. At present such an approach within the oral cavity for either gingivitis or caries is perhaps within the realms of science fiction.

Conclusions
- At present most antiplaque agents are antimicrobial and prevent the bacterial proliferation phase of plaque development.
- Plaque formation could be controlled by antiadhesive or plaque removal agents, but these are not, as yet, available or safe for oral use.
- Alteration of bacterial plaque pathogenicity through chemical agents or bacterial modification would require a greater understanding of the bacterial etiology of gingivitis.

Vehicles for the delivery of chemical agents

The carriage of chemical agents into the mouth for supragingival plaque control has involved a small but varied range of vehicles (for reviews see Addy 1994, Cummins 1997).

Toothpaste
By virtue of common usage the ideal vehicle for the carriage of plaque control agents is toothpaste. A number of ingredients go to make up toothpaste and each has a role in either influencing the consistency and stability of the product or its function (for reviews see Davis 1980, Forward et al. 1997).

The major ingredients may be classified under the following headings:

1. *Abrasives*, such as silica, alumina, dicalcium phosphate and calcium carbonate either alone, or more usually today, in combination. Abrasives affect the consistency of the toothpaste and assist in the control of extrinsic dental staining.
2. *Detergents*: the most common detergent used in toothpaste is sodium lauryl sulfate, which imparts the foaming and "feel" properties to the product. Additionally, detergents may help dissolve active ingredients and the anionic detergent sodium lauryl sulfate has both antimicrobial and plaque inhibitory properties (Moran et al. 1988, Jenkins et al. 1991a,b). Certain toothpaste products cannot employ anionic detergents as they interact with cationic substances that may be added to the product such as chlorhexidine or polyvalent metal salts such as strontium used in the treatment of dentine hypersensitivity.
3. *Thickeners*, such as silica and gums.
4. *Sweeteners*, including saccharine.
5. *Humectants*, notably glycerine and sorbitol to prevent drying out of the paste once the tube has been opened.
6. *Flavors*, of which there are many but mint or peppermint are popular in the western world although rarely found in toothpaste in the Indian subcontinent where herbal flavors are more popular.
7. *Actives*, notably fluorides for caries prevention, but for plaque control triclosan and stannous fluoride have been the most common examples.

As stated, the addition of cationic antiseptics to toothpastes is difficult but chlorhexidine has been formulated into toothpastes and shown to be effective (Gjermo & Rolla 1970, 1971, Yates et al. 1993, Sanz et al. 1994).

Mouthrinses

Despite the ideal nature of the toothpaste vehicle, most chemical plaque control agents have been evaluated and later formulated in the mouthrinse vehicle. Mouthrinses vary in their constituents but are usually considerably less complex than toothpastes. They can be simple aqueous solutions, but the need for products, purchased by the general public, to be stable and acceptable in taste usually requires the addition of flavoring, coloring and preservatives such as sodium benzoate. Anionic detergents are included in some products but, again, cannot be formulated with cationic antiseptics such as cetylpyridinium chloride or chlorhexidine (Barkvoll et al. 1989). Ethyl alcohol is commonly used both to stabilize certain active ingredients and to improve the shelf-life of the product. Concerns over the possible association of alcohol intake and pharyngeal cancer have been extended to include alcohol-containing mouthrinses. Whether these concerns are scientifically valid has not been established. Also, since at present there seems little support for the long-term chronic use of mouthrinses for gingival health benefits, when correctly prescribed

the risk from contained alcohol is probably minuscule. This, however, does not obviate the possible risk from self-prescription, the chronic use of mouthrinses, or the ingestion of alcoholic mouthrinses by children. The proportion of alcohol is usually less than 10% but some rinses have in excess of 20% alcohol. Some manufacturers are now producing alcohol-free mouthrinses.

Spray

Spray delivery of chemical plaque control agents has attracted both research interest and the development of products by some manufacturers in some countries. Sprays have the advantage of focusing delivery on the required site. The dose is clearly reduced and for antiseptics such as chlorhexidine this has taste advantages. When correctly applied chlorhexidine sprays were as effective as mouthrinses for plaque inhibition although there was no reduction in staining (Francis et al. 1987a, Kalaga et al. 1989a). Chlorhexidine sprays were found particularly useful for plaque control in physically and mentally handicapped groups (Francis et al. 1987a,b, Kalaga et al. 1989b).

Irrigators

Irrigators were designed to spray water, under pressure, around the teeth. As such they only removed debris, with little effect on plaque deposits (for review see Frandsen 1986). Antiseptics and other chemical plaque control agents, such as chlorhexidine, have been added to the reservoir of such devices. A variety of dilutions of chlorhexidine have been employed to good effect (Lang & Raber 1981).

Chewing gum

Over a relatively short period there has been interest in employing chewing gum to deliver a variety of agents for oral health benefits. Also, there appear to be significant benefits to dental health through the use of sugar-free chewing gum. Unfortunately, chewing gums alone appear to have little in the way of plaque control benefits particularly at sites prone to gingivitis (Addy et al. 1982a). Nonetheless, the vehicle has been used to deliver chemical agents such as chlorhexidine and, when used as an adjunct to normal toothbrushing, reduced plaque and gingivitis levels have been shown (Ainamo & Etemadzadeh 1987, Ainamo et al. 1990, Smith et al. 1996).

Varnishes

Varnishes have been employed to deliver antiseptics including chlorhexidine, but the purpose has been to prevent root caries rather than as a reservoir for plaque control throughout the mouth.

Conclusions

- Many vehicles may be used to deliver antiplaque agents but most information relates to mouthrinses and toothpaste.
- Toothpaste appears the most practical and cost ef-

fective method for chemical plaque control for most individuals.

- In formulating antiplaque agents into toothpaste, potential inactivation by other ingredients must be considered.
- Minority groups, such as the handicapped, may benefit from other delivery systems.

CHEMICAL PLAQUE CONTROL AGENTS

Over a period of more than three decades there has been quite intense interest in the use of chemical agents to control supragingival plaque and thereby gingivitis. The number and variation of chemical agents evaluated are quite large but most have antiseptic or antimicrobial actions and success has been variable at the extreme. It is important to emphasize that formulations based on antimicrobial agents provide a considerably greater preventive than therapeutic action. The most effective agents inhibit the development of plaque and gingivitis but are limited or slow to affect established plaque and gingivitis. Were they available, antiadhesive agents would similarly be expected to provide preventive rather than therapeutic effects, although plaque removal agents would almost certainly provide both preventive and therapeutic actions. Chemical plaque control agents have been the subject of many detailed reviews since 1980 (Hull 1980, Addy 1986, Kornman 1986, Mandel 1988, Gjermo 1989, Addy et al. 1994, Heasman & Seymour 1994, Jackson 1997). Based on knowledge derived from chlorhexidine, the most effective plaque inhibitory agents in the antiseptic or antimicrobial group are those showing persistence of action in the mouth measured in hours. Such persistence of action, sometimes termed substantivity (Kornman 1986), appears dependent on several factors:

1. Adsorption and prolonged retention on oral surfaces including, importantly, pellicle coated teeth.
2. Maintenance of antimicrobial activity once adsorbed primarily through a bacteriostatic action against the primary plaque forming bacteria.
3. Minimal or slow neutralization of antimicrobial activity within the oral environment or slow desorption from surfaces.

The latter concepts will be discussed later under chlorhexidine.

Antimicrobial activity *in vitro* of antiseptics *per se* is not a reliable predictor of plaque inhibitory activity *in vivo* (Gjermo et al. 1970, 1973). Early studies on a number of antiseptics revealed similar antimicrobial profiles but a large variation in clinical effects. For example, compared to chlorhexidine, the cationic quaternary ammonium compound, cetylpyridinium chloride, has a similar antimicrobial profile *in vitro*

(Gjermo et al. 1970, 1973, Roberts & Addy, 1981) and is initially adsorbed in the mouth to a considerably greater extent (Bonesvoll & Gjermo 1978). However, the persistence of action of cetylpyridinium chloride is much shorter than chlorhexidine (Schiott et al. 1970, Roberts & Addy, 1981), and plaque inhibition considerably less (for review see Mandel 1988). Several reasons may explain these apparent anomalies, including poor retention of cetylpyridinium chloride within the oral cavity (Bonesvoll & Gjermo 1978), reduced activity once adsorbed, and neutralization in the oral environment (Moran & Addy 1984), or a combination of these factors. Attempts to improve efficacy of cetylpyridinium chloride can, of course, include increasing the frequency of use, but this is likely to incur compliance problems and side effects (Bonesvoll & Gjermo 1978). Alternatively, substantivity could be improved by combining antimicrobials or using agents to increase the retention of antimicrobials (for review see Cummins 1992, Gaffar et al. 1992). Individual groups of compounds, together with the specific agents within the group, are listed in Table 22-1 and discussed under the following headings.

Antibiotics (for reviews see Addy 1986, Kornman 1986)
Despite evidence for efficacy in preventing caries and gingivitis or resolving gingivitis, the opinion today is that antibiotics should not be used either topically or systemically as preventive agents against these diseases. The risk-to-benefit ratio is high and even antibiotic use in the treatment of adult periodontitis is open to debate (for reviews see Genco 1981, Slots & Rams 1990, Addy & Renton-Harper 1996b and Chapter 23). Thus, antibiotics have their own specific side effects not all of which can be avoided by topical application. Perhaps of greatest importance is the development of bacterial resistance within human populations, for example the methycillin-resistant *Staphylococcus aureas* (MRSA), which causes serious and life-threatening wound infections, particularly within hospitalized patients.

Enzymes (for reviews see Addy 1986)
Enzymes fall into two groups. Those in the first group are not truly antimicrobial agents but more plaque removal agents in that they have the potential to disrupt the early plaque matrix, thereby dislodging bacteria from the tooth surface. In the late 1960s/early 1970s enzymes such as dextranase, mutanase and various proteases were thought to be a major breakthrough in dental plaque control that might prevent the development of both caries and gingivitis. Such agents, unfortunately, had poor substantivity and were not without unpleasant local side effects, notably mucosal erosion. The second group of enzymes employed glucose oxidase and amyloglucosidase to enhance the host defense mechanism. The aim was to catalyse the conversion of endogenous and exogenous thiocyanate to hypothiocyanite via the salivary lactoperoxydase system. The hypothiocyanite produces

Table 22-1. Groups of agents used in the control of dental plaque and/or gingivitis

Group	Examples of agents	Action	Used now/product
Antibiotics	Penicillin Vancomycin Kanamycin Niddamycin Spiromycin	Antimicrobial	No
Enzymes	Protease Lipase Nuclease Dextranase Mutanase *Glucose oxidase *Amyloglucosidase	Plaque removal Antimicrobial	No *Yes Toothpaste
Bisbiguanide antiseptics	*Chlorhexidine Alexidine Octenidine	Antimicrobial	*Yes Mouthrinse Spray Gel Toothpaste Chewing gum Varnish
Quaternary ammonium compounds	*Cetylpyridinium chloride *Benzalconium chloride	Antimicrobial	*Yes Mouthrinse
Phenols & essential oils	*Thymol *Hexylresorcinol *Ecalyptol *Triclosan+	*Antimicrobial +Anti-inflammatory	*Yes Mouthrinse Toothpaste
Natural products	*Sanguinarine	Antimicrobial	*Yes Mouthrinse Toothpaste
Fluorides	(*)Sodium Fluoride (*)Sodium monofluoro- phosphate *Stannous fluoride+ +Amine fluoride	*Antimicrobial ( )minimal +?	+*Yes Toothpaste Mouthrinse +Gel
Metal salts	*Tin+ *Zinc Copper	Antimicrobial	*Yes Toothpaste Mouthrinse +Gel
Oxygenating agents	*Hydrogen peroxide *Sodium peroxyborate *Sodium peroxycarbonate	Antimicrobial ?Plaque removal	*Yes Mouthrinse
Detergents	*Sodium lauryl sulfate	Antimicrobial ?plaque removal	*Yes Toothpaste Mouthrinse
Amine alcohols	Octapinol Delmopinol	Plaque matrix Inhibition	No

inhibitory effects upon oral bacteria, particularly streptococci, to interfere with their metabolism. This approach is a theoretical possibility and the chemical processes can be produced in the laboratory. Tooth-paste products containing the enzymes and thiocyanate were produced but equivocal results for benefits to gingivitis were obtained and there are no convincing long-term studies of efficacy.

Bisbiguanide antiseptics (for review see Addy et al. 1986, 1994, Kornman 1986, Gjermo 1989, Jones 1997)
Chlorhexidine is thus far the most studied and effective antiseptic for plaque inhibition and the prevention of gingivitis. Consequent upon the original publication (Löe & Schiott 1970), chlorhexidine, arguably perhaps, represents the nearest that research has come to identifying a chemical agent that could be used as a replacement for, rather than an adjunct to, mechanical oral hygiene practices. Other bisbiguanides such as alexidine and octenidine have less or similar activity, respectively, to chlorhexidine but bring with them no improvement in local side effects and have less toxicity data available. Chlorhexidine has thus remained the only bisbiguanide used in a number of vehicles and available in commercial products. In view of the importance of this antiseptic within preventive dentistry, a separate section later in the chapter will be devoted to considering its activity and usage in the mouth.

Quaternary ammonium compounds (for review see Mandel 1988)
Benzylconium chloride and, more particularly, cetylpyridinium chloride are the most studied of this family of antiseptics. Cetylpyridinium chloride is used in a wide variety of antiseptic mouthrinse products usually at a concentration of 0.05%. At oral pH these antiseptics are monocationic and adsorb readily and quantitatively, to a greater extent, than chlorhexidine to oral surfaces (Bonesvoll & Gjermo 1978). However, the substantivity of cetylpyridinium chloride appears to be only 3-5 hours (Roberts & Addy 1981) due either to loss of activity once adsorbed or rapid desorption. Cetylpyridinium chloride in mouthrinses has some chemical plaque inhibitory action but evidence for gingivitis benefits is equivocal, particularly when formulations are used alongside toothbrushing with toothpaste. Long-term home use studies, given the large number of rinse products containing this antiseptic, are surprisingly few. Those that are available, with one exception, failed to demonstrate any adjunctive benefits to toothbrushing with toothpaste, of cetylpyridinium chloride mouthrinses. The one exception (Allen et al. 1998) was peculiar in that there was a lack of the expected Hawthorne effect in the control group (see section "Evaluation of chemical agents and products" later in this chapter) and the plaque reduction in the active group, 28%, was as great as seen in chemical plaque inhibition studies. As will be discussed, it is not unusual to find chemicals that provide modest, even moderate, plaque inhibition in no brushing studies but fail to show effects in adjunctive home use studies. This occurs because the range over which to show a benefit of the chemical is limited by the mechanical oral hygiene practices of the study subjects. The efficacy of cetylpyridinium chloride can be increased by doubling the frequency of rinsing to four times per day (Bonsvoll & Gjermo 1978), but this increases local side effects, including tooth staining, and would affect compliance. Mouthrinses combining cetylpyridinium chloride with chlorhexidine are available and compare well with established chlorhexidine products (Quirynen et al. 2001). Whether the cetylpyridinium chloride actually contributed to the activity of the chlorhexidine cannot be assessed. There is limited information on quaternary ammonium compounds in toothpastes and very few products are available.

Phenols and essential oils (for review see Mandel 1988)
Phenols and essential oils have been used in mouthrinses and lozenges for many years. One mouthrinse formulation dates back more than 100 years and although not as efficacious as chlorhexidine, has antiplaque activity supported by a number of short and long-term home use studies. Combining essential oils with cetylpyridinium chloride has been attempted and with promising results from initial studies (Hunter et al. 1994).

The non-ionic antimicrobial triclosan is usually considered to belong to the phenol group and has been widely used over many years in a number of medicated products including antiperspirants and soaps. More recently, it has been formulated into toothpaste and mouthrinses and, for the former, has accumulated an impressive amount of literature, some of which is conflicting. In simple solutions, at relatively high concentrations (0.2%) and dose (20 mg twice per day), triclosan has moderate plaque inhibitory action and antimicrobial substantivity of around 5 hours (Jenkins et al. 1991a,b). The dose response against plaque of triclosan alone is relatively flat (Jenkins et al. 1993) although significantly greater benefits are obtained at 20 mg doses twice daily compared to 10 mg doses. In terms of plaque inhibition, a 0.1% triclosan concentration (10 mg dose twice per day) was considerably less effective than a 0.01% chlorhexidine mouthrinse (1 mg twice per day) (Jenkins et al. 1994).

The activity of triclosan appears to be enhanced by the addition of zinc citrate or the co-polymer, polyvinylmethyl ether maleic acid (for reviews see Cummins 1992, Gaffar et al. 1992). The co-polymer appears to enhance the retention of triclosan whereas the zinc is thought to increase the antimicrobial activity. Only triclosan toothpastes with the co-polymer or zinc citrate have shown antiplaque activity in long-term home use studies (Svatun et al. 1989, Garcia-Gadoy et al. 1990, Stephen et al. 1990, for review see Jackson 1997). Some home use studies showed little or no effect for one or other of the products on plaque alone, gingivitis alone or both (Palomo et al. 1994, Kanchanakamol et al. 1995, Renvert & Birkhed 1995, Binney et al. 1996, Owens et al. 1997). Triclosan toothpastes appear to provide greater gingivitis benefits in some studies than plaque reductions and this could be explained by a possible anti-inflammatory action for this agent (Barkvoll & Rolla 1994).

More recently, long-term studies have suggested

that triclosan-containing toothpaste can reduce the progress of periodontitis, although the effects were so small as to be of questionable clinical relevance (Rosling et al. 1997, Ellwood et al. 1998). Mouthrinses containing triclosan and the co-polymer are available, with some evidence of adjunctive benefits to oral hygiene and gingival health when used alongside normal tooth cleaning (Worthington et al. 1993). This latter study was again interesting with, unusually, no clear Hawthorne effect in the control group. Other studies on the plaque inhibitory properties of a triclosan/co-polymer mouthrinse showed effects significantly less than an essential oil mouthrinse product (Moran et al. 1997).

Natural products (for review see Mandel 1988)
Herb and plant extracts have been used in oral hygiene products for many years if not centuries. Unfortunately, there are few data available and such toothpaste products provide no greater benefits to oral hygiene and gingival health than conventional fluoride toothpaste does (Moran et al. 1991). The plant extract sanguinarine has been used in a number of formulations. Zinc salts are also incorporated, which makes it difficult to evaluate the efficacy of sanguinarine alone. However, even when it is combined with zinc, data are equivocal for benefits (Moran et al. 1988a, 1992a, Quirynen et al. 1990). Some positive findings were reported for the combined use of sanguinarine/zinc toothpaste and mouthrinses (Kopczyk et al. 1991), but the benefit-to-cost ratio must be low. Importantly and very recently, sanguinarine-containing mouthrinses have been shown to increase the likelihood of oral precancerous lesions almost ten-fold even after cessation of mouthrinse use. The manufacturer of the most well-known product has replaced sanguinarine in the mouthrinses with an alternative agent.

Fluorides
The caries preventive benefits for a number of fluoride salts are well established but the fluoride ion has no effect against the development of plaque and gingivitis. Amine fluoride and stannous fluoride provide some plaque inhibitory activity, particularly when combined; however, the effects appear to be derived from the non-fluoride portion of the molecules. A mouthrinse product containing amine fluoride and stannous fluoride is available and there is some evidence from home use studies of efficacy against plaque and gingivitis (Brecx et al. 1990, 1992), but less so than chlorhexidine.

Metal salts (for reviews see Addy et al. 1994, Jackson 1997)
Antimicrobial actions including plaque inhibition by metal salts have been appreciated for many years, with most research interest centered on copper, tin and zinc. Results have been somewhat contradictory but appear dependent on the metal salt used, its concentration and use. Essentially, polyvalent metal salts alone are effective plaque inhibitors at relatively high concentration when taste and toxicity problems may arise. Stannous fluoride is an exception but is difficult to formulate into oral hygiene products because of stability problems, with hydrolysis occurring in the presence of water (Miller et al. 1969). Stable anhydrous gel and toothpaste products are available with evidence of efficacy against plaque and gingivitis (Beiswanger et al. 1995, Perlich et al. 1995). Stannous pyrophosphate at 1% has been added to some stannous fluoride toothpaste to good effect (Svatun et al. 1978). Indeed, it appears that the concentration of available stannous ions is the most significant factor in determining efficacy (Addy et al. 1997). Dental staining, however, occurs with stannous formulations and appears to occur by the same mechanism as for chlorhexidine and other cationic antiseptics, involving interaction with dietary chromogens (for reviews see Addy & Moran 1995, Watts & Addy 2001). Combining metal salts with other antiseptics produces added plaque and gingivitis inhibitory effects, for example zinc and hexetidine (Saxer & Muhlemann 1983) and, as already described, zinc and triclosan. Copper also causes dental staining but is not available in oral hygiene products. Zinc, at low concentration, has no side effects and is used in a number of toothpastes and mouthrinses; however, alone it has little effect on plaque (Addy et al. 1980) except at higher concentrations.

Oxygenating agents (for review see Addy et al. 1994)
Oxygenating agents have been used as disinfectants in various disciplines of dentistry, including endodontics and periodontics. Hydrogen peroxide has been employed for supragingival plaque control and more recently has become important as a bleach in tooth whitening. Similarly, peroxyborate may be used in the treatment of acute ulcerative gingivitis (Wade et al. 1966). Products containing peroxyborate and peroxycarbonate are available in Britain and Europe with evidence of antimicrobial and plaque inhibitory activity (Moran et al. 1995). There are little data from long-term home use studies and such evaluations would seem warranted before conclusions about true antiplaque activity can be drawn.

Detergents
Detergents, such as sodium lauryl sulfate, are common ingredients in toothpaste and mouthrinse products. Besides other qualities and, for that matter, side effects, detergents such as sodium lauryl sulfate have antimicrobial activity (Moran et al. 1988b) and probably provide most of the modest plaque inhibitory action of toothpaste (Addy et al. 1983). Alone, sodium lauryl sulfate was shown to have moderate substantivity measured at between 5 and 7 hours and plaque inhibitory action similar to triclosan (Jenkins et al. 1991a,b). Detergent only formulations are not avail-

able and no long-term evaluations have been performed.

Amine alcohols

This group of compounds does not truly fit into an antimicrobial or antiseptic category; indeed they exhibit minimal effects against microbes. Octopenol was first shown to be effective as an antiplaque agent but was withdrawn for toxicological reasons. Delmopinol followed and at 0.1% and 0.2% in mouthrinses was shown to be effective as a plaque inhibitor and antigingivitis agent in short-term no oral hygiene and long-term home use studies (Collaert et al. 1992, Moran et al. 1992b, Claydon et al. 1996). Side effects include tooth discoloration, transient numbness of the mucosa, particularly the tongue, and burning sensations in the mouth. The mode of action of delmopinol can be debated but, in part, appears to be the inhibition in formation or disruption of the matrix of early plaque forming bacteria. No products are available at present.

Acidified sodium chlorites (for review see Yates et al. 1997)

This agent does not sit well with any particular group listed in Table 22-1; however, depending on the acid chosen and the conditions of the reaction between the acid and the sodium chlorite, a varied and complex range of reaction products can ensue. Under ideal conditions for antimicrobial benefits sodium chlorite is reacted with a protic acid to produce chlorous acid, which then liberates a range of higher oxidant species but contains minimal amounts of chlorine dioxide. These higher oxidant species have a broad range of antimicrobial action against bacteria, fungi, yeast and viruses and products are available in the US within the veterinary and food industry, both as a preventive for mastitis in cows and for the preservation of frozen poultry. Experimental mouthrinses have been tested in short-term plaque regrowth studies and salivary bacterial count investigations (Yates et al. 1997). Surprisingly, given that the acid and sodium chlorite are mixed immediately before rinsing, and that the duration of the chemical reaction would be limited to the rinsing time, three experimental formulations were shown to be as good as chlorhexidine against plaque regrowth and showed the same substantivity as chlorhexidine. Although not tested in longer-term studies, side effects, particularly staining and alternation of taste, would appear unlikely with the acidified sodium chlorite mouthrinses. Unfortunately, the low pH of the formulations would be expected to cause some dental erosion and this has been proven in studies *in situ* (Pontefract et al. 2001). Such erosion, which was found comparable to that of orange juice *in situ*, would tend to obviate the long-term continuous use of such agents. However, acidified sodium chlorite mouthrinses could find application in preventive dentistry

similar to those to be described for chlorhexidine (see the section "Clinical uses of chlorhexidine" later in this chapter). The erosive effects would not, in short to medium-term use, reach clinically significant levels. To date no commercial products are available.

Other antiseptics (for review see Addy 1986)

A number of antiseptics/antimicrobial agents have been studied for plaque inhibition. Most have been found to have little or no effect *in vivo*; a few have been formulated in mouthrinse products including povidone iodine and hexetidine. Povidone iodine at 1% has a substantivity of only 60 minutes (Addy & Wright 1978) and lacks appreciable plaque inhibitory activity (Addy et al. 1977) or action in acute infections such as acute ulcerative gingivitis (Addy & Llewelyn 1978), for which it is recommended. Povidone iodine is largely without side effects but as a rinse has potential to affect thyroid function adversely (Wray et al. 1978). Hexetidine, a saturated pyrimidine, at 0.1% was shown to have limited plaque inhibitory action (Bergenholtz & Hanstrom 1974) and no evidence for antiplaque activity when used as an adjunct for oral hygiene (Chadwick et al. 1991). The action of hexetidine against plaque appears enhanced by zinc salts (Saxer & Muhlemann 1983) but data are derived only from short-term studies. Side effects for hexetidine include tooth staining and mucosal erosion, although both are uncommon (Bergenholtz & Hanstrom 1974). Nevertheless, mucosal erosion is markedly increased in incidence if the concentration is raised to 0.14% (Bergenholtz & Hanstrom 1974). A mouthrinse product containing 0.1% hexetidine is available in some European countries.

Conclusions

- Effective antimicrobial antiplaque agents show prolonged persistence of action in the mouth (substantivity). Chlorhexidine is the most effective antiplaque agent to date. Stannous fluoride and triclosan oral hygiene products are available with proven antiplaque activity. The long established mouthrinse, based on essential oils, has some evidence for adjunctive antiplaque activity.
- The limited information on natural products, for example herbal formulations, is not encouraging and the root extract sanguinarine has been withdrawn because of the potential to cause precancerous oral lesions.
- The amine alcohol, delmopinol, appears effective but products are not available.
- Acidified sodium chlorite appears as effective as chlorhexidine but the acidic nature of the rinse may obviate oral hygiene products ever coming to the marketplace.
- Combinations of agents sometimes provide additive or synergistic action, but with the exception of triclosan, few products are available.

NH   NH
‖   ‖
Cl ⟨ ⟩ NH. C NH. C. NH. (CH₂)₆ NH. C. NH. C. NH ⟨ ⟩ Cl   Fig. 22-2. Chlorhexidine molecule.
        ‖   ‖
        NH   NH

1,6–di (4–chlorophenyldiguanido) hexane

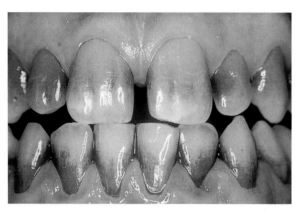

Fig. 22-3. Brown discoloration of the teeth of an individual rinsing twice a day for 3 weeks with a 0.2% chlorhexidine mouthrinse.

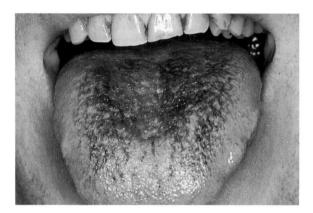

Fig. 22-4. Brown discoloration of the tongue of an individual rinsing twice a day for 2 weeks with a 0.2% chlorhexidine mouthrinse.

CHLORHEXIDINE

Chlorhexidine is available in three forms, the digluconate, acetate and hydrochloride salts. Most studies and most oral formulations and products have used the digluconate salt, which is manufactured as a 20% V/V concentrate. Digluconate and acetate salts are water-soluble but hydrochloride is very sparingly soluble in water. Chlorhexidine was developed in the 1940s by Imperial Chemical Industries, England, and marketed in 1954 as an antiseptic for skin wounds. Later, the antiseptic was more widely used in medicine and surgery including obstetrics, gynecology, urology and presurgical skin preparation for both patient and surgeon. Use in dentistry was initially for presurgical disinfection of the mouth and in endodon-

tics. Plaque inhibition by chlorhexidine was first investigated in 1969 (Schroeder 1969), but the definitive study was performed by Löe and Schiott (1970). This study showed that rinsing for 60 seconds twice per day with 10 ml of a 0.2% (20 mg dose) chlorhexidine gluconate solution in the absence of normal tooth cleaning, inhibited plaque regrowth and the development of gingivitis. Numerous studies followed, such that chlorhexidine was one of the most investigated compounds in dentistry (for review see Jones 1997). Chlorhexidine is a bisbiguanide antiseptic, being a symmetrical molecule consisting of four chlorophenyl rings and two biguanide groups connected by a central hexamethylene bridge (Fig. 22-2). The compound is a strong base and dicationic at pH levels above 3.5, with two positive charges on either side of a hexamethylene bridge (Albert & Sargeant 1962). Indeed, it is the dicationic nature of chlorhexidine, making it extremely interactive with anions, which is relevant to its efficacy, safety, local side effects and difficulties with formulation in products.

Toxicology, safety and side effects

The cationic nature of chlorhexidine minimizes absorption through the skin and mucosa, including from the gastrointestinal tract. Systemic toxicity from topical application or ingestion is therefore not reported, nor is there evidence of teratogenicity in the animal model. Even in intravenous infusion in animals, chlorhexidine is well tolerated and has occurred accidentally in humans without serious consequences. Hypersensitivity reactions including anaphylaxis have been reported in fewer than 10 people in Japan and resulted from the application of non-proprietary chlorhexidine products to sites other than the mouth. There was insufficient information to confirm that the reactions were actually due to chlorhexidine. Neurosensory deafness can occur if chlorhexidine is introduced into the middle ear and the antiseptic should not be placed in the outer ear in case the eardrum is perforated. The antiseptic has a broad antimicrobial action, including a wide range of Gram-positive and Gram-negative bacteria (Wade & Addy 1989). It is also effective against some fungi and yeasts including candida, and some viruses including HBV and HIV. Bacterial resistance has not been reported with long-term, oral use, or evidence of supra-infection by fungi, yeasts or viruses. Long-term oral use resulted in a small shift in the flora towards the less sensitive organisms but this was rapidly reversible at the end of the 2-year study (Schiott et al. 1976).

In oral use as a mouthrinse, chlorhexidine has been reported to have a number of local side effects (Flotra et al. 1971). These side effects are:

1. Brown discoloration of the teeth and some restorative materials and the dorsum of the tongue (to be discussed further) (Figs. 22-3 and 22-4).
2. Taste perturbation where the salt taste appears to be preferentially affected (Lang et al. 1988) to leave food and drinks with a rather bland taste.
3. Oral mucosal erosion (Fig. 22-5). This appears to be an idiosyncratic reaction and concentration dependent. Dilution of the 0.2% formulation to 0.1%, but rinsing with the whole volume to maintain dose, usually alleviates the problem. Erosions are rarely seen with 0.12% rinse products used at 15 ml volume.
4. Unilateral or bilateral parotid swelling (Fig. 22-6). This is an extremely rare occurrence and an explanation is not available.
5. Enhanced supragingival calculus formation. This effect may be due to the precipitation of salivary proteins on to the tooth surface, thereby increasing pellicle thickness and/or precipitation of inorganic salts on to the pellicle layer. Certainly pellicle forming under the influence of chlorhexidine shows an early and highly calcified structure (Leach 1977).

Chlorhexidine also has a bitter taste, which is difficult to mask completely.

Chlorhexidine staining

The mechanisms proposed for chlorhexidine staining can be debated (Eriksen et al. 1985, Addy & Moran 1995, Watts & Addy 2001) but have been proposed as:

1. Degradation of the chlorhexidine molecule to release parachloraniline
2. Catalysis of Maillard reactions
3. Protein denaturation with metal sulfide formation
4. Precipitation of anionic dietary chromogens.

Degradation of chlorhexidine to release parachloraniline appears not to occur on storage or as a result of metabolic processes. Also, alexidine, a related bisbiguanide, does not have parachloraniline groups, yet causes staining identical to that of chlorhexidine (Addy & Roberts 1981). Non-enzymatic browning reactions (Maillard reactions) catalysed by chlorhexidine are a theoretical possibility (Nordbo 1979); however, evidence is indirect, circumstantial or inconclusive (Eriksen et al. 1985). The theory does not consider the fact that other antiseptics and metals such as tin, iron and copper also produce dental staining. Protein denaturation produced by chlorhexidine with the interaction of exposed sulfide radicals with metal

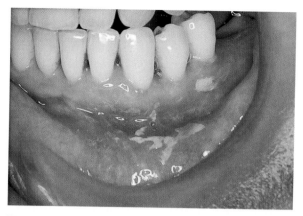

Fig. 22-5. Mucosal erosion occurring following a few days of rinsing twice a day with a 0.2% chlorhexidine mouthrinse.

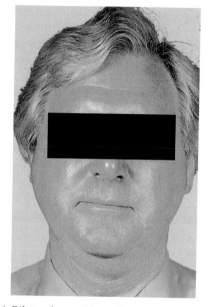

Fig. 22-6. Bilateral parotid swelling following a few days of rinsing with a 0.2% chlorhexidine mouthrinse.

ions is also theoretically possible (Ellingsen et al. 1982, Nordbo et al. 1982) but there is no direct evidence to support this concept. Again, the theory does not take into account similar staining by other antiseptics and metal ions. Laboratory and clinical studies also could not reproduce this process (Addy et al. 1985, Addy & Moran 1985). Precipitation of anionic dietary chromogens by cationic antiseptics, including chlorhexidine and polyvalent metal ions as an explanation for the phenomenon of staining by these substances, is supported by a number of well-controlled laboratory and clinical studies (for reviews see Addy & Moran 1995, Watts & Addy 2001). Thus, the locally bound antiseptics or metal ions on mucosa or teeth can react with polyphenols in dietary substances to produce staining. Beverages such as tea, coffee and red wine are particularly chromogenic, but other foods and beverages will interact to produce various colored stains. These reactions between chlorhexidine and other cationic antiseptics and polyvalent metal ions with chromogenic beverages can be performed within the test tube. Interestingly, most of the precipitates formed between polyvalent metal ions and chromogens have the same color as their sulfide salts. It is for this reason that original theories considered that staining, seen in individuals exposed to these polyvalent metal ions, usually in the workplace, was due to metal sulfide formation. Again, laboratory and clinical experiments have failed to produce such interactions.

It is perhaps the staining side effect that limits long-term use of chlorhexidine in preventive dentistry (Flotra et al. 1971) and occurs with all correctly formulated products including gels, toothpastes and sprays. Indeed, the staining side effect can be used to assess patient compliance in the use and activity of formulations. In the latter case laboratory and clinical studies on staining have revealed a proprietary chlorhexidine mouthrinse product to be inactive (Addy & Wade 1995, Renton-Harper et al. 1995). Interestingly, this particular chlorhexidine product was reformulated in the UK to produce an active formulation (Addy et al. 1991), but the manufacturers maintained the original formulation within France when both laboratory and clinical studies confirmed markedly reduced potential of the product to cause staining in the laboratory, and plaque inhibition in the clinic (Addy & Wade 1995, Renton-Harper et al. 1995).

Mechanism of action

Chlorhexidine is a potent antibacterial substance but this alone does not explain its antiplaque action. The antiseptic binds strongly to bacterial cell membranes. At low concentration this results in increased permeability with leakage of intracellular components including potassium (Hugo & Longworth 1964, 1965). At high concentration, chlorhexidine causes precipitation of bacterial cytoplasm and cell death (Hugo & Longworth 1966). In the mouth chlorhexidine readily adsorbs to surfaces including pellicle-coated teeth. Once adsorbed, and unlike some other antiseptics, chlorhexidine shows a persistent bacteriostatic action lasting in excess of 12 hours (Schiott et al. 1970). Radio-labelled chlorhexidine studies suggest a slow release of the antiseptic from surfaces (Bonesvoll et al. 1974a,b) and this was suggested to produce a prolonged antibacterial milieu in the mouth (Gjermo et al. 1974). However, the methods could not determine the activity of the chlorhexidine, which was almost certainly attached to the salivary proteins and desquamating epithelial cells and therefore unavailable for action. Consistent with the original work and conclusions (Davies et al. 1970), a more recent study and review suggested that plaque inhibition is derived only from the chlorhexidine adsorbed to the tooth surface (Jenkins et al. 1988). It is possible that the molecule attaches to pellicle by one cation leaving the other free to interact with bacteria attempting to colonize the tooth surface. This mechanism would, therefore, be similar to that associated with tooth staining. It would also explain why anionic substances such as sodium lauryl sulfate based toothpastes reduce the plaque inhibition of chlorhexidine if used shortly after rinses with the antiseptic (Barkvoll et al. 1989). Indeed, a more recent study has demonstrated that plaque inhibition by chlorhexidine mouthrinses is reduced if toothpaste is used immediately before or immediately after the rinse (Owens et al. 1997). These inhibitory effects on chlorhexidine activity by substances such as toothpastes can be modeled using the chlorhexidine tea staining method, which shows reduced staining activity by the chlorhexidine solutions resulting from an interaction with toothpaste (Sheen et al. 2001).

Plaque inhibition by chlorhexidine mouthrinses appears to be dose related (Cancro et al. 1973, 1974, Jenkins et al. 1994) such that similar effects to that seen with the more usual 10 ml, 0.2% solution (20 mg) can be achieved with high volumes of low concentration solutions (Cumming & Löe 1973, Lang & Ramseier-Grossman 1981). It is worth noting, however, that not inconsiderable plaque inhibition is obtained with doses as low as 1–5 mg twice daily (Jenkins et al. 1994). Also, and relevant to the probable mechanism of action, topically applying 0.2% solutions of chlorhexidine only to the tooth surface, including by the use of sprays, produces the same level of plaque inhibition as rinsing with the full 20 mg dose (Addy & Moran 1983, Francis et al. 1987a, Jenkins et al. 1988, Kalaga et al. 1989a).

Chlorhexidine products

Chlorhexidine has been formulated into a number of products.

Mouthrinses
Aqueous alcohol solutions of 0.2% chlorhexidine were first made available for mouthrinse products for twice daily use in Europe in the 1970s. A 0.1% mouthrinse product also became available; however questions were raised over the activity of the 0.1% product and in some countries the efficacy of this product is less than would be expected from a 0.1% solution (Jenkins et al. 1989). Later, in the US, a 0.12% mouthrinse was manufactured but to maintain the almost optimum 20 mg doses derived from 10 ml of 0.2% rinses, the product was recommended as a 15 ml rinse (18 mg dose). The studies revealed equal efficacy for 0.2% and 0.12% rinses when used at appropriate similar doses (Segreto et al. 1986).

Gel
A 1% chlorhexidine gel product is available and can be delivered on a toothbrush or in trays. The distribution of the gel by toothbrush around the mouth appears to be poor and preparations must be delivered to all tooth surfaces to be effective (Saxen et al. 1976).

In trays the chlorhexidine gel was found to be particularly effective against plaque and gingivitis in handicapped individuals (Francis et al. 1987a). The acceptability of this tray delivery system to the recipients and the carers was found to be poor (Francis et al. 1987b). More recently, 0.2% and 0.12% chlorhexidine gels have become available.

Sprays

0.1% and 0.2% chlorhexidine in sprays are commercially available in some countries. Studies with the 0.2% spray have revealed that small doses of approximately 1-2 mg delivered to all tooth surfaces produces similar plaque inhibition to a rinse with 0.2% mouthrinses (Kalaga et al. 1989a). Sprays appear particularly useful for the physically and mentally handicapped groups, being well received by individuals and their carers (Francis et al 1987a,b, Kalaga et al. 1989b).

Toothpaste

Chlorhexidine is difficult to formulate into toothpaste for reasons already given and early studies produced variable outcomes for benefits to plaque and gingivitis (Gjermo & Rolla 1970, 1971, Johansen et al. 1972, 1975). More recently, a 1% chlorhexidine toothpaste with and without fluoride was found to be superior to the control product for the prevention of plaque and gingivitis in a 6-month home use study (Yates et al. 1993). However, stain scores were markedly increased as was supragingival calculus formation, and the manufacturer did not produce a commercial product. For a short time a commercial product was available, having been shown to be efficacious for both plaque and gingivitis (Sanz et al. 1994). Although effective, chlorhexidine products based on toothpaste and sprays produce similar tooth staining to mouthrinses and gels; taste disturbance, mucosal erosion and parotid swellings tend to be less or have never been reported.

Varnishes

Chlorhexidine varnishes have been used mainly for prophylaxis against root caries rather than an antiplaque depot for chlorhexidine in the mouth.

Conclusions

- Chlorhexidine to date is the proven most effective antiplaque agent for which commercial products are available to the public.
- Chlorhexidine is free from systemic toxicity in oral use, and microbial resistance and supra-infection do not occur.
- Local side effects are reported which are mainly cosmetic problems.
- The antiplaque action of chlorhexidine appears dependent on prolonged persistence of antimicrobial action in the mouth (substantivity).
- A number of vehicles for delivering chlorhexidine are available, but mouthrinses are most commonly recommended.
- Extrinsic dental staining and perturbation of taste are variably the two side effects of chlorhexidine mouthrinse usage which limit acceptability to users and the long-term employment of this antiseptic in preventive dentistry.

CLINICAL USES OF CHLORHEXIDINE

Despite the excellent plaque inhibitory properties of chlorhexidine, widespread and prolonged use of the agent is limited by local side effects. Moreover, because of the cationic nature of the chlorhexidine and therefore its poor penetrability, the antiseptic is of limited value in the therapy of established oral conditions including gingivitis, and is much more valuable in the preventive mode. A number of clinical uses, some well researched, have been recommended for chlorhexidine (for reviews see Gjermo 1974, Addy 1986, Addy & Renton-Harper 1996a, Addy & Moran 1997).

As an adjunct to oral hygiene and professional prophylaxis

Oral hygiene instruction is a key factor in the treatment plan for patients with periodontal disease and as part of the maintenance program following treatment. Adequate plaque control by periodontal patients is therefore essential to successful treatment and the prevention of re-occurrence of the disease. Chlorhexidine should therefore increase the improvement in gingival health through plaque control, particularly following a professional prophylaxis to remove existing supra and immediately subgingival plaque. There is, however, a potential disadvantage of using such an effective chemical plaque control agent at this stage of the periodontal treatment plan. Thus, following oral hygiene instruction, it is normal, usually by the use of indices, to quantify the improvement in plaque control by patients so instructed and, in particular, the improvement at specific sites which previously had been missed by individual patients. By virtue of the excellent plaque control effects of chlorhexidine, the response to oral hygiene instruction cannot be accurately assessed since the antiseptic will overshadow any deficiencies in mechanical cleaning. Indeed, as the original research demonstrated, patients could maintain close to zero levels of plaque following a professional prophylaxis without using any form of mechanical oral hygiene (Löe & Schiott 1970).

Postoral surgery including periodontal surgery or root planing

Chlorhexidine may be used postoperatively since it offers the advantage of reducing the bacterial load in the oral cavity and preventing plaque formation at a time when mechanical cleaning may be difficult because of discomfort. In periodontal surgery, periodontal dressings have largely been replaced by the use of chlorhexidine preparations, in particular mouthrinses, since healing is improved and discomfort reduced (Newman & Addy 1978, 1982). Regimens vary but chlorhexidine should be used immediately post treatment and for periods of time until the patient can re-institute normal oral hygiene. Depending on the appointment schedule, chlorhexidine could be used throughout the treatment phase and for periods of weeks after completion of the treatment plan. If dressings are used, chlorhexidine is of limited value to the postoperative site since it does not penetrate beneath the periodontal dressings (Pluss et al. 1975). The idea of full mouth disinfection using chlorhexidine both supra and subgingivally has recently been assessed by one group of researchers (Quirynen et al. 1995). In the event, few adjunctive benefits could be shown and it appeared that the more dominant factor was the time over which the non-surgical treatment plan was completed. Thus, root planing performed totally within 24 hours was more effective than root planing completed over more conventional periods of several weeks (for review see Quirynen et al. 2001).

For patients with jaw fixation
Oral hygiene is particularly difficult when jaws are immobilized by such methods as intermaxillary fixation. Chlorhexidine has been shown to reduce markedly the bacterial load, which tends to increase during jaw immobilization, and improve plaque control (Nash & Addy 1979).

For oral hygiene and gingival health benefits in the mentally and physically handicapped
Chlorhexidine has been found particularly useful in institutionalized mentally and physically handicapped groups, improving both oral hygiene and gingival health (Storhaug 1977). Spray delivery of 0.2% solutions was found particularly useful and acceptable to patients and care workers (Francis et al. 1987a,b, Kalaga et al. 1989b).

Medically compromised individuals predisposed to oral infections
A number of medical conditions predispose individuals to oral infections, notably candidiasis. Chlorhexidine is effective as an anticandidal agent but is most useful when combined with specific anticandidal drugs, such as nystatin or amphoteracin B (Simonetti et al. 1988). Indications for chlorhexidine use combined with anticandidal drugs have been for the prevention of oral and systemic infections in the immunocompromised, including those with blood dyscrasias, those receiving chemotherapy and/or radiotherapy and notably bone marrow transplant patients (Ferretti et al. 1987, 1988, Toth et al. 1990). The value of chlorhexidine appears greatest when initiated before oral or systemic complications arise. A chlorhexidine spray was also found to produce symptomatic/psychological oral care benefits in the terminally ill (Jobbins et al. 1992).

High-risk caries patients
Chlorhexidine rinses or gels can reduce considerably the streptococcus mutans counts in individuals who are caries prone. Additionally, and interestingly, chlorhexidine appears synergistic with fluoride and combining chlorhexidine and fluoride rinses appears beneficial to such at risk individuals (Dolles & Gjermo 1980, Lindquist et al. 1989).

Recurrent oral ulceration
Several studies have shown that chlorhexidine mouthrinses and chlorhexidine gels reduce the incidence, duration and severity of recurrent minor aphthous ulceration (Addy et al. 1974, 1976, Hunter & Addy 1987). The mechanism of action is unclear but may relate to a reduction in contamination of ulcers by oral bacteria, thereby reducing the natural history of the ulceration. Regimens have included three times daily use of chlorhexidine products for several weeks. Interestingly, one study showed that triclosan rinses reduce the incidence of recurrent mouth ulcers (Skaare et al. 1996). There have been no controlled studies of chlorhexidine in the management of major aphthous ulceration or other oral erosive or ulcerative conditions, although anecdotally chlorhexidine appears ineffective. Again, this may reflect the low therapeutic potential of this and other antiseptics.

Removal and fixed orthodontic appliance wearers
Plaque control in the early stages of orthodontic appliance therapy may be compromised and chlorhexidine can be prescribed for the first 4-8 weeks. Additionally, chlorhexidine has been shown to reduce the number and severity of traumatic ulcers during the first 4 weeks of fixed orthodontic therapy (Shaw et al. 1984).

In denture stomatitis
Chlorhexidine has been recommended in the treatment of candidal associated infections; however, in practice even applying chlorhexidine gel to the fitting surfaces of denture produces, in many cases, slow and incomplete resolution of the condition. Again, chlorhexidine is less effective in the therapeutic mode and it is more advantageous to treat denture stomatitis with specific anticandidal drugs and then employ chlorhexidine to prevent recurrence. The denture itself can be usefully sterilized from candida by soaking in chlorhexidine solutions (Olsen et al. 1975a,b).

Immediate preoperative chlorhexidine rinsing and irrigation
This technique can be used immediately prior to operative treatment, particularly when ultrasonic polishing or high-speed instruments are to be used. Such preoperative rinsing markedly reduces the bacterial load and contamination of the operative area and operator and staff (Worral et al. 1987). Additionally, in susceptible patients, irrigation of chlorhexidine around the gingival margin reduces the incidence of

THE USE OF ANTISEPTICS IN PERIODONTAL THERAPY • 481

bacteremia (MacFarlane et al. 1984). However, this should be seen only as an adjunct to appropriate systemic antimicrobial prophylaxis.

Subgingival irrigation

Numerous antimicrobial agents have been used as subgingival irrigants in the management and treatment of periodontal diseases (for reviews see Wennstrom 1992, 1997). Alone, irrigation with antimicrobial agents produces effects little different from using saline and of short duration, suggesting that the action is a washing-out effect. Irrigation combined with root planing appears to provide no adjunctive benefits.

Conclusions

- There are a significant number of indications for the use of chlorhexidine in preventive dentistry, most of which rely on the antimicrobial properties of the antiseptic and its duration of action.
- The most valuable chemical plaque control uses of chlorhexidine are in the short to medium term when mechanical tooth cleaning is not possible, difficult or inadequate and during which time local side effects are likely to be minimized.
- Chlorhexidine is more effective as a preventive rather than a therapeutic agent and therefore must be of questionable value as a subgingival adjunct in the treatment of periodontitis (see next chapter).

EVALUATION OF CHEMICAL AGENTS AND PRODUCTS

(for reviews see Addy et al. 1992, Addy 1995, Moss et al. 1995, Addy & Moran 1997)

The number and use of oral hygiene products has grown enormously in recent years and, as an example, hundreds of millions of pounds per year are spent on oral hygiene products in the UK. There can be no doubt that the oral hygiene industries, through their collaboration and research with the dental profession and their promotion of their products have, in no small way, contributed to the improvement in dental health seen in many countries. However, claims for efficacy of oral hygiene products are frequently made and it is essential that these are supported by scientific evidence. Without such evidence the profession and the public may be confused or misled. The dental profession is, however, faced with a large number of oral hygiene products supported by huge quantities of varied promotional literature and media advertising, which makes impossible, in many cases, any valid judgement or assessment of the efficacy or value of individual products to specific patient groups or the public as a whole. Even those with specialized interest, and research experience in specific aspects of oral hygiene product evaluation, must find validation

based on published literature a daunting task. This is made all the more difficult since what constitutes proof of efficacy is not generally agreed even amongst so-called experts. Few countries of the world have central control over what evidence is required before efficacy clearance can be made and there are very few guidelines suggesting requirements for proof of efficacy for oral hygiene products.

The scientific evaluation of dental products, and for that matter preventive and therapeutic agents in medicine as a whole, is a relatively modern concept but today must be the backbone on which to base claims of efficacy. Anecdotal and case reports, uncontrolled studies and data listed as "held on file" by manufacturers, whilst interesting, should not be used as the basis for efficacy claims. Blind, randomized, controlled clinical and laboratory studies must be the methods used today to obtain data on the activity of agents, formulations and products. Terminology and phraseology in product claims also needs to be carefully reviewed and assessed. Perhaps the greatest area for criticism must be the implied claim by the manufacturer and/or the inferences left to be drawn from promotional material by the dental profession or public. A classic scenario for which there is precedence can be stated as follows: A is the cause of B, C reduces A, leaving the inference to be drawn that C can control B. Perhaps nowhere is this more apparent than in the use of agents which are known to control plaque, and therefore it can be implied, without evidence, they must control gingivitis. The now familiar claim would be "this product reduces plaque, the major cause of gum disease". Similarly, creative arithmetic is not infrequently used to give inflated impressions of efficacy. Proportional differences, rather than actual differences, are not infrequently quoted, as are percentages of percentages giving hundreds of percent improvements over another product or control, yet the actual benefit is a fraction of the scoring index used. Finally, "piggy back" claims are not uncommon, when a known active ingredient is formulated into a new product and equivalent efficacy to established products is assumed. In respect of terminology for oral hygiene products, the European Workshop on Periodontology in 1996 defined certain terms (Lang & Newman 1997):

- *Antimicrobial agents*: Chemicals that have a bacteriostatic or bacteriocidal effect *in vitro* that alone cannot be extrapolated to a proven efficacy *in vivo* against plaque.
- *Plaque reducing/inhibitory agents*: Chemicals that have only been shown to reduce the quantity and/or affect quality of plaque, which may or may not be sufficient to influence gingivitis and/or caries.
- *Antiplaque agents*: Chemicals that have an effect on plaque sufficient to benefit gingivitis and/or caries.
- *Antigingivitis agents*: Chemicals which reduce gingival inflammation without necessarily influ-

encing bacterial plaque (includes anti-inflammatory agents).

Thus the fact that antimicrobial agents such as antiseptics kill or inhibit the growth of bacteria does not necessarily mean they will be effective plaque inhibitors (Gjermo et al. 1970). Also, the mere incorporation of a known antiplaque agent into a formulation is not a guarantee of efficacy because inactivation by other ingredients may occur.

This section looks at methods that have been used to test oral hygiene products both in the laboratory and the clinic. No one protocol can provide all the answers, and research and development of agents into products is a step-by-step process, hopefully culminating in a body of evidence proving efficacy, beyond doubt, of a final product. Methods *in vitro* and *in vivo* will be summarized but animal testing will not be discussed except to acknowledge that the use of animals is still necessary in drug development, in understanding the mode of action of drugs and, particularly, in evaluating safety from a toxicological point of view. However, the evaluation of oral hygiene products on animals, particularly for efficacy, must be questioned on a number of scientific and moral grounds.

Most laboratory and clinical methods have been developed to test antimicrobial agents but methodologies are available, or present ones could be modified, to study potential antiadhesive and plaque removal chemicals. (For reviews see Addy et al. 1992, 1995a,b, Addy & Moran, 1997.)

Studies in vitro

Bacterial tests
Antimicrobial tests including minimum inhibitory concentration (MIC), minimum bactericidal concentration (MBC) and kill curves can be determined. These tests indicate the antibacterial activity and antimicrobial spectrum of agents and formulations against a range of oral bacteria. Continuous culture techniques can also be used but they may not provide more meaningful data. It is likely that, with technological advances, laboratory models to accurately replicate the plaque biofilm will become available to test chemical plaque control agents. At present, antimicrobial tests *in vitro* primarily only indicate activity, or lack of it, and they are very poor predictors *per se* of plaque action *in vivo*. This is because, so far, methods do not provide particularly reliable information on the substantivity of the antimicrobial agent. Nevertheless, antimicrobial tests are valuable for a variety of reasons. With few exceptions, agents without activity *in vitro* will not provide activity *in vivo*. The additive or negative effects of ingredient mixtures can be determined. The availability of active ingredients incorporated in the product can be assessed. The adverse influence of the oral environment can be modeled; for example, the influence of saliva or proteins on the antibacterial activity of agents can be tested.

Uptake measurements
One aspect of substantivity is adsorption of antimicrobials and other potential plaque inhibitory agents on to surfaces. This can be quantified using a variety of substrates such as hydroxyapatite, dentine, enamel, acrylic and other polymers. The influence of other factors or agents on the uptake of a particular agent can also be assessed. Such data are of interest but must be interpreted with caution since they only measure uptake, not activity once adsorbed. Nevertheless, desorbtion of an agent from such surfaces can be measured by a variety of analytical techniques thereby giving some indication of both the adsorption profile and the subsequent substantivity of the agent to the substrate surface.

Other methods
Activity or availability of an ingredient in a formulation can be measured or assessed. Methods include chemical analyses; however, some methods chemically extract the agent from the formulation in its entirety and therefore do not necessarily demonstrate that it is freely available and active within the formulation. For the cationic antiseptics and polyvalent metal salts, their potential to bind dietary chromogens from beverages such as tea can be used to assess the possibility that they may cause staining *in vivo*. More usefully, the test method can be employed to determine and compare the availability of the same ingredient in different formulations. Such methods have shown considerable differences in availability of chlorhexidine and cetylpyridinium chloride in apparently similar mouthrinses (Addy et al. 1995b). Moreover, how other oral hygiene products might interfere with the activity of chemical plaque control agents, such as toothpaste with chlorhexidine and cetylpyridinium chloride, has given surprisingly accurate predictions of clinical outcome (Owens et al. 1997, Sheen et al. 2001, 2002). Again, these methods give little indication of substantivity and therefore the staining method *in vitro* cannot be used to compare different agents for propensities to cause staining *in vivo*. For example, a 0.05% cetylpyridinium chloride mouthrinse produces comparable tea staining on a substrate surface to a 0.2% chlorhexidine mouthrinse, yet clinically the amount of staining reported for chlorhexidine is considerably greater than that for cetylpyridinium chloride and this can be explained by the fact that the substantivity of the former is greater than the latter.

Study methods *in vivo*
A considerable number of protocols have been developed to evaluate potential antiplaque agents and products. Ideally, because of the number of ingredients and more particularly formulations, a step-by-step pyramid approach is taken. Thus initially, study

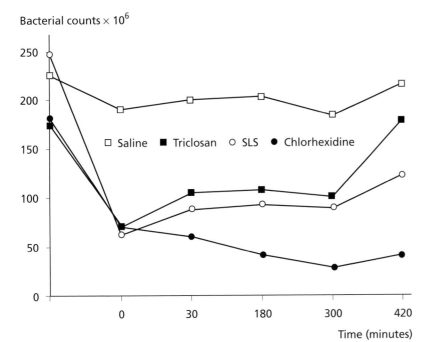

Bacterial counts × 10^6

□ Saline   ■ Triclosan   ○ SLS   ● Chlorhexidine

Time (minutes)

Fig. 22-7. Salivary bacterial counts over time following mouthrinsing with chlorhexidine, saline, sodium lauryl sulfate and triclosan. Following a single rinse with chlorhexidine, sodium lauryl sulfate and triclosan there is an immediate large reduction in bacterial counts. This continues and persists to the 420-minute endpoint of the study for chlorhexidine (positive control) with a tendency for counts to revert towards baseline for triclosan and sodium lauryl sulfate. With saline (placebo control) there is little change in counts over time.

designs are used which permit, if necessary, the screening of relatively large numbers of agents and formulations and on relatively small numbers of subjects.

Depot studies

Retention of agents in the mouth may be measured by determining the amount expectorated versus the known dose (the buccal retention test) or by measuring plaque and saliva levels of the agent over time. Such retention assessments can be misleading because retention is only one aspect of substantivity and the measurement techniques do not provide information on the activity of the retained agents. Moreover, the buccal retention test does not distinguish drug absorption from adsorption nor determine how much is swallowed. Thus, for example, studies using radio-labeled chlorhexidine purported to demonstrate slow release from oral surfaces and this occurred over a protracted period of time. However, saliva derived from subjects following rinsing with chlorhexidine only provided antimicrobial activity for up to 3 hours following rinsing (Addy & Wright 1978). This is clearly markedly less than the known substantivity or persistence of action of chlorhexidine in the mouth of at least 12 hours (Schiott et al. 1970). It is likely, therefore, that the initial desorption studies using a radio-label were merely detecting chlorhexidine adsorbed to desquamating oral surfaces, particularly the mucosa.

Antimicrobial tests

For antimicrobial agents only, salivary bacterial count assessments are much more indicative of substantivity and are predictive of antiplaque action for the same agents. The method involves measuring salivary bacterial counts before and at time points after a single rinse with the agent (Fig. 22-7) and was first described for chlorhexidine (Schiott et al. 1970). In the case of toothpaste, the product can be either brushed or rinsed as an aqueous slurry (Addy et al, 1983, Jenkins et al. 1990). Agents and products produce variable reductions in counts ranging from none, as with water, to greater than 90% as with chlorhexidine. More importantly, the duration of reduction from baseline varies from minutes to hours. Thus, povidone iodine only reduces counts for approximately 1 hour, cetylpyridinium chloride for 3 hours (Roberts & Addy 1981), whereas chlorhexidine produces such effects for over 12 hours (Schiott et al. 1970). Toothpastes generally show reductions in counts between 3 and 5 hours, probably largely due to contained detergents and/or specific ingredients such as triclosan (Addy et al. 1989).

Experimental plaque studies

Short-term plaque regrowth studies are perhaps the most commonly used clinical experiments to screen chemical oral hygiene products. They have the advantage of assessing the chemical action of the formulation divorced from the indeterminate variable of toothbrushing. Typically, plaque regrowth from a zero baseline and the influence of the test agent is recorded. Originally used for mouthrinses, the method has been modified for toothpaste by delivering the formulation in a tray applied to the teeth (Gjermo & Rolla 1970, 1971, Etemadzadeh et al. 1985) or as a slurry rinse (Addy et al.1983). Studies are usually cross-over, allowing many formulations to be evaluated against suitable controls. Study periods range from 24 hours to several days, usually 4-5 (Harrap 1974, Addy et al. 1983). A negative control such as water and a positive

Plaque Area (sp cm)

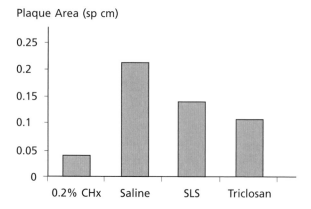

Fig. 22-8. Plaque area following the use of chlorhexidine, saline, sodium lauryl sulfate and triclosan mouthrinses after 4-day periods. Considerable plaque inhibition was afforded by chlorhexidine (positive control) when toothcleaning was suspended. Both sodium lauryl sulfate and triclosan show significant plaque inhibitory action compared to saline (placebo control) albeit significantly less than chlorhexidine.

Plaque index

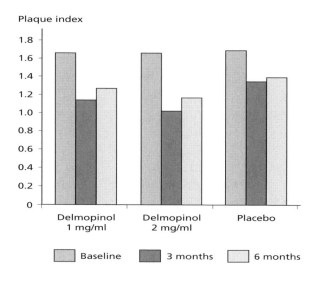

Fig. 22-9. A 6-month study of delmopinol rinses as adjuncts to oral hygiene. Significant improvements in plaque scores are seen in the delmopinol mouthrinse groups at 3 and 6 months compared to placebo. A Hawthorne effect of improved toothcleaning irrespective of the treatment is apparent in the placebo group, particularly at 3 months, although this is still present at 6 months.

control such as chlorhexidine may be used (Fig. 22-8). These help to position the activity of the test formulations between the extremes. Also, because the results from these controls can be predicted, their use tends to confirm or otherwise the conduct of these blind, randomized study designs.

Experimental gingivitis studies

Experimental gingivitis studies (Löe & Schiott, 1970) are based on the original experimental gingivitis in man protocol first used to demonstrate the direct etiological relationship between plaque and gingivitis (Löe et al. 1965). This latter original study did not return subjects to zero baseline plaque scores or gingival health, whereas most subsequent methods, to evaluate oral hygiene products, have taken this approach with baseline parameters. Study periods usually range from 12, but more particularly 19–28 days. In the absence of normal tooth cleaning, the development of plaque and gingivitis are recorded under the influence of test and control formulations. Studies may be either cross-over or parallel.

Home use studies

For chemical oral hygiene products and usually tooth-

pastes and mouthrinses, the final evaluation requires that they are shown to be effective against plaque and, more particularly, gingivitis when used along with normal mechanical tooth cleaning. Studies can be over days or weeks but usually, in accordance with guidelines such as those for the American Dental Association (Council of Dental Therapeutics 1985) they need to be 6 months or longer, particularly since safety needs to be assessed (Fig. 22-9). Most studies are parallel in design. Protocols have used two approaches. One is perhaps more therapeutic in concept whereby subjects have to exhibit a certain level of plaque and/or gingivitis before entry (Johansen et al. 1975). The other is more preventive in concept and there is a prestudy period in which subjects with gingivitis receive prophylaxis and instruction to improve their gingival health. Those satisfactorily responding are entered, and change in gingival health is monitored in the test and control groups (Stephen et al. 1990). Several factors tend to confound home use studies of oral hygiene products and may mask a proven chemical antiplaque action determined from short-term plaque and experimental gingivitis studies. Most important is the so-called Hawthorne effect where subjects knowingly involved in oral hygiene studies improve their tooth cleaning (Fig. 22-9). Secondly, baseline prophylaxes are commonly given and the influence of this on the subsequent gingivitis levels is not known. In mouthrinse studies used as adjuncts to tooth cleaning, there is the potential of interaction between toothpaste and mouthrinse, which could be additive but in most cases is more likely negative for effects on mouthrinse ingredients (Owens et al. 1997, Sheen et al. 2001, 2002). Compliance in home use studies can also be a problem and difficult to accurately determine. In short-term studies compliance can be guaranteed through supervision but this is difficult if not impossible in home use studies. Finally, particularly in toothpaste studies, the control product will have some inherent plaque inhibitory action consequent upon ingredients such as detergents (Addy et al. 1983). If the appropriate control products have been used in the screening plaque inhibitory and experimental gingivitis models this should not pose a problem. However, there is no doubt, and this will be discussed, that the choice of control toothpaste, whereby to compare an active toothpaste, could considerably influence the outcome and therefore the conclusions concerning a potential antiplaque toothpaste.

CLINICAL TRIAL DESIGN CONSIDERATIONS

Clinical trials involving human patients, subjects or healthy volunteers should conform to the Guidelines for Good Clinical Practice (ICH 1996) including the Declaration of Helsinki (World Medical Association 1996). These guidelines were introduced not only to protect the well-being of the participants but also the interest of those organizing, supporting and conducting the trials. An additional purpose for the guidelines was to limit the possibility for falsification of data. Broadly, the guidelines are concerned with all aspects of a clinical trial and, in particular, the ethical requirements, the design and conduct of the trial, data collection and record keeping, data analysis and reporting of the findings. Requirements of ethical committees will vary locally, nationally and internationally; however, common to all is a need for a detailed protocol covering all aspects of the clinical trial, subject or patient information and consent. Written indemnification and/or insurance cover from the appropriate source or sources for the subjects or patients is required, although the details may vary both nationally and internationally. For example, in the UK most ethical committees would adopt the indemnification principles as set out by the Association of British Pharmaceutical Industries.

The basic requirements of a clinical trial are that it should be blind, randomized and suitably controlled. These three aspects of clinical trial design are intimately related and are there to remove, limit or allow adjustment for possible influences that might confound the outcome of a clinical trial and thereby reduce or completely obviate the scientific value of any particular study. These three design features will be discussed individually.

Blindness

All clinical studies must be, at least, single, examiner blind. Single blindness requires that any investigator collecting data from the patients or subjects should not know the identity of the treatments used by any particular individual. Single blindness should eliminate bias in data collection. Examiner blindness, however, can be compromised to a variable degree if a particular treatment produces changes within the oral cavity, which can be perceived by the examiner. Such an example could be extrinsic staining of the teeth and/or oral mucosa like chlorhexidine formulations. The use of objective measures, which reduce or remove the requirement for the subjective judgement of the examiner, can improve the likelihood of single blindness but such objective methods are not common to the recording of plaque, gingivitis and periodontal disease parameters. Double blindness is the ideal when neither the examiner nor subject or patient is aware of the treatment being used by the individual. Numerous factors will influence whether the subjects or patients can be maintained totally blind to their treatment(s), including whether the study is parallel or cross-over (to be discussed later), prior experience with treatments and the presentation, taste and appearance of the treatments, particularly controls. Subject blindness, although ideal, is less important where the treatment outcome measures are out of the immediate control of the subject, e.g. plaque accumulation and gingivitis; assuming, that is, that lack of subject blindness does not influence compliance. Subject blindness becomes highly important where the subject is required to make a valid judgement of the effects of the treatment, for example the effects of treatments on symptoms such as pain.

Randomization

The order in which treatments are received by each subject in a cross-over study, or into which treatment group subjects are placed in a parallel study, should be according to a randomized schedule. Randomization provides several important safety aspects to the study design in that firstly it is an essential part of examiner blindness, secondly in a cross-over study randomization should remove the potential confounding effects of the order of product use, the so-called period effects. Thirdly, the use of balanced randomization designs allows for potential carry-over in cross-over design studies (Newcombe 1992, Newcombe et al. 1995). Finally, where the effects of a treatment on a disease state are to be assessed, randomization improves the chances that parallel treatment groups should be as similar as possible in baseline disease levels and, if relevant, demographic data. Randomization schedules, which use subject matching for demographic and disease status or stratification for level of disease, can be employed to improve balancing of parallel groups.

Controls

The use of appropriate control treatments is essential to the evaluation of the benefits of a particular agent or product. Without such controls, studies essentially become no more than case report data at best and anecdotal at worst, particularly when a particular treatment is evaluated alone for effects on particular parameters. However, the choice of controls can vary depending on the aim of the study and the level of evaluation of an agent or product within a program of research. The choice of controls could therefore be one or more of the following.

Placebo control

Here the control is a substance without any expected pharmacological action, e.g. water. This is useful when assessing a new agent or positioning an agent or formulation between a positive or benchmark control. Placebo controls are particularly valuable where a condition or symptom may be perceived by the subject or patient to have improved, so-called placebo response, or where a condition appears to improve naturally over time, the so-called regression to the mode. Both of these phenomena are common to studies of the treatment of dentine hypersensitivity where pain is a primary outcome measure, but they are of course unlikely to occur in studies where the outcome measure are levels of plaque and gingivitis.

Minus active control (negative control)

This type of control is commonly employed to determine whether an agent provides activity over and above its vehicle. It is particularly useful in the initial assessment of formulations such as toothpastes which have included a new active. In the later stages of development, perhaps at the product level, the use of minus active controls in home use studies is of less value since minus active controls are not normally used by the general public.

Bench mark control

This term is usually used to define a control which is a commercially available product commonly used by the general public. Such controls would appear more sensible for home use studies rather than minus active products when, for example, a new toothpaste product is formulated to promote gingival health benefits. In this case it would seem reasonable to determine whether efficacy is superior to conventional fluoride toothpaste rather than the minus active toothpaste.

Positive control

Positive control is an agent or formulation presently considered the most effective agent available. In this case chlorhexidine mouthrinses are arguably considered the standard antiplaque agent and are frequently used as the positive control by which to compare and position the efficacy of agents and formulations. Usually chlorhexidine mouthrinses as positive controls are used in the early no oral hygiene study protocols.

Depending on the aims and constraints of a clinical study, more than one of the aforementioned controls may be used; for example, in the short-term studies it is not unusual to position an agent or formulation for plaque and gingivitis efficacy between a positive control, chlorhexidine, and a placebo, water.

Study groups

Study designs for oral hygiene products are usually either parallel or cross-over. Parallel group studies require that each individual uses only one of the formulations (active or control) during the duration of the study. Parallel designs can be used for any of the previously described oral hygiene study methods; however they are more commonly used when the study duration is protracted to weeks or months. Parallel designs require that the study groups are large in number to provide sufficient power for statistical analysis. Indeed, the power of any particular study to demonstrate a statistically significant difference between treatments should be calculated prior to the study, although this may be compromised by lack of data as to the likely outcome or by difficulty in deciding the clinical relevance of any difference found. Advice from a statistician is important and group sizes can be calculated based on expected differences between test and control formulations. It must be remembered that small differences can be found statistically significant merely by using large group sizes.

Cross-over studies randomly allocate subjects to use all of the agents or formulations under test. Since each individual acts as their own control, paired statistical analytical techniques mean that the power to detect differences is markedly increased compared to parallel designs, and thereby the total study cohort of subjects can be relatively small. Furthermore, a considerable number of formulations can be compared, although this will be limited by the duration of each study period which, in itself, will have a knock-on effect to acceptability to and compliance of the subjects. Cross-over studies require a wash-out period between each treatment period and this will depend on the known, or expected, carry-over effect of a treatment or a condition into the next period. Random incomplete block designs can be used, in which each subject only uses so many of the agents under test.

The relationship between statistical significance and clinical significance is always difficult to resolve. Statistical significance is a mathematical concept which, with varying levels of probability, supports the idea that any difference between treatments is not due to chance. Clinical significance, on the other hand, is conceptual and attempts to define the benefit to the patient of any particular treatment. Clinical significance could be:

1. *Bench mark equivalent*: when a formulation performs as well as an established formulation or product.
2. *Bench mark superior*: when a formulation performs significantly better than an established formulation.
3. *Disease related*: when a formulation has an effect on an etiological factor such that the related signs or symptoms of the associated disease are reduced to a significantly greater extent than the control, e.g. plaque reduction which reduced gingivitis to a greater extent than control.
4. *Positive*: when a formulation produced the effect significantly greater than the most effective agent today, e.g. the antiplaque effect is greater than chlorhexidine.
5. *Proportional superiority*: when from the outset of a study a minimum percentage improvement over the control group is set down as clinically significant.

Conclusions

- Terminology concerning oral hygiene products needs to be standardized and defined.
- Claims for efficacy, which are implied or rely on inferences to be drawn, should be avoided.
- Studies *in vitro* can provide supportive data to clinical investigations but cannot stand alone as proof of efficacy *in vivo*.
- Research and development of oral hygiene products needs to be step-by-step processed, making available a body of knowledge supporting the efficacy of a final formulation.
- Clinical proof should be largely dependent on data from blind, randomized, controlled, clinical trials conducted to the Guideline for Good Clinical Practice (GCP).
- In reporting clinical trials the clinical significance of the finding should be considered.
- Statistical significance should not necessarily be taken as proof *per se* of the benefit of an oral hygiene product to the general public.
- Clinical outcome, when possible, should be evaluated against side effects and the cost-benefit ratio should be determined.

REFERENCES

Addy, M. (1986). Chlorhexidine compared with other locally delivered anti-microbials. A short review. *Journal of Clinical Periodontology* **13**, 957-964.

Addy, M. (1994). Local delivery of anti-microbial agents to the oral cavity. *Advanced Drug Delivery Reviews* **13**, 123-134.

Addy, M. (1995). Evaluation of clinical trials of agents and procedures to prevent caries and periodontal disease: choosing products and recommending procedures. *International Dental Journal* **45**, 185-196.

Addy, M. & Adriaens, P. (1998). Consensus report of Group A: Epidemiology and aetiology of periodontal diseases and the role of plaque control in dental caries. In: Lang, N.P., Attstrom, R. & Löe, H., eds. *Proceedings of the European Workshop on Mechanical Plaque Control*. Berlin: Quintessence Publishing Company, pp. 98-101.

Addy, M., Carpenter, R. & Roberts, W.R. (1976). Management of recurrent aphthous ulceration. *British Dental Journal* **141**, 118-120.

Addy, M., Dummer, P.M.H., Griffiths, G., Hicks, R., Kingdon, A. & Shaw, W.C. (1986). Prevalence of plaque, gingivitis, and caries in 11-12 year old children in South Wales. *Community Dentistry and Oral Epidemiology* **14**, 115-118.

Addy, M., Greenman, J., Renton-Harper, P., Newcombe, R.G. & Doherty, F.M. (1997). Studies on stannous fluoride toothpaste and gel 2: Effects on salivary bacterial counts and plaque re-growth *in vivo*. *Journal of Clinical Periodontology* **24**, 86-91.

Addy, M., Griffiths, C. & Isaac, R. (1977). The effect of povidone iodine on plaque and salivary bacteria. A double blind cross-over trial. *Journal of Periodontology* **48**, 730-732.

Addy, M., Hassan, H., Moran, J., Wade, W. & Newcombe, R. (1988). A 3 month follow up study of anti-microbial containing acrylic strips used in the treatment of chronic periodontal disease. *Journal of Periodontology* **59**, 557-564.

Addy, M., Jenkins, S. & Newcombe, R. (1989). Toothpastes containing 0.3% and 0.5% triclosan. II. Effects of single brushings on salivary bacterial counts. *American Journal of Dentistry* **2**, 215-220.

Addy, M. & Langeroudi, M. (1984). Comparison of the immediate effects on the subgingival micro-flora of acrylic strips containing 40% chlorhexidine, metronidazole or tetracycline. *Journal of Clinical Periodontology* **11**, 379-386.

Addy, M. & Llewelyn, J. (1978). Use of chlorhexidine gluconate and povidone iodine mouthwashes in the treatment of acute ulcerative gingivitis. *Journal of Clinical Periodontology* **5**, 272-277.

Addy, M., Mahdavi, S.A. & Loyn T. (1995b). Dietary staining *in vitro* by mouthrinses as a comparative measure of antiseptic activity and predictor of staining *in vivo*. *Journal of Dentistry* **22**, 95-99.

Addy, M. & Moran, J. (1983). Comparison of plaque accumulation after topical application and mouth rinsing with chlorhexidine gluconate. *Journal of Clinical Periodontology* **10**, 69-71.

Addy, M. & Moran, J.M. (1985). Extrinsic tooth discoloration by metals and chlorhexidine. 2. Clinical staining produced by chlorhexidine iron and tea. *British Dental Journal* **159**, 331-334.

Addy, M. & Moran, J.M. (1995). Mechanisms of stain formation on teeth, in particular associated with metal ions and antiseptics. *Advances in Dental Research* **9**, 450-456.

Addy, M. & Moran, J.M. (1997). Clinical indications for the use of chemical adjuncts to plaque control: chlorhexidine formulations. In: Addy, M. & Moran, J.M., eds. Toothpaste, mouth rinse and other topical remedies in periodontics. *Periodontology 2000* **15**, 52-54.

Addy, M., Moran, J.M., Griffiths, A.A. & Wills-Wood, N.J. (1985). Extrinsic tooth discolouration. I. Surface protein denaturation or dietary precipitation. *British Dental Journal* **159**, 281-285

Addy, M., Moran, J.M. & Newcombe, R. (1991). A comparison of 0.12% and 0.1% chlorhexidine mouth-rinses in the development of plaque and gingivitis. *Clinical Preventive Dentistry* **13**, 26-29.

Addy, M., Moran, M., Newcombe, R. & Warren, P. (1995a). The comparative tea staining potential of phenolic, chlorhexidine and antiadhesive mouth-rinses. *Journal of Clinical Periodontology* **22**, 929-934.

Addy, M., Moran, J. & Wade, W. (1994). Chemical plaque control in the prevention of gingivitis and periodontitis. In: Lang, N.E. & Karring, T., eds. *Proceedings of the 71st European Workshop on Periodontology.* London: Quintessence Publishing, pp. 244-257.

Addy, M., Moran, J., Wade, W. & Jenkins, S. (1992). The evaluation of toothpaste products in promoting gingival health. In: Embery, G. & Rolla, G., eds. *Clinical and Biological Aspects of Dentifrices.* Oxford: Oxford University Press, pp. 249-262.

Addy, M., Perriam, E. & Sterry, A. (1982a). Effects of sugared and sugar-free chewing gum on the accumulation of plaque and debris on the teeth. *Journal of Clinical Periodontology* 9, 346-354.

Addy, M., Rawle, L., Handley, R., Newman, H.N. & Coventry, J.F. (1982b). The development and *in vitro* evaluation of acrylic strips and dialysis tubing for local drug delivery. *Journal of Periodontology* 53, 693-699.

Addy, M. & Renton-Harper, P (1996b). Local and systemic chemotherapy in the management of periodontal disease: an opinion and review of the concept. *Journal of Oral Rehabilitation* 23, 219-231.

Addy, M. & Renton-Harper, P. (1996a). The role of antiseptics in secondary prevention. In: Lang, N.P., Karring, T. & Lindhe, J., eds. *Proceedings of the 2nd European Workshop on Periodontology, Chemicals in Periodontics.* Berlin: Quintessence, pp. 152-173.

Addy, M., Richards, J. & Williams, G. (1980). Effects of a zinc citrate mouthwash on dental plaque and salivary bacteria. *Journal of Clinical Periodontology* 7, 309-315.

Addy, M. & Roberts, W.R. (1981) Comparison of the bisguanide antiseptics alexidine and chlorhexidine II. Clinical and *in vitro* staining properties. *Journal of Clinical Periodontology* 8, 220-230.

Addy, M., Tapper-Jones, L. & Seal, M. (1974). Trial of astringent and antibacterial mouthwashes in the management of recurrent aphthous ulceration. *British Dental Journal* 136, 452-455.

Addy, M. & Wade, W.G. (1995). An approach to efficacy screening of mouth rinses: studies on a group of French products (I). Staining and anti-microbial properties in vitro. *Journal of Clinical Periodontology* 22, 718-722.

Addy, M., Willis, L. & Moran, J. (1983). The effect of toothpaste and chlorhexidine rinses on plaque accumulation during a 4 day period. *Journal of Clinical Periodontology* 10, 89-98.

Addy, M. & Wright, R. (1978). Comparison of the *in vivo* and *in vitro* antibacterial properties of povidone iodine and chlorhexidine gluconate mouthrinses. *Journal of Clinical Periodontology* 5, 198-205.

Ainamo, J. & Etemadzadeh, H. (1987). Prevention of plaque growth with chewing gum containing chlorhexidine acetate. *Journal of Clinical Periodontology* 14, 524-527.

Ainamo, J., Nieminen, A. & Westerlund, U. (1990). Optimal dosage of chlorhexidine acetate in chewing gum. *Journal of Clinical Periodontology* 17, 729-733.

Albert, A. & Sargeant, E.R. (1962). In: *Ionization Constants of Acids and Bases.* London: Methuen, p. 173.

Allen, D.R., Davies, R., Bradshaw, B., Ellwood, R., Simone, A.J., Robinson, R., Mukerjee, C., Petrone, M.E., Chaknis, P., Volpe, A.R. & Proskin, H.M. (1998). Efficacy of a mouth rinse containing 0.05% cetylpyridinium chloride for the control of plaque and gingivitis: a 6-month clinical study in adults. *Compendium of Continuing Education in Dentistry* 19, 20-26.

Ash, M., Gitlin, B.N. & Smith, N.A. (1964). Correlation between plaque and gingivitis. *Journal of Periodontology* 35, 425-429.

Axelsson, P. (1994). Mechanical plaque control. In: Lang, N.E & Karring, T., eds. *Proceedings of the 1st European Workshop on Periodontology.* London: Quintessence, pp. 219-243.

Axelsson, P. & Lindhe, J. (1981a). Effect of controlled oral hygiene procedures on caries and periodontal disease in adults. Results after 6 yrs. *Journal of Clinical Periodontology* 8, 239-248.

Axelsson, P. & Lindhe, J. (1981b). The significance of maintenance care in the treatment of periodontal disease. *Journal of Clinical Periodontology* 8, 281-294.

Baehni, P.C. & Bourgeois, D.M. (1998). Epidemiology of periodontal health and disease. In: Lang, N.P., Attstrom, R. & Löe,

H., eds. *Proceedings of the European Workshop on Mechanical Plaque Control.* Berlin: Quintessence Publishing Company, pp. 19-34.

Baelum, V., Fejerskov, O. & Karring, T. (1986). Oral hygiene, gingivitis and periodontal breakdown in adult Tanzanians. *Journal of Periodontal Research* 21, 221-232.

Barkvoll, P. & Rolla, C. (1994). Triclosan protects the skin against dermatitis caused by sodium lauryl sulfate exposure. *Journal of Clinical Periodontology* 21, 717-719.

Barkvoll, P., Rolla, G. & Svendsen, A. (1989). Interaction between chlorhexidine digluconate and sodium lauryl sulphate *in vivo. Journal of Clinical Periodontology* 16, 593-598.

Beiswanger, B.B., Doyle, P.M., Jackson, R.D., Mallatt, M.E., Mau, M.S., Bollmer, B.W., Crisanti, M.M., Guay, C.B., Lanzalaco, A.C., Lukacovic, M.F., Majeti, S. & McClanahan, T. (1995). The clinical effect of dentifrices containing stabilised stannous fluoride on plaque formation and gingivitis 97, a six-month study with *ad libitum* brushing. *Journal of Clinical Dentistry* 6, 46-53.

Bergenholtz, A. & Hanstrom, L. (1974). The plaque inhibiting effect of hexetidine (Oraldene) mouthwash compared to that of chlorhexidine. *Community Dentistry and Oral Epidemiology* 2, 70-74.

Binney, A., Addy, M., Owens, J., Faulkner, J., McKeown, S. & Everatt, L. (1996). A 3-month home use study comparing the oral hygiene and gingival health benefits of triclosan and conventional fluoride toothpastes. *Journal of Clinical Periodontology* 23, 1020-1024.

Bonesvoll, P. & Gjermo, P. (1978). A comparison between chlorhexidine and some quaternary ammonium compounds with regard to retention, salivary concentration and plaque inhibiting effect in the human mouth after mouthrinses. *Archives of Oral Biology* 23, 289-294.

Bonesvoll, P., Lokken, P. & Rolla, G. (1974a). Influence of concentration, time, temperature and pH on the retention of chlorhexidine in the human oral cavity after mouth rinses. *Archives of Oral Biology* 19, 1025-1029.

Bonesvoll, P., Lokken, P., Rolla, G. & Paus, P.N. (1974b). Retention of chlorhexidine in the human oral cavity after mouth rinses. *Archives of Oral Biology* 19, 209-212.

Brecx, M., Brownstone, E., MacDonald, L., Gelskey, S. & Cheang, M. (1992). Efficacy of Listerine, Meridol and chlorhexidine mouth rinses as supplements to regular tooth-cleaning measures. *Journal of Clinical Periodontology* 19, 202-207.

Brecx, M., Netuschil, I., Reichert, B. & Schreil, C. (1990). Efficacy of Listerine, Meridol and chlorhexidine mouth rinses on plaque, gingivitis and plaque bacteria vitality. *Journal of Clinical Periodontology* 17, 292-297.

British Standards Institution (1981). Specification for Toothpastes, BS 5136.

Cancro, L.P., Klein, K. & Picozzi, A. (1973). Dose response of chlorhexidine gluconate in a model *in vivo* plaque system. *Journal of Dental Research* 52, Spec. issue, Abstr 659, 223.

Cancro, L.P., Paulovich, D.B., Bolton, S. & Picozzi, A. (1974). Dose response of chlorhexidine gluconate in a model *in vivo* plaque system. *Journal of Dental Research* 53, 765.

Chadwick, B., Addy, M. & Walker, D.M. (1991). The use of a hexetidine mouthwash in the management of minor aphthous ulceration and as an adjunct to oral hygiene. *British Dental Journal* 171, 83-87.

Claydon, N., Hunter. L., Moran, J., Wade, W., Kelty, F., Movert, R. & Addy, M. (1996). A 6-month home-usage trial of 0.1% and 0.2% delmopinol mouthwashes. 1. Effects on plaque, gingivitis, supragingival calculus and tooth staining. *Journal of Clinical Periodontology* 23, 220-228.

Collaert, B., Attstrom, R., de Bruyn, N. & Movert, R. (1992). The effect of delmopinol rinsing on dental plaque formation and gingivitis healing. *Journal of Clinical Periodontology* 19, 274-280.

Cooke, B.E.D. & Armitage, P. (1960). Recurrent Mikuliczs aphthae treated with topical hydrocortisone hemisuccinate sodium. *British Medical Journal* 1, 764-766.

Council of Dental Therapeutics (1985). Guidelines for acceptance of chemotherapeutic products for the control of supragingival dental plaque and gingivitis. *Journal of the American Dental Association* **112**, 529-532.

Coventry, J. & Newman, H.N. (1982). Experimental use of a slow release device employing chlorhexidine gluconate in areas of acute periodontal inflammation. *Journal of Clinical Periodontology* **9**, 129-1 33.

Cumming, B.R. & Löe, H. (1973). Optimal dosage and method of delivering chlorhexidine solutions for the inhibition of dental plaque. *Journal of Periodontal Reserarch* **8**, 57-62.

Cummins, D. (1992). Mechanisms of actions of clinically proven antiplaque agents. In: Embery, G. & Rolla, G., eds. *Clinical and Biological Aspects of Dentifrices*. Oxford: Oxford University Press, pp. 205- 228.

Cummins, D. (1997). Vehicles: how to deliver the goods. In: Addy, M. & Moran, J.M., eds. Toothpaste, mouthrinse and other topical remedies in periodontics. *Periodontology 2000* **15**, 84-99.

Dahlen, C., Lindhe, J., Sato, K., Hanamura, H. & Okamoto, H. (1992). The effect of supragingival plaque control on the subgingival microbiota in subjects with periodontal disease. *Journal of Clinical Periodontology* **19**, 802-809.

Davies, R.M., Jensen, S.B., Schiott, C.R. & Löe, H. (1970). The effect of topical application of chlorhexidine on the bacterial colonization of the teeth and gingiva. *Journal of Periodontal Research* **5**, 96-101.

Davis, W.B. (1980). Cleaning and polishing the teeth by brushing. *Community Dentistry and Oral Epidemiology* **8**, 237-243.

de la Rosa, M.R., Guerra, J.Z., Johnson, D.A. & Radike, A.W. (1979). Plaque growth and removal with daily tooth brushing. *Journal of Periodontology* **50**, 661-664.

Dilling, W.J. & Hallam, S. (1936). *Dental Materia Medica, Pharmacology and Therapeutics*, 3rd edn. London: Cassell & Company.

Dolles, O.K. & Gjermo, P. (1980). Caries increment and gingival status during two years of chlorhexidine and fluoride containing dentifrices. *Scandinavian Journal of Dental Research* **88**, 22-27.

Egelberg, J. & Claffey, N. (1998). Consensus Report of Group B: Role of mechanical plaque removal in the prevention and therapy of caries and periodontal disease. In: Lang, N.P., Attstrom, R. & Loe, H., eds. *Proceedings of the European Workshop on Mechanical Plaque Control*. Berlin: Quintessence Publishing Company, pp. 169-172.

Ellingsen, J.E., Rolla, G. & Eriksen, H.M. (1982). Extrinsic dental stain caused by chlorhexidine and other denaturing agents. *Journal of Clinical Periodontology* **9**, 317-322.

Ellwood, R.P., Worthington, H.V., Blinkhorn, A.S.B., Volpe, A.R. & Davies, R.M. (1998). Effect of a triclosan/copolymer dentifrice on the incidence of periodontal attachment loss in adolescents. *Journal of Clinical Periodontology* **25**, 363-367.

Eriksen, H.M., Nordbo, H., Kantanen, H. & Ellingsen, J.E. (1985). Chemical plaque control and extrinsic tooth discoloration. A review of possible mechanisms. *Journal of Clinical Periodontology* **12**, 345-350.

Etemadzadeh, H., Ainamo, J. & Murtoma, H. (1985). Plaque growth inhibiting effects of an abrasive fluoride-chlorhexidine toothpaste and a fluoride toothpaste containing oxidative enzymes. *Journal of Clinical Periodontology* **12**, 607-616.

Ferretti, G., Ash, R.C., Brown, A.T., Largent, B.M., Kaplan, A. & Lillich, T.T. (1987). Chlorhexidine for prophylaxis against oral infections and associated complications in patients receiving bone marrow transplants. *Journal of the American Dental Association* **114**, 461-467.

Ferretti, G., Ash, R.C., Brown, A.T., Parr, M.D., Romand, E.H. & Lillich, T.T. (1988). Control of oral mucositis and candidiasis in marrow transplantation: a prospective double blind trial of chlorhexidine digluconate oral rinse. *Bone Marrow Transplantation* **3**, 483-493.

Fischman, S.L. (1992). Hare's teeth to fluorides; historical aspects of dentifrice use. In: Embery, G. & Rolla, G., eds. *Clinical and Biological Aspects of Dentifrices*. Oxford: Oxford University Press, pp. 1-7.

Fischman, S. (1997). Oral hygiene products: How far have we come in 6000 years. *Periodontology 2000* **15**, 7-14.

Flotra, L., Gjermo, P., Rolla, G. & Waerhaug, J. (1971). Side effects of chlorhexidine mouthwashes. *Scandinavian Journal of Dental Research* **79**, 119-125.

Forward, G.C., James, A.H., Barnett, P. & Jackson, R.J. (1997). Gum health product formulations: what is in them and why? *Periodontology 2000* **15**, 32-39.

Francis, J.R., Addy, M. & Hunter, B. (1987b). A comparison of three delivery methods of chlorhexidine in institutionalised physically handicapped children. *Journal of Periodontology* **58**, 456-459.

Francis, J.R., Hunter, B. & Addy, M. (1987a). A comparison of three delivery methods of chlorhexidine in handicapped children. I. Effects on plaque, gingivitis and tooth staining. *Journal of Periodontology* **58**, 451-454.

Frandsen, A. (1986). Mechanical oral hygiene practices In: Löe, H. & Kleinman, D.V., eds. *Dental Plaque Control Measures and Oral Hygiene Practices*. Oxford: IRL Press, pp. 93-116.

Gaffar, A., Volpe, A. & Lindhe, J. (1992). Recent advances in plaque/gingivitis control. In: Embery, G. & Rolla, C., eds. *Clinical and Biological Aspects of Dentifrices*. Oxford: Oxford University Press, pp. 229-248.

Garcia-Gadoy, F., Garcia-Gadoy, F., DeVizio, W., Volpe, A.R., Ferlauto, R.J. & Miller, J.M. (1990). Effect of a triclosan/copolymer/fluoride dentifrice on plaque formation and gingivitis: a 7-month clinical study. *American Journal of Dentistry* **3**, 15-26.

Genco, R. J. (1981). Antibiotics in the treatment of human periodontal diseases. *Journal of Periodontology* **52**, 545-558.

Gjermo, P. (1974). Chlorhexidine in dental practice. *Journal of Clinical Periodontology* **1**, 143-152.

Gjermo, P. (1989). Chlorhexidine and related compounds. *Journal of Dental Research* **68**, 1602-1608.

Gjermo, P. & Rolla, G. (1970). Plaque inhibition by antibacterial dentifrices. *Scandinavian Journal of Dental Research* **78**, 464-470.

Gjermo, P. & Rolla, G. (1971). Plaque inhibiting effect of chlorhexidine containing dentifrices. *Scandinavian Journal of Dental Research* **79**, 126-132.

Gjermo, P., Rolla, C. & Arskaug, L. (1973). Effect on dental plaque formation and some in vitro properties of 12 bisbiguanides. *Journal of Periodontal Research* **8**, Supplement 12, 81-88.

Gjermo, P., Baastad, K.L. & Rolla, C. (1970). The plaque inhibitory capacity of 11 antibacterial compounds. *Journal of Periodontal Research* **5**, 102-109.

Gjermo, P., Bonesvoll, P. & Rolla, C. (1974). The relationship between plaque inhibiting effect and retention of chlorhexidine in the human oral cavity. *Archives of Oral Biology* **19**, 1031-1034.

Haffajee, A.D. & Socransky, S.S. (1994). Microbial etiological agents of periodontal destruction. *Periodontology 2000* **5**, 78-111.

Hancock, E.B. (1996). Prevention. World Workshop in Periodontics. *Annals of Periodontology* **1**, 223-249.

Harrap, G.J. (1974). Assessment of the effect of dentifrices on the growth of dental plaque. *Journal of Clinical Periodontology* **1**, 166-174.

Heasman, P.A. & Seymour, R.A. (1994). Pharmacological control of periodontal disease. 1. Anti-plaque agents. *Journal of Dentistry* **22**, 323-326.

Hodge, P.J., Riggio, M.P. & Kinane, D.F. (2001). Failure to detect an association with IL1 genotypes in European Caucasians with generalised early onset periodontitis. *Journal of Clinical Periodontology* **28**, 430-436.

Hofer, K. (1978). Try Hippocrates home made tooth powder. CAL (Chicago) **42**, 27-28.

Hugo, W.B. & Longworth, A.R. (1964). Some aspects of the mode of action of chlorhexidine. *Journal of Pharmacy and Pharmacology* **16**, 655-662.

Hugo, W.B. & Longworth, A.R. (1965). Cytological aspects of the mode of action of chlorhexidine diacetate. *Journal of Pharmacy and Pharmacology* **17**, 28-32.

Hugo, W.B. & Longworth, A.R. (1966). The effects of chlorhexidine on the electrophoretic mobility, cytoplasmic constituents, dehydrogenase activity and cell walls of *Escherichia coli and Staphylococcus aureus. Journal of Pharmacy and Pharmacology* **18**, 569-578.

Hugoson, A. & Jordan, T. (1982). Frequency distribution of individuals aged 20-70 years according to severity of periodontal disease. *Community Dentistry and Oral Epidemiology* **10**, 187-192.

Hugoson, A., Norderyd, O., Slotte, C. & Thorstensson, H. (1998a). Oral hygiene and gingivitis in a Swedish adult population 1973, 1983, 1993. *Journal of Clinical Periodontology* **25**, 807-812.

Hugoson, A., Norderyd, O., Slotte, C. & Thorstensson, H. (1998b). Distribution of periodontal disease in a Swedish adult population 1973, 1983, 1993. *Journal of Clinical Periodontology* **25**, 542-548.

Hull, P.S. (1980). Chemical inhibition of plaque. *Journal of Clinical Periodontology* **7**, 431-442.

Hunter, L., Addy, M., Moran, J., Kohut, B., Hovliaras, C. & Newcombe, R. (1994). A study of a pre-brushing as an adjunct to oral hygiene. *Journal of Periodontology* **65**, 762-765.

Hunter, M.L. & Addy, M. (1987). Chlorhexidine gluconate mouthwash in the management of minor aphthous ulceration. A double-blind, placebo-controlled cross-over trial. *British Dental Journal* **162**, 106-108.

ICH (1996). Topic 6 Guidelines for Good Clinical Practice, CPMP/ICH/135/95. Geneva: International Conference on Harmonization.

ISO 11609 (1995). International Standard: Dentistry-Toothpaste-Requirements, test methods and marking. Geneva: International Standards Organization.

Jackson, R.J. (1997). Metal salts, essential oils and phenols-old or new? In: Addy, M. & Moran, J.M., eds. Toothpaste, mouth rinse and other topical remedies in periodontics. *Periodontology 2000* **15**, 63-73.

Jenkins, S., Addy, M. & Newcombe, R. (1989). Comparison of two commercially available chlorhexidine mouth rinses. II. Effects on plaque reformation, gingivitis and tooth staining. *Clinical Preventive Dentistry* **11**, 12-16.

Jenkins, S., Addy, M. & Newcombe, R. (1990). Comparative effects of toothpaste brushing and toothpaste rinsing on salivary bacterial counts. *Journal of Periodontal Research* **25**, 316-319.

Jenkins, S., Addy, M. & Newcombe, R. (1991a). Triclosan and sodium lauryl sulphate mouth rinses. II. Effects on 4-day plaque re-growth. *Journal of Clinical Periodontology* **18**, 145-148.

Jenkins, S., Addy, M. & Newcombe, R.G. (1991b). Triclosan and sodium lauryl sulphate mouthrinses. I. Effects on salivary bacterial counts. *Journal of Clinical Periodontology* **18**, 140-144.

Jenkins, S., Addy, M. & Newcombe, R.G. (1993). A dose response study of triclosan mouth rinses on plaque re-growth. *Journal of Clinical Periodontology* **20**, 609-612.

Jenkins, S., Addy, M. & Newcombe, R. (1994). Dose response of chlorhexidine against plaque and comparison with triclosan. *Journal of Clinical Periodontology* **21**, 250-255.

Jenkins, S., Addy, M. & Wade, W. (1988). The mechanism of action of chlorhexidine: a study of plaque growth on enamel inserts *in vivo. Journal of Clinical Periodontology* **15**, 415-424.

Jepsen, S. (1998). The role of manual toothbrushes in effective plaque control: advantages and limitations. In: Lang, N.P., Attstrom, R. & Löe, H., eds. *Proceedings of the European Workshop on Mechanical Plaque Control.* Berlin: Quintessence Verlag, pp. 121-137.

Jobbins, J., Addy, M., Bagg, J., Finlay, I., Parsons, K. & Newcombe, R. (1992). A double blind, single phase placebo controlled clinical trial of 0.2% chlorhexidine gluconate oral spray in terminally ill cancer patients. *Palliative Medicine* **6**, 299-307.

Johansen, J.R., Gjermo, P. & Eriksen, H.M. (1972). A longitudinal study on the effect of chlorhexidine containing dentifrices. *Journal of Periodontal Research* **7**, (Suppl. 10), 36-37.

Johansen, J.R., Gjermo, P. & Eriksen, H.M. (1975). Effect of two years' use of chlorhexidine containing dentifrices on plaque, gingivitis and caries. *Scandinavian Journal of Dental Research* **83**, 288-292.

Johnson, N.W. (1994). Risk factors and diagnostic tests for destructive periodontitis. In: Lang, N.P & Karring, T., eds. *Proceedings of the* 1st *European Workshop on Periodontology.* London: Quintessence, pp. 90-119.

Jones, C.G. (1997). Chlorhexidine: is it still the gold standard? In: Addy, M. & Moran, J.M., eds. Toothpaste, mouth rinse and other topical remedies in periodontics, *Periodontology 2000* **15**, 55-62.

Kalaga, A., Addy, M. & Hunter, B. (1989a). Comparison of chlorhexidine delivery by mouthwash and spray on plaque accumulation. *Journal of Periodontology* **60**, 127-130.

Kalaga, A., Addy, M. & Hunter, B. (1989b). The use of 0.2% chlorhexidine as an adjunct to oral health in physically and mentally handicapped adults. *Journal of Periodontology* **60**, 38 1-385.

Kanchanakamol, U., Umpriwan, R., Jotikasthira, N., Srisilapanan, P., Tuongratanaphan, S., Sholitkul, W. & Chat-Uthai, T. (1995). Reduction of plaque formation and gingivitis by a dentifrice containing triclosan and copolymer. *Journal of Periodontology* **66**, 109-112.

Kelly, A., Restaghini, R., Williams, B. & Dolby, A.E. (1985). Pressures recorded during periodontal pocket irrigation. *Journal of Periodontology* **56**, 297-299.

Kelner, R.M., Wohl, B.R., Deasy, M.J. & Formicola, A.J. (1974). Gingival inflammation as related to frequency of plaque removal. *Journal of Periodontology* **45**, 303-307.

Kieser, J.B. (1994). Non-surgical periodontal therapy. In: Lang, N.P & Karring, T., eds. *Proceedings of the1st European Workshop on Periodontology.* London: Quintessence, pp. 131-158.

Kinane, D.F. (1998). The role of interdental cleaning in effective plaque control: need for inter-dental cleaning in primary and secondary prevention. In: Lang, N.P., Attstrom, R. & Löe, H., eds. *Proceedings of the European Workshop on Mechanical Plaque Control.* Berlin: Quintessence Publishing Company, pp. 156-168.

Kopczyk, R.A., Abrams, H., Brown, A.T., Matheny, J.L. & Kaplan, A.L. (1991). Clinical and microbiological effects of a sanguinarine containing mouth-rinse and dentifrice with and without fluoride during 6 months use. *Journal of Periodontology* **62**, 617-622.

Kornman, K.S. (1986). Anti-microbial agents. In: Löe, H. & Kleinman, D.V., eds. *Dental Plaque Control Measures and Oral Hygiene Practices.* Oxford: IRL Press, pp. 121-142.

Kornman, K.S., Crane, A., Wang, H.Y., di Giovine, F.S., Newman, M.G., Pirk, F.W., Wilson, T.G., Higginbottom, F.L. & Duff, G.W. (1997). The interleukin-1 genotype as a severity factor in adult periodontal disease. *Journal of Clinical Periodontology* **24**, 72-77.

Lang, N.P., Catalanotto, P.A., Knopfli, R.U. & Antczak, A.A.A. (1988). Quality specific taste impairment following the application of chlorhexidine gluconate mouthrinses. *Journal of Clinical Periodontology* **15**, 43-48.

Lang, N.P., Cumming, B.R. & Löe, H. (1973). Toothbrush frequency as it's related to plaque development and gingival health. *Journal of Periodontology* **44**, 396-405.

Lang, N.P. & Newman, H.N. (1997). Consensus report of session II. In: Lang, N.P., Karring, T. & Lindhe, J., eds. *Proceedings of the 2nd European Workshop on Periodontology. Chemicals in Periodontics.* Berlin: Quintessence Verlag, pp. 192-200.

Lang, N.P & Raber, K. (1981). Use of oral irrigators as vehicles for the application of anti-microbial agents in chemical plaque control. *Journal of Clinical Periodontology* **8**, 177-188.

Lang, N.P & Ramseier-Grossman, I.C. (1981). Optimal dosage of chlorhexidine gluconate in chemical plaque control when delivered by an oral irrigator. *Journal of Clinical Periodontology* **8**, 189-202.

Lavstedt, S., Modeer, T. & Welander, F. (1982). Plaque and gingivitis in a group of Swedish school children with particular reference to tooth brushing habits. *Acta Odontologica Scandinavica* **40**, 307-311.

Leach, S.A. (1977). Mode of action of chlorhexidine in the mouth. In: Lehner, T., ed. *The Borderland between Caries and Periodontal Disease.* London: Academic Press, pp. 105-128.

Lindhe, J. (1986). In: Gingivitis, General Discussion. *Journal of Clinical Periodontology* **13**, 395.

Lindquist, B., Edward, S., Torell, P & Krasse, B. (1989). Effect of different caries preventive measures in children highly infected with mutans streptococci. *Scandinavian Journal of Dental Research* **97**, 330-337.

Löe, H. (1986). Progression of natural untreated periodontal disease in man. In: *Borderland between Caries and Periodontal Disease,* 3rd edn. Geneve: Medecin et Hygiene.

Löe, H. & Schiott, C.R. (1970). The effect of mouth rinses and topical application of chlorhexidine on the development of dental plaque and gingivitis in man. *Journal of Periodontal Research* **5**, 79-83.

Löe, H., Theilade, E. & Jensen S.B. (1965). Experimental gingivitis in man. *Journal of Periodontology* **36**, 177-187.

MacFarlane, T.W., Ferguson, M.M. & Mulgrew, C.J. (1984). Post extraction bacteraemia: role of antiseptics and antibiotics. *British Dental Journal* **156**, 179-181.

MacGregor, D.M. & Rugg-Gunn, A.J. (1979). A survey of tooth brushing sequence in children and young adults. *Journal of Periodontal Research* **14**, 225-230.

Mandel, I.D. (1988). Chemotherapeutic agents for controlling plaque and gingivitis. *Journal of Clinical Periodontology* **15**, 488-496.

McNabb, H., Mombelli, A. & Lang, N.P. (1992). Supragingival cleaning 3 times a week. *Journal of Clinical Periodontology* **19**, 348-356.

Miller, J.T., Shannon, I., Kilgore, W. & Bookman, J. (1969). Use of water free stannous fluoride containing gel in the control of dentine hypersensitivity. *Journal of Periodontology* **40**, 490-491.

Moore, W.E.C. & Moore, L.V.H. (1994). The bacteria of periodontal diseases. *Periodontology 2000* **5**, 66-77.

Moran, J. & Addy, M. (1984). The effect of surface adsorption and staining reactions on the anti-microbial properties of some cationic antiseptic mouthwashes. *Journal of Periodontology* **55**, 278-282.

Moran, J., Addy, M. & Newcombe, R. (1988a). A clinical trial to assess the efficacy of sanguinarine mouth rinse (Veadent) compared with a chlorhexidine mouth rinse (Corsodyl). *Journal of Clinical Periodontology* **15**, 612-616.

Moran, J., Addy, M. & Newcombe, R. (1988b). The antibacterial effect of toothpastes on the salivary flora. *Journal of Clinical Periodontology* **15**, 193-199.

Moran, J., Addy, M. & Newcombe, R. (1991). Comparison of a herbal toothpaste with a fluoride toothpaste on plaque and gingivitis. *Clinical Preventive Dentistry* **13**, 12-15.

Moran, J., Addy, M., Newcombe, R. & Warren, P (1995). The comparative effects on plaque re-growth of phenolic, chlorhexidine and anti-adhesive mouthrinses. *Journal of Clinical Periodontology* **22**, 923-928.

Moran, J., Addy, M. & Newcombe, R.G. (1997). A 4-day plaque re-growth study comparing an essential oil mouth rinse with a triclosan mouth rinse. *Journal of Clinical Periodontology* **24**, 636-639.

Moran, J., Addy, M. & Roberts, S. (1992a). A comparison of natural product, triclosan and chlorhexidine mouthrinses on 4-day plaque re-growth. *Journal of Clinical Periodontology* **19**, 578-582.

Moran, J., Addy, M., Wade, W.G., Maynard, J.H., Roberts, S.F., Astrom, M. & Movert, R. (1992b). A comparison of delmopinol and chlorhexidine on plaque re-growth over a 4-day period and salivary bacterial counts. *Journal of Clinical Periodontology* **19**, 749-753.

Moran, J., Addy, M., Wade, W., Milsom, S., McAndrew, R. & Newcombe, R. (1995). The effect of oxidising mouth rinses compared with chlorhexidine on salivary bacterial counts and plaque re-growth. *Journal of Clinical Periodontology* **22**, 750-755.

Moss, S., Holmgren, C. & Addy, M. (1995). A reader's and writer's guide to the publication of clinical trials. *International Dental Journal* **45**, 177-184.

Nash, E.S. & Addy, M. (1979). The use of chlorhexidine gluconate mouth rinses in patients with inter-maxillary fixation. *British Journal of Oral Surgery* **17**, 251-255.

Newcombe, R.G. (1992). Crossover trials comparing several treatments. *Journal of Clinical Periodontology* **19**, 785-788.

Newcombe, R.G., Addy, M. & McKeown, S. (1995). Residual effect of chlorhexidine gluconate in 4 day plaque regrowth trials and its implications for study design. *Journal of Periodontal Research* **30**, 319-324.

Newman, P.S. & Addy, M. (1978). A comparison of a periodontal dressing and chlorhexidine gluconate mouthwash after the internal bevel flap procedure. *Journal of Periodontology* **49**, 576-579.

Newman, P.S. & Addy, M. (1982). Comparison of hypertonic saline and chlorhexidine mouthrinses after the inverse bevel flap procedure. *Journal of Periodontology* **52**, 315-318.

Nordbo, H. (1979). Ability of chlorhexidine and benzalkonium chloride to catalyse browning reactions *in vitro. Journal of Dental Research* **58**, 1429.

Nordbo, H., Eriksen, H.M., Attramadal, A. & Solheim, H. (1982). Iron staining of the acquired enamel pellicle after exposure to tannic acid or chlorhexidine. *Scandinavian Journal of Dental Research* **90**, 11 7-123.

Norton, M.R. & Addy, M. (1989). Chewing sticks versus toothbrushes in West Africa. A pilot study. *Clinical Preventive Dentistry* **11**, 11-13.

Olsen, I. (1975a). Denture stomatitis. Effects of chlorhexidine and Amphotericin B on the mycotic flora. *Acta Odontologica Scandinavica* **33**, 41-46.

Olsen, I. (1975b). Denture stomatitis. The clinical effects of chlorhexidine and Amphotericin B. *Acta Odontologica Scandinavica* **33**, 47-52.

Owens, J., Addy, M. & Faulkner, J. (1997). An 18 week home use study comparing the oral hygiene and gingival health benefits of triclosan and fluoride toothpaste. *Journal of Clinical Periodontology* **24**, 626-631.

Palomo, F., Wantland, L., Sanchez, A., Volpe, A.R., McCool, J. & DeVizio, W. (1994). The effect of three commercially available dentifrices containing triclosan on supragingival plaque formation and gingivitis: a six month clinical study. *International Dental Journal* **44**, 75-81.

Papapanou, R.N. (1994). Epidemiology and natural history of periodontal disease. In: Lang, N.P. & Karring, T., eds. *Proceedings of the 1st European Workshop on Periodontology.* London: Quintessence, pp. 23-41.

Perlich, M.A., Bacca, L.A., Bolimer, B.W., Lanzalaco, A.C., McClanahan, L.K., Sewak, L.K., Beiswanger, B.B., Eichold, W.A., Hull, J.R., Jackson, R.D. & Mau, M.S. (1995). The clinical effect of dentifrices containing stabilised stannous fluoride on plaque formation and gingivitis and gingival bleeding – a six-month study. *Journal of Clinical Dentistry* **6**, 54-58.

Pluss, E.M., Engelberg, P.R. & Rateitschak, K.H. (1975). Effect of chlorhexidine on plaque formation under a periodontal pack. *Journal of Clinical Periodontology* **2**, 136-142,

Pontefract, H., Hughes, J., Kemp, K., Yates, R., Newcombe, R.G. & Addy, M. (2001). The erosive effects of some mouth rinses on enamel. A study *in situ. Journal of Clinical Periodontology* **28**, 319-324.

Porter S.R. & Scully, C. (1994). Periodontal aspects of systemic disease classifications. In: Lang, N.P. & Karring, T., eds. *Proceedings of the 1st European Workshop on Periodontology.* London: Quintessence, pp. 375-414.

Quirynen, M., Aventroodt, P., Peeters, W., Pauwels, M., Coucke, W. & Van Steenberge, D. (2001). Effect of different chlorhexidine formulations in mouthrinses on de novo plaque formation. *Journal of Clinical Periodontology* **28**, 1127-1136.

Quirynen, M., Bollen, C., Vandekerckhove, B., Dekeyser, C., Papaioannou, W. & Eyssen, H. (1995). Full vs partial mouth disinfection in the treatment of periodontal infections: short term clinical and microbiological observations. *Journal of Dental Research* **74**, 1459-1467.

Quirynen, M., De Soete, M., Dierickx, K. & van Steenberghe, D. (2001). The intra-oral translocation of periodontopathogens jeopardises the outcome of periodontal therapy. A review of the literature. *Journal of Clinical Periodontology* **28**, 499-507.

Quirynen, M., Marachal, M. & van Steenberghe, D. (1990). Comparative anti-plaque activity of sanguinarine and chlorhexidine in man. *Journal of Clinical Periodontology* **17**, 223-227.

Renton-Harper, P.R., Milsom, S., Wade, W.G., Addy, M., Moran, J. & Newcombe, R.G. (1995). An approach to efficacy screening of mouth rinses: studies on a group of French products (II). Inhibition of salivary bacteria and plaque *in vivo*. *Journal of Clinical Periodontology* **22**, 723-727..

Renvert, S. & Birkhed, D. (1995). Comparison between 3 triclosan dentifrices on plaque, gingivitis and salivary microflora. *Journal of Clinical Periodontology* **22**, 63-70.

Roberts, W.R. & Addy, M. (1981). Comparison of *in vitro* and *in vivo* antibacterial properties of antiseptic mouth rinses containing chlorhexidine, alexidine, CPC and hexetidine. Relevance to mode of action. *Journal of Clinical Periodontology* **8**, 295-310.

Rolla, G., Kjaerheim, V. & Waaler, S.M. (1997). The role of antiseptics in secondary prevention. In: Lang, N.P., Karring, T. & Lindhe, J., eds. *Proceedings of the 2nd European Workshop on Periodontology, Chemicals in Periodontics*. Berlin: Quintessence, pp. 120-130.

Rosling, B., Wannfors, B., Volpe, A.R., Furuichi, Y., Ramberg, P. & Lindhe, J. (1997). The use of a triclosan/copolymer dentifrice may retard the progression of periodontitis. *Journal of Clinical Periodontology* **24**, 873-880.

Rugg-Gunn, A.J. & MacGregor, D.M. (1978). A survey of tooth brushing behaviour in children and young adults. *Journal of Periodontal Research* **13**, 382-388.

Sanz, M., Vallcorba, N., Fabregues, S., Muller, I. & Herkstroter, F. (1994). The effect of a dentifrice containing chlorhexidine and zinc on plaque, gingivitis, calculus and tooth staining. *Journal of Clinical Periodontology* **21**, 431-437.

Saxen, L., Niemi, M.L. & Ainamo, J. (1976). Intra-oral spread of the antimicrobial effect of a chlorhexidine gel. *Scandinavian Journal of Dental Research* **84**, 304-307.

Saxer, U.P. & Muhlemann, H. (1983). Synergistic anti-plaque effects of a zinc fluoride/hexetidine containing mouthwash. A review. *Helvetica Odontologica Acta* **27**, 1-16.

Schiott, C.R., Löe, H. & Briner, W.N. (1976). Two years use of chlorhexidine in man. 4. Effect on various medical parameters. *Journal of Periodontal Research* **11**, 158-164.

Schiott, C., Löe, H., Jensen, S.B., Kilian, M., Davies, R.M. & Glavind, K. (1970). The effect of chlorhexidine mouthrinses on the human oral flora. *Journal of Periodontal Research* **5**, 84-89.

Schroeder, H.E. (1969). In: *Formation and Inhibition of Dental Calculus*. Berlin: Hans Huber, pp.145-172.

Segreto, V.A., Collins, E.M., Beiswanger, B.B., de la Rosa, M., Isaacs, R.L., Lang, N.P., Mallet, M.E. & Meckel, A.H. (1986). A comparison of mouthwashes containing two concentrations of chlorhexidine. *Journal of Periodontal Research* **21**, Suppl. 16, 23-32.

Shaw, W.C., Addy, M., Griffiths, S. & Price, C. (1984). Chlorhexidine and traumatic ulcers in orthodontic patients. *European Journal of Orthodontics* **6**, 137-140.

Sheen, S., Eisenburger, M. & Addy, M. (2002). The effect of toothpaste on the plaque inhibitory properties of a cetylpyridinium chloride mouth rinse. *Journal of Clinical Periodontology* (in press).

Sheen, S., Owens, J. & Addy, M. (2001). The effect of toothpaste on the propensity of chlorhexidine and cetylpyridinium chloride to produce staining *in vitro*: a possible predictor of inactivation. *Journal of Clinical Periodontology* **28**, 46-51.

Simonetti, N., D'Aurin, F.D., Strippoli, V. & Lucchetti, G (1988). Itraconazole: increased activity of chlorhexidine. *Drugs and Experimental Clinical Research* **14**, 19-23.

Skaare, A.B., Herlofson, B.B. & Barkvoll, P (1996). Mouthrinses containing triclosan reduce the incidence of recurrent aphthous ulcers (RAU). *Journal of Clinical Periodontology* **23**, 778-782.

Slots, J. & Rams, T.E. (1990). Antibiotics in periodontal therapy: advantages and disadvantages. *Journal of Clinical Periodontology* **17**, 479-493.

Smith, A., Moran, J., Dangler, L.V., Leight, R.S. & Addy, M. (1996). The efficacy of an anti-gingivitis chewing gum. *Journal of Clinical Periodontology* **23**,19-24.

Soskolne, A., Golomb, G., Friedman, M. & Sela, M.N. (1983). New sustained release dosage form of chlorhexidine for dental use. II. Use in periodontal therapy. *Journal of Periodontol Research* **18**, 330-336.

Stephen, K.W., Saxton, C.A., Jones, C.L., Ritchie, J.A. & Morrison, T. (1990). Control of gingivitis and calculus by a dentifrice containing a zinc salt and triclosan. *Journal of Periodontology* **61**, 674-679.

Storhaug, K. (1977). Hibitane in oral disease in handicapped patients. *Journal of Clinical Periodontology* **4**, 102-107.

Stralfors, A. (1961). In: Muhlemann, H.R. & Konig, K.G., eds. Caries Symposium. Berne: Hans Huber, p. 154.

Svatun, B. (1978). Plaque inhibitory effect of dentifrices containing stannous fluoride. *Acta Odontologica Scandinavica* **36**, 205-210.

Svatun, B., Saxton, C.A., Rolla, G. & van der Ooderaa, F. (1989). A one year study on the maintainance of gingival health by a dentifrice containing a zinc salt and a non-ionic anti-microbial agent. *Journal of Clinical Periodontology* **16**, 75-80.

Toth, B.B., Martin, J.W. & Fleming, T.J. (1990). Oral complications associated with cancer therapy. A MD Anderson Cancer Center experience. *Journal of Clinical Periodontology* **17**, 508-515.

Van der Weijden, G.A., Timmerman, M.F., Danser, M.M. & van der Velden, U. (1998). The role of electric toothbrushes: advantages and limitations. In: Lang, N.P., Attstrom, R. & Löe, H. *Proceedings of the European Workshop on Mechanical Plaque Control*. Berlin: Quintessence Verlag, pp. 138-155.

Wachtel, H. (1994). Surgical periodontal therapy: In: Lang, N.P. & Karring, T., eds. *Proceedings of the 1st European Workshop on Periodontology*. London: Quintessence, pp. 159-171.

Wade, W. & Addy, M. (1989). *In vitro* activity of a chlorhexidine containing mouth-rinse against subgingival bacteria. *Journal of Periodontology* **60**, 521-525.

Wade, A.B., Blake, G.C. & Mirza, K.B. (1966). Effectiveness of metronidazole in treating the acute phase of ulcerative gingivitis. *Dental Practice* **16**, 440-443.

Wade, W.G. & Slayne, M.A. (1997). Controlling plaque by disrupting the process of plaque formation. *Periodontology 2000* **15**, 25-31.

Watts, A. & Addy, M. (2001). Tooth discolouration and staining: A review of the literature. *British Dental Journal* **190**, 309-316.

Wennstrom, J.L. (1992). Subgingival irrigation systems for the control of oral infections. *International Dental Journal* **42**, 281-285.

Wennstrom, J.L. (1997). Rinsing, irrigation and sustained delivery. In: Lang, N.P., Karring, T. & Lindhe, J., eds. *Proceedings of the 2nd European Workshop on Periodontology, Chemicals in Periodontics*. Berlin: Quintessence, pp. 131-151.

World Medical Association (1996). *Declaration of Helsinki*. 48th World Medical Assembly, Somerset West, Republic of South Africa.

World Workshop in Periodontics (1996a). Consensus report on prevention. *Annals of Periodontology* **1**, 250-255.

World Workshop on Periodontics (1996b). Consensus report on periodontal disease: pathogenesis and microbial factors. *Annals of Periodontology* **1**, 926-932.

Worral, S.F., Knibbs, P.J. & Glenwright, H.D. (1987). Methods of reducing contamination of the atmosphere from use of an air polisher. *British Dental Journal* **163**, 118-119.

Worthington, H.V., Blinkhorn, A.S., Petrone, M. & Volpe, A.R.

(1993). A six month clinical study of the effect of a pre-brush rinse on plaque removal and gingivitis. *British Dental Journal* **175**, 322-329.

Wray, D., Ferguson, M.M. & Geddes, D.A.M. (1978). The effect of povidone iodine mouthwash on plaque accumulation and thyroid function. *British Dental Journal* **144**, 14-16.

Yates, R., Jenkins, S., Newcombe, R.G., Wade, W.G., Moran, J. & Addy, M. (1993). A 6-month home usage trial of a 1% chlorhexidine toothpaste. 1. Effects on plaque, gingivitis, calculus and tooth staining. *Journal of Clinical Periodontology* **20**, 130-138.

Yates, R., Moran, J., Addy, M., Mullan, P.J., Wade, W. & Newcombe, R. (1997). The comparative effect of acidified sodium chlorite and chlorhexidine mouthrinses on plaque regrowth and salivary bacterial counts. *Journal of Clinical Periodontology* **24**, 603-609.

Zambon, J.J. (1996). Periodontal Diseases: Microbial factors. Proceedings of the 1996 World Workshop in Periodontics. *Annals of Periodontology* **1**, 879-925.

CHAPTER 23

The Use of Antibiotics in Periodontal Therapy

Andrea Mombelli

Principles for antibiotic therapy
    The limitations of mechanical therapy
    Specific characteristics of the periodontal infection
    Infection concepts and treatment goals
    Drug delivery routes

Evaluation of antimicrobial agents for periodontal therapy
    Systemic antimicrobial therapy in clinical trials
    Local antimicrobial therapy in clinical trials
    Comparison of treatment methods

Overall conclusion

PRINCIPLES FOR ANTIBIOTIC THERAPY

The limitations of mechanical therapy. Can antimicrobial agents help?

Accumulation of bacteria on hard oral surfaces is the primary cause of gingivitis and periodontitis. Therefore, regular mechanical removal of bacterial plaque from all non-shedding oral surfaces is considered the primary means to prevent and stop the progression of periodontal disease. Longitudinal studies have shown the efficacy of the standard treatment approach consisting of the combination of systematic scaling and planing of the root surfaces, the patient's daily meticulous oral hygiene and regular maintenance visits to remove newly formed subgingival deposits. In most cases, periodontal disease can be treated successfully in this way and results can be maintained over prolonged periods of time. The main adverse effects of this approach are irreversible hard tissue damage and gingival recession, ensuing from repetitive mechanical brushing and scraping of tooth surfaces. Substantial hard tissue trauma may occasionally arise from repeated treatment of sites that are locally unresponsive or have recurrent disease (Fig. 23-1).

A closer look at the composition of plaque reveals that mechanical treatment is targeted at a variable mixture of different bacteria. Although the number of different species and subspecies occasionally identified in samples from human plaque by far exceeds one hundred, only relatively few organisms show a distinctive pattern of association with disease. Possible pathogens have been suggested among these organisms based on their animal pathogenicity and the demonstration of virulence factors (for review see Chapter 4). Certain species, notably *Actinobacillus actinomycetemcomitans* and *Porphyromonas gingivalis*, have attracted particular attention because longitudinal and retrospective studies have indicated an increased risk for periodontal breakdown in positive sites and because results of treatment have been better if the organisms could no longer be detected at follow-up (Bragd et al. 1987, Carlos et al. 1988, Haffajee et al. 1991, Grossi et al. 1994, Haffajee & Socransky 1994). *If periodontal disease is in fact caused by a limited number of bacterial species, then non-specific continuous plaque suppression is not the only possibility for prevention and therapy. Specific elimination or reduction of pathogenic bacteria from plaque becomes a valid alternative.*

Mechanical treatment may not predictably eliminate putative pathogens, such as *A. actinomycetemcomitans*, from the subgingival area. The pathogens may be inaccessible by mechanical interventions due to their ability to invade periodontal tissues or dentin tubules (Adriaens et al. 1988) or because they reside in sites inaccessible for periodontal instruments. This may be the case in the presence of root concavities or in furcations. In addition, successfully treated sites may be recolonized by periodontal pathogens persisting in non-dental areas such as the dorsum of the tongue or the tonsils. Although we know that mechanical periodontal therapy may be clinically successful in many patients even if all putative pathogens

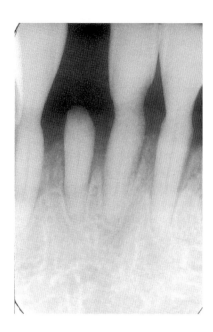

Fig. 23-1. Conventional periodontal therapy and maintenance imply repeated treatment of sites with localized unresponsive or recurrent disease, resulting in sometimes substantial hard tissue trauma.

are not completely eradicated, persistence or regrowth of certain microorganisms in treated sites should be considered the main cause of unsatisfactory treatment outcomes. *Can antimicrobial agents, delivered either locally or systemically, enhance the effect of root instrumentation, limit its side effects, or could they even be a substitute in some cases?*

In the late 1930s and early 1940s the appearance of potent chemotherapeutic agents selectively active against bacteria, revolutionized the treatment of bacterial infections. The discovery of such drugs – sulfonamides, penicillin and streptomycin – led many to believe that bacterial infections were about to vanish. After six decades of experience with these and hundreds of additionally developed chemotherapeutic drugs, the potential and limitation of antimicrobial therapy are better understood. Emerging problems, resulting from the widespread use of antibiotics have modified the general perception of the capabilities of antimicrobial agents. Over the years, bacteria have developed a remarkable ability to withstand or repel many antibiotic agents and are increasingly resistant to formerly potent agents. The use of antibiotics may disturb the delicate ecologic equilibrium of the body, allowing the proliferation of resistant bacteria or nonbacterial organisms. Sometimes this may initiate new infections that are worse than the ones originally treated. In addition, no antibacterial drug is absolutely non-toxic and the use of any antimicrobial agent carries with it accompanying risks.

Before any antimicrobial agent can be recommended for periodontal therapy a number of conditions need to be fulfilled. First, the drug must show *in vitro* activity against the organisms considered most important in the etiology of the disease. Next it should be demonstrated that a dose sufficient to kill the target organisms can be reached within the subgingival environment. At this dose the drug should not have major local or systemic adverse effects. It should be safe to maintain the required concentration over a

long enough period to significantly affect the microbiota. Well-controlled longitudinal studies then need to be carried out in patients with periodontal disease, demonstrating a favorable clinical outcome of therapy with the agent. Finally, one would like to see a practical advantage over conventional treatment alternatives (better outcome, less adverse effects, simpler to perform, cheaper, faster).

Specific characteristics of the periodontal infection

In discussing the potential usefulness of chemotherapeutic agents to treat periodontal diseases, one should be clear that antibiotics and antiseptics can kill living bacteria, but will neither eliminate calculus nor remove bacterial debris. The recognition of periodontitis as an infection caused by living microorganisms is thus a fundamental issue for any chemotherapeutic treatment concept. The term infection refers to the presence and multiplication of microorganisms in or on body tissues. The uniqueness of plaque-associated dental diseases as infections relates to the lack of massive bacterial invasion of tissues. Although there is evidence for bacterial penetration in severely diseased periodontal tissues, notably in periodontal abscesses and in acute necrotizing ulcerative lesions (Listgarten 1965, Saglie et al. 1982a,b, Allenspach-Petrzilka & Guggenheim 1983, Carranza et al. 1983), it has not been generally accepted that true bacterial invasion (including multiplication of bacteria within tissues) is crucial for periodontal disease progression. Bacteria in the subgingival plaque obviously interact with host tissues even without direct tissue penetration. Thus, for any antimicrobial agent used in periodontal therapy to have an effect there is the requirement that the agent is available at a sufficiently high concentration not only within, but also in the subgingival environment outside the periodontal tissues

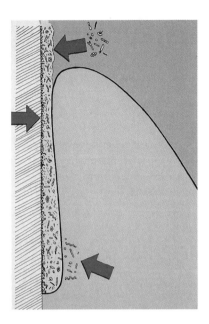

Fig. 23-2. Specific conditions for the use of antimicrobial agents in periodontal therapy. The periodontal pocket as an open site is subject to recolonization after therapy (top arrow). The subgingival bacteria are protected from antimicrobial agents in a biofilm (middle arrow). The agent must be available at a sufficiently high concentration not only within, but also in the subgingival environment outside, the periodontal tissues (bottom arrow).

(Fig. 23-2). Periodontal pockets may actually contain an enormous amount of bacteria. This may cause problems for antimicrobial agents to work properly because they may be inhibited, inactivated or degraded by non-target microorganisms.

In addition, the subgingival microbiota accumulate on the root surface to form an adherent layer of plaque. Accumulation of bacteria on solid surfaces can be observed on virtually all surfaces immersed in natural aqueous environments and is called "biofilm" formation. Extensive bacterial growth, accompanied by excretion of copious amounts of extracellular polymers, is a typical phenomenon in biofilms. Biofilms effectively protect bacteria from antimicrobial agents (Anwar et al. 1990, 1992). Bacteria involved in adhesion-mediated infections that develop on permanently or temporarily implanted materials such as intravascular catheters, vascular prostheses or heart valves are notoriously resistant to systemic antimicrobial therapy and tend to persist until the device is removed (Gristina 1987, Marshall 1992). Several mechanisms leading to this increased resistance of bacteria in biofilms have been proposed. Due to limited diffusion, antimicrobial agents may simply not reach deeper parts of a biofilm at sufficiently high levels during a given time of exposure. Within biofilms an unequal distribution of electrical charge may develop. Intrusion may thus be further complicated in certain areas of the biofilm depending on the charge of the penetrating molecule. Because of a limited availability of nutrients within the biofilm, bacteria may also reduce their metabolism, rendering them less susceptible to killing by agents interfering with protein, DNA or cell wall synthesis. Most interesting are the results from recent *in vitro* experiments, indicating that the attachment of bacteria to surfaces may trigger genes which activate specific resistance mechanisms. Since these mechanisms are switched on upon contact, they may occur already in newly forming, very thin biofilms (Costerton et al. 1995).

The above described problems suggest that treatment of periodontal diseases by antimicrobial agents alone will probably not suffice and indicate that mechanical instrumentation to disrupt the biofilm and to remove the bulk of bacterial deposits must precede antimicrobial therapy.

Infection concepts and treatment goals

Infections may be divided into exogenous and endogenous on the basis of the source of the infecting agent. While *exogenous infections* are caused by organisms acquired from an external source (primary pathogens), *endogenous infections* are caused by organisms present already in the healthy host (commensal organisms). Infections caused by endogenous microbes are called *opportunistic infections* if they occur in the usual habitat of the organisms. They may be the result of changing ecologic conditions or may be due to a decrease in host resistance. Exogenous infections are caused by organisms that are not part of the normal flora. They are transmitted to healthy subjects from diseased humans or animals, or from carriers that show no signs of disease. *A. actinomycetemcomitans* and *P. gingivalis* are regarded as true infectious agents in periodontal disease by some researchers. This view is based on findings of low prevalence of these microorganisms in periodontally healthy individuals in North America and Europe, evidence for transmission, such as from parent to child or between spouses, findings of immune responses towards these bacteria that markedly exceed those expected for endogenous infections and on clinical studies showing that *A. actinomycetemcomitans* and *P. gingivalis* can be eliminated with appropriate mechanical treatment and adjunctive antibiotic therapy (for review see van Winkelhoff et al. 1996).

The majority of organisms associated with periodontal disease can, however, also be detected fre-

Table 23-1. Comparison of local and systemic antimicrobial therapy

Issue	Systemic administration	Local administration
Drug distribution	Wide distribution	Narrow effective range
Drug concentration	Variable levels in different body compartments	High dose at treated site, low levels elsewhere
Therapeutic potential	May reach widely distributed microorganisms better	May act better locally on biofilm associated bacteria
Problems	Systemic side effects	Reinfection from non-treated sites
Clinical limitations	Requires good patient compliance	Infection limited to the treated site
Diagnostic problems	Identification of pathogens, choice of drug	Distribution pattern of lesions and pathogens, identification of sites to be treated

quently at low numbers in the absence of periodontal disease, and the view that *A. actinomycetemcomitans* and *P. gingivalis* cause true infections has been opposed on the basis of cross-sectional studies showing a high prevalence of the two organisms in certain populations, particularly those from developing countries. If *A. actinomycetemcomitans* and *P. gingivalis* are truly exogenous pathogens, the elimination of these organisms should be a primary objective of therapy. In the therapy of opportunistic infections, however, elimination is not a realistic goal. Successfully suppressed putative pathogens may grow back if favorable ecologic conditions (e.g. deep pockets) persist. Continuous control of ecologic factors will be necessary after initial treatment. Thus, therapy will not have an unambiguously defined endpoint.

The periodontal flora never consists of one single species. Frequently, several potential pathogens can be identified at the same time, suggesting that interactions between microorganisms play an important role in the development of periodontal disease. The pathogenicity of simultaneously present organisms could be enhanced in an additive or synergistic way. Antagonistic relationships between microorganisms could, however, also occur. Based on the concept that the presence of beneficial bacterial species may suppress the pathogenic impact of pathogens, one can speculate that it may be advantageous to specifically eliminate target bacteria only and to allow the growth of potentially beneficial microorganisms. Such contemplations have been used as an argument to propagate narrow spectrum antibiotics for periodontal therapy.

Drug delivery routes

Antimicrobial agents may be delivered by direct placement into the periodontal pocket or via the systemic route. Each method of delivery has specific advantages and disadvantages (Table 23-1). Local therapy may allow the application of antimicrobial agents at levels that cannot be reached by the systemic route. Local therapy may be particularly successful if the presence of target organisms is confined to the clinically visible lesions. On the other hand, systemically administered antibiotics may reach widely distributed microorganisms. Studies have shown that periodontal bacteria may be distributed throughout the whole mouth in some patients (Mombelli et al. 1991a, 1994), including non-dental sites, such as the dorsum of the tongue or tonsillary crypts (Zambon et al. 1981, Van Winkelhoff et al. 1988, Müller et al. 1993, 1995, Pavicic et al. 1994). Disadvantages of systemic antibiotic therapy relate to the fact that the drug is dissolved by dispersal over the whole body, and only a small portion of the total dose actually reaches the subgingival microflora in the periodontal pocket. Adverse drug reactions are a greater concern and more likely to occur if drugs are distributed via the systemic route. Even mild forms of unwanted effects may severely decrease patient compliance (Loesche et al. 1993). Local delivery is independent of patient compliance.

Local drug delivery systems are means of drug application to confined areas. For the treatment of periodontal disease, local delivery of antimicrobial drugs ranges from simple pocket irrigation, over the placement of drug-containing ointments and gels, to sophisticated devices for sustained release of antibacterial agents. In order to be effective, the drug should not only reach the entire area affected by the disease, including the base of the pocket, but should also be maintained at a sufficiently high local concentration for some time. With a mouthrinse or supragingival irrigation it is not possible to predictably deliver an agent to the deeper parts of a periodontal defect (Pitcher et al. 1980, Eakle et al. 1986). Agents brought into periodontal pockets by subgingival irrigation are washed out rapidly by the gingival fluid. Based on an assumed pocket volume of 0.5 ml and a gingival fluid flow rate of 20 µl/h, Goodson (1989) estimated that the half-time of a non-binding drug placed into a pocket is about 1 minute. Even a highly concentrated, highly potent agent would thus be diluted below a minimal inhibitory concentration (MIC) for oral microorganisms within minutes. If an agent can bind to surfaces and be released in active form, a prolonged

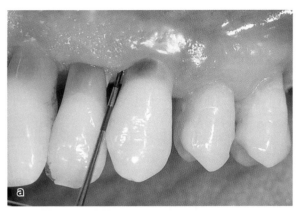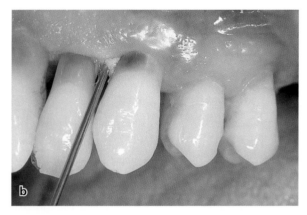

Fig. 23-3. An antimicrobial gel is applied with a syringe inserted into a residual pocket (a). For retention of the agent in the site, the viscosity of the carrier should change immediately. A large portion of the product may otherwise be expelled from the pocket quickly (b).

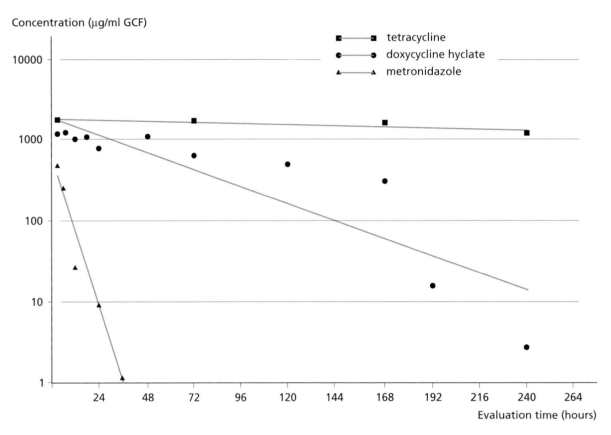

Fig. 23-4. Mean concentration of tetracycline in gingival crevicular fluid (GCF) during tetracycline fiber treatment (Tonetti et al. 1990), of doxycycline hyclate after application in a biodegradable polymer (Stoller et al. 1998), and of metronidazole after application of 25% metronidazole dental gel (Stoltze 1992).

time of antibacterial activity could be expected. Such an effect has in fact been noted for salivary concentrations of chlorhexidine after use of chlorhexidine mouthrinse (Bonesvoll & Gjermo 1978). Although there are indications that this may also occur to a certain extent within the periodontal pocket, for instance after prolonged subgingival irrigation with tetracycline (Tonetti et al. 1990), the potential to create a drug reservoir of significant size on the small surface area available in a periodontal pocket is limited. To maintain a high concentration over a prolonged period of time, the flushing action of the crevicular fluid

flow has to be counteracted by a steady release of the drug from a larger reservoir. Considering the small volume of a periodontal pocket and the pressure exerted by the tonus of the periodontal tissues on anything inserted, it appears unlikely that this task can be completed by a carrier that does not maintain its physical stability for some time and that cannot be secured against premature loss. Gels, for instance, rapidly disappear after instillation into periodontal pockets (Fig. 23-3a,b), unless they change their viscosity immediately after placement (Oostervaal et al. 1990, Stoltze 1995). Viscous and/or biodegradable de-

Table 23-2. Characteristics of antimicrobial agents used in the treatment of periodontal disease (adapted from Lorian 1986, Slots & Rams 1990)

Antimicrobial agent	Dose (mg)	c Serum (μg/ml)	c Crevicular fluid (μg/ml)	t_{max} Serum (h)	Half-life (h)
Penicillin	500	3	ND	1	0.5
Amoxicillin	500	8	3-4	1.5-2	0.8-2
Doxycycline	200	2-3	2-8	2	12-22
Tetracycline	500	3-4	5-12	2-3	2-3
Clindamycin	150	2-3	1-2	1	2-4
Metronidazole	500	6-12	8-10	1-2	6-12
Ciprofloxacin	500	1.9-2.9	ND	1-2	3-6

c: concentration.
t_{max}: hours to reach peak serum concentration.
ND: not determined.

vices show an exponential decrease of their concentration in gingival fluid. Depending on the physical and chemical nature of the carrier, the drug reservoir in the periodontal pocket will be depleted within hours to days after placement. Controlled delivery of an antimicrobial agent over several days has been shown for tetracycline released from non-degradable monolithic ethylene vinyl acetate fibers (Fig. 23-4).

EVALUATION OF ANTIMICROBIAL AGENTS FOR PERIODONTAL THERAPY

In the large range of antimicrobial agents, a limited number have been tested thoroughly for use in periodontal therapy. The drugs more extensively investigated for systemic use include tetracycline, minocycline and doxycycline, erythromycin, clindamycin, ampicillin, amoxicillin, and the nitro-imidazole compounds metronidazole and ornidazole. The drugs investigated for local application include tetracycline, minocycline, doxycycline, metronidazole and chlorhexidine.

The first antibiotics used in periodontal therapy were mainly systemically administered penicillins. The choice was initially based on empirical evidence exclusively. Penicillins and cephalosporins act by inhibition of cell wall synthesis. They are narrow-spectrum and bactericidal. Among the penicillins, amoxicillin has been favored for treatment of periodontal disease because of its considerable activity against several periodontal pathogens at levels available in gingival fluid. The molecular structure of penicillins includes a β-lactam ring that may be cleaved by bacterial enzymes. Some bacterial β-lactamases have a high affinity for clavulanic acid, a β-lactam molecule without antimicrobial activity. To inhibit bacterial β-

lactamase activity, clavulanic acid has been added successfully to amoxicillin. This combination (Augmentin®) has been tested for periodontal therapy in clinical studies. Tetracycline-HCl became popular in the 1970s due to its broad spectrum antimicrobial activity and low toxicity. The tetracyclines, clindamycin and erythromycin are inhibitors of protein synthesis. They have a broad-spectrum of activity and are bacteriostatic. In addition to their antimicrobial effect, tetracyclines are capable of inhibiting collagenase (Golub et al. 1985). This inhibition may interfere with tissue breakdown in periodontal disease. Furthermore they bind to tooth surfaces, from where they may be released slowly over time (Stabholz et al. 1993). The nitro-imidazoles (metronidazole and ornidazole) and the quinolone antibiotics (e.g. ciprofloxacin) act by inhibiting DNA synthesis. Metronidazole is known to convert into several short-lived intermediates after diffusion into an anaerobic organism. These products react with the DNA and other bacterial macromolecules, resulting in cell death. The process involves reductive pathways characteristic of strictly anaerobic bacteria and protozoa, but not aerobic or microaerophilic organisms. Thus, metronidazole affects specifically the obligately anaerobic part of the oral flora, including *P. gingivalis* and other black-pigmenting Gram-negative organisms, but not *A. actinomycetemcomitans*, a facultative anaerobe.

The concentrations following systemic administration of the most common antimicrobial agents used in the treatment of periodontal disease are listed in Table 23-2. The *in vitro* susceptibility of *A. actinomycetemcomitans* to selected antimicrobial agents is given in Table 23-3 and the susceptibility of *P. gingivalis* is listed in Table 23-4. The data given in these tables may serve as a base for the choice of an appropriate agent. However, it is important to remember that *in vitro* tests do not reflect the true conditions found in periodontal pockets. In particular, they do not account for the biofilm effect. One should add that MIC values de-

Table 23-3. Susceptibility of *A. actinomycetemcomitans* to selected antimicrobial agents. MIC90: minimal inhibitory concentration for 90% of the strains (adapted from Mombelli & van Winkelhoff 1997)

Antimicrobial agent	MIC90 µg/ml	Reference
Penicillin	4.0	Pajukanta et al. (1993b)
	1.0	Walker et al. (1985)
	6.25	Höffler et al. (1980)
Amoxicillin	1.0	Pajukanta et al. (1993b)
	2.0	Walker et al. (1985)
	1.6	Höffler et al. (1980)
Tetracycline	0.5	Pajukanta et al. (1993b)
	8.0	Walker et al. (1985), Walker (1992)
Doxycycline	1.0	Pajukanta et al. (1993b)
	3.1	Höffler et al. (1980)
Metronidazole	32	Pajukanta et al. (1993b)
	32	Jousimies-Somer et al. (1988)
	12.5	Höffler et al. (1980)

Table 23-4. Susceptibility of *P. gingivalis* to selected antimicrobial agents (adapted from Mombelli & van Winkelhoff 1997)

Antimicrobial agent	MIC90 µg/ml	Reference
Penicillin	0.016	Pajukanta et al. (1993a)
	0.29	Baker et al. (1983)
Amoxicillin	0.023	Pajukanta et al. (1993a)
	< 1.0	Walker (1992)
Doxycycline	0.047	Pajukanta et al. (1993a)
Metronidazole	0.023	Pajukanta et al. (1993a)
	2.1	Baker et al. (1983)
	2.0	Walker (1992)
Clindamycin	0.016	Pajukanta et al. (1993a)
	< 1.0	Walker (1992)

Table 23-5. Adverse effects of antibiotics used in the treatment of periodontal diseases

Antimicrobial agent	Frequent effects	Infrequent effects
Penicillin	hypersensitivity (mainly rashes), nausea, diarrhea	hematological toxicity, encephalopathy, pseudomembranous colitis (ampicillin)
Tetracycline	gastrointestinal intolerance, Candidiasis, dental staining and hypoplasia in childhood, nausea, diarrhea, interaction with oral contraceptives	photosensitivity, nephrotoxicity, intracranial hypertension
Metronidazole	gastrointestinal intolerance, nausea, antabus effect, diarrhea, unpleasant metallic taste	peripheral neuropathy, furred tongue
Clindamycin	rashes, nausea, diarrhea	pseudomembranous colitis, hepatitis

pend on technical details that may vary between laboratories. As a consequence, demonstration of *in vitro* susceptibility is no proof that an agent will work in treatment of periodontal disease.

Since the subgingival microbiota in periodontitis often harbors several putative periodontopathic species with different antimicrobial susceptibility, combination drug therapy may be useful. A combination of antimicrobial drugs may have a wider spectrum of activity than a single agent. Overlaps of the antimicrobial spectrum may reduce the possible development of bacterial resistance. For some combinations of drugs there may be synergy in action against target organisms, allowing a lower dose of the single agents. A synergistic effect against *A. actinomycetemcomitans* has been noted *in vitro* between metronidazole and its hydroxy metabolite (Jousimies-Somer et al. 1988, Pavicic et al. 1991) and between these two compounds and amoxicillin (Pavicic et al. 1992). With some drug combinations there may, however, also be antagonistic drug interaction. For instance, bacteriostatic agents such as tetracyclines, which suppress cell division, decrease the antimicrobial effect of bactericidal antibiotics such as β-lactam drugs or metronidazole, which act during bacterial cell division. Combination drug therapy may also lead to increased adverse reactions.

Table 23-5 lists common adverse reactions to systemic antibiotic therapy (for a detailed overview the reader is referred to Walker 1996). The penicillins are among the least toxic antibiotics. Hypersensitivity reactions are by far the most important and most common adverse effects of these drugs. Most reactions are mild and limited to a rash or skin lesion in the head or neck region. More severe reactions may induce swelling and tenderness of joints. In highly sensitized patients a life-threatening anaphylactic reaction may develop. The systemic use of tetracyclines may lead to epigastric pain, vomiting or diarrhea. Tetracyclines can induce changes in the intestinal flora, and superinfections with non-bacterial microorganisms (i.e. *Candida albicans*) may emerge. Tetracyclines are deposited in calcifying areas of teeth and bones where they cause yellow discoloration. Systemic administration of clindamycin may be accompanied by gastrointestinal disturbances, leading to diarrhea or cramps and may cause mild skin rashes. The suppression of the normal intestinal flora increases the risk for colonization of *Clostridium difficile*, which may cause a severe colon infection. Although not related to *C. difficile*, gastrointestinal problems are also the most frequent adverse event of systemic metronidazole therapy. Nausea, headache, anorexia, vomiting may be experienced. Symptoms may be more pronounced with alcohol consumption, because imidazoles affect the activity of liver enzymes. Because some cases have developed permanent peripheral neuropathies (numbness or paresthesia), patients should be advised to immediately stop therapy if such symptoms occur.

Systemic antimicrobial therapy in clinical trials

As mentioned before, the ultimate evidence for the efficacy of systemic antibiotics must be obtained from treatment studies in humans with periodontitis. Because compromises are often necessary to conduct an investigation under given clinical, technical or financial circumstances, a large number of studies reported in the literature can be criticized using the basic study quality criteria for evidence-based medicine. Studies may be difficult to interpret and compare due to an unclear status of patients at baseline (treatment history, disease activity, composition of subgingival microbiota), insufficient or non-standardized maintenance after therapy, short observation periods, or lack of randomization and controls. Studies not only vary with regard to the treatment provided, but also in the selection of subjects, sample size, range of study parameters, outcome variables, the duration of the study, and the controls to which the test procedure is compared. In most studies, systemic antibiotics have been used as an adjunct to scaling and root planing. Typically, the effect of mechanical therapy plus the antimicrobial agent has been compared to mechanical treatment alone. In studies evaluating the effect of antimicrobial therapy in patients with refractory periodontitis or with recurrent abscess formation, placebo control is often lacking for ethical reasons.

Chronic and aggressive periodontitis in the adult patient

Several case reports claimed clinical success with *tetracycline* therapy; however, in placebo controlled trials, only slight differences were noted in the change of mean probing depths and attachment levels between patients receiving tetracycline or placebo as an adjunct to mechanical therapy (Listgarten et al. 1978, Helldén et al. 1979, Slots et al. 1979, Scopp et al. 1980, Lindhe et al. 1983).

Systemic *metronidazole* in conjunction with scaling and root planing yielded slightly better results than scaling alone (Clark et al. 1983, Lekovic et al. 1983, Lindhe et al. 1983, Joyston-Bechal et al. 1984, 1986, Loesche et al. 1984, Söder et al. 1990). No improvement in clinical effects of therapy was found in patients receiving metronidazole in conjunction with periodontal surgery over surgery alone (Sterry et al. 1985, Mahmood & Dolby 1987). In rapidly progressive periodontitis, metronidazole seemed to improve clinical conditions for up to 6 months compared to periodontal scaling alone (Söder et al. 1989, 1990).

A limited number of patients with advanced adult periodontitis were treated with *clindamycin* without concurrent mechanical therapy, except oral hygiene instructions. Despite this limited treatment regimen, clinical and microbiologic parameters improved over the following 6 months. *P. gingivalis* appeared to be particularly susceptible to clindamycin therapy; this species was no longer detected at 6 months. Other organisms, however, were resistant to clindamycin and were found at slightly higher levels after 6 months (Ohta et al. 1986).

Haffajee et al. (1995) examined the effects of systemic amoxicillin plus clavulanic acid, tetracycline HCl, or placebo therapy, given for 30 days in conjunction with subgingival debridement and modified Widman flap surgery, in adults with progressive periodontitis. Significantly greater mean gains in clinical periodontal attachment and decreased probing depths were measured at 10 months post-treatment in subjects receiving adjunctive systemic amoxicillin plus clavulanic acid or tetracycline therapy as compared to the placebo regimen. Although decreases in numbers of subgingival putative periodontal pathogens paralleled the marked clinical improvements, no pathogen was eliminated from the subgingival microbiota.

Metronidazole plus amoxicillin, Augmentin or ciprofloxacin have been used successfully in the treatment of advanced *A. actinomycetemcomitans* associated periodontitis (Christersson et al. 1989, Kornman et al. 1989, van Winkelhoff et al. 1989, 1992, Goené et al. 1990, Pavicic et al. 1992, 1994, Rams et al. 1992). These combinations markedly suppressed or even eliminated *A. actinomycetemcomitans* and other subgingival organisms from periodontitis lesions and other oral sites.

Serial drug regimens studied to date in periodontics include systemic *doxycycline* administered initially and followed by either *amoxicillin* plus clavulanic acid or *metronidazole* (Aitken et al. 1992, Matisko & Bissada 1992). The sequential use of drugs overcomes the potential risk of antagonism between bacteriostatic and bactericidal antibiotics. The value of serial antibiotic therapy in the management of advanced periodontitis merits further investigation.

Conclusion

In general, adult periodontitis can and should be treated without systemic antibiotics. The adjunctive use of antibiotics in adult periodontitis should be limited to cases with advanced or progressive disease. *A. actinomycetemcomitans* associated periodontitis may be treated with adjunctive metronidazole plus amoxicillin.

"Refractory" periodontitis

A beneficial effect of *tetracycline* therapy was reported in several studies in adult patients with "refractory" periodontitis. Double blind studies showed significant reductions in probing pocket depth with systemic tetracycline (Rams & Keyes 1983, McCulloch et al. 1989, 1990).

McCulloch et al. (1990) selected patients on the basis of periodontal disease activity; active disease was defined as loss of clinical attachment or abscess formation. In this study, *doxycycline*, administered for 3 weeks, reduced probing pocket depths significantly more than placebo and resulted in more gain of clinical attachment, however, only at sites with evidence of recent disease activity. The doxycycline regimen reduced the relative risk for subsequent periodontal breakdown over a 7-month period by 43%. Even though adjunctive doxycycline therapy was effective in some active periodontitis patients, it failed to prevent periodontal breakdown in 13 of 29 individuals. Recurrent disease activity after systemic tetracycline therapy was also reported by other authors (van Winkelhoff et al. 1989, Goené et al. 1990, Aitken et al. 1992, Walker et al. 1993). Disease progression may have been caused by subgingival organisms not sufficiently suppressed by the doxycycline therapy. *A. actinomycetemcomitans* and *E. corrodens* were not markedly suppressed in the doxycycline treated patients (McCulloch et al. 1990) and the difference in the composition of the subgingival microbiota between the placebo and doxycycline patients was not significant after 7 months (McCulloch et al. 1990, Kulkarni et al. 1991). Other studies have also pointed to a possible failure of systemic tetracycline in the suppression of subgingival *A. actinomycetemcomitans* (Müller et al. 1989, 1993, van Winkelhoff et al. 1989). In some instances an increase of this organism was even noted (Müller et al. 1990). Furthermore, systemic tetracycline therapy may lead to colonization of superinfecting and opportunistic pathogens (Bragd et al. 1985, Haffajee et al. 1988, Hull et al. 1989). It may thus be speculated that non-antimicrobial effects, such as collagenase inhibition, may have been more important for the observed outcome than the antibiotic action (Golub et al. 1983, 1985).

Systemic *clindamycin* and scaling yielded a significant improvement in patients treated for active periodontal disease despite previous conventional periodontal treatment and systemic tetracycline therapy (Gordon et al. 1985). The clinical effects were associated with significant reductions of spirochetes, motile rods and Gram-negative anaerobic rods, including *P. gingivalis* and *P. intermedia*, and an increase of Gram-positive rods and cocci over 1-2 years (Walker & Gordon 1990). However, clindamycin did not perma-

nently suppress subgingival *P. gingivalis*, which may explain the recurrence of disease activity in some patients. It should also be mentioned that one study patient developed pseudomembraneous colitis, a gastrointestinal superinfection by *Clostridium difficile* which may be life-threatening.

In one study, refractory adult periodontitis patients, who in the past had been subjected to periodontal surgery, systemic tetracycline administration and supportive periodontal therapy, were retreated with scaling and root planing in conjunction with either clindamycin or amoxicillin plus clavulanic acid (Magnusson et al. 1994). The two systemic antimicrobial therapies were prescribed on the basis of the susceptibility of the whole subgingival microbiota (Walker et al. 1983). Over a 2-year evaluation period, the difference in the proportions of sites losing attachment following either clindamycin or amoxicillin plus clavulanic acid therapy was not significant.

Statistically significant improvements in clinical parameters have also been observed after mechanical debridement combined with systemic metronidazole and ornidazole in patients with recurrent periodontal disease (Gusberti et al. 1988, Mombelli et al. 1989).

Conclusion

Various antibiotic regimens have been tested for the treatment of patients not responding to conventional periodontal therapy. Favorable short term effects have been reported; however, a great variability in treatment response among patients has been noted. Re-emergence of putative pathogens has been observed and has been considered the reason for recurrence of disease.

Aggressive localized periodontitis

Reduced gingival inflammation, gain of clinical attachment and alveolar bone were reported following tetracycline therapy in juvenile patients with aggressive localized periodontitis (Slots et al. 1979, Genco et al. 1981, Lindhe 1982, Slots & Rosling 1983). However, as many as 25% of juvenile periodontitis patients treated with tetracycline may experience a reactivation of disease, even if their dentition is professionally cleaned every 3 months after therapy (Lindhe 1982). Further destruction of periodontal attachment was noted in sites with high post-treatment levels of *A. actinomycetemcomitans* (Slots & Rosling 1983, Kornman & Robertson 1985, Mandell & Socransky 1988, Asikainen et al. 1990, Saxén & Asikainen 1993). Suppression of *A. actinomycetemcomitans* does not seem possible in all aggressive localized periodontitis lesions with scaling and root planing and adjunctive systemic tetracycline.

Suppression of *A. actinomycetemcomitans* has been reported for up to 18 months in juvenile patients with aggressive localized periodontitis after mechanical debridement plus metronidazole (200 mg TID, 10 days). In comparison, systemic tetracycline therapy or mechanical treatment alone eliminated *A. actinomy-*

cetemcomitans in only 44% and 67% of the juvenile periodontitis patients, respectively (Saxén & Asikainen 1993). Considering the limited effect of metronidazole on facultative organisms, documented in *in vitro* susceptibility tests (Walker et al. 1985), these results are quite surprising. The hydroxy metabolite of metronidazole may be responsible for the suppression of subgingival *A. actinomycetemcomitans* (Jousimies-Somer et al. 1988, Pavicic et al. 1992). The successful use of metronidazole plus amoxicillin in the treatment of various cases with advanced *A. actinomycetemcomitans* associated periodontitis suggests the adjunctive use of this combination may also be a good choice for aggressive localized periodontitis in juvenile patients (Christersson et al. 1989, Kornman et al. 1989, van Winkelhoff et al. 1989, 1992, Goené et al. 1990, Pavicic et al. 1994).

Conclusion

Several regimens including the adjunctive administration of tetracyclines or metronidazole have been tested for the treatment of localized juvenile periodontitis. Again, re-emergence of putative pathogens, in this case of *A. actinomycetemcomitans,* has been observed and has been considered the reason for recurrence of disease. Metronidazole in combination with amoxicillin may suppress *A. actinomycetemcomitans* more efficiently than single antibiotic regimens.

Implications for clinical practice

Overall, it can be stated that systemic antibiotic therapy may improve the microbiologic and clinical conditions of periodontal patients under certain circumstances. Monotherapy with systemic antibiotics as an adjunct to mechanical periodontal treatment can suppress the total subgingival bacterial load and may induce a significant change in the composition of the subgingival microbiota. However, antibiotic therapy with single antimicrobial agents cannot predictably eliminate periodontal organisms such as *A. actinomycetemcomitans*. To reach this goal, combination therapy, i.e. metronidazole plus amoxicillin, seems to be more appropriate. There is evidence to support the use of systemic antibiotic therapy in cases of *P. gingivalis* and/or *A. actinomycetemcomitans* associated early onset forms of periodontitis. Systemic antibiotic therapy is also indicated in generalized refractory periodontitis patients with evidence of ongoing disease despite optimal mechanical therapy.

It is biologically sound and good medical practice to base systemic antimicrobial therapy on appropriate microbiologic data. In addition, antibiotics should not be administered systemically before completion of thorough mechanical debridement (patients with acute signs of disease such as periodontal abscesses, or acute necrotizing gingivitis, with fever and malaise, may be the exception). Therefore, in most cases, the initial mechanical therapy should be carried out and evaluated before microbiologic testing. The original treatment plan, may be modified six to twelve weeks after initial therapy, taking into account how the periodontal tissues reacted to the non-specific reduction of the bacterial mass by root instrumentation and oral hygiene. Microbial samples from the deepest pocket in each quadrant can give a good picture of the presence and relative importance of putative pathogens in the oral flora (Mombelli et al. 1991b, 1994). Microbial testing should be comprehensive and sensitive enough to determine the presence and relative proportion of the most important periodontal organisms. Since the antimicrobial profiles of most putative periodontal pathogens are quite predictable, susceptibility testing is not routinely performed. One should keep in mind, however, that some important microorganisms may demonstrate resistance to tetracyclines, β-lactam drugs or metronidazole. It is recommended to start drug administration immediately following a mechanical re-instrumentation. In practical terms this often means that the patient commences antibiotic therapy in the evening after the last surgical procedure. Even if no further mechanical therapy is indicated from a clinical point of view, the pockets should be re-instrumented to reduce the subgingival bacterial deposits as much as possible and to disrupt the subgingival biofilm.

After resolution of the periodontal infection, the patient should be placed on an individually tailored maintenance care program. Optimal plaque control by the patient is of paramount importance for a favorable clinical and microbiologic response to systemic antimicrobial therapy (Kornman et al. 1994).

Local antimicrobial therapy in clinical trials

A variety of methods to deliver antimicrobial agents into periodontal pockets have been devised and subjected to numerous kinds of experiments. The pharmacokinetic shortcomings of rinsing, irrigating and similar forms of drug placement, and the lack of significant clinical effects have already been discussed. This section will deal with clinically tested drug delivery systems that fulfill at least the basic pharmacokinetic requirements of sustained drug release. Much of what has been stated about difficulties in the interpretation of studies dealing with the systemic use of antibiotics applies to the studies conducted with local delivery devices. Again, comparison of various forms of therapy is complicated because studies vary with regard to sample size, selection of subjects, range of parameters, controls, duration of the study, and the inclusion of only one form of local drug delivery. Most of the evidence for a therapeutic effect of local delivery devices comes from trials involving patients with previously untreated adult periodontitis. Some protocols compare local drug delivery to a negative control, such as the application of only the carrier without the drug. These studies may be able to show a net effect of the drug, but they are not able to demonstrate a benefit over the most obvious alternative – scaling and root planing – and the question remains as to how much value the procedure has in *addition* to mechanical treatment. If a study is unable to demonstrate a significant difference between local drug delivery and scaling and root planing, this is not automatically a proof of equivalence of the two treatments. Equivalence testing requires statistical testing of the power of the data, taking into account the size of the study sample. Only very few studies have addressed the use of local drug delivery in recurrent or persistent periodontal lesions – the potentially most valuable area for their application. The following paragraphs discuss the predominant products available today for local antimicrobial therapy. Further developments currently under way will undoubtedly lead to the commercial availability of additional products in the future.

Minocycline ointment and microspheres

A 2% *minocycline* ointment (Dentomycin; Cyanamid, Lederle Division, Wayne, NJ, US) has been distributed commercially in some countries for several years. The efficacy of this product has been assessed in a series of clinical trials mainly conducted in adult patients in Japan. In a randomized, double-blind study of 103 adults with moderate to severe periodontitis, the safety and efficacy of subgingivally applied 2% minocycline ointment was tested at four Belgian universities (van Steenberghe et al. 1993). All patients were treated by conventional scaling and root planing at baseline. In addition, the patients received either the test or a control ointment in four consecutive sessions at an interval of two weeks (baseline and 2, 4, 6). Assessment of clinical response was made at weeks 4 and 12. A significantly greater reduction of probing depth was observed in the test group. An additional multicenter study evaluated the long-term safety and efficacy of subgingivally administered minocycline ointment when used intermittently as an adjunct to subgingival debridement in chronic periodontitis. The repeated subgingival administration of minocycline ointment yielded an adjunctive improvement after subgingival instrumentation in both clinical and microbiologic variables over a 15-month period (van Steenberghe et al. 1999). One study assessed the effect of a weekly repeated local application of minocycline ointment for 8 weeks after placement of expanded polytetrafluoroethylene membranes to guide regeneration of periodontal tissue. Although bacterial colonization of treated sites could not be prevented, the mean clinical attachment gain of the test group was significantly greater than that of the control group (Yoshinari et al. 2001).

The subgingival delivery of minocycline in different forms, for example in bioabsorbable 10% minocycline-loaded microcapsules, has also been investigated. Proof of principle studies involving relatively small numbers of patients with chronic periodontitis indicated that such local subgingival delivery systems may reduce bleeding on probing better than scaling

and root planing alone and may induce a microbial response more favorable for periodontal health than scaling and root planing (Yeom et al. 1997). The efficacy and safety of locally administered microencapsulated minocycline was assessed in a multicenter trial including 748 patients with moderate to advanced periodontitis. Minocycline microspheres plus scaling and root planing provided substantially more probing depth reduction than either scaling and root planing alone or SRP plus vehicle. The difference reached statistical significance after the first month and was maintained throughout the 9 months of the trial (Williams et al. 2001).

Doxycycline hyclate in a biodegradable polymer

A two syringe mixing system for the controlled release of *doxycycline* (Atridox; Block Drug, Jersey City, NJ, US) has been evaluated in a number of investigations, and has become available commercially in several countries. Syringe A contains the delivery vehicle, which is a bioabsorbable, flowable polymeric formulation composed of poly(DL-lactide) dissolved in N-methyl-2-pyrrolidone, and syringe B contains 50 mg of doxycycline hyclate. The constituted product contains 10% w/w doxycycline hyclate. The clinical efficacy and safety of Atridox was compared to placebo control, oral hygiene, and scaling and root planing in two multicenter studies. Each study entered 411 patients who demonstrated moderate to severe adult periodontitis. Comparisons showed the treatment to be statistically superior to placebo control and oral hygiene and equally effective as scaling and root planing in reducing the clinical signs of adult periodontitis over a 9-month period (Garrett et al. 1999). Clinical changes resulting from local delivery of doxycycline hyclate or traditional scaling and root planing were evaluated in a group of patients undergoing supportive periodontal therapy. Attachment level gains and probing depth reductions were similar at 9 months after therapy (Garrett et al. 2000).

The effect of Atridox, applied after no more than 45 minutes of debridement without analgesia in subjects with moderately advanced chronic periodontitis, was compared to 4 hours of thorough deep scaling and root planing in a study involving 105 patients at three centers. Interestingly, clinical parameters indicated a better result for the pharmaco-mechanical treatment approach after 3 months, although considerably less time had been invested than for conventional mechanical therapy (Wennström et al. 2001).

Metronidazole gel

Dialysis tubing, acrylic strips, and poly-OH-butyric acid strips have been tested as solid devices for delivery of *metronidazole*. The most extensively used device for metronidazole application is a gel consisting of a semi-solid suspension of 25% metronidazole benzoate in a mixture of glyceryl mono-oleate and sesame oil (Elyzol Dental Gel; Dumex, Copenhagen, Denmark). Applied with a syringe inserted into the pocket, the

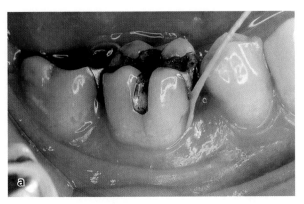 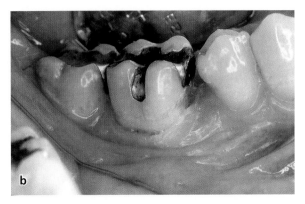

Fig. 23-5. Tetracycline fiber is packed into the periodontal pocket (a), secured with a thin layer of cyanoacrylate adhesive (b), and left in place for 7 to 12 days.

gel is expected to increase in viscosity after placement. It has been reported that 40% of the applied gel remained in place, while 60% was immediately lost and normally would probably be swallowed (Stoltze & Stellfeld 1992). After treating an average number of 18 teeth in 14 patients, a mean peak metronidazole plasma concentration of 0.6 g/ml was reached within 2 to 8 hours. The estimated mean dose of metronidazole per treated tooth was 3 mg. The drug concentration determined in crevicular fluid was below 1 g/ml in half of the sampled sites after one day and in 92% of the sites after 36 hours (Fig. 23-4). The clinical response to subgingival application of the metronidazole gel was compared to the effect of subgingival scaling in a large multicenter study of 206 patients with untreated adult periodontitis (Ainamo et al. 1992). Two randomly selected quadrants were treated with the gel twice within one week; the other two quadrants were treated with two episodes of subgingival scaling. Differences between gel application and scaling were considered clinically insignificant by the authors. Using a similar design, the microbiological outcome of two gel applications versus scaling was compared in 24 subjects during a 6-month observation period (Pedrazzoli et al. 1992). The total bacterial cultivable count and the proportions of anaerobic bacteria were affected in a similar way in the two groups, and no difference could be detected in terms of reduced probing depth and bleeding on probing. Although in theory the antimicrobial action of metronidazole is bactericidal and independent of time, in practice a sufficient period of drug presence is important irrespective of whether a substance has been determined bactericidal or bacteriostatic in the laboratory.

A subsequent controlled, randomized, blind study extended the previous observations to include clinical attachment level measurements. The results from a total of 164 subjects indicated no significant difference between metronidazole gel application and scaling and root planing (Grossi et al. 1995). The fact that no significant difference between the two treatments was observed opened the question of equivalence between the two treatment modalities. From a practical stand-

point, one form of treatment may be preferred to another of equal efficacy if it offers better tolerability for the patient, lower costs, etc. Equivalence between scaling and root planing and metronidazole gel therapy has been evaluated using the lower bounds of confidence intervals in a parallel arm, multicenter, controlled clinical trial including 84 subjects (Pihlstrom et al. 1995). The estimates provided by this study indicated that metronidazole gel therapy is 82% as good as mechanical debridement at the 95% confidence level.

Tetracycline in a non-resorbable plastic co-polymer

Hollow devices such as dialysis tubing, and solid devices such as acrylic strips, collagen, or poly-OH-butyric acid strips have been tested for *tetracycline* delivery in several experiments. Semi-solid viscous media include white petrolatum and poloxamer or carbopol gels. The most extensively tested tetracycline releasing device is the Actisite periodontal fiber (ALZA, Palo Alto, CA, US; Solco, Birsfelden, Switzerland), a monolithic thread of a biologically inert, non-resorbable plastic co-polymer (ethylene and vinylacetate) containing 25% tetracycline hydrochloride powder. The fiber is packed into the periodontal pocket, secured with a thin layer of cyanoacrylate adhesive (Fig. 23-5), and left in place for 7 to 12 days (Goodson et al. 1983, 1991a). By continuous delivery of tetracycline, a local concentration of the active drug in excess of 1000 mg/l can be maintained throughout that period (Fig. 23-4). The drug is also deposited on the root surface and penetrates into the soft periodontal tissues. Salivary tetracycline concentrations ranging from 8 to 51 mg/l have been measured when treating multiple sites, while serum concentrations remained below detection level (Goodson et al. 1985, Rapley et al. 1992). Many clinical studies have been performed with Actisite, among them three large multicenter trials, which we will discuss briefly. The safety and efficacy of tetracycline fiber therapy were investigated in a 60-day multicenter study conducted in 107 periodontitis patients after supragingival scaling and prophylaxis. Four non-adjacent teeth with pockets in the range of 6-10 mm were selected. They were ran-

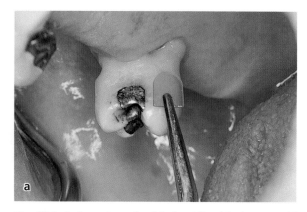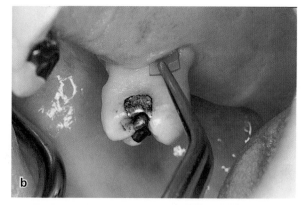

Fig. 23-6a,b. Insertion of a chlorhexidin chip into a residual pocket mesial of an upper molar with a furcation involvement.

domly assigned to either tetracycline or placebo fiber placement, scaling, or were left untreated. The analysis showed that fiber therapy significantly decreased pocket depth, increased attachment levels, and decreased the bleeding tendency to a greater extent than the control procedures (Goodson et al. 1991b). A second multicenter study is of particular interest for two reasons: first, because it was conducted in periodontal maintenance patients needing treatment of localized recurrent periodontitis, and secondly, because the effect of fiber therapy was evaluated as an adjunct to scaling and root planing (Newman et al. 1994). After 6 months, sites treated with scaling and root planing plus tetracycline fiber showed a significantly higher attachment level, significantly more pocket depth reduction and less bleeding on probing than scaling and root planing alone. A third large-scale multicenter study demonstrated that the results obtained within 3 months after therapy were maintained over 1 year and that the combined treatment with fiber and scaling had a significantly lower incidence of disease recurrence than any of the other tested treatment modalities (Michalowicz et al. 1995).

Chlorhexidine gluconate in a gelatin chip

Several attempts have been made to develop local delivery devices for the subgingival application of antiseptic, rather than antibiotic agents. Acrylic strips and ethyl-cellulose compounds have been tested for this purpose. PerioChip (Perio Products, Jerusalem, Israel), a degradable gelatin chip containing 2.5 mg chlorhexidine, is the most extensively tested delivery device of this category (Fig. 23-6). Safety and efficacy of PerioChip were evaluated in a multicenter study of 118 patients with moderate periodontitis (Soskolne et al. 1997). A split-mouth design was used to compare the treatment outcomes of scaling and root planing alone with the combined use of scaling and root planing and PerioChip in pockets with probing depths of 5-8 mm. The average pocket depth reduction in the treated sites with the chip was significantly greater than in the sites receiving mechanical treatment only (mean difference of 0.42 mm at 6 months). The efficacy of the chlorhexidine chip when used as an adjunct to

scaling and root planing on reducing probing depth and improving clinical attachment level in adult periodontitis was evaluated in two double-blind, randomized, placebo-controlled multicenter clinical trials. At 9 months significant reductions from baseline were shown with the chlorhexidine chip compared with mechanical control treatments (Jeffcoat et al. 1998).

Conclusion

To treat periodontal disease successfully, local delivery devices must provide therapeutic levels of antimicrobial agents in the subgingival area over prolonged periods. Clinical trials show the efficacy of topical antibiotic therapy under these conditions.

Comparison of treatment methods

Few studies have addressed the problem of incorporating local or systemic antimicrobial therapy into an overall treatment strategy. Most studies have tested a single form of local drug delivery or systemic administration, instead of comparing various forms of therapy. Understandably, developers and distributors have an intrinsic interest to register and promote their own product for the broadest possible usage. As little direct evidence for a comparison of various methods of treatment is available so far, well-founded decision algorithms to choose specific methods of intervention for distinct clinical situations are not yet available.

In patients with persistent periodontal lesions the efficacy of three commercially available local delivery systems as adjuncts to scaling and root planing was tested (Radvar et al. 1996, Kinane & Radvar 1999). Treatment modalities included scaling and root planing alone and in conjunction with the application of 25% tetracycline fibers, or 2% minocycline gel, or 25% metronidazole gel. Although all three locally applied antimicrobial systems seemed to offer some benefit over scaling and root planing alone, a treatment regimen of scaling and root planing plus tetracycline fiber placement gave the greatest reduction in probing depth over the 6 months after treatment. Suppuration was most effectively reduced in the scaling plus tetracycline fiber group, followed by the minocycline group. The clinical and microbiological effects of three sustained-release biodegradable polymers delivered into periodontal pockets following initial periodontal therapy, were assessed in a single-blind, randomized, parallel-designed controlled clinical trial (Salvi et al. 2002). Forty-seven patients were randomly assigned to receive either Atridox, Elyzol Dental Gel or Perio-Chip at residual periodontal pockets > 5 mm. Therapy resulted in a statistically significant gain in mean probing attachment levels for Atridox and a significant reduction in probing depth for all three devices during the study period. Furthermore, significantly more probing attachment level was gained in sites treated with Atridox when compared to sites treated with Elyzol.

A key issue requiring clarification refers to the selection of a local or a systemic delivery approach whenever the use of an antibiotic is indicated. One investigation addressed this question in patients with rapidly progressing periodontitis (Bernimoulin et al. 1995). Overall, no significant differences were noted between systemic administration of amoxicillin-clavulanic acid and tetracycline fibers as an adjunct to mechanical therapy. For patients with adult periodontitis, two studies reported better results of scaling and root planing supplemented with locally applied metronidazole than adjunctive systemic metronidazole (Paquette et al. 1994, Noyan et al. 1997).

As different oral distribution patterns can be recognized in periodontitis patients for microorganisms such as *P. gingivalis* (Mombelli et al. 1991a,b), local therapy may be less successful in patients where these organisms are widespread than in patients where the presence of pathogens is confined to isolated areas. This hypothesis was tested in a study comparing two extremes of local therapy. In one group of patients, a combination of measures including full mouth scaling and root planing, application of tetracycline fibers, and chlorhexidine rinse, was applied. In the other group, only two teeth were treated locally and no attempt was made to interfere with the overall condi-

tions of the oral environment. Major clinical differences were found in the local healing response, depending on whether the rest of the dentition was left untreated or was also subjected to therapy (Mombelli et al. 1997). These findings agree with earlier studies, showing the importance of general oral hygiene after mechanical periodontal therapy. From these studies we have learned that clinical outcomes of scaling and root planing and various forms of surgical intervention depend on the general level of oral hygiene (Rosling et al. 1976, Nyman et al. 1977, Magnusson et al. 1984). A more recent study has underscored the importance of oral hygiene, showing differences in outcomes attributable to the level of postoperative oral hygiene, also after a combination therapy including mechanical debridement and administration of various systemic antibiotics (Kornman et al. 1994). The available evidence presently suggests that local delivery may be most beneficial in the control of localized ongoing disease in otherwise stable patients. Maintenance patients with a few non-responding sites may therefore benefit most from local antimicrobial therapy.

Overall conclusion

Although mechanical periodontal treatment alone improves clinical conditions sufficiently in most cases, adjunctive antimicrobial agents, delivered either locally or systemically, can enhance the effect of therapy in certain situations. Systemic antibiotics may be a useful adjunct to the mechanical treatment of progressive adult and early onset periodontitis. Patients with evidence of generalized ongoing disease despite optimal mechanical therapy may also benefit from systemic antibiotics. Localized non-responding sites and localized recurrent disease may be treated with locally delivered antibiotics. Mechanical debridement before the application of antimicrobial agents, and mechanical plaque control after therapy, are essential for treatment success.

REFERENCES

Adriaens, P.A., De Boever, J.A. & Loesche, W.J. (1988). Bacterial invasion in root cementum and radicular dentin of periodontally diseased teeth in humans. *Journal of Periodontology* **59**, 222-230.

Ainamo, J., Lie, T., Ellingsen, B.H., Hansen, B.F., Johansson, L.-Å., Karring, T., Kirsch, J., Paunio, K. & Stoltze, K. (1992). Clinical responses to subgingival placement of a metronidazole 25% gel compared to the effect of subgingival scaling in adult periodontitis. *Journal of Clinical Periodontology* **19**, 723-729.

Aitken, S., Birek, P., Kulkarni, G.V., Lee, W. & McCulloch, C.A.G. (1992). Serial doxycycline and metronidazole in prevention of recurrent periodontitis in high risk patients. *Journal of Periodontology* **63**, 87-92.

Allenspach-Petrzilka, G.E. & Guggenheim, B. (1983). Bacterial invasion of the periodontum; an important factor in the

pathogenesis of periodontitis? *Journal of Clinical Periodontology* **10**, 609-617.

Anwar, H., Dasgupta, M.K. & Costerton, J.W. (1990). Testing the susceptibility of bacteria in biofilms to antibacterial agents. *Antimicrobial Agents and Chemotherapy* **34**, 2043-2046.

Anwar, H., Strap, J.L. & Costerton, J.W. (1992). Establishment of aging biofilms: possible mechanism of bacterial resistance to antibiotic therapy. *Antimicrobial Agents and Chemotherapy* **36**, 1347-1351.

Asikainen, S., Jousimies-Somer, H., Kanervo, A. & Saxén, L. (1990). The immediate efficacy of adjunctive doxycycline in treatment of localized juvenile periodontitis. *Archives of Oral Biology* **35**, 231S-234S.

Baker, P.J., Slots, J., Genco, R.J. & Evans, R.T. (1983). Minimal inhibitory concentrations of various antimicrobial agents for human oral anaerobic bacteria. *Antimicrobial Agents and Chemotherapy* **24**, 420-424.

Bernimoulin, P., Purucker, H., Mertes, B. & Krüger, B. (1995). Local versus systemic adjunctive antibiotic therapy in RPP patients. *Journal of Dental Research* **74**, 481.

Bonesvoll, P. & Gjermo, P. (1978). A comparison between chlorhexidine and some quaternary ammonium compounds with regard to retention, salivary concentration and plaque-inhibiting effect in the human mouth after mouth rinses. *Archives of Oral Biology* **23**, 289-294.

Bragd, L., Dahlén, G., Wikström, M. & Slots, J. (1987). The capability of *Actinobacillus actinomycetemcomitans*, *Bacteroides gingivalis* and *Bacteroides intermedius* to indicate progressive periodontitis; a retrospective study. *Journal of Clinical Periodontology* **14**, 95-99.

Bragd, L., Wikström, M. & Slots, J. (1985). Clinical and microbiological study of "refractory" adult periodontitis. *Journal of Dental Research* **64**, 234.

Carlos, J.P., Wolfe, M.D., Zambon, J.J. & Kingman, A. (1988). Periodontal disease in adolescents: Some clinical and microbiologic correlates of attachment loss. *Journal of Dental Research* **67**, 1510-1514.

Carranza, F.A. Jr., Saglie, R., Newman, M.G. & Valentin, P.L. (1983). Scanning and transmission electron microscopic study of tissue-invading microorganisms in localized juvenile periodontitis. *Journal of Periodontology* **54**, 598-617.

Christersson, L., van Winkelhoff, A.J., Zambon, J.J., de Graaff, J. & Genco, R.J. (1989). Systemic antibiotic combination therapy in recalcitrant and recurrent localized juvenile periodontitis. *Journal of Dental Research* **68**, 197.

Clark, D.C., Shenker, S., Stulginsky, P. & Schwartz, S. (1983). Effectiveness of routine periodontal treatment with and without adjunctive metronidazole therapy in mentally retarded adolescents. *Journal of Periodontology* **54**, 658-665.

Costerton, J.W., Lewandowski, Z., Caldwell, D.E., Korber, D.R. & Lappin-Scott, H.M. (1995). Microbial biofilms. *Annual Reviews in Microbiology* **49**, 711-745.

Eakle, W., Ford, C. & Boyd, R. (1986). Depth of penetration in periodontal pockets with oral irrigation. *Journal of Clinical Periodontology* **13**, 39-44.

Garrett, S., Adams, D.F., Bogle, G., Donly, K., Drisko, C.H., Hallmon, W.W., Hancock, E.B., Hanes, P., Hawley, C.E., Johnson, L., Kiger, R., Killoy, W., Mellonig, J.T., Raab, F.J., Ryder, M., Stoller, N., Polson, A., Wang, H-L., Wolinsky, L.E., Yukna, R.A., Harrold, C.Q., Hill, M., Johnson, V.B. & Southard, G.L. (2000). The effect of locally delivered controlled-release doxycycline or scaling and root planing on periodontal maintenance patients over 9 months. *Journal of Periodontology* **71**, 22-30.

Garrett, S., Johnson, L., Drisko, C.H., Adams, D.F., Bandt, C., Beiswanger, B., Bogle, G., Donly, K., Hallmon, W.W., Hancock, E.B., Hanes, P., Hawley, C.E., Kiger, R., Killoy, W., Mellonig, J.T., Polson, A., Raab, F.J., Ryder, M., Stoller, N.H., Wang, H.L., Wolinsky, L.E., Evans, G.H., Harrold, C.Q., Arnold, R.M., Atack, D.F., Fitzgerald, B., Hill, M., Isaacs, R.L., Nasi, H.F., Newell, D.H., MacNeil, R.L., MacNeill, S., Spolsky, V.W., Duke, S.P., Polson, A. & Southard, G.L. (1999). Two multicenter studies evaluating locally delivered doxycycline hyclate, placebo control, oral hygiene, and scaling and root planing in the treatment of periodontitis. *Journal of Periodontology* **70**, 490-503.

Genco, R.J., Cianciola, L.J. & Rosling, B.G. (1981). Treatment of localized juvenile periodontitis. *Journal of Dental Research* **60**, 527.

Goené, R.J., Winkel, E.G., Abbas, F., Rodenburg, J.P., Van Winkelhoff, A.J. & De Graaff, J. (1990). Microbiology in diagnosis and treatment of severe periodontitis. A report of four cases. *Journal of Periodontology* **61**, 61-64.

Golub, L.M., Lee, H.M., Lehrer, G., Nemitroff, A., McNamara, T.F., Kaplan, R. & Ramamurthy, N.S. (1983). Minocycline reduces gingival collagenolytic activity during diabetes. *Journal of Periodontal Research* **18**, 516-526.

Golub, L.M., Wolff, M., Lee, H.M., McNamara, T.F., Ramamurthy, N.S., Zambon, J. & Ciancio, S. (1985). Further evidence that tetracyclines inhibit collagenase activity in human crevicular fluid and other mammalian sources. *Journal of Periodontal Research* **20**, 12-23.

Goodson, J., Cugini, M., Kent, R., Armitage, G., Cobb, C., Fine, D., Fritz, M., Green, E., Imoberdorf, M., Killoy, W., Mendieta, C., Niederman, R., Offenbacher, S., Taggart, E. & Tonetti, M. (1991a). Multicenter evaluation of tetracycline fiber therapy: I. Experimental design, methods and baseline data. *Journal of Periodontal Research* **26**, 361-370.

Goodson, J., Cugini, M., Kent, R., Armitage, G., Cobb, C., Fine, D., Fritz, M., Green, E., Imoberdorf, M., Killoy, W., Mendieta, C., Niederman, R., Offenbacher, S., Taggart, E. & Tonetti, M. (1991b). Multicenter evaluation of tetracycline fiber therapy: II. Clinical response. *Journal of Periodontal Research* **26**, 371-379.

Goodson, J., Holborow, D., Dunn, R., Hogan, P. & Dunham, S. (1983). Monolithic tetracycline containing fibers for controlled delivery to periodontal pockets. *Journal of Periodontology* **54**, 575-579.

Goodson, J., Offenbacher, S., Farr, D. & Hogan, P. (1985). Periodontal disease treatment by local drug delivery. *Journal of Periodontology* **56**, 265-272.

Goodson, J.M. (1989). Pharmacokinetic principles controlling efficacy of oral therapy. *Journal of Dental Research* **68**, 1625-1632.

Gordon, J., Walker, C., Lamster, I., West, T., Socransky, S., Seiger, M. & Fasciano, R. (1985). Efficacy of clindamycin hydrochloride in refractory periodontitis. 12 month results. *Journal of Periodontology* Suppl, 75-80.

Gristina, A.G. (1987). Biomaterial-centered infection: Microbial adhesion versus tissue integration. *Science* **237**, 1588-1595.

Grossi, S.G., Zambon, J.J., Ho, A.W., Koch, G., Dunford, R.G., Machtei, E.E., Norderyd, O.M. & Genco, R.J. (1994). Assessment of risk for periodontal disease. I. Risk indicators for attachment loss. *Journal of Periodontology* **65**, 260-267.

Grossi, S., Dunford, R., Genco, R.J., Pihlstrom, B., Walker, C., Howell, H. & Thorøe, U. (1995). Local application of metronidazole dental gel. *Journal of Dental Research* **74**, 468.

Gusberti, F.A., Syed, S.A. & Lang, N.P. (1988). Combined antibiotic (metronidazole) and mechanical treatment effects on the subgingival bacterial flora of sites with recurrent periodontal disease. *Journal of Clinical Periodontology* **15**, 353-359.

Haffajee, A.D., Dibart, S., Kent, R.L.J. & Socransky, S.S. (1995). Clinical and microbiological changes associated with the use of 4 adjunctive systemically administered agents in the treatment of periodontal infections. *Journal of Clinical Periodontology* **22**, 618-627.

Haffajee, A.D., Dzink, J.L. & Socransky, S.S. (1988). Effect of modified Widman flap surgery and systemic tetracycline on the subgingival microbiota of periodontal lesions. *Journal of Clinical Periodontology* **15**, 255-262.

Haffajee, A.D. & Socransky, S.S. (1994). Microbial etiological agents of destructive periodontal diseases. *Periodontology 2000* **5**, 78-111.

Haffajee, A.D., Socransky, S.S., Smith, C. & Dibart, S. (1991). Relation of baseline microbial parameters to future periodontal attachment loss. *Journal of Clinical Periodontology* **18**, 744-750.

Helldén, L.B., Listgarten, M.A. & Lindhe, J. (1979). The effect of tetracycline and/or scaling on human periodontal disease. *Journal of Clinical Periodontology* **6**, 222-230.

Höffler, U., Niederau, W. & Pulverer, G. (1980). Susceptibility of *Bacterium actinomycetemcomitans* to 45 antibiotics. *Antimicrobial Agents and Chemotherapy* **17**, 943-946.

Hull, P.S., Abu-Fanas, S.H. & Drucker, D.B. (1989). Evaluation of two antibacterial agents in the management of rapidly progressive periodontitis. *Journal of Dental Research* **68**, 564.

Jeffcoat, M.K., Bray, K.S., Ciancio, S.G., Dentino, A.R., Fine, D.H., Gordon, J.M., Gunsolley, J.C., Killoy, W.J., Lowenguth, R.A., Magnusson, N.I., Offenbacher, S., Palcanis, K.G., Proskin, H.M., Finkelman, R.D. & Flashner, M. (1998). Adjunctive use of a subgingival controlled-release chlorhexidine chip reduces probing depth and improves attachment level compared with scaling and root planing alone. *Journal of Periodontology* **69**, 989-997.

Jousimies-Somer, H., Asikainen, S., Suomala, P. & Summanen, P. (1988). Activity of metronidazole and its hydroxymetabolite. *Oral Microbiology and Immunology* **3**, 32-34.

Joyston-Bechal, S., Smales, F.C. & Duckworth, R. (1984). Effect of metronidazole on chronic periodontal disease in subjects using topically applied chlorhexidine gel. *Journal of Clinical Periodontology* **11**, 53-62.

Joyston-Bechal, S., Smales, F.C. & Duckworth, R. (1986). A follow-up study 3 years after metronidazole therapy for chronic periodontal disease. *Journal of Clinical Periodontology* **13**, 944-949.

Kinane, D.F. & Radvar, M. (1999). A six-month comparison of three periodontal local antimicrobial therapies in persistent periodontal pockets. *Journal of Periodontology* **70**, 1-7.

Kornman, K.S., Newman, M.G., Flemmig, T., Alvarado, R. & Nachnani, S. (1989). Treatment of refractory periodontitis with metronidazole plus amoxicillin or Augmentin. *Journal of Dental Research* **68**, 917.

Kornman, K.S., Newman, M.G., Moore, D.J. & Singer, R.E. (1994). The influence of supragingival plaque control on clinical and microbial outcomes following the use of antibiotics for the treatment of periodontitis. *Journal of Periodontology* **65**, 848-854.

Kornman, K.S. & Robertson, P.B. (1985). Clinical and microbiological evaluation of therapy for juvenile periodontitis. *Journal of Periodontology* **56**, 443-446.

Kulkarni, G.V., Lee, W.K., Aitken, S., Birek, P. & McCulloch, C.A.G. (1991). A randomised placebo-controlled trial of doxycycline. Effects on the microflora of recurrent periodontitis lesions in high risk patients. *Journal of Periodontology* **62**, 197-202.

Lekovic, V., Kenney, E.B., Carranza, F.A. & Endres, B. (1983). The effect of metronidazole on human periodontal disease. A clinical and bacteriological study. *Journal of Periodontology* **54**, 476-480.

Lindhe, J. (1982). Treatment of localized juvenile periodontitis. In: Genco, R.J. & S.E. Mergenhagen, eds. *Host-parasite interactions in periodontal diseases*. Washington, D.C: American Society for Microbiology, pp. 382-394.

Lindhe, J., Liljenberg, B. & Adielson, B. (1983). Effect of long term tetracycline therapy on human periodontal disease. *Journal of Clinical Periodontology* **10**, 590-601.

Listgarten, M.A. (1965). Electron microscopic observations on the bacterial flora of acute necrotizing ulcerative gingivitis. *Journal of Periodontology* **36**, 328-339.

Listgarten, M.A., Lindhe, J. & Helldén, L. (1978). Effect of tetracycline and/or scaling on human periodontal disease. *Journal of Clinical Periodontology* **5**, 246-271.

Loesche, W.J., Grossman, N. & Giordano, J. (1993). Metronidazole in periodontitis (IV). The effect of patient compliance on treatment parameters. *Journal of Clinical Periodontology* **20**, 96-104.

Loesche, W.J., Syed, S.A., Morrison, E.C., Kerry, G.A., Higgins, T. & Stoll, J. (1984). Metronidazole in periodontitis. I. Clinical and bacteriological results after 15 to 30 weeks. *Journal of Periodontology* **55**, 325-335.

Lorian, V. (1986). *Antibiotics in laboratory medicine*, 2nd edn., Baltimore: Williams and Wilkins.

Magnusson, I., Lindhe, J., Yoneyama, T. & Liljenberg, B. (1984). Recolonization of a subgingival microbiota following scaling in deep pockets. *Journal of Clinical Periodontology* **11**, 193-207.

Magnusson, I., Low, S.B., McArthur, W.P., Marks, R.G., Walker, C.B., Maruniak, J., Taylor, M., Padgett, P., Jung, J. & Clark, W.B. (1994). Treatment of subjects with refractory periodontal disease. *Journal of Clinical Periodontology* **21**, 628-637.

Mahmood, M.M. & Dolby, A.E. (1987). The value of systemically administered metronidazole in the modified Widman flap procedure. *Journal of Periodontology* **58**, 147-152.

Mandell, R.L. & Socransky, S.S. (1988). Microbiological and clinical effects of surgery plus doxycycline on juvenile periodontitis. *Journal of Periodontology* **59**, 373-379.

Marshall, K.C. (1992). Biofilms: An overview of bacterial adhesion, activity, and control at surfaces. *ASM News* **58**, 202-207.

Matisko, M. & Bissada, N. (1992). Short-term systemic administration of Augmentin and doxycycline in the treatment of recurrent progressive periodontitis. *Journal of Dental Research* **71**, 319.

McCulloch, C.A.G., Birek, P., Aitken, S. & Lee, W. (1989). Efficacy of doxycycline in prevention of recurrent periodontitis. *Journal of Dental Research* **68**, 916.

McCulloch, C.A.G., Birek, P., Overall, C., Aitken, S., Lee, W. & Kulkarni, G. (1990). Randomised controlled trial of doxycycline in prevention of recurrent periodontitis in high risk patients: antimicrobial activity and collagenase inhibition. *Journal of Clinical Periodontology* **17**, 616-622.

Michalowicz, B.S., Pihlstrom, B.L., Drisko, C.L. et al. (1995). Evaluation of periodontal treatments using controlled release tetracycline fibers: maintenance response. *Journal of Periodontology* **66**, 708-715.

Mombelli, A., Gmür, R., Gobbi, C. & Lang, N.P. (1994). *Actinobacillus actinomycetemcomitans* in adult periodontitis. I. Topographic distribution before and after treatment. *Journal of Periodontology* **65**, 820-826.

Mombelli, A., Gusberti, F.A. & Lang, N.P. (1989). Treatment of recurrent periodontal disease by root planing and Ornidazole (Tiberal®). Clinical and microbiological findings. *Journal of Clinical Periodontology* **16**, 38-45.

Mombelli, A., McNabb, H. & Lang, N.P. (1991a). Black-pigmenting Gram-negative bacteria in periodontal disease. I. Topographic distribution in the human dentition. *Journal of Periodontal Research* **26**, 301-307.

Mombelli, A., McNabb, H. & Lang, N.P. (1991b). Black-pigmenting Gram-negative bacteria in periodontal disease. II. Screening strategies for *P. gingivalis*. *Journal of Periodontal Research* **26**, 308-313.

Mombelli, A. & van Winkelhoff, A.J. (1997). The systemic use of antibiotics in periodontal therapy. In: Lang, N.P., Karring, T. & Lindhe, J., eds. *Proceedings of the Second European Workshop on Periodontology*, London: Quintessence, pp. 38-77.

Müller, H.P., Eickholz, P., Heinecke, A., Pohl, S., Müller, R.F. & Lange, D.E. (1995). Simultaneous isolation of *Actinobacillus actinomycetemcomitans* from subgingival and extracrevicular locations of the mouth. *Journal of Clinical Periodontology* **22**, 413-419.

Müller, H., Lange, D.E. & Müller, R.F. (1990). Konzentrierung von *A. actinomycetemcomitans* in subgingivaler Plaque nach kurzfristiger Minocyclin-Therapie. *Deutsche Zahnärztliche Zeitschrift* **45**, 462-465.

Müller, H., Lange, D.E. & Müller, R.F. (1993). Failure of adjunctive minocycline-HCl to eliminate oral *Actinobacillus actinomycetemcomitans*. *Journal of Clinical Periodontology* **20**, 498-504.

Müller, H.P., Müller, R.F. & Lange, D.E. (1989). Die Reduktion von *A. actinomycetemcomitans* bei der profunden Parodontitis. *Deutsche Zahnärztliche Zeitschrift* **44**, 293-297.

Newman, M.G., Kornman, K.S. & Doherty, F.M. (1994). A 6-month multi-center evaluation of adjunctive tetracycline fiber therapy used in conjunction with scaling and root planing in maintenance patients: Clinical results. *Journal of Periodontology* **65**, 685-691.

Noyan, Ü., Yilmaz, S., Kuru, B., Kadir, T., Acar, O. & Büget, E. (1997). A clinical and microbiological evaluation of systemic and local metronidazole delivery in adult periodontitis patients. *Journal of Clinical Periodontology* **24**, 158-165.

Nyman, S., Lindhe, J. & Rosling, B. (1977). Periodontal surgery in plaque-infected dentitions. *Journal of Clinical Periodontology* **4**, 240-249.

Ohta, Y., Okuda, K. & Takazoe, I. (1986). Microbiological and clinical effects of systemic antibiotic administration in advanced periodontitis. *Bulletin of the Tokyo Dental College* **27**, 139-148.

Oostervaal, P.J., Mikx, F.H. & Renggli, H.H. (1990). Clearance of a topically applied fluorescein gel from periodontal pockets. *Journal of Clinical Periodontology* **17**, 613-615.

Pajukanta, R., Asikainen, S., Forsblom, B., Saarela, M. & Jousimies-Somer, H. (1993a). β-Lactamase production and *in vitro* antimicrobial susceptibility of *Porphyromonas gingivalis*. *FEMS Immunology and Medical Microbiology* **6**, 241-244.

Pajukanta, R., Asikainen, S., Saarela, M., Alaluusua, S. & Jousimies-Somer, H. (1993b). *In vitro* antimicrobial suscepti-bility of different serotypes of *Actinobacillus actinomycetem-comitans*. *Scandinavian Journal of Dental Research* **101**, 299-303.

Paquette, D., Ling, S., Fiorellini, J., Howell, H., Weber, H. & Williams, R. (1994). Radiographic and BANA test analysis of locally delivered metronidazole: a phase I/II clinical trial. *Journal of Dental Research* **73**, 305.

Pavicic, M.J.A.M.P., van Winkelhoff, A.J. & de Graaff, J. (1991). Synergistic effects between amoxicillin, metronidazole, and the hydroxymetabolite of metronidazole against *Actinobacil-lus actinomycetemcomitans*. *Antimicrobial Agents and Chemo-therapy* **35**, 961-966.

Pavicic, M.J.A.M.P., van Winkelhoff, A.J. & de Graaff, J. (1992). *In vitro* susceptibilities of *Actinobacillus actinomycetemcomitans* to a number of antimicrobial combinations. *Antimicrobial Agents and Chemotherapy* **36**, 2634-2638.

Pavicic, M.J.A.M.P., van Winkelhoff, A.J., Douqué, N. H., Steures, R.W.R. & de Graaff, J. (1994). Microbiological and clinical effects of metronidazole and amoxicillin in *Actinobac-illus actinomycetemcomitans*-associated periodontitis. *Journal of Clinical Periodontology* **21**, 107-112.

Pedrazzoli, V., Kilian, M. & Karring, T. (1992). Comparative clinical and microbiological effects of topical subgingival ap-plication of metronidazole 25% dental gel and scaling in the treatment of adult periodontitis. *Journal of Clinical Periodontol-ogy* **19**, 715-722.

Pihlstrom, B., Michalowicz, B., Aeppli, D., Genco, R., Walker, C., Howell, H. & Mørup-Jenson, A. (1995). Equivalence in clinical trials. *Journal of Dental Research* **74**, 530.

Pitcher, G., Newman, H. & Strahan, J. (1980). Access to subgingi-val plaque by disclosing agents using mouthrinsing and di-rect irrigation. *Journal of Clinical Periodontology* **7**, 300-308.

Radvar, M., Pourtaghi, N. & Kinane, D.F. (1996). Comparison of three periodontal local antibiotic therapies in persistent peri-odontal pockets. *Journal of Periodontology* **67**, 860-865.

Rams, T.E., Feik, D. & Slots, J. (1992). Ciprofloxacin/metronida-zole treatment of recurrent adult periodontitis. *Journal of Den-tal Research* **71**, 319.

Rams, T.E. & Keyes, P.H. (1983). A rationale for the management of periodontal diseases: effects of tetracycline on subgingival bacteria. *Journal of the American Dental Association* **107**, 37-41.

Rapley, J.W., Cobb, C.M., Killoy, W.J. & Williams, D.R. (1992). Serum levels of tetracycline during treatment with tetracy-cline-containing fibers. *Journal of Periodontology* **63**, 817-820.

Rosling, B., Nyman, S., Lindhe, J. & Jern, B. (1976). The healing potential of the periodontal tissues following different tech-niques of periodontal surgery in plaque-free dentitions. A 2-year clinical study. *Journal of Clinical Periodontology* **3**, 233-250.

Saglie, F.R., Carranza, F.A. Jr., Newman, M.G., Cheng, L. & Lewin, K.J. (1982a). Identification of tissue-invading bacteria in human periodontal disease. *Journal of Periodontal Research* **17**, 452-455.

Saglie, R., Newman, M.G., Carranza, F.A. & Pattison, G.L. (1982b). Bacterial invasion of gingiva in advanced periodon-titis in humans. *Journal of Periodontology* **53**, 217-222.

Salvi, G.E., Mombelli, A., Mayfield, L., Rutar, A., Suvan, J., Garrett, S. & Lang, N.P. (2002). Local antimicrobial therapy after initial periodontal treatment. A randomized controlled clinical trial comparing three biodegradable sustained release polymers. *Journal of Clinical Periodontology* **69**, 540-550.

Saxén, L. & Asikainen, S. (1993). Metronidazole in the treatment

of localized juvenile periodontitis. *Journal of Clinical Periodon-tology* **20**, 166-171.

Scopp, I.W., Froum, S.J., Sullivan, M., Kazandjian, G., Wank, D. & Fine, A. (1980). Tetracycline: a clinical study to determine its effectiveness as long-term adjuvant. *Journal of Periodontol-ogy* **51**, 328-330.

Slots, J., Mashimo, P., Levine, M.J. & Genco, R.J. (1979). Periodon-tal therapy in humans. I. Microbiological and clinical effects of a single course of periodontal scaling and root planing, and of adjunctive tetracycline therapy. *Journal of Periodontology* **50**, 495-509.

Slots, J. & Rams, T.E. (1990). Antibiotics in periodontal therapy: advantages and disadvantages. *Journal of Clinical Periodontol-ogy* **17**, 479-493.

Slots, J. & Rosling, B.G. (1983). Suppression of the periodontopa-thic microflora in localized juvenile periodontitis by systemic tetracycline. *Journal of Clinical Periodontology* **10**, 465-486.

Söder, P.O., Frithiof, L., Wikner, S., Wouters, F.R., Nedlich, V., Söder, B. & Rubin, B. (1989). The effects of metronidazole in treatment of young adults with severe periodontitis. *Journal of Dental Research* **68**, 710.

Söder, P.O., Frithiof, L., Wikner, S., Wouters, F.R., Nedlich, V., Söder, B. & Rubin, B. (1990). The effect of systemic metroni-dazole after non-surgical treatment in moderate and ad-vanced periodontitis. *Journal of Periodontology* **61**, 281-288.

Soskolne, W.A., Heasman, P.A., Stabholz, A., Smart, G.J., Palmer, M., Flashner, M. & Newman, H.N. (1997). Sustained local delivery of chlorhexidine in the treatment of periodontitis: a multicenter study. *Journal of Periodontology* **68**, 32-38.

Stabholz, A., Kettering, J., Aprecio, R., Zimmerman, G., Baker, P.J. & Wikesjö, U.M.E. (1993). Antimicrobial properties of human dentin impregnated with tetracycline HCl or chlor-hexidine. An *in vitro* study. *Journal of Clinical Periodontology* **20**, 557-562.

Sterry, K.A., Langeroudi, M. & Dolby, A.E. (1985). Metronidazole as an adjunct to periodontal therapy with subgingival curet-tage. *British Dental Journal* **158**, 176-178.

Stoller, N.H., Johnson, L.R., Trapnell, S., Harrold, C.Q. & Garrett, S. (1998). The pharmacokinetic profile of a biodegradable controlled-release delivery system containing doxycycline compared to systemically delivered doxycycline in gingival crevicular fluid, saliva, and serum. *Journal of Periodontology* **69**, 1085-1091.

Stoltze, K. (1992). Concentration of metronidazole in periodontal pockets after application of a metronidazole 25% dental gel. *Journal of Clinical Periodontology* **19**, 698-701.

Stoltze, K. (1995). Elimination of Elyzol® 25% Dentalgel matrix from periodontal pockets. *Journal of Clinical Periodontology* **22**, 185-187.

Stoltze, K. & Stellfeld, M. (1992). Systemic absorbtion of metroni-dazole after application of a metronidazole 25% dental gel. *Journal of Clinical Periodontology* **19**, 693-697.

Tonetti, M., Cugini, M.A. & Goodson, J.M. (1990). Zero-order delivery with periodontal placement of tetracycline loaded ethylene vinyl acetate fibers. *Journal of Periodontal Research* **25**, 243-249.

van Steenberghe, D., Bercy, P., Kohl, J., De Boever, J., Adriaens, P., Vanderfaeillie, A., Adriaenssen, C., Rompen, E., De Vree, H., McCarthy, E.F. & Vandenhoven, G. (1993). Subgingival minocycline hydrochloride ointment in moderate to severe chronic adult periodontitis: A randomized, double-blind, ve-hicle-controlled, multicenter study. *Journal of Periodontology* **64**, 637-644.

van Steenberghe, D., Rosling, B., Soder, P.O., Landry, R.G., van der Velden, U., Timmerman, M.F., McCarthy, E.F., Vanden-hoven, G., Wouters, C., Wilson, M., Matthews, J. & Newman, H.N. (1999). A 15-month evaluation of the effects of repeated subgingival minocycline in chronic adult periodontitis. *Jour-nal of Periodontology* **70**, 657-667.

van Winkelhoff, A.J., Rams, T.E. & Slots, J. (1996). Systemic antibiotic therapy in periodontics. *Periodontology 2000* **10**, 45-78.

van Winkelhoff, A.J., Rodenburg, J.P., Goené, R.J., Abbas, F., Winkel, E.G. & de Graaff, J. (1989). Metronidazole plus amoxicillin in the treatment of *Actinobacillus actinomycetemcomitans* associated periodontitis. *Journal of Clinical Periodontology* **16**, 128-131.

van Winkelhoff, A.J., Tijhof, C.J. & de Graaff, J. (1992). Microbiological and clinical results of metronidazole plus amoxicillin therapy in *Actinobacillus actinomycetemcomitans*-associated periodontitis. *Journal of Periodontology* **63**, 52-57.

van Winkelhoff, A.J., Van der Velden, U., Clement, M. & De Graaff, J. (1988). Intra-oral distribution of black-pigmented *Bacteroides* species in periodontitis patients. *Oral Microbiology and Immunology* **3**, 83-85.

Walker, C.B. (1992). Antimicrobial agents and chemotherapy. In: Slots, J. & Taubmann, M., eds. *Contemporary oral microbiology and immunology*. St. Louis: Mosby Yearbook, pp. 242-264.

Walker, C.B. (1996). Selected antimicrobial agents: mechanisms of action, side effects and drug interactions. *Periodontology 2000* **10**, 12-28.

Walker, C.B. & Gordon, J.M. (1990). The effect of clindamycin on the microbiota associated with refractory periodontitis. *Journal of Periodontology* **61**, 692-698.

Walker, C.B., Gordon, J.M., Magnusson, I. & Clark, W. B. (1993). A role for antibiotics in the treatment of refractory periodontitis. *Journal of Periodontology* **64**, 772-781.

Walker, C.B., Gordon, J.M. & Socransky, S.S. (1983). Antibiotic susceptibility testing of subgingival plaque samples. *Journal of Clinical Periodontology* **10**, 422-432.

Walker, C.B., Pappas, J.D., Tyler, K.Z., Cohen, S. & Gordon, J.M. (1985). Antibiotic susceptibilities of periodontal bacteria. *In vitro* susceptibilities to eight antimicrobial agents. *Journal of Periodontology* **56**, 67-74.

Wennström, J., Newman, MacNeil, Killoy, Griffiths, Gillam, Krok, Needleman, Weiss & Garrett (2001). Utilization of locally delivered doxycycline in non-surgical treatment of chronic periodontitis. A comparative multicenter trial of two treatment approaches. *Journal of Clinical Periodontology* **28**, 753-761.

Williams, R.C., Paquette, D.W., Offenbacher, S., Adams, D.F., Armitage, G.C., Bray, K., Caton, J., Cochran, D.L., Drisko, C.H., Fiorellini, J.P., Giannobile, W.V., Grossi, S., Guerrero, D.M., Johnson, G.K., Lamster, I.B., Magnusson, I., Oringer, R.J., Persson, G.R., Van Dyke, T.E., Wolff, L.F., Santucci, E.A., Rodda, B.E. & Lessem, J. (2001). Treatment of periodontitis by local administration of minocycline microspheres: a controlled trial. *Journal of Periodontology* **72**, 1535-1544.

Yeom, H.R., Park, Y.J., Lee, S.J., Rhyu, I.C., Chung, C.P. & Nisengard, R.J. (1997). Clinical and microbiological effects of minocycline-loaded microcapsules in adult periodontitis. *Journal of Periodontology* **68**, 1102-1109.

Yoshinari, N., Tohya, T., Kawase, H., Matsuoka, M., Nakane, M., Kawachi, M., Mitani, A., Koide, M., Inagaki, K., Fukuda, M. & Noguchi, T. (2001). Effect of repeated local minocycline administration on periodontal healing following guided tissue regeneration. *Journal of Periodontology* **72**, 284-295.

Zambon, J.J., Reynolds, H.S. & Slots, J. (1981). Black-pigmented *Bacteroides* spp. in the human oral cavity. *Infection and Immunity* **32**, 198-203.

CHAPTER 24

Breath Malodor

DANIEL VAN STEENBERGHE AND MARC QUIRYNEN

Breath malodor means an unpleasant odor of the expired air, whatever the origin may be. Oral malodor specifically refers to such odor originating from the oral cavity itself. A term like halitosis is synonymous with breath malodor but is not always understood by the general population. Breath malodor has long been a matter of concern. There are references to it in the Bible and in the Koran. Surprisingly enough, until recently breath malodor has not been a matter of much interest in periodontology, although its most frequent causes are plaque-related gingivitis and periodontitis.

Even the literature concerning this subject is scarce. There was only one book on this topic in the nineteenth century (Howe 1898) and it was not until the end of the twentieth century that two more books were devoted to the subject (Rosenberg 1995, van Steenberghe & Rosenberg 1996). Joe Tonzetich from the University of British Columbia unfolded the biologic basis for oral malodor (Tonzetich 1977) but his observations received only limited attention from clinicians, even if oral or breath malodor is frequently encountered in any dental and especially periodontal office.

SOCIO-ECONOMIC ASPECTS

A transient breath malodor is noticed when waking up in the morning in more than half the adult population (Morris & Read 1949). It does not deserve special attention since it is due to the xerostomia developed during sleep, i.e. when salivary flow is reduced to a minimum. This with the ongoing intra-oral putrefaction explains the malodor when waking up. Morning breath odor disappears soon after the intake of food or fluid. The intra-oral placement of a toothpaste containing zinc salts and triclosan has the capacity to reduce the odor for several hours, even in the absence of toothbrushing (Hoshi & van Steenberghe 1996).

The real concern of the population is the breath malodor which remains during the day and which can cause social and/or relational problems. Unsubstantiated press releases claim that breath malodor may concern as many as 25 million people in the US alone. Everyone has sometimes experienced, when a person is speaking to them at close proximity, breath odor that is unpleasant if not unbearable. Subjects who believe they produce malodor can adopt avoidance patterns such as keeping a distance when speaking to others or holding their hand in front of the mouth while speaking. There is also a tendency to constantly use rinses, sprays, chewing gums or pills to mask the breath odor, although many such items have no effect whatsoever or at least no lasting effect.

Even more disturbing is the fact that a number of subjects imagine they have breath malodor when they may not have. This imaginary breath odor, also called halitophobia (Oxtoby & Field 1994), has been associated with obsessive-compulsive disorders or hypochondria. It has even led to suicide (Yaegaki 1995). There are well-established personality disorder questionnaires such as the SCL-90 (Derogatis et al. 1973) which allow the clinician to assess the tendency for illusionary breath malodor among those where no objective diagnosis of breath malodor can be made (Eli et al. 1996). For such patients, the presence of a psychologist/psychiatrist at the multidisciplinary malodor consultation is essential.

Epidemiological investigations concerning breath malodor are rare. There is a large-scale Japanese study involving more than 2500 subjects aged 18 to 64 years in which the malodor was measured by a portable sulfide monitor (see section on diagnosis later in this chapter) at several times during the day. The volatile sulfur components reached high levels several hours after food intake and increased with age, tongue coating and periodontal inflammation. About one out of four subjects exhibited volatile sulfur components (VSC) values higher than 75 ppb, which is considered the limit for social acceptance.

Thus one can conclude that the socio-economic impact of breath malodor is considerable.

ETIOLOGY AND PATHOPHYSIOLOGY

Findings from different investigations have documented that the vast majority of causes of malodor relate to the oral cavity, with gingivitis (Persson et al. 1989, 1990), periodontitis (Yaegaki & Sanada 1992a) and tongue coating (Yaegaki & Sanada 1992b) as predominant factors. On the other hand, since more than 90% of the population suffers from gingivitis and periodontitis, there is a risk that such plaque-related inflammatory conditions are always considered to be the cause, while in fact more important pathologies, such as a hepatic or renal insufficiency or a bronchial carcinoma, may be the main etiological factor.

In a multidisciplinary breath odor clinic, it appeared that 87% of the etiologies were intra-oral, 8% in the oto-rhino-laryngological field and 5% from elsewhere in the body or unknown (Delanghe et al. 1997)

Members of the oral anaerobic microbiota, especially species such as *Treponema denticola, Porphyromonas gingivalis* and *Prevotella intermedia*, can produce hydrogen sulfide and methylmercaptan from L-cysteine or serum (Tonzetich 1977), i.e. proteins which are consistently present in the oral cavity and in the crevicular fluid. Chromatography (see section on diagnosis later in this chapter) revealed that crevicular fluid contains hydrogen sulfide, methylmercaptan and also dimethyl sulfide and even dimethyl disulfide (Coil 1996). When deep pockets are present the relationship with methylmercaptan/H_2S increases (Coil 1996).

One should never forget that many components besides sulfide components, e.g. diamines (putrescine, cadaverine) in the crevicular fluid and in saliva can be malodorous (Goldberg et al. 1995). It is important to realize that the latter odor-inducing components cannot be detected by a portable sulfide monitor (see section on diagnosis later in this chapter), which is often used in breath odor consultations. All such malodor-inducing components can only be perceived when they become volatile. This means that as long as they are dissolved in the saliva, they will not be expressed – just as a perfume only evaporates when the skin becomes dry. This explains why xerostomia reveals a strong breath malodor, which otherwise might only be a faint odor.

While on the one hand periodontitis favors the production of malodorous components, the latter may in their turn play a role in the ongoing periodontitis.

Volatile sulfur components, such as methylmercaptan, enhance the interstitial collagenase production, the IL-1 production by mononuclear cells and the cathepsin B production (Lancero et al. 1996, Ratkay et al. 1996) and thus mediate connective tissue breakdown. Brunette et al. (1996) found that human gingival fibroblasts grown *in vitro* showed an affected cytoskeleton when exposed to CH_3SH. The same gas altered cell proliferation and migration. These potent biologic effects can be blocked by Zn^{++}, at least for the influence of VSC on protein synthesis.

The tongue dorsum, because of its large surface, is a prominent host for products that can cause malodor. Desquamated cells, food remnants, bacteria, etc. accumulate on the tongue and putrefy under the action of bacteria (Bosy et al. 1994). There is six times more tongue coating in patients with periodontitis than in subjects with a healthy periodontium (Yaegaki & Sanada 1992b).

Saliva plays a predominant role in the control/expression of malodorous components. After drying, sulfur and non-sulfur-containing gases such as cadaverine, skatole, indole, etc. are released (Kleinberg & Codipilly 1995). The oral microbiology involved in VSC production is well identified; *Porphyromonas gingivalis, Prevotella intermedia, Fusobacterium nucleatum, Porhyromonas endodontalis, Prevotella loeschii, Haemophilus para influenzae, Treponema denticola, Enterobacter cloacae* and many others have been associated with malodoros gas production (Persson et al. 1990, Kleinberg & Codipilly 1995, Niles & Gaffar 1995). The above are members of the oral microbiota, are anaerobic and are Gram-negative.

The *ear-nose-throat* causes include chronic pharyngitis, purulent sinusitis and postnasal drip. The latter, rather frequent condition is associated with regurgitation oesophagitis and is perceived by patients as a liquid flow in the throat which originates from the nasal cavity (Rosenberg 1996). Ozena, which is an atrophic condition of the nasal mucosa with the appearance of crusts, leads to a very strong breath malodor but is a rare disease.

Pulmonary causes include chronic bronchitis, bronchiectasis, and bronchial carcinoma (Lorber 1975, McGregor et al. 1982).

Gastro-intestinal tract causes include:

- The Zenker diverticle: the accumulation of food and debris in the pouch of the esophagus, not separated from the oral cavity by any sphincter, can cause a significant breath odor (Crescenzo et al. 1998).
- A gastric hernia can, especially when reflux esophagitis occurs, lead to a disturbing breath odor. Otherwise, the stomach never causes breath malodor, contrary to a common opinion among the public and even some clinicians (Norfleet 1993).
- Intestinal gas production can also play a role, probably because some gases such as dimethylsulfide are poorly resorbed by the intestinal endothelium and when transported by the blood they can reach

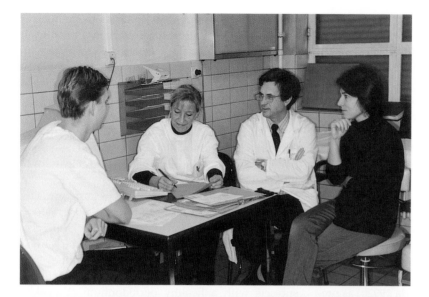

Fig. 24-1 The periodontologist, the oto-rhino-laryngologist and the psychologist listen to the patient.

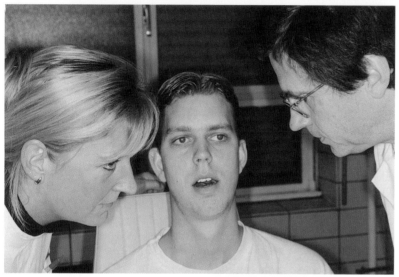

Fig. 24-2. Two calibrated judges evaluate the expired air and compare their rating.

the lung tissue and be exhaled in the breath air (Suarez et al. 1999).

Other *systemic* causes (Leopold et al. 1990, Preti et al. 1995) of breath malodor include renal (uremia) (Simenhoff et al. 1977), pancreatic (acetone) (Booth & Ostenson 1966) and liver (ammonium) (Chen et al. 1970) insufficiencies which appear as breath malodors with different characteristics that can be detected by experienced clinicians.

Some medications such as metronidazole can by themselves cause some breath malodor.

Periodontologists should keep these possible non-oral causes in mind. Their role may be masked to the clinician by the fact that a patient with such a disease may also present, as the vast majority of adults do, with gingivitis or periodontitis.

DIAGNOSIS

Patient history

There is a saying "Listen to the patient and he will tell you the diagnosis". This is very true for patients with breath odor complaints. Besides what is spontaneously told, the clinician should question about the frequency of odor (e.g. does it happen only some weeks), the time of appearance within the day (e.g. after meals, which can indicate a hernia), whether others (non-confidants) have identified the problem (imaginary breath odour?), what kind of medications are taken, whether dryness of the mouth is noticed, etc. (Fig. 24-1).

Several of the points retrieved from this case history, which because of the emotional character of the matter cannot be obtained by a written questionnaire, must be used in the (differential) diagnosis of the problem.

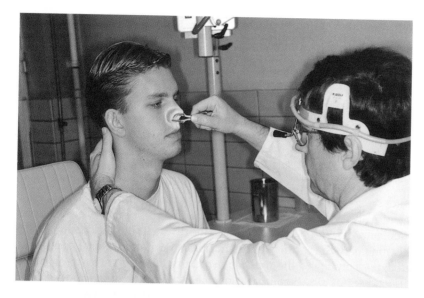

Fig. 24-3. Nasal examination should be done routinely when the air expired through the nose is malodorous.

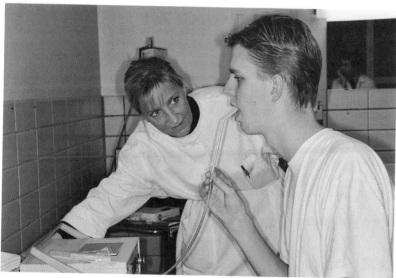

Fig. 24-4. The oropharyngeal air is sampled by an electronic apparatus which measures the volatile sulfur components.

Clinical and laboratory examination

Organoleptic

Even though some instruments are now available, the best method in the examination of breath malodor is still the organoleptic assessment made by a judge, who has been tested and calibrated for his/her smelling acuity. This testing is done by determining the threshold level for detecting a series of dilutions of a malodorous compound such as isovaleric acid. The discrimination power of the judge is evaluated by presenting to him/her a series of odors for identification (Doty et al. 1984).

The use of any fragance, shampoo or body lotion, and smoking, alcohol consumption or garlic intake are strictly forbidden 12 hours before the assessment is made. This involves both the patient and the judge. The judge will not wear rubber gloves, the odor of which may interfere with the organoleptic assessments. Assessments should be performed at several appointments on different days, since breath odor fluctuates dramatically from one day to the next. The patient should be encouraged to bring a confidant to the consultations to help him/her identify the odor

causing the problem. The judge will smell a series of different air samples (Fig. 24-2):

- *Oral cavity odor*: the subject opens his/her mouth and refrains from breathing; the judge places his nose close to the mouth opening.
- *Breath odor*: the subject breathes out through the mouth; the judge smells both the beginning (determined by the oral cavity and systemic factors) and the end (originating from the bronchi and lungs) of the expired air.
- *Tongue coating scraping*: the judge smells the tongue scraping and also presents it to the patient or the accompanying confidant to evaluate whether they associate the smell from the scraping with the malodor complaint.
- *Breath odor when breathing out through the nose*: when the air expired through the nose is malodorous, but the air expired through the mouth is not, a nasal/paranasal etiology should be suspected.

In the oro-pharyngeal examination, the clinician must look for inflammation of the gingiva, or in the mucosa under a prosthesis. Fresh extraction wounds or interdental food entrapment can cause breath malodor. The pharynx should be thoroughly inspected for the presence of inflamed tonsils. The tonsils often present with crypts which may harbor anaerobic bacteria, pus and even calculus (tonsilloliths).

Less obvious for a dentist is the examination of the nostrils, although this is essential if the breath malodor is noticed more clearly when the subject breathes out through the nostrils (Fig. 24-3).

Portable volatile sulfide monitor

This is an electronic device that aspirates the air of the mouth or expired air through a straw and analyses the concentration of H_2S (hydrogen sulfide) and CH_3SH (methylmercaptan), without discriminating between the two (Fig. 24-4). It can also be used to measure the headspace above incubated saliva (Rosenberg et al. 1991). The monitor is good for the detection of hydrogen sulfide but less good for methyl mercaptan. It needs regular calibrations.

It should be stressed that this machine will not detect malodorous components such as cadaverine, putrescine, urea, indole, skatole and several others which have been described in salivary headspace (Kostelc 1981). Cadaverine (produced by bacteria through decarboxylation of lysine to counteract the unfavorable acidic growth conditions during glycolysis) and putrescine (from decarboxylation of ornithine or arginine) are both diamines the level of which in air expired from the mouth does not, evidence shows, correlate with VSC scores (Goldberg et al. 1994) but does correlate to a certain extent with tongue coating and/or periodontitis.

Gas chromatography

This can analyse air or incubated saliva or crevicular fluid for any volatile component (Goldberg et al. 1994). Some hundred components were isolated, and mostly identified, from saliva and/or tongue coating, from ketones to alkanes and from sulfur-containing compounds to phenyl compounds (Claus et al. 1996). Gas chromatography is only available in specialized centers and for identifying non-oral causes such as intestinal (Suarez et al. 1999) or bronchial/pulmonary causes.

TREATMENT

An etiologic treatment is to be preferred. The treatment of oral malodor consists of the elimination of the pathology present, such as deepened and inflamed periodontal pockets and/or tongue coating. If another underlying disease is suspected, or if clinical experts in the different disciplines (internal medicine, periodontology, ENT, psychology, etc.) are not available, it is possible to rapidly (within 1-2 weeks) make a differential diagnosis by performing a full-mouth one-stage disinfection of the oro-pharynx, including the

use of chlorhexidine spray to deal with the pharynx (Quirynen et al. 2000). Since all oral diseases which cause malodor relate to microorganisms, this one-stage professional approach reinforced by stringent home care will dramatically reduce the oro-pharyngeal microbiota and the putrefraction they cause and thus the malodour (Quirynen et al. 1998). If the symptoms do not disappear, the patient should be referred to a specialized multidisciplinary center where gas chromatography can help in the differential diagnosis.

Masking of breath malodor should be distinguished from etiological treatment. It is well established that zinc-containing mouthrinses have the property to complex the divalent sulfur radicals, reducing this important cause of malodor. Thus it appears that the application of a zincchloride/triclosan-containing toothpaste on the tongue dorsum reduces the oral malodor for some 4 hours (Hoshi & van Steenberghe 1996). Baking soda containing dentifrices (> 20%) confers a significant odor-reducing benefit for up to 3 hours (Brunette et al. 1998). The use of hydrogen peroxide rinse also offers positive perspectives (Suarez et al. 2000). To deal with the tongue coating it appears that tongue brushing with chlorhexidine, besides oral rinses with the same antiseptic, reduces the organoleptic scores significantly (Loesche & De Boever 1996). Whether the beneficial effect of tongue brushing is related to the removal of bacteria and/or to the reduction of their substratum, remains an open question.

Hardly efficient are mints and other short acting "anti-breath" odor components. Most of them have not been properly tested in a blind way against a placebo. A recent review compared the efficiency of oral rinses, toothpastes and cosmetics for breath odor therapy (Quirynen et al. 2002).

When dryness is at stake, any measure to increase the salivary flow may be beneficial. This can mean a proper fluid intake or the use of chewing gum to trigger the periodontal-parotid reflex, which originates from the mechanoreceptors in the periodontal ligament of molar teeth (lower) and has the parotid gland as a target (Hector & Linden 1987). The presence of these molars is therefore crucial before advocating the use of chewing gum to enhance salivary secretion. The pH of the saliva can also be reduced to increase the solubility of malodorous components (Reingewirtz et al. 1999). Evidence shows that the effect is short-lived.

CONCLUSIONS

Breath malodor has important socio-economic consequences. A proper diagnosis and determination of the etiology allows the proper etiological treatment to be instituted quickly. Although gingivitis, periodontitis and tongue coating are by far the most common causes, other more challenging diseases should not be overlooked. This can be dealt with either by a trial therapy to deal quickly with intra-oral causes (the full-mouth one-stage disinfection) or by a multidisciplinary consultation.

REFERENCES

Booth, G. & Ostenson, S. (1966). Acetone to alveolar air, and the control of diabetes. *Lancet* **II**, 1102-1105.

Bosy, A., Kulkarni, G.V., Rosenberg, M. & McCulloch, C.A.G. (1994). Relationship of oral malodor to periodontitis: evidence of independence in discrete subpopulations. *Journal of Periodontology* **65**, 37-46.

Brunette, D.M., Ouyang, Y., Glass-Brudzinski, J. & Tonzetich, J. (1996). Effects of methyl mercaptan on human gingival fibroblast shape, cytoskeleton and protein synthesis and the inhibition of its effect by Zn^{++}. In: van Steenberghe, D. & Rosenberg, M., eds. *Bad Breath: a multidisciplinary approach.* Leuven: Leuven University Press, pp. 47-62.

Brunette, D.M., Proskin, H.M. & Nelson, B.J. (1998). The effects of dentifrice systems on oral malodor. *Journal of Clinical Dentistry* **9**, 76-82.

Chen, S., Zieve, L. & Mahadevan, V. (1970). Mercaptans and dimethyl sulfide in the breath of patients with cirrhosis of the liver. Effect of feeding methionine. *The Journal of Laboratory and Clinical Medicine* **75**, 628-635.

Claus, D., Geypens, B., Rutgeers, P., Ghyselen, J., Hoshi, K., van Steenberghe, D. & Ghoos, Y. (1996). Where gastroenterology and periodontology meet: determination of oral volatile organic compounds using closed-loop trapping and high-resolution gas chromatography-ion trap detection. In: van Steenberghe, D. & Rosenberg, M., eds. *Bad Breath: a multidisciplinary approach.* Leuven: Leuven University Press, pp. 15-27.

Coil, J.M. (1996). Characterization of volatile sulphur compounds production at individual crevicular sites. In: van Steenberghe, D. & Rosenberg, M., eds. *Bad Breath: a multidisciplinary approach.* Leuven: Leuven University Press, pp. 31-38.

Cresecenzo, D.G., Trastek, V.F., Allen, M.S., Descamps, C. & Pairolero, P.C. (1998). Zenker's diverticulum in the elderly: is operation justified? *Annals of Thoracic Surgery* **66**, 347-350.

Delanghe, G., Ghyselen, J., van Steenberghe, D. & Feenstra, L. (1997). Multidisciplinary breath-odour clinic. *The Lancet* **350**, 187.

Derogatis, L.R., Lipman, R.S. & Covi, L. (1973). SCL-90: an outpatient psychiatric rating scale – preliminary report. *Psychopharmacology Bulletin* **9**, 13-28.

Doty, R.L., Shaman, P., Dann, M. (1984). Development of the University of Pennsylvania Smell Identification Test: a standardized microencapsulated test of olfactory function. *Physiological Behaviour* **32**, 489-502.

Eli, I., Baht, R., Kozlovsky, A. & Rosenberg, M. (1996). The complaint of oral malodor: possible psychopathological aspects. *Psychosomatic Medicine* **58**, 156-159.

Goldberg, S., Kozlovsky, A., Gordon, D., Gelernter, I., Sintov, A. & Rosenberg, M. (1994). Cadaverine as a putative component of oral malodor. *Journal of Dental Research* **73**, 1168-1172.

Goldberg, S., Kozlovsky, A. & Rosenberg, M. (1995). Association of diamines with oral malodor. In: Rosenberg, M., ed. *Bad Breath: Research perspectives.* Tel-Aviv: Ramot Publishing, Tel-Aviv University, pp. 71-85.

Hector, M.P. & Linden, R.W. (1987). The possible role of periodontal mechanoreceptors in the control of parotid secretion in man. *The Quarterly Journal of Experimental Physiology* **72**, 285-301.

Hoshi, K. & van Steenberghe, D. (1996). The effect of tongue brushing or toothpaste application on oral malodor reduction. In: van Steenberghe, D. & Rosenberg, M., eds. *Bad Breath: a multidisciplinary approach.* Leuven: Leuven University Press, pp. 255-264.

Howe, J.W. (1898). *The breath and the diseases which give it a fetid odor*, 4th edn. New York: D. Appleton and Co.

Kleinberg, I. & Codipilly, M. (1995). The biological basis of oral malodor formation. In: Rosenberg M, ed. *Bad Breath: Research perspectives.* Tel-Aviv: Ramot Publishing, Tel-Aviv University, pp. 13-39.

Kostelc, J.G. (1981). Volatiles of exogenous origin from the human oral cavity. *Journal of Chromatography* **226**, 315-323.

Lancero, H., Niu, J. & Johnson, P.W. (1996). Thiols modulate metabolism of gingival fibroblasts and periodontal ligament cells. In: van Steenberghe, D. & Rosenberg, M., eds. *Bad Breath: a multidisciplinary approach.* Leuven: Leuven University Press, pp. 63-78.

Leopold, D.A., Preti, H.J., Monzell, Youngentob, S.L. & Wright, H.N. (1990). Fish-odor syndrome presenting as dysosmia. *Archives of Otolaryngology – Head and Neck Surgery* **116**, 354-355.

Loesche, W. J. & De Boever, E. (1996). Strategies to identify the main microbial contributors to oral malodor. In: van Steenberghe, D. & Rosenberg, M., eds. *Bad Breath: a multidisciplinary approach.* Leuven: Leuven University Press, pp. 41-54.

Lorber, B. (1975). Bad breath. Presenting manifestation of anaerobic pulmonary infection. *American Reviews of Respiratory Diseases* **112**, 875-877.

McGregor, I.A., Watson, J.D., Sweeney, G. & Sleigh, J.D. (1982). Tinidazole in smelly oropharyngeal tumours. *Lancet* **I**, 110.

Morris, P.P. & Read, R.R. (1949). Halitosis: variations in mouth and total breath odor intensity resulting from prophylaxis and antisepsis. *Journal of Dental Research* **28**, 324-333.

Niles, H. & Gaffar, A. (1995). Advances in mouth odor research. In: Rosenberg, M., ed. *Bad Breath: Research perspectives.* Tel-Aviv: Ramot Publishing, Tel-Aviv University, pp. 55-69.

Norfleet, R.G. (1993). *Helicobacter* halitosis. *Journal of Clinical Gastroenterology* **16**, 274.

Oxtoby, A. & Field, E.A. (1994). Delusional symptoms in dental patients: a report of four cases. *British Dental Journal* **176**, 140-142.

Persson, S., Claesson, R. & Carlsson, J. (1989). The capacity of subgingival microbiotas to produce volatile sulfur compounds in human serum. *Oral Microbiology & Immunology* **4**, 169-172.

Persson, S., Edlund, M.B., Claesson, R. & Carlsson, J. (1990). The formation of hydrogen sulfide and methylmercaptan by oral bacteria. *Oral Microbiology & Immunology* **5**, 195-201.

Preti, G., Lawley, H.J. & Hormann, C.A. (1995). Non-oral and oral aspects of oral malodor. In: Rosenberg, M., ed. *Bad Breath: Research perspectives.* Tel-Aviv: Ramot Publishing, Tel-Aviv University, pp. 149-173.

Quirynen, M., Mongardini, C., De Soete, M., Pauwels, M., Coucke, W. & van Steenberghe, D. (2000). The role of chlorhexidine in the one-stage full-mouth disinfection treatment of patients with advanced adult periodontitis. Long-term clinical and microbiological observations. *Journal of Clinical Periodontology* **27**, 578-589.

Quirynen, M., Mongardini, C. & van Steenberghe, D. (1998). The effect of a 1-stage full-mouth disinfection on oral malodor and microbial colonization of the tongue in periodontitis patients. A pilot study. *Journal of Periodontology* **69**, 374-382.

Quirynen, M., Zhao, H. & van Steenberghe, D. (2002). Review of the treatment strategies for oral malodour. *Clinical Oral Investigations* (in press).

Ratkay, L.G., Tonzetich, J. & Waterfield, J.D. (1996). The effect of methyl mercaptan on the enzymatic and immunological activity leading to periodontal tissue destruction. In: van Steenberghe, D. & Rosenberg, M., eds. *Bad Breath: a multidisciplinary approach.* Leuven: Leuven University Press, pp. 35-46.

Reingewirtz, Y., Girault, O., Reingewirtz, N., Senger, B. & Tenenbaum, H. (1999). Mechanical effects and volatile sulfur compound-reducing effects of chewing gums: comparison between test and base gums and a control group. *Quintessence International* **30**, 319-323.

Rosenberg, M. (1995). *Bad Breath: Research Perspectives.* Tel-Aviv: Ramot Publishing, Tel-Aviv University, Tel-Aviv, pp. 237.

Rosenberg, M. (1996). Clinical assessment of bad breath: current concepts. *Journal of American Dental Association* **127**, 475-482.

Rosenberg, M., Kulkarni, G.V., Bosy, A. & McCulloch, C.A.G. (1991). Reproducibility and sensitivity of oral malodor measurements with a portable sulfide monitor. *Journal of Dental Research* **11**, 1436-1440.

Simenhoff, M.L., Burke, J.F., Saukkonen, J.J., Ordinario, A.T. & Doty, R.L. (1977). Biochemical profile of uremic breath. *New England Journal of Medicine* **297**, 132-135.

Suarez, F.L., Furne, J.K., Springfield, J. & Levitt, M.D. (2000). Morning breath odor: influence of treatments on sulfur gases. *Journal of Dental Research* **79**, 1773-1777.

Suarez, F., Springfield, J., Furne, J. & Levitt, M. (1999). Differentiation of mouth versus gut as site of origin of odoriferous breath gases after garlic ingestion. *The American Journal of Physiology* **276**, G425-430.

Tonzetich, J. (1977). Production and origin of oral malodor: a review of mechanisms and methods of analysis. *Journal of Periodontology* **48**, 13-20.

van Steenberghe, D. (1997). Breath malodor. *Current Opinion in Periodontology* **4**, 137-143.

van Steenberghe, D. & Rosenberg, M. (1996). *Bad Breath: a multidisciplinary approach.* Leuven: Leuven University Press, p. 287.

Yaegaki, K. (1995). Oral malodor and periodontal disease. In: Rosenberg, M., ed. *Bad Breath: Research perspectives.* Tel-Aviv: Ramot Publishing, Tel-Aviv University, pp. 88-108.

Yaegaki, K. & Sanada, K. (1992a). Biochemical and clinical factors influencing oral malodor in periodontal patients. *Journal of Periodontology* **63**, 783-789.

Yaegaki, K. & Sanada, K. (1992b). Volatile sulfur compounds in mouth air from clinically healthy subjects and patients with periodontal disease. *Journal of Periodontal Research* **27**, 233-238.

CHAPTER 25

Periodontal Surgery: Access Therapy

JAN L. WENNSTRÖM, LARS HEIJL AND JAN LINDHE

Since most forms of periodontal disease are plaque-associated disorders, it is obvious that surgical access therapy can only be considered as adjunctive to cause-related therapy (see Chapter 20). Therefore, the various surgical methods described below should be evaluated on the basis of their potential to facilitate removal of subgingival deposits and self-performed plaque control and thereby enhance the long-term preservation of the periodontium.

The decision concerning what type of periodontal surgery should be performed and how many sites should be included is usually made after the effect of initial cause-related measures has been evaluated. The time lapse between termination of the initial cause-related phase of therapy and this evaluation may vary from 1 to 6 months. This routine has the following advantages:

- The removal of calculus and bacterial plaque will eliminate or markedly reduce the inflammatory cell infiltrate in the gingiva (edema, hyperemia, flabby tissue consistency), thereby making assessment of the "true" gingival contours and pocket depths possible.
- The reduction of gingival inflammation makes the soft tissues more fibrous and thus firmer, which facilitates surgical handling of the soft tissues. The propensity for bleeding is reduced, making inspection of the surgical field easier.

- A better basis for a proper assessment of the prognosis has been established. The effectiveness of the patient's home care, which is of decisive importance for the long-term prognosis, can be properly evaluated. Lack of effective self-performed care will often mean that the patient should be excluded from surgical treatment.

TECHNIQUES IN PERIODONTAL POCKET SURGERY

Over the years, several different surgical techniques have been described and used in periodontal therapy. A superficial review of the literature in this area may give the reader a somewhat confusing picture of the specific objectives and indications relevant for various surgical techniques. It is a matter of historical interest that the first surgical techniques used in periodontal therapy were described as means of gaining access to diseased root surfaces. Such access could be accomplished without excision of the soft tissue pocket ("open-view operations"). Later, procedures were described by which the "diseased gingiva" was excised (gingivectomy procedures).

The concept that not only inflamed soft tissue but also "infected and necrotic bone" had to be eliminated called for the development of surgical techniques by

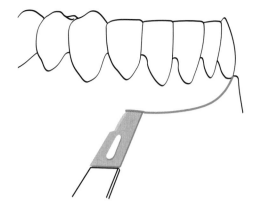

Fig. 25-1. *Gingivectomy*. The straight incision technique (Robicsek 1884).

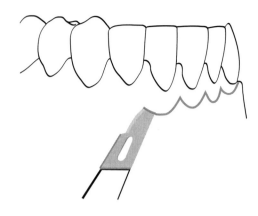

Fig. 25-2. *Gingivectomy*. The scalloped incision technique (Zentler 1918).

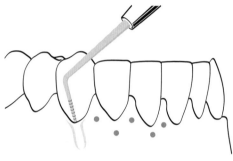

a

b

Fig. 25-3. *Gingivectomy*. Pocket marking. (a) An ordinary periodontal probe is used to identify the bottom of the deepened pocket. (b) When the depth of the pocket has been assessed, an equivalent distance is delineated on the outer aspect of the gingiva. The tip of the probe is then turned horizontally and used to produce a bleeding point at the level of the bottom of the probeable pocket.

which the alveolar bone could be exposed and resected (flap procedures). Other concepts such as (1) the importance of maintaining the mucogingival complex (i.e. a wide zone of gingiva) and (2) the possibility for regeneration of periodontal tissues have also prompted the introduction of "tailor-made" surgical techniques.

In the following, surgical procedures will be described which represent important steps in the development of the surgical component of periodontal therapy.

Gingivectomy procedures

The surgical approach as an alternative to subgingival scaling for pocket therapy was already recognized in the latter part of the nineteenth century, when Robicsek (1884) pioneered the so-called *gingivectomy* procedure. Gingivectomy was later defined by Grant et al. (1979) as being "the excision of the soft tissue wall of a pathologic periodontal pocket". The surgical procedure, which aimed at "pocket elimination", was usu-

ally combined with recontouring of the diseased gingiva to restore physiologic form.

Robicsek (1884) and, later, Zentler (1918) described the gingivectomy procedure in the following way: The line to which the gum is to be resected is determined first. Following a straight (Robicsek; Fig. 25-1) or scalloped (Zentler; Fig. 25-2) incision, first on the labial and then on the lingual surface of each tooth, the diseased tissue should be loosened and lifted out by means of a hook-shaped instrument. After elimination of the soft tissue, the exposed alveolar bone should be scraped. The area should then be covered with some kind of antibacterial gauze or be painted with disinfecting solutions. The result obtained should include eradication of the deepened periodontal pocket and a local condition which could be kept clean more easily.

Technique
The gingivectomy procedure as it is employed today was described in 1951 by Goldman.

- When the dentition in the area scheduled for surgery has been properly anesthetized, the depths of the pathologic pockets are identified with a conven-

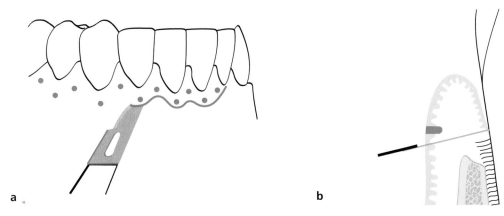

Fig. 25-4. *Gingivectomy*. (a) The primary incision. (b) The incision is terminated at a level apical to the "bottom" of the pocket and is angulated to give the cut surface a distinct bevel.

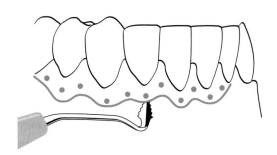

Fig. 25-5. *Gingivectomy*. The secondary incision through the interdental area is performed with the use of a Waerhaug knife.

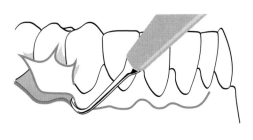

Fig. 25-6. *Gingivectomy*. The detached gingiva is removed with a scaler.

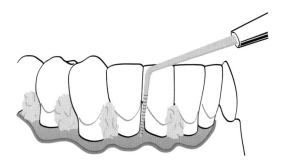

Fig. 25-7. *Gingivectomy*. Probing for residual pockets. Gauze packs have been placed in the interdental spaces to control bleeding.

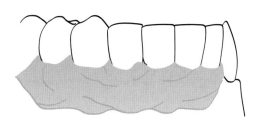

Fig. 25-8. *Gingivectomy*. The periodontal dressing has been applied and properly secured.

tional periodontal probe (Fig. 25-3a). At the level of the bottom of the pocket, the gingiva is pierced with the probe and a bleeding point is produced on the outer surface of the soft tissue (Fig. 25-3b). The pockets are probed and bleeding points produced at several location points around each tooth in the area. The series of bleeding points produced describes the depth of the pockets in the area scheduled for treatment and is used as a guideline for the incision.

• The primary incision (Fig. 25-4), which may be made by a scalpel (blade No. 12B or 15; Bard-

Parker®) in either a Bard-Parker handle or an angulated handle (e.g. a Blake's handle), or a Kirkland knife No. 15/16, should be planned to give a thin and properly festooned margin of the remaining gingiva. Thus, in areas where the gingiva is bulky, the incision must be placed at a level more apical to the level of the bleeding points than in areas with a thin gingiva, where a less accentuated bevel is needed. The beveled incision is directed towards the base of the pocket or to a level slightly apical to the apical extension of the junctional epithelium. In areas where the interdental pockets are deeper than the buccal or lingual pockets, additional amounts of buccal and/or lingual (palatal) gingiva must be removed in order to establish a "physiologic" contour of the gingival margin. This is often accomplished by initiating the incision at a more apical level.

- Once the primary incision is completed on the buccal and lingual aspects of the teeth, the interproximal soft tissue is separated from the interdental periodontium by a secondary incision using an Orban knife (No. 1 or 2) or a Waerhaug knife (No. 1 or 2; a saw-toothed modification of the Orban knife; Fig. 25-5).
- The incised tissues are carefully removed by means of a curette or a scaler (Fig. 25-6). Remaining tissue tabs are removed with a curette or a pair of scissors. Pieces of gauze packs often have to be placed in the interdental areas to control bleeding. When the field of operation is properly prepared, the exposed root surfaces are carefully scaled and planed.
- Following meticulous debridement, the dentogingival regions are probed again to detect any remaining pockets (Fig. 25-7). The gingival contour is checked and, if necessary, corrected by means of knives or rotating diamond burs.
- To protect the incised area during the period of healing, the wound surface must be covered by a periodontal dressing (Fig. 25-8). The dressing should be closely adapted to the buccal and lingual wound surfaces as well as to the interproximal spaces. Care should be taken not to allow the dressing to become too bulky, since this is not only uncomfortable for the patient, but also facilitates dislodgement of the dressing.
- The dressing should remain in position for 10-14 days. After removal of the dressing, the teeth must be cleaned and polished. The root surfaces are carefully checked and remaining calculus removed with a curette. Excessive granulation tissue is eliminated with a curette. The patient is instructed to properly clean the operated segments of the dentition, which now have a different morphology as compared to the preoperative situation.

Flap procedures

The original Widman flap
One of the first detailed descriptions of the use of a flap procedure for pocket elimination was published in 1918 by *Leonard Widman*. In his article "The operative treatment of pyorrhea alveolaris" Widman described a mucoperiosteal flap design aimed at removing the pocket epithelium and the inflamed connective tissue, thereby facilitating optimal cleaning of the root surfaces.

Technique
- Sectional releasing incisions were first made to demarcate the area scheduled for surgery (Fig. 25-9).

These incisions were made from the mid-buccal gingival margins of the two peripheral teeth of the treatment area and were continued several millimeters out into the alveolar mucosa. The two releasing incisions were connected by a gingival incision which followed the outline of the gingival margin and *separated the pocket epithelium and the inflamed connective tissue from the non-inflamed gingiva*. Similar releasing and gingival incisions were, if needed, made on the lingual aspect of the teeth.

- A mucoperiosteal flap was elevated to expose at least 2-3 mm of the marginal alveolar bone. The collar of inflamed tissue around the neck of the teeth was removed with curettes (Fig. 25-10) and the exposed root surfaces were carefully scaled. Bone recontouring was recommended in order to achieve an ideal anatomic form of the underlying alveolar bone (Fig. 25-11).
- Following careful debridement of the teeth in the surgical area, the buccal and lingual flaps were laid back over the alveolar bone and secured in this position with interproximal sutures (Fig. 25-12). Widman pointed out the importance of placing the soft tissue margin at the level of the alveolar bone crest, so that no pockets would remain. The surgical procedure resulted in the exposure of root surfaces. Often the interproximal areas were left without soft tissue coverage of the alveolar bone.

The main advantages of the *"original Widman flap"* procedure in comparison to the gingivectomy procedure included, according to Widman (1918):

- less discomfort for the patient, since healing occurred by primary intention and
- that it was possible to reestablish a proper contour of the alveolar bone in sites with angular bony defects.

The Neumann flap
Only a few years later, *Neumann* (1920, 1926) suggested the use of a flap procedure which in some respects was different from that originally described by Widman.

Technique
- According to the technique suggested by Neumann, an intracrevicular incision was made through the base of the gingival pockets, and the entire gingiva (and part of the alveolar mucosa) was elevated in a mucoperiosteal flap. Sectional releasing incisions were made to demarcate the area of surgery.
- Following flap elevation, the inside of the flap was curetted to remove the pocket epithelium and the granulation tissue. The root surfaces were subsequently carefully "cleaned". Any irregularities of the alveolar bone were corrected to give the bone crest a horizontal outline.
- The flaps were then trimmed to allow both an optimal adaptation to the teeth and a proper coverage

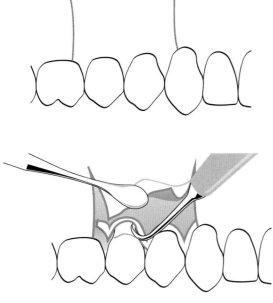

Fig. 25-9. *Original Widman flap*. Two releasing incisions demarcate the area scheduled for surgical therapy. A scalloped reverse bevel incision is made in the gingival margin to connect the two releasing incisions.

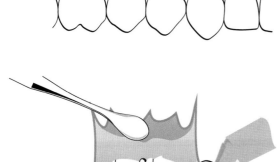

Fig. 25-10. *Original Widman flap*. The collar of inflamed gingival tissue is removed following the elevation of a mucoperiosteal flap.

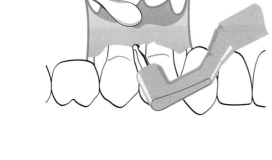

Fig. 25-11. *Original Widman flap*. By bone recontouring, a "physiologic" contour of the alveolar bone may be reestablished.

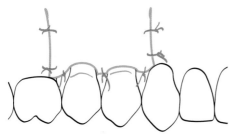

Fig. 25-12. *Original Widman flap*. The coronal ends of the buccal and lingual flaps are placed at the alveolar bone crest and secured in this position by interdentally placed sutures.

of the alveolar bone on both the buccal/lingual (palatal) and the interproximal sites. With regard to pocket elimination, Neumann (1926) pointed out the importance of removing the soft tissue pockets, i.e. replacing the flap at the crest of the alveolar bone.

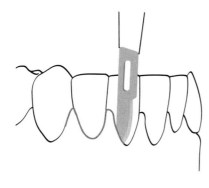

Fig. 25-13. *Modified flap operation (The Kirkland flap)*. Intracrevicular incision.

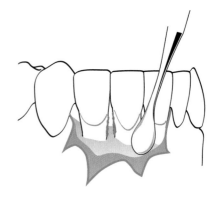

Fig. 25-14. *Modified flap operation (The Kirkland flap)*. The gingiva is retracted to expose the "diseased" root surface.

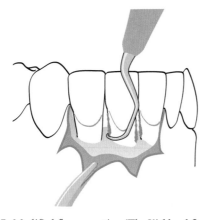

Fig. 25-15. *Modified flap operation (The Kirkland flap)*. The exposed root surfaces are subjected to mechanical debridement.

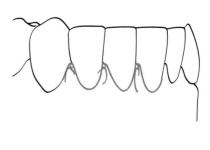

Fig. 25-16. *Modified flap operation (The Kirkland flap)*. The flaps are replaced to their original position and sutured.

The modified flap operation

In a publication from 1931 *Kirkland* described a surgical procedure to be used in the treatment of "periodontal pus pockets". The procedure was called the *modified flap operation,* and is basically an access flap for proper root debridement.

Technique

- In this procedure incisions were made intracrevicularly through the bottom of the pocket (Fig. 25-13) on both the labial and the lingual aspects of the interdental area. The incisions were extended in a mesial and distal direction.
- The gingiva was retracted labially and lingually to expose the diseased root surfaces (Fig. 25-14), which were carefully debrided (Fig. 25-15). Angular bony defects were curetted.
- Following the elimination of the pocket epithelium and granulation tissue from the inner surface of the flaps, these were *re-placed* to their original position and secured with interproximal sutures (Fig. 25-16). Thus, no attempt was made to reduce the preoperative depth of the pockets.

In contrast to the *original Widman flap* as well as the *Neumann flap,* the *modified flap operation* did not include (1) extensive sacrifice of non-inflamed tissues and (2) apical displacement of the gingival margin. Since the root surfaces were not markedly exposed thereby, the method could for esthetic reasons be useful in the anterior regions of the dentition. Another advantage of the *modified flap operation* was the potential for bone regeneration in intrabony defects which, according to Kirkland (1931), in fact frequently occurred.

The main objectives of the flap procedures so far described were to:

- facilitate the debridement of the root surfaces as well as the removal of the pocket epithelium and the inflamed connective tissue,
- eliminate the deepened pockets (the *original Widman flap* and the *Neumann flap*) and
- cause a minimal amount of trauma to the periodontal tissues and discomfort to the patient.

The apically repositioned flap

In the 1950s and 1960s new surgical techniques for the removal of soft and, when indicated, hard tissue periodontal pockets were described in the literature. The importance of maintaining *an adequate zone of attached gingiva* after surgery was now emphasized. One of the first authors to describe a technique for the preservation of the gingiva following surgery was *Nabers* (1954). The surgical technique developed by Nabers was originally denoted "repositioning of attached gingiva" and was later modified by Ariaudo & Tyrrell (1957). In 1962 *Friedman* proposed the term *apically repositioned flap* to more appropriately describe the surgical technique introduced by Nabers. Friedman emphasized the fact that, at the end of the surgical procedure, the entire complex of the soft tissues (gingiva and alveolar mucosa) rather than the gingiva alone was displaced in an apical direction. Thus, rather than excising the amount of gingiva which would be in excess *after* osseous surgery (if performed), the whole mucogingival complex was maintained and apically repositioned. This surgical technique was used on buccal surfaces in both maxillas and mandibles and on lingual surfaces in the mandible, while an excisional technique had to be used on the palatal aspect of maxillary teeth.

Technique

According to Friedman (1962) the technique should be performed in the following way:

- A reverse bevel incision is made using a scalpel with a Bard-Parker blade (No. 12B or No. 15). How far from the buccal/lingual gingival margin the incision should be made is dependent on the pocket depth as well as the thickness and the width of the gingiva (Fig. 25-17). If the gingiva preoperatively is thin and only a narrow zone of keratinized tissue is present, the incision should be made close to the tooth. The beveling incision should be given a scalloped outline to ensure maximal interproximal coverage of the alveolar bone, when the flap subsequently is repositioned. Vertical releasing incisions extending out into the alveolar mucosa (i.e. past the mucogingival junction) are made at each of the end points of the reverse incision, thereby making possible the apical repositioning of the flap.
- A full thickness mucoperiosteal flap including buccal/lingual gingiva and alveolar mucosa is raised by means of a mucoperiosteal elevator. The flap has to be elevated beyond the mucogingival line in order to later be able to reposition the soft tissue apically. The marginal collar of tissue, including pocket epithelium and granulation tissue, is removed with curettes (Fig. 25-18), and the exposed root surfaces are carefully scaled and planed.

- The alveolar bone crest is recontoured with the objective of recapturing the normal form of the alveolar process but at a more apical level (Fig. 25-19). The osseous surgery is performed using burs and/or bone chisels.
- Following careful adjustment, the buccal/lingual flap is repositioned to the level of the newly recontoured alveolar bone crest and secured in this position (Fig. 25-20). The incisional and excisional technique used means that it is not always possible to obtain proper soft tissue coverage of the denuded interproximal alveolar bone. A periodontal dressing should therefore be applied to protect the exposed bone and to retain the soft tissue at the level of the bone crest (Fig. 25-21). After healing, an "adequate" zone of gingiva is preserved and no residual pockets should remain.

To handle periodontal pockets on the palatal aspect of the teeth, Friedman described a modification of the "apically repositioned flap", which he termed the *beveled flap*. Since there is no alveolar mucosa present on the palatal aspect of the teeth, it is not possible to reposition the flap in an apical direction.

- In order to prepare the tissue at the gingival margin to properly follow the outline of the alveolar bone crest, a conventional mucoperiosteal flap is first resected (Fig. 25-22).
- The tooth surfaces are debrided and osseous recontouring is performed (Fig. 25-23).
- The palatal flap is subsequently replaced and the gingival margin is prepared and adjusted to the alveolar bone crest by a secondary scalloped and beveled incision (Fig. 25-24). The flap is secured in this position with interproximal sutures (Fig. 25-25).

Among a number of suggested advantages of the *apically repositioned flap* procedure, the following have been emphasized:

- Minimum pocket depth postoperatively.
- If optimal soft tissue coverage of the alveolar bone is obtained, the postsurgical bone loss is minimal.
- The postoperative position of the gingival margin may be controlled and the entire mucogingival complex may be maintained.

The sacrifice of periodontal tissues by bone resection and the subsequent exposure of root surfaces (which may cause esthetic and root hypersensitivity problems) were regarded as the main disadvantages of this technique.

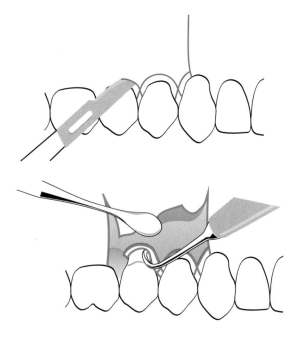

Fig. 25-17. *Apically repositioned flap*. Following a vertical releasing incision, the reverse bevel incision is made through the gingiva and the periosteum to separate the inflamed tissue adjacent to the tooth from the flap.

Fig. 25-18. *Apically repositioned flap*. A mucoperiosteal flap is raised and the tissue collar remaining around the teeth, including the pocket epithelium and the inflamed connective tissue, is removed with a currette.

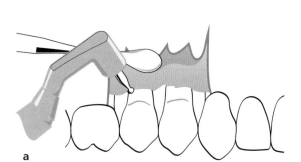

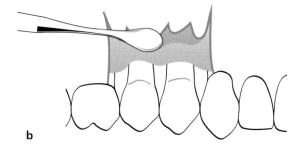

Fig. 25-19. *Apically repositioned flap*. Osseous surgery is performed with the use of a rotating bur (a) to recapture the physiologic contour of the alveolar bone (b).

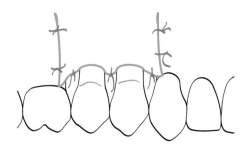

Fig. 25-20. *Apically repositioned flap*. The flaps are repositioned in an apical direction to the level of the recontoured alveolar bone crest and retained in this position by sutures.

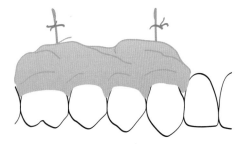

Fig. 25-21. *Apically repositioned flap*. A periodontal dressing is placed over the surgical area to ensure that the flaps remain in the correct position during healing.

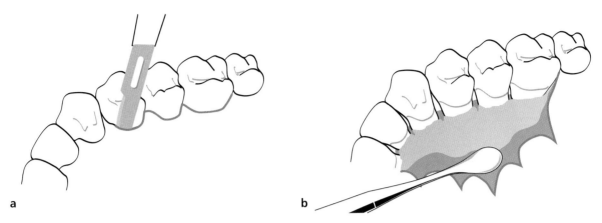

a

b

Fig. 25-22. *Beveled flap*. A primary incision is made intracrevicularly through the bottom of the periodontal pocket (a) and a conventional mucoperiosteal flap is elevated (b).

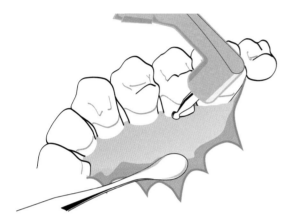

Fig. 25-23. *Beveled flap*. Scaling, root planing and osseous recontouring is performed in the surgical area.

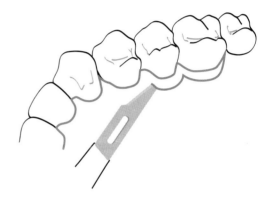

Fig. 25-24. *Beveled flap*. The palatal flap is replaced and a secondary, scalloped, reverse bevel incision is made to adjust the length of the flap to the height of the remaining alveolar bone.

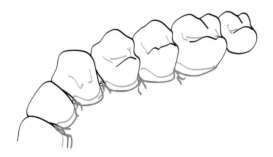

Fig. 25-25. *Beveled flap*. The shortened and thinned flap is replaced over the alveolar bone and in close contact with the root surfaces.

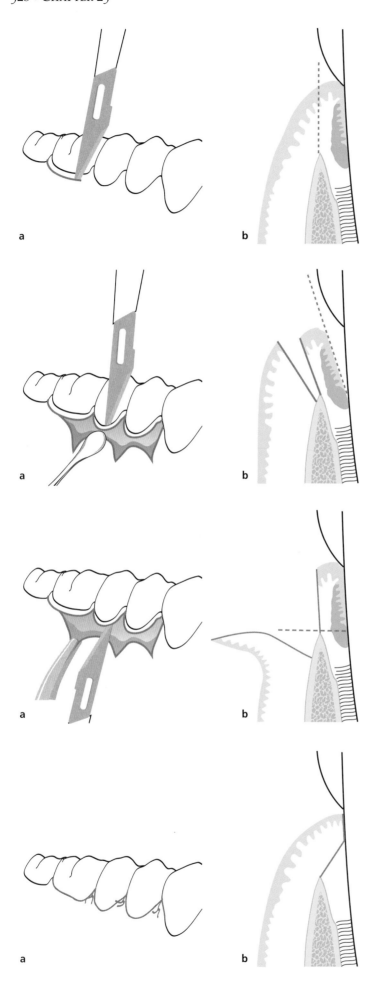

Fig. 25-26. *Modified Widman flap.* The initial incision is placed 0.5-1 mm from the gingival margin (a) and parallel to the long axis of the tooth.

Fig. 25-27. *Modified Widman flap.* Following careful elevation of the the flaps, a second intracrevicular incision (a) is made to the alveolar bone crest (b) to separate the tissue collar from the root surface.

Fig. 25-28. *Modified Widman flap.* The third incision is made perpendicular to the root surface (a) and as close as possible to the bone crest (b), thereby separating the tissue collar from the alveolar bone.

Fig. 25-29. *Modified Widman flap.* (a) Following proper debridement and currettage of angular bone defects, the flaps are carefully adjusted to cover the alveolar bone and sutured. (b) Complete coverage of the interdental bone as well as close adaptation of the flaps to the tooth surfaces should be accomplished.

The modified Widman flap

Ramfjord & Nissle (1974) described the *modified Widman flap* technique, which is also recognized as the *open flap curettage* technique. It should be noted that, while the *original Widman flap* technique included both apical displacement of the flaps and osseous recontouring (elimination of bony defects) to obtain proper pocket elimination, the *modified Widman flap* technique is not intended to meet these objectives.

Technique

• According to the description by Ramfjord & Nissle (1974) the *initial incision* (Fig. 25-26), which may be performed with a Bard-Parker knife (No. 11), should be parallel to the long axis of the tooth and placed approximately 1 mm from the buccal gingival margin in order to properly separate the pocket epithelium from the flap. If the pockets on the buccal aspects of the teeth are less than 2 mm deep or if esthetic considerations are important, an intracrevicular incision may be made. Furthermore, the scalloped incision should be extended as far as possible in between the teeth, to allow maximum amounts of the interdental gingiva to be included in the flap. A similar incision technique is used on the palatal aspect. Often, however, the scalloped outline of the initial incision may be accentuated by placing the knife at a distance of 1-2 mm from the midpalatal surface of the teeth. By extending the incision as far as possible in between the teeth sufficient amounts of tissue can be included in the palatal flap to allow for proper coverage of the interproximal bone when the flap is sutured. Vertical releasing incisions are not usually required.

• Buccal and palatal full thickness flaps are carefully elevated with a mucoperiosteal elevator. The flap elevation should be limited and allow only a few millimeters of the alveolar bone crest to become exposed. To facilitate the gentle separation of the collar of pocket epithelium and granulation tissue from the root surfaces, an intracrevicular incision is made around the teeth (*second incision*) to the alveolar crest (Fig. 25-27).

• A *third incision* (Fig. 25-28) made in a horizontal direction and in a position close to the surface of the alveolar bone crest separates the soft tissue collar of the root surfaces from the bone.

• The pocket epithelium and the granulation tissues are removed by means of curettes. The exposed roots are carefully scaled and planed, except for a narrow area close to the alveolar bone crest in which remnants of attachment fibers may be preserved. Angular bony defects are carefully curetted.

• Following the curettage, the flaps are trimmed and adjusted to the alveolar bone to obtain complete coverage of the interproximal bone (Fig. 25-29). If this adaptation cannot be achieved by soft tissue recontouring, some bone may be removed from the outer aspects of the alveolar process in order to facilitate the all-important flap adaptation. The flaps are sutured together with individual interproximal sutures. Surgical dressing may be placed over the area to ensure close adaptation of the flaps to the alveolar bone and root surfaces. The dressing, as well as the sutures, are removed after 1 week.

The main advantages of the *modified Widman flap* technique in comparison with other procedures previously described are, according to Ramfjord & Nissle (1974):

• the possibility of obtaining a close adaptation of the soft tissues to the root surfaces,

• the minimum of trauma to which the alveolar bone and the soft connective tissues are exposed and

• less exposure of the root surfaces, which from an esthetic point of view is an advantage in the treatment of anterior segments of the dentition.

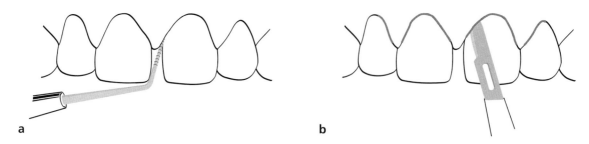

a
b

Fig. 25-30. *Papilla preservation flap*. Intrasulcular incisions are made at the facial and proximal aspects of the teeth.

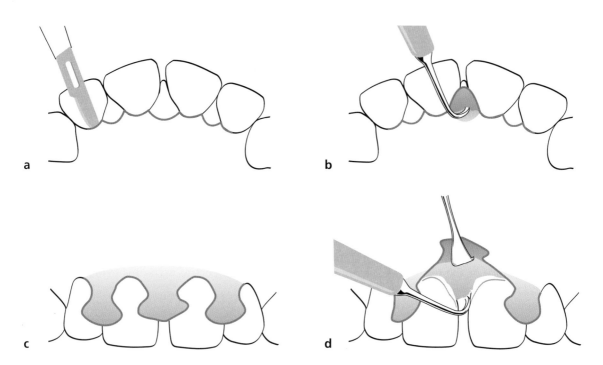

a
b

c
d

Fig. 25-31. *Papilla preservation flap*. (a) An intrasulcular incision is made along the lingual/palatal aspect of the teeth with a semi-lunar incision made across each interdental area. (b) A curette or interproximal knife is used to carefully free the interdental papilla from the underlying hard tissue. (c-d) The detached interdental tissue is pushed through the embrasure with a blunt instrument to be included in the facial flap.

The papilla preservation flap

In order to preserve the interdental soft tissues for maximum soft tissue coverage following surgical intervention involving treatment of proximal osseous defects, Takei et al. (1985) proposed a surgical approach called *papilla preservation technique*. Later, Cortellini et al. (1995b, 1999) described modifications of the flap design to be used in combination with regenerative procedures. For esthetic reasons, the papilla preservation technique is often utilized in the surgical treatment of anterior tooth regions.

Technique

- According to the description by Takei et al. (1985) the *papilla preservation flap technique* is initiated by an intrasulcular incision at the facial and proximal aspects of the teeth without making incisions through the interdental papillae (Fig. 25-30a,b). Subsequently, an intrasulcular incision is made along the lingual/palatal aspect of the teeth with a semi-lunar

incision made across each interdental area (Fig. 25-31a). The semi-lunar incision should dip apically at least 5 mm from the line-angles of the teeth, which will allow the interdental tissue to be dissected from the lingual/palatal aspect so that it can be elevated intact with the facial flap. In situations where an osseous defect has a wide extension into the lingual/palatal area, the semi-lunar incision may be placed on the facial aspect of the interdental area to have the papillae included with the lingual/palatal flap.

- A curette or interproximal knife is used to carefully free the interdental papilla from the underlying hard tissue (Fig. 25-31b). The detached interdental tissue is pushed through the embrasure with a blunt instrument (Fig. 25-31c,d).

- A full-thickness flap is reflected with a periosteal elevator on both facial and lingual/palatal surfaces. The exposed root surfaces are thoroughly scaled

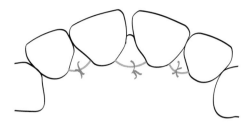

Fig. 25-32. *Papilla preservation flap*. The flap is replaced and sutures are placed on the palatal aspect of the interdental areas.

and root planed and bone defects carefully curetted (Fig. 25-31d).

- While holding the reflected flap, the margins of the flap and the interdental tissue are scraped to remove pocket epithelium and excessive granulation tissue. In anterior areas, the trimming of granulation tissue should be limited in order to maintain the maximum thickness of tissue.
- The flaps are repositioned and sutured using cross mattress sutures (Fig. 25-32). Alternatively, a direct suture of the semi-lunar incisions can be done as the only means of flap closure. A surgical dressing may be placed to protect the surgical area. The dressing and sutures are removed after 1 week.

Regenerative procedures

In the 1980s treatment of periodontal pockets was given a new dimension when it was shown that with specific surgical handling of the periodontal wound a significant amount of new connective tissue attachment is achievable following surgical treatment (Nyman et al. 1982, Bowers et al. 1989).

To obtain periodontal regeneration has always been a major challenge to the periodontist and several approaches to periodontal regeneration have been used throughout the years. The earliest attempts involved various bone grafting procedures, such as the use of autogenous grafts from both extraoral and intraoral donor sites, allogenic marrow grafts and non-decalcified/decalcified lyophilized bone grafts, or "implant" procedures utilizing slowly resorbable tri-calcium-phosphate and non-resorbable, non-porous hydroxy-apatite. Other approaches to periodontal regeneration involved the use of citric acid for root surface demineralization or the use of methods for improved root surface biocompatibility or to enhance cellular responses.

The use of physical barriers, such as membranes (non-biodegradable or biodegradable), to retard or prevent apical migration of epithelium as well as exclude gingival connective tissue from the healing wound, formed the basis for the concept known as "guided tissue regeneration" (Gottlow et al. 1986). The procedure can be described as a coronally reposi-

tioned flap procedure without bone recontouring, with the adjunctive use of a membrane tightened to the tooth to cover the exposed root surface and adjacent intrabony defect before repositioning of the soft tissue flaps.

In the late 1990s a new approach to periodontal regeneration was presented, which involves the use of a derivate of enamel matrix proteins (Hammarström 1997, Heijl et al. 1997). These proteins are involved in the embryogenesis of cementum, periodontal ligament and supporting bone, and when applied to the exposed root surface facing an intrabony periodontal defect they mediate regeneration of a new attachment apparatus. The surgical procedure is performed as a coronally repositioned flap procedure without bone recontouring. Before repositioning of the soft tissue flaps, the exposed roots are treated with EDTA for removal of the "smear layer", followed by the application of the derivate of enamel matrix proteins.

Various regenerative procedures for surgical treatment of periodontal lesions, as well as the biological basis for periodontal regeneration, are discussed in detail in Chapter 28.

DISTAL WEDGE PROCEDURES

In many cases the treatment of periodontal pockets on the distal surface of distal molars is complicated by the presence of bulbous tissues over the tuberosity or by a prominent retromolar pad. The most direct approach to pocket elimination in such cases in the maxilla is the gingivectomy procedure. The incision is started on the distal surface of the tuberosity and carried forward to the base of the pocket of the distal surface of the molar (Fig. 25-33).

However, when only limited amounts of keratinized tissue are present, or none at all, or if a distal angular bony defect has been diagnosed, the bulbous tissue should be reduced in size rather than being removed *in toto*. This may be accomplished by the *distal wedge procedure* (Robinson 1966). This technique facilitates access to the osseous defect and makes it possible to preserve sufficient amounts of gingiva and mucosa to achieve soft tissue coverage.

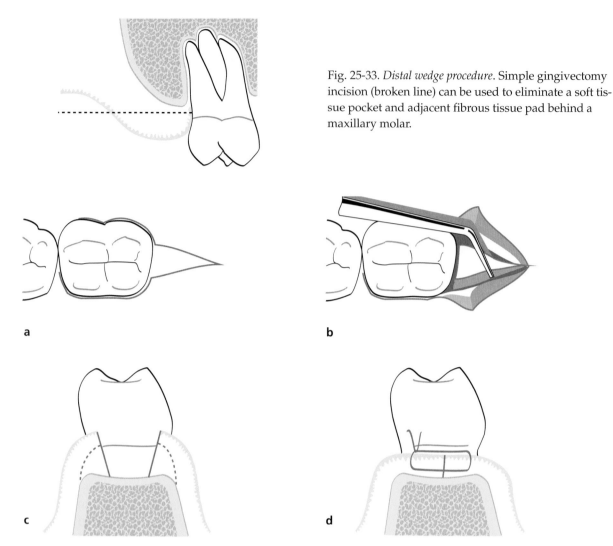

Fig. 25-33. *Distal wedge procedure*. Simple gingivectomy incision (broken line) can be used to eliminate a soft tissue pocket and adjacent fibrous tissue pad behind a maxillary molar.

a

b

c

d

Fig. 25-34. *Distal wedge procedure*. (a) Buccal and lingual vertical incisions are made through the retromolar pad to form a triangle behind a mandibular molar. (b) The triangular-shaped wedge of tissue is dissected from the underlying bone and removed. (c) The walls of the buccal and lingual flaps are reduced in thickness by undermining incisions (broken lines). (d) The flaps, which have been trimmed and shortened to avoid overlapping wound margins, are sutured.

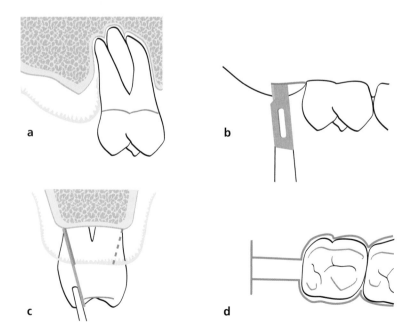

a

b

c

d

Fig. 25-35. *Modified distal wedge procedure*. A deep periodontal pocket combined with an angular bone defect at the distal aspect of a maxillary molar (a). Two parallel reverse bevel incisions, one buccal and one palatal, are made from the distal surface of the molar to the posterior part of the tuberosity (b-d), where they are connected with a buccolingual incision (d). The buccal and palatal incisions are extended in a mesial direction along the buccal and palatal surfaces of the molar to facilitate flap elevation.

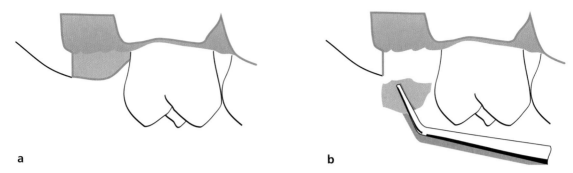

Fig. 25-36. *Modified distal wedge procedure*. Buccal and palatal flaps are elevated (a) and the rectangular wedge is released from the tooth and underlying bone by sharp dissection and removed (b).

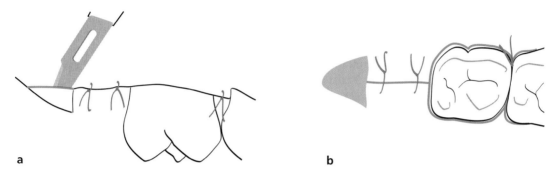

Fig. 25-37. *Modified distal wedge procedure*. Following bone recontouring and root debridement, the flaps are trimmed and shortened to avoid overlapping wound margins and sutured (a). A close soft tissue adaptation should be accomplished to the distal surface of the molar. The remaining fibrous tissue pad distal to the buccolingual incision line is "leveled" by the use of a gingivectomy incision (b, c).

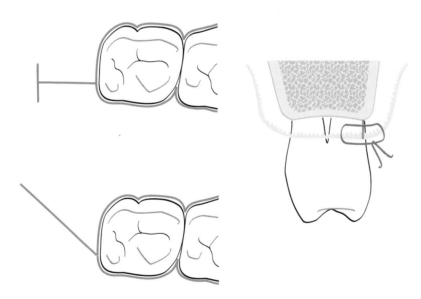

Fig. 25-38. *Modified incision techniques in distal wedge procedures*. To ensure optimal flap adaptation at the furcation site the incision technique may be modified. The amount of attached keratinized tissue present as well as the accessibility to the retromolar area has to be considered when placing the incision.

Technique

- Buccal and lingual incisions are made in a vertical direction through the tuberosity or retromolar pad to form a triangular wedge (Fig. 25-34a). The facial and lingual incisions should be extended in a mesial direction along the buccal and lingual surfaces of the distal molar to facilitate flap elevation.
- The facial and lingual walls of the tuberosity or retromolar pad are deflected and the incised wedge of tissue is dissected and separated from the bone (Fig. 25-34b).

- The walls of the facial and lingual flaps are then reduced in thickness by undermining incisions (Fig. 25-34c). Loose tags of tissue are removed and the root surfaces are scaled and planed. If necessary, the bone is recontoured.
- The buccal and lingual flaps are replaced over the exposed alveolar bone, and the edges trimmed to avoid overlapping wound margins. The flaps are secured in this position with interrupted sutures (Fig. 25-34d). The sutures are removed after approximately 1 week.

The original distal wedge procedure may be modified according to individual requirements. Some commonly used modifications of the incision technique are illustrated in Figs. 25-35 to 25-38, all having as a goal to eliminate the deep pocket and to achieve mucosal coverage of the remaining periodontium.

OSSEOUS SURGERY

The principles of osseous surgery in periodontal therapy were outlined by Schluger (1949) and Goldman (1950). They pointed out that alveolar bone loss caused by inflammatory periodontal disease often results in an uneven outline of the bone crest. Since, according to these authors, the gingival contour is closely dependent on the contour of the underlying bone as well as the proximity and anatomy of adjacent tooth surfaces, the elimination of soft tissue pockets often has to be combined with osseous reshaping and the elimination of osseous craters and angular bony defects to establish and maintain shallow pockets and optimal gingival contour after surgery.

Osteoplasty
The term *osteoplasty* was introduced by Friedman in 1955. The purpose of osteoplasty is to create a physiologic form of the alveolar bone *without* removing any "supporting" bone. Osteoplasty therefore is a technique analogous to gingivoplasty. Examples of osteoplasty are the thinning of thick osseous ledges and the establishment of a scalloped contour of the buccal (lingual and palatal) bone crest (Fig. 25-39). In flap surgery without bone recontouring, interdental morphology may sometimes preclude optimal mucosal coverage of the bone postsurgically, even if pronounced scalloping of soft tissue flaps is performed. In such a situation, removal of non-supporting bone by vertical grooving to reduce the faciolingual dimension of the bone in the interdental areas may facilitate flap adaptation, thereby reducing the risk of bone denudation as well as reducing the risk of ischemic necrosis of unsupported mucosal flaps due to flap margin deficiencies.

Removal of non-supporting bone may sometimes also be required to gain access for intrabony root surface debridement. The leveling of interproximal craters and the elimination (or reduction) of bony walls of circumferential osseous defects are often referred to as "osteoplasty" since usually no resection of supporting bone is required (Fig. 25-40).

Ostectomy
By *ostectomy*, supporting bone, i.e. bone directly involved in the attachment of the tooth, is removed to reshape deformities caused by periodontitis in the

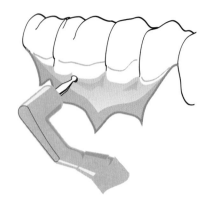

Fig. 25-39. *Osteoplasty*. Thick osseous ledges in a mandibular molar region area are eliminated with the use of a round bur to facilitate optimal flap adaptation.

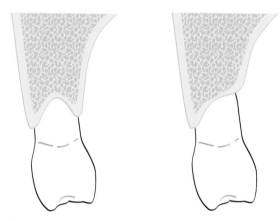

Fig. 25-40. *Osteoplasty*. Leveling of an interproximal bone crater through the removal of the palatal bone wall. For esthetic reasons the buccal bone wall is maintained to support the height of the soft tissue.

marginal and interdental bone. Ostectomy is considered to be an important part of surgical techniques aimed at pocket elimination. As a general rule, however, care must be exercised when supporting bone is to be removed.

After exposing the alveolar bone by elevation of a flap, buccal and/or lingual crater walls are reduced to the base of the osseous defect using bone chisels and bone rongeurs (Fig. 25-41). A round bur or a diamond stone under continuous saline irrigation can also be used. If bone resection has been carried out in the interdental area, the buccal and lingual/palatal bone margins may subsequently have to be recontoured to compensate for discrepancies in bone height resulting from the interdental bone resection (Fig. 25-41b). It is considered important to remove the small peaks of bone which often remain in the area of the line angles. The objective of bone surgery is thus to establish a "physiologic" anatomy of the alveolar bone, but at a more apical level.

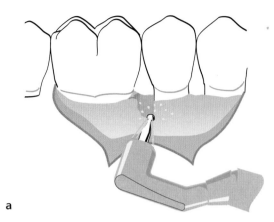
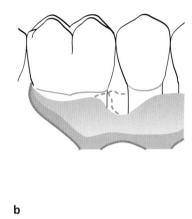

a

b

Fig. 25-41. *Ostectomy*. (a) A combined one- and two-wall osseous defect on the distal aspect of a mandibular premolar has been exposed following reflection of mucoperiosteal flaps. Since esthetics is not a critical factor to consider in the posterior tooth region of the mandible, the bone walls are reduced to a level close to the base of the defect using rotating round burs under continuous saline irrigation. (b) The osseous recontouring completed. Note that some supporting bone has to be removed from the buccal and lingual aspect of both the second premolar and the first molar in order to provide a hard tissue topography which allows a close adaptation of the covering soft tissue flap.

GENERAL GUIDELINES FOR PERIODONTAL SURGERY

Objectives of surgical treatment

Traditionally, *pocket elimination* has been a main objective of periodontal therapy. The removal of the pocket by surgical means served two purposes: (1) the pocket, which established an environment conducive to progression of periodontal disease, was eliminated and (2) the root surface was made accessible for scaling and, after healing, for self-performed toothcleaning.

While these objectives cannot be entirely discarded today, the necessity for pocket elimination in periodontal therapy has been challenged. During recent years our understanding of the biology of the periodontium, the pathogenesis of periodontal disease and the healing capacity of the periodontium has markedly increased. This new information has thus formed the basis for a more differentiated understanding of the role played by periodontal surgery in the preservation of teeth.

In the past, *increased pocket depth* was the main indication for periodontal surgery. However, pocket depth is no longer as unequivocal a concept as it used to be. The *probeable depth*, i.e. the distance from the gingival margin to the point where further periodontal probe penetration is stopped by tissue resistance, may only rarely correspond to the "true" depth of the pocket (see Chapter 18). Furthermore, regardless of the accuracy with which pockets can be measured, there is no established correlation between probeable pocket depth and the presence or absence of active

disease. This means that symptoms other than increased probing depth should be present to justify surgical therapy. These include clinical signs of inflammation, especially exudation and bleeding on probing (to the bottom of the pockets), as well as aberrations of gingival morphology. Finally, the fact that proper plaque control, maintained by the patient, is a decisive factor for a good prognosis (Rosling et al. 1976a, Nyman et al. 1977, Axelsson & Lindhe 1981) must be considered prior to the initiation of surgery.

In conclusion, the main objective of periodontal surgery is to contribute to the long-term preservation of the periodontium by facilitating plaque removal and plaque control, and periodontal surgery can serve this purpose by:

- creating accessibility for proper professional scaling and root planing
- establishing a gingival morphology which facilitates the patient's self-performed plaque control.

In addition to this, periodontal surgery may aim at:

- regeneration of periodontal attachment lost due to destructive disease. (New attachment procedures in periodontal therapy are discussed in Chapter 28.)

Indications for surgical treatment

Impaired access for scaling and root planing

Scaling and root planing are methods of therapy which are difficult to master. The difficulties in accomplishing proper debridement increase with (1) increasing depth of the periodontal pockets, (2) increasing

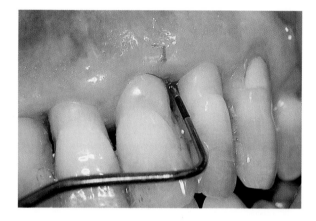

Fig. 25-42. Evaluation following non-surgical instrumentation reveals persistent signs of inflammation, bleeding following pocket probing and probing depth ≥ 6 mm. Flap elevation to expose the root surface for proper cleaning should be considered.

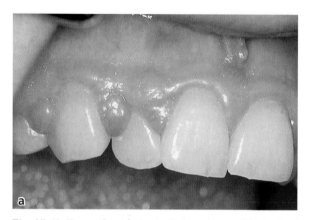
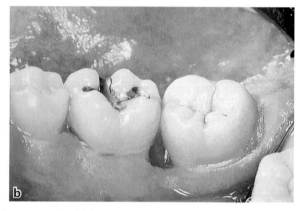

Fig. 25-43. Examples of gingival aberrations, (a) gingival enlargement and (b) proximal soft tissue crater, which favor plaque retention and thereby impede the patient's plaque control.

width of the tooth surfaces, (3) the presence of root fissures, root concavities, furcations, and defective margins of dental restorations in the subgingival area.

Provided a correct technique and suitable instruments are used, it is usually possible to properly debride pockets up to 5 mm deep (Waerhaug 1978, Caffesse et al. 1986). However, this 5 mm limit cannot be used as a universal rule-of-thumb. Reduced accessibility and the presence of one or several of the above-mentioned impeding conditions may prevent proper debridement of shallow pockets, whereas at sites with good accessibility and favorable root morphology, proper debridement can be accomplished even in deeper pockets (Badersten et al. 1981, Lindhe et al. 1982).

It is often difficult to ascertain by clinical means whether subgingival instrumentation has been properly performed. Following scaling, the root surface should be smooth – roughness will often indicate the presence of remaining subgingival calculus. It is also important to monitor carefully the gingival reaction to subgingival debridement. If inflammation persists and if bleeding is elicited by gentle probing in the subgingival area, the presence of subgingival deposits should be suspected (Fig. 25-42). If such symptoms are not resolved by repeated subgingival instrumentation, surgical treatment should be performed to expose the root surfaces for proper cleaning.

Impaired access for self-performed plaque control

The level of plaque control which can be maintained by the patient is determined not only by his/her interest and dexterity but also, to some extent, by the morphology of the dentogingival area.

The patient's responsibility in a plaque control program must obviously include the cleansing of the supragingival tooth surfaces and the marginal part of the gingival sulcus. This means that the tooth area coronal to the gingival margin and at the entrance to the gingival sulcus should be the target for the patient's home care efforts.

Pronounced gingival hyperplasia and gingival craters (Fig. 25-43) are examples of morphologic aberrations which may impede proper home care. Likewise, the presence of restorations with defective marginal fit or adverse contour and surface characteristics at the gingival margin may seriously compromise plaque removal.

By the professional treatment of periodontal disease, the dentist prepares the dentition in such a way that home care can be effectively managed. At the completion of treatment, the following objectives should have been met:

• no sub or supragingival dental deposits
• no pathologic pockets (no bleeding on probing to the bottom of the pockets)

- no plaque-retaining aberrations of gingival morphology
- no plaque-retaining parts of restorations in relation to the gingival margin

These requirements lead to the following indications for periodontal surgery:

- accessibility for proper scaling and root planing
- establishment of a morphology of the dento-gingival area conducive to plaque control
- pocket depth reduction
- correction of gross gingival aberrations
- shift of the gingival margin to a position apical to plaque-retaining restorations
- facilitate proper restorative therapy

Contraindications for periodontal surgery

Patient cooperation

Since optimal postoperative plaque control is decisive for the success of periodontal treatment (Axelsson & Lindhe 1981), a patient who fails to cooperate during the cause-related phase of therapy should not be exposed to surgical treatment.

Even though short-term postoperative plaque control entails frequent professional treatments, the long-term responsibility for maintaining good oral hygiene must rest with the patient. Theoretically, even the poorest oral hygiene performance by a patient may be compensated for by frequent recall visits for supportive therapy (e.g. once a week), but it is unrealistic to consider larger groups of patients being maintained in this manner. A typical recall schedule for periodontal patients involves professional consultations for supportive periodontal therapy once every 3-6 months. Patients who cannot maintain satisfactory oral hygiene over such a period should normally be considered unsuited for periodontal surgery.

Cardiovascular disease

Arterial hypertension does not normally preclude periodontal surgery. The patient's medical history should be checked for previous untoward reactions to local anesthesia. Local anesthetics free from or low in adrenaline may be used and an aspirating syringe should be adopted to safeguard against intravascular injection.

Angina pectoris does not normally preclude periodontal surgery. The drugs used and the number of episodes of angina may indicate the severity of the disease. Premedication with sedatives and the use of local anesthesia low in adrenaline are often recommended. Safeguards should be adopted against intravascular injection.

Myocardial infarction patients should not be subjected to periodontal surgery within 6 months following hospitalization, and thereafter only in cooperation with the physician responsible for the patient.

Anticoagulant treatment implies increased propensity for bleeding. Periodontal surgery should be scheduled first after consultation with the patient's physician to determine whether modification of the anticoagulant therapy is indicated. In patients on moderate levels of anticoagulation and only requiring minor surgical treatment no alteration of their anticoagulant therapy may be required. To keep the prothrombin time within a safety level for hemorrhage control during surgery in patients with higher levels of anticoagulation, adjustments of the anticoagulant drug therapy usually need to be initiated 2-3 days prior to the dental appointment. Anticoagulation may be safely resumed immediately after the periodontal surgical procedure since several days are needed for full anticoagulation to return. Aspirin and other non-steroidal anti-inflammatory drugs should not be used for postoperative pain control since they increase bleeding tendency. Furthermore, tetracyclines are contraindicated in patients on anticoagulant drugs due to interference with prothrombin formation (Fay & O'Neil 1984).

Rheumatic endocarditis, congenital heart lesions and heart/vascular implants involve risk for transmission of bacteria to heart tissues and heart implants during the transient bacteremia that follows manipulation of infected periodontal pockets. Surgical treatment (including tooth extractions) of patients with these conditions, as well as of patients at risk of hematogenous prosthetic joint infection (for the first 2 years following joint placement) (American Dental Association and American Academy of Orthopedic Surgeons 1997), should be preceded by antiseptic mouthrinsing (0.2 % chlorhexidine) and prescription and administration of an appropriate antibiotic in a high dose. According to the recommendations by the American Heart Association (Dajani et al. 1997), 2 g of amoxicillin administered 1 hour before the treatment is an adequate regimen. In case the patient is allergic to penicillin, clindamycin (600 mg) is recommended as an alternative. No second doses are recommended for any of the above dosing regimens. Tetracyclines and erythromycin are not recommended for prophylactic cardiovascular antibiotic coverage.

Organ transplantation

In organ transplantation, medications are used to prevent transplant rejection. The drug of choice today is cyclosporin A, a potent immunosuppressant drug. The adverse effects seen following cyclosporin A treatment include an increased risk for gingival enlargement as well as hypertension. In addition, hypertension seen in renal transplant recipients is often treated with calcium channel blockers. These antihypertensive agents have also been associated with gingival enlargement. As in patients on phenytoin therapy, gingival enlargement in patients on cyclosporin A therapy or on antihypertensive therapy with calcium blockers may be corrected by means of periodontal surgery. However, due to the strong propensity for recurrence, the use of intensified conservative periodontal therapy to prevent gingival enlargement in susceptible patients should be encouraged.

Prophylactic antibiotics are recommended in transplant patients taking immunosuppressive drugs, and the patient's physician should be consulted before any periodontal therapy is performed. In addition, antiseptic mouthrinsing (0.2% chlorhexidine) should precede the surgical treatment.

Blood disorders
If the medical history includes blood disorders, the exact nature of these should be ascertained.

Patients suffering from *acute leukemias, agranulocytosis* and *lymphogranulomatosis* must *not* be subjected to periodontal surgery.

Anemias in mild and compensated forms do not preclude surgical treatment. More severe and less compensated forms may entail lowered resistance to infection and increased propensity for bleeding. In such cases, periodontal surgery should only be performed after consultation with the patient's physician.

Hormonal disorders
Diabetes mellitus entails lowered resistance to infection, propensity for delayed wound healing and predisposition for arteriosclerosis. Well compensated patients may be subjected to periodontal surgery provided precautions are taken not to disturb dietary and insulin routines.

Adrenal function may be impeded in patients receiving large doses of corticosteroids over an extended period. These conditions involve reduced resistance to physical and mental stress, and the doses of corticosteroid may have to be altered during the period of periodontal surgery. The patient's physician should be consulted.

Neurologic disorders
Multiple sclerosis and Parkinson's disease may in severe cases make ambulatory periodontal surgery impossible. Paresis, impaired muscular function, tremor, and uncontrollable reflexes may necessitate treatment under general anesthesia.

Epilepsy is often treated with *phenytoin* which, in approximately 50% of cases, may mediate the formation of gingival enlargement. These patients may, without special restrictions, be subjected to periodontal surgery for correction of the enlargement. There is, however, a strong propensity for recurrence of the enlargement, which in many cases can be countered by intensifying the plaque control.

Smoking
Although smoking negatively affects wound healing (Siana et al. 1989), it may not be considered a contraindication for surgical periodontal treatment. The clinician should be aware, however, that less resolution of probing pocket depth and smaller improvement in clinical attachment may be observed in smokers than in non-smokers (Preben & Bergström 1990, Ah et al. 1994, Scabbia et al. 2001).

Local anesthesia in periodontal surgery

Traditional views of pain and discomfort as an inevitable consequence of dental procedures, in particular surgical procedures (including scaling and root planing) and extractions, are no longer accepted by patients. Pain management is an ethical obligation and will improve patient satisfaction in general (e.g. increased confidence and improved cooperation) as well as patient recovery and short-term functioning after oral/periodontal surgical procedures.

In order to prevent pain during the performance of a periodontal surgical procedure, the entire area of the dentition scheduled for surgery, the teeth as well as the periodontal tissues, requires proper local anesthesia.

Mechanism of action
Local anesthesia is defined as a loss of feeling or sensation that is confined to a certain area of the body. All local anesthetics have a common mechanism of action. To produce their effect they block the generation and propagation of impulses along nerve fibers. Such impulses are transmitted by the rapid depolarization and repolarization within the nerve axons. These changes in polarity are due to the passage of sodium and potassium ions across the nerve membrane through ionic channels within the membrane. Local anesthetics prevent the inward movement of sodium ions which initiate depolarization and as a consequence the nerve fiber cannot propagate any impulse. The potassium efflux, on the other hand, is influenced very little and there is no change in the resting potential. The mechanisms behind the activity of the local anesthetics are not fully understood, but the most plausible theory is that the lipid-soluble free base form of the local anesthetic, which is the form that penetrates biologic membranes most easily, penetrates the connective tissue to reach the axons and diffuses across the lipid membrane into the axon. Inside the axon the drug interacts with specific receptor sites on or within the sodium channels to exert an inhibitory effect on sodium influx and, consequently, on impulse conduction.

Dental local anesthetics
Anesthetics from the chemical group amino-amides, for example lidocaine, mepivacaine, prilocaine and articaine, are more potent and significantly less allergenic than amino-esters (e.g. procaine and tetracaine)

and have therefore replaced esters as the "gold standard" for dental local anesthetics.

Due to the specific need for bone penetration, dental local anesthetics contain high concentrations of the active agent. Although most amide local anesthetics may cause local vasoconstriction in low concentrations, the clinically used concentrations in dental solutions will cause an increase in the local blood flow. Significant clinical effects of this induced vasodilation are an increased rate of absorption, thus decreasing the duration of anesthesia. Major benefits can therefore be obtained by adding relatively high concentrations of vasoconstrictors (e.g. epinephrine > 1:200 000 or > 5 mg/ml) to dental local anesthetic solutions; the duration is considerably prolonged, the depth of anesthesia may be enhanced and the peak concentrations of the local anesthetic in blood can be reduced. Furthermore, in periodontal surgery, incorporation of adrenergic vasoconstrictors into the local anesthetic is of considerable value in keeping bleeding to a minimum during surgery (avoiding considerable blood loss, making it possible to visualize the surgical site and thus with intact surgical quality shorten the time spent on the procedure). As a matter of fact, the use of a dental local anesthetic without a vasoconstrictor during a periodontal surgical procedure is counterproductive because the vasodilating properties of such a local anesthetic will increase the bleeding in the area of surgery.

Vasoconstrictors and local hemostasis

Epinephrine is the vasoconstrictor of choice for local hemostasis and is most commonly used in a concentration of 1:80 000 (12.5 mg/ml). However, 1:100 000 epinephrine also provides excellent hemostasis and most periodontists are unable to detect a clinical difference between the two concentrations. It therefore seems prudent to use the least concentrated form of epinephrine that provides clinically effective hemostasis (i.e. the 1:100 000 concentration).

Although the cardiovascular effects of the usually small amounts of epinephrine used during a periodontal surgical procedure are of little practical concern in most individuals, accidental intravascular injections, unusual patient sensitivity and unanticipated drug interactions (or excessive doses) can result in potentially serious outcomes. It must also be understood that the use of epinephrine for hemostasis during periodontal surgery has some potential drawbacks. Epinephrine will produce a rebound vasodilation after the vasoconstriction has worn off, leading to increased risk for bleeding in the immediate postoperative period. There is a greater potential for such undesirable delayed hemorrhage following the use of 1:80 000 epinephrine than after the use 1:100 000.

Postoperative pain may increase and wound healing may be delayed when adrenergic vasoconstrictors are used because of local ischemia with subsequent tissue acidosis and accumulation of inflammatory mediators. Furthermore, the possibility of an ischemic

necrosis of surgical flaps infiltrated with an adrenergic vasoconstrictor (especially if norepinephrine is used instead of epinephrine) cannot be discounted. For these reasons as well as because of the possibility of systemic reactions alluded to above, dental local anesthetics containing adrenergic vasoconstrictors for hemostasis should be infiltrated *only* as needed and *not* merely from habit.

Felypressin, another commonly used vasoconstrictor, appears to act preferentially on the venous side of the microcirculation and is not very active in constricting the arteriolar circulation. Felypressin is therefore not nearly as effective as adrenergic vasoconstrictors in limiting hemorrhage during a surgical procedure.

Individual variability in response to dental local anesthetics

Although it is possible for the periodontist to choose from a broad spectrum of dental local anesthetics to achieve the expected clinical action, there are a number of other factors (i.e. not related to the drug) that can affect the drug action in a single patient.

During clinical conditions the variability in response to dental local anesthetics administered can be expected to be great, for example with regard to depth and duration of anesthesia. The reason for the great variation has not been adequately explained but has to be accepted as it may have significant implications in periodontal surgical procedures. A list of possible factors that may cause anesthetic failures include:

- Accuracy in administration of the drug
- Anatomic variation between patients (e.g. in elderly patients with bone resorption)
- Status of the tissues at the site of injection (vascularity, inflammation)
- General condition of patient
- Psychologic factors

Inaccuracy in administration is a major factor causing anesthetic failures. Although not particularly significant in infiltration anesthesia, the mandibular block is a prime example of a technique in which duration of anesthesia is greatly influenced by accuracy of injection.

The general condition of the patient as well as psychologic factors may also affect the anticipated duration of action. Infection, stress or pain will usually lead to decreased duration of anesthesia, while an increase in the patient's own defense mechanisms against pain perception by, for example, release of endogenous endorphins, may provide improved depth and/or duration of anesthesia.

Techniques for anesthesia in periodontal surgery

Injections of dental local anesthetics prior to a periodontal surgical procedure may be routine for the dentist, but are often a most unpleasant experience for the patient. Reassurance and psychologic support are essential and will increase the patient's confidence in his dentist. To create a relaxed atmosphere and to decrease the patient's fear of an unusual situation is of course also a useful way of increasing the patient's own defense mechanisms against pain perception (e.g. release of endogenous endorphins).

Anesthesia for periodontal surgery is obtained by nerve block and/or by local infiltration. In cases of flap surgery, complete anesthesia must be attained before commencing the operation, as it may be difficult to supplement the anesthesia after the bone surface has been exposed. In addition, the pain elicited by needle insertion can be significantly reduced if the mucosa at the puncture site is anesthetized in advance by the use of a suitable topical ointment or spray.

Local infiltration may have a greatly decreased rate of success in areas where inflammation, in spite of optimal conservative periodontal therapy and good oral hygiene, remains in the periodontal tissues. The suggested reason for this is that tissue pH tends to be low in inflamed areas and anesthetic solutions are less potent at low pH because there is a greater proportion of charged cation molecules than of the uncharged base molecules. Because of this, diffusion of the local anesthetic into the axoplasm is slower, with subsequent delayed onset and decreased efficacy. Another more recent hypothesis suggests that NGF (Nerve Growth Factor) released during tissue inflammation will induce sprouting or proliferation of sensory nerve endings, expressing a different (sub-)type of sodium channel than in normal tissues. The dental local anesthetics used at present may not be selective enough for proper interaction with these sodium channel subtypes to induce anticipated anesthesia.

Local anesthesia in the mandible

As a rule, analgesia of the teeth and the soft and hard tissues of the mandible should be obtained by a mandibular block and/or a mental block. In the anterior region of the mandible, canines and incisors can often be anesthetized by infiltration, but there are often anastomoses over the midline. These anastomoses must be anesthetized by bilateral infiltration, or by bilateral mental blocks. The buccal soft tissues of the mandible are anesthetized by local infiltration or by blocking the buccal nerve. Local infiltration, performed as a series of injections in the buccal fold of the treatment area, has of course the added advantage of providing a local ischemic effect if a suitable anesthetic is used.

The lingual periodontal tissues must also be anesthetized. This is accomplished by blocking the lingual nerve and/or by infiltration in the floor of the mouth close to the site of operation. If necessary to obtain proper ischemia, and only then, supplementary injections may be made in the interdental papillae (intraseptal injections).

Local anesthesia in the maxilla

Local anesthesia of the teeth and buccal periodontal tissues of the maxilla can easily be obtained by injections in the mucogingival fold of the treatment area. If larger areas of the maxillary dentition are scheduled for surgery, repeated injections (in the mucogingival fold) have to be performed, e.g. at the central incisor, canine, second premolar and second molar. In the posterior maxillary region a tuberosity injection can be used to block the superior alveolar branches of the maxillary nerve. However, because of the vicinity to the pterygoid venous plexus, this type of block anesthesia is not recommended due to the risk of intravenous injection and/or hematoma formation.

The palatal nerves are most easily anesthetized by injections made at right angles to the mucosa and placed around 10 mm apical to the gingival margin adjacent to teeth included in the operation. In cases of advanced bone loss, the pain produced by injecting into the non-resilient palatal mucosa can be minimized if the injections are performed from the buccal aspect, i.e. through the interdental gingiva. Sometimes blocks of the nasopalatine nerves and/or the greater palatine nerves can be applied. Especially for periodontal surgery involving molars, supplementary blocking of the greater palatine nerve should be considered.

Instruments used in periodontal surgery

General considerations

Surgical procedures used in periodontal therapy often involve the following measures (instruments):

- Incision and excision (periodontal knives)
- Deflection and readaptation of mucosal flaps (periosteal elevators)
- Removal of adherent fibrous and granulomatous tissue (soft tissue rongeurs and tissue scissors)
- Scaling and root planing (scalers and curettes)
- Removal of bone tissue (bone rongeurs, chisels and files)
- Root sectioning (burs)
- Suturing (sutures and needle holders, suture scissors)
- Application of wound dressing (plastic instruments)

The set of instruments used for the various periodontal surgical procedures should have a comparatively simple design. As a general rule, the number and varieties of instruments should be kept to a minimum. In addition to particular instruments used for periodontal treatment modalities, equipment and instruments generally used in oral surgery are often needed.

Within each category of surgical instruments used for periodontal therapy there are usually several

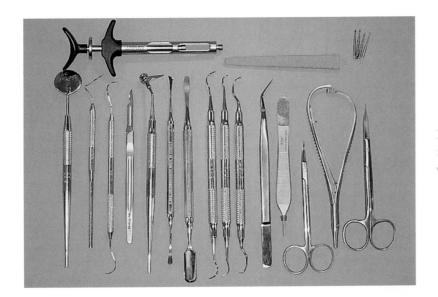

Fig. 25-44. Set of instruments used for periodontal surgery and included in a standard tray.

brands available, varying in form and quality, leaving ample room for individual preferences.

The instruments should be stored in sterile "ready-to-use" packs or trays. Handling, storing and labeling of surgical instruments and equipment must be managed in such a way that interchanging of sterile and non-sterile items is prevented.

It is also important that the instruments are kept in good working condition. The maintenance routine should ensure that scalers, curettes, knives with fixed blades, etc., are sharp and that the hinges of scissors, rongeurs and needle holders are properly lubricated. Spare instruments (sterile) should always be available to replace instruments found to be defective or accidentally contaminated.

The instrument tray

Instrument trays for periodontal surgery may be arranged in several ways. Different trays can be used for different procedures or a standard tray can be used for all procedures supplemented with the particular instruments that are needed for a specific procedure.

A commonly used standard tray combines the basic set of instruments used in oral surgery and a few periodontal instruments. The instruments listed below are often found on such a standard tray (Fig. 25-44):

- Mouth mirrors
- Graduated periodontal probe/Explorer
- Handles for disposable surgical blades (e.g. Bard-Parker handle)
- Mucoperiosteal elevator and tissue retractor
- Scalers and curettes
- Cotton pliers
- Tissue pliers (*ad modum* Ewald)
- Tissue scissors
- Needle holder
- Suture scissors
- Plastic instrument
- Hemostat
- Burs

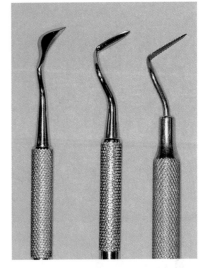

Fig. 25-45. Examples of gingivectomy knifes with fixed blades. From left to right: Kirkland $^{15}/_{16}$, Orban ½, and Waerhaug ½.

Additional equipment may include:

- Syringe for local anesthesia
- Syringe for irrigation
- Aspirator tip
- Physiologic saline
- Drapings for the patient
- Surgical gloves, surgical mask, surgeon's hood

Surgical instruments

Knives

Knives are available with fixed or replaceable blades. The advantage of the fixed blade versions is that the blade can be given any desired shape and orientation in relation to the handle. A disadvantage is that such instruments need frequent resharpening. Fig. 25-45 shows examples of knives with fixed blades.

New disposable blades are always sharp. They can be rapidly replaced if found defective. The cutting edge of the blades normally follows the long axis of

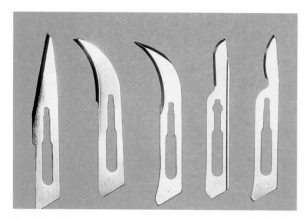

Fig. 25-46. Disposable blades which can be mounted in various types of handles. The shape of the blades are from left to right: No. 11, No. 12, No. 12D, No. 15 and No. 15C.

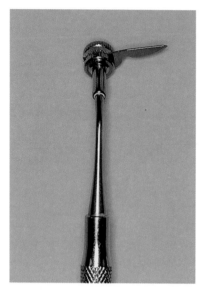

Fig. 25-47. A universal 360° handle for disposable blades, which allows the mounting of the blade in any angulated position of choice.

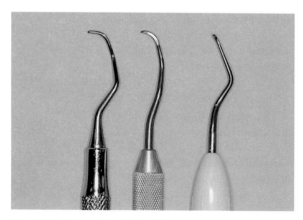

Fig. 25-48. Examples of double-ended sickle scalers and curettes useful for root debridement in conjunction with periodontal surgery. From left to right: Curette SG 215/16C Syntette, Sickle 215-216 Syntette and mini-curette SG 215/16MC.

the handle, which limits their use. However, knives with disposable blades fitted at an angle to the handle are also available.

The disposable blades are manufactured in different shapes (Fig. 25-46). When mounted in ordinary handles (Bard-Parker®), they are used for releasing incisions in flap operations and mucogingival surgery and for reverse bevel incisions where access is obtainable. Special handles (Fig. 25-47) make it possible to mount blades in angulated positions, which facilitates the use of such knives for both gingivectomy excisions and reverse bevel incisions.

Scalers and curettes

Scaling and root planing in conjunction with periodontal surgery take place on exposed root surfaces. Therefore access to the root surfaces for debridement may be obtained also with the use of comparatively sturdy instruments (Fig. 25-48). Tungsten carbide curettes and scalers with durable cutting edges are often used when "access" is not a problem. Rotating fine-grained diamond stones (Fig. 25-49) may be used within infrabony pockets, root concavities and entrances to furcations.

Instruments for bone removal

Sharp bone chisels or bone rongeurs (Fig. 25-50) cause the least tissue damage and should be employed whenever access permits. With reduced access, surgical burs or files may be used. The burs should operate at low speed and ample rinsing with sterile physiologic saline should ensure cooling and removal of tissue remnants.

Instruments for handling flaps

The proper healing of the periodontal wound is critical for the success of the operation. It is therefore important that the manipulations of the soft tissue flaps are performed with the minimum of tissue damage. Care should be exercised in the use of periosteal elevators when flaps are deflected and retracted for optimal visibility. Surgical pliers and tissue retractors which pierce the tissues should not be used in the marginal area of the flaps. Needle holders with small beaks and atraumatic sutures should be used.

Additional equipment

Hemorrhage is rarely a problem in periodontal surgery. The characteristic oozing type of bleeding can normally be controlled by a pressure pack (sterile gauze moistened with saline). Bleeding from small vessels can be stopped by clamping and tying using a hemostat and resorbable sutures. If the vessel is surrounded by bone, bleeding may be stopped by crushing the nutrient canal in which the vessel runs with a blunt instrument.

Sterile physiologic saline is used for rinsing and moistening the field of operation and for cooling when burs are employed. The saline solution may be kept in a sterile metal cup on the instrument tray and may be

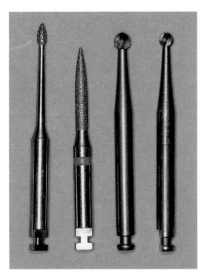

Fig. 25-49. A set of burs which may be useful in peri-odontal surgery. The rotating fine-grained diamond stones may be used for debridement of infrabony defects. The round burs are used for bone recontouring.

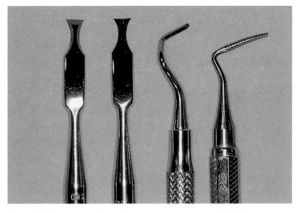

Fig. 25-50. Examples of instruments used for bone re-contouring. From left to right: Bone chisels Ochsenbein no. 1 and 2 (Kirkland 13K/13KL), Bone chisel Ochsenbein no. 3 and Schluger curved file no. 9/10.

applied to the wound by means of a sterile disposable plastic syringe and a needle with rounded tip.

Visibility in the field of operation is secured by using effective suction. The lumen of the aspirator tip should have a smaller diameter than the rest of the tube, in order to prevent clogging.

The patient's head may be covered by autoclaved cotton drapings or sterile disposable plastic/paper drapings. The surgeon and all assistants should wear sterile surgical gloves, surgical mask and surgeon's hood.

Selection of surgical technique

Many of the technical problems experienced in peri-odontal surgery stem from the difficulties in assessing accurately the degree and type of breakdown that has occurred prior to surgery. Furthermore, at the time of surgery, previously undiagnosed defects may be rec-ognized or some defects may have a more complex outline than initially anticipated. Since each of the surgical procedures described above is designed to deal with a specific situation or to meet a certain objective, it must be understood that in most patients no single standardized technique alone can be applied when periodontal surgery is undertaken. Therefore, in each surgical field, different techniques are often used and combined in such a way that the overall objectives of the surgical part of the periodontal ther-apy are met. As a general rule, surgical modalities of therapy which preserve or induce the formation of periodontal tissue should be preferred over those which resect or eliminate tissue.

General indications for various surgical techniques
Gingivectomy
The obvious indication for gingivectomy is the pres-ence of deep supra-alveolar pockets. In addition, the gingivectomy technique can be used to reshape abnor-mal gingival contours such as gingival craters and

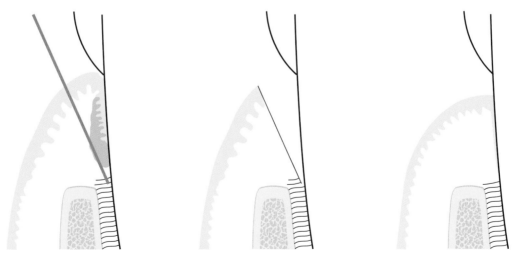

Fig. 25-51. *Internal beveled gingivectomy*. Schematic illustration of the incision technique in case of the presence of only a minimal zone of gingiva.

gingival hyperplasias (Fig. 25-43). In such cases the technique is often termed *gingivoplasty*.

Gingivectomy is not considered suitable in situations where the incision will lead to the removal of the entire zone of gingiva. This is the case when the bottom of the probeable pocket to be excised is located at or below the mucogingival junction. As an alternative in such a situation, an *internal beveled gingivectomy* may be performed (Fig. 25-51). Furthermore, since the gingivectomy procedure is aimed at the complete elimination of the periodontal pocket, the procedure cannot be used in periodontal sites where infrabony lesions or bony craters are present.

These limitations, combined with the development in recent years of surgical methods which have a broader field of application, have led to less frequent use of gingivectomy in the treatment of periodontal disease.

Flap operation with or without osseous surgery
Flap operations can be used in all cases where surgical treatment of periodontal disease is indicated. Flap procedures are particularly useful at sites where pockets extend beyond the mucogingival border and/or where treatment of bony lesions and furcation involvements is required.

The advantages of flap operations include:

- existing gingiva is preserved
- the marginal alveolar bone is exposed whereby the morphology of bony defects can be identified and the proper treatment rendered
- furcation areas are exposed, the degree of involvement and the "tooth-bone" relationship can be identified
- the flap can be repositioned at its original level or shifted apically, thereby making it possible to adjust the gingival margin to the local conditions
- the flap procedure preserves the oral epithelium and often makes the use of surgical dressing superfluous
- the postoperative period is usually less unpleasant for the patient when compared to gingivectomy.

Treatment decisions for soft and hard tissue pockets in flap surgery
Classifications of different flap modalities used in the treatment of periodontal disease often make distinctions between methods involving the marginal tissues and those involving the mucogingival area and, further, between tissue eliminating/resective varieties and tissue preserving/reconstructive types (access flaps for debridement). Such classifications appear less than precise since several techniques are often combined in the treatment of individual cases, and since there is no clear-cut relationship between disease characteristics and selection of surgical methods. From a didactic point of view it seems more appropriate to discuss surgical therapy with regard to how to deal with (1) the soft tissue component and (2) the hard tissue component of the periodontal pocket at a specific tooth site (Fig. 25-52).

Soft tissue pockets
The description of the various flap procedures reveals that, depending on the surgical technique used, the soft tissue flap should either be apically positioned at the level of the bone crest (original Widman flap, Neumann flap and apically repositioned flap) or maintained in a coronal position (Kirkland flap, modified Widman flap and papilla perservation flap) at the completion of the surgical intervention. The maintenance of the presurgical soft tissue height is of importance from an esthetic point of view, particularly in the anterior tooth region. However, long-term results from clinical trials have shown that major differences in the final position of the soft tissue margin are not evident between surgical procedures involving coronal and apical positioning of the flap margin. The reported difference in final positioning of the gingival margin between surgical techniques is attributed to osseous recontouring (Townsend-Olsen et al. 1985, Lindhe et al. 1987, Kaldahl et al. 1996, Becker et al. 2001). In many patients, however, it may be of significance to position the flap coronally in the anterior tooth region in order to give the patient a prolonged period of adaptation to the inevitable soft tissue reces-

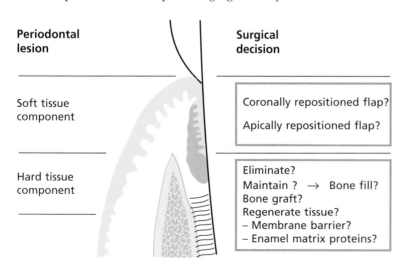

Fig. 25-52. *Surgical decisions*. Treatment decisions with respect to the soft and the hard tissue component of a periodontal pocket.

sion. In the posterior tooth region, an apical positioning should be the standard.

Independent of flap positioning the goal should be to achieve complete soft tissue coverage of the alveolar bone, not only at buccal/lingual sites but also in proximal sites. It is therefore of utmost importance to carefully plan the incisions in such a way that this goal can be achieved at the termination of the surgical intervention.

Hard tissue pockets

During conventional periodontal surgery one would usually opt for the conversion of an intrabony defect into a suprabony defect, which then is eliminated by an apical repositioning of the soft tissues. Osseous recontouring of angular bony defects and craters involves excisional techniques which should be used with caution and discrimination. However, the therapist is often faced with the dilemma of deciding whether or not to eliminate an angular bony defect. There are a number of factors that should be considered in the treatment decision, such as:

- esthetics
- tooth/tooth site involved
- defect morphology
- amount of remaining periodontium

Since alveolar bone supports the soft tissue, an altered bone level through recontouring will result in recession of the soft tissue margin. For esthetic reasons one may therefore be conservative in eliminating proximal bony defects in the anterior tooth region. For example, in the case of an approximal crater it may often be sufficient to reduce/eliminate the bone wall on the lingual side of the crater, thereby maintaining the bone support for the soft tissue on the facial aspect (Fig. 25-40). In favor of esthetics one may even have to compromise the amount of bone removal and accept that some pocket depth will remain in certain situations. In addition to esthetics, the presence of furcations may limit the extent to which bone recontouring can be performed.

Defect morphology is a variable of significance for repair/regeneration during healing (Rosling et al. 1976a, Cortellini et al. 1993, 1995a). While two and, especially, three-wall defects may show great potential for repair/regeneration, one-wall defects and approximal craters will rarely result in such a healing. Further, the removal of intrabony connective tissue/granulation tissue during a surgical procedure will always lead to crestal resorption of bone, especially in sites with thin bony walls. This results in reduction of the vertical dimensions of the bone tissue at the site (Fig. 25-53). Thus, the potential for bone fill following a compromise in regard to osseous surgery is greater in areas with thick, non-supporting bone.

The various treatment options available for the hard tissue defect may include:

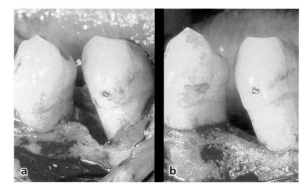

Fig. 25-53. Illustration of the amount of crestal bone resorption that may take place following a modified Widman flap procedure without bone recontouring. (a) View of the area at time of initial surgical treatment. (b) At the re-entry operation performed after 6 months of healing.

- elimination of the osseous defect by resection of bone (osteoplasty and/or ostectomy)
- maintenance of the area without osseous resection (hoping for some type of periodontal repair, e.g. bone fill leading to gain of clinical attachment),
- compromising the amount of bone removal and accepting that a certain pocket depth will remain
- an attempt to improve healing through the use of a regenerative procedure or
- extraction of the involved tooth if the bony defect is considered too advanced.

After careful consideration, indications for osseous surgery in conjunction with apical repositioning of flaps may also include subgingival caries, perforations or root fractures in the coronal third of the root as well as inadequate retention for fixed prosthetic restorations due to a short clinical crown (crown-lengthening procedures). The "crown lengthening" needed in such cases is performed by removing often significant amounts of supporting bone and by recontouring. A "biologic width" of approximately 3 mm is needed between the alveolar bone crest to be established and the anticipated restoration margin for successful results (Brägger et al. 1992, Herrero et al. 1995, Pontoriero & Carnevale 2001).

Root surface instrumentation

Before incisions are made to excise or elevate the soft tissue, a careful examination should be carried out to identify at which tooth sites periodontal lesions remain. Only tooth sites with signs of pathology (bleeding following pocket probing) should be subjected to root instrumentation following surgical exposure. Further, at these sites, root surface instrumentation should be limited to that part of the root that will be covered by the soft tissue following flap replacement and suturing. This is an important consideration since instrumentation of the supragingival portion of the root may lead to postsurgical dentin hypersensitivity, which in turn may impede proper oral hygiene measures. Hence, before root instrumentation is executed, remaining granulation tissue must be removed, bone recontouring carried out, if indicated, and the postsurgical soft tissue level determined. If the intention is to apically reposition the flap at the level of the bone crest, only approximately 3 mm of the root surface coronal to the bone crest has to be carefully scaled and root planed, whereas if the flap is to be coronally positioned the entire exposed root often has to be instrumented.

The root instrumentation can be performed with hand or ultrasonic instruments according to the operator's preferences. Ultrasonic (sonic) instrumentation offers the additional benefits of improved visibility due to the irrigating effect of the cooling water. For root instrumentation within intrabony defects, root concavities and entrances to furcations, the use of rotating fine-grained diamond stones may be used.

Root surface conditioning / biomodification

An important consideration in periodontal surgery is to make the exposed root surface biologically compatible with a healthy periodontium. This so-called conditioning includes removing bacteria, endotoxins and other antigens found within the cementum-dentin of a pathologically exposed root. In addition to scaling and root planing, agents such as citric acid/orthophosphoric acid, tetracycline and EDTA are used for root surface conditioning. Root surface conditioning/biomodification by means of an etching procedure may serve several purposes:

- removal of the smear layer following mechanical debridement
- demineralization of the root surface (citric acid)
- selective removal of hydroxyapatite and exposure of the collagenous matrix of the root surface (EDTA)
- local delivery of antimicrobial compound (tetracycline HCL)
- inhibition of collagenolytic activity (tetracycline HCL)
- enhancing cellular responses (migration and attachment)
- preventing epithelial down-growth
- improving retention of different biomolecules to exposed collagen
- expressing a cementoblast phenotype for colonizing cells.

It should be noted that etching of a root surface with an agent operating at a low pH, e.g. citric acid or orthophosphoric acid, might exert immediate necrotizing effects on the surrounding periodontal ligament and other periodontal tissues, whereas agents operating at a neutral pH (e.g. EDTA) do not seem to have this negative effect (Blomlöf & Lindskog 1995a,b).

Although *in vitro* results have indicated possible benefits of the use of root surface conditioning/biomodification agents through enhanced cellular responses during wound healing, the usefulness of acids as well as other chemical agents for conditioning of root surfaces in conjunction with conventional periodontal surgery has been questionned (Blomlöf et al. 2000). Histological evidence indicates that healing following root surface conditioning with acids or other chemical agents is generally dominated by a long junctional epithelium or connective tissue attachment without evidence of new cementum formation. However, root surface biomodification must still be regarded as an important method to facilitate regeneration. Thus, in this treatment the root represents one of the wound margins and must provide an appropriate surface for cell attachment, colonization and proliferation.

Suturing

When a flap procedure has been employed it is important to ensure that, at the end of surgery, the flaps are placed in the intended position and that the flaps are properly adapted to each other and to the tooth surfaces. Preferably, full coverage of the buccal/lingual (palatal) and interdental alveolar bone should be obtained by full (primary) closure of the soft tissue flaps. If this can be achieved, healing by first intention results and the postoperative bone resorption becomes minimal. Therefore, prior to suturing, the flap margins should be trimmed to properly fit the buccal and lingual (palatal) bone margin as well as the interproximal areas; excessive soft tissue must be removed. If the amount of flap tissue present is insufficient to cover the interproximal bone, the flaps at the buccal or lingual aspects of the teeth must be recontoured and, in some cases, even coronally displaced.

Following proper trimming, the flaps are secured in the correct position by sutures. The materials most commonly used as sutures in periodontal surgery are fabricated of silk and various synthetic materials. The dimensions usually preferred are 3-0 or 4-0. These materials are non-resorbable and should be removed after 7-14 days. If the sutures need to be maintained in place for several weeks, Teflon® suture material is preferable due to minimal tissue reactions to the material.

Since the flap tissue following the final preparation is thin, non-traumatic needles (eyeless), either curved or straight, with a small diameter should be used. Such needles are available as rounded (non-cutting) or with different cutting edges.

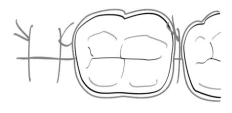
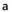

a

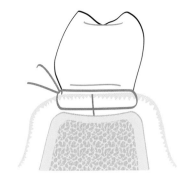

b

Fig. 25-54a,b. *Suturing*. Interrupted interdental suture.

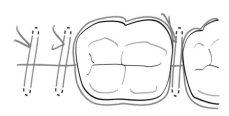

a

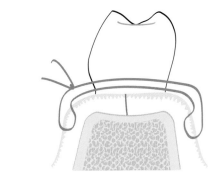

b

Fig. 25-55a,b. *Suturing*. Modified interrupted interdental suture. Note that with this suturing technique the suture is lying on the surface of the interdental tissue keeping the soft tissue flaps in close contact with the underlying bone.

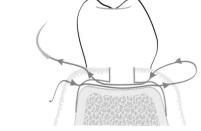

a

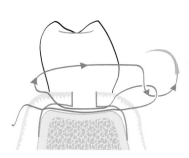

b

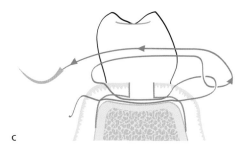

c

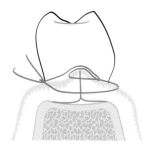

d

Fig. 25-56a-d. *Suturing*. Modified mattress suture.

Suturing technique

The three most frequently used sutures in periodontal flap surgery are:

- interrupted interdental sutures,
- suspensory sutures and
- continuous sutures.

The *interrupted interdental suture* (Fig. 25-54) provides a close interdental adaptation between the buccal and lingual flaps with equal tension on both units. This type of suture is therefore not recommended when the buccal and lingual flaps are repositioned at different levels. When this technique of suturing is employed,

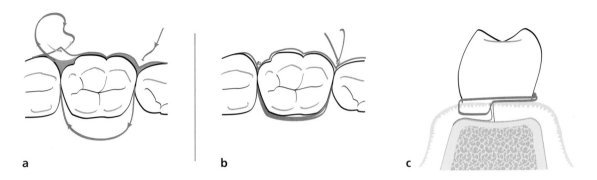

Fig. 25-57a-c. *Suturing*. Suspensory suture.

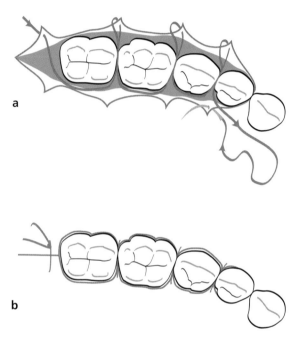

Fig. 25-58a,b. *Suturing*. Continuous suture.

the needle is passed through the buccal flap from the external surface, across the interdental area and through the lingual flap from the internal surface, or vice versa. When closing the suture, care must be taken to avoid tearing the flap tissues.

In order to avoid having the suture material between the mucosa and the alveolar bone in the interdental area, an alternative technique for the use of the interrupted interdental suture can be used if the flaps have not been elevated beyond the mucogingival line (Fig. 25-55). With the use of a curved needle the suture is anchored in the attached tissue on the buccal aspect of the proximal site, the suture brought to the lingual side through the proximal sites, and anchored in the attached tissue on the lingual side. The suture is then brought back to the starting point and tied (Fig. 25-55b). Hence, the suture will be lying on the surface of the interdental tissue, keeping the soft tissue flaps in close contact with the underlying bone.

In regenerative procedures, which usually require a coronal advancing of the flap, a *modified mattress suture* may be used to secure close flap adaptation (Fig. 25-56). The needle is passed through the buccal flap from the external surface, across the interdental area and through the lingual flap from the internal surface. The suture is run back to the buccal side by passing the needle through the lingual and buccal flaps. Thereafter, the suture is brought through the approximal site coronally to the tissue, passed through the loop of the suture on the lingual aspect, and then brought back to the starting point on the buccal side and tied.

The *suspensory suture* (Fig. 25-57) is used primarily when the surgical procedure is of limited extent and involves only the tissue of the buccal or lingual aspect of the teeth. It is also the suture of choice when the buccal and lingual flaps are repositioned at different levels. The needle is passed through the buccal flap from its external surface at the mesial side of the tooth, the suture placed around the lingual surface of the tooth and the needle passed through the buccal flap on the distal side of the tooth (Fig. 25-57a). The suture is brought back to the starting point via the lingual surface of the tooth and tied (Fig. 25-57b,c). If a lingual flap has been elevated as well, this is secured in the intended position using the same technique.

The *continuous suture* (Fig. 25-58) is commonly used when flaps involving several teeth are to be apically repositioned. When flaps have been elevated on both sides of the teeth, one flap at a time is secured in its correct position. The suturing procedure is started at the mesial/distal aspect of the buccal flap by passing the needle through the flap and across the interdental area. The suture is laid around the lingual surface of the tooth and returned to the buccal side through the next interdental space. The procedure is repeated tooth by tooth until the distal/mesial end of the flap is reached. Thereafter, the needle is passed through the lingual flap (Fig. 25-58a), with the suture laid around the buccal aspect of each tooth and through each interproximal space. When the suturing of the lingual flap is completed and the needle has been brought back to the first interdental area, the positions of the flaps are adjusted and secured in their proper positions by closing the suture (Fig. 25-58b). Thus, only one knot is needed.

Periodontal dressings

Periodontal dressings are mainly used:

- to protect the wound postsurgically,
- to obtain and maintain a close adaptation of the mucosal flaps to the underlying bone (especially when a flap has been apically repositioned) and
- for the comfort of the patient.

In addition, periodontal dressings can, during the initial phase of healing, prevent postoperative bleeding and, if properly placed in the operated segment (especially interproximally), prevent the formation of excessive granulation tissue.

Periodontal dressings should have the following properties:

- The dressing should be soft, but still have enough plasticity and flexibility to facilitate its placement in the operated area and to allow proper adaptation.
- The dressing should harden within a reasonable time.
- After setting, the dressing should be sufficiently rigid to prevent fracture and dislocation.
- The dressing should have a smooth surface after setting to prevent irritation to the cheeks and lips.
- The dressing should preferably have bactericidal properties to prevent excessive plaque formation.
- The dressing must not detrimentally interfere with healing.

It has been suggested that antibacterial agents should be incorporated in periodontal dressings to prevent bacterial growth in the wound area during healing. Results from clinical studies and *in vitro* evaluation of the antibacterial properties of various periodontal dressings, however, suggest that the antibacterial activity of most commercial dressings probably is exhausted long before the end of the 7-14-day period during which the dressing is frequently maintained in the operated segment (O'Neil 1975, Haugen et al. 1977).

Mouth rinsing with antibacterial agents such as chlorhexidine does not prevent the formation of plaque *under* the dressing (Plÿss et al. 1975) and should therefore not be regarded as a means to improve or shorten the period of wound healing. On the other hand, results from clinical studies as well as clinical experience suggest that a periodontal dressing may often be unnecessary or even undesirable after periodontal flap procedures and may be usefully re-

placed by rinsing with chlorhexidine only (Sanz et al. 1989, Vaughan & Garnick 1989).

A commonly used periodontal dressing is Coe-Pak™ (Coe Laboratories Inc., Chicago, IL, US), which is supplied in two tubes. One tube contains oxides of various metals (mainly zinc-oxide) and lorothidol (a fungicide). The second tube contains non-ionizing carboxylic acids and chlorothymol (a bacteriostatic agent). Equal parts from both tubes are mixed together immediately prior to insertion. The setting time can be prolonged by adding a retarder.

A light curing dressing, e.g. Barricaid™ (Dentsply International Inc., Milford, DE, US), is useful in the anterior tooth region and particularly following mucogingival surgery, because it has a favorable esthetic appearence and it can be applied without dislocating the soft tissue. However, the light curing dressing is not the choice of dressing to be used in situations where the flap has to be apically retained, due to its soft state before curing.

Cyanoacrylates have also been used as periodontal dressings with varying success. Dressings of the cyanoacrylate type are applied in a liquid directly onto the wound, or sprayed over the wound surface. Although the application of this kind of dressing is simple, its properties often do not meet clinical demands, which is why its use is rather limited at present.

Application technique

- Ensure that bleeding from the operated tissues has ceased before the dressing material is inserted.
- Carefully dry teeth and soft tissue before the application for optimal adherence of the dressing.
- Moisten the surgical gloves to avoid the material sticking to the fingertips.
- When using the Coe-Pak™' dressing material, the interproximal areas are filled first. Thin rolls of the dressing, adjusted in length to cover the entire field of operation, are then placed against the buccal and lingual surfaces of the teeth. The rolls are pressed against the tooth surfaces and the dressing material is forced into the interproximal areas. Coe-Pak™ may also be applied to the wound surfaces by means of a plastic syringe. It is important to ensure that dressing material is never introduced between the flap and the underlying bone or root surface.
- The surface of the dressing is subsequently smoothed and excess material is removed with a suitable instrument. The dressing should not cover more than the apical third of the tooth surfaces. Furthermore, interferences of the dressing with mucogingival structures (e.g. the vestibular fold, frenula) should be carefully checked to avoid displacement of the dressing during normal function.

The light curing dressing (Barricaid™) is preferably applied with the supplied syringe, adjusted and then cured by light. It is important to carefully dry teeth and soft tissue before the application for optimal adherence. Excess of dressing material can easily be removed following the curing with a knife or finishing burs in a low-speed handpiece.

Postoperative pain control

In order to minimize postoperative pain and discomfort for the patient, the surgical handling of the tissues should be as atraumatic as possible. Care should be taken during surgery to avoid unnecessary tearing of the flaps, to keep the bone moistened and to ensure complete soft tissue coverage of the alveolar bone at suturing. With a carefully performed surgical procedure most patients will normally experience only minimal postoperative problems. The pain experience is usually limited to the first days following surgery and is of a level that in most patients can be adequately controlled with normally used drugs for pain control. However, it is important to recognize that the pain threshold level is subjective and may vary between individuals. It is also important to give the patient information about the postsurgical sequence and that uncomplicated healing is the common event. Further, during the early phase of healing, the patient should be instructed to avoid chewing in the area subjected to surgical treatment.

Postsurgical care

Postoperative plaque control is the most important variable in determining the long-term result of periodontal surgery. Provided proper postoperative plaque control levels are established, most surgical treatment techniques will result in conditions which favor the maintenance of a healthy periodontium.

Although there are other factors of a more general nature affecting surgical outcome (e.g. the systemic status of the patient at time of surgery and during healing), disease recurrence is an inevitable complication, regardless of surgical technique used, in patients not given proper postsurgical and maintenance care.

Since self-performed oral hygiene is often associated with pain and discomfort during the immediate postsurgical phase, regularly performed professional toothcleaning is a more effective means of mechanical plaque control following periodontal surgery. In the immediate postsurgical patient management self-performed rinsing with a suitable antiplaque agent, e.g. twice daily rinsing with 0.1-0.2% chlorhexidine solution, is recommended. Although an obvious disadvantage with the use of chlorhexidine is the staining of teeth and tongue, this is usually not a deterrent for compliance. Nevertheless, it is important to return to and maintain good mechanical oral hygiene measures as soon as possible. This is especially important since rinsing with chlorhexidine, in contrast to properly performed mechanical oral hygiene, is not likely to have any influence on subgingival recolonization of plaque.

Maintaining good postsurgical wound stability is another important factor affecting the outcome of some types of periodontal flap surgery. If wound stability is judged an important part of a specific procedure, the procedure itself as well as the postsurgical care must include measures to stabilize the healing wound (e.g. adequate suturing technique, protection from mechanical trauma to the marginal tissues during the initial healing phase). If a mucoperiosteal flap is replaced rather than apically repositioned, early apical migration of gingival epithelial cells will occur as a consequence of a break between root surface and healing connective tissue. Hence, a maintained tight adaptation of the flap to the root surface is essential and one may therefore consider keeping the sutures in place for a longer period of time than the 7-10 days usually prescribed following standard flap surgery.

Following suture removal, the surgically treated area is thoroughly irrigated with a dental spray and the teeth are carefully cleaned with a rubber cup and polishing paste. If the healing is satisfactory for starting mechanical toothcleaning, the patient is instructed in gentle brushing of the operated area using a toothbrush that has been softened in hot water. For cleaning of the interdental area, toothpicks are prescribed. At this early phase following the surgical treatment the use of interdental brushes is abandoned due to the risk of traumatizing the interdental tissues. Visits are scheduled for supportive care at 2-week intervals to closely monitor the patient's plaque control. During this postoperative maintenance phase, adjustments of the methods for optimal self-performed mechanical cleaning are made depending on the healing status of the tissues. Dictated by the patient's plaque control standard, the time interval between visits for supportive care may gradually be increased.

OUTCOME OF SURGICAL PERIODONTAL THERAPY

Healing following surgical pocket therapy

Gingivectomy (Fig. 25-59): Within a few days following excision of the inflamed gingival soft tissues coronal to the base of the periodontal pocket, epithelial cells start to migrate over the wound surface. The epithelialization of the gingivectomy wound is usually complete within 7 to 14 days following surgery (Engler et al. 1966, Stahl et al. 1968). During the following weeks a new dento-gingival unit is formed. The fibroblasts in the supra-alveolar tissue adjacent to the tooth surface proliferate (Waerhaug 1955) and new connective tissue is laid down. If the wound healing occurs in the vicinity of a plaque-free tooth surface, a

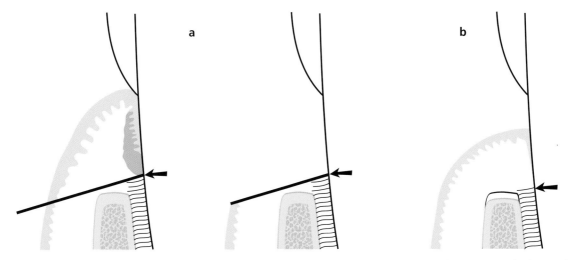

Fig. 25-59. *Gingivectomy*. Dimensional changes as a result of therapy. (a) The preoperative dimensions. The line indicates the location of the primary incision, i.e. the suprabony pocket is eliminated with the gingivectomy technique. (b) Dimensions following proper healing. Minor resorption of the alveolar bone crest as well as some loss of connective tissue attachment has occurred.

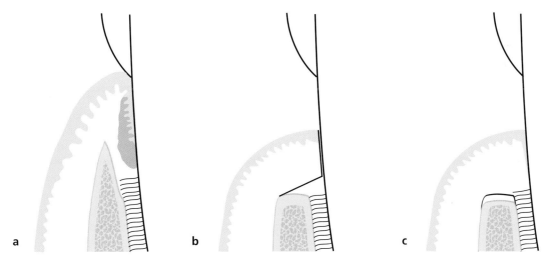

Fig. 25-60. *Apically repositioned flap*. Dimensional changes. (a) The preoperative dimensions. The broken line indicates the site from which the mucoperiosteal flap is reflected. (b) Bone recontouring has been completed and the flap repositioned to cover the alveolar bone. (c) Dimensions following healing. Minor resorption of the marginal alveolar bone has occurred as well as some loss of connective tissue attachment.

free gingival unit will form which has all the characteristics of a normal free gingiva (Hamp et al. 1975). The height of the newly formed free gingival unit may vary not only between different parts of the dentition but also from one tooth surface to another due to primarily anatomical factors.

The re-establishment of a new, free gingival unit by coronal regrowth of tissue from the line of the "gingivectomy" incision implies that sites with so-called "zero pockets" only occasionally occur following gingivectomy. Complete healing of the gingivectomy wound takes 4-5 weeks, although the surface of the gingiva may appear by clinical inspection to be healed already after approximately 14 days (Ramfjord et al. 1966). Minor remodeling of the alveolar bone crest may also occur postoperatively.

The apically repositioned flap (Fig. 25-60): Following osseous surgery for elimination of bony defects and the establishment of "physiologic contours" and repositioning of the soft tissue flaps to the level of the alveolar bone, healing will occur primarily by first intention, especially in areas where proper soft tissue coverage of the alveolar bone has been obtained. During the initial phase of healing, bone resorption of varying degrees almost always occurs in the crestal area of the alveolar bone (Ramfjord & Costich 1968). The extent of the reduction of the alveolar bone height resulting from this resorption is related to the thickness of the bone in each specific site (Wood et al. 1972, Karring et al. 1975).

During the phase of tissue regeneration and maturation a new dento-gingival unit will form by coronal growth of the connective tissue. This regrowth occurs in a manner similar to that which characterized healing following gingivectomy.

The modified Widman flap (Fig. 25-61): If a "modified

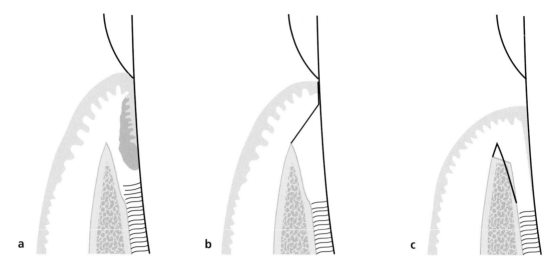

Fig. 25-61. *Modified Widman flap*. Dimensional changes. (a) The preoperative dimensions. The broken line indicates the site from which the mucoperiosteal flap is reflected. (b) Surgery (including curettage of the angular bone defect) is completed with the mucoperiosteal flap repositioned as close as possible to its presurgical position. (c) Dimensions following healing. Osseous repair as well as some crestal bone resorption can be expected during healing with the establishment of a "long" junctional epithelium interposed between the regenerated bone tissue and the root surface. An apical displacement of the soft tissue margin has occurred.

Widman flap" is carried out in an area with a deep infrabony lesion, bone repair may occur within the boundaries of the lesion (Rosling et al. 1976a, Polson & Heijl 1978). However, crestal bone resorption is also seen. The amount of bone fill obtained is dependent upon (1) the anatomy of the osseous defect (e.g. a three-walled infrabony defect often provides a better mould for bone repair than two-walled or one-walled defects), (2) the amount of crestal bone resorption, and (3) the extent of chronic inflammation, which may occupy the area of healing. Interposed between the regenerated bone tissue and the root surface, a long junctional epithelium is always found (Caton & Zander 1976, Caton et al. 1980). The apical cells of the newly formed junctional epithelium are found at a level on the root that closely coincides with the presurgical attachment level.

Soft tissue recession will take place during the healing phase following a modified Widman flap procedure. Although the major apical shift in the position of the soft tissue margin will occur during the first 6 months following the surgical treatment (Lindhe et al. 1987), the soft tissue recession may often continue for more than 1 year. Among factors influencing the degree of soft tissue recession, besides the period for soft tissue remodeling, are the initial height and thickness of the supracrestal flap tissue and the amount of crestal bone resorption.

Clinical outcome of surgical access therapy in comparison to non-surgical therapy

Surgical treatment of periodontal lesions mainly serves the purpose of (1) creating accessibility for proper professional debridement of the infected root surfaces and (2) establishing a gingival morphology that facilitates the patient's self-performed plaque control, in order to enhance the long-term preservation of the dentition. Hence, the amount of tooth loss would be the most relevant criterion in an evaluation of the relative importance of surgical access therapy in the overall treatment of periodontal disease. However, since the rate of tooth loss is comparatively low, this would require studies with extremely long periods of follow-up. Other criteria, such as resolution of gingivitis (bleeding on probing), probing pocket depth reduction and clinical attachment level change, have therefore commonly been used to evaluate the efficacy of periodontal therapy, even if these may only be considered as surrogate end points. An additional variable often of concern is gingival recession, since this outcome variable may affect the patient's overall appreciation of the treatment result. With regard to changes in probing attachment levels, it should be recalled that healing following conventional surgical access therapy consistently results in the formation of a junctional epithelium to a level on the root that closely coincides with the presurgical attachment level. Hence, when evaluating the outcome of various therapeutic approaches the magnitude of *gain* of clinical attachment may be of less importance since it mainly is a measure of "pocket closure". Instead, maintained probing attachment levels or further loss should be focused on as the pertinent outcome variable.

Pioneering contributions to the understanding of the relative importance of the surgical component of periodontal therapy were generated by the classic longitudinal studies by the Michigan group (Ramfjord and co-workers) and the Gothenburg group (Lindhe and co-workers). Subsequently, several other clinical research centers contributed with important data regarding the efficacy of surgical access therapy in com-

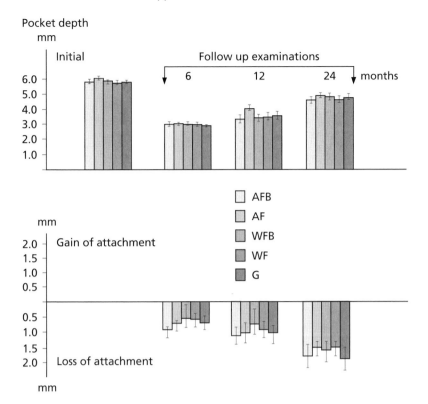

Fig. 25-62. Average *approximal* pocket depths at the initial examination and 6, 12 and 24 months after surgery (top) and alterations in *approximal* attachment levels from the initial examination immediately prior to surgery to the reexaminations 6, 12 and 24 months postoperatively (bottom). Note that only areas with pockets which at the initial examination had a depth of 3 mm or more are included in the analysis. I = standard error. AFB = apically repositioned flap with bone recontouring. AF = apically repositioned flap. WFB = modified Widman flap with bone recontouring. WF = modified Widman flap. G = gingivectomy including curettage of bone defects. (Data from Nyman et al. 1977.)

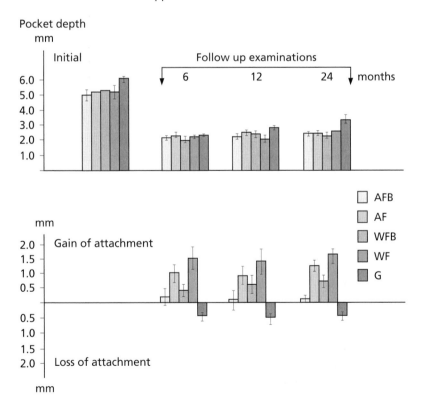

Fig. 25-63. Average approximal pocket depths at the initial examination and 6, 12 and 24 months after surgery (top), and alterations in approximal attachment levels from the initial examination immediately prior to surgery to the reexaminations 6, 12, and 24 months postoperatively (bottom). Note that only areas with pockets which at the initial examination had a depth of 3 mm or more have been included in the statistical analysis. I = standard error. AFB = apically repositioned flap and bone correction. AF = apically repositioned flap. WFB = Widman flap and bone correction. WF = Widman Flap. G = gingviectomy, including curettage of the bony defects. (Data from Rosling et al. 1976.)

parison to non-surgical periodontal therapy. The topic has been extensively reviewed in several publications (e.g. Kaldahl et al. 1993, Palcanis 1996) and some of the general conclusions from these reviews will be highlighted below.

Plaque accumulation

An important factor to consider in the evaluation of the relative effect of the surgical component of periodontal therapy is the standard of postoperative plaque control. Nyman et al. (1977) reported on a clinical study in which the patients received only a

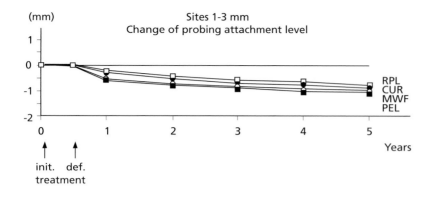

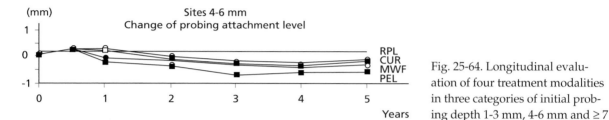

Fig. 25-64. Longitudinal evaluation of four treatment modalities in three categories of initial probing depth 1-3 mm, 4-6 mm and ≥ 7 mm. RPL = scaling and root planing.
CUR = subgingival curettage.
MWF = Modified Widman Flap.
PEL = pocket elimination surgery.
(Data from Ramfjord et al. 1987, presented by Egelberg 1995.)

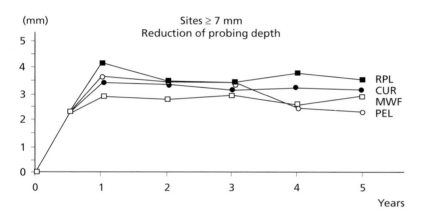

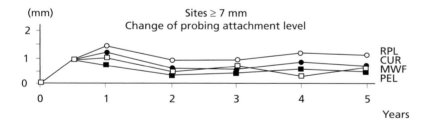

single episode of oral hygiene instruction before the surgical treatment and no specific postoperative supportive care. As a consequence both plaque and gingival indices remained relatively high during the 2 years of postoperative follow-up. Independent of surgical technique used, the patients showed a rebound of pocket depths to more or less pretreatment levels and further deterioration of clinical attachment levels at both proximal and lingual tooth sites (Fig. 25-62). In contrast, in a parallel study in which the patients received repeated oral hygiene instructions and professional tooth-cleaning once every 2 weeks during the postoperative period (Rosling et al. 1976b), the patients maintained the surgically reduced pocket depth throughout the 2-year follow-up period and

clinical attachment level gains were observed for most of the surgical procedures evaluated (Fig. 25-63). The fact that the standard of postoperative oral hygiene is decisive for the outcome of surgical pocket therapy is further underlined by data from a 5-year longitudinal study by Lindhe et al. (1984), which showed that patients with a high standard of plaque control maintained clinical attachment levels and probing depth reductions following treatment more consistently than patients with poor plaque control. On the other hand, professional tooth cleaning including subgingival scaling every 3 months may partly compensate for the negative effects of variations in self-performed plaque control (Ramfjord et al. 1982, Isidor & Karring 1986).

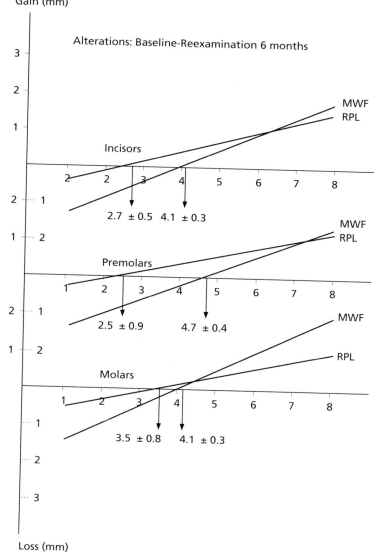

Fig. 25-65. Diagram illustrating the gain and loss of clinical attachment (Y-axis) in relation to initial probing depth (X-axis) at *incisors, premolars and molars,* calculated from measurements made at the baseline examination and after 6 months. RPL = non-surgical scaling and root planing. MWF = modified Widman flap surgery. The non-surgical approach (RPL) consistently yielded lower critical probing depth (CPD) values than the surgical approach. (Data from Lindhe et al. 1982b.)

With regard to post-treatment plaque accumulation, there is no evidence to suggest that differences exist between non-surgical or surgical treatment or between various surgical procedures. In addition, most studies have shown that the magnitude of gingivitis resolution is not influenced by the treatment modality.

Probing pocket depth reduction
All surgical procedures result in a decrease in probing pocket depths with greater reduction occurring at initially deeper sites (Knowles et al. 1979, Lindhe et al. 1984, Ramfjord et al. 1987, Kaldahl et al. 1996, Becker et al. 2001). Furthermore, surgical therapy generally creates greater short-term reduction of probing depth than non-surgically performed scaling and root planing. Flap surgery with bone recontouring (pocket elimination surgery) usually results in the most pronounced short-term pocket reduction. Long-term (5-8 years) results show various outcomes. Some studies reported greater probing depth reduction following surgery while others reported no differences in relation to non-surgical therapy. Also, the magnitude of

the initial probing depth reduction shows a tendency to decrease with time, independent of treatment modality.

Clinical attachment level change
In sites with initially shallow probing depth, both short-term and long-term data demonstrate that surgery creates a greater loss of clinical attachment than non-surgical treatment, whereas in sites with initially deep pockets (≥ 7 mm), a greater gain of clinical attachment is generally obtained (Knowles et al. 1979, Lindhe et al. 1984, Ramfjord et al. 1987, Kaldahl et al. 1996, Becker et al. 2001) (Fig. 25-64). When clinical attachment levels following surgery with and without osseous resection were compared, either no difference was found between therapies or flap surgery without osseous resection produced a greater gain. In addition, there was no difference in the longitudinal maintenance of clinical attachment levels between sites treated non-surgically and those treated surgically, with or without osseous resection.

Based on data generated from a clinical trial comparing non-surgical and surgical (modified Widman

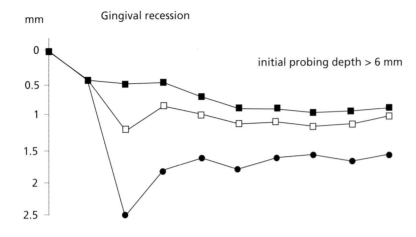

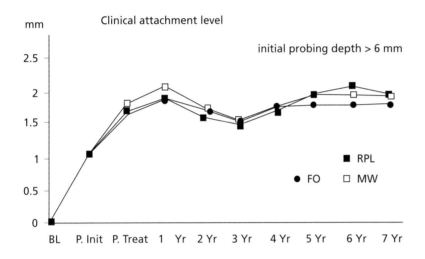

Fig. 25-66. Longitudinal changes in recession (REC) and clinical attachment levels (CAL) at sites with initial probing depth of 6 mm following three periodontal treatment modalities. RPL = scaling and root planing. MWF = modified Widman flap procedure. FO = flap and osseous surgery. (Data from Kaldahl et al. 1996.)

flap) approaches to root debridement, Lindhe et al. (1982b) developed the concept of *critical probing depth* in relation to clinical attachment level change. For each treatment approach, the clinical attachment change was plotted against the initial pocket depth and regression lines were calculated (Fig. 26-65). The point where the regression line crossed the horizontal axis (initial probing depth) was defined as the *critical probing depth* (CPD), i.e. the level of pocket depth below which clinical attachment loss would occur as the result of the treatment procedure performed. The CPD was consistently found to be greater for the surgical approach than for the non-surgical treatment. Furthermore, at incisors and premolars the surgical therapy showed superior outcome only when the initial probing depth was greater than 6-7 mm, while at molars the corresponding cut-off point was 4.5 mm. The interpretation of the latter finding would be that, in the molar tooth regions, the surgical approach to root debridement offers advantages over the non-surgical approach. This interpretation is supported by the observation that inferior results are obtained by non-surgical therapy in molars compared to single-rooted teeth (Nordland et al. 1987, Loos et al. 1988). Also, data generated from studies comparing closed and open root debridement in furcation sites favor surgical ac-

cess therapy in the treatment of molar tooth regions (Matia et al. 1986).

The removal of the pocket epithelium and the soft tissue lesion by curettage (Echeverria & Caffesse 1983, Ramfjord et al. 1987) or surgical excision (Lindhe & Nyman 1985) is not a prerequisite for proper healing of the treated periodontal site. In the study by Lindhe & Nyman (1985), three treatment modalities were used, i.e. excision of the soft tissue lesion during flap surgery (modified Widman flap procedure), surgery without removal of the soft tissue lesion (Kirkland flap) and non-surgical scaling and root planing. The 1-year follow-up examination revealed about 1 mm of gain in clinical attachment level for all three procedures. Thus, deliberate excision of the soft tissue lesion did not improve the healing result.

Gingival recession

Gingival recession is an inevitable consequence of periodontal therapy. Since it occurs primarily as a result of resolution of the inflammation in the periodontal tissues, it is seen following both non-surgical and surgical therapy. Irrespective of treatment modality used, initially deeper pocket sites will experience more pronounced signs of recession of the gingival margin than sites with initial shallow probing depths

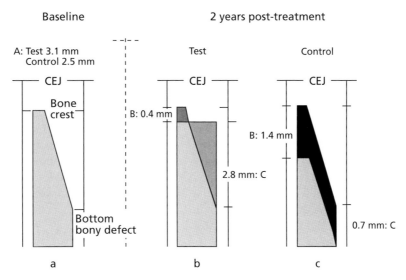

Fig. 25-67. Schematic drawing illustrating alterations in the level of the marginal bone crest and the level of the bottom of the bone defects in the test and control groups. Distance A denotes the depth of the bone defects at the initial examination; test group 3.1 mm, control group 2.5 mm. Distance B denotes resorption of the marginal alveolar crest (b,c), which anounted to 0.4 mm in the test patients (a) and 1.4 mm in the controls (c). Distance C denotes gain or loss of bone in the apical portion of the defect. There was a refill of bone in test patients amounting to 2.8 mm (b), whereas a further 0.7 mm loss of bone occurred in the control patients (c). (Data from Rosling et al. 1976a.)

(Badersten et al. 1984, Lindhe et al. 1987, Becker et al. 2001).

A general finding in short-term follow-up studies of periodontal therapy is that non-surgically performed scaling and root planing cause less gingival recession than surgical therapy, and that surgical treatment involving osseous resection results in the most pronounced recession. However, data obtained from long-term studies reveal that the initial differences seen in amount of recession between various treatment modalities diminish over time due to a coronal rebound of the soft tissue margin following surgical treatment (Kaldahl et al. 1996, Becker et al. 2001) (Fig. 25-66). Lindhe & Nyman (1980) found that after apically repositioned flap procedure the buccal gingival margin shifted to a more coronal position (about 1 mm) during 10-11 years of maintenance. In interdental areas denuded following surgery, Van der Velden (1982) found an upgrowth of around 4 mm of gingival tissue 3 years after surgery, while no significant change in attachment levels was observed. A similar finding was reported by Pontoriero & Carnevale (2001) 1 year after apical positioned flap procedure for crown lengthening.

Bone fill in angular bone defects
The potential for bone formation in angular defects following surgical access therapy has been demonstrated in a number of studies. Rosling et al. (1976a) studied the healing of two-wall and three-wall angular bone defects following a modified Widman flap procedure, including careful curettage of the bone defect and proper root debridement, in 24 patients with multiple osseous defects. Following active treatment, patients assigned to the test group received supportive periodontal care once every 2 weeks for a 2-year period, while the patients in the control group were only recalled once a year for prophylaxis. Re-examination carried out 2 years after therapy demonstrated that the patients who had been subjected to the intensive professional tooth-cleaning regimen had experienced a mean gain of clinical attachment in the angular bone defects amounting to 3.5 mm. Measurements performed on radiographs revealed a marginal bone loss of 0.4 mm, but that the remaining portion of the original bone defect (2.8 mm) was refilled with bone (Fig. 25-67). All the 124 bone defects treated were completely resolved. In the control group most of the sites treated showed signs of recurrent periodontitis, including further loss of clinical attachment and alveolar bone. Similar healing results were reported by Polson & Heijl (1978). They treated 15 defects (two-wall and three-wall) in 9 patients using a modified Widman flap procedure. Following curettage of the bone defect and root planing, the flaps were closed to achieve complete soft tissue coverage of the defect area. All patients were enrolled in a professional tooth-cleaning program. The healing was evaluated at a re-entry operation 6-8 months after the initial surgery. Eleven of the 15 defects had resolved completely. The healing was characterized by a combination of coronal bone regeneration (77% of the initial depth of the defects) and marginal bone resorption (18%). The authors concluded that intrabony defects may predictably remodel after surgical debridement and establishment of optimal plaque control.

The results from the studies referred to demonstrate that a significant bone fill may be obtained in two-wall and three-wall intrabony defects at single-rooted teeth, provided the postoperative supportive care is of very high quality. Two recent reviews (Laurell et al. 1998, Lang 2000), focusing on the outcome of surgical access therapy in angular bone defects, give additional information regarding expected bone regeneration in angular defects following open flap debridement (modified Widman flap). In the review by Laurell et al. (1998), 13 studies were included representing a total of 278 treated defects with a mean depth of 4.1 mm. The weighted mean bone fill in the angular defects amounted to 1.1 mm. Lang (2000) reported an analysis of 15 studies providing data generated from radiographic assessments of the healing of 523 angular bone defects. Their analysis yielded a weighted mean of 1.5 mm of bone gain. Since the included studies in these reviews showed great variability in bone fill, one may assume that the standard of post-surgical plaque control varied between the studies. As shown in the study by Rosling et al. (1976a), a meticulous postsurgical plaque control and the close professional supervision of the patients are critical for optimal healing conditions. One also has to consider that the potential for bone fill may differ depending on the morphology of the angular bone defect. Most angular defects appear as combinations of one-wall, two-wall and three-wall defects and whereas the two-wall and three-wall component of an angular bone defect may show great potential for bone fill during healing, the one-wall component will rarely demonstrate this type of healing.

References

Ah, M.K.B., Johnson, G.K., Kaldahl, W.B., Patil, K.D. & Kalkwarf, K.L. (1994). The effect of smoking on the response to periodontal therapy. *Journal of Clinical Periodontology* **21**, 91-97.

American Dental Association and American Academy of Orthopaedic Surgeons (1997). Advisory statement. Antibiotic prophylaxis for dental patients with total joint replacements. *Journal of the American Dental Association* **128**, 1004-1008.

Ariaudo, A.A. & Tyrell, H.A. (1957). Repositioning and increasing the zone of attached gingiva. *Journal of Periodontology* **28**, 106-110.

Axelsson, P. & Lindhe, J. (1981). The significance of maintenance care in the treatment of periodontal disease. *Journal of Clinical Periodontology* **8**, 281-294.

Badersten, A., Nilveus, R. & Egelberg, J. (1981). Effect of nonsurgical periodontal therapy. I. Moderately advanced periodontitis. *Journal of Clinical Periodontology* **8**, 57-72.

Badersten, A., Nilveus, R. & Egelberg, J. (1984). Effect of nonsurgical periodontal therapy. II. Severely advanced periodontitis. *Journal of Clinical Periodontology* **11**, 63-76.

Becker, W., Becker, B.E., Caffesse, R., Kerry, G., Ochsenbein, C., Morrison, E. & Prichard, J. (2001). A longitudinal study comparing scaling, osseous surgery and modified Widman procedures: Results after 5 years. *Journal of Peridontology* **72**, 1675-1684.

Blomlöf, J. & Lindskog, S. (1995a). Root surface texture and early cell and tissue colonization after different etching modalities. *European Journal Oral Sciences* **103**, 17-24.

Blomlöf, J. & Lindskog, S. (1995b). Periodontal tissue-vitality after different etching modalities. *Journal of Clinical Peridontology* **22**, 464-468.

Blomlöf, L., Jonsson, B., Blomlöf, J. & Lindskog, S. (2000). A clinical study of root surface conditioning with an EDTA gel. II. Surgical periodontal treatment. *International Journal of Periodontics and Restorative Dentistry* **20**, 566-573.

Bowers, G.M., Chadroff, B., Carnevale, R., Mellonig, J.T., Corio, R., Emerson, J., Stevens, M. & Romberg, E. (1989). Histologic evaluation of new human attachment apparatus formation in humans, Part III. *Journal of Periodontology* **60**, 683-693.

Brägger, U., Lauchenauer, D. & Lang, N.P. (1992). Surgical lengthening of the clinical crown. *Journal of Clinical Periodontology* **19**, 58-63.

Caffesse, R.G., Sweeney, P.L. & Smith, B.A. (1986). Scaling and root planing with and without periodontal flap surgery. *Journal of Clinical Periodontology* **13**, 205-210.

Caton, J., Nyman, S. & Zander, H. (1980). Histometric evaluation of periodontal surgery. II. Connective tissue attachment levels after four regenerative procedures. *Journal of Clinical Periodontology* **7**, 224-231.

Caton, J.G. & Zander, H.A. (1976). Osseous repair of an infrabony pocket without new attachment of connective tissue. *Journal of Clinical Periodontology* **3**, 54-58.

Cortellini, P., Pini Prato, G. & Tonetti, M.S. (1993). Periodontal regeneration of human infrabony defects. I. Clinical measures. *Journal of Periodontology* **64**, 254-260.

Cortellini, P., Pini Prato, G. & Tonetti, M.S. (1995a). Periodontal regeneration of human intrabony defects with titanium reinforced membranes. A controlled clinical trial. *Journal of Periodontology* **66**, 797-803.

Cortellini, P., Pini Prato, G. & Tonetti, M. (1995b). The modified papilla preservation technique. A new surgical approach for interproximal regenerative procedures. *Journal of Periodontology* **66**, 261-266.

Cortellini, P., Pini Prato, G. & Tonetti, M. (1999). The simplified papilla preservation flap. A novel surgical approach for the management of soft tissues in regenerative procedures. *International Journal of Periodontics and Restorative Dentistry* **19**, 589-599.

Dajani, A.S., Taubert, K.A., Wilson, W., Bolger, A.F., Bayer, A., Ferrieri, P., Gewitz, M.H., Shulman, S.T., Nouri, S., Newburger, J.W., Hutto, C., Pallasch, T.J., Gage, T.W., Levison, M.E., Peter, G. & Zuccaro, G. Jr. (1997). Prevention of bacterial endocarditis: recommendations by the American Heart Association. *Journal of the American Dental Association* **128**, 1142-1151.

Echeverria, J.J. & Caffesse, R.G. (1983). Effects of gingival curettage when performed 1 month after root instrumentation. A biometric evaluation. *Journal of Clinical Periodontology* **10**, 277-286.

Egelberg, J. (1995). *Periodontics the scientific way. Synopsis of human clinical studies*, 2nd edn. Malmö: Odonto Science, p. 113.

Engler, W.O., Ramfjord, S.P. & Hiniker, J.J. (1966). Healing following simple gingivectomy. A tritiated thymidine radioautographic study. I. Epithelialization. *Journal of Periodontology* **37**, 298-308.

Fay, J.T. & O'Neal, R.B. (1984). Dental responsibility for the medically compromised patient. *Journal of Oral Medicine* **39**, 218-255.

Friedman, N. (1955). Periodontal osseous surgery: Osteoplasty and ostectomy. *Journal of Periodontology* **26**, 257-269.

Friedman, N. (1962). Mucogingival surgery. The apically repositioned flap. *Journal of Periodontology* **33**, 328-340.

Goldman, H.M. (1950). Development of physiologic gingival contours by gingivoplasty. *Oral Surgery, Oral Medicine and Oral Pathology* **3**, 879-888.

Goldman, H.M. (1951). Gingivectomy. *Oral Surgery, Oral Medicine and Oral Pathology* **4**, 1136-1157.

Gottlow, J., Nyman, S., Lindhe, J., Karring, T. & Wennström, J. (1986). New attachment formation in the human periodontium by guided tissue regeneration. *Journal of Clinical Periodontology* **13**, 604-616.

Grant, D.A., Stern, I.B. & Everett, F.G. (1979). *Periodontics in the tradition of Orban and Gottlieb.* 5th edn. St. Louis: C.V. Mosby Co.

Hammarström, L. (1997). Enamel matrix, cementum development and regeneration. *Journal of Clinical Periodontology* **24**, 658-668.

Hamp, S.E., Rosling, B. & Lindhe, J. (1975). Effect of chlorhexidine on gingival wound healing in the dog. A histometric study. *Journal of Clinical Periodontology* **2**, 143-152.

Haugen, E., Gjermo, P. & Ørstavik, D. (1977). Some antibacterial properties of periodontal dressings. *Journal of Clinical Periodontology* **4**, 62-68.

Heijl, L., Heden, G., Svärdström, G. & Östgren, A. (1997). Enamel matrix derivative (Emdogain®) in the treatment of intrabony periodontal defects. *Journal of Clinical Periodontology* **24**, 705-714.

Herrero, F., Scott, J.B., Maropis, P.S. & Yukna, R.A. (1995). Clinical comparison of desired versus actual amount of surgical crown lengthening. *Journal of Periodontology* **66**, 568-571.

Isidor, F. & Karring, T. (1986). Long-term effect of surgical and non-surgical periodontal treatment. A 5-year clinical study. *Journal of Periodontal Research* **21**, 462-472.

Kaldahl, W.B., Kalkwarf, K.L. & Patil, K.D. (1993). A review of longitudinal studies that compared periodontal therapies. *Journal of Periodontology* **64**, 243-253.

Kaldahl, W.B., Kalkwarf, K.L., Patil, K.D., Molvar, M.P. & Dyer, J.K. (1996). Long-term evaluation of periodontal therapy: I. Response to 4 therapeutic modalities. *Journal of Periodontology* **67**, 93-102.

Karring, T., Cumming, B.R., Oliver, R.C. & Löe, H. (1975). The origin of granulation tissue and its impact on postoperative results of mucogingival surgery. *Journal of Periodontology* **46**, 577-585.

Kirkland, O. (1931). The suppurative periodontal pus pocket; its treatment by the modified flap operation. *Journal of the American Dental Association* **18**, 1462-1470.

Knowles, J.W., Burgett, F.G., Nissle, R.R., Schick, R.A., Morrison, E.C. & Ramfjord, S.P. (1979). Results of periodontal treatment related to pocket depth and attachment level. Eight years. *Journal of Periodontology* **50**, 225-233.

Lang, N.P. (2000). Focus on intrabony defects – conservative therapy. *Periodontology 2000* **22**, 51-58.

Laurell, L., Gottlow, J., Zybutz, M. & Persson, R. (1998). Treatment of intrabony defects by different surgical procedures. A literature review. *Journal of Periodontology* **69**, 303-313.

Lindhe, J. & Nyman, S. (1980). Alterations of the position of the marginal soft tissue following periodontal surgery. *Journal of Clinical Periodontology* **7**, 525-530.

Lindhe, J. & Nyman, S. (1985). Scaling and granulation tissue removal in periodontal therapy. *Journal of Clinical Periodontology* **12**, 374-388.

Lindhe, J., Nyman, S., Socransky, S.S., Haffajee, A.D. & Westfelt, E. (1982b). "Critical probing depth" in periodontal therapy. *Journal of Clinical Periodontology* **9**, 323-336.

Lindhe, J., Socransky, S.S., Nyman, S. & Westfelt, E. (1987). Dimensional alteration of the periodontal tissues following therapy. *International Journal of Periodontics & Restorative Dentistry* **7**(2), 9-22.

Lindhe, J., Westfelt, E., Nyman, S., Socransky, S.S. & Haffajee, A.D. (1984). Long-term effect of surgical/non-surgical treatment of periodontal disease. *Journal of Clinical Periodontology* **11**, 448-458.

Lindhe, J., Westfelt, E., Nyman, S., Socransky, S.S., Heijl, L. & Bratthall, G. (1982a). Healing following surgical/non-surgical treatment of periodontal disease. *Journal of Clinical Periodontology* **9**, 115-128.

Loos, B., Claffey, N. & Egelberg, J. (1988). Clinical and microbiological effects of root debridement in periodontal furcation pockets. *Journal of Clinical Periodontology* **15**, 453-463.

Matia, J.I., Bissada, N.F., Maybury, J.E. & Ricchetti, P. (1986).

Efficiency of scaling of the molar furcation area with and without surgical access. *International Journal of Periodontics and Restorative Dentistry* **6**, 24-35.

Nabers, C.L. (1954). Repositioning the attached gingiva. *Journal of Periodontology* **25**, 38-39.

Neuman, R. (1920). *Die Alveolar-Pyorrhöe und ihre Behandlung.* 3rd edn. Berlin: Herman Meusser.

Nordland, P., Garrett, S., Kiger, R., Vanooteghem, R., Hutchens, L.H. & Egelberg, J. (1987). The effect of plaque control and root debridement in molar teeth. *Journal of Clinical Periodontology* **14**, 231-236.

Nyman, S., Lindhe, J., Karring, T. & Rylander, H. (1982). New attachment following surgical treatment of human periodontal disease. *Journal of Clinical Periodontology* **9**, 290-296.

Nyman, S., Lindhe, J. & Rosling, B. (1977). Periodontal surgery in plaque-infected dentitions. *Journal of Clinical Periodontology* **4**, 240-249.

O'Neil, T.C.A. (1975). Antibacterial properties of periodontal dressings. *Journal of Periodontology* **46**, 469-474.

Palcanis, K.G. (1996). Surgical pocket therapy. *Annals of Periodontology* **1**, 589-617.

Plüss, E.M., Engelberger, P.R. & Rateitschak, K.H. (1975). Effect of chlorhexidine on dental plaque formation under periodontal pack. *Journal of Clinical Periodontology* **2**, 136-142.

Polson, A.M. & Heijl, L. (1978). Osseous repair in infrabony periodontal defects. *Journal of Clinical Periodontology* **5**, 13-23.

Pontoriero, R. & Carnevale, G. (2001). Surgical crown lengthening: A 12-month clinical wound healing study. *Journal of Periodontology* **72**, 841-848.

Preber, H. & Bergström, J. (1990). Effect of cigarette smoking on periodontal healing following surgical therapy. *Journal of Clinical Periodontology* **17**, 324-328.

Ramfjord, S.P., Caffesse, R.G., Morrison, E.C., Hill, R.W., Kerry, G.J., Appleberry, E.A., Nissle, R.R. & Stults, D.L. (1987). Four modalities of periodontal treatment compared over 5 years. *Journal of Periodontology* **14**, 445-452.

Ramfjord, S.P. & Costich, E.R. (1968). Healing after exposure of periosteum on the alveolar process. *Journal of Periodontology* **38**, 199-207.

Ramfjord, S.P., Engler, W.O. & Hiniker, J.J. (1966). A radioautographic study of healing following simple gingivectomy. II. The connective tissue. *Journal of Periodontology* **37**, 179-189.

Ramfjord, S.P., Morrison, E.C., Burgett, F.G., Nissle, R.R., Schick, R.A., Zann, G.J. & Knowles, J.W. (1982). Oral hygiene and maintenance of periodontal support. *Journal of Periodontology* **53**, 26-30.

Ramfjord, S.P. & Nissle, R.R. (1974). The modified Widman flap. *Journal of Periodontology* **45**, 601-607.

Robicsek, S. (1884). Ueber das Wesen und Entstehen der Alveolar-Pyorrhöe und deren Behandlung. The 3rd Annual Report of the Austrian Dental Association (Reviewed in *Journal of Periodontology* **36**, 265, 1965).

Robinson, R.E. (1966). The distal wedge operation. *Periodontics* **4**, 256-264.

Rosling, B., Nyman, S. & Lindhe, J. (1976a). The effect of systemic plaque control on bone regeneration in infrabony pockets. *Journal of Clinical Periodontology* **3**, 38-53.

Rosling, B., Nyman, S., Lindhe, J. & Jern, B. (1976b). The healing potential of the periodontal tissue following different techniques of periodontal surgery in plaque-free dentitions. A 2-year clinical study. *Journal of Clinical Peridontology* **3**, 233-255.

Sanz, M., Newman, M.G., Anderson, L., Matoska, W., Otomo-Corgel, J. & Saltini, C. (1989). Clinical enhancement of post-periodontal surgical therapy by a 0.12% chlorhexidine gluconate mouthrinse. *Journal of Periodontology* **60**, 570-576.

Scabbia, A., Cho, K.S., Sigurdsson, T.J., Kim, C.K. & Trombelli, L. (2001). Cigarette smoking negatively affects healing response following flap debridement surgery. *Journal of Periodontology* **72**, 43-49.

Schluger, S. (1949). Osseous resection – a basic principle in periodontal surgery? *Oral Surgery, Oral Medicine and Oral Pathology* **2**, 316-325.

Siana, J. E., Rex, S. & Gottrup, F. (1989). The effect of cigarette smoking on wound healing. *Scandinavian Journal of Plastic and Reconstructive Surgery and Hand Surgery* **23**, 207-209.

Stahl, S.S., Witkin, G.J., Cantor, M. & Brown, R. (1968). Gingival healing. II. Clinical and histologic repair sequences following gingivectomy. *Journal of Periodontology* **39**, 109-118.

Takei, H.H., Han, T.J., Carranza, F.A., Kennedy, E.B. & Lekovic, V. (1985). Flap technique for periodontal bone implants. Papilla preservation technique. *Journal of Periodontology* **56**, 204-210.

Townsend-Olsen, C., Ammons, W.F. & Van Belle, C.A. (1985). A longitudinal study comparing apically repositioned flaps with and without osseous surgery. *International Journal of Periodontics & Restorative Dentistry* **5**(4), 11-33.

Van der Velden, U. (1982). Regeneration of the interdental soft tissues following denudation procedures. *Journal of Clinical Periodontology* **9**, 455-459.

Vaughan, M.E. & Garnick, J.J. (1989). The effect of a 0.125% chlorhexidine rinse on inflammation after periodontal surgery. *Journal of Periodontology* **60**, 704-708.

Wachtel, H.C. (1994). Surgical periodontal therapy. In: Lang, N.P. & Karring, T., eds. *Proceedings of the 1st European Workshop on Periodontology*. London: Quintessence, pp. 159-171.

Waerhaug, J. (1955). Microscopic demonstration of tissue reaction incident to removal of subgingival calculus. *Journal of Periodontology* **26**, 26-29.

Waerhaug, J. (1978). Healing of the dentoepithelial junction following subgingival plaque control. II. As observed on extracted teeth. *Journal of Periodontology* **49**, 119-134.

Widman, L. (1918). The operative treatment of pyorrhea alveolaris. A new surgical method. *Svensk Tandläkaretidskrift* (reviewed in *British Dental Journal* **1**, 293, 1920).

Wood, D.L., Hoag, P.M., Donnenfeld, O.W. & Rosenfeld, L.D. (1972). Alveolar crest reduction following full and partial thickness flaps. *Journal of Periodontology* **42**, 141-144.

Zentler, A. (1918). Suppurative gingivitis with alveolar involvement. A new surgical procedure. *Journal of the American Medical Association* **71**, 1530-1534.

Chapter 26

The Effect of Therapy on the Microbiota in the Dentogingival Region

Anne D. Haffajee, Sigmund S. Socransky and Jan Lindhe

INTRODUCTION

The information in Chapter 4 indicated that the biofilms that colonize tooth surfaces and oral soft tissues are complex and the resident bacteria have intriguing interactions with each other and with the surfaces that they colonize. The data indicated that organisms in biofilms are "worthy" adversaries for control and/or eradication. Of concern to the therapist in treating such dental infections is the fact that the pathogenic species exist in very large numbers, are widely distributed within the oral cavity and exist in community structures (biofilms) that provide protection against host defense mechanisms and antimicrobial agents. Further, the organisms can rapidly multiply and have a talent for attaching to new surfaces of the host or to other organisms that are already attached to the host; thus, spread and recolonization are a persistent threat. Given this formidable opponent, it is worth remembering that periodontal therapies, by and large, have a beneficial effect in terms of arresting progression of periodontal disease and maintaining the periodontium. The "by and large" is a phrase that certainly indicates that conventional, i.e mechanical therapies, are not always successful and that alternative or adjunctive methods are sometimes essential. The purpose of this chapter is to examine the microbiological changes that are brought about by therapies of different types, alone and in combination, and the effect that these changes have on clinical outcomes in both the short and longer-term.

The goals of periodontal infection control

The desired clinical outcomes of periodontal therapy have been clearly defined. These include reduction in (1) probing pocket depth, (2) the percentage of sites that exhibit bleeding on probing, (3) suppuration, (4) overt gingivitis, and (5) visible plaque accumulation. Even more critical is maintaining the stability of the periodontal attachment level as measured by probing attachment and alveolar bone level assessments. Given the complexity of the periodontal microbiota, microbial therapeutic endpoints are less well defined. Ideally, putative periodontal pathogens would be eliminated from the oral cavity. However, this is rarely achieved since many periodontal pathogens appear to be indigenous species and can frequently be found in periodontally healthy subjects albeit in lower numbers and proportions. Thus, the therapist is left with the problem of lowering the numbers of pathogenic species while maintaining or raising the level of host compatible species. Further, these changes in the microbiota must be maintained for the life of the patient if future disease episodes are to be prevented.

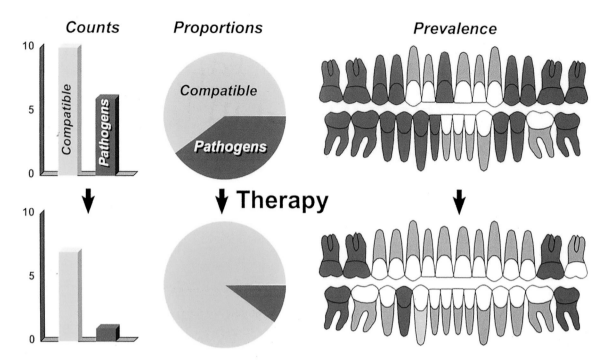

Fig. 26-1. Diagrammatic representation of methods of describing microbial changes in plaque samples. The left panel depicts changes in counts, the middle panel changes in proportions and the right panel changes in the percentage of sites colonized (in this instance percentage of teeth colonized).

Measurement of microbiological endpoints

Changing the composition of the subgingival microbiota in a directed fashion is not easy and if the microbiota is altered, how would the change be measured? Fig. 26-1 presents three microbiological parameters that have been used to describe changes in the composition of the subgingival microbiota after periodontal therapy. The first is a measure of the change in counts (numbers) of one or more pathogenic species. In this method, the plaque samples are taken at one or more sites before and after therapy, using, for instance, scalers or paper points. The test species in the sample(s) are enumerated by cultural, microscopic, DNA probe or immunologic techniques. In some studies, the counts at multiple sites in a subject are averaged prior to and after therapy and reductions identified. In the second example, the proportion of each species in the total sample is computed. From these data, changes in the proportions of each species resulting from therapy can then be determined. The third method requires sample taking from multiple sites within each subject. The percentage of sites colonized by each of the pathogens is computed and the difference in prevalence determined before and after therapy. Each of these measures provides different information. Counts indicate pathogen load at the sampled site(s) and usually are the most easily changed by therapy. The change in proportions at a site indicates the shifts in the composition of the sampled microbiota. If such shifts occur, one or more species would be reduced in proportion, while other species increase.

The prevalence (percentage of sites colonized) is usually the most difficult parameter to change as a result of therapy. This parameter indicates the extent of the distribution of a species in the oral cavity and reduction in this parameter requires "elimination" of the species from one or more sites. It must be understood that "elimination" is dependent on the sensitivity of the microbiological method used. Thus, cultural or DNA probe techniques that indicate elimination of a species really mean reduction of the species to below detection limits of the method.

The first two techniques of microbial assessment, i.e. change in counts and change in proportions of test species, are commonly employed in therapeutic studies. The change in prevalence (percentage of sites colonized) is less frequently employed because multiple sites in the same subject must be individually sampled and analyzed.

TREATMENT OF PERIODONTAL BIOFILMS

At the present time, periodontal therapies designed to affect the composition of the subgingival microbiota can be grouped in three broad categories:

- Physically removing microorganisms, often called mechanical debridement
- Attempting to kill or affect the metabolism of the organism, such as antiseptics and antibiotics

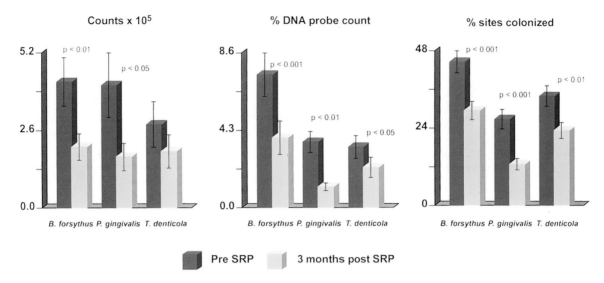

Fig. 26-2. Bar charts of the mean counts ($\times 10^5 \pm$ SEM) (left panel), mean proportions ($\pm$ SEM) (middle panel) and mean percentage of sites colonized ($\pm$ SEM) (right panel) pre and 3 months post SRP for red complex species in 71 subjects (N samples = 3546). The red bar of each pair summarizes pretherapy values and the yellow bar post-therapy values. The significance of differences in mean counts, prevalence and percentage of sites colonized between pre and post-therapy was determined using the Wilcoxon signed ranks test after adjusting for multiple comparisons (Socransky et al. 1991).

- Affecting the environment (habitat) of the organisms.

Other types of therapy are on the horizon, such as possible vaccines against oral pathogens or replacement therapy in which a species is introduced to the biofilm in order to control potentially pathogenic microorganisms. These two approaches will not be discussed further, although their addition to the therapist's armamentarium may eventually become real.

The physical removal of microorganisms – mechanical debridement

Given the remarkable resistance of organisms in biofilms to host defense mechanisms and antimicrobial agents, the logical first step in the control of these organisms would be their removal by physical means. Fortunately, biofilms in the oral cavity, unlike many other biofilms, are readily accessible, allowing their physical removal. Indeed, the most common form of periodontal therapy is the removal of supragingival and subgingival plaque by procedures such as self-performed oral hygiene, scaling and root planing (SRP), sometimes combined with periodontal surgery. Although many studies have documented the clinical effects of SRP, few have evaluated comprehensively the microbiological changes associated with SRP. Studies in the earlier years emphasized use of dark-field or phase contrast microscopy and indicated that the proportion of spirochetes and motile rods declined after SRP, while cocci and non-motile rods increased (Listgarten et al. 1978, Mousques et al. 1980, Lindhe et

al. 1983a,b, Muller et al. 1986, Lavanchy et al. 1987). Other studies employed cultural techniques generally on small numbers of sites and subjects, largely because of the cost in terms of labor and time. Such studies indicated a decrease in groups of microorganisms such as "black pigmented *Bacteroides*" (Pedrazzoli et al. 1991) or specific species such as *Porphyromonas gingivalis* (Sbordone et al. 1990, Ali et al. 1992) and *Actinobacillus actinomycetemcomitans* (Ali et al. 1992). However, other studies found minimal long-term effects of SRP on the subgingival microbiota (Sbordone et al. 1990) particularly for species such as *A. actinomycetemcomitan* (Sato et al. 1993, Saxen & Asikainen 1993, Gunsolley et al. 1994, Mombelli et al. 1994, Nieminen et al. 1995). Other long-term studies reported a decrease in the levels and prevalence of certain species including *Bacteroides forsythus*, *Treponema gingivalis*, *Prevotella intermedia* and *T. denticola* (Simonson et al. 1992, Rawlinson et al. 1993, Shiloah & Patters 1994, Lowenguth et al. 1995, Takamatsu et al. 1999, Darby et al. 2001)

The use of DNA probe techniques has permitted larger scale studies of the effect of therapies on the composition of the subgingival microbiota. The following data demonstrate the effect of SRP on the composition of the subgingival plaque. In this study, an extension of the study described by Haffajee et al. (1997), 71 subjects with chronic periodontitis were monitored clinically at six sites per tooth. Subgingival plaque samples were taken from the mesiobuccal surface of each tooth and individually analyzed for their content of 40 bacterial species using a checkerboard DNA-DNA hybridization technique. Clinical measurements and microbial samples were taken at base-

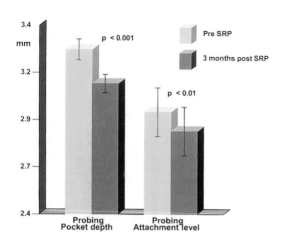

Fig. 26-3. Bar chart of the mean pocket depth and attachment level (± SEM) at baseline and 3 months post SRP (N subjects = 71). The significance of differences between pre and post-therapy visits was determined using the Wilcoxon signed ranks test. Note that the y-axis does not start at 0.

line and 3 months after treatment, which consisted of full mouth SRP accompanied by oral hygiene instruction. The data indicated that 37 out of 40 species monitored did not change significantly. However, three species of the "red" complex (see Chapter 4), *B. forsythus*, *P. gingivalis* and *T. denticola* were signifi-

cantly decreased in counts, proportions and percentage of sites colonized 3 months post SRP (Fig. 26-2). These microbial changes were accompanied by improved clincial parameters such as a significant decrease in mean probing pocket depth and mean probing attachment level (Fig. 26-3).

The data of this and other investigations are of interest in the light of the discussion in Chapter 4 on biofilms. The mechanical procedures undoubtedly removed major proportions (90%) of the organisms that colonized the tooth surface. However, given the rapid multiplication rates of bacteria, it is not surprising that the majority of the species returned to almost baseline levels at 3 months. Data in the literature suggest that the return to baseline *total counts* of microorganisms may occur within 4-8 days after treatment (Sharawy et al. 1966, Furuichi et al. 1992). However, certain species were affected by SRP. These bacterial species might have been diminished by the mechanical procedures and returned more slowly, in part because of their fastidious nature, and in part because the environment presented by the healing tissues may have been changed.

Few studies have evaluated the effect of periodontal surgery on the composition of the subgingival microbiota. Rosenberg et al. (1984) used dark field microscopy to examine the composition of the subgingival microbiota after a procedure that included open flap curettage with some osseous recontouring and apical repositioning of the flaps. After surgery, the

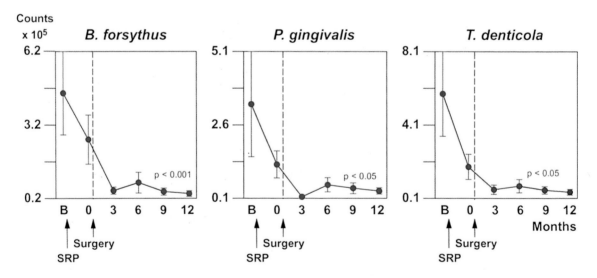

Fig. 26-4. Plots of the mean counts (× 10^5 ± SEM) of red complex species, *B. forsythus*, *P. gingivalis* and *T. denticola* at baseline (B), 3 months post SRP (0 on the x-axis) and at 3, 6, 9 and 12 months post apically repositioned flap surgery. 18 patients with chronic periodontitis were monitored clinically and sampled microbiologically at baseline (B). They then received full mouth SRP and instruction in proper home care procedures. 3 months after SRP, the subjects were clinically and microbiologically monitored again (at time 0) to determine the effect of SRP on clinical and microbiological parameters and to determine which areas of the mouth required periodontal surgery. The time 0 monitoring also served as the starting values for the surgical phase of treatment. The subjects then received apically repositioned flap surgery at sites with PPD > 5 mm. Subjects were remonitored clinically and microbiologically at 3, 6, 9 and 12 months after the surgical treatment phase. The vertical dotted lines indicate the time of periodontal surgery. Significance of differences over time was tested using the Quade test and adjusted for multiple comparisons (Socransky et al. 1991).

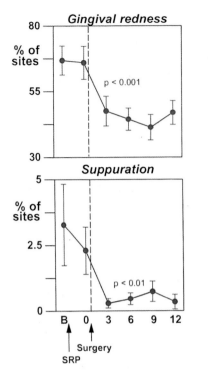

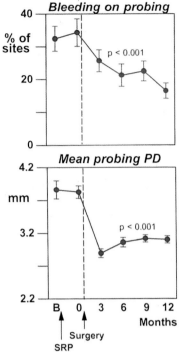

Fig. 26-5. Plots of the change in clinical parameters at surgically treated sites from baseline (B) to 3 months post SRP (0 on the x-axis) and 3, 6, 9 and 12 months post apically repositioned flap surgery. The experimental design was described in Fig. 26-4. The circles represent the mean values and the whiskers represent the standard error of the mean. Values for each parameter were measured at all surgically treated sites in each subject, averaged within a subject and then averaged across subjects for each time point. The vertical dotted lines indicate the time of periodontal surgery. Significance of differences over time was tested using the Quade test.

proportions of spirochetes and motile rods decreased while the proportions of cocci increased. Rawlinson and co-workers (1995) used cultural techniques to examine the effects of a modified Widman flap surgery or SRP on the microbiota in periodontal pockets. *P. intermedia* was reduced at 3 and 6 months, but began to increase at 1 year following therapy. Overall, Gram-negative species were not affected significantly by SRP, but became virtually eradicated in surgically treated subjects during the year of the study. Mombelli et al. (1995) performed a similar study using cultural techniques, in which they monitored the levels of subgingival species in plaque samples for 1 year post therapy. There was a decrease in total anaerobic viable bacteria along with a decrease in Gram-negative rod species. *P. gingivalis*, *Fusobacterium* sp. and *Campylobacter rectus* were lower, while *Capnocytophaga* sp. and *Actinomyces odontolyticus* were detected in higher numbers at the 1 year examination. More recently, a similar study was performed at the Forsyth Institute with essentially identical conclusions to the Rawlinson and Mombelli studies. Eighteen patients with chronic periodontitis received initial SRP, followed at 3 months by apically repositioned flap surgery at sites with PPD > 5 mm. Subjects were monitored clinically and microbiologically at baseline (B), 3 months post SRP (0) and at 3, 6 and 12 months post-surgery. Subgingival plaque samples were examined using checkerboard DNA-DNA hybridization. Treatment resulted in a decrease in the mean counts of, among others, *B. forsythus*, *P. gingivalis* and *T. denticola* (Fig. 26-4) as well as members of the orange complex (Socransky et al. 1998). The clinical changes at the surgically treated sites are presented in Fig. 26-5. There was a significant decrease in the percentage of sites

exhibiting gingival redness, bleeding on probing and suppuration as well as a marked decrease in mean PPD. It seems likely that the decrease in PPD led to a decrease in the levels of pathogenic species and that the decrease in pathogenic species resulted in an improved clinical status as measured by changes in gingival inflammation and the continued decrease in PPD over time.

Antibiotics in the treatment of periodontal infections

Since periodontal diseases are infections, it is not surprising that antibiotics have been used and continue to be used in their treatment. Given the discussion on increased antibiotic resistance that occurs in organisms growing in biofilms, as well as the difficulty of some antibiotics in effectively penetrating a biofilm, one might of course question the use of such agents in the treatment of periodontal diseases.

Antibiotics have been successfully employed, however, as adjuncts in the treatment of periodontitis (Lindhe et al. 1983b, Joyston-Bechal et al. 1984a,b, Loesche et al. 1984, 1987, 1991, 1992, 1996, van Oosten et al. 1987, Asikainen 1989, Hull et al. 1989, Jenkins et al. 1989, Soder et al. 1990, Eisenberg et al. 1991, Paquette et al. 1992, Haffajee et al. 1995, van Winkelhoff et al. 1996, Noyan et al. 1997). The expectation that one might have of the results of treatment by a systemically administered antibiotic can vary widely. On the one hand, the expectation might be that the agent would kill all of the sensitive species and leave hopefully host-compatible species to emerge. On the other hand, from the discussion in Chapter 4, one might

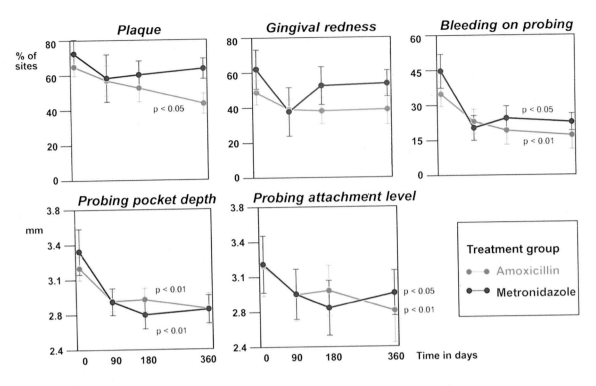

Fig. 26-6. Plots of the full mouth mean values (± SEM) for clinical parameters at baseline, 90, 180 and 360 days for subjects treated with SRP and metronidazole or SRP and amoxicillin. The circles represent the mean values and the whiskers represent the standard error of the mean. Values for each parameter were measured at up to 168 sites in each subject, averaged within a subject and then averaged across subjects in each treatment group for each time point. Significance of differences over time was tested using the Quade test.

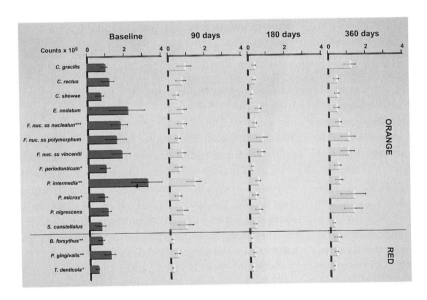

Fig. 26-7. Bar charts of the mean counts ($\times 10^5 \pm$ SEM) of red and orange complex species at baseline, 90, 180 and 360 days for the amoxicillin treated subjects. Mean levels of each species were computed for each subject and then averaged across subjects at each time point. Significance of differences over time was tested using the Quade test (*p < 0.05, **p < 0.01, ***p < 0.001). Seven of the 15 species were significantly reduced.

surmise that the antibiotic might have virtually no effect on organisms grown in biofilms. The "truth" lies somewhere in between. Systemically administered antibiotics do have certain effects on segments of the subgingival microbiota, but usually do not completely eliminate the bacterial species sensitive to the administered antibiotic.

The appropriate use of antibiotics in the treatment of periodontal diseases was discussed in more detail in Chapter 23. In the current chapter the effects of these agents on the composition of the subgingival micro-

biota will be described. The following study provides examples of two popularly employed systemic antibiotics, amoxicillin and metronidazole, used as adjuncts to SRP (Feres et al. 2001). After baseline clinical monitoring and microbial sampling, 17 chronic periodontitis subjects received full mouth SRP. Subjects were then randomly assigned to treatment groups receiving either systemically administered amoxicillin (500 mg tid) or systemically administered metronidazole (250 mg tid) for 14 days. Post-therapy, full mouth clinical monitoring and bacterial sampling was per-

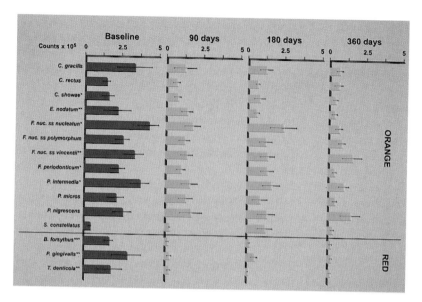

Fig. 26-8. Bar charts of the mean counts ($\times 10^5 \pm$ SEM) of red and orange complex species at baseline, 90, 180 and 360 days for the metronidazole treated subjects. The presentation of the data and significance testing was as described in Fig. 26-7. Nine of the 15 species were significantly reduced.

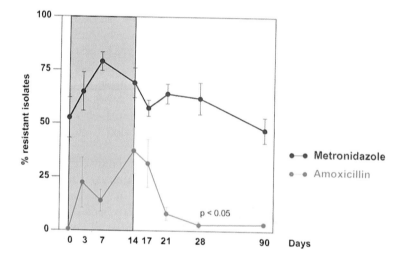

Fig. 26-9. Percentage of isolates resistant to amoxicillin or metronidazole in the plaque samples from subjects receiving those agents. Samples were plated on enriched blood agar plates with or without either 2 µg/ml metronidazole or 2 µg/ml amoxicillin. Colonies were counted at 7 days. Data were averaged within a subject at each time point and then across subjects separately in the two groups. The circles represent the mean and the whiskers the standard error of the mean. The shaded area represents the period of antibiotic administration in the test subjects. Significant differences in the percentage of resistant organisms over time were determined by the Quade test.

formed at 3, 6 and 12 months. Additional subgingival plaque samples were taken, from pairs of randomly selected posterior teeth, at 3, 7 and 14 days during antibiotic administration as well as at 3, 7 and 14 days after completion of the antibiotic therapy to determine antibiotic resistance of isolates. Both therapies produced a significant improvement in clinical parameters (Fig. 26-6). Figs. 26-7 and 26-8 present the counts of the red complex species at baseline, 3, 6 and 12 months in the two treatment groups. Both amoxicillin and metronidazole produced significant decreases in counts of many of the bacterial species, particularly those in the red and orange complexes. The decrease in counts of red complex species was particularly marked and the initial decreases were maintained to 12 months, most noticeably in the subjects treated with metronidazole.

The proportion of organisms that were resistant to the two agents before, during and after their administration are shown in Fig. 26-9. More than half of the cultivable organisms were resistant to metronidazole at baseline. This number increased to about 81% during metronidazole administration and decreased to baseline levels at 90 days. Only about 0.5% of the isolates were resistant to amoxicillin at baseline. The resistant proportion rose to about 41% at the end of amoxicillin administration and declined to close to baseline levels at 90 days. Thus, 19% of organisms in the biofilms were sensitive to metronidazole and 59% were sensitive to amoxicillin, even when the subjects had taken the prescribed agent for 14 days. These figures attest to the protection afforded to organisms in biofilms that was discussed in Chapter 4. The microbial count data and the antibiotic resistance data suggest the possibility that the systemically administered antibiotics may have affected, primarily, the organisms in the epithelial cell associated biofilms and the loosely adherent adjacent cells. These organisms might be more accessible to the administered agents, in part, because of their proximity to the host tissues and, in part, because of a less developed glycocalyx. Conceivably, organisms in this area were reduced to very low levels. However, the same species may also have been resident in the tooth associated biofilms but at much lower levels. The species in the tooth associated biofilms may have been more resistant to the antibiotics due to mechanisms described in Chapter 4 and thus, the potential for regrowth from this source was perpetuated.

The data from the study outlined above indicate that systemically administered antibiotics do affect microorganisms located within biofilms. Many of the test species were significantly reduced in numbers even up to 1 year after the initial therapy, although no species was eliminated. It was also clear that the two agents had different effects on the subgingival microbiota. While both agents reduced, at least initially, the red complex, metronidazole appeared to have a more pronounced and long-lasting effect. Further, amoxicillin produced a significant decrease in the proportion of *Actinomyces* species with a concomitant increase in the proportion of yellow complex species. This potentially undesirable effect was not seen in the subjects treated with metronidazole. It was also apparent, within the limitations of the study, that short-term use of these two agents did not affect the proportion of antibiotic resistant species long term.

The effect of an antibiotic can go beyond its direct effects on individual species. For example, the *counts* of *Actinomyces* species were found to be decreased 3 months after metronidazole administration. The *Actinomyces* are not sensitive to metronidazole, suggesting that this reduction was due to a decrease in other bacterial species that affected the inflammatory status of the habitat which in turn lowered levels of all colonizing species (Ramberg et al. 1994, 1995).

Therapies that affect the microbial environment – supragingival plaque removal

While it is widely recognized that bacteria can affect the tissues that they colonize, it is less appreciated that the environment of the bacteria has a major effect on their growth and activities. It is axiomatic in microbial ecology that colonizing species affect the environment in which they live (habitat) and the habitat affects the colonizing organisms. This is clearly the case in the oral environment where species have specific tissue tropisms with certain species flourishing on certain surfaces and others in other locations. The subgingival pocket is clearly an environment in which many species, including those of the red and orange complexes, flourish (Chapter 4). This habitat provides an environment conducive to their multiplication and perhaps to their ability to mediate tissue destruction. If the environment surrounding the subgingival microbiota was altered, then changes in numbers, proportions and prevalence of species would be likely to be affected. The two major environmental factors that impact on

subgingival plaque are the tissues of the periodontal pocket and the supragingival plaque. Changes in either of these factors are likely to lead to changes in the composition of the subgingival microbiota. It has been recognized for a long time that meticulous removal of supragingival plaque leads to an improvement in the parameters associated with gingival inflammation. Indeed, clinicians have urged and continue to urge patients to carefully and regularly remove supragingival deposits. What is less appreciated is the effect of regular supragingival plaque removal on subgingival plaque composition. A few studies have suggested that supragingival plaque removal can decrease putative periodontal pathogens (Tabita et al. 1981, Smulow et al. 1983, Dahlen et al. 1992, Al-Yahfoufi et al. 1995, Hellstrom et al. 1996). These effects were examined further in a study of 18 chronic periodontitis subjects who were in a periodontal maintenance program (Ximenez-Fyvie et al. 2000). After baseline clinical and microbiological examination, the subjects received full mouth SRP followed by weekly professional removal of supragingival plaque for 3 months. The subjects performed their improved home care procedures for the 12 months of the study. The subjects were monitored at 3, 6 and 12 months, at which points they also received maintenance subgingival scaling. Fig. 26-10 presents the mean total counts of supra and subgingival plaque at baseline, 3, 6 and 12 months. Total counts of both supra and subgingival plaque decreased significantly at 3 months, immediately after completion of the professional supragingival plaque removal phase. It was of interest, however, that the counts continued to decrease at the 6 and 12 month visits, even though professional cleaning had not been employed for 3 and 9 months respectively. Similar findings were seen in both supra and subgingival samples for the 40 species examined. Fig. 26-11 presents the mean counts of the 40 test species at baseline, 3, 6 and 12 months; 34 species were significantly reduced over time. These included periodontal pathogens such as *B. forsythus, P. gingivalis* and *A. actinomycetemcomitans*. This suggests that meticulous removal of supragingival plaque after initial periodontal therapy, such as SRP, can lead to a microbiota that is remarkably similar to that observed in periodontal health.

The meticulous repeated removal of supragingival plaque not only lowers the counts of subgingival pathogens but has a clear beneficial clinical effect. This procedure is critical to a predictable, successful outcome after periodontal surgery (Lindhe & Nyman 1975, Nyman et al. 1975, Rosling et al. 1976b, Axelsson & Lindhe 1981, Lindhe et al. 1982, Westfelt et al. 1985) and for bone regeneration in infrabony pockets (Rosling et al. 1976a). Further, repeated professional tooth cleaning every 2 weeks reduced dental plaque, gingivitis and the caries increment in children (Axelsson & Lindhe 1974, Axelsson et al. 1976), while similar programs had comparable results in adults (Axelsson & Lindhe 1978, 1981).

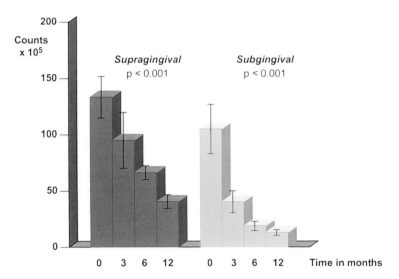

Fig. 26-10. Mean total DNA probe counts ($\times 10^5 \pm$ SEM) in supra and subgingival plaque samples taken at baseline, 3, 6 and 12 months. Professional supragingival plaque control was performed weekly between baseline and 3 months. Mean counts were computed for a subject for each visit and then values were averaged across the 18 subjects at each time point. The whiskers indicate the SEM. Significance of differences over time was sought using the Quade test.

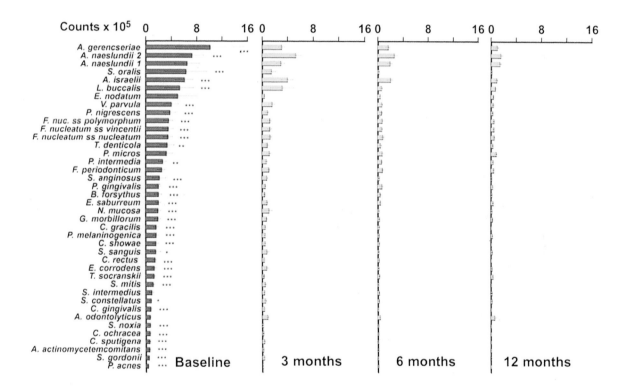

Fig. 26-11. Bar charts of the mean counts ($\times 10^5 \pm$ SEM) of the 40 test species in subgingival plaque samples taken at baseline, 3, 6 and 12 months. Professional supragingival plaque control was performed weekly between baseline and 3 months. Mean counts for each species were computed for a subject for each visit and then values were averaged across the 18 subjects at each time point. The whiskers indicate the SEM. Significance of differences over time was sought using the Quade test. * $p < 0.05$, ** $p < 0.01$, *** $p < 0.001$ after adjusting for multiple comparisons.

The above studies demonstrated that repeated professional removal of supragingival plaque has major beneficial effects on altering the composition of the subgingival microbiota and the clinical status of the patient. However, repeated professional plaque removal may be somewhat impractical for most patients since it requires frequent visits to the dental office. Effective, self-performed plaque removal would be a more practical means of removing supragingival plaque providing the patient is proficient in the techniques employed.

The effects of self-performed plaque removal by either the use of manual or powered toothbrushes on clinical and microbiological parameters were examined in a study of 48 periodontal maintenance subjects (Haffajee et al. 2001a,b). After assignment to either the manual or powered toothbrushing group, subjects received instruction in the use of the assigned brush,

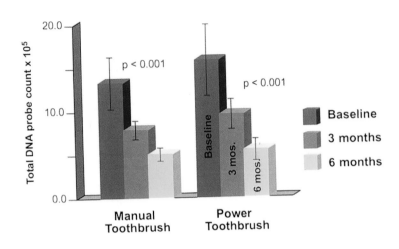

Fig. 26-12. Bar charts of the mean total DNA probe counts ($\times 10^5 \pm$ SEM) for subgingival plaque samples at baseline, 3 and 6 months in subjects using either the manual or power toothbrush. The bars indicate the means and the whiskers the SEM. The total counts were computed at each site, averaged within a subject for each time point. Significance of differences over time was sought using the Quade test.

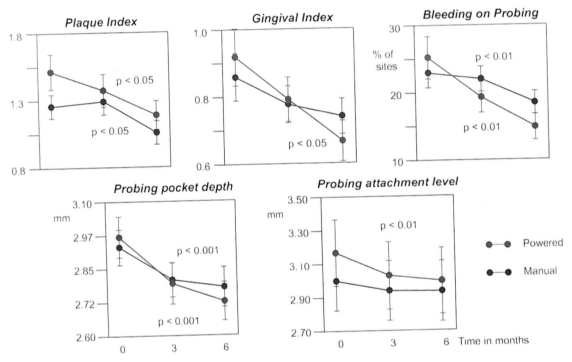

Fig. 26-13. Plots of the full mouth mean values ($\pm$ SEM) for clinical parameters at baseline, 3 and 6 months for subjects in the manual and powered brushing groups. The circles represent the mean values and the whiskers represent the standard error of the mean. Values for each parameter were measured at up to 168 sites in each subject, averaged within a subject and then averaged across subjects in each brushing group for each time point. Significance of differences over time was tested using the Quade test.

which they used for 6 months. Clinical and microbiological parameters were measured at baseline and at 3 and 6 months. Mean total bacterial counts were significantly reduced for subgingival plaque samples in both groups (Fig 26-12). In addition, virtually all of 18 test species examined were reduced in mean counts and prevalence in subgingival plaque samples. The decrease in microorganisms was accompanied by improvements in clinical parameters. Both manual and powered toothbrushes significantly reduced PPD, plaque index and BOP, while the powered toothbrush also significantly reduced mean gingival index and probing attachment level (Fig. 26-13). Although the benefits of repeated professional supragingival plaque removal may be superior, these data suggest

that careful self-performed plaque control is of benefit to the patient in terms of lowering subgingival species and improving clinical status.

In controlling infectious diseases, there are usually two types of procedures employed. The first is to control the level of the organism in the environment, usually by "sanitation" procedures. The second is to target the organism in an infected host who is exhibiting disease. On a population basis, the first might be the more important in that epidemic disease has been markedly reduced in first world countries by improvements in sewage systems, water supplies, food handling, etc. Supragingival plaque control may be thought of as a "sanitary" procedure that lowers the levels of potentially pathogenic species that colonize the individual and the community. As such, this reduction in the reservoir of potentially pathogenic organisms is of major importance in lowering the risk of new disease or recurrence of disease in infected individuals. However, supragingival plaque removal has an added benefit in that it appears to affect the numbers and composition of the subgingival microbiota. Clearly, the removal of the biofilm from the supragingival area affects the composition of the subgingival biofilm on the same surface. This may be due to a direct effect of the supragingival colonizers on subgingival organisms or an effect on the adjacent periodontal tissues which might lead to reduction in subgingival species. Most likely the effect is due to both phenomena. Supragingival organisms and also the adjacent periodontal tissues provide both nutrients and physical-chemical environments for proliferation of the subgingival species. Removal of the supragingival colonizers would diminish this source, while diminished inflammation and improved barrier function of the epithelium would decrease a second source of growth requirements (Ramberg et al. 1994, 1995). In essence, the subgingival biofilm numbers decrease because the essential requirements for growth have been cut off or decreased. Alteration of the habitat may be one of the most important mechanisms for the long-term control of subgingival pathogens. If our treatment or prevention efforts diminish nutrient availability and maintain epithelial barrier function, then the numbers of organisms in the subgingival environment will diminish and the proportions of organisms that appear to be pathogenic will be decreased. Further, decreasing reservoirs of pathogenic species by systematic removal from tooth surfaces, perhaps accompanied by suppression on soft tissue surfaces, should lead to long-term stability in the majority of periodontal patients. In a similar fashion, altering the habitat by pocket reduction, whether by SRP or by surgery, also affects the composition of the subgingival microbiota and thus the risk of periodontal disease progression.

Combined antimicrobial therapies

The use of combined therapies has been shown to be effective in treatment of several medically important infections. For example, the treatment of HIV infections currently employs two or three therapeutic agents providing better outcomes than the single therapies employed previously. Treatment of stomach ulcers caused by *Helicobacter pylori* is usually best accomplished by the combined use of two or more agents such as metronidazole with amoxicillin and protein pump blocking agents. The combination of systemically administered amoxicillin and metronidazole for the treatment of certain periodontal infections has been quite effective (van Winkelhoff et al. 1989, 1992, Pavicic et al. 1994, Berglundh et al. 1998, Winkel et al 1998, 2001, Rudiger et al. 1999). For exam-

ple, this treatment in combination with SRP significantly reduced the detection of *A. actinomycetemcomitans* in subjects with *A. actinomycetemcomitans*-associated adult periodontitis (Pavicic et al. 1994), localized juvenile periodontitis, as well as rapidly progressive and refractory periodontitis (van Winkelhoff et al. 1989, 1992). Other studies have shown that the combination of these two agents was also effective in controlling the levels of other pathogens such as *P. gingivalis*, *B. forsythus* and *P. intermedia* (Pavicic et al. 1994, Winkel et al. 1997, 1998, 2001, Berglundh et al. 1998, Lopez & Gamonal 1998, Rudiger et al. 1999).

Long-term effects of antimicrobial therapy

The above sections focused on the effects of different periodontal therapies alone or in combination on clinical and microbiological parameters of periodontal diseases. The majority of the cited studies were relatively short term running from 3 months to 1-2 years. They leave unanswered the question, what are the effects of the various treatment procedures long term? Recently, a series of long-term studies have been reported from the University of Gothenburg in which the effect of different therapeutic procedures has been followed for large numbers of subjects for periods over 13 years. These studies suggested that different forms of periodontal therapy followed by careful maintenance care can maintain alveolar bone and periodontal attachment levels in patients with normal or high susceptibility to periodontal disease (Rosling et al. 2001). Periodontal surgery provided a better long-term reduction in mean probing pocket depth and percentage of subjects exhibiting deterioration of periodontal sites (Serino et al. 2001b). Adjunctive, systemically administered antibiotics such as tetracycline (Ramberg et al. 2001) or amoxicillin plus metronidazole (Serino et al. 2001a) may have provided a short-term clinical benefit which appeared to diminish over time. The nature of the microbial shifts that took place over time in these long-term treatment studies is not known. However, it may be speculated that a shift would have occurred in the subgingival microbiota toward that present before therapy, and this may have been delayed by rigorous removal of supragingival plaque accompanied by periodic subgingival instrumentation. Further studies of long-term microbial changes resulting from periodontal therapy are warranted.

CONCLUDING REMARKS

Many different biofilms exist in nature, some of which are useful (to the human) while others are associated with potentially harmful effects. Dental plaque is a naturally occurring biofilm that has the potential to cause disease. Dental plaques have many properties

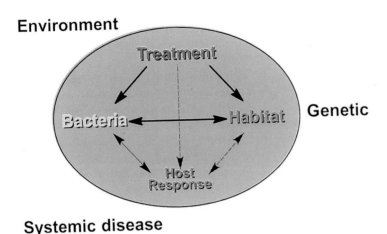

Fig. 26-14. Diagrammatic representation of the effect of therapy on colonizing bacteria, the host and the habitat. Treatment can affect the composition of the bacterial plaque directly, can affect the host response or can alter the habitat. Alterations of any of these factors can impact on the remaining factors in this triad. As indicated, treatment effects are influenced by the genetic background of the subject, environmental influences such as smoking and the systemic well-being of the patient.

in common with biofilms found in other locations. However, they have certain characteristics that are important in terms of control of disease. They are easily accessible and thus allow direct removal and application of antimicrobial agents. However, they are microbiologically very complex. This complexity helps the therapist in one way and presents problems in another. The complexity helps to assure the therapist that treatment will usually lead to the return of a relatively similar, diverse microbial plaque, hopefully with pathogenic species reduced or eliminated. If treatment virtually eliminated all or most species, the potential for colonization by even more harmful organisms would be very high. On the other hand, the complexity can present difficulties for the therapist. The first is knowing which of several potential pathogens in an individual is causing that individual's disease. The second is that the network provided by the community structure of the biofilm may help to "rescue" a suppressed species by providing the essential factors needed for rapid recolonization. Nonetheless, as indicated in this chapter and as described in greater detail in other chapters, dental biofilms can be altered by various therapies, providing a beneficial outcome to the patient. Treatment can affect bacteria directly by physical removal and/or chemotherapeutic agents (Fig. 26-14). Treatment can also affect the habitat, for example by eliminating or by meticulously removing supragingival plaque. As discussed earlier, the bacteria affect their habitat and the habitat affects the bacteria so that the elimination of pockets or the removal of supragingival plaque will provide a less favorable environment for the growth of subgingival species, particularly those associated with disease. Treatment can also affect host response, possibly by "vaccination" during mechanical debridement procedures or by using anti-inflammatory or host modifying local or systemic agents. Modification of host response affects the habitat and also affects the colonizing microbiota. Thus, the therapist can potentially affect periodontal infections at several levels, improving the possibility for long-term periodontal stability. For certain periodontal patients, combinations of therapy may be required in order to control the infection via different antimicrobial strategies.

By and large, the currently available treatment procedures do not eliminate periodontal pathogens. They often lower the numbers, perhaps proportions, or even prevalence of pathogenic species for various periods of time. The mechanical debridement procedures seem essential in any rational treatment protocol since they can directly remove the biofilms which provide the major survival mechanism for tooth associated bacterial species. Antimicrobial agents do affect pathogenic species in subgingival plaque and can be used judiciously to lower the number of such species when disease is extensive, rapidly progressive or refractory to conventional therapy. Ultimately, long-term control of pathogenic species resides primarily in habitat change. The control of subgingival pathogens can be markedly improved by minimizing supragingival plaque, decreasing gingival inflammation that provides nutrients to pathogenic species, decreasing periodontal pocket depth which also fosters pathogen reservoirs, and decreasing pernicious habits such as cigarette smoking. These procedures have been utilized for years in successfully controlling periodontal disease in the majority of patients. When these procedures prove inadequate, it seems likely that carefully selected combinations of therapeutic procedures will diminish pathogen loads to levels that are tolerated by the host.

REFERENCES

Ali, R.W., Lie, T. & Skaug, N. (1992). Early effects of periodontal therapy on the detection frequency of four putative periodontal pathogens in adults. *Journal of Periodontology* **63**, 540-547.

Al-Yahfoufi, Z., Mombelli, A., Wicki, A. & Lang, N.P. (1995). The effect of plaque control in subjects with shallow pockets and high prevalence of periodontal pathogens. *Journal of Clinical Periodontology* **22**, 78-84.

Asikainen, S. (1989). The efficacy of nitroimidazoles on moderate or deep periodontal pockets. *Journal of Dental Research* **68**, 411, abstract 1839.

Axelsson, P. & Lindhe, J. (1974). The effect of a preventive programme on dental plaque, gingivitis and caries in schoolchildren. Results after one and two years. *Journal of Clinical Periodontology* **1**, 126-138.

Axelsson, P. & Lindhe, J. (1978). Effect of controlled oral hygiene procedures on caries and periodontal disease in adults. *Journal of Clinical Periodontology* **5**, 133-151.

Axelsson, P. & Lindhe, J. (1981). The significance of maintenance care in the treatment of periodontal disease. *Journal of Clinical Periodontology* **8**, 281-294.

Axelsson, P., Lindhe, J. & Waseby, J (1976). The effect of various plaque control measures on gingivitis and caries in schoolchildren. *Community Dentistry & Oral Epidemiology* **4**, 232-239.

Berglundh, T., Krok, L., Liljenberg, B., Westfelt, E., Serino, G. & Lindhe, J. (1998). The use of metronidazole and amoxicillin in the treatment of advanced periodontal disease. A prospective, controlled clinical trial. *Journal of Clinical Periodontology* **25**, 354-362.

Dahlen, G., Lindhe, J., Sato, K., Hanamura, H. & Okamoto, H. (1992). The effect of supragingival plaque control on the subgingival microbiota in subjects with periodontal disease. *Journal of Clinical Periodontology* **19**, 802-809.

Darby, I.B., Mooney, J. & Kinane, D.F. (2001). Changes in subgingival microflora and humoral immune response following periodontal therapy. *Journal of Clinical Periodontology* **28**, 796-805.

Eisenberg, L., Suchow, R., Coles, R.S. & Deasy, M.J. (1991). The effects of metronidazole administration on clinical and microbiologic parameters of periodontal disease. *Clinical Preventive Dentistry* **13**, 28-34.

Feres, M., Haffajee, A.D., Allard, K.A., Som, S. & Socransky S.S. (2001). Change in subgingival microbial profiles in adult periodontitis subjects receiving either systemically administered amoxicillin or metronidazole. *Journal of Clinical Periodontology* **28**, 597-609.

Furuichi, Y., Lindhe, J., Ramberg, P. & Volpe, A.R. (1992). Patterns of de novo plaque formation in the human dentition. *Journal of Clinical Periodontology* **19**, 423-433.

Gunsolley, J.C., Zambon, J.J., Mellott, C.A., Brooks, C.N. & Kaugars, C.C. (1994). Periodontal therapy in young adults with severe generalized periodontitis. *Journal of Periodontology* **65**, 268-273.

Haffajee, A.D., Cugini, M.A., Dibart, S., Smith, C., Kent, R.L. Jr. & Socransky, S.S. (1997). The effect of SRP on the clinical and microbiological parameters of periodontal diseases. *Journal of Clinical Periodontology* **24**, 324-334.

Haffajee, A.D., Dibart, S., Kent, R.L. Jr. & Socransky, S.S. (1995). Clinical and microbiological changes associated with the use of four adjunctive systemically administered agents in the treatment of periodontal infections. *Journal of Clinical Periodontology* **22**, 618-627.

Haffajee, A.D., Smith, C., Thompson, M., Torresyap, G., Guerrero, D. & Socransky, S.S. (2001a). Efficacy of manual and powered toothbrushes: II. Effect on microbial parameters. *Journal of Clinical Periodontology* **28**, 947-954.

Haffajee, A.D., Thompson, M., Torresyap, G., Guerrero, D. & Socransky, S.S. (2001b). Efficacy of manual and powered toothbrushes: I. Effect on clinical parameters. *Journal of Clinical Periodontology* **28**, 937-947.

Hellstrom, M-K., Ramberg, P., Krok, L. & Lindhe, J. (1996). The effect of supragingival plaque control on the subgingival microflora in human periodontitis. *Journal of Clinical Periodontology* **23**, 934-940.

Hull, P.S., Abu, F.S. & Drucker, D.B. (1989). Evaluation of two antibacterial agents in the management of rapidly progressive periodontitis. *Journal of Dental Research* **68**, 564, abstract 46.

Jenkins, W.M., MacFarlane, T.W., Gilmour, W.H., Ramsay, I. & MacKenzie, D. (1989). Systemic metronidazole in the treatment of periodontitis. *Journal of Clinical Periodontology* **16**, 443-450.

Joyston-Bechal, S., Smales, F.C. & Duckworth, R. (1984a). Effect of metronidazole on chronic periodontal disease in subjects using a topically applied chlorhexidine gel. *Journal of Clinical Periodontology* **11**, 53-62.

Joyston-Bechal, S., Smales, F.C. & Duckworth R. (1984b). A follow-up study 3 years after metronidazole therapy for chronic periodontal disease. *Journal of Clinical Periodontology* **13**, 944-949.

Lavanchy, D.L., Bickel, M. & Baehni, P.C. (1987). The effect of plaque control after scaling and root planing on the subgingival microflora in human periodontitis. *Journal of Clinical Periodontology* **14**, 295-299.

Lindhe, J., Liljenberg, B. & Adielsson, B. (1983a). Effect of long-term tetracycline therapy on human periodontal disease. *Journal of Clinical Periodontology* **10**, 590-601.

Lindhe, J., Liljenberg, B., Adielsson, B. & Borjesson, I. (1983b). Use of metronidazole as a probe in the study of human periodontal disease. *Journal of Clinical Periodontology* **10**, 100-112.

Lindhe, J. & Nyman, S. (1975). The effect of plaque control and surgical pocket elimination on the establishment and maintenance of periodontal health. A longitudinal study of periodontal therapy in cases of advanced disease. *Journal of Clinical Periodontology* **2**, 67-79.

Lindhe, J., Westfelt, E., Nyman, S., Socransky, S.S., Heijl, L. & Bratthall, G. (1982). Healing following surgical/non-surgical treatment of periodontal disease. *Journal of Clinical Periodontology* **9**, 115-128.

Listgarten, M.A., Lindhe, J. & Hellden, L. (1978). Effect of tetracycline and/or scaling on human periodontal disease. Clinical, microbiological and histological observations. *Journal of Clinical Periodontology* **5**, 246-271.

Loesche, W.J., Giordano, J., Soehren, S., Hutchinson, R., Rau, C.F., Walsh, L. & Schork, M.A. (1996). Non-surgical treatment of patients with periodontal disease. *Oral Surgery Oral Medicine Oral Pathology Oral Radiology and Endodontics* **81**, 533-543.

Loesche, W.J., Giordano, J.R., Hujoel, P.P., Schwarcz, J. & Smith, B.A. (1992). Metronidazole in periodontitis: reduced need for surgery. *Journal of Clinical Periodontology* **19**, 103-112.

Loesche, W.J., Schmidt, E., Smith, B.A., Caffesse, R. & Stoll, J. (1987). Metronidazole therapy for periodontitis. *Journal of Periodontal Research* **22**, 224-226.

Loesche, W.J., Schmidt, E., Smith, B.A., Morrison, E.C., Caffesse, R. & Hujoel, P.P. (1991). Effects of metronidazole on periodontal treatment needs. *Journal of Periodontology* **62**, 247-257.

Loesche, W.J., Syed, S.A., Morrison, E.C., Kerry, G.A., Higgins, T. & Stoll, J. (1984). Metronidazole in periodontitis. I. Clinical and bacteriological results after 15 to 30 weeks. *Journal of Periodontology* **55**, 325-335.

Lopez, N.J. & Gamonal, J.A. (1998). Effects of metronidazole plus amoxicillin in progressive untreated adult periodontitis: results of a single 1-week course after 2 and 4 months. *Journal of Periodontology* **69**, 1291-1298.

Lowenguth, R.A., Chin, I., Caton, J.G., Cobb, C.M., Drisko, C.L.,

Killoy, W.J., Michalowicz, B.S., Pihlstrom, B.L. & Goodson, J.M. (1995). Evaluation of periodontal treatments using controlled-release tetracycline fibers: microbiological response. *Journal of Periodontology* **66**, 700-707.

Mombelli, A., Gmur, R., Gobbi, C. & Lang, N. P. (1994). *Actinobacillus actinomycetemcomitans* in adult periodontitis. II. Characterization of isolated strains and effect of mechanical periodontal treatment. *Journal of Periodontology* **65**, 827-834.

Mombelli, A., Nyman, S., Bragger, U., Wennstrom, J. & Lang, N,P. (1995). Clinical and microbiologic changes associated with an altered subgingival environment induced by periodontal pocket reduction. *Journal of Clinical Periodontology* **22**, 780-787.

Mousques, T., Listgarten, M.A. & Phillips, R.W. (1980). Effect of scaling and root planing on the composition of the human subgingival microbial flora. *Journal of Periodontal Research* **15**, 144-151.

Muller, H.P., Hartmann, J. & Flores-de-Jacoby, L. (1986). Clinical alterations in relation to the morphological composition of the subgingival microflora following scaling and root planing. *Journal of Clinical Periodontology* **13**, 825-832.

Nieminen, A., Siren, E., Wolf, J. & Asikainen, S. (1995). Prognostic criteria for the efficiency of non-surgical periodontal therapy in advanced periodontitis. *Journal of Clinical Periodontology* **22**, 153-161.

Noyan, U., Yilmaz, S., Kuru, B., Kadir, T., Acar, O. & Buget, E. (1997). A clinical and microbiological evaluation of systemic and local metronidazole delivery in adult periodontitis patients. *Journal of Clinical Periodontology* **24**, 158-165.

Nyman, S., Rosling, B. & Lindhe, J. (1975). Effect of professional tooth cleaning on healing after periodontal surgery. *Journal of Clinical Periodontology* **2**, 80-86.

Paquette, D.W., Fiorellini, J.P. & Howell, T.H. (1992). Effects of systemic metronidazole on human periodontal disease progression and BANA test results. *Journal of Dental Research* **71**, 757, abstract 1934.

Pavicic, M.J., van Winkelhoff, A.J., Douque, N.H., Steures, R.W. & de Graaff, J. (1994). Microbiological and clinical effects of metronidazole and amoxicillin in *Actinobacillus actinomycetemcomitans*-associated periodontitis. A 2-year evaluation. *Journal of Clinical Periodontology* **21**, 107-112.

Pedrazzoli, V., Kilian, M., Karring, T. & Kirkegaard, E. (1991). Effect of surgical and non-surgical periodontal treatment on periodontal status and subgingival microbiota. *Journal of Clinical Periodontology* **18**, 598-604.

Ramberg, P., Axelsson, P. & Lindhe, J. (1995). Plaque formation at healthy and inflamed gingival sites in young individuals. *Journal of Clinical Periodontology* **22**, 85-88.

Ramberg, P., Lindhe, J., Dahlen, G. & Volpe, A.R. (1994). The influence of gingival inflammation on de novo plaque formation. *Journal of Clinical Periodontology* **21**, 51-56.

Ramberg, P., Rosling, B., Serino, G., Socransky, S.S. & Lindhe, J. (2001). The long-term effect of systemic tetracycline used as an adjunct to non-surgical treatment of advanced periodontitis. *Journal of Clinical Periodontology* **28**, 446-452.

Rawlinson, A., Duerden, B. I. & Goodwin, L. (1993). Effects of root planing on the distribution of microorganisms at adult periodontitis sites. *European Journal of Prosthodontics & Restorative Dentistry* **1**, 103-110.

Rawlinson, A., Duerden, B.I. & Goodwin, L. (1995). Effects of surgical treatment on the microbial flora in residual periodontal pockets. *European Journal of Prosthetics and Restorative Dentistry* **3**, 155-161.

Rosenberg, E.S., Evian, C.I. & Listgarten, M.A. (1984). The composition of the subgingival microbiota after periodontal treatment. *Journal of Periodontology* **52**, 435-441.

Rosling, B., Nyman, S. & Lindhe, J. (1976a). The effect of systematic plaque control on bone regeneration in infrabony pockets. *Journal of Clinical Periodontology* **3**, 38-53.

Rosling, B., Nyman, S., Lindhe, J. & Jern, B. (1976b). The healing potential of the periodontal tissues following different techniques of periodontal surgery in plaque-free dentitions. A 2-year clinical study. *Journal of Clinical Periodontology* **3**, 233-250.

Rosling, B., Serino, G., Hellstrom, M-K., Socransky, S.S. & Lindhe, J. (2001). Longitudinal periodontal tissue alterations during supportive therapy. Findings from subjects with normal and high susceptibility to periodontal disease. *Journal of Clinical Periodontology* **28**, 241-249.

Rudiger, S., Petersilka, G. & Flemmig, T.F. (1999). Combined systemic and local antimicrobial therapy of periodontal disease in Papillon-LeFevre syndrome. A report of four cases. *Journal of Clinical Periodontology* **26**, 847-854.

Sato, K., Yoneyama, T., Okamoto, H., Dahlen, G. & Lindhe, J. (1993). The effect of subgingival debridement on periodontal disease parameters and the subgingival microbiota. *Journal of Clinical Periodontology* **20**, 359-365.

Saxen, L. & Asikainen, S. (1993). Metronidazole in the treatment of localized juvenile periodontitis. *Journal of Clinical Periodontology* **20**, 166-171.

Sbordone, L., Ramaglia, L., Gulletta, E. & Iacono, V. (1990). Recolonization of the subgingival microflora after scaling and root planing in human periodontitis. *Journal of Periodontology* **61**, 579-584P.

Serino, G., Rosling, B., Ramberg, P., Hellstrom, M-K., Socransky, S.S. & Lindhe, J. (2001a). The effect of systemic antibiotics in the treatment of patients with recurrent periodontitis. *Journal of Clinical Periodontology* **28**, 411-418.

Serino, G., Rosling, B., Ramberg, P., Socransky, S.S. & Lindhe, J. (2001b). Initial outcome and long-term effect of surgical and non-surgical treatment of advanced periodontal disease. *Journal of Clinical Periodontology* **28**, 910-916.

Sharawy, A.M., Sabharwal, K., Socransky, S.S. & Lobene, R.R. (1966). A quantitative study of plaque and calculus formation in normal and periodontally involved mouths. *Journal of Periodontology* **37**, 495-501.

Shiloah, J. & Patters, M. R. (1994). DNA probe analyses of the survival of selected periodontal pathogens following scaling, root planing, and intra-pocket irrigation. *Journal of Periodontology* **65**, 568-575.

Simonson, L.G., Robinson, P.J., Pranger, R.J., Cohen, M.E. & Morton, H. E. (1992). *Treponema denticola* and *Porphyromonas gingivalis* as prognostic markers following periodontal treatment. *Journal of Periodontology* **63**, 270-273.

Smulow, J., Turesky, S.S. & Hill, R.G. (1983). The effect of supragingival plaque removal on anaerobic bacteria in deep periodontal pockets. *Journal of American Dental Association* **107**, 737-742.

Socransky, S.S., Haffajee, A.D., Cugini, M.A., Smith, C. & Kent, R.L. Jr. (1998). Microbial complexes in subgingival plaque. *Journal of Clinical Periodontology* **25**, 134-144.

Socransky, S.S., Haffajee, A.D., Smith, C. & Dibart. S. (1991). Relation of counts of microbial species to clinical status at the sampled site. *Journal of Clinical Periodontology* **18**, 766-775.

Soder, P.O., Frithiof, L., Wikner, S., Wouters, F., Engstrom, P.E., Rubin, B., Nedlich, U. & Soder, B. (1990). The effect of systemic metronidazole after non-surgical treatment in moderate and advanced periodontitis in young adults. *Journal of Periodontology* **61**, 281-288.

Tabita, P.V., Bissada, N.F. & Mayberry, J.E. (1981). Effectiveness of supragingival plaque control on the development of subgingival plaque and gingival inflammation in patients with moderate pocket depth. *Journal of Periodontology* **52**, 88-93.

Takamatsu, N., Yano, K., Umeda, M. & Ishikawa, I. (1999). Effect of initial periodontal therapy on the frequency of detecting *Bacteroides forsythus*, *Porphyromonas gingivalis* and *Actinobacillus actinomycetemcomitans*. *Journal of Periodontology* **70**, 574-580.

van Oosten, M.A., Mikx, F.H. & Renggli, H.H. (1987). Microbial and clinical measurements of periodontal pockets during sequential periods of non-treatment, mechanical debridement and metronidazole therapy. *Journal of Clinical Periodontology* **14**, 197-204.

van Winkelhoff, A.J., Rams, T.E. & Slots, J. (1996). Systemic antibiotic therapy in periodontics. *Periodontology 2000* **10**, 45-78.

van Winkelhoff, A.J., Rodenburg, J.P., Goene, R.J., Abbas, F., Winkel, E.G. & de Graaff, J. (1989). Metronidazole plus amoxicillin in the treatment of *Actinobacillus actinomycetemcomitans* associated periodontitis. *Journal of Clinical Periodontology* **16**, 128-131.

van Winkelhoff, A.J., Tijhof, C.J. & deGraaff, J. (1992). Microbiological and clinical results of metronidazole plus amoxicillin therapy in *Actinobacillus actinomycetemcomitans*-associated periodontitis. *Journal of Periodontology* **63**, 52-57.

Westfelt, E., Bragd, L., Socransky, S.S., Haffajee, A.D., Nyman, S. & Lindhe, J. (1985). Improved periodontal conditions following therapy. *Journal of Clinical Periodontology* **12**, 283-293.

Winkel, E.G., van Winkelhoff, A.J., Timmerman, M., Vangsted, T. & van der Velden, U. (1997). Effects of metronidazole in patients with "refractory" periodontitis associated with *Bacteroides forsythus*. *Journal of Clinical Periodontology* **24**, 573-579.

Winkel, E.G., van Winkelhoff, A.J., Timmerman, M.F., van der Velden, U. & van der Weijden, G.A. (2001). Amoxicillin and metronidazole in the treatment of adult periodontitis patients. A double-blind placebo-controlled study. *Journal of Clinical Periodontology* **28**, 296-305.

Winkel, E.G., van Winkelhoff, A. & van der Velden, U. (1998). Additional clinical and microbiological effects of amoxicillin and metronidazole after initial periodontal therapy. *Journal of Clinical Periodontology* **25**, 857-864.

Ximenez-Fyvie, L.A., Haffajee, A.D., Som, S., Thompson, M., Torresyap, G. & Socransky, S.S. (2000). The effect of repeated professional supragingival plaque removal on the composition of the supra and subgingival microbiota. *Journal of Clinical Periodontology* **27**, 637-647.

Chapter 27

Mucogingival Therapy – Periodontal Plastic Surgery

Jan L. Wennström and Giovan P. Pini Prato

Gingival augmentation
   Marginal tissue recession
   Orthodontic therapy
   Restorative dentistry
   Procedures
   Healing

Root coverage
   Clinical outcome
   Healing

Interdental papilla reconstruction

Crown lengthening procedures
   Excessive gingival display
   Exposure of sound tooth structure
   Ectopic tooth eruption

The deformed edentulous ridge

Mucogingival therapy is a general term used to describe non-surgical and surgical treatment procedures for correction of defects in morphology, position and/or amount of soft tissue and underlying bone support at teeth and implants. Accordingly, mucogingival therapy may involve not only traditional periodontal treatment procedures but also, for example, orthodontic therapy.

A more specific term, *mucogingival surgery*, was introduced in the 1950s by Friedman (1957) and was defined as "surgical procedures designed to preserve gingiva, remove aberrant frenulum or muscle attachments, and increase the depth of the vestibule". Frequently, however, the term "mucogingival surgery" was used to describe all surgical procedures which involved both the gingiva and the alveolar mucosa. Consequently, not only were techniques designed (1) to enhance the width of the gingiva and (2) to correct particular soft tissue defects regarded as mucogingival procedures but (3) certain pocket elimination approaches were also included in this group of periodontal treatment modalities. According to the *Glossary of Periodontal Terms* (1992) mucogingival surgery is defined as "plastic surgical procedures designed to correct defects in the morphology, position and/or amount of gingivae surrounding the teeth". Miller (1993) proposed that the term *periodontal plastic surgery*

is more appropriate, since mucogingival surgery has moved beyond the traditional treatment of problems associated with the amount of gingivae and recession type defects to also include correction of ridge form and soft tissue esthetics. *Periodontal plastic surgery* would accordingly be defined as "surgical procedures performed to prevent or correct anatomic, developmental, traumatic or disease induced defects of the gingiva, alveolar mucosa or bone" (Proceedings of the World Workshop in Periodontics 1996). Among treatment procedures that may fall within this definition are various soft and hard tissue procedures aiming at:

- gingival augmentation
- root coverage
- correction of mucosal defects at implants
- crown lengthening
- gingival preservation at ectopic tooth eruption
- removal of aberrant frenulum
- prevention of ridge collapse associated with tooth extraction
- augmentation of the edentulous ridge.

This chapter will discuss mainly treatment procedures for corrections of soft tissue defects in relation to the tooth and the edentulous ridge, while bone augmentation procedures are covered in Chapters 38 and 39.

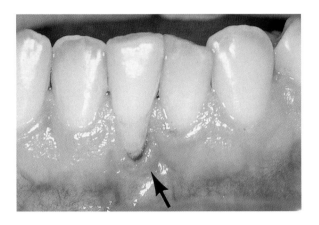

Fig. 27-1. A clinical photograph of a mandibular front tooth region. The gingiva on the buccal aspect of tooth 41 has a narrow width and shows more pronounced signs of inflammation than adjacent gingival units with a wider zone of gingiva.

GINGIVAL AUGMENTATION

A review of the large number of articles published on surgical, mucogingival therapy reveals that the rationale for increasing the width of gingiva as a means to promote gingival health and to improve attachment levels has been poorly supported by scientific data. Usually clinical impressions, case reports and anecdotal information have been used as the main reference to justify surgical intervention. Research performed during the earlier decades, however, has established a better understanding of the role played by the gingiva in the protection of the periodontium proper.

Gingival dimensions and periodontal health

For many years the presence of an "adequate" zone of gingiva was considered critical for the maintenance of marginal tissue health and for the prevention of continuous loss of connective tissue attachment (Nabers 1954, Ochsenbein 1960, Friedman & Levine 1964, Carranza & Carraro 1970, Hall 1981, Matter 1982). Clinicians had the "impression" that sites with a narrow zone of gingiva (Fig. 27-1) were often inflamed while the wide zone of gingiva found at neighboring teeth remained healthy. The prevailing concept was thus that a narrow zone of gingiva was insufficient (1) to protect the periodontium from injury caused by friction forces encountered during mastication and (2) to dissipate the pull on the gingival margin created by the muscles of the adjacent alveolar mucosa (Friedman 1957, Ochsenbein 1960, Friedman & Levine 1964). Moreover, it was believed that an "inadequate" zone of gingiva would (1) facilitate subgingival plaque formation because of improper pocket closure resulting from the movability of the marginal tissue (Friedman 1962) and (2) favor attachment loss and soft tissue recession because of less tissue resistance to apical spread of plaque-associated gingival lesions (Stern 1976, Ruben 1979). It was also believed that a narrow gingiva in combination with a shallow vestibular fornix might favor (1) the accumulation of food particles during mastication and (2) impede proper oral hy-

giene measures (Gottsegen 1954, Rosenberg 1960, Corn 1962, Carranza & Carraro 1970).

The opinions expressed concerning what could be regarded as being an "adequate" or "sufficient" dimension of the gingiva varied. While some authors suggested that less than 1 mm of gingiva may be sufficient (Bowers 1963), others claimed that the apicocoronal height of keratinized tissue ought to exceed 3 mm (Corn 1962). A third category of authors had a more biologic approach to the question and stated that an adequate amount of gingiva is any dimension of gingiva which (1) is compatible with gingival health or (2) prevents retraction of the gingival margin during movements of the alveolar mucosa (Friedman 1962, De Trey & Bernimoulin 1980).

One of the first studies in which attempts were made to evaluate the significance of the gingival zone for the maintenance of periodontal health was carried out by Lang & Löe (1972) on dental students who had their teeth professionally cleaned once a day for 6 weeks. All buccal and lingual sites were examined for plaque, gingival conditions and apicocoronal height of gingiva. The results showed that despite the fact that the tooth surfaces were free from plaque, all sites with less than 2 mm of gingiva exhibited persisting clinical signs of inflammation. Based on this observation the authors suggested that 2 mm of gingiva is an adequate width for maintaining gingival health. Findings reported from controlled clinical trials by Miyasato et al. (1977) and Grevers (1977), on the other hand, failed to support the concept of a required minimum dimension of gingiva. In these clinical trials it was in fact demonstrated that it is possible to maintain clinically healthy marginal tissue even in areas with less than 1 mm of keratinized tissue. Furthermore, when the individuals participating in the study by Miyasato et al. (1977) ceased oral hygiene for a period of 25 days, there was no difference in the development of clinical signs of gingival inflammation between areas with a minimal (≤ 1 mm) and those with an appreciable (≥ 2 mm) width of the gingiva.

The question whether a firmly attached marginal tissue, i.e. attached gingiva, is critical for the protection of the periodontium proper was addressed by Wennström & Lindhe (1983a,b) utilizing the beagle dog model. In these studies dentogingival units with

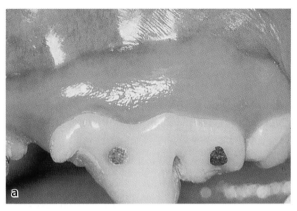
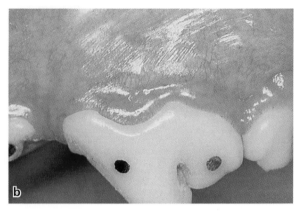

Fig. 27-2. Two teeth in a dog with varying dimensions of the marginal gingiva. A buccal tooth site with a wide zone of attached gingiva (a) and a site with an unattached, narrow band of gingiva (b).

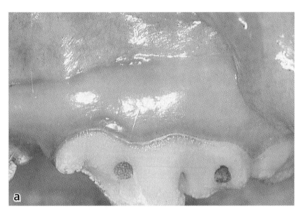
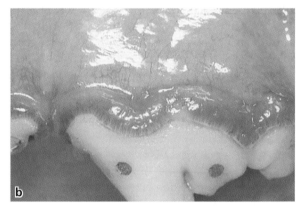

Fig. 27-3. The same teeth as in Fig. 27-2a,b after 40 days of plaque accumulation. The clinical signs of inflammation are more pronounced at the site with the narrow band of gingiva (b) than at the site with the wide zone of attached gingiva (a).

different clinical characteristics were experimentally established: (1) units with only a narrow and mobile zone of keratinized tissue and (2) units with a wide, firmly attached gingiva (Fig. 27-2). With daily performed mechanical plaque control measures, the gingival units could be maintained free from clinical as well as histologic signs of inflammation irrespective of the presence or absence of an attached portion of gingiva. When bacterial plaque was allowed to accumulate (for 40 days), clinical signs of inflammation (redness and swelling) developed which were more pronounced in tooth regions with mobile gingiva (Fig. 27-3b) than in areas with a wide and firmly attached gingival zone (Fig. 27-3a). However, histologic analysis revealed that the size of the inflammatory cell infiltrate and its extension in apical direction (an assessment which indirectly may be used as an estimate of the apical migration of the bacterial plaque) were similar in the two categories of dentogingival units. Compared to the gingival units with firmly attached tissue, it was found that the units lacking attached gingiva were thinner in the buccolingual dimension and that the covering oral epithelium had a thinner keratin layer. Presumably these morphologic differences in the marginal tissue made the vascular system more readily visible from the buccal aspect of the

gingiva, and may thus explain why areas with only a narrow gingival zone clinically appeared more inflamed than those with a wide and properly attached gingiva.

The observation that the clinical signs of gingival inflammation did not correspond with the size of the inflammatory cell infiltrate illustrates the difficulties inherent in the interpretation of data from clinical examinations made in areas with varying width of gingiva. This should be kept in mind when interpreting the data by Lang & Löe (1972) showing that clinically visible signs of inflammation, such as redness and swelling, were more frequent in areas with less than 2 mm of gingiva than in areas with a wider zone of gingiva.

The necessity for and effectiveness of gingival augmentation in maintaining periodontal attachment was examined by Dorfman et al. (1980). Ninety-two patients with bilateral facial tooth surfaces exhibiting minimal keratinized tissue (i.e. less than 2 mm) had a free gingival graft placed on one side, while the contralateral side served as the untreated control. Prior to and after surgery the patients were subjected to scaling and root planing and instruction in oral hygiene measures. Not surprisingly, the investigators found a significant increase (approximately 4 mm) in the width of keratinized tissue at the grafted sites. This increased width of gingiva was maintained for a 2-year follow-up period. The attachment level was also maintained throughout this time period. In the control sites the width of gingiva was less than 2 mm and did not vary significantly during the 2 years of observation. However, the attachment level was maintained unchanged also in the non-grafted areas. Thus, a narrow zone of gingiva apparently has the same resistance to continuous attachment loss as a wider zone of gingiva. Subsequent 4 and 6-year follow-up reports of this patient material (Dorfman et al. 1982, Kennedy et al. 1985) confirmed the 2-year follow-up findings.

Hangorsky & Bissada (1980), who evaluated the long-term clinical effect of free soft tissue grafts on the periodontal condition in 34 patients, also failed to observe any difference between grafted and non-grafted sites after 1-8 years with regard to gingival health and pocket depth. They concluded that while the free gingival graft is an effective means to widen the zone of the gingiva, there is no indication that this increase has a direct influence upon periodontal health. This conclusion is in agreement with the findings of De Trey & Bernimoulin (1980), who examined the effect of free gingival grafts in 12 patients with less than 1 mm of attached gingiva on homologous contralateral pairs of mandibular teeth. The authors found no significant differences in gingival health when test and control sites were compared longitudinally.

Further support for the conclusion that a certain quantity of gingiva is not essential for the maintenance of the integrity of the periodontium is found in a number of longitudinal clinical studies (Lindhe & Nyman 1980, Kennedy et al. 1985, Schoo & van der Velden 1985, Kisch et al. 1986, Salkin et al. 1987, Wennström 1987, Freedman et al. 1999) showing that a minimal zone of gingiva may not compromise periodontal health.

Conclusion

Gingival health can be maintained independent of its dimensions. Furthermore, there is evidence from both experimental and clinical studies that, in the presence of plaque, areas with a narrow zone of gingiva possess the same "resistance" to continuous attachment loss as teeth with a wide zone of gingiva. Hence, the traditional dogma of the need of an "adequate" width (in millimeters) of gingiva, or attached portion of gingiva, for prevention of attachment loss, is not scientifically supported.

Marginal tissue recession

Marginal tissue recession, i.e. displacement of the soft tissue margin apical to the cemento-enamel junction with exposure of the root surface, is a common feature in populations with high standards of oral hygiene (Sangnes & Gjermo 1976, Murtomaa et al. 1987, Löe et al. 1992, Serino et al. 1994), as well as in populations with poor oral hygiene (Baelum et al. 1986, 1988, Yoneyama et al. 1988, Löe et al. 1992). In populations maintaining high standards of oral hygiene, loss of attachment and marginal tissue recession are predominantly found at buccal surfaces (Källestål et al. 1990, Löe et al. 1992, Serino et al. 1994), and are frequently associated with the presence of a "wedge-shaped defect in the crevicular area of one or several teeth" (Sangnes & Gjermo 1976). In contrast, all tooth surfaces are usually affected with soft tissue recession in periodontally untreated populations (Löe et al. 1978, 1992, Miller et al. 1987, Okamoto et al. 1988, Yoneyama et al. 1988). However, buccal recessions seem to be more common and more advanced at single-rooted teeth than at molars (Yoneyama et al. 1988).

Tissue trauma caused by vigorous toothbrushing is considered to be a dominating causative factor for the development of recessions, particularly in young individuals. Traumatizing toothbrushing and tooth malposition are the factors most frequently found to be associated with marginal tissue recession (Gorman 1967, Modéer & Odenrick 1980, Vekalahti 1989, Källestål & Uhlin 1992, Checci et al. 1999). In addition, Khocht et al. (1993) showed that recessions are related to the use of hard toothbrushes. Among other factors that have been associated with marginal tissue reces-

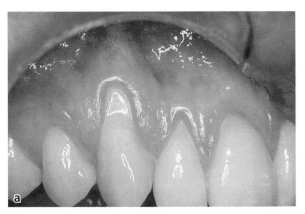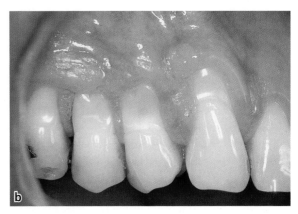

Fig. 27-4a,b. Recessions associated with toothbrushing trauma. The marginal gingiva is clinically healthy and abrasion defects of various extension can be noted in the exposed roots.

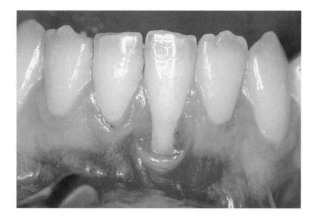

Fig. 27-5. A recession associated with localized plaque-induced inflammatory lesion.

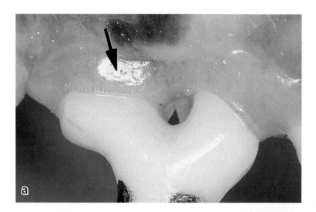

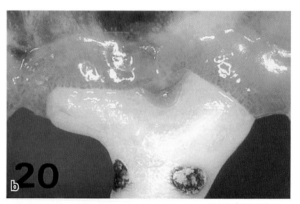

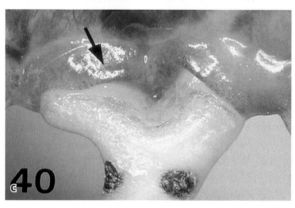

Fig. 27-6. Clinical photographs illustrating the development of a soft tissue recession as a result of plaque-induced inflammation in a beagle dog. Note the thin but healthy gingiva (arrow) at the start of the plaque accumulation period (a). Pronounced clinical signs of inflammation are seen after 20 days (b), and after 40 days of no toothcleaning, the gingival margin has receded (c).

sion are (1) alveolar bone dehiscences (Bernimoulin & Curilivic 1977, Löst 1984), (2) inadequate gingival dimensions (Maynard 1987), (3) high muscle attachment and frenal pull (Trott & Love 1966), (4) calculus (van Palenstein Helderman et al. 1998) and (5) iatrogenic factors related to restorative and periodontal treatment procedures (Gorman 1967, Lindhe & Nyman 1980, Valderhaug 1980).

It seems reasonable to suggest that at least three different types of marginal tissue recessions may exist:

• *Recessions associated with mechanical factors, predominantly toothbrushing trauma* (Fig 27-4). Recessions resulting from improper toothbrushing techniques are often found at sites with clinically healthy

gingiva and where the exposed root has a wedge-shaped defect, the surface of which is clean, smooth and polished.

• *Recessions associated with localized plaque-induced inflammatory lesions* (Fig. 27-5). Such recessions may be found at teeth that are prominently positioned, i.e. the alveolar bone is thin or absent (bone dehiscence), and where in addition the gingival tissue is thin (delicate). An inflammatory lesion that develops in response to subgingival plaque occupies an area of the connective tissue adjacent to the dentogingival epithelium. Measurements made by Waerhaug (1952) suggest that the distance between the periphery of microbial plaque on the tooth surface and the lateral and apical extension of the

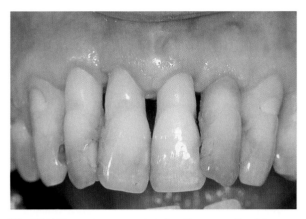

Fig. 27-7. Recessions associated with generalized forms of destructive periodontal disease. Recession of the soft tissue is found not only at the facial aspect of the teeth but also at proximal sites.

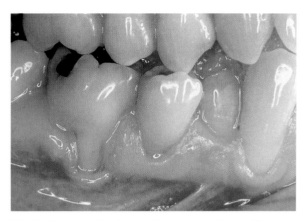

Fig. 27-8. A mandibular tooth segment with multiple buccal recessions illustrating the association proposed between recession depth and height of gingiva.

inflammatory cell infiltrate seldom exceeds 1-2 mm. Thus, if the free gingiva is voluminous the infiltrate will occupy only a small portion of the connective tissue. In a thin and delicate gingiva, on the other hand, the entire connective tissue portion may be engaged. Proliferation of epithelial cells from the oral as well as the dento-gingival epithelium into the thin and degraded connective tissue may bring about a subsidence of the epithelial surface, which clinically becomes manifest as recession of the tissue margin (Baker & Seymour 1976) (Fig. 27-6).

• *Recessions associated with generalized forms of destructive periodontal disease* (Fig. 27-7). The loss of periodontal support at proximal sites may result in compensatory remodeling of the support at the buccal/lingual aspect of the teeth leading to an apical shift of the soft tissue margin (Serino et al. 1994).

Cross-sectional studies showing that a correlation exists between the presence of recession defects and the height (width) of the gingiva (e.g. Stoner & Mazdyasna 1980, Tenenbaum 1982) have often been interpreted as evidence that a narrow zone of gingiva is a contributing factor in the development of soft tissue recessions (Fig. 27-8). It should be realized, however, that data derived from cross-sectional studies can neither prove nor disprove a cause-effect relationship. Consequently, the data reported from such studies may equally well be interpreted to demonstrate that the formation of a recession defect results in a reduced height of the gingiva. Fig. 27-1 illustrates a mandibular incisor tooth region with a localized gingival recession at the buccal aspect of tooth 41. The gingiva apical to the recession defect is narrow – "insufficient" – while at neighboring teeth the gingival height may be considered "adequate". It is reasonable to assume that the gingiva at tooth 41, *before the recession defect developed*, had a height that was similar to that found at tooth 31 and tooth 42. In other words, the narrow zone of gingiva found at tooth 41 may be the result of *loss of gingival tissue during the period of*

recession development, rather than being the cause of the formation of the defect. If this interpretation is valid, the rationale for increasing the height of the gingiva in an area *apical to the existing defect* as a means of preventing further recession may appear somewhat obscure. In fact, data obtained from prospective, longitudinal studies of patients showing areas with only a minimal zone of gingiva favor the conclusion that a certain quantity of gingiva is not essential for the preclusion of soft tissue recessions. Lindhe & Nyman (1980) examined the alterations of the position of the gingival margin following periodontal surgery in 43 patients with advanced periodontal breakdown. Following active treatment, all patients were recalled once every 3-6 months for maintenance care. The position of the soft tissue margin in relation to the cemento-enamel junction was assessed on the facial aspect of all teeth after initial healing and after 10-11 years of maintenance. The presence or absence of keratinized tissue after surgical treatment was also determined. The results showed that in areas both with and without visible keratinized tissue after healing, a small coronal regrowth (~ 1 mm) of the soft tissue margin had occurred during the period of maintenance. In other words, no recession was observed in this group of patients maintained on a careful prophylaxis program.

Dorfman et al. (1982) reported a 4-year follow-up study including 22 patients with bilateral tooth areas exhibiting gingival recession and lack of firmly attached marginal soft tissue. In conjunction with scaling and root planing a free gingival graft was placed on one side, while the contralateral control side was treated by scaling and root planing only. All patients were recalled for prophylaxis once every 3-6 months during a 4-year period. The data obtained from the examinations of the non-grafted control areas revealed that no further recession of the soft tissue margin or loss of probing attachment had occurred despite the lack of attached marginal tissue. In fact, there was a slight gain of probing attachment. The authors con-

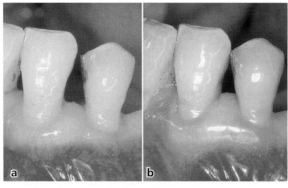

Fig. 27-9. Clinical photographs of a canine and a first premolar in the mandible with < 1 mm of attached portion of gingiva 6 months after surgical treatment (a). Note the increase of the width of the gingiva at the facial aspect of the teeth and the more coronally positioned gingival margin 5 yrs later (b).

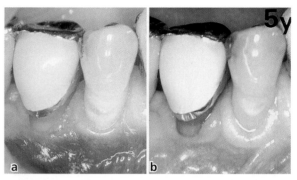

Fig. 27-10. A mandibular canine and first premolar tooth region showing a very narrow zone of gingiva 6 months following surgical therapy (a). No major change in the position of the soft tissue margin has occurred during a 5-year period despite the lack of attached gingiva (b).

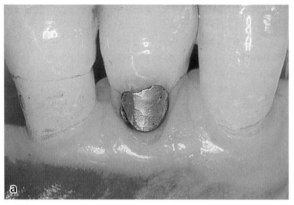

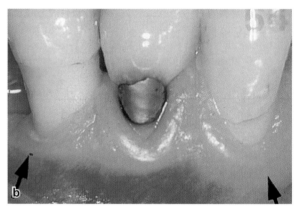

Fig. 27-11. Clinical photographs of the right mandibular canine-premolar tooth region in the patient showing several sites with apical displacement of the soft tissue margin during the 5 years of observation. At the initial examination the two premolars had < 1 mm and the canine > 1 mm of attached portion of gingiva (a). After 5 years (b) recession and loss of keratinized tissue can be seen on the buccal aspect of the canine, which initially had a broad zone of gingiva (black arrow). The second premolar also showed further apical displacement of the soft tissue margin.

cluded that recession sites with lack of attached gingiva will not develop further attachment loss and recession if the inflammation is controlled, a conclusion which was also valid in their 6-year report on the same patient material (Kennedy et al. 1985). The latter report also included data on 10 patients who had not participated in the maintenance phase of treatment for a period of 5 years. In these patients plaque and clinical signs of inflammation as well as some further recession were noted at the 5-year examination as compared with the data obtained after termination of active treatment. However, except for the clinical signs of inflammation, which were more pronounced in non-grafted sites, no differences were observed between control sites with < 1 mm or complete lack of attached gingiva and grafted sites.

In a controlled animal study Gould et al. (1992) evaluated whether placing a gingival graft to augment the apicocoronal height of keratinized tissue would prevent development of recession. Despite an almost 6 mm mean increase of the gingival height at grafted sites, recession continued to develop to a similar degree as in non-grafted contralateral control sites. The authors concluded that augmenting the width of gingiva does not prevent or retard naturally occurring recession.

The lack of relationship between the height of gingiva and the development of soft tissue recession is further validated by results from longitudinal clinical studies reported by Schoo & van der Velden (1985), Kisch et al. (1986), Salkin et al. (1987), Wennström (1987) and Freedman et al. (1999). The study by Wennström (1987) reports observations made at 26 buccal sites surgically deprived of all keratinized tissue. A baseline examination carried out 6 months after treatment revealed that these sites had regained a zone of gingiva which was, however, not attached or had only a minimal (< 1 mm) portion attached to the underlying hard tissues (Figs. 27-9a and 27-10a). Adjacent teeth with a broad zone of attached gingiva were also included in the examinations. In most sites the position of the soft tissue margin had been maintained unchanged over the 5 years of follow-up (Figs. 27-9b and 27-10b). A further apical displacement of the soft tissue margin had occurred at two out of 26 sites with no/minimal attached gingiva and at three out of 12 adjacent control sites with a wide attached zone of gingiva. Since four of these five sites were found in one patient (Fig. 27-11), and all sites were free from clinical signs of inflammation, excessive toothbrushing was considered to be the causative factor, and following correction of the brushing technique no further progression was observed. Furthermore, the development of soft tissue recession at the control sites resulted in a decreased height of the gingiva, an observation that supports the concept that a narrow zone of gingiva apical to a localized recession is a consequence rather than a cause of the recession.

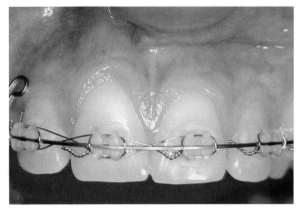

Fig. 27-12. Soft tissue recession at tooth 11 observed during the course of active orthodontic treatment.

Conclusion

Marginal soft tissue recession is a common feature in populations with good as well as poor standards of oral hygiene. There is evidence to suggest that the predominant cause for localized recessions in young individuals is toothbrushing trauma, while periodontal disease may be the primary cause in older adults. Evidence from prospective longitudinal studies shows that the gingival height is not a critical factor for the prevention of marginal tissue recession, but that the development of a recession will result in loss of gingival height.

Marginal tissue recession and orthodontic treatment

Results from clinical and experimental research have documented that most forms of orthodontic therapy are innocuous to the periodontium (see Chapter 31). The clinician may experience, however, that some patients respond to frontal movements of incisors and lateral movements of posterior teeth by gingival recession and loss of attachment (Pearson 1968, Maynard & Ochsenbein 1975, Coatoam et al. 1981, Foushee et al. 1985) (Fig. 27-12). Based on the clinical observation that recession may occur during orthodontic therapy involving sites which have an "insufficient" zone of gingiva, it has been suggested that a grafting procedure to increase the gingival dimensions should precede the initiation of orthodontic therapy in such areas (Boyd 1978, Hall 1981, Maynard 1987).

As discussed previously, the presence of an alveolar bone dehiscence is considered to be a prerequisite for the development of a marginal tissue recession, i.e. a root dehiscence may establish an environment which, for one reason or another, is conducive to loss of gingival tissue. With respect to orthodontic therapy, this would imply that as long as a tooth is moved exclusively within the alveolar bone, soft tissue recession will not develop (Wennström et al. 1987). On the other hand, "predisposing" alveolar bone dehiscences may be induced by uncontrolled facial expansion of teeth through the cortical plate, thereby rendering the teeth liable to development of soft tissue recession. In this context it is interesting to note that experimental

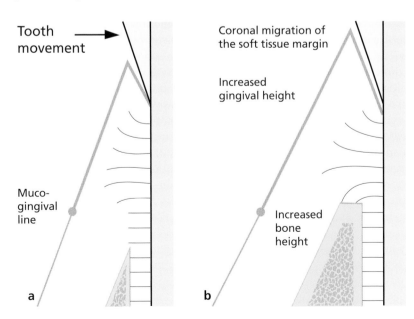

Fig. 27-13. Schematic drawing illustrating alterations occurring in the marginal periodontal tissues following lingual movement of a tooth prominently positioned in the arch and having a bone dehiscence (a). An increase in bone height and gingival height will be seen as well as a coronal migration of the soft tissue margin following lingual positioning of the tooth (b).

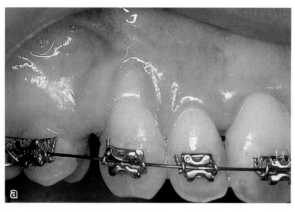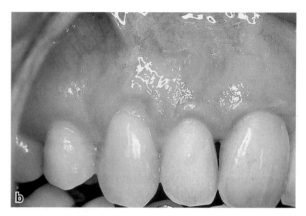

Fig. 27-14. A prominently positioned 13 showing soft tissue recession (a). The same tooth following the completion of the orthodontic tooth movement (b). Note the reduction of the recession that has taken place as a consequence of the changed position of the tooth.

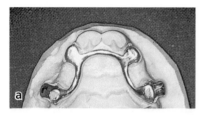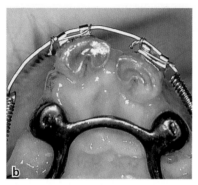

Fig. 27-15. Occlusal view of the maxilla in a monkey showing the position of the central incisors before (a) and after (b) bodily movement in labial direction. The canines and lateral incisors were joined in an individual fabricated silver splint and used as anchorage teeth.

studies have shown that labial bone will reform in the area of a dehiscence when the tooth is retracted towards a proper positioning of the root within the alveolar process (Engelking & Zachrisson 1982, Karring et al. 1982) (Fig. 27-13). It is therefore likely that the reduction in recession seen at a previously prominently positioned tooth which has been moved into a more proper position within the alveolar process, is also accompanied by bone formation (Fig. 27-14).

Alterations occurring in gingival dimensions and marginal tissue position in conjunction with orthodontic therapy are related to the direction of tooth movement. Facial movement results in reduced facial gingival dimensions, while an increase is observed following lingual movement (Coatoam et al. 1981, Andlin-Sobocki & Brodin 1993). Batenhorst et al. (1974) and Steiner et al. (1981) used the monkey as an experimental animal and studied soft tissue alterations following either tipping and extrusion movements or bodily movements of incisors. It was reported that such tooth movements resulted in recession of the labial gingival margin and loss of attachment. However, similarly designed studies carried out in dogs (Karring et al. 1982, Nyman et al. 1982) and

humans (Rateitschak et al. 1968) failed to demonstrate that labial tooth movement is accompanied by marginal tissue recession and attachment loss. This discrepancy in the response of the marginal soft tissue to orthodontic therapy in the studies referred to is difficult to understand but may be related to differences with respect to (1) the amount of labial tooth displacement, (2) the magnitude of force applied, (3) the presence/absence of plaque and gingival inflammation in the regions subjected to tooth movement and/or (4) differences in gingival dimensions. Steiner et al. (1981) speculated on mechanisms by which gingival tissue could be lost as a result of labial tooth movement and suggested that tension in the marginal tissue created by the forces applied to the teeth could be an important factor. If this hypothesis is valid, obviously the volume (thickness) of the gingival tissue at the pressure side rather than its apicocoronal height would determine whether or not marginal tissue recession develops during orthodontic therapy.

Support for this hypothesis is obtained from an experimental study in monkeys (Wennström et al. 1987) in which teeth were orthodontically moved into areas with varying thickness and quality of the mar-

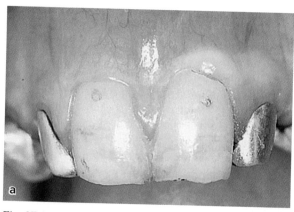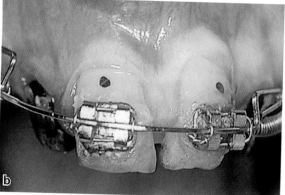

Fig. 27-16. The buccal aspect of the central incisors in the same monkey as in Fig. 27-15, before (a) and after (b) the labial tooth movement. No obvious change in the location of the gingival margin has occurred despite the pronounced labial displacement of the incisors.

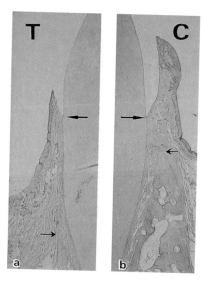

Fig. 27-17. Histologic specimens showing (a) reduced alveolar bone height at an incisor bodily moved in labial direction and (b) normal alveolar bone height at a non-moved control tooth. Note the maintained level of connective tissue attachment and the reduced height of the free gingiva at the labially displaced incisor (a). Large arrows indicate the position of the cemento-enamel junction and small arrows the position of the alveolar bone crest.

ginal soft tissue. Following extensive bodily movement of incisors in labial direction through the alveolar bone (Fig. 27-15), most teeth showed a small apical displacement of the soft tissue margin but no loss of connective tissue attachment (Fig. 27-16). In other words, the apical displacement of the gingival margin was the result of a reduced height of the free gingiva (Fig. 27-17), which in turn may be related to tension – "stretching" – in the soft tissues during the facial tooth movement and reduced buccolingual tissue thickness. Similar to results presented by Foushee et al. (1985) from a study in humans, no relationship was found between the initial apicocoronal width (height) of the gingiva and the degree of apical displacement of the soft tissue margin during orthodontic therapy. Hence, the findings do not lend support to the hypothesis that a certain zone of gingiva is essential for the prevention of recession during orthodontic therapy, but rather corroborate clinical observations reported by Coatoam et al. (1981) suggesting that the integrity of the periodontium can be maintained during orthodontic therapy also in areas which have only a minimal zone of gingiva.

Both Steiner et al. (1981) and Wennström et al. (1987) reported that teeth which experienced loss of connective tissue attachment when orthodontically moved facially showed obvious clinical signs of inflammation throughout the experimental period. Since it has been demonstrated that, in the presence of plaque-induced suprabony lesions, orthodontic forces generating bodily tooth movement are incapable of causing accelerated destruction of the connective tissue attachment (Ericsson et al. 1978), it can be assumed that "stretching" of the facial gingiva may favor the destructive effect of the plaque-associated inflammatory lesion due to the decreased buccolingual dimension of the border tissue. This assumption is validated by the observations that, in the presence of plaque-induced gingivitis, a thin marginal soft tissue is more susceptible to complete breakdown than a thick one (Baker & Seymour 1976). Furthermore, since attachment loss was found to be similar for plaque-infected teeth which had been bodily moved *within the alveolar bone* irrespective of the type of soft tissue (gingiva or lining mucosa) (Wennström et al. 1987), the thickness rather than the quality of the marginal soft tissue on the pressure side of the tooth seems to be the determining factor for the development of recession defects during orthodontic therapy in plaque-infected dentitions. Hence, the observations made in the studies discussed strongly emphasize the importance of adequate plaque control during orthodontic treatment.

Conclusion

The clinical implication of the results from the studies discussed is that labial tooth movement should be preceded by careful examination of the dimensions of the tissues covering the facial aspect of the teeth to be moved. As long as the tooth can be moved within the envelope of the alveolar process, the risk of harmful side-effects in the marginal tissue is minimal, irrespective of the dimensions and quality of the soft tissue. If, however, the tooth movement is expected to result in the establishment of an alveolar bone dehiscence, the volume (thickness) of the covering soft tissue should be considered as a factor that may influence the development of soft tissue recession during and/or after the phase of active orthodontic therapy. A thin gingiva may serve as a *locus minorus resistentiae* to developing soft tissue defects in the presence of plaque-induced inflammation or toothbrushing trauma.

Gingival dimensions and restorative therapy

The claim has been made that in segments of the dentition involved in restorative therapy there is a particular demand for gingiva (Maynard & Wilson 1979, Nevins 1986). The placement of restoration margins subgingivally may not only create a direct operative trauma to the tissues (Donaldson 1974), but may also facilitate subgingival plaque accumulation, with resultant inflammatory alterations in the adjacent gingiva and recession of the soft tissue margin (Valderhaug 1980, Parma-Benfenati et al. 1985). Valderhaug (1980) evaluated longitudinally over a 10-year period the soft tissue alterations taking place at facial sites of 286 teeth with subgingivally or supragingivally placed crown margins in 82 patients. The re-examination performed 1 year after insertion of the restorations revealed that the gingivae at teeth with subgingival restoration margins were more inflamed than at those with supragingivally placed borders. Of the 150 teeth which at the time of cementation had the facial crown margin located subgingivally, 40% showed supragingival exposure of the crown margin already after 1 year and at the 10-year examination as many as 71% had become supragingivally positioned due to recession of the soft tissue margin. Compared to teeth with supragingivally placed crown margins, the amount of recession and clinical attachment loss was greater at sites with subgingivally placed restoration margins.

Stetler & Bissada (1987) evaluated the periodontal conditions at teeth with subgingivally placed restoration margins on teeth with varying apicocoronal height of gingiva and found that teeth having a narrow (< 2 mm) band of gingiva showed more pronounced clinical signs of inflammation than restored teeth with a wide gingival zone, but that there was no difference in loss of probing attachment. However, if subgingivally placed restorations facilitate plaque accumulation and the adjacent gingiva is thin, there may be a potential risk for the development of soft tissue recession. An experimental study in the beagle dog (Ericsson & Lindhe 1984), in which metallic strips were inserted subgingivally in areas with varying width of gingiva, showed that in sites with a thin gingival margin, recession was a more likely consequence of the combined tissue trauma caused by the insertion of the strip and subsequent plaque accumulation during a 6-month period than in sites with a broad gingival zone. The authors suggested that the placement of restorations in a subgingival position at sites with a thin gingiva may in the presence of subgingival plaque favor an inflammatory tissue reaction which results in loss of tissue height, i.e. in apical displacement of the soft tissue margin. Accordingly, if such an apical displacement as a consequence of plaque-induced inflammation is to be prevented, either the plaque control standard has to be improved or the *thickness* of the gingival margin has to be increased. However, an increased gingival dimension will not reduce the apical propagation of the plaque-associated lesion and the associated loss of periodontal attachment.

Conclusion

Subgingival placement of the margin of a restoration is likely to result in soft tissue recession over time. Experimental and clinical data suggest that the thickness of the marginal gingiva, but not the apicocoronal width of the gingiva, is influencing the magnitude of recession taking place as a result of direct mechanical trauma during tooth preparation and bacterial plaque retention.

Indications for gingival augmentation

Scientific data obtained from well-controlled clinical and experimental studies have unequivocally demonstrated that the apicocoronal width of gingiva and the presence of an attached portion of gingiva are not of decisive importance for the maintenance of gingival health and the height of the periodontal tissues. Consequently, the presence of a narrow zone of gingiva *per se* cannot justify surgical intervention (Proceedings of the 1st European Workshop on Periodontology 1994, Proceedings of the World Workshop on Periodontics 1996). However, gingival augmentation should be considered in situations where the patient experiences discomfort during toothbrushing and/or chewing due to an interfering lining mucosa. Furthermore, when orthodontic tooth movement is planned and the final positioning of the tooth can be expected to result in an alveolar bone dehiscence, an increase of the *thickness* of the covering soft tissue may reduce the risk for development of soft tissue recession. An increase of the *thickness* of the gingival margin may in certain

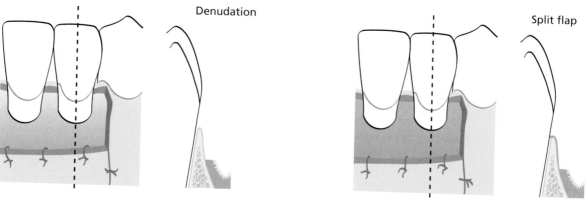

Denudation

Split flap

Fig. 27-18. The use of vestibular extension operations for increasing the width of the gingiva involves the production of a wound extending from the gingival margin to a level some mm apical to the mucogingival junction. With the "denudation" technique all soft tissue is removed, leaving the alveolar bone exposed. With the "split flap" procedure only the superficial portion of the oral mucosa is removed, leaving the bone covered with connective tissue.

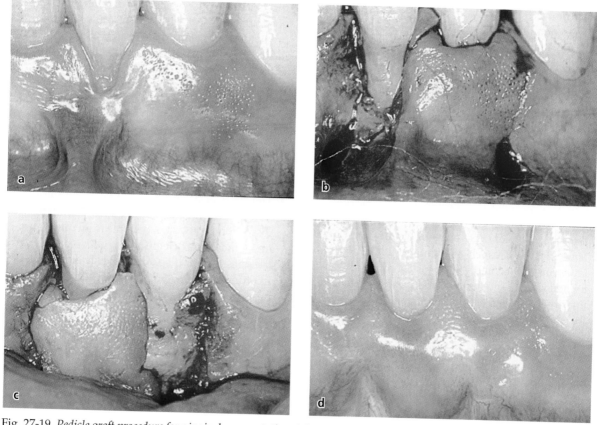

Fig. 27-19. *Pedicle graft procedure for gingival augmentation.* A lower central incisor with facial soft tissue recession associated with high attachment of a frenulum (a). The frenulum is released and a split flap of keratinized tissue is dissected from the area of the neighboring tooth (b). The mobilized soft tissue flap is laterally moved and secured in position at the recipient site (c). The healing result 1-year post-treatment shows the establishment of a broad zone of keratinized tissue without interfering frenulum (d).

situations also be considered when subgingival restorations are placed in areas with a thin marginal tissue.

Gingival augmentation procedures

The gingival augmentation operations comprise a number of surgical techniques, the majority of which have been developed mainly on an empirical basis and without sufficient knowledge of the biology of the involved tissues. The earliest of these techniques are the "vestibular extension operations", which were designed mainly with the objective of extending the depth of the vestibular sulcus (Bohannan 1962a,b). In recent years, however, pedicle or free soft tissue grafts have become the most commonly used techniques in the management of "insufficient" gingival dimensions, because of higher predictability of the healing result.

Vestibular/gingival extension procedures

The "denudation techniques" included the removal of all soft tissue within an area extending from the gingival margin to a level apical to the mucogingival junction, leaving the alveolar bone completely exposed (Ochsenbein 1960, Corn 1962, Wilderman 1964) (Fig. 27-18). Healing following this type of treatment resulted often in an increased height of the gingival zone, although in some cases only a very limited effect was observed. However, the exposure of alveolar bone produced severe bone resorption with permanent loss of bone height (Wilderman et al. 1961, Costich & Ramfjord 1968). In addition, the recession of marginal gingiva in the surgical area often exceeded the gain of gingiva obtained in the apical portion of the wound (Carranza & Carraro 1963, Carraro et al. 1964). Due to these complications and severe postoperative pain for the patient, the use of the "denudation technique" can hardly be justified.

With the "periosteal retention" procedure or "split flap" procedure (Fig. 27-18) only the superficial portion of the oral mucosa within the wound area is removed, leaving the bone covered by periosteum (Staffileno et al. 1962, Wilderman 1963, Pfeifer 1965, Staffileno et al. 1966). Although the preservation of the periosteum implies that less severe bone resorption will occur than following the "denudation technique", loss of crestal bone height was observed also following this type of operation unless a relatively thick layer of connective tissue was retained on the bone surface (Costich & Ramfjord 1968). If a thick layer was not secured, the periosteal connective tissue tended to undergo necrosis and the subsequent healing closely resembled that following the "denudation technique" described above.

Other described gingival extension procedures may be regarded as modifications of the "denudation" and "split flap" techniques or combinations of these procedures. The apically repositioned flap procedure (Friedman 1962), for instance, involved the elevation of soft tissue flaps and their displacement during suturing in an apical position, often leaving 3-5 mm of alveolar bone denuded in the coronal part of the surgical area. This resulted in the same risk for extensive bone resorption as other "denudation techniques". It was proposed by Friedman (1962) that a postsurgical increase of the width of the gingiva can be predicted with the "apically repositioned flap", but several studies indicated that the presurgical width most often was retained or became only slightly increased (Donnenfeld et al. 1964, Carranza & Carraro 1970).

The described vestibular/gingival extension procedures were based on the assumption that it is the frictional forces encountered during mastication which determine the presence of keratinized tissue adjacent to the teeth (Orban 1957, Pfeifer 1963). Therefore, it was believed that by the displacement of muscle attachments and the extension of vestibular depth, the regenerating tissue in the surgical area would be subjected to physical impacts and adapt to the same functional requirements as those met by "normal" gingiva (Ivancie 1957, Bradley et al. 1959, Pfeifer 1963). Later studies, however, showed that the characteristic features of the gingiva are determined by some inherent factors in the tissue rather than being the result of functional adaptation, and that the differentiation (keratinization) of the gingival epithelium is controlled by morphogenetic stimuli from the underlying connective tissue (see Chapter 1).

Grafting procedures

The gingival and palatal soft tissues will maintain their original characteristics after transplantation to areas of the alveolar mucosa (see Chapter 1). Hence, the use of transplants offers the potential to predict the postsurgical result. The type of transplants used can be divided into (1) pedicle grafts, which after placement at the recipient site maintain their connection with the donor site (Fig 27-19), and (2) free grafts, which have no connection with the donor area (Fig. 27-20). Free grafts have most commonly been used for gingival augmentation (Haggerty 1966, Nabers 1966, Sullivan & Atkins 1968a, Hawley & Staffileno 1970, Edel 1974).

Technique
- The surgical procedure is initiated with the preparation of the recipient site (Fig. 27-20a,b). By sharp dissection a periosteal bed free from muscle attachment and of sufficient size is prepared. The partial thickness flap is displaced apically and sutured.
- In order to ensure that a graft of sufficient size and proper contour is removed from the donor area, usually the palatal mucosa in the region of the premolars, it is recommended to produce a foil template over the recipient site. The template is transferred to the donor site where it is outlined by a shallow incision (Fig. 27-20c). A graft with a thickness of approximately 1.5-2 mm is then dissected from the donor area (Fig. 27-20d). It is advocated to place the sutures in the graft before it is cut completely free from the donor area, since this may facilitate its transfer to the recipient site.
- The graft is immediately transferred to the prepared recipient bed and sutured (Fig. 27-20e). In order to immobilize the graft at the recipient site the sutures must be placed in the periosteum or the adjacent attached gingiva. After suturing, pressure is exerted against the graft for 5 min in order to eliminate blood and exudate between the graft and the recipient bed. The graft as well as the palatal wound is protected with a periodontal dressing. To retain the dressing in the palatal site, a stent usually has to be used.

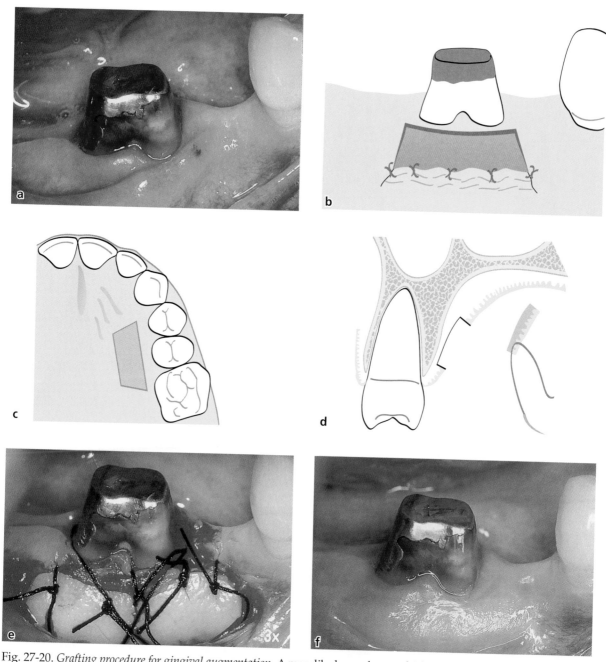

Fig. 27-20. *Grafting procedure for gingival augmentation.* A mandibular molar at which the patient experiences discomfort during toothbrushing due to interfering lining mucosa and high attachment of a frenulum (a). The decision was made to apically displace the attachment of the frenulum and augment the gingival zone through the placement of a free graft. A partial thickness flap is dissected to prepare a recipient bed. The flap is apically displaced and sutured (b). A graft with a thickness of 1.5-2 mm and of sufficient size and contour (a foil template of the recipient site may be used) is dissected from the palatal mucosa in the region of the premolars (c-d). The graft is immediately transferred to the prepared recipient bed and anchored by sutures to secure a close adaptation of the graft to the recipient bed (e). A periodontal dressing is applied to protect the graft. Following healing, a broad zone of keratinized tissue has been established (f).

- The sutures and periodontal dressing are removed after 1-2 weeks.

For a description of the pedicle graft procedure, see "Root coverage procedures" later in the chapter.

Healing following gingival augmentation procedures

Vestibular/gingival extension procedures
Since the specificity of the gingiva is determined by some inherent factor in the tissues, the postoperative results of vestibular extension procedures depend on the degree to which the various tissues contribute to the formation of granulation tissue in the wound area

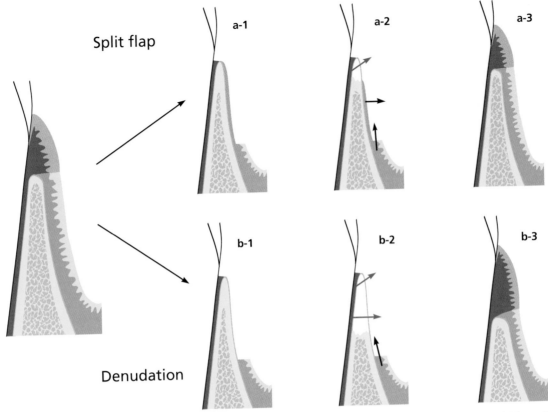

Fig. 27-21. Schematic drawing illustrating different stages of healing following the "split flap" (a) and "denuda-tion" (b) techniques. Cells from the oral mucosa, bone and periodontal ligament (arrows) participate in granulation tissue formation. Due to the difference in the degree of bone resorption (a-2, b-2), a larger area of the coronal por-tion of the wound is filled with granulation tissue from the periodontal ligament following "denudation" than fol-lowing the "split flap" technique. Since granulation tissue from the periodontal ligament possesses the ability to in-duce a keratinized epithelium, "denudation" usually results in a wider zone of keratinized tissue than is the case following the "split flap" technique (a-3, b-3).

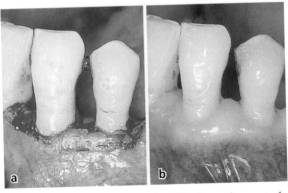

Fig. 27-22. Clinical photographs of the buccal aspect of a canine and a premolar following the removal of the entire zone of gingiva by a gingivectomy procedure (a). The healing result 9 months after surgery (b) shows the regain of keratinized tissue.

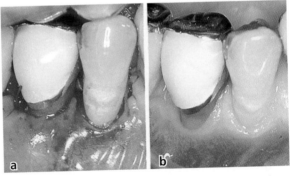

Fig. 27-23. Clinical photographs of a tooth region sub-jected to excision of the entire zone of gingiva by a flap procedure. The alveolar mucosa has been coronally dis-placed to achieve complete coverage of the surgically exposed alveolar bone (a). Healing has resulted in the reformation of a narrow zone of gingiva on the buccal aspect of the teeth, 9 months post-surgery (b).

(Karring et al. 1975). Following the "denudation" or "split flap technique", the wound area is filled with granulation tissue derived from the periodontal liga-ment, the tissue of the bone marrow spaces, the re-tained periosteal connective tissue, and the surround-ing gingiva and lining mucosa (Fig. 27-21). The degree of bone resorption induced by the surgical trauma influences the relative amount of granulation tissue which grows into the wound from these various tissue sources. The resorption of crestal bone exposes vary-ing amounts of the periodontal ligament tissue in the marginal area allowing granulation tissue from the periodontal ligament to fill out the coronal portion of the wound. The greater the bone loss, the greater the portion of the wound which becomes filled with granulation tissue from the periodontal ligament. This particular tissue possesses the capability to induce keratinization of the covering epithelium. This means that the widening of the keratinized tissue following "denudation" and "split flap" operations is achieved at the expense of a reduced bone height. The "denudation technique" results usually in more bone loss than the "split flap technique". Therefore, a greater amount of granulation tissue with the capability of inducing a keratinized epithelium develops in the marginal area following the "denudation technique" than following the "split flap technique". This is in accordance with the clinical observation that the "denudation technique" usually is superior to the "split flap technique" in increasing the width of keratinized tissue (Bohannan 1962a,b).

In a clinical study by Wennström (1983) periodontal pockets were eliminated by the use of a "gingivectomy" or a "flap" procedure, both of which involved the complete removal of the keratinized tissue. In the "gingivectomy" procedure the wounded area was left to heal by second intention, while in the "flap" procedure the alveolar mucosa was repositioned to achieve complete coverage of the surgically exposed alveolar bone (Figs. 27-22a & 27-23a). Irrespective of the surgical technique used, healing resulted in the reformation of keratinized tissue, the width of which, however, was greater following the "gingivectomy" procedure than following the "flap" procedure (Figs. 27-22b & 27-23b). The gingiva was formed because granulation tissue from the periodontal ligament with the capacity of inducing a keratinized epithelium had proliferated coronally along the root surface. This granulation tissue formation was obviously favored by a more pronounced bone resorption during the healing following the "gingivectomy" procedure.

It can be concluded that the success or failure in extending the width of keratinized tissue by the "denudation" or "split flap" techniques rests with the origin of granulation tissue, which is related to the extent of bone loss induced by the surgical trauma. This in turn means that the result with respect to increasing the gingival width by methods involving periosteal exposure or denudation of the alveolar bone is unpredictable. The use of such methods is therefore not justified in periodontal therapy. The procedures discussed merely represent examples of how lack of knowledge about basic biologic principles may

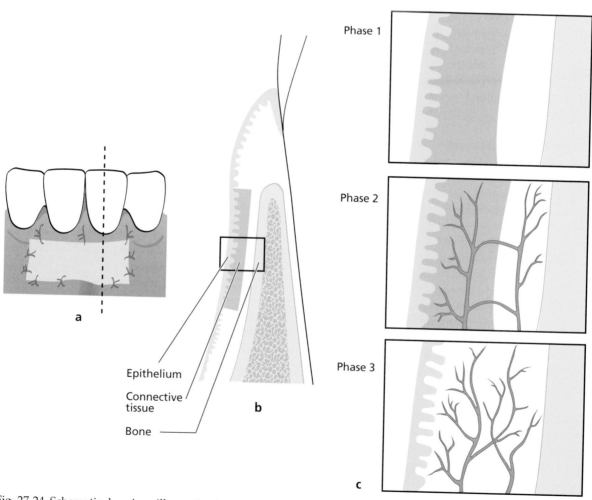

Fig. 27-24. Schematic drawings illustrating healing of a free gingival graft placed entirely on a connective tissue recipient bed (a). A cross-section through the area is shown in (b). The framed areas (c) illustrate the three phases into which the healing process can be divided.

lead to the development of inappropriate therapeutic methods.

Grafting procedures

Healing of free soft tissue grafts placed entirely on a connective tissue recipient bed has been studied in monkeys by Oliver et al. (1968) and Nobuto et al. (1988). According to these authors, healing can be divided into the following three phases (Fig. 27-24).

The initial phase (from 0 to 3 days)

In these first days of healing a thin layer of exudate is present between the graft and the recipient bed. During this period the grafted tissue survives with an avascular "plasmatic circulation" from the recipient bed. Therefore, it is essential for the survival of the graft that a close contact is established to the underlying recipient bed at the time of operation. A thick layer of exudate or a blood clot may hamper the "plasmatic circulation" and result in the rejection of the graft. The epithelium of the free graft degenerates early in the initial healing phase, and subsequently it becomes desquamated. In placing a graft over a recession, part of the recipient bed will be the avascular root surface. Since the graft is dependent on the nature of its bed for diffusion of plasma and subsequent revascularization, the utilization of free grafts in the treatment of gingival recessions involves a great risk of failure. The area of the graft over the avascular root surface must receive nutrients from the connective tissue bed that surrounds the recession. Thus, the amount of tissue that can be maintained over the root surface is limited by the size of the avascular area.

Revascularization phase (from 2 to 11 days)

After 4-5 days of healing, anastomoses are established between the blood vessels of the recipient bed and those in the grafted tissue. Thus, the circulation of blood is re-established in the preexisting blood vessels of the graft. The subsequent time period is characterized by capillary proliferation, which gradually results in a dense network of blood vessels in the graft. At the same time a fibrous union is established between the graft and the underlying connective tissue bed. The re-epithelialization of the graft occurs mainly by proliferation of epithelium from the adjacent tissues. If a free graft is placed over the denuded root surface, apical migration of epithelium along the tooth-facing surface of the graft may take place at this stage of healing.

Tissue maturation phase (from 11 to 42 days)

During this period the number of blood vessels in the transplant becomes gradually reduced, and after approximately 14 days the vascular system of the graft appears normal. Also, the epithelium gradually matures with the formation of a keratin layer during this stage of healing.

The establishment and maintenance of a "plasmatic circulation" between the recipient bed and the graft

during the initial phase of healing is critical for the result of this kind of therapy. Therefore, in order to ensure ideal conditions for healing, blood between the graft and the recipient site must be removed by exerting pressure against the graft following suturing.

ROOT COVERAGE

The main indications for root coverage procedures are esthetic/cosmetic demands (Fig. 27-25) and root hypersensitivity and management of shallow root caries lesions and cervical abrasions. Changing the topography of the marginal soft tissue in order to facilitate plaque control is also a common indication for root coverage procedures (Fig. 27-26).

It should be recalled that the two major causative factors in the development of marginal tissue recessions are plaque-induced periodontal inflammation and trauma caused by toothbrushing. The control of these factors will in most cases prevent further progression of the recession. This means that in tooth regions with a thin covering soft tissue, with or without an incipient recession, the patient should be encouraged to carry out effective but at the same time non-traumatic plaque control measures. With respect to toothbrushing, the Bass' method (Chapter 21) should be avoided and the patient should be instructed to use a technique creating as little apically directed pressure on the soft tissue margin as possible. A soft toothbrush should, of course, be used.

Miller (1985a) described a useful classification of recession defects, taking into consideration the anticipated root coverage that it is possible to obtain (Fig. 27-27):

- Class I: Marginal tissue recession not extending to the mucogingival junction. No loss of interdental bone or soft tissue.
- Class II: Marginal tissue recession extends to or beyond the mucogingival junction. No loss of interdental bone or soft tissue.
- Class III: Marginal tissue recession extends to or beyond the mucogingival junction. Loss of interdental bone or soft tissue is apical to the cemento-enamel junction, but coronal to the apical extent of the marginal tissue recession.
- Class IV: Marginal tissue recession extends beyond the mucogingival junction. Loss of interdental bone extends to a level apical to the extent of the marginal tissue recession.

While complete root coverage can be achieved in Class I and II defects, only partial coverage may be expected in Class III. Class IV recession defects are not amenable to root coverage. Consequently, the critical clinical variable to assess in order to determine the possible outcome of a root coverage procedure is the level of

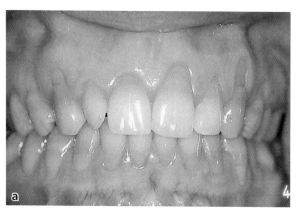
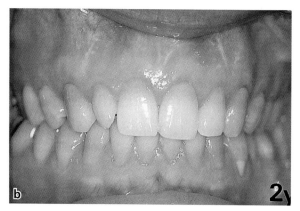

Fig. 27-25. A 25-year-old woman having esthetic concerns due to multiple soft tissue recessions in the maxilla and a high lip line (a). The gingiva is healthy and several of the exposed root surfaces show abrasion defects, indicating toothbrushing trauma as the causative factor for the development of the recessions. The brushing technique was altered and root coverage was surgically achieved. The 2-year post-treatment view (b).

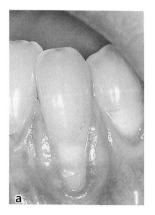
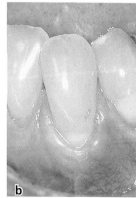

Fig. 27-26. A mandibular canine with a deep recession, which offers problems with respect to self-performed plaque control (a). To facilitate plaque control the position of the soft tissue margin was altered surgically (b).

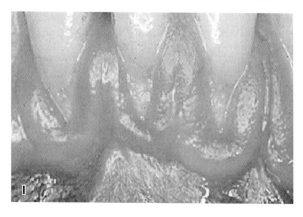
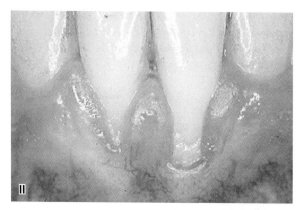
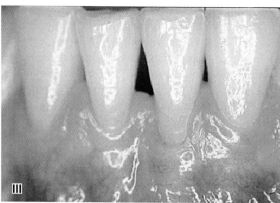
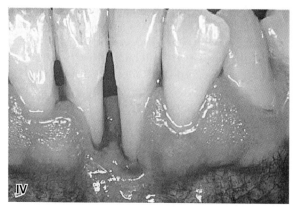

Fig. 27-27. The Miller classification of recession defects (see text).

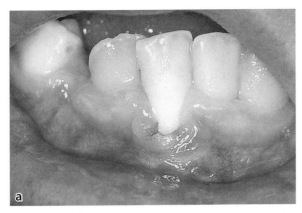
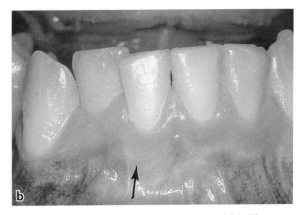

Fig. 27-28. A 9-year-old boy showing recession at tooth 41. The tooth is rotated and buccally positioned (a). The minimal amount of gingiva found apical to the recession shows pronounced signs of inflammation. The plaque control in the region was improved but surgical intervention was postponed. (b) The same tooth area at the age of 14 years. Note the spontaneous soft tissue repair that has taken place at tooth 41 as a consequence of the improved plaque control and the growth in the alveolar process.

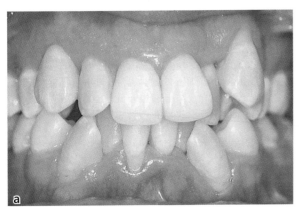
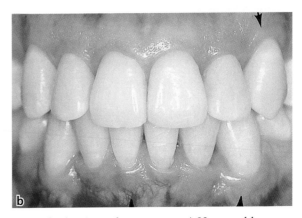

Fig. 27-29. Spontaneous repair of soft tissue recessions following orthodontic tooth movement. A 22-year-old woman showing recessions and thin marginal tissues at prominently positioned teeth, particularly 23, 33, 41 and 43 (a). Following proper alignment of the teeth (b), the recessions have spontaneously been resolved and an increased gingival height can be noted.

periodontal tissue support at the proximal surfaces of the tooth.

Recession defects in the child need particular attention. In the growing child, recession defects may be eliminated spontaneously, provided an adequate plaque control is established and maintained (Fig. 27-28). Andelin-Sobocki et al. (1991) reported from a 3-year prospective study that 25 out of 35 recessions with an initial depth of 0.5-3.0 mm spontaneously healed following improvement of the oral hygiene standard. Furthermore, all but three of remaining recessions showed a decrease and no site demonstrated an increase in depth. Hence, reparative surgical treatment of soft tissue recessions in the developing dentition may not be necessary and should preferably be postponed until the growth has been completed.

Furthermore, in an orthodontic case showing a recession defect and a thin (delicate) gingiva due to prominent position of the tooth (Fig. 27-29a), surgical treatment for root coverage should be postponed until the orthodontic therapy is completed. The recession, as well as the dehiscence, will decrease as a conse-

quence of the lingual movement of the tooth into a more proper position within the alveolar bone (Fig. 27-29b) and, if still indicated, the root coverage procedure will show higher predictability if performed after than before the tooth movement.

Root coverage procedures

Surgical procedures used in the treatment of recession defects may basically be classified as (1) pedicle soft tissue graft procedures and (2) free soft tissue graft procedures.

The pedicle graft procedures are, depending on the direction of transfer, grouped as (1) rotational flap procedures (e.g. laterally sliding flap, double papilla flap, oblique rotated flap) or (2) advanced flap procedures (e.g. coronally repositioned flap, semilunar coronally repositioned flap). The latter procedures do not include rotation or lateral movement of the pedicle graft. Within the group of pedicle graft procedures, guided tissue regeneration procedures may also be

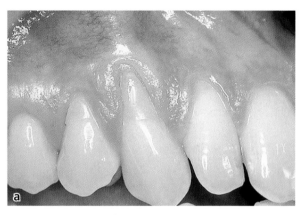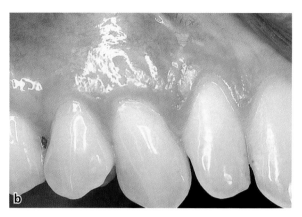

Fig. 27-30. A canine showing pronounced recession and a composite resin restoration in the exposed root (a). Following removal of the restoration the exposed root was surgically covered with soft tissue (pedicle graft). (b) 2-year postoperative healing result.

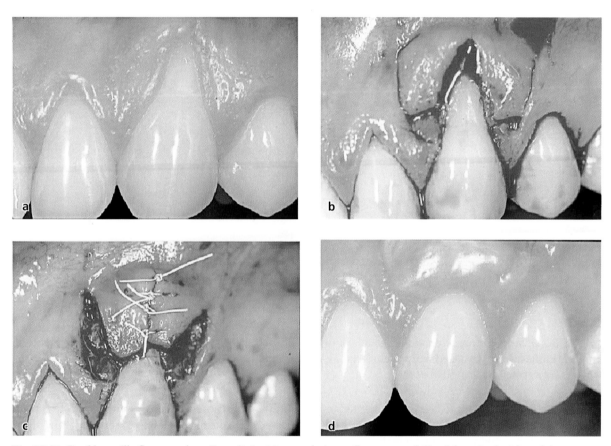

Fig. 27-31. *Double papilla flap procedure*. By split incisions soft tissue flaps are mobilized from both sides of the recession (b) and sutured together for coverage of the exposed root (c). The healing result 6 months postoperatively shows complete root coverage (d).

included, i.e. rotational and advanced flap procedures involving the placement of a membrane barrier between the graft and the root.

The autogenous free soft tissue graft procedure may be performed as (1) an epithelialized graft or as (2) a subepithelial connective tissue graft (non-epithelialized graft), both usually taken from the area of the masticatory mucosa in the palate.

In the selection of treatment procedure factors such as depth and width of recession, availability of donor tissue, presence of muscle attachments and esthetics have to be taken into consideration.

Treatment of the exposed root surface

Before root coverage is attempted the exposed portion of the root should be rendered free from bacterial plaque. Preferably, this is achieved by the use of a rubber cup and a polishing paste, particularly on root surfaces that have been exposed due to toothbrushing trauma. Controlled clinical trials have shown no differences in terms of root coverage or residual probing

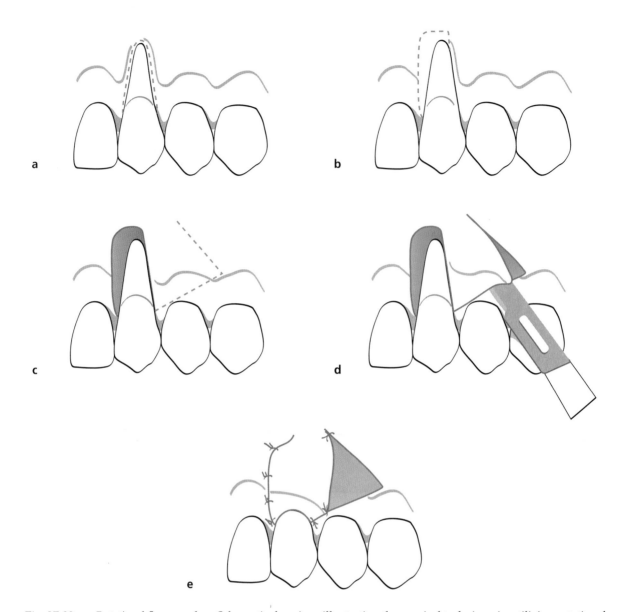

Fig. 27-32a-e. *Rotational flap procedure*. Schematic drawings illustrating the surgical technique in utilizing rotational pedicle grafts to cover localized recession defects (see text for explanation).

depth between teeth that had been instrumented (root planed) or polished only (Oles et al. 1985, Pini Prato et al. 1999). Extensive root planing may therefore only be performed in situations where a reduced root prominence would be considered beneficial for graft survival or tissue regeneration, or if a shallow root caries lesion is diagnosed. The presence of a filling in the root does not preclude the possibility for root coverage (Fig. 27-30), but the filling should be removed before the root is covered with soft tissue.

Miller (1985b) advocated the use of root surface demineralization agents to be an important treatment component in the free soft tissue graft procedure. In addition to the removal of the smear layer, the use of acid demineralization of the root surface is intended to facilitate the formation of a new fibrous attachment through exposure of collagen fibrils of the dentine matrix and allow subsequent interdigitation of these

fibrils with those in the covering connective tissue. However, controlled clinical trials comparing the effect of free gingival graft procedures with and without root conditioning (Ibbott et al. 1985, Bertrand & Dunlap 1988, Laney et al. 1992, Bouchard et al. 1997, Caffesse et al. 2000) have failed to demonstrate a beneficial clinical effect from the use of acid root biomodification. Also, controlled studies comparing the effect of laterally positioned flap with and without root conditioning showed no statistically significant positive effect of the use of acid root conditioning (Oles et al. 1985, Caffesse et al. 1987). Gottlow et al. (1986) evaluated the healing following treatment of localized gingival recessions with coronally positioned flaps and citric acid root biomodification in a controlled study in dogs. The histological analysis after 3 months of healing disclosed no differences in the amount of root coverage or new connective tissue attachment between citric acid treated sites and saline treated control sites. Although root resorption was a common finding among the citric acid treated teeth in this dog model, such a finding has not been commonly reported in humans. Hence, the literature clearly indicates that the inclusion of root conditioning does not improve the healing outcome of root coverage procedures.

Pedicle soft tissue graft procedures

Rotational flap procedures
The use of a laterally repositioned flap to cover areas with localized recession was introduced by Grupe & Warren (1956). This technique, which was called *the laterally sliding flap* operation, involved the reflection of a full thickness flap in a donor area adjacent to the defect and the subsequent lateral displacement of this flap to cover the exposed root surface (Fig. 27-19). In order to reduce the risk for recession on the donor tooth, Grupe (1966) suggested that the marginal soft tissue should not be included in the flap. Staffileno (1964) and Pfeifer & Heller (1971) advocated the use of a split thickness flap to minimize the potential risk for development of dehiscence at the donor tooth. Other modifications of the procedure presented are *the double papilla flap* (Fig. 27-31) (Cohen & Ross 1968), *the oblique rotational flap* (Pennel et al. 1965), *the rotation flap* (Patur 1977), and *the transpositioned flap* (Bahat et al. 1990).

Technique
- The rotational flap procedure (Fig. 27-32) is initiated with the preparation of the recipient site. A reverse bevel incision is made all along the soft tissue margin of the defect (Fig. 27-32a). After removal of the dissected pocket epithelium, the exposed root surface is thoroughly curetted.
- At a distance of approximately 3 mm from the wound edge which delineates the defect at the side opposite the donor area, a superficial incision is made extending from the gingival margin to a level approximately 3 mm apical to the defect (Fig. 27-32b). Another superficial incision is placed horizontally from this incision to the opposite wound edge. The epithelium together with the outer portion of the connective tissue within the area delineated by these incisions and the wound edges is removed by sharp dissection (Fig. 27-32c). In this way a 3-mm-wide recipient bed is created at the one side of the defect, as well as apically to the defect.
- A tissue flap to cover the recession is then dissected

in the adjacent donor area. The preparation of this flap is initiated by a vertical superficial incision placed parallel to the wound edge of the recession and at a distance which exceeds the width of the recipient bed and the exposed root surface of approximately 3 mm (Fig. 27-32c). This incision is extended beyond the apical level of the recipient bed and is terminated within the lining mucosa with an oblique releasing incision directed towards the recession site. An incision connecting the vertical incision and the incision previously made around the recession is placed approximately 3 mm apical to the gingival margin of the donor site.
- A split thickness flap is then prepared by sharp dissection within the area delineated by these incisions so that a layer of connective tissue is left covering the bone in the donor area when the flap is laterally displaced over the denuded root surface (Fig. 27-32d). It is important that the oblique releasing incision is made so far apically that the tissue flap can be placed on the recipient bed without being subjected to tearing forces when adjacent soft tissues are moved. The prepared tissue flap is rotated about 90° when sutured at the recipient bed (Fig. 27-32e).

The suturing of the flap should secure a close adaptation of the pedicle graft to the underlying recipient bed. Pressure is applied against the flap for 2-3 min in order to further secure a good adaptation. To protect the surgical area during the initial phase of healing, a periodontal dressing is applied. A light curing dressing material, e.g. Barricaid™ (Dentsply International Inc., Milford, DE, US), is preferably used since this can be applied without dislocating the flap and has a favorable esthetic appearance.
- Following removal of the dressing and the sutures, usually after 10-14 days, the patient is instructed to avoid mechanical toothcleaning for a further 2 weeks, but to use twice daily rinsing with a chlorhexidine solution as a means of plaque control.

Advanced flaps
Since the lining mucosa is elastic, a mucosal flap raised beyond the mucogingival junction can be stretched in coronal direction to cover exposed root surfaces (Harvey 1965, Sumner 1969, Brustein 1979, Allen & Miller 1989, Wennström & Zucchelli 1996, Pino Prato et al. 1999). The coronally advanced flap can be used for root coverage of a single tooth as well as multiple teeth, provided suitable donor tissue is available. In situations with only shallow recession defects and minimal probing pocket depth labially, the *"semilunar*

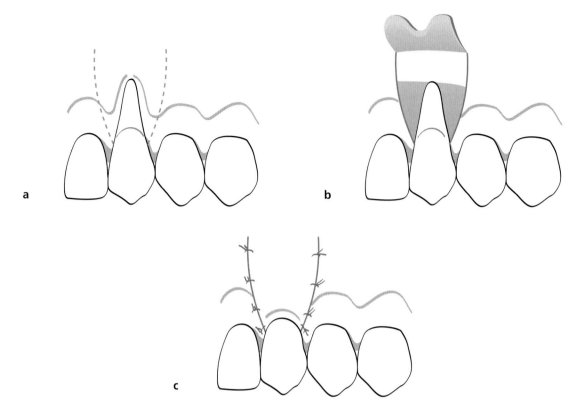

Fig. 27-33a-c. *Coronally advanced flap procedure*. Schematic drawings illustrating the surgical technique in utilizing coronally advanced pedicle grafts to cover localized recession defects (see text for explanation).

coronally repositioned flap" may offer an alternative approach (Harlan 1907, Tarnow 1986).

Technique
Coronally advanced flap procedure (Fig. 27-33)

- The coronally advanced flap procedure is initiated with the placement of two apically divergent vertical releasing incisions, extending from a point coronal to the cemento-enamel junction at the mesial and distal line axis of the tooth and apically into the lining mucosa (Fig. 27-33a).
- A split thickness flap is prepared by sharp dissection mesial and distal to the recession and connected with an intracrevicular incision. Apical to the receded soft tissue margin on the facial aspect of the tooth, a full thickness flap is elevated to maintain maximal thickness of tissue flap to be used for root coverage (Fig. 27-33b). Approximately 3 mm apical

to the bone dehiscence, a horizontal incision is made through the periosteum, followed by a blunt dissection into the vestibular lining mucosa to release muscle tension. The blunt dissection is extended buccally and laterally to such an extent that the mucosal graft can be easily positioned coronally at the level of the cemento-enamel junction.

- The tissue flap is coronally advanced, adjusted for optimal fit to the prepared recipient bed, and secured at the level of the cemento-enamel junction by suturing the flap to the connective tissue bed in the papilla regions (Fig. 27-33c). Additional lateral sutures are placed to carefully close the wound of the releasing incisions. A light curing dressing may be applied to protect the area during initial healing.

Fig. 27-34 illustrates the treatment of a recession defect with the use of the coronally advanced flap procedure.

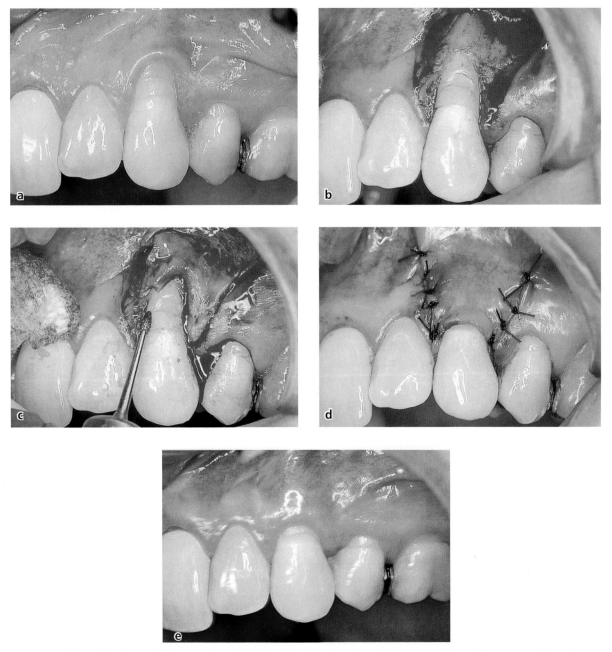

Fig. 27-34. *Coronally advanced flap procedure*. A deep and wide recession defect on a canine with a composite resin restoration in the exposed root portion (a). Before preparation of the pedicle graft, the root is polished with pumice and a rubber cup. A split flap has been dissected mesial and distal to the root, and a full thickness flap apical to the recession (b). Approximately 4 mm apical to the bone dehiscence the periosteum has been cut and a blunt dissection performed to facilitate the coronal positioning of the pedicle graft. The composite resin restoration is removed (c) followed by a close suturing of the pedicle graft to cover the exposed root surface (d). Healing outcome 1-year postoperatively (e).

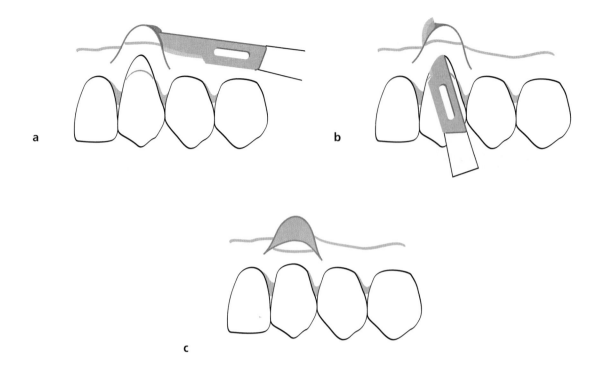

Fig. 27-35a-c. *Semi-lunar coronally repositioned flap procedure.* Schematic drawings illustrating the surgical technique in utilizing coronally displaced pedicle grafts to cover shallow localized recession defects (see text for explanation).

Semi-lunar coronally repositioned flap procedure (Fig. 27-35)

- A semi-lunar incision is placed apically to the recession and at a distance from the soft tissue margin, which should be approximately 3 mm greater than the depth of the recession. The outline of the incision should be parallel to the curvature of the gingival margin (Fig. 27-35a). The incision is extended into the papilla region on each side of the tooth, but care should be taken to maintain a broad base of anchorage to secure a collateral blood supply to the pedicle graft.
- A split thickness dissection of the facially located tissue is then made by an intracrevicular incision extending apically to the level of the semi-lunar incision (Fig. 27-35b). The mid-facial soft tissue graft is coronally repositioned to the level of the cemento-enamel junction (Fig. 27-35c) and stabilized by light pressure for 5 min.
- No suturing is needed but a light curing dressing is applied for wound protection.

Coronally advanced flap procedure for multiple recessions (Fig. 27-36)

Zucchelli and De Sanctis (2000) described a flap design for the treatment of multiple recessions, which allows for optimal adaptation of the flap following its coronal advancement without placement of vertical releasing incisions.

- Oblique submarginal incisions are placed in the interdental areas and connected with intracrevicular incisions at the recession defects. The incisions are extended to include one tooth on each side of the teeth to be treated to facilitate a coronal repositioning of the flap. The oblique incisions over the interdental areas are placed in such a manner that the "surgically created papillae" mesial to the midline of the surgical field are dislocated apically and distally, while the papillae of the flap distal to the mid-line are shifted in a more apical and mesial position (27-36a).
- Starting at the oblique interdental incisions, a split-thickness flap is dissected (Fig. 27-36c). Apical to the level of the root exposures, a full-thickness flap is raised to provide maximum soft tissue thickness of the flap to be coronally positioned over the roots (Fig. 27-36d).
- At the most apical portion of the flap, the periosteum is incised and followed by dissection into the vestibular lining mucosa to eliminate all muscle tension. The mobilized flap should be able to passively reach a level coronal to the CEJ at each single tooth in the surgical field.
- The remaining facial portion of the interdental papillae is de-epithelialized to create connective tissue beds to which the flap can be sutured.
- Sutures are placed to accomplish a precise adaptation of the coronally advanced flap against the teeth and to the interdental connective tissue beds (Fig.

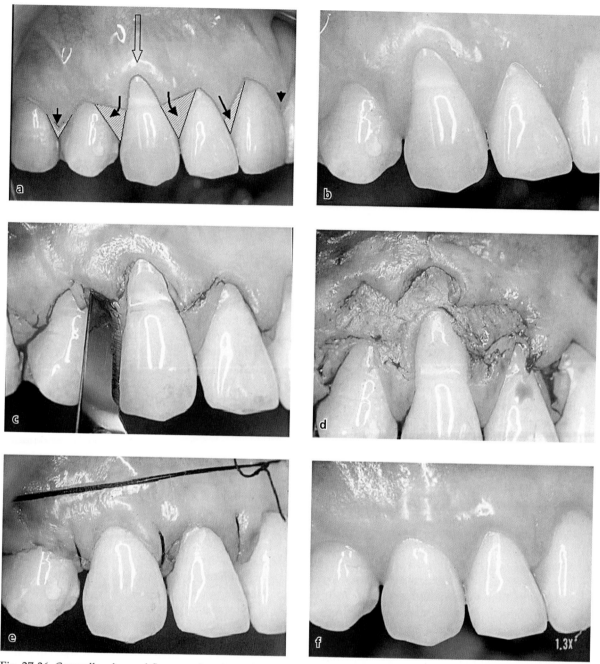

Fig. 27-36. *Coronally advanced flap procedure for multiple recessions.* (a-e) The oblique incisions over the interdental areas are placed in such a manner that the "surgically created papillae" mesial to the midline of the surgical field are dislocated apically and distally, while the papillae of the flap distal to the mid-line are shifted in a more apical and mesial position (see text for explanation). (f) The 1-year post-treatment view.

27-36e). In addition, a horizontal double mattress suture is placed to reduce lip tension on the marginal portion of the flap.

Pedicle soft tissue graft procedures combined with membrane barriers

The use of a membrane barrier, according to the principles of guided tissue regeneration (GTR, see Chapter 28), in conjunction with pedicle soft tissue graft procedures was introduced as a treatment modality for root coverage (Pini Prato et al. 1992). A membrane barrier is placed between the graft and the root in order to favor the regeneration of the periodontium.

According to the concept of the GTR, a critical factor for the outcome of the treatment procedure is that a space for tissue formation is established between the facial root surface and the membrane and maintained during the healing. In order to create such a space, Pini Prato et al. (1992) suggested that extensive root planing should be carried out to produce a concave root morphology. In addition, bending of the membrane by the placement of a Teflon suture (Fig. 27-37) in mesiodistal direction through the membrane could facilitate the maintenance of an adequate space. Specially designed membranes for the treatment of recession type defects are also available, such as non-absorbable tita-

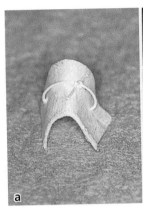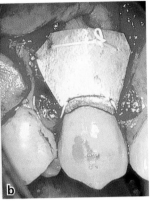

Fig. 27-37a,b. Membrane barrier for treatment of recession defects. A Teflon suture has been placed in mesiodistal direction through an expanded polytetrafluorethylene (ePTFE) membrane in order to establish adequate space between the barrier and the root surface.

nium-reinforced expanded polytetrafluorethylene (ePTFE) membranes (Fig. 27-38). In addition, a variety of bioabsorbable membranes are commercially available, but many of these may not be rigid enough for maintaining required space during healing.

Technique

The principles of using a GTR procedure in the treatment of recessions were originally outlined by Pini Prato et al. (1992). Commonly, the pedicle graft used in the GTR procedure is generated through a coronally advanced flap (Fig. 27-38).

- Apically divergent vertical releasing incisions are made at the mesial and distal line axis of the tooth, extending from a point coronal to the cemento-enamel junction and apically into the lining mucosa (Fig. 27-38b). A trapezium-shaped full-thickness flap is raised beyond the bone dehiscence. A horizontal incision is then made through the periosteum at the base of the raised mucoperiosteal flap, followed by a blunt supraperiosteal dissection to such a depth that the trapezoidal flap can be easily advanced coronally to the desired position. Depending on the degree of coronal repositioning, the facial portion of the interdental papillae may need to be de-epithelialized to prepare proper recipient beds for the pedicle graft.
- The root is extensively planed or ground to obtain a concave profile of the root surface, thereby providing space for tissue formation. If a titanium-reinforced membrane is used, the root profile may not need to be changed to establish the required space between the root and the membrane.

- The membrane barrier to be used is trimmed to cover the exposed root and approximately 3 mm of the bone laterally and apically of the dehiscence (Fig. 27-38c). Following trimming, the membrane is positioned over the root and anchored to the tooth by a sling suture placed at the level of the cemento-enamel junction.
- The mobilized flap is coronally positioned and secured by interdentally placed interrupted sutures (Fig. 27-38d). The membrane should be completely covered by the flap to reduce the risk for bacterial contamination during the healing. Additional sutures are placed to close the lateral wound of the releasing incisions.
- To avoid the risk of collapse of the membrane over the root, which may limit the space for blood clot formation, a periodontal dressing should not be applied.
- The patient is advised to use a chlorhexidine mouthrinse for plaque control and not to use any mechanical cleaning devices for at least 6 weeks in the tooth region subjected to surgery.
- The use of non-biodegradable membrane barriers requires a second surgery for membrane removal, usually after 5-6 weeks (Fig. 27-38e-f). A partial thickness trapezoidal flap is raised to expose the membrane. Following its removal, the flap is repositioned at the level of the cemento-enamel junction to completely cover the newly formed tissue. Mechanical plaque control is reinstituted 4 weeks after membrane removal.

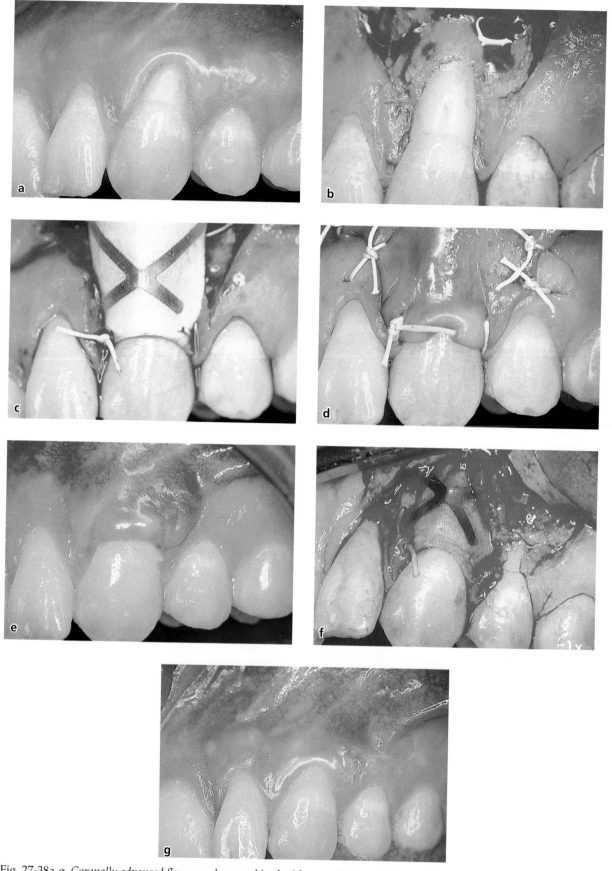

Fig. 27-38a-g. *Coronally advanced flap procedure combined with a non-biodegradable membrane barrier.* A recession defect at tooth 23 requiring treatment due to the patient's esthetic demands (see text for explanation). (g) The 1-yr postoperative healing result.

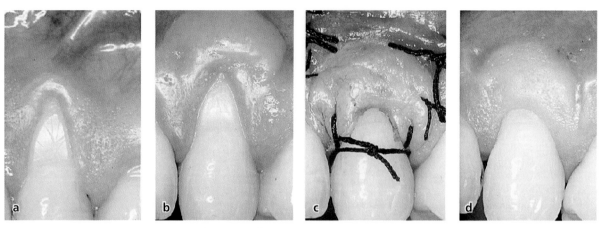

Fig. 27-39. *Two-stage epithelialized free soft tissue graft procedure.* (a-c) An epithelialized soft tissue graft is placed apical to the recession and allowed to heal. At a second stage surgery a coronally advanced flap procedure is performed to achieve coverage of the denuded root. (d) The 1-year postoperative healing result.

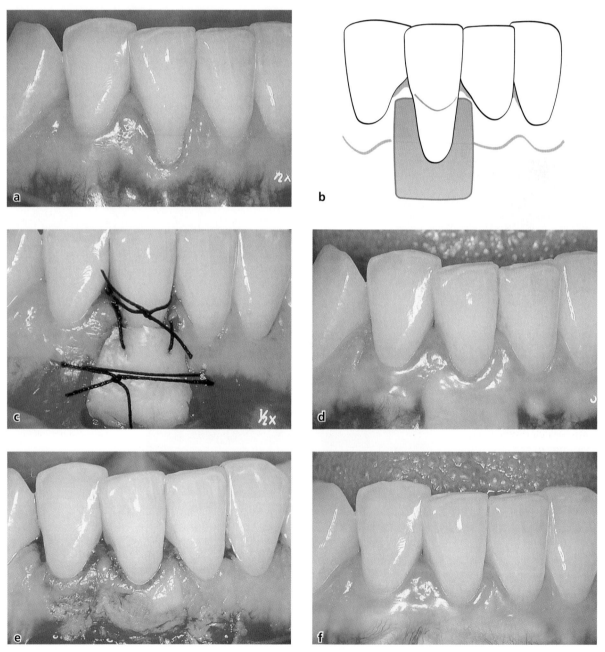

Fig. 27-40a-f. *Epithelialized free soft tissue graft procedure.* A recession defect at a mandibular central incisor treated with the free graft procedure (see text for explanation).

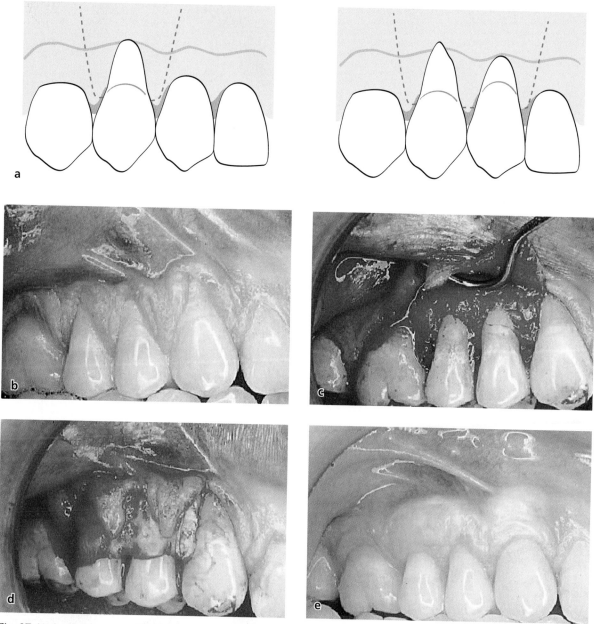

Fig. 27-41. (a-d) *Free connective tissue graft combined with a coronally advanced flap procedure* (see text for explanation). (e) The 1-year post-treatment result.

Free soft tissue graft procedures

A free soft tissue graft of masticatory mucosa is usually selected when there is no acceptable donor tissue present in the area adjacent to the recession defect or when a thicker marginal tissue is desirable. The procedure can be used for the treatment of a single tooth as well as for groups of teeth. The graft used may either be (1) an epithelialized graft or (2) a subepithelial connective tissue graft of palatal masticatory mucosa.

Epithelialized soft tissue graft

The epithelialized free soft tissue graft procedure can be performed either as a two-step surgical technique, where an epithelialized free soft tissue graft is placed apical to the recession and following healing is coronally positioned over the denuded root (Fig. 27-39) (Bernimoulin et al. 1975, Guinard & Caffesse 1978),

or as a one-step technique, in which the graft is placed directly over the root surface (Fig. 27-40) (Sullivan & Atkins 1968a,b, Miller 1982). The latter technique has been the one most commonly used.

Technique

The principles of utilizing free mucosal grafts were outlined by Sullivan & Atkins (1968a,b) and later modified by Miller (1982).

• Before any incisions the exposed root surface is carefully scaled and root planed (Fig. 27-40a). The convexity of the root may be reduced to minimize the mesiodistal avascular recipient bed.
• As in the treatment with pedicle grafts, the preparation of *the recipient bed* is crucial for the success of free graft procedure. A 3-4-mm-wide recipient connective tissue bed apical as well as lateral of the

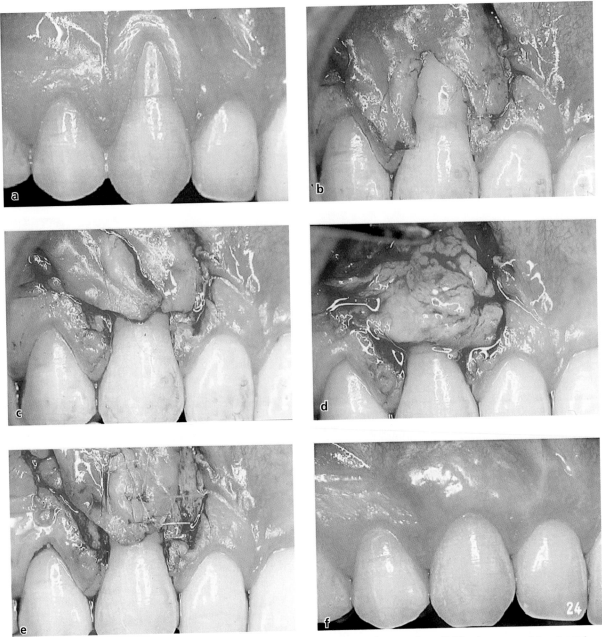

Fig. 27-42. (a-e) *Free connective tissue graft combined with a double papilla flap procedure.* (f) The 1-year post-treatment result.

recession defect should be prepared (Fig. 27-40b). The area is demarcated by first placing a horizontal incision, at the level of the cemento-enamel junction, in the interdental tissue on each side of the tooth to be treated. Subsequently, two vertical incisions, extending from the incision line placed in the interdental tissue to a level approximately 4-5 mm apical of the recession, are placed. A horizontal incision is then made, connecting the two vertical incisions at their apical termination. Starting from an intracrevicular incision, a split incision is made to sharply dissect the epithelium and the outer portion of the connective tissue within the demarcated area.

- To ensure that a graft of sufficient size and proper contour is removed from the donor area, a foil template of the recipient site is prepared. This template

is transferred to the donor site, the palatal mucosa in the region of the premolars, and the required size of the graft is outlined by a shallow incision. A graft with a thickness of 2-3 mm is then dissected from the donor area (Fig. 27-20c-d). It is advocated to place sutures in the graft before it is cut completely free from the donor area since this may facilitate its transfer to the recipient site. Following the removal of the graft, pressure is applied to the wound area for control of bleeding.

- The graft is immediately placed on the prepared recipient bed. In order to immobilize the graft at the recipient site the sutures must be anchored in the periosteum or in the adjacent attached gingiva. Adequate numbers of sutures are placed to secure a close adaptation of the graft to the underlying connective tissue bed and root surface (Fig. 27-40c).

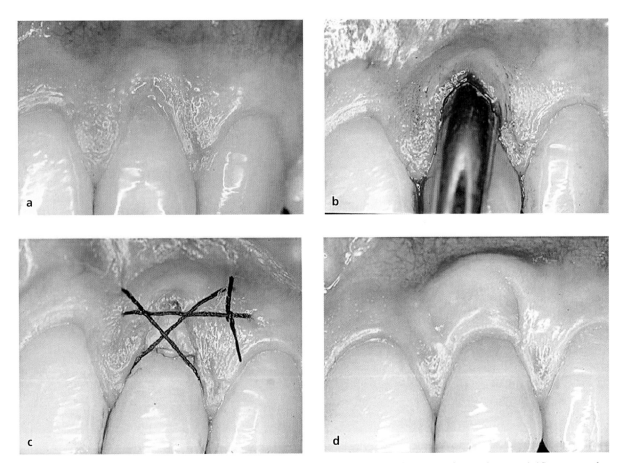

Fig. 27-43. (a-c) *Free connective tissue graft procedure – the "envelope technique"* (see text for explanation) (Courtesy of Dr M. Cattabriga). (d) The 1-year post-treatment result (Courtesy of Dr P. Cortellini).

Before the placement of a periodontal dressing, pressure is exerted against the graft for some minutes in order to eliminate blood between the graft and the recipient bed. The wound in the donor area in the palate is, following the control of the bleeding, covered by a periodontal dressing. To maintain the dressing in place during the healing phase, the use of an acrylic plate may often be required.

- The sutures and periodontal dressing are usually maintained for 2 weeks. The appearance of a grafted area after 3-month healing is shown in Fig. 27-40d. A gingivoplasty may sometimes be indicated to achieve a satisfactory esthetic appearance of the grafted area (Fig. 27-40e-f).

Connective tissue graft
The technique utilizing a subepithelial soft tissue graft, i.e. the connective tissue, involves the placement of the graft directly over the exposed root and the mobilization of a mucosal flap to be coronally (Fig. 27-41) or laterally (Fig. 27-42) moved for coverage of the graft (Langer & Langer 1985, Nelson 1987, Harris 1992, Bruno 1994). An alternative technique is to place the base of the connective tissue graft within an "envelope" prepared by an undermining partial thickness incision from the soft tissue margin, i.e. part of the graft will rest on the root surface coronal to the soft tissue margin (Fig. 27-43) (Raetzke 1985, Allen 1994). For the treatment of multiple adjacent recessions, a multi-envelope recipient bed ("tunnel") may be prepared (Zabalegui et al. 1999). The subepithelial connective graft is harvested from the palate or the retromolar pad by the use of a "trap door" approach (Fig. 27-44d-f). Compared to the epithelialized graft, the connective tissue graft is preferable due to less invasive palatal wound and improved esthetic result.

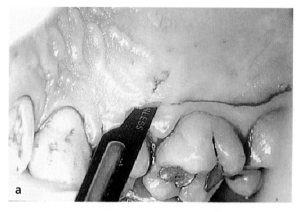

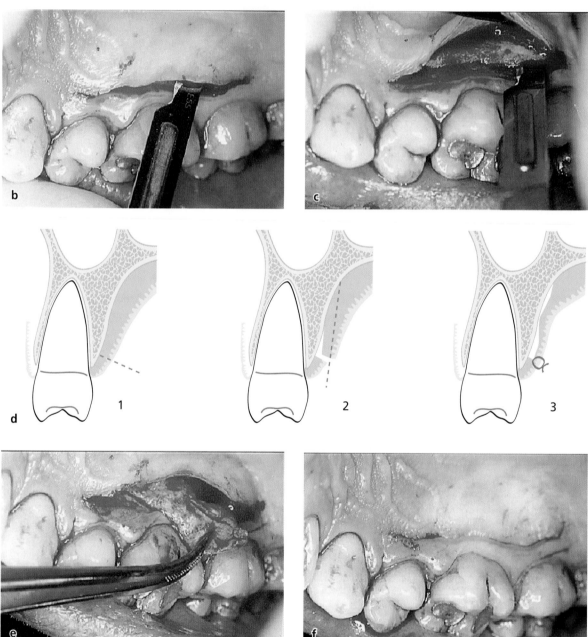

Fig. 27-44a-f. *"Trap-door" technique for harvest of a free connective tissue graft* (see text for explanation).

Technique
Connective tissue graft covered by a coronally advanced flap
(Fig. 27-41)
• A horizontal incision is first made in the facial sur-

face of the interdental tissue on each side of the teeth to be treated (Fig. 27-41a). The incision should be placed just coronal to the intended level of root coverage. Care should be taken not to decrease the

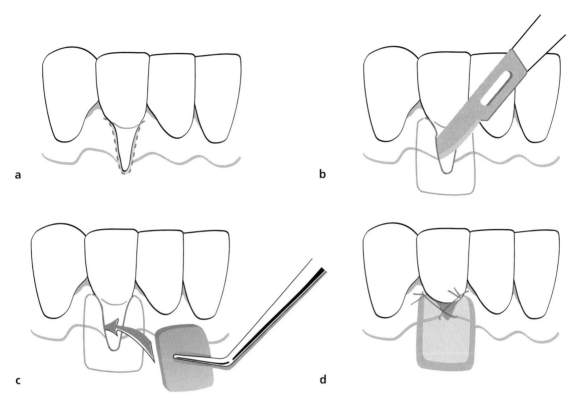

Fig. 27-45a-c. *Free connective tissue graft procedure – the "envelope technique"*. Schematic drawings illustrating the surgical technique (see text for explanation).

height of the papillae. Subsequently, starting from the line of incision in the interdental area at the mesial and distal termination of the surgical area, two divergent, vertical incisions are placed and extended well beyond the mucogingival line.

- A split thickness flap is then prepared by sharp dissection and elevated to such an extent that it can be coronally repositioned at the level of the cemento-enamel junction without tension (Fig. 27-41c).

- A subepithelial connective tissue graft of masticatory mucosa is harvested on the palatal aspect of the maxillary premolars (or from the retromolar pad) by the use of a "trap door" approach (Fig. 27-44). Before incisions are placed, the available thickness of the mucosa is estimated by the use of the tip of the syringe. A horizontal incision, perpendicular to the underlying bone surface, is made approximately 3 mm apical to the soft tissue margin (Fig. 27-44a). The mesiodistal extension of the incision is determined by the graft size required. To facilitate the removal of the graft, a vertical releasing incision can be made at the mesial termination of the primary incision. An incision is then placed from the line of the first incision and directed apically to perform a split incision of the palatal mucosa (Fig. 27-44b-f). A small periosteal elevator or the scalpel is used to release the connective tissue graft from the bone. Sutures may be placed in the graft before it is released completely free from the donor area to facilitate its placement at the recipient site.

- The graft is immediately placed in the recipient site (Fig. 27-41d) and secured in position with interrupted sutures or a sling suture. The mucosal flap is then sutured to cover the connective tissue graft. Interrupted sutures are placed in the papilla regions as well as along the wound of the vertical incisions. A surgical dressing may be applied for protection of the area during the first week of healing.

The "envelope" technique (Fig. 27-45)

- With the use of the "envelope" technique the recipient site is prepared by first eliminating the sulcular epithelium by an internal beveled incision (Fig. 27-45a). Secondly, an "envelope" is prepared apically and laterally of the recession by split incisions (Fig. 27-45b). The depth of the preparation should be 3-5 mm in all directions. In apical direction, the preparation of the site should extend beyond the mucogingival junction to facilitate the placement of the connective tissue graft and to allow for coronal advancement of the mucosal flap at time of suturing.

- A foil template may be used for the harvest of an appropriately sized connective tissue graft. The graft, which is obtained by the "trap door" approach described above (Fig. 27-44), is inserted into the prepared "envelope" and positioned to cover the exposed root surface (Fig. 27-45c-d).

- Sutures are placed to secure graft position (Fig. 27-45d). A crossed sling suture may be placed to coronally advance the mucosal flap. Pressure is ap-

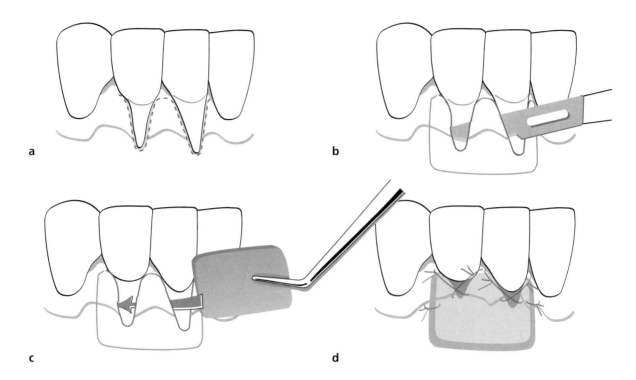

Fig. 27-46a-d. *Free connective tissue graft procedure – the "tunnel technique"*. Schematic drawings illustrating the surgical technique (see text for explanation).

plied for 5 min to closely adapt the graft to the root surface and covering soft tissue. Application of a periodontal dressing is usually not required.

Fig. 27-43 shows the treatment of a recession defect with the "envelope" technique.

The "tunnel" technique (Fig. 27-46)
- In case multiple adjacent recessions are to be treated, "envelopes" are prepared for each tooth as described above. However, the lateral split incisions are extended so that the multi-envelopes are connected mesially and distally to form a mucosal tunnel. Care should be taken to avoid detachment of the papillae.
- The graft is gently positioned inside the tunnel and its mesial and distal extremities are fixed with two interrupted sutures. Sling sutures may be placed to coronally advance the mucosal flap over the exposed portions of the connective tissue graft. Pressure is applied for 5 min to closely adapt the graft to the root surface and covering soft tissue. Application of a periodontal dressing is often not required.

Clinical outcome of root coverage procedures

Independent of the modality of surgical procedure used to obtain soft tissue root coverage, shallow residual probing depths, gain in clinical attachment and an increase in gingival height are the common characteristics of treatment outcome. Although the major indication for performing root coverage procedures is esthetic demands by the patient, almost no studies have included assessments of esthetics as an endpoint of success. Instead, the common outcome variable used is the amount of root coverage achieved, expressed as a percentage of the initial depth of the recession. In some studies also the proportion of treated sites showing complete root coverage is reported.

Root coverage
An overall comparison of the treatment outcome of root coverage procedures is hampered by the fact that comparatively few studies have presented well-documented clinical results. A summary of published studies providing data for calculation of the average amount of the initial recession defect that has been successfully covered following treatment (Table 27-1) shows that an average of 63-86% root coverage may be expected, depending on the treatment procedure used. However, the variation (range) in treatment outcome for the various procedures, both within and between studies, is large. This indicates that the procedures are operator sensitive and/or that factors influencing the treatment outcome have not been adequately considered. Complete coverage of the recession defect is the ultimate goal of the therapy. Table 27-2 summarizes available data on the predictability of complete root coverage with the use of the various

Table 27-1. Summary of the data available in the literature on the amount of root coverage obtainable with various procedures

Root coverage procedure			Root coverage	
	No. of studies	No. of patients/ teeth	Mean % of initial recession	Range
Rotational flaps	10	222/235	68%	41-74
Coronally advanced flap	12	216/416	80%	55-99
Guided tissue regeneration	34	576/682	75%	48-94
Free connective tissue graft	30	589/796	86%	53-98
Epithelialized free soft tissue graft	16	335/491	63%	11-87

Table 27-2. Summary of the data available in the literature on the predictability of complete root coverage following the use of various procedures

Root coverage procedure			Complete root coverage	
	No. of studies	No. of patients/ teeth	Mean % of teeth	Range
Rotational flaps	1	30/30	43%	-
Coronally advanced flap	10	188/388	50%	9-95
Guided tissue regeneration	23	344/440	36%	0-75
Free connective tissue graft	25	532/715	61%	0-93
Epithelialized free soft tissue graft	10	253/380	28%	0-90

procedures. The average percentage of complete root coverage following pedicle or free graft procedures varies between 28% and 61%; the lowest figure for the epithelialized soft tissue graft and the highest for the connective tissue graft procedure. The lower predictability of complete root coverage with the GTR procedure, compared to the coronally advanced flap procedure, has been associated with the problem of membrane exposure during healing (Trombelli et al. 1995), but whether a bioabsorbable or a non-biodegradable barrier membrane is used does not seem to affect the treatment outcome (Roccuzzo et al. 1996).

Short-term clinical trials comparing the treatment outcome of the two modalities of free soft tissue grafts (Sbordone et al. 1988, Daniel & Cheru 1990, Jahnke et al. 1993) have shown that the connective tissue graft results in superior root coverage compared to the epithelialized free soft tissue graft. The color match of the connective tissue grafted area to the adjacent gingiva is esthetically also more favorable with the connective tissue graft than that of an epithelialized free graft.

Factors influencing the degree of root coverage

Patient-related factors
As with other surgical periodontal treatment procedures, poor oral hygiene following the procedure will negatively influence the success of root coverage procedures (Caffesse et al. 1987). Also, the predominant causative factor in the development of gingival recession is toothbrushing trauma, and hence this factor has to be corrected to secure an optimal outcome of any root coverage procedure. Whether smoking may negatively influence the outcome of root coverage procedures is still a controversial issue. Some studies have reported less favorable outcome in terms of root coverage following free graft and GTR procedures in smokers (Miller 1987, Trombelli & Scabbia 1997, Müller et al. 1998, Zucchelli et al. 2000), while other studies have shown no differences between smokers and non-smokers (Tolmie et al. 1991, Harris 1994).

Site-related factors
Among site specific factors, the level of interdental periodontal support may be of greatest significance for the outcome of root coverage procedures. From a biological point of view complete root coverage is achievable in Class I and II type recession defects (Fig.

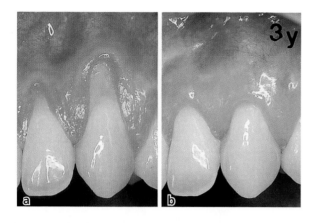

Fig. 27-47a-b. Buccal recession defects but no loss of periodontal support at proximal surfaces (a). Complete root coverage can be achieved. (b) 3-year follow-up.

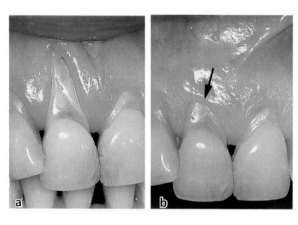

Fig. 27-48. A deep buccal recession at tooth 11 (a). The tooth has loss of support at proximal sites (Miller Class III) and complete root coverage is not achievable. Also neighboring teeth show recessions at all tooth surfaces. (b) 2-year healing result following attempted root coverage at the facial aspect of tooth 11. The coronal position of the soft tissue margin is defined by the extension of proximal loss of periodontal support.

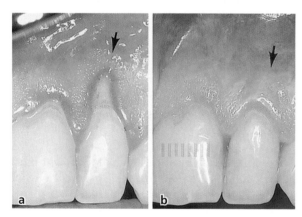

Fig. 27-49. Increased dimension of keratinized tissue 1 year following root coverage with a coronally advanced flap procedure. Before (a) and 1-year postoperatively (b). Arrows indicate the position of the mucogingival line.

27-47), while when loss of connective tissue attachment also involves proximal tooth sites (Class III-IV recession defects), only partial facial root coverage is obtainable (Miller 1985b) (Fig. 27-48).

An additional factor shown to influence the degree of attainable root coverage is the dimensions of the recession defect. Less favorable treatment outcome has been reported at sites with wide (> 3 mm) and deep (≥ 5 mm) recessions (Holbrook & Ochsenbein 1983, Pini Prato et al. 1992, Trombelli et al. 1995). Wennström & Zucchelli (1996) reported in a study comparing the treatment effect of coronally advanced flap and free connective tissue graft procedures that complete root coverage was observed in only 50% of the defects with an initial depth of ≥ 5 mm compared to 96% in shallower defects. In a controlled clinical trial Pini Prato et al. (1992) treated 50 teeth with a coronally advanced flap procedure, either with or without the use of a non-degradable membrane barrier. The mean percentage root coverage at the 18-month follow-up examination was 73% with and 71% without the use of a barrier, and a subsequent 4-year follow-up report revealed long-term stability of achieved root coverage for both procedures (Pini Prato et al. 1996). The authors suggested that a more favorable result with respect to root coverage might be obtained with the GTR procedure in sites with deep (≥ 5 mm) recession defects as compared to the coronally advanced flap. At the 18-month examination the coverage was 77% with and 66% without the inclusion of a membrane barrier in the treatment procedure. However, the data presented in Table 27-2, showing that the predictability of complete root coverage is markedly reduced with the use of barrier membranes, limit the justification to utilize the GTR procedure in the treatment of recession defects.

The pretreatment gingival height apical to the recession defect is not correlated to the amount of root coverage obtained (Romanos et al. 1993, Harris 1994).

Technique-related factors
Several technique-related factors may influence the treatment outcome of a pedicle graft procedure. A positive association between recession reduction and the thickness of the flap was shown by Baldi et al. (1999). Complete root coverage at sites with Miller Class I-II recessions was obtained only when the flap thickness was 0.8 mm. However, whether a full or split thickness pedicle graft is used for root coverage was not found to influence the treatment outcome (Espinel & Caffesse 1981).

Flap tension has been reported to be an important factor for the outcome of the coronally advanced flap procedure. The best clinical result is achieved if the flap is passively adapted to the root surface (Allen & Miller 1989, Pini Prato et al. 2000a). In the study by Pini Prato et al. (2000a) the tension in coronally advanced flaps was measured to compare the amount of recession reduction in sites with and without residual flap tension. At the test sites, which had an average residual tension of 6.5 g, the root coverage amounted to 78% 3 months post-surgically and 18% of the treated sites showed complete root coverage, whereas the control sites without or with only minimal remaining tension demonstrated a mean root coverage of 87% and complete root coverage in 45% of the cases. Furthermore, in the test group a statistically significant negative association was shown between the magnitude of residual tension in the flap and the amount of recession reduction.

Although the connective tissue areas lateral to the recession defect may be considered important for the retention of the advanced flap when positioned over the root surface, the dimension of the interdental papilla is not a prognostic factor for the clinical outcome of the root coverage procedure (Saletta et al. 2001).

With regard to free graft procedures, the thickness of the graft is a factor influencing the success of treatment procedure (Borghetti & Gardella 1990). A thickness of the free graft of about 2 mm is recommended.

Increased gingival height
An increased apicocoronal height of gingiva is found following all procedures in which pedicle grafts of adjacent gingiva or free grafts from the palate have been placed over the recession defect. It is interesting to note, however, that an increased gingival height is also a common finding following a coronally advanced flap procedure only involving the existing gingiva apical to the recession (Fig. 27-49). This finding may be explained by several events taking place during the healing and maturation of the marginal tissue. Granulation tissue formation derived from the periodontal ligament tissue will form a connective tissue similar to the one of gingiva and with the potential to induce keratinization of the covering epithe-

lium (Karring et al. 1971, Lundberg & Wennström 1988). A second factor to consider is the tendency of the mucogingival line to regain its "genetically" defined position following its coronal "dislocation" with the coronally advanced flap procedure used to achieve root coverage. Support for the concept that the mucogingival line over time will regain its original position is generated from a study by Ainamo et al. (1992). The authors performed an apically repositioned flap procedure in the mandibular anterior tooth region, which resulted in a 3-mm apical displacement of the mucogingival line. The re-examination after 18 years showed no differences in position of the mucogingival line between sites treated with the apically repositioned flap and contralateral control sites treated with a procedure not interfering with the mucogingival line, indicating that the mucogingival line had regained its original position.

Soft tissue healing against the covered root surface

Although successful treatment outcome of gingival recessions by pedicle grafts or free grafts has been reported in a number of publications (for review see Wennström 1996), it is debated to which extent this type of treatment results in new connective tissue attachment or epithelial attachment. However, independent of the quality of attachment formed, the root coverage procedures evidently rarely result in the formation of a deep periodontal pocket.

Healing of pedicle soft tissue grafts
In the areas surrounding the recession defect, i.e. where the recipient bed consists of bone covered by connective tissue, the pattern of healing is similar to that observed following a traditional flap operation. Cells and blood vessels from the recipient bed as well as from the tissue graft invade the fibrin layer, which gradually becomes replaced by connective tissue. As early as 1 week later a fibrous reunion is established between the graft and the underlying tissue.

Healing in the area where the pedicle graft is in contact with the denuded root surface was studied by Wilderman & Wentz (1965) in dogs. According to these authors the healing process can be divided into four different stages (Fig. 27-50).

The adaptation stage (from 0 to 4 days)
The laterally repositioned flap is separated from the exposed root surface by a thin fibrin layer. The epithelium covering the transplanted tissue flap starts to proliferate and reaches contact with the tooth surface at the coronal edge of the flap after a few days.

The proliferation stage (from 4 to 21 days)
In the early phase of this stage the fibrin layer between the root surface and the flap is invaded by connective tissue proliferating from the subsurface of the flap. In

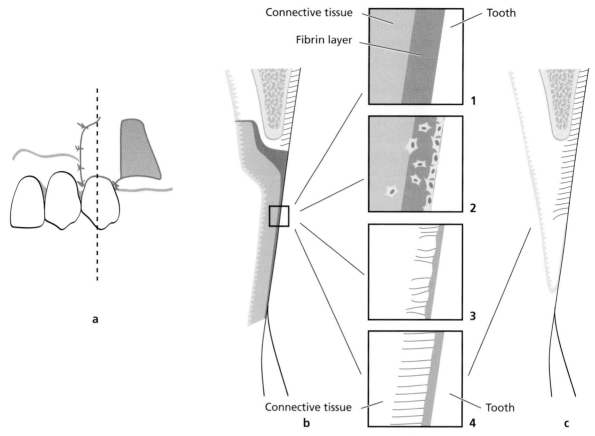

Fig. 27-50. Schematic drawing illustrating healing following treatment of a localized soft tissue recession with a pedicle graft (a). (b) Cross-section through the area immediately after operation. The framed areas (1-4) illustrate the four stages into which the healing process can be divided. (c) Area after healing. Approximately 50% of the successfully covered defect may show new connective tissue attachment.

contrast to areas where healing occurs between two connective tissue surfaces, growth of connective tissue into the fibrin layer can only take place from one surface. After 6-10 days a layer of fibroblasts is seen in apposition to the root surface. These cells are believed to differentiate into cementoblasts at a later stage of healing. At the end of the proliferation stage, thin collagen fibers are formed adjacent to the root surface, but a fibrous union between the connective tissue and the root has not been observed. From the coronal edge of the wound, epithelium is proliferating apically along the root surface. According to Wilderman & Wentz (1965), the apical proliferation of epithelium may stop within the coronal half of the defect, although further downgrowth of epithelium was also frequently observed.

The attachment stage (from 27 to 28 days)
During this stage of healing thin collagen fibers become inserted in a layer of new cementum formed at the root surface in the apical portion of the recession.

The maturation state
This last stage of healing is characterized by continuous formation of collagen fibers. After 2-3 months, bundles of collagen fibers are inserting into the cemen-

tum layer on the curetted root surface in the apical portion of the recession.

Results of experimental studies in monkeys and dogs on the healing characteristics of the periodontal wound have been interpreted to indicate that gingival connective tissue lacks the ability to form a new connective tissue attachment, but may induce root resorption (see Chapter 28). This finding is of particular interest when considering the rationale for the treatment of recession defects by free or pedicle soft tissue grafts. Since in these surgical procedures gingival connective tissue is placed in contact with a denuded root surface, root resorption should be expected to occur. The reason why it is not a common complication following this type of treatment can be explained by two possible events. Either cells from the periodontal ligament form a fibrous attachment to the root surface or epithelial cells proliferate apically, forming a root protective barrier (long junctional epithelium) towards the gingival connective tissue.

Histologic studies on whether it is the one or the other type of attachment that results following treatment of recessions with pedicle grafts indicate that new connective tissue attachment with cementum formation may be formed in part of the defect. In the study by Wilderman & Wentz (1965) a new connective tissue attachment of around 2 mm and an epithelial

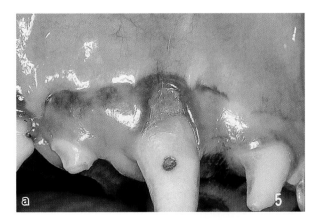
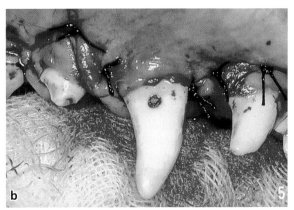
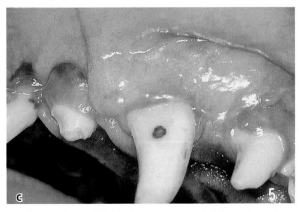

Fig. 27-51. Clinical photographs illustrating the treatment of an experimentally induced localized recession defect in a dog with a coronally displaced flap. Presurgical appearance of the localized recession defect (a). The site following flap closure of the defect (b) and after 3 months of healing (c).

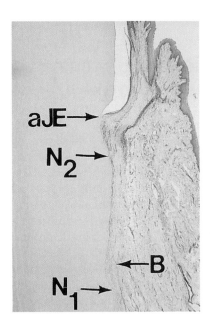

Fig. 27-52. Microphotograph of the healing following a coronally displaced flap in the dog as illustrated in Fig. 27-51. A new connective tissue attachment is formed and extends coronally from the apical border of the notch prepared at the bottom of the bone dehiscence (N_1) to the apical termination of the epithelium (aJE) located within the notch indicating the presurgical level of the soft tissue margin (N_2). B: alveolar bone crest.

attachment of the same height had formed in the soft tissue covered portion of the defect, i.e. about 50% of the successfully covered defect showed new connective tissue attachment.

Gottlow et al. (1986) examined the result of healing following treatment of experimentally produced recession type defects with a coronally advanced flap in dogs (Fig. 27-51). The histologic analysis after 3 months of healing disclosed that on average 20% of

the apicocoronal length of the original defect had been exposed due to recession during healing (i.e. about 80% root coverage was achieved), 40% was covered by epithelium and 40% demonstrated new connective tissue attachment (Fig. 27-52). Determining factors for the type of healing result were the size and the shape of the defect. The possibility of achieving a new connective tissue attachment in the apical portion of the defect seemed to be considerably better in narrow recession defects than in wider ones, most likely because the periodontal ligament at the lateral parts of the defect will serve as a source of granulation tissue from which a new connective tissue attachment can develop.

The healing following pedicle graft procedures has also been histologically studied in monkeys (Caffesse et al. 1984, Gottlow et al. 1990), and in these studies 38-44% of the successfully covered recession defects demonstrated formation of new connective tissue attachment. The study by Gottlow et al. (1990) also showed that the use of a GTR membrane between the root surface and the pedicle graft generated significantly more new connective tissue attachment (79% of the covered recession defect).

Some case reports with human block sections provide evidence that new connective tissue attachment with cementum formation may be formed following pedicle graft procedures. Histologic evaluation of two teeth treated with a laterally positioned flap revealed that connective tissue attachment was re-established in the apical fourth of the successfully covered portion of the root (Sugerman 1969). Cortellini et al. (1993) examined histologically a tooth treated with the GTR procedure and showed that connective tissue faced 74% of the length of the recession defect. New cementum with inserting collagen fibers, i.e. new connective tissue attachment, covered 48% of the distance between the apical border of the root instrumentation and the soft tissue margin.

Healing of free soft tissue grafts

Survival of a free soft tissue graft placed over a denuded root surface depends on diffusion of plasma and subsequent revascularization from those parts of the graft that are resting on the connective tissue bed surrounding the dehiscence. The establishment of collateral circulation from adjacent vascular borders of the bed allows the healing phenomenon of "bridging" (Sullivan & Atkins 1968a,b). Hence, the amount of tissue that can be maintained over the root surface is limited by the size of the avascular area (Oliver et al. 1968, Sullivan & Atkins 1968). Other factors considered critical for the survival of the tissue graft placed over the root surface are that a sufficient vascular bed is prepared around the dehiscence and that a thick graft is used (Miller 1985b).

Another healing phenomenon frequently observed following free graft procedures is "creeping attachment", i.e. a coronal migration of the soft tissue margin. This occurs as a consequence of tissue maturation during a period of about 1 year post-treatment.

Histologic evaluations of the nature of the attachment established to the root surface following the use of free grafts for root coverage are few. Sugerman (1969) reported from a histologic evaluation of a human tooth treated with a free soft tissue graft that new connective tissue attachment was found in the apical fourth of the successfully covered recession defect. Pasquinelli (1995) harvested a human block biopsy of a premolar for histologic evaluation 42 weeks after treatment of a narrow recession defect with root biomodification (tetracycline HCl) and an epithelialized free soft tissue graft. The root coverage amounted to 5 mm, or 83% of the original recession. The epithelial lining was found to terminate 2.6 mm below the gingival margin, and the most coronally positioned new cementum with inserting connective tissue fibers was seen 3.4 mm apical to the gingival margin. No histologic reference for the apical extension of the original defect was available, but the author estimated, based on extrapolations from pre-treatment probing assessments, that 3.6 mm of new attachment had formed, corresponding to 51% of the apicocoronal height of the covered, previously detached root portion.

On the other hand, Harris (1999) and Majzoub et al. (2001), each reporting the histological outcome of free connective tissue grafts in two cases, found only minimal amounts of new cementum formation in the most apical part of the recession defect and that healing resulted in a long junctional epithelium occupying the interface between the covering soft tissue and the root.

Thus, the limited histological information available from humans on the healing of free soft tissue grafts indicates that a healing pattern similar to the one discussed above following pedicle graft procedures may result, namely that connective tissue attachment may be established in the most apical and lateral parts of the recession defect, but that an epithelial attachment is formed along the major portion of the root.

INTERDENTAL PAPILLA RECONSTRUCTION

There may be several factors contributing to the loss of papilla height and the establishment of "black triangles" between teeth. The most common reason in the adult individual is loss of periodontal support due to plaque-associated lesions. However, abnormal tooth shape, improper contours of prosthetic restorations and traumatic oral hygiene procedures may also negatively influence the outline of the interdental soft tissues.

Nordland & Tarnow (1998) proposed a classification system regarding the papillary height adjacent to natural teeth, based on three anatomical landmarks: the interdental contact point, the apical extent of the facial cemento-enamel junction (CEJ), and the coronal extent of the proximal CEJ (Fig. 27-53).

- *Normal*: the interdental papilla occupies the entire embrasure space apical to the interdental contact point/area.
- *Class I*: the tip of the interdental papilla is located between the interdental contact point and the level of the CEJ on the proximal surface of the tooth.
- *Class II*: the tip of the interdental papilla is located

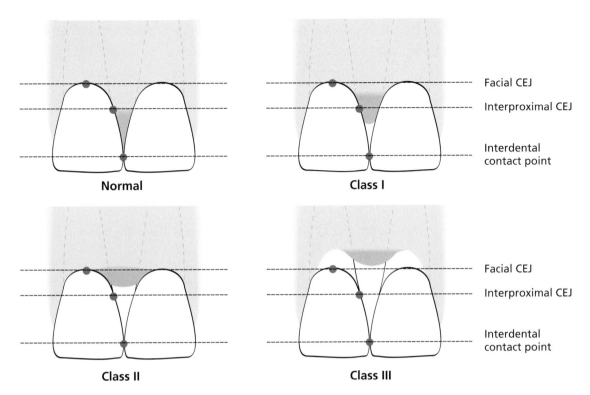

Fig. 27-53. Schematic drawing illustrating the classification system for papilla height (Nordland & Tarnow 1998),

at or apical to the level of the CEJ on the proximal surface of the tooth but coronal to the level of the CEJ mid-buccally.

- *Class III*: the tip of the interdental papilla is located at or apical to the level of the CEJ mid-buccally.

In an observational study in humans, Tarnow et al. (1992) analyzed the correlation between the presence of interproximal papillae and the vertical distance between the contact point and the interproximal bone crest. When the vertical distance from the contact point to the crest of bone was 5 mm or less, the papilla was present almost 100% of the time, whereas if the distance was 6 mm or more most commonly only partial papilla fill of the embrasure between the teeth was found. Considering that a supracrestal connective tissue attachment zone of approximately 1 mm is normally found (Gargiulo 1961), the observation indicates that the biological height of the interdental papilla may be limited to about 4 mm. This interpretation is supported by the observation that in interdental areas denuded following an apically repositioned flap procedure, an up-growth of around 4 mm of soft tissue had taken place 3 years after surgery (Van der Velden 1982). Hence, before attempts are made to surgically reconstruct an interdental papilla, it is important to carefully assess both (1) the vertical distance between the bone crest and the apical point of the contact area between the crowns, and (2) the soft tissue height in the interdental area. If the distance bone crest-contact point is ≤ 5 mm and the papilla height is less than 4 mm, surgical intervention for increasing the volume of the papilla could be justified in order to solve the

problem of an interdental "black triangle". However, if the contact point is located > 5 mm from the bone crest, because of loss of periodontal support and/or an inappropriate interdental contact relationship between the crowns, means to apically lengthen the contact area between the teeth should be selected rather than a surgical attempt to improve the topography of the papilla.

If loss of papilla height is caused by soft tissue damage only from oral hygiene devices, the interproximal hygiene procedures must be initially discontinued to allow soft tissue recovery and then successively modified in order to eliminate/minimize the traumatic injury to the papillae.

Surgical techniques

Several case reports have been published regarding surgical techniques for reconstruction of deficient papillae (e.g. Beagle 1992, Han & Takei 1996, Azzi et al. 1998). However, the predictability of the various procedures has not been documented and no data are available in the literature providing information on the long-term stability of surgically regained interdental papillae.

Beagle (1992) described a pedicle graft procedure utilizing the soft tissues palatal of the interdental area.

Technique (Fig. 27-54): A split-thickness flap is dissected on the palatal aspect of the interdental area. The flap is elevated labially, folded and sutured to create the new papilla at the facial part of the indental area. A periodontal dressing is applied on the palatal aspect only, in order to support the papilla.

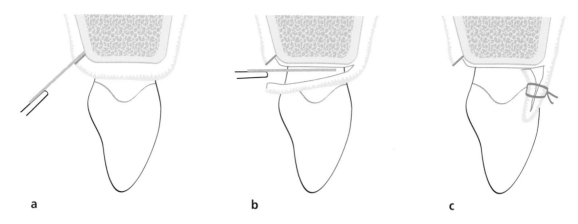

a   b   c

Fig. 27-54a-c. *Papilla reconstruction – pedicle graft technique*. Schematic drawings illustrating the surgical technique (see text for explanation).

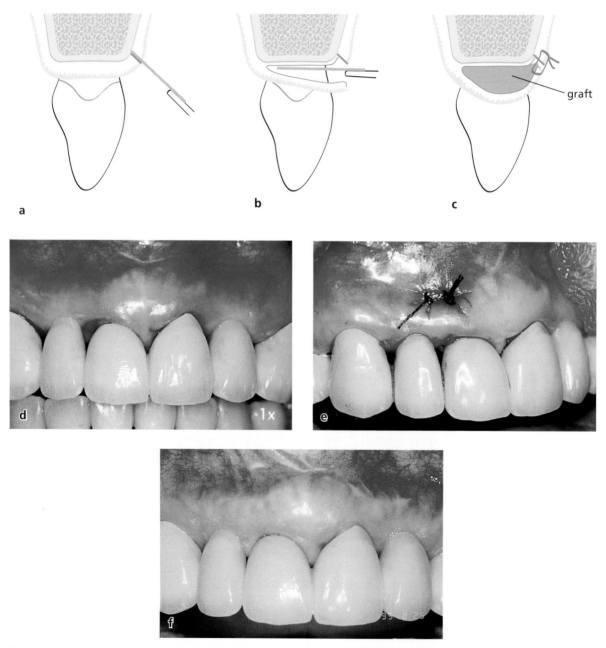

Fig. 27-55. *Papilla reconstruction – the "semi-lunar coronally repositioned papilla" technique*. (a-c) Schematic drawings illustrating the surgical technique (see text for explanation). (d-f) Reconstruction of papillae distal to the central incisors with the use of the semi-lunar coronally repositioned papilla technique in a patient with a fixed bridge reconstruction.

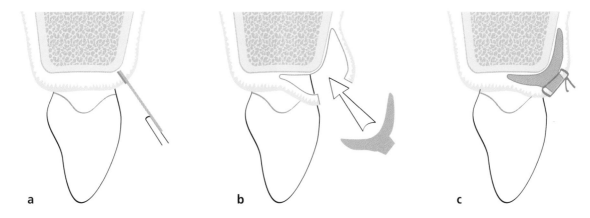

Fig. 27-56a-c. *Papilla reconstruction – "envelope" technique.* Schematic drawings illustrating the surgical technique (see text for explanation).

Han and Takei (1996) proposed an approach for papilla reconstruction ("semi-lunar coronally repositioned papilla") based on the use of a free connective tissue graft.

Technique (Fig. 27-55): A semi-lunar incision is placed in the alveolar mucosa facial to the interdental area and a pouch-like preparation is performed into the interdental area. Intrasulcular incisions are made around the mesial and distal half of the two adjacent teeth to free the connective tissue from the root surfaces to allow a coronal displacement of the gingival-papillary unit. A connective tissue graft, taken from the palate, is placed into the pouch to support the coronally positioned interdental tissue.

Azzi et al. (1998) described a technique in which an envelope-type flap was prepared for coverage of a connective tissue graft.

Technique (Fig. 27-56): An intrasulcular incision is made at the tooth surfaces facing the interdental area to be reconstructed. Subsequently, an incision is placed across the facial aspect of the interdental area and an envelope-type, split-thickness flap is elevated into the proximal site as well as apically to a level beyond the mucogingival line. A connective tissue graft is harvested from the tuberosity area, trimmed to adequate size and shape and placed under the flaps in the interdental papilla area. The flaps are brought together and sutured with the connective tissue graft underneath.

CROWN LENGTHENING PROCEDURES

Excessive gingival display

In most patients, the lower edge of the upper lip assumes a "gum-wing" profile which limits the amount of gingiva that is exposed when a person smiles. Patients who have a high lip line expose a broad zone of gingival tissue and may often express concern about their "gummy smile" (Fig. 27-57a). The form of the lips and the position of the lips during speech and smiling cannot be easily changed, but the dentist may, if necessary, modify/control the form of the teeth and interdental papillae as well as the position of the gingival margins and the incisal edges of the teeth. In other words, it is possible by a combination of periodontal and prosthetic treatment measures to improve dentofacial esthetics in this category of patient.

As a base for treatment decisions, a careful analysis of the dentofacial structures and how they may affect esthetics should be performed and should include the following features:

- Facial symmetry
- Interpupillary line – even or uneven
- Smile line – low, median or high
- Dental midline in relation to facial midline
- Gingival display during speech and during broad, relaxed smile
- Harmony of gingival margins
- Location of gingival margins in relation to the cemento-enamel junctions
- Tooth size and proportions/harmony
- Incisal plane/occlusal plane.

If excessive gingival exposure is due to insufficient length of the clinical crowns, a crown lengthening procedure is indicated to reduce the amount of gingiva exposed, which in turn will favorably alter the shape and form of the anterior teeth. To select the proper treatment approach for crown lengthening, an analysis of the individual case with regard to crown-root-alveolar bone relationships should also be included.

In the young adult with an intact periodontium the gingival margin normally resides about 1 mm coronal to the cemento-enamel junction. However, some patients may have a height of free gingiva that is greater than 1 mm, resulting in an unproportional appearance

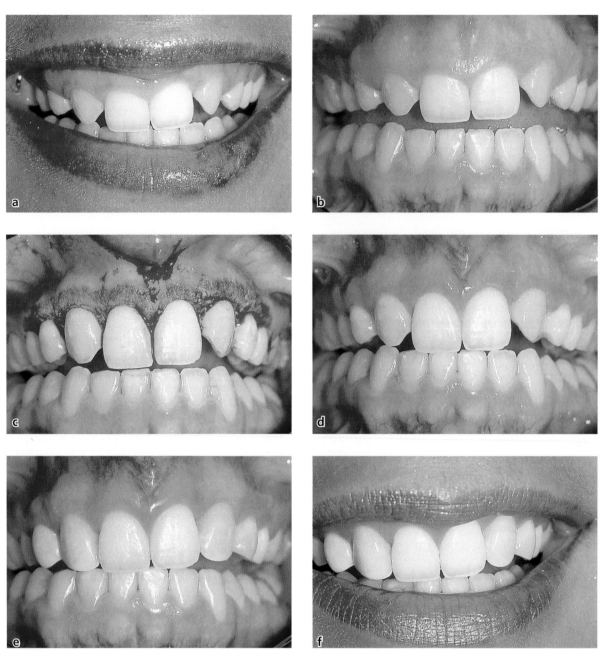

Fig. 27-57. *Crown lengthening procedure.* (a-b) Pretreatment views. The clinical crowns are considerably shorter than the anatomical crowns. The lateral incisors were congenitally missing and orthodontic treatment had been carried out to move the posterior teeth anteriorly. The canine teeth in the position of the lateral incisors added to the esthetic disharmony. (c) A gingivectomy was performed to expose the anatomical crowns of the teeth. (d) One month post-surgery. At this appointment, the canine and first premolar teeth were reshaped and bonded. (e) Tooth form and proportional balance were improved by bonding. (f) At 3 years post-treatment, the gingival tissues exhibited no rebound and retained the architectural form sculpted into the tissue at the time of the surgical procedure. Courtesy of Dr J. Seibert, US.

of the clinical crown. If such a patient complains about their "small front teeth" and the periodontium is of a thin biotype, full exposure of the anatomical crown can be accomplished by a gingivecomy/gingivoplasty procedure (Fig. 27-57).

An assessment should also be made regarding the amount and pattern of pigmentation existing within the gingival tissues, and the patient's desire to maintain or lessen the pigmentation contained within the tissues. The externally beveled path of incision that is usually employed in a gingivectomy procedure will

remove the pigmentation and produce pink gingival tissue upon initial healing (Fig. 27-58). The surgically induced color change in the tissues comes about rapidly, and markedly affects esthetic values. For this reason, an externally beveled gingivectomy procedure should not be terminated at the midline in patients that have pigmented gingival tissues. It should be extended across the midline to the premolar area to avoid a color mismatch in the esthetic zone of the anterior teeth. The color change may be permanent or the pigmentation may slowly return over a period of

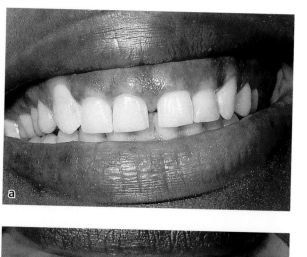
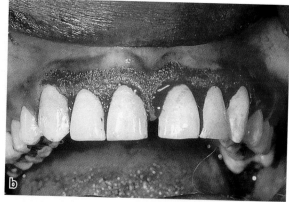
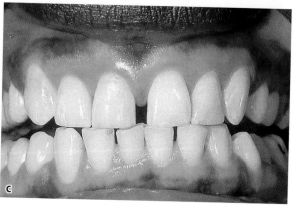
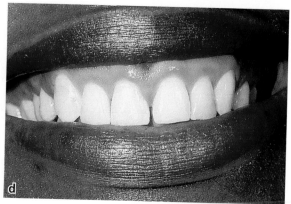

Fig. 27-58. (a) Pretreatment view. The patient disliked her "small front teeth" and diastema. Radiographs and probing indicated the gingival tissues were covering the cervical one third of the crowns. Crestal bone was thin and in normal relationship to the cemento-enamel junctions. The patient preferred "pink gums" if she could possibly have them. (b) A long externally beveled path of incision was used to accomplish the gingivectomy. (c) This view shows the color changes and pleasing architecture produced in the anterior gingiva at 2 months post-surgery. The diastema was partially closed by direct bonding at this time. (d) Post-treatment view showing the enhancement of esthetic values for the patient. Courtesy of Dr J. Seibert, US.

a year or more. Patients should be informed of the changes in tissue color that will occur and should be allowed to make a choice as to the color of the tissue they will have postsurgically. If they wish to maintain their pigmentation, an internally beveled path of incision (internal gingivectomy) should be employed (Fig. 27-59).

If the periodontium is of the thick biotype and there is a bony ledge at the osseous crest, an apically positioned flap procedure (see Chapter 25) should be performed. This will allow for osseous recontouring (Fig. 27-60).

More extensive bone recontouring is required to solve esthetic problems found in patients who do indeed have short anatomical crowns in the anterior section of the dentition. In this category of patients, prosthetic measures must be used after resective periodontal therapy to increase the apicocoronal dimension of the crowns (Fig. 27-61). Patients who are candidates for this kind of resective therapy can be divided into two categories:

1. Subjects who have normal occlusal relationships and incisal guidance. In this category the incisal line of the front teeth must remain unaltered but the clinical crowns can be made longer by surgically exposing root structure and by locating the cervical margins of the restorations apical to the cemento-enamel junction (Fig. 27-61).

2. Subjects who have abnormal occlusal relationships with excessive interocclusal space in the posterior dentition when the anterior teeth are in edge-to-edge contact. In this category of patients the length of the maxillary front teeth can be reduced without inducing posterior occlusal interferences. In addition, the marginal gingiva can be resected or relocated to an apical position before crown restorations are made.

In some individuals having excessive display of gingiva, the size and shape of the teeth and the location of the gingival margins may be perfectly normal. The excessive display of gingiva in these cases is often caused by vertical maxillary excess and a long midface (Fig. 27-62). Periodontal crown lengthening procedures will not suffice to solve their problems, but rather the maxilla must be impacted by major maxillofacial surgical procedure. The risk-benefits and cost ratios must be thoroughly evaluated before recom-

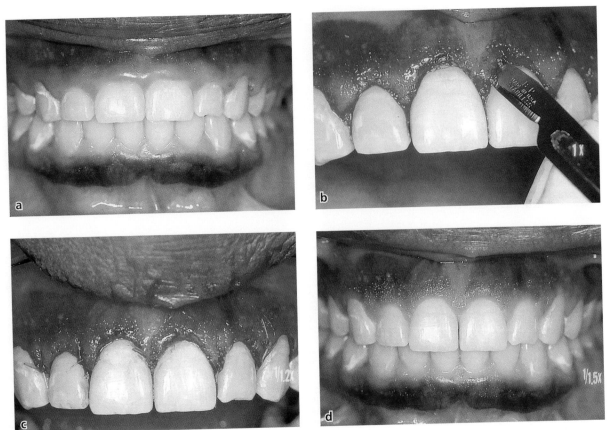

Fig. 27-59. Pretreatment view. This patient disliked the looks of her "small front teeth"; she sought consultation to have her teeth made longer by crowning them. Probing and radiographs revealed normal osseous morphology and a wide zone of attached gingiva that covered the cervical one third of the incisors. It was explained to the patient that a surgical solution was preferred to restorative procedures to make her teeth longer. The patient made a request that the color of her gingival tissues remain unchanged. (b) An internally beveled path of incision was used to effect an "internal gingivectomy" to maintain the pigmentation in the tissues. This created mini flaps in the areas of the papillae. (c) 5-0 gut sutures were used to stabilize the papillae. (d) The crown lengthening that was achieved with maintenance of color harmony can be seen in this view at 3 months post-surgery. Courtesy of Dr E. Saacks, Pennsylvania, PA.

mending this type of surgical therapy to correct esthetic problems.

Exposure of sound tooth structure

Crown lengthening procedures may be required to solve problems such as (1) inadequate amount of tooth structure for proper restorative therapy, (2) subgingival location of fracture lines, and (3) subgingival location of carious lesions.

The techniques used to accomplish crown lengthening include (1) apically positioned flap procedure including bone resection, and (2) forced tooth eruption with or without fiberotomy.

Apically positioned flap with bone recontouring

The apically positioned flap technique with bone recontouring (resection) may be used to expose sound tooth structure. As a general rule, at least 4 mm of sound tooth structure must be exposed at time of surgery. During healing the supracrestal soft tissues will proliferate coronally to cover 2-3 mm of the root (Herrero et al. 1995, Pontoriero & Carnevale 2001), thereby leaving only 1-2 mm of supragingivally located sound tooth structure. When this technique is used for crown lengthening it must also be realized

Fig. 27-61. *Crown lengthening by surgical and prosthetic procedures.* (a) Pretreatment view. The patient displayed "short front teeth" and a broad exposure of gum tissue. The full anatomical crown is exposed in this case and the surgically induced recession will expose root structure. (b) The patient had an unusually wide zone of attached gingiva. The gingival margins were positioned apically by making an internally beveled flap with a submarginal entrance incision as outlined in red ink. The crest of the bone was reduced in height. (c) After the tissues had matured following surgery, individual crowns were prepared for each of the anterior teeth. Crown lengthening was achieved and the patient no longer exposed a broad expanse of gum tissue. Courtesy of Dr D. Garber, Atlanta, GA.

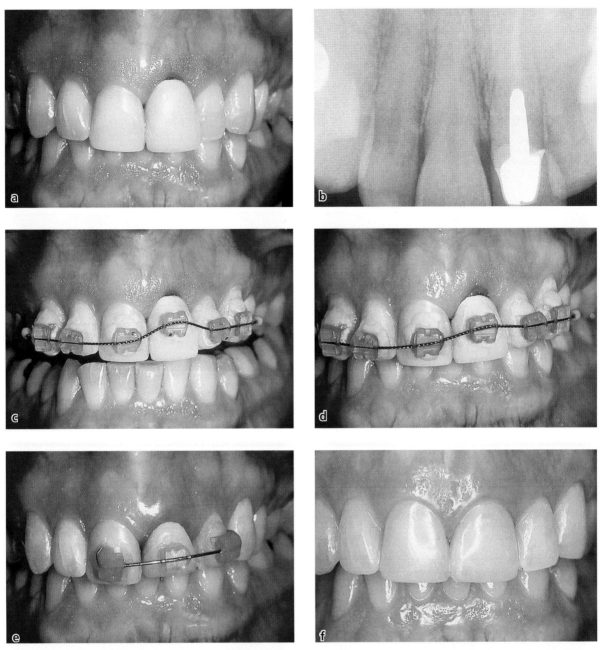

Fig. 27-65. Forced tooth eruption (slow method) used to level gingival margins, treat recession on a single tooth and create esthetic harmony. (a-b) Recession on the left central incisor exposed the root surface darkened from root canal treatment. The uneven gingival margins and dark root surface detracted from an otherwise attractive smile. (c) A nitol wire with an offset bracket was used to slowly extrude the incisor. (d) Occlusal adjustment was done on the lingual side of the crown to create room for the tooth to erupt. This view, at 1 month in tooth movement, shows the gingival tissues moving with the root of the tooth. (e) Sufficient eruption had occurred by 3 months to level the gingival margins. The orthodontic brackets were used for temporary stabilization and a new crown was prepared. (f) The new crown masked the show-through of the dark root. The even gingival margins and beautiful crown created esthetic harmony. Courtesy of Dr J. Ingber, Philadelphia, PA.

Forced tooth eruption

Orthodontic tooth movement can be used to erupt teeth in adults (Reitan 1967, Ingber 1974, 1976, Potashnick & Rosenberg 1982). If moderate eruptive forces are used, the entire attachment apparatus will move in unison with the tooth. The tooth must be extruded a distance equal to or slightly longer than the portion of sound tooth structure that will be exposed in the subsequent surgical treatment. After the tooth has reached the intended position and has been stabilized, a full thickness flap is elevated and bone recontouring is performed to expose sound root structure. For esthetic reasons it is important that the bone and soft tissue levels at adjacent teeth remain unchanged.

Forced tooth eruption can also be used to level and align gingival margins and the crowns of teeth to obtain esthetic harmony. Instead of using surgical procedures to apically position the gingival margins

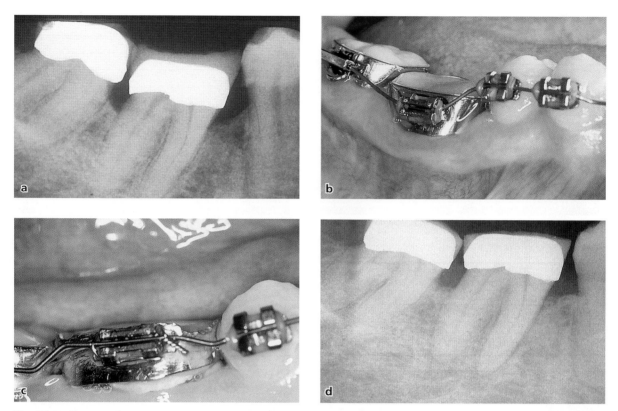

Fig. 27-66. Slow tooth eruption procedure used to level cemento-enamel junctions and angular bone crests. (a) Pre-treatment radiograph. (b) A nitol wire was used to erupt the molar. (c) The crown was shortened over a period of 4 months by selective grinding. (d) Radiograph taken 8 months after the start of treatment. The angular bone defects were leveled. Courtesy of Dr J. Seibert, US.

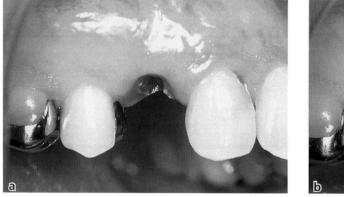
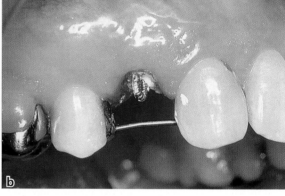

Fig. 27-67a-b. Rapid tooth eruption procedure in conjunction with fiberotomy procedure. (a) Buccal view, the fracture on the first premolar extended subgingivally. (b) Soft tooth structure was excavated and a twisted wire with an occlusal hook was temporarily cemented in the root canal. A bar was placed into the amalgam restoration on the premolar and bonded to the lingual surface of the canine.

of unaffected normal teeth to the level of a tooth with recession or orthodontic malalignment, the tooth that is malpositioned or has sustained recession is erupted to the level of the normally positioned teeth. The entire attachment apparatus and dentogingival junction will follow the root of the tooth as it is moved coronally (Fig. 27-65).

Indication: Crown lengthening at sites where removal of attachment and bone from adjacent teeth must be avoided. The forced eruption technique can also be used as a means of reducing pocket depth at sites with

angular bony defects (Brown 1973, Ingber 1974, 1976). The angular bony defect at the problem tooth can be reduced while the attachment level at the adjacent tooth surface remains unchanged (Fig. 27-66).

Contraindication: The forced eruption technique requires the use of fixed orthodontic appliances. Thus, in patients who have only a few teeth remaining, an alternative approach for crown lengthening has to be selected.

Technique: Orthodontic brackets are bonded to the pro-

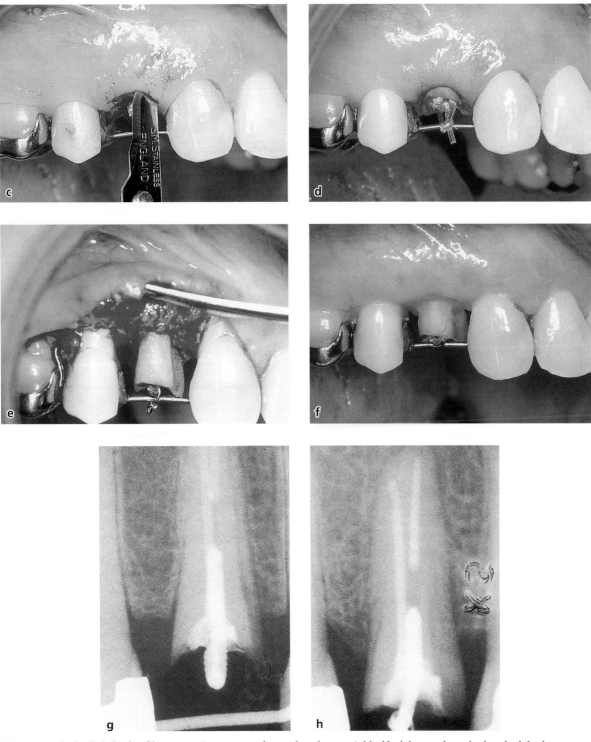

Fig. 27-67c-h. (c-d) Sulcular fiber resection was performed at the mesial half of the tooth to the level of the bone crest. The distal half remained as a control surface. The fiber resection was repeated once a week during the 3-week eruption phase. (e) The tooth was stabilized for 6 weeks, and at that time a full-thickness flap was raised. The bone crest had a "positive" angulation at the distal surface and remained unchanged at the "test" mesial surface. Osseous resection was used to level the bony septum on the distal surface. (f) Ample crown lengthening was obtained and the gingival margins healed to their former shape and location. (g) Pretreatment radiograph enlarged to show the normal shape of the crests of the interdental septae. (h) Enlargement of the posteruption radiograph (3 weeks of rapid eruption and 6 weeks of stabilization) to show the "positive" angular crest on the "control" distal side and the unchanged crest on the mesial "test" side. Courtesy of Dr R. Pontoriero, Milan, Italy.

blem tooth and to adjacent teeth and are combined with an arch wire. Another type of mechanical system can be utilized by placing a heavy gauge bar or wire in grooves prepared in the adjacent teeth and over the problem tooth. A power elastic is tied from the bracket to the arch wire (or the bar), which pulls to tooth coronally. If most of the crown structure is lost, root canal therapy is required. A post placed in the root

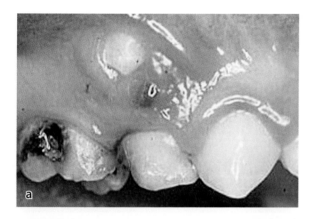

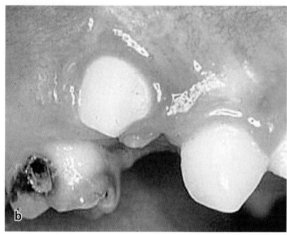

Fig. 27-68. Ectopic tooth eruption. The permanent tooth is erupting close to the mucogingival junction.

canal is fitted with a power elastic, which is also joined with the arch wire. The direction of the tooth movement must be carefully checked to ensure that the problem tooth is not tilted or moved toward the adjacent tooth surfaces.

Forced tooth eruption with fiberotomy

If fiberotomy is performed during the forced tooth eruption procedure the crestal bone and the gingival margin are retained at their pretreatment locations, and the tooth-gingiva interface at adjacent teeth is unaltered. Fiberotomy is performed by the use of a scalpel at 7 to 10-day intervals during the forced eruption to sever the supracrestal connective tissue fibers, thereby preventing the crestal bone from following the root in coronal direction. In the case presented in Fig. 27-67, fiberotomy was performed only at the mesial half of the root. Radiographs obtained after 9 weeks demonstrate that crestal bone migration has occurred at the distal but not at the mesial surface of the erupted tooth (Pontoriero et al. 1987).

Indication: Crown lengthening at sites where it is important to maintain unchanged the location of the gingival margin at adjacent teeth.

Contraindication: Fiberotomy should not be used at teeth associated with angular bone defects.

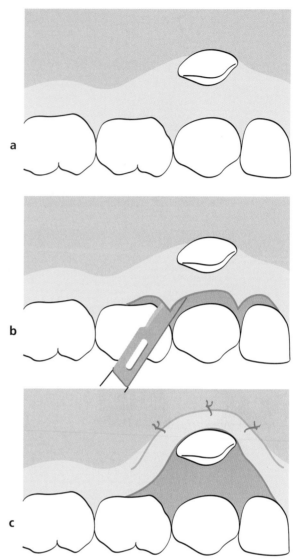

Fig. 27-69a-c. *Ectopically erupting tooth – double pedicle graft.* Schematic drawings illustrating the surgical technique (see text for explanation).

Technique: Similar to the technique described for the forced tooth eruption procedure. Fiberotomy is performed once every 7-10 days during the phase of forced tooth eruption.

Ectopic tooth eruption

Surgical intervention is often indicated for teeth erupting ectopically, i.e. having an eruption position facial to the alveolar ridge (Fig. 27-68). To create a satisfactory width of the gingiva for the permanent tooth, the tissue entrapped between the erupting tooth and the deciduous tooth is usually utilized as donor tissue (Agudio et al. 1985, Pini Prato et al. 2000b).

Three different techniques have been described for the interceptive mucogingival treatment of buccally erupting teeth, depending on the distance from the donor site (entrapped gingiva) to the recipient site

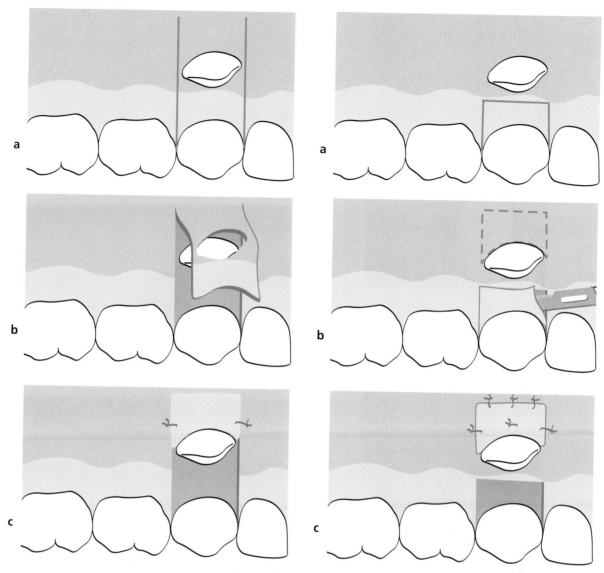

Fig. 27-70a-c. *Ectopically erupting tooth – apically positioned flap*. Schematic drawings illustrating the surgical technique (see text for explanation).

Fig. 27-71a-c. *Ectopically erupting tooth – free gingival graft*. Schematic drawings illustrating the surgical technique (see text for explanation).

(area located facially-apically to the erupting permanent tooth) (Agudio et al. 1985, Pini Prato et al. 2000b):

Double pedicle graft (Fig. 27-69): This flap procedure is indicated when the permanent tooth erupts within the zone of keratinized tissue but close to the mucogingival junction. An intrasulcular incision is performed at the deciduous tooth and extended laterally to the gingival crevice of the adjacent teeth and apically to the erupting permanent tooth. By mobilization of the flap apical to the mucogingival line, the entrapped gingiva can be elevated and transposed for positioning apically to the erupting tooth. Sutures may be placed to secure the position of the gingival tissue facial to the erupting tooth.

Apically positioned flap (Fig. 27-70): When the permanent tooth is erupting apical to the mucogingival junction, vertical releasing incisions have to be placed to allow for apical positioning of the keratinized tissue.

Two lateral releasing incisions are made and extended apically beyond the mucogingival junction. An intrasulcular incision is performed at the deciduous tooth and a partial thickness flap is elevated beyond the ectopically erupting tooth. The mobilized gingival flap is moved apical to the erupting tooth and secured in position by sutures.

Free gingival graft (Fig. 27-71): If the tooth is erupting within the alveolar mucosa distant to the mucogingival junction, a free gingival graft procedure may be selected. The entrapped gingiva is removed by a split incision and used as an epithelialized connective tissue graft. The free gingival graft is placed at a prepared recipient site facial/apical of the erupting tooth. Careful suturing is performed to secure a close adaptation of the graft to the underlying connective tissue bed.

All the described procedures have been proven to be effective in establishing a facial zone of gingiva

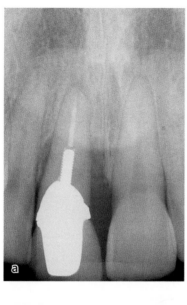
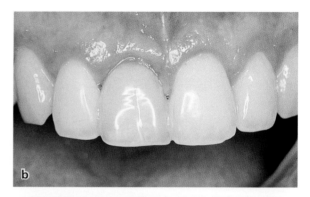
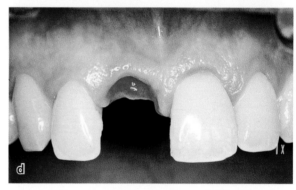
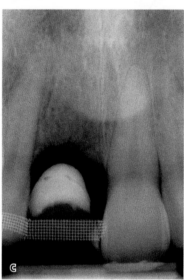
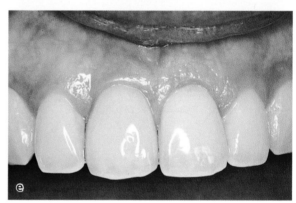

Fig. 27-72. (a) A central incisor that cannot be maintained because of root fracture which also caused pronounced periodontal destruction. (b) Immediately following tooth extraction, an ovate pontic was inserted to support the facial and proximal soft tissues. (c-d) Radiographic and clinical view of the area 6 weeks after tooth extraction. (e) Follow-up 1 year after the placement of permanent prosthetic recontruction (single implant).

following the alignment of teeth erupting in an ectopic position (Pino Prato et al. 2000b,c).

THE DEFORMED EDENTULOUS RIDGE

A partially edentulous ridge may retain the general shape of the alveolar process. Such a ridge is traditionally refered to as a normal ridge. Even though this normal ridge has retained the buccolingual and apicocoronal dimensions of the alveolar process, it is not normal in many other respects; the eminences that existed in the bone over the roots are no longer present and the interdental papillae are missing.

The smooth contours of the normal ridge create problems for the restorative dentist. In a fixed bridge the pontics (1) frequently give the impression that they rest on the top of the ridge rather than emerge from within the alveolar process, (2) lack a root eminence, and (3) lack marginal gingivae and interdental papillae. Dark triangles, which almost always interfere with dentofacial esthetics, are present in the embrasure area between the pontics and between the abutments and the pontics. In other words, in the presence of a normal ridge it may be difficult or impossible to produce a fixed prosthesis which truly restores the esthetics and function of the natural dentition.

Prevention of soft tissue collapse following tooth extraction

Following extraction of a tooth, the topography of the surrounding soft and hard tissues will be altered. The

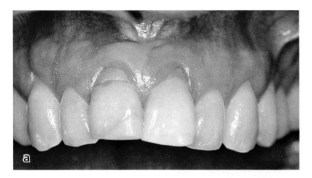
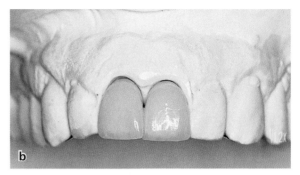
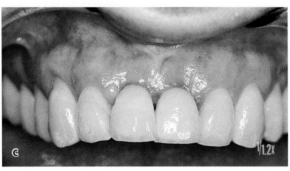

Fig. 27-73. (a) A 26-year-old female patient who had a trauma against the maxillary central incisors. Due to root fracture and endodontic complications both central incisors had to be extracted. (b) A Rochette bridge with ovate pontics was fabricated as a temporary replacement for the incisors. (c) Clinical view of the front tooth region 8 weeks after tooth extraction and placement of the resin bonded temporary bridge.

soft tissue margin will collapse and the height of the adjacent papillae will be reduced. This soft tissue collapse may be prevented by immediate post-extraction placement of an ovate pontic to support the soft tissues. Fig. 27-72 illustrates such a situation where a central incisor had to be extracted due to root fracture. With the immediate placement of the pontic the facial soft tissue margin and the papillae were maintained almost unchanged following the healing of the extraction site. Also, in situations where several adjacent teeth have to be extracted, insertion of ovate pontics may facilitate the preservation of the outline of the soft tissue ridge (Fig. 27-73).

Prevention of ridge collapse due to alveolar bone resorption following tooth extractions must also be considered. Borghetti & Laborde (1996) recommended means for prevention of bone ridge collapse after tooth extraction in any case of:

1. fracture of the vestibular osseous plate during tooth extraction or due to trauma
2. resorption of the vestibular osseous plate
3. presence of a thin vestibular bone plate.

Among procedures proposed for prevention of ridge collapse in conjunction with tooth extractions are (1) flap elevation for complete soft tissue closure of the extraction sites (Borghetti & Glise 2000), (2) placement of connective tissue grafts over the extraction sites (Nevins & Mellonig 1998), (3) placement of bone grafts (Becker et al. 1994), and (4) utilization of barrier membranes (Lekovic et al. 1997). Procedures for preserva-

tion of the bone dimensions following tooth extraction are discussed in Chapter 28.

Correction of ridge defects by the use of soft tissue grafts

A deformed ridge may result from tooth extractions, advanced periodontal disease, abscess formations, etc. The deformity that exists in the ridge is directly related to the volume of root structure and associated bone that is missing or has been destroyed. According to Seibert (1983), ridge defects can be divided into three classes:

Class I: Loss of buccolingual width but normal apicocoronal height
Class II: Loss of apicocoronal height but normal buccolingual width
Class III: A combination of loss of both height and width of the ridge.

Ridge augmentation procedures should be preceded by a careful surgical-prosthetic treatment planning by joint consultations involving the surgeon and the restorative dentist in order to attain an optimal esthetic result. The following factors should be determined prior to the initiation of therapy:

• Volume of tissue required to eliminate the ridge deformity
• Type of graft procedure to be used
• Timing of various treatment procedures

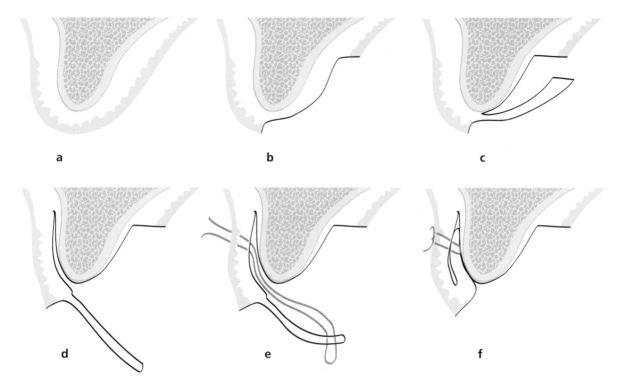

Fig. 27-74. Sequence of steps in the *"roll flap procedure"*. (a) Cross section of the residual edentulous ridge prior to treatment. (b) The removal of the epithelium. (c) The elevation of the pedicle. (d) The pouch is created. (e) Sutures are placed at the mucogingival junction to catch the tip of the pedicle flap and pull it into place in the pouch. (f) The flap is secured. A convexity in the ridge was created.

- Design of the provisional restoration
- Potential problems with tissue discolorations and matching tissue color.

Ideally, a provisional restoration should be made prior to surgery. The shape of the teeth in the provisional restoration, the axial inclination and emergence profile of the teeth and the embrasure form should be an exact prototype of the final prosthesis that is to be constructed. It is the task of the clinician performing the surgery to augment the tissues to meet the provisional prosthesis in the most exact manner possible. If a gingival flange of pink-colored acrylic is used around single or multiple pontics on a temporary removable partial denture, the flange must be cut away in order to avoid pressure on the graft and give the tissues room to swell during the immediate post-surgical phase of healing. The soft tissue at the surgically treated recipient site for a graft will undergo considerable swelling during the early phase of healing and the tissues will conform to the tissue-facing surfaces of the bridge or partial denture. The prosthesis is thus used to help in shaping the outline of the augmented ridge to the desired form. The location and shape of interproximal embrasure areas in the provisional bridge will determine where the "papillae" created in the ridge will be located.

Surgical procedures for ridge augmentation
Numerous surgical graft and implant procedures with the attempt to reconstruct a partially edentulous ridge or ridge defect have been described in the literature

over the years. The procedures may be grouped according to the means used for ridge augmentation as (1) soft tissue augmentation procedures and (2) hard tissue augmentation procedures. In this chapter only soft tissue augmentation procedures will be addressed, while hard tissue augmentation procedures are covered in Chapter 28. To illustrate various approaches for utilization of soft tissues for ridge augmentation, the following procedures will be discussed:

Pedicle graft procedure
- Roll flap procedure
Free graft procedures
- Pouch graft procedure
- Interpositional graft procedure
- Onlay graft procedure

Studer et al. (1997) proposed the use of the pedicle graft procedure for correction of a single-tooth ridge defect with minor horizontal and vertical loss, whereas in cases of larger defects submerged free connective tissue graft procedures should be selected. The onlay full thickness graft procedure is indicated for ridge augmentation primarily in the presence of additional mucogingival problems such as insufficient gingival width, high frenum, gingival scarring, or tattoo. These recommendations were based on short-term evaluation of the obtained volumetric increase of the edentulous ridge following various augmentation procedures, which demonstrated superior results with the use of submerged connective tissue

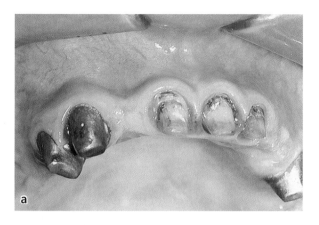
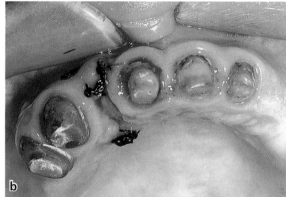
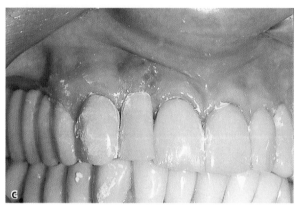
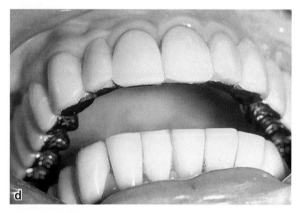

Fig. 27-75. *"Roll flap procedure"*. (a) Pretreatment view of a Class I ridge defect in the area of the right lateral incisor. Note the marked concavity in the ridge. (b) This view shows the surgical site 1 week after surgery and prior to the removal of the sutures. (c) The tissue surface of the pontic was relined with autopolymerizing resin. (d) Final prosthesis in place. Note the illusion of a root eminence and a free gingival margin apical to the lateral incisor pontic tooth. Courtesy of Dr L. Abrams, Philadelphia, PA.

grafts compared to the use of full-thickness grafts (Studer et al. 2000).

The "roll flap procedure"

Surgical concept: The "roll flap procedure" (Abrams 1980) involves the preparation of a de-epithelialized connective tissue pedicle graft, which is subsequently placed in a subepithelial pouch (Fig. 27-74). This procedure is used in the treatment of small to moderate Class I ridge defects, primarily in cases with a single-tooth space. The technique enables the surgeon to augment tissue apically and labially to the cervical area of a pontic and to give the recipient site the appearance of a normal tooth-gingiva interface. Hence, a buccolingual ridge concavity can be converted into a ridge convexity resembling the eminence produced by the roots of the adjacent teeth (Fig. 27-75).

Technique (Fig. 27-74): A rectangular pedicle of connective tissue is prepared on the palatal side of the defect. The length of the pedicle must match the amount of apicocoronal augmentation that is planned. This, in turn, is related to the amount of root eminence that exists on either side of the defect. If a two or three-tooth pontic space is treated with the "roll technique", two or three separate pedicles are raised. Each of these pedicles will form a new "root-cervical margin".

The epithelium on the palatal surface of the donor site is first removed. A maximum amount of supraperiosteal connective tissue is raised from the palate using sharp dissection. The void that is produced at the donor site will gradually fill in with granulation tissue. Caution must be exercised in dissecting the pedicle flap so that tissue perforation is avoided when the plane of dissection approaches the facial (labial) surface. A pouch is made in the supraperiosteal connective tissue at the facial (labial) surface of the ridge. In order to preserve as much connective tissue and blood supply as possible at the recipient site, the dissection must be made as close as possible to the periosteum of the facial bone.

The pedicle is tucked into the pouch as a try-in procedure. Adjustment of pedicle size should now be made. Once the pedicle fits as desired, it is made ready for the stabilizing suture. The suturing scheme is illustrated in Fig. 27-74. The suture must be positioned close to the mucobuccal fold. This enables the surgeon to pull the pedicle to the apical portion of the pouch. The suture should not be tightly tied, since it only serves as a positioning and stabilizing device. The use of a resorbable suture material is recommended.

Adjustment of pontic contours: Measures used to adapt the tissue surface of the pontic to the contour of the

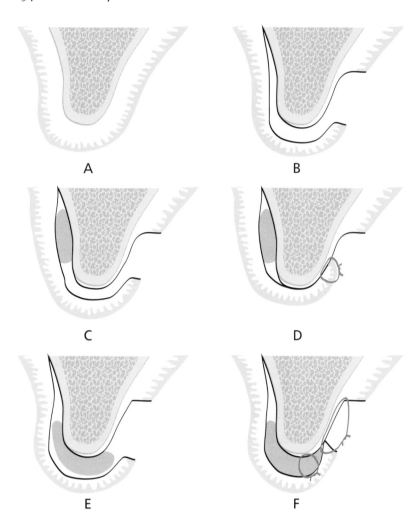

A

B

C

D

E

F

Fig. 27-76. Sequence of steps in the *"pouch graft procedure"* utilizing a free graft of connective tissue (CT) to expand the ridge. (A) Cross-section of the residual edentulous ridge prior to treatment. (B) The horizontal incision to create the pouch is made well to the palatal side of the defect. The incision is started partial-thickness to leave CT to suture to when the flap is closed. The dissection is made supraperiosteal on the labial side of the ridge to (1) ensure an adequate blood supply within the pedicle and (2) permit the flap to expand labially or labially and coronally free of tension. (C-D) The CT graft can be placed as shown for maximal buccolingual augmentation. (E-F) If vertical augmentation is desired, the CT implant can be placed closer to the crest of the ridge. As is shown in D and F, the more the flap is stretched or expanded to gain augmentation, the more difficult it is to gain primary flap closure.

surgically treated ridge are common to all soft tissue ridge augmentation procedures in patients with fixed bridgework. A light contact is maintained between the pedicle graft and the tissue surface of the pontics. The postoperative swelling will cause the tissue to conform to the shape of the pontic. This enables the clinician to shape the soft tissue into a form that is intended for the augmented site. Autopolymerizing resin is added to the tissue surface of the pontics and is allowed to cure until the resin reaches a dough-like state. The bridge is then seated and pressed into the grafted site. When the resin has set to a firm consistency, the bridge is removed and placed in hot water to complete the process of polymerization (Fig. 27-75). The tissue surface of the pontics and the embrasure areas are then carved to the shape that is intended for the final bridge. The surface of the pontic is polished and the bridge put in place using an appropriate temporary cement.

Postoperative care: A periodontal dressing is placed over the donor site. No dressing should be placed over the facial (labial) surface of the grafted area where swelling will occur. The dressing at the donor site should be changed at weekly intervals and maintained until wound healing has progressed to a point where the tissue is no longer tender to touch.

Pouch graft procedures

Surgical concept: A subepithelial pouch is prepared in the area of the ridge deformity, into which a free graft of connective tissue is placed and molded to create the desired contour of the ridge. The entrance incision and the plane of dissection may be made in different ways (Kaldahl et al. 1982, Seibert 1983, Allen et al. 1985, Miller 1986, Cohen 1994):

• Coronal-apically: the horizontal incision is made on the palatal or lingual side of the defect and the plane of dissection carried in an apical direction (Fig. 27-76)

• Apical-coronally: the horizontal incision is made high in the vestibule near the mucobuccal fold and the plane of dissection is carried coronally to the crest of the ridge

• Laterally: one or two vertical entrance incisions are started from either side of the defect (Fig. 27-77). The plane of dissection is made laterally across the span of the deformity.

Indication: The technique is used to correct Class I defects. Patients with large volume defects may have thin palatal tissues which are insufficient to provide the volume of the donor tissue necessary to fill the deformity. In such cases, various procedures for hard tissue augmentation may be selected (see Chapter 28).

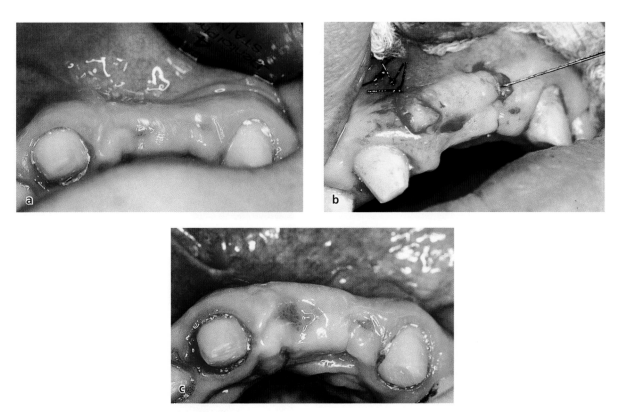

Fig. 27-77. *Pouch graft procedure*. (a) Pretreatment view of a Class I ridge deformity. (b) Placement of the free connective tissue graft in a tunnel prepared by split incision between the two vertical incisions. The graft is brought into position by the use of a suture placed in one end of the free graft. (c) 4 months post-treatment showing restored facial dimension of the edentulous ridge.

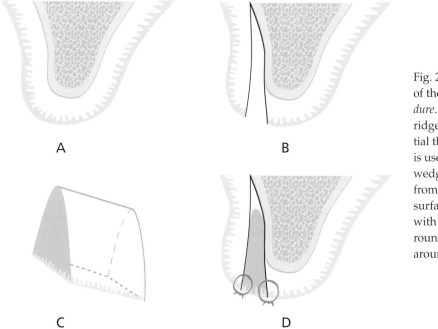

A

B

C

D

Fig. 27-78. Schematic illustrations of the *interpositional graft procedure*. (A) Cross-section of Class I ridge defect. (B) A labial flap (partial thickness dissection preferred) is used to create the pouch. (C) A wedge-shaped graft is removed from the palate. (D) The epithelial surface of the graft is placed flush with the surface of the tissue surrounding the pouch and sutured around its circumference.

Technique (Fig. 27-76): The pouch is prepared as described above. The mesiodistal entrance incision for the edge of the pouch should be made with a long bevel and must be started well to the palatal (lingual) side of the defect. After the pouch has been filled with graft, the facial tissue will be stretched. The long bevel

of the entrance incision permits the palatal edge of the flap to slide toward the facial surface without opening a gap at the incision line. Sometimes vertical releasing incisions have to be made lateral to the border of the defect.

A suitable donor site is selected in the palate, the tuberosity area, or in an edentulous area and a free

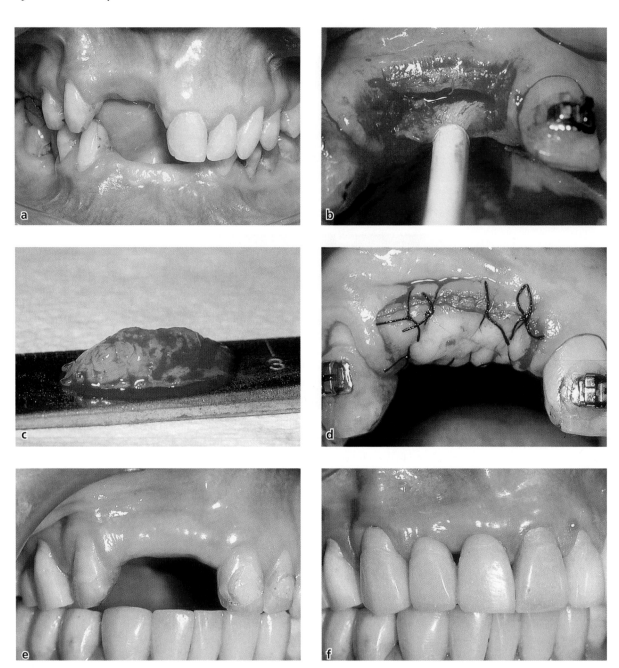

Fig. 27-79. (a) Pretreatment view, Class III ridge defect. A 2-stage procedure will be used to augment the ridge. (b) A pouch was prepared to receive an interpositional graft. Epithelium was removed from the borders of the recipient site to permit some of the graft to be placed above the level of the surrounding tissue in order to gain apico-coronal augmentation. (c) The wedge-shaped graft was 10 mm thick at its center. (d) The interpositional graft is both displacing the labial surface of the pouch in the labial direction as well as gaining height to the ridge. (e) Two months post-treatment. Additional augmentation is needed apicocoronally. (f) A second-stage onlay graft will be used to create a papilla and fill the dark triangle between the pontics.

graft of connective tissue is excised by the use of a "trap-door" approach. The graft is immediately transferred to the recipient site and properly positioned. The palatal entrance incision and the releasing incisions are closed with sutures.

Interpositional graft procedure
Surgical concept: Interpositional grafts are not completely submerged and covered in the manner that a subepithelial connective tissue graft is placed (Fig. 27-78) (Seibert 1991, 1993a,b). Therefore, there is no

need to remove the epithelium from the surface of the donor tissue. If augmentation is required not only in the buccolingual but also in the apicocoronal direction, a portion of the graft must be positioned above the surface of the tissue surrounding the recipient site (Fig. 27-79). A certain amount of the grafted connective tissue will thus be exposed in the oral cavity.

Indications: Interpositional graft procedures are used to correct Class I as well as small and moderate Class II defects.

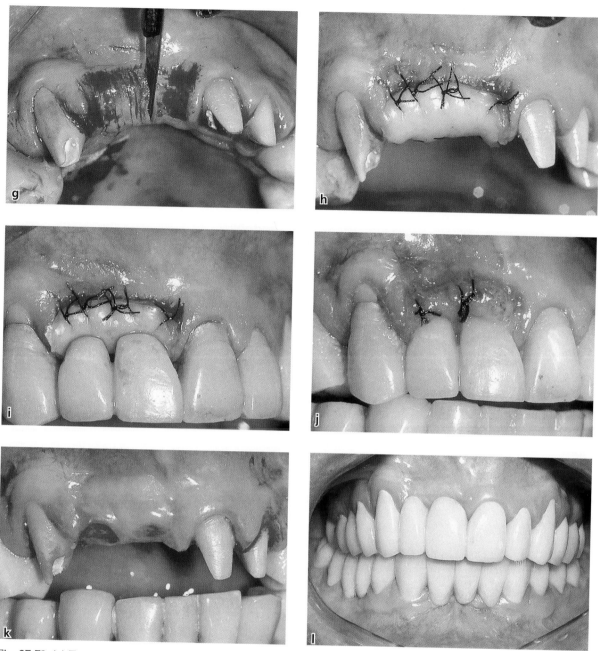

Fig. 27-79. (g) Two months after the first surgical procedure, the ridge was de-epithelialized and cuts were made into the connective tissue prior to placing the second-stage onlay graft into position. (h) The onlay graft was sutured into position. (i) The pontics were adjusted and brought into light contact with the graft. (j) Marked swelling occurred within the graft at 14 days post-surgery. (k) Two months following the second surgical procedure, a gingivoplasty was performed to deepen the pontic receptacle sites for the ovate pontics. (l) Post-treatment view 1 year after the final surgical procedure. Courtesy of Dr J. Seibert and Dr P. Malpeso, US.

Technique (Fig. 27-78): An envelope flap, or a split thickness flap with releasing incisions, is prepared at the facial surface of the defect area. The provisional bridge is placed in position to serve as a reference when estimates are made regarding the amount of tissue that has to be grafted to fill the defect. A periodontal probe may be used to measure the length, width and depth of the void of the pouch. A suitable donor site is selected in the palate or the tuberosity area, and a free graft of epithelium-connective tissue is excised.

The donor tissue is transferred to the recipient site and placed in position. If gain in ridge height is not intended, the epithelial surface for the graft is placed flush with the surrounding epithelium. The graft is sutured along its entire circumference to the tissues of the recipient site. The provisional bridge is placed in position and the pontics are trimmed and adjusted as discussed above. No dressing is used to cover the recipient site.

If gain in ridge height is also intended, a certain portion of the graft has to be kept above the surface of the surrounding tissue (Fig. 27-79d). Granulation tissue formed during healing will eventually make the

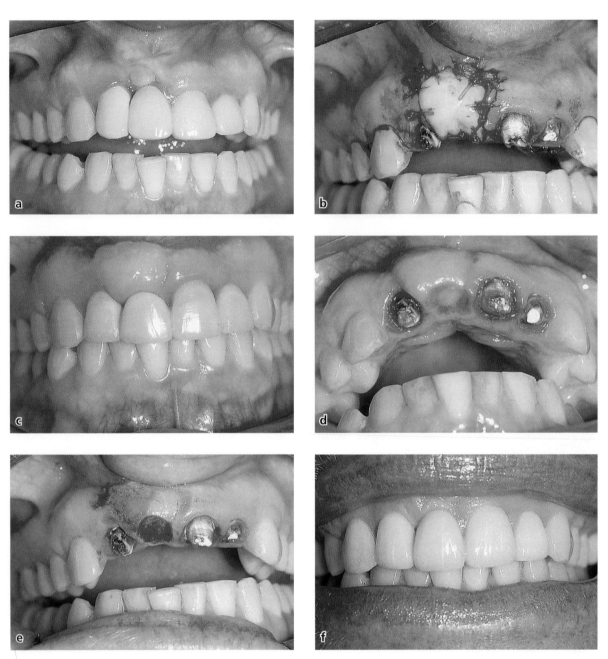

Fig. 27-80. *Onlay graft procedure.* (a) Pretreatment view. The gingival tissues were distorted from previous attempts at esthetic reconstruction. The patient wished to have a papilla between the right maxillary lateral and central incisor and a natural looking bridge. (b) The pontic area, including the papilla on the mesial of the right lateral incisor, was de-epithelialized and a thick (5 mm) onlay graft was sutured into position. (c) The pontic was shortened at the time of surgery to accommodate the thick graft. At 3 months post- surgery the graft had undergone maximum shrinkage and gingivoplasty could now be done. (d) Incisal view at 3 months post-surgery. Note the "papilla" that has been created. The indentation in the ridge was naturally created by the tissue swelling against the pontic tooth. (e) Rotary diamond point gingivoplasty was done to reshape the bulky graft to normal contours, deepen the receptacle site for the ovate pontic and level the gingival margins. (f) This view shows the esthetic harmony that was obtained in the soft tissues and tooth form at 2 years post-treatment. Courtesy of Dr J. Seibert and Dr C. Williams, US.

Fig. 27-81a-h. *Onlay graft procedures* utilized to augment ridge and create papillae. (a) Pretreatment view. The left lateral incisor was extracted after a traumatic injury. The patient detested the dark triangle on the mesial of the pontic, the poor tooth form in the bridge and the irregular contours in her gingival tissue. (b-c) An onlay graft was used to gain apicocoronal and buccolingual ridge augmentation as well as to develop papillae. Note how the graft was extended to the palatal side of the ridge to gain greater blood supply from a larger connective tissue base. (d-e) At 2 months post-surgery, a second-stage veneer graft was used to eliminate the surface irregularities on the surface of the gingiva and gain greater buccolingual augmentation. (f) At 4 months post second-stage surgery, gingivoplasty was done to prepare the area for an ovate form pontic. (g-h) One year post-treatment, esthetics have been restored for this patient. Courtesy of Dr J. Seibert and Dr D. Garber, US.

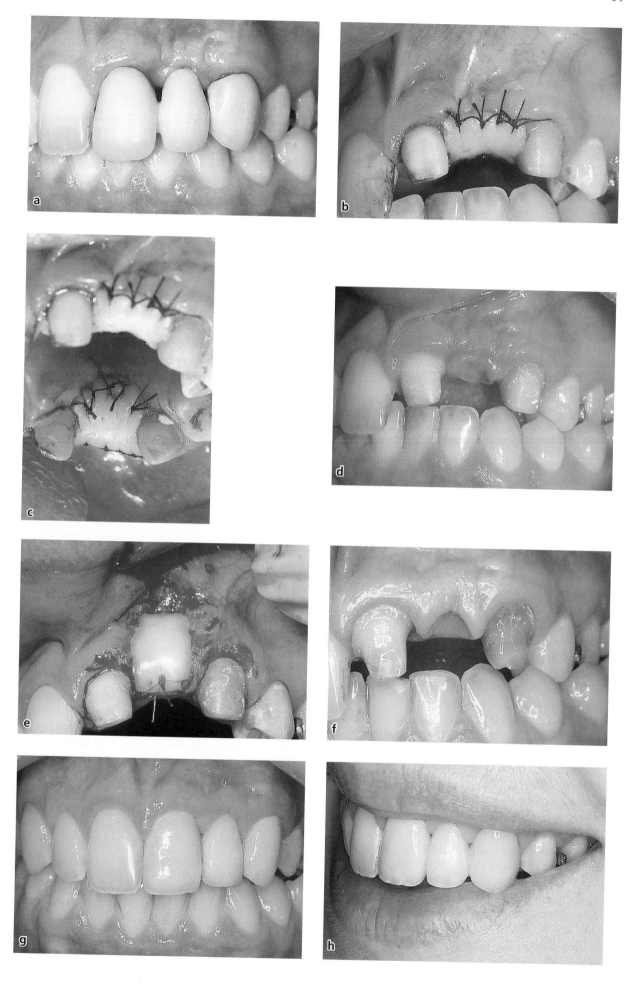

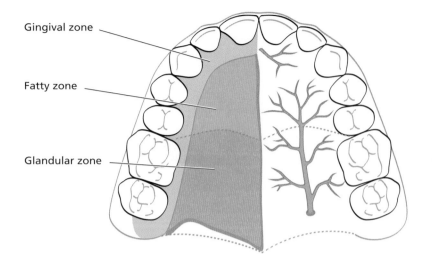

Gingival zone

Fatty zone

Glandular zone

Fig. 27-82. Basic anatomical-histological zones of the palate. Note the normal location of the greater palatine foramen.

border between the graft and the adjacent tissue smooth and properly epithelialized. The swelling, which occurs postoperatively, will assist in sculpting the contour of the ridge.

Onlay graft procedures
Surgical concept: The onlay procedure was designed to augment ridge defects in the apicocoronal plane, i.e. to gain ridge height (Meltzer 1979, Seibert 1983). Onlay grafts are epithelialized free grafts which, following placement, receive their nutrition from the de-epithelialized connective tissue of the recipient site. The amount of apicocoronal augmentation that can be obtained is related to the initial thickness of the graft, the events of the wound healing process and the amount of graft tissue that survives (Figs. 27-79, 27-80 and 27-81). If necessary, the grafting procedure can be repeated at 2-month intervals to gradually increase the ridge height.

Indications: Onlay graft procedures are used in the treatment of large Class II and III defects. They are not suitable in areas where the blood supply at the recipient site has been compromised by scar tissue formation from previous wound healing.

Technique (Fig. 27-79g-i): An attempt must be made to retain as much as possible the lamina propria of the recipient site. The anesthetic solution should be placed high in the vestibular fornix and in the palate, thus keeping vasoconstriction in the recipient site to a minimum. A scalpel blade is used to remove the epithelium. The scalpel is moved with short, saw-like strokes across the recipient site at a level approximately 1 mm below the outer surface of the epithelium. The least amount of connective tissue possible should be excised. The margins of the recipient site can be prepared with either a butt-joint or a beveled margin. The prepared recipient site should be covered with a surgical gauze moistened with isotonic saline while the donor tissue is dissected.

Selection of donor site: Onlay graft procedures, as well as frequently interpositional graft procedures, require large amounts of donor tissue. The palatal vault region of premolars and first molars, midway between the gingival margin and the midline raphae, is as a general rule the only area in the maxilla that contains the necessary volume of tissue required to augment large size ridge defects. During the presurgical planning phase, the tissue of the palate should be probed with a 30-gauge syringe needle to ensure that an acceptable volume of tissue can be obtained at the time of surgery.

The major palatine artery emerges from the posterior palatine foramen located adjacent to the distal surface of the maxillary second molar, midway between the gingival margin and the midline raphae (Fig. 27-82). The artery passes in an anterior direction close to the surface of the palatal bone. It is important therefore that the second and third molar regions are not used as donor sites for large volume grafts.

Planning in graft preparation: As a rule the graft should be made a few mm wider and longer than the dimensions required at the recipient site. The dimensions of the graft are outlined on the palate with the use of a scalpel and light bleeding is provoked to define the surface borders. In order to avoid interference with the palatine artery, the borders of the graft must be planned in such a way that its thinner portions are located high in the palatal vault or in the first molar area. The thicker portions should be harvested from the premolar areas.

Dissection of donor tissue: The base of the graft should be V or U-shaped to match the shape of the defect in the ridge. The different planes of incision prepared in the palate must therefore converge towards an area under the center or toward one edge of the donor site. It is comparatively easy, with the use of a scalpel, to dissect in an anteroposterior direction or from an area high in the palate in a lateral direction towards the teeth. It is, however, difficult to dissect in an anterior

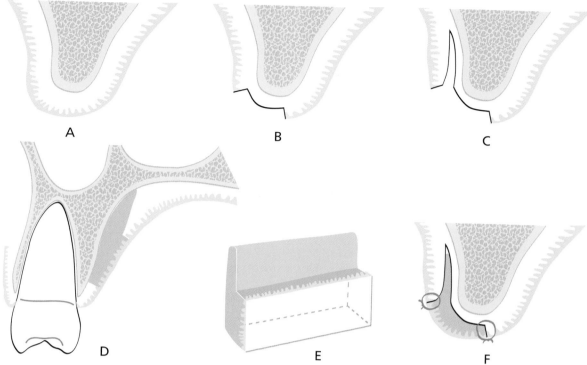

Fig. 27-83. Diagram of the *combination onlay-interpositional graft procedure*. (A) Cross-section of a Class III ridge defect. (B) Epithelium is removed on the labial-crestal side of the ridge to prepare the recipient bed for the onlay segment of the graft. (C) Partial-thickness dissection was then used to create a pouch for the interpositional section of the graft. (D) The dissection for the graft is started at right angles to the surface of the palate. The scalpel blade is then angled to remove a long connective tissue segment for the graft. (E) Three-dimensional view of the onlay section of the graft (including epithelium) and the connective tissue segment for buccolingual augmentation. (F) Graft sutured into position. Reprinted with permission, *International Journal of Periodontics and Restorative Dentistry*.

direction from the distal edge of the donor site. There are a variety of blade holders available which permit the scalpel blade to be positioned at different angles to the holder and which enable the surgeon to cut with a back-action. When the donor tissue has been removed, it must at all times be stored in pieces of surgical gauze moistened in isotonic saline.

Treatment of the donor site: Since it is difficult to anchor and maintain a periodontal dressing at the donor site in the palatal vault, an acrylic stent should be fabricated prior to surgery. The stent should be made with wrought wire clasps on each side to add retention and to aid the patient in removing and inserting the device.

The donor site must be inspected carefully for signs of arterial bleeding. If any small-vessel bleeding is observed, a circumferential suture must be placed around the vessel distal to the bleeding point. Immediately thereafter, the void at the donor site should be packed with a suitable hemostatic agent and the edges of the wound should be brought closer together with sutures. The stent is then put into position.

Try-in and stabilization of graft: The graft is transferred with tissue forceps to the recipient site for a try-in. The graft is trimmed to the proper shape and adjusted to fit the connective tissue surface of the prepared ridge. A series of parallel cuts may be made deep into the exposed lamina propria of the recipient site to sever

large blood vessels (Fig. 27-79g) immediately before suturing. A series of interrupted sutures is placed along the borders of the graft. The dental assistant should stabilize the onlay graft against the surface of the recipient site, while the surgeon completes the placement of sutures.

Wound healing in the recipient site: Considerable postoperative swelling often occurs during the first week after pouch and onlay augmentation procedures. The epithelium of the graft will slough to form a white film on the surface of the graft. Patients should rinse two to four times per day with an antimicrobial mouthwash during the first week after surgery and should refrain from mechanical cleaning measures in the area until a new epithelial covering has formed over the graft, which will not occur until a functional capillary circulation has been re-established in the graft (4-7 days after the surgery). The grafted tissue will assume a normal color as the epithelium thickens via stratification. Tissue form is usually stable after 3 months, but further shrinkage may occur over a period of several months. Final restorative measures should therefore not be initiated until after 6 months.

Wound healing in the donor site: Granulation tissue will gradually fill the donor site. Initial healing is usually complete within 3-4 weeks after the removal of a 4-5 mm thick graft. Patients should wear the surgical stent

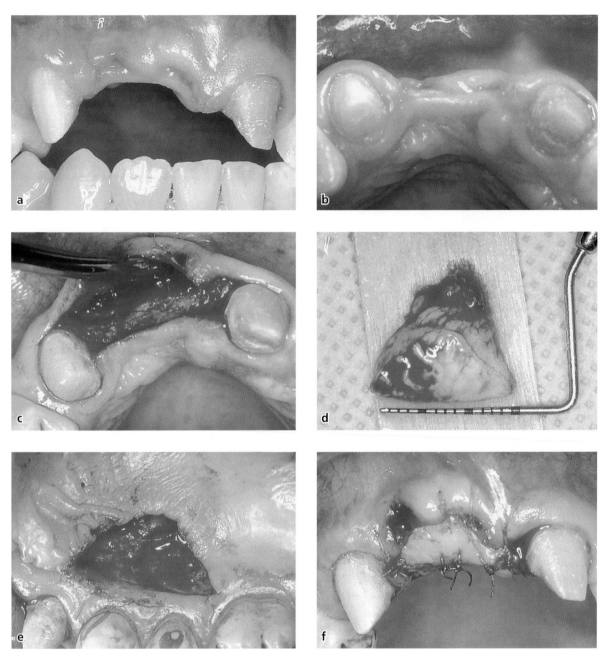

Fig. 27-84. (a-b) The right maxillary lateral and central incisors were lost due to trauma. These views show the horizontal and vertical loss of ridge tissue 10 months after the extractions. (c) A partial-thickness path of incision was extended labially and apically to create a pouch. The amount of space created within the pouch and the degree of relaxation of the flap was then tested with a periosteal elevator. (d) The epithelialized section of the graft can be seen in this view. (e) The premolar area, maxillary right side, was used as the donor area. The area of exposed connective tissue corresponds to the onlay section of the graft. The incisions were extended another 5-7 mm towards the midline on a long bevel to obtain the interpositional segment of the graft. (f) The graft was tucked into the labial pouch and sutured first along its palatal border. The labial flap was then sutured along the epithelial connective border of the graft. The residual labial socket defect in the flap created a soft tissue discontinuity defect along the labial margin of the flap.

for about 2 weeks to protect the healing wound. The palate returns to its presurgical contour after about 3 months.

Combined onlay – interpositional graft procedures
Class III ridge defects pose a major challenge to the clinician since the ridge has to be augmented in both vertical and horizontal dimensions. The combined

onlay-interpositional graft procedure (Figs. 27-83 and 27-84) may successfully be used in such a situation (Seibert & Louis 1996). The combined graft procedure may offer the following advantages:

- The submerged connective tissue section of the interpositional graft aids in the revascularization of

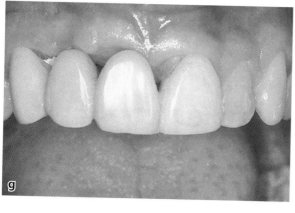
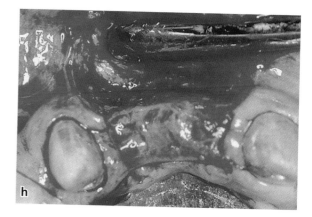
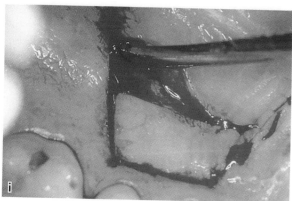
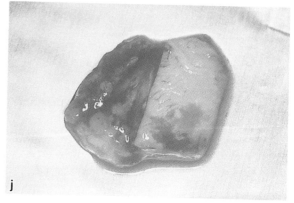

Fig. 27-84. (g) At 6 weeks postsurgery, it can be seen that further augmentation would be required to gain additional soft tissue in both the vertical and horizontal planes. A second-stage procedure was done at this time. (h) An incision 1.5 mm in depth was utilized to de-epithelialize the crestal surface of the ridge. Note that the papillae were not included within the surgical field. The mesial and distal borders of the onlay section of the recipient site were then extended apically to create vertical releasing incisions. The overall recipient site was to be trapezoidal in shape. A labial flap to create the pouch section of the recipient site was made using partial-thickness dissection. (i) The left maxillary premolar area was used as the donor site for the second-stage surgery. (j) This side view perspective clearly shows the epithelialized onlay section of the graft and the de-epithelialized connective tissue section of the graft, as well as tissue thickness.

the onlay section of the graft, thereby gaining a greater percentage of take of the overall graft

• A smaller postoperative open wound in the palate donor site

• Faster healing in the palate donor site with less patient discomfort

• Greater latitude or ability to control the degree of buccolingual and apicocoronal augmentation within a single procedure

• Vestibular depth is not decreased and the mucogingival junction is not moved coronally, thereby eliminating the need for follow-up corrective procedures.

Refinement of pontic contours and gingivoplasty soft tissue sculpting procedures

It is desirable, when reconstructing defects within a partially edentulous ridge, to moderately overcorrect the ridge in the area of the deformity. This will compensate for wound contraction and provide the necessary bulk of tissue within the ridge to sculpt the ridge to its final form. Gingivoplasty techniques using rotary coarse diamond stones in an ultraspeed handpiece with copious water spray are used to smooth out incision lines and perfect the fit and shape of the pontic teeth to the crest of the ridge (Figs. 27-80 and 27-84). Adjustments are made to shape the cervical contour and emergence profile of the pontic teeth to match that of the contralateral teeth. The tissue-contacting surfaces of the pontic teeth are immediately rebased with autopolymerizing resin and polished. This final tissue sculpting procedure and reshaping of the provisional prothesis is minor in nature but aids greatly in defining the shape of the papillae and creating the illusion of the presence of a cuff of free gingiva at the pontic/ridge interface.

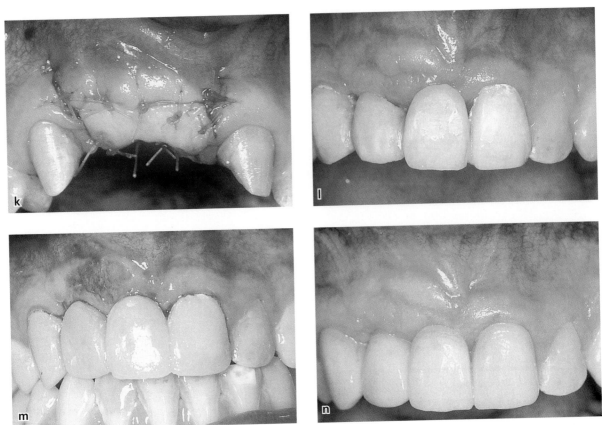

Fig. 27-84. (k) The graft was sutured first along the fixed palatal border to gain initial stabilization. Then the connective tissue interpositional section was sutured along the lateral borders. The flap was then sutured over the interpositional section of the graft at the epithelialized edge of the onlay section of the graft and along the vertical incisions. (l) At 6 weeks postsurgery, the provisional prosthesis was modified to bring the tissue surface of the pontics into contact with the healing ridge. (m) At 2 months postsurgery, tooth form was further modified on the provisional prosthesis and gingivoplasty was done to sculpt the tissues to final form and smooth out surface irregularities. (n) The final ceramo-metal prosthesis was inserted 4 months later. The life-like reconstruction of the soft tissues and dentition restored dentofacial esthetics for the patient. Courtesy of Dr J. Seibert, Dr J. Louis & Dr D. Hazzouri, US. Reprinted with permission from *International Journal of Periodontics and Restorative Dentistry*.

REFERENCES

Abrams, L. (1980). Augmentation of the residual edentulous ridge for fixed prosthesis. *Compendium of Continuing Education in General Dentistry* **1**, 205-214.

Agudio, G., Pini Prato, G., De Paoli, S. & Nevins, M. (1985). Mucogingival interceptive therapy. *International Journal of Periodontics and Restorative Dentistry* **5**, 49-59.

Ainamo, A., Bergenholtz, A., Hugoson, A. & Ainamo, J. (1992). Location of the mucogingival junction 18 years after apically repositioned flap surgery. *Journal of Clinical Periodontology* **19**, 49-52.

Allen, A.L. (1994). Use of the supraperiosteal envelope in soft tissue grafting for root coverage. I. Rationale and technique. *International Journal of Periodontics and Restorative Dentistry* **14**, 217-227.

Allen, E.P., Gainza, C.S., Farthing, G.G., et al. (1985). Improved technique for localized ridge augmentation. *Journal of Periodontology* **56**, 195-199.

Allen, E.P. & Miller, P.D. (1989). Coronal positioning of existing gingiva. Short term results in the treatment of shallow marginal tissue recession. *Journal of Periodontology* **60**, 316-319.

Andlin-Sobocki, A. & Bodin, L. (1993). Dimensional alterations of the gingiva related to changes of facial/lingual tooth position in permanent anterior teeth of children. A 2-year longitudinal study. *Journal of Clinical Periodontology* **20**, 219-224.

Andlin-Sobocki, A., Marcusson, A. & Persson, M. (1991). 3-year observation on gingival recession in mandibular incisors in children. *Journal of Clinical Periodontology* **18**, 155-159.

Azzi, R., Etienne, D. & Carranza, F. (1998). Surgical reconstruction of the interdental papilla. *International Journal of Periodontics and Restorative Dentistry* **18**, 467-473.

Baelum, V., Fejerskov, O. & Karring T. (1986). Oral hygiene, gingivitis and periodontal breakdown in adult Tanzanians. *Journal of Periodontal Research* **21**, 221-232.

Baelum, V., Fejerskov, O. & Manji, F. (1988). Periodontal diseases in adult Kenyans. *Journal of Clinical Periodontology* **15**, 445-452.

Bahat, O., Handelsman, M. & Gordon, J. (1990). The transpositional flap in mucogingival surgery. *International Journal of Periodontics and Restorative Dentistry* **10**, 473-482.

Baker, D.L. & Seymour, G.J. (1976). The possible pathogenesis of gingival recession. A histological study of induced recession in the rat. *Journal of Clinical Periodontology* **3**, 208-219.

Baldi, C., Pini Prato, G., Pagliaro, U., Nieri, M., Saletta, D., Muzzi, L. & Cortellini P. (1999). Coronally advanced flap procedure for root coverage. Is flap thickness a relevant predictor to achieve root coverage? A 19-case series. *Journal of Periodontology* **70**, 1077-1084.

Batenhorst, K.F., Bowers, G.M. & Williams, J.E. (1974). Tissue changes resulting from facial tipping and extrusion of incisors in monkeys. *Journal of Periodontology* **45**, 660-668.

Beagle, J.R. (1992). Surgical reconstruction of the interdental papilla: Case report. *The International Journal of Periodontics and Restorative Dentistry* **12**, 144-151.

Becker, W., Becker, B.E. & Caffesse, R. (1994). A comparison of demineralized freeze-dried bone and autologous bone to induce bone formation in human extraction sockets. *Journal of Periodontology* **65**, 1128-1133.

Bernimoulin, J.P. & Curilivic, Z. (1977). Gingival recession and tooth mobility. *Journal of Clinical Periodontology* **4**, 208-219.

Bernimoulin, J.P., Lüscher, B. & Mühlemann, H.R. (1975). Coronally repositioned periodontal flap. Clinical evaluation after one year. *Journal of Clinical Periodontology* **2**, 1-13.

Bertrand, P.M. & Dunlap, R.M. (1988). Coverage of deep, wide gingival clefts with free gingival autografts: Root planing with and without citric acid demineralization. *International Journal of Periodontics and Restorative Dentistry* **8** (1), 65-77.

Bohannan, H.M. (1962a). Studies in the alteration of vestibular depth. I. Complete denudation. *Journal of Periodontology* **33**, 120-128.

Bohannan, H.M. (1962b). Studies in the alteration of vestibular depth. II. Periosteum retention. *Journal of Periodontology* **33**, 354-359.

Borghetti, A. & Gardella, J-P. (1990). Thick gingival autograft for the coverage of gingival recession: A clinical evaluation. *International Journal of Periodontics and Restorative Dentistry* **10**, 217-229.

Borghetti, A. & Glise, J.M. (2000). Aménagement de la crête édentée pour la prothèse fixéesur pilers naturales. In: Borghetti, A. & Monnet-Corti, V. eds. *Chirurgie plastique parodontale*. Rueil-Malmaison Cedex: Editions CdP Groupe Liaisons SA, pp. 391-422.

Borghetti, A. & Laborde, G. (1996). La chirurgie parodontale pro-prothétique. *Actualités Odonto-Stomatologiques* **194**, 193-227.

Bouchard, P., Nilveus, R. & Etienne, D. (1997). Clinical evaluation of tetracycline HCL conditioning in the treatment of gingival recessions. A comparative study. *Journal of Periodontology* **68**, 262-269.

Bowers, G.M. (1963). A study of the width of attached gingiva. *Journal of Periodontology* **34**, 201-209.

Boyd, R.L. (1978). Mucogingival considerations and their relationship to orthodontics. *Journal of Periodontology* **49**, 67-76.

Bradley, R.E., Grant, J.C. & Ivancie, G.P. (1959). Histologic evaluation of mucogingival surgery. *Oral Surgery* **12**, 1184-1199.

Brown, S.I. (1973). The effect of orthodontic therapy on certain types of periodontal defects. I. Clinical findings. *Journal of Periodontology* **44**, 742-756.

Bruno, J.F. (1994). Connective tissue graft technique assuring wide root coverage. *International Journal of Periodontics and Restorative Dentistry* **14**, 127-137.

Brustein, D. (1979). Cosmetic periodontics. Coronally repositioned pedicle graft. *Dental Survey* **46**, 22.

Caffesse, R.G., Alspach, S.R., Morrison, E.C. & Burgett, F.G. (1987). Lateral sliding flaps with and without citric acid. *International Journal of Periodontics and Restorative Dentistry* **7** (6), 43-57.

Caffesse, R.G., De LaRosa, M., Garza, M., Munne-Travers, A., Mondragon, J.C. & Weltman, R. (2000). Citric acid demineralization and subepithelial connective tissue grafts. *Journal of Periodontology* **71**, 568-572.

Caffesse, R.G., Kon, S., Castelli, W.A. & Nasjleti, C.E. (1984). Revascularization following the lateral sliding flap procedure. *Journal of Periodontology* **55**, 352-359.

Carranza, F.A. & Carraro, J.J. (1963). Effect of removal of periosteum on post-operative results of mucogingival surgery. *Journal of Periodontology* **34**, 223-226.

Carranza, F.A. & Carraro, J.J. (1970). Mucogingival techniques in periodontal surgery. *Journal of Periodontology* **41**, 294-299.

Carraro, J.J., Carranza, F.A., Albano, E.A. & Joly, G.G. (1964).

Effect of bone denudation in mucogingival surgery in humans. *Journal of Periodontology* **35**, 463-466.

Checchi, L., Daprile, G., Gatto, M.R. & Pelliccioni, G.A. (1999). Gingival recession and toothbrushing in an Italian School of Dentistry: a pilot study. *Journal of Clinical Periodontology* **26**, 276-280.

Coatoam, G.W., Behrents, R.G. & Bissada, N.F. (1981). The width of keratinized gingiva during orthodontic treatment: its significance and impact on periodontal status. *Journal of Periodontology* **52**, 307-313.

Cohen, D. & Ross, S. (1968). The double papillae flap in periodontal therapy. *Journal of Periodontology* **39**, 65-70.

Cohen, E.S. (1994). Ridge augmentation utilizing the subepithelial connective tissue graft: Case reports. *Practical Periodontics and Aesthetic Dentistry* **6**, 47-53.

Corn, H. (1962). Periosteal separation – its clinical significance. *Journal of Periodontology* **33**, 140-152.

Cortellini, P., Clauser, C. & Pini Prato, G.P. (1993). Histologic assessment of new attachment following the treatment of a human buccal recession by means of a guided tissue regeneration procedure. *Journal of Periodontology* **64**, 387-391.

Costich, E.R. & Ramfjord, S.F. (1968). Healing after partial denudation of the alveolar process. *Journal of Periodontology* **39**, 5-12.

Daniel, A. & Cheru, R. (1990). Treatment of localised gingival recession with subpedicle connective tissue graft and free gingival auto graft – a comparative clinical evaluation. *Journal of Indian Dental Association* **61**, 294-297.

De Trey, E. & Bernimoulin, J. (1980). Influence of free gingival grafts on the health of the marginal gingiva. *Journal of Clinical Periodontology* **7**, 381-393.

Donaldson D. (1974). The etiology of gingival recession associated with temporary crowns. *Journal of Periodontology* **45**, 468-471.

Donnenfeld, O.W., Marks, R.M. & Glickman, I. (1964). The apically repositioned flap – a clinical study. *Journal of Periodontology* **35**, 381-387.

Dorfman, H.S., Kennedy, J.E. & Bird, W.C. (1980). Longitudinal evaluation of free autogenous gingival grafts. *Journal of Clinical Periodontology* **7**, 316-324.

Dorfman, H.S., Kennedy, J.E. & Bird, W.C. (1982). Longitudinal evaluation of free gingival grafts. A four-year report. *Journal of Periodontology* **53**, 349-352.

Edel, A. (1974). Clinical evaluation of free connective tissue grafts used to increase the width of keratinized gingiva. *Journal of Clinical Periodontology* **1**, 185-196.

Engelking G. & Zachrisson B.U. (1982). Effects of incisor repositioning on monkey periodontium after expansion through the cortical plate. *American Journal of Orthodontics* **82**, 23-32.

Ericsson, I. & Lindhe, J. (1984). Recession in sites with inadequate width of the keratinized gingiva. An experimental study in the dog. *Journal of Clinical Periodontology* **11**, 95-103.

Ericsson, I., Thilander B. & Lindhe J. (1978). Periodontal condition after orthodontic tooth movement in the dog. *Angle Orthodontics* **48**, 210-218.

Espinel, M.C. & Caffesse, R.G. (1981). Lateral positioned pedicle sliding flap – revised technique in the treatment of localized gingival recession. *International Journal of Periodontics and Restorative Dentistry*, **1** (1), 43-51.

Foushee, D.G., Moriarty, J.D. & Simpson, D.M. (1985). Effects of mandibular orthognatic treatment on mucogingival tissue. *Journal of Periodontology* **56**, 727-733.

Freedman, A.L., Green, K., Salkin, L.M., Stein, M.D. & Mellado, J.R. (1999). An 18-year longitudinal study of untreated mucogingival defects. *Journal of Periodontology* **70**, 1174-1176.

Friedman, N. (1957). Mucogingival surgery. *Texas Dental Journal* **75**, 358-362.

Friedman, N. (1962). Mucogingival surgery: the apically repositioned flap. *Journal of Periodontology* **33**, 328-340.

Friedman, N. & Levine, H.L. (1964). Mucogingival surgery: current status. *Journal of Periodontology* **35**, 5-21.

Gargiulo, A.W. (1961). Dimensions and relations of the dentogingival junction in humans. *Journal of Periodontology* **32**, 261-267.

Glossary of Terms in Periodontology. (1992). The American Academy of Periodontology, Chicago, US.

Gorman, W.J. (1967). Prevalence and aetiology of gingival recession. *Journal of Periodontology* **38**, 316-322.

Gottlow, J., Karring, T. & Nyman, S. (1990). Guided tissue regeneration following treatment of recession-type defects in the monkey. *Journal of Periodontology* **61**, 680-685.

Gottlow, J., Nyman, S., Karring, T. & Lindhe, J. (1986). Treatment of localized gingival recessions with coronally displaced flaps and citric acid. An experimental study in the dog. *Journal of Clinical Periodontology* **13**, 57-63.

Gottsegen, R. (1954). Frenulum position and vestibular depth in relation to gingival health. *Oral Surgery* **7**, 1069-1078.

Gould, T.R.L., Robertson, P.B. & Oakley, C. (1992). Effect of free gingival grafts on naturally-occurring recession in miniature swine. *Journal of Periodontology* **63**, 593-597.

Grevers, A. (1977). *Width of attached gingiva and vestibular depth in relation to gingival health*. Thesis. University of Amsterdam.

Grupe, J. (1966). Modified technique for the sliding flap operation. *Journal of Periodontology* **37**, 491-495.

Grupe, J. & Warren, R. (1956). Repair of gingival defects by a sliding flap operation. *Journal of Periodontology* **27**, 290-295.

Guinard, E.A. & Caffesse, R.G. (1978). Treatment of localized gingival recessions. III. Comparison on results obtained with lateral sliding and coronally repositioned flaps. *Journal of Periodontology* **49**, 457-461.

Haggerty, P.C. (1966). The use of a free gingival graft to create a healthy environment for full crown preparation. *Periodontics* **4**, 329-331.

Hall, W.B. (1981). The current status of mucogingival problems and their therapy. *Journal of Periodontology* **52**, 569-575.

Han, T.J. & Takei, H.H. (1996). Progress in gingival papilla reconstruction. *Periodontology 2000* **11**, 65-68.

Hangorsky, U. & Bissada, N.B. (1980). Clinical assessment of free gingival graft effectiveness on maintenance of periodontal health. *Journal of Periodontology* **51**, 274-278.

Harlan, A.W. (1907). Discussion of paper: restoration of gum tissue. *Dental Cosmos* **49**, 591-598.

Harris, R.J. (1992). The connective tissue and partial thickness double pedicle graft: a predictable method of obtaining root coverage. *Journal of Periodontology* **63**, 477-486.

Harris, R.J. (1994). The connective tissue with partial thickness double pedicle graft: the results of 100 consecutively-treated defects. *Journal of Periodontology* **65**, 448-461.

Harris, R.J. (1999). Human histologic evaluation of root coverage obtained with a connective tissue with partial thickness double pedicle graft: a case report. *Journal of Periodontology* **70**, 813-821.

Harvey, P. (1965). Management of advanced periodontitis. Part I. Preliminary report of a method of surgical reconstruction. *New Zealand Dental Journal* **61**, 180-187.

Hawley, C.E. & Staffileno, H. (1970). Clinical evaluation of free gingival grafts in periodontal surgery. *Journal of Periodontology* **41**, 105-112.

Herrero, F., Scott, J.B., Maropis, P.S. & Yukna, R.A. (1995). Clinical comparison of desired versus actual amount of surgical crown lengthening. *Journal of Periodontology* **66**, 568-571.

Holbrook, T. & Ochsenbein, C. (1983). Complete coverage of the denuded root surface with a one-stage gingival graft. *International Journal of Periodontics and Restorative Dentistry*, **3** (3), 9-27.

Ibbott, C.G., Oles, R.D. & Laverty, W.H. (1985). Effects of citric acid treatment on autogenous free graft coverage of localized recession. *Journal of Periodontology* **56**, 662-665.

Ingber, J.S. (1974). Forced eruption: Part I. A method of treating isolated one and two wall infrabony osseous defects – rationale and case report. *Journal of Periodontology* **45**, 199-206.

Ingber, J.S. (1976). Forced eruption: Part II. A method of treating non-restorable teeth – periodontal and restorative considerations. *Journal of Periodontology* **47**, 203-216.

Ivancie, G.P. (1957). Experimental and histological investigation of gingival regeneration in vestibular surgery. *Journal of Periodontology* **28**, 259-263.

Jahnke, P.V., Sandifer, J.B., Gher, M.E., Gray, J.L. & Richardson, A.C. (1993). Thick free gingival and connective tissue autografts for root coverage. *Journal of Periodontology* **64**, 315-322.

Kaldahl, W.B., Tussing, G.J., Wentz, F.M. & Walker, J.A. (1982). Achieving an esthetic appearance with a fixed prosthesis by submucosal grafts. *Journal of the American Dental Association* **104**, 449-452.

Karring, T., Cumming, B.R., Oliver, R.C. & Löe, H. (1975). The origin of granulation tissue and its impact on postoperative results of mucogingival surgery. *Journal of Periodontology* **46**, 577-585.

Karring, T., Nyman, S., Thilander, B., Magnusson, I. & Lindhe, J. (1982). Bone regeneration in orthodontically produced alveolar bone dehiscences. *Journal of Periodontal Research* **17**, 309-315,1982

Karring, T., Ostergaard, E. & Löe, H. (1971). Conservation of tissue specificity after heterotopic transplantation of gingiva and alveolar mucosa. *Journal of Periodontal Research* **6**, 282-293.

Kennedy, J.E., Bird, W.C., Palcanis, K.G. & Dorfman, H.S. (1985). A longitudinal evaluation of varying widths of attached gingiva. *Journal of Clinical Periodontology* **12**, 667-675.

Khocht, A., Simon, G., Person, P. & Denepitiya, J.L. (1993). Gingival recession in relation to history of hard toothbrush use. *Journal of Periodontology* **64**, 900-905.

Kisch, J., Badersten, A. & Egelberg, J. (1986). Longitudinal observation of "unattached", mobile gingival areas. *Journal of Clinical Periodontology* **13**, 131-134.

Källestål, C., Matsson, L. & Holm, A-K. (1990). Periodontal conditions in a group of Swedish adolescents. I. A descriptive epidemiologic study. *Journal of Clinical Periodontology* **17**, 601-608.

Källestål, C. & Uhlin, S. (1992). Buccal attachment loss in Swedish adolescent. *Journal of Clinical Periodontology* **19**, 485-491.

Laney, J.B., Saunders, V.G. & Garnick, J.J. (1992). A comparison of two techniques for attaining root coverage. *Journal of Periodontology* **63**, 19-23.

Lang, N.P. (1995). Periodontal considerations in prosthetic dentistry. *Periodontology 2000* **9**, 118-131.

Lang, N.P. & Löe, H. (1972). The relationship between the width of keratinized gingiva and gingival health. *Journal of Periodontology* **43**, 623-627.

Langer, B. & Langer, L. (1985). Subepithelial connective tissue graft technique for root coverage. *Journal of Periodontology* **56**, 715-720.

Lekovic, V., Kenney, E.B., Weinlaender, M., Han, T., Klokkevold, P., Nedic, M. & Orsini, M. (1997). A bone regenerative approach to alveolar ridge maintenance following tooth extraction. Report of 10 cases. *Journal of Periodontology* **68**, 563-570.

Lindhe, J. & Nyman, S. (1980). Alterations of the position of the marginal soft tissue following periodontal surgery. *Journal of Clinical Periodontology* **7**, 525-530.

Lundberg, M. & Wennström, J.L. (1988). Development of gingiva following surgical exposure of a facially positioned unerupted incisor. *Journal of Periodontology* **59**, 652-655.

Löe, H., Änerud, A., Boysen, H. & Smith, M. (1978). The natural history of periodontal disease in man. The rate of periodontal destruction before 40 years of age. *Journal of Periodontology* **49**, 607-620.

Löe, H., Änerud, Å. & Boysen H. (1992). The natural history of periodontal disease in man: prevalence, severity, extent of gingival recession. *Journal of Periodontology* **63**, 489-495.

Löst, C. (1984). Depth of alveolar bone dehiscences in relation to gingival recessions. *Journal of Clinical Periodontology* **11**, 583-589.

Majzoub, Z., Landi, L., Grusovin, G. & Cordioli, G. (2001). Histology of connective tissue graft. A case report. *Journal of Periodontology* **72**, 1607-1615.

Matter, J. (1982). Free gingival grafts for the treatment of gingival recession. A review of some techniques. *Journal of Clinical Periodontology* **9**, 103-114.

Maynard, J.G. (1987). The rationale for mucogingival therapy in the child and adolescent. *International Journal of Periodontics and Restorative Dentistry*, **7** (1), 37-51.

Maynard, J.G. & Ochsenbein, D. (1975). Mucogingival problems, prevalence and therapy in children. *Journal of Periodontology* **46**, 543-552.

Maynard, J.G. & Wilson, R.D. (1979). Physiologic dimensions of the periodontium significant to the restorative dentist. *Journal of Periodontology* **50**, 170-174.

Meltzer, J.A. (1979). Edentulous area tissue graft correction of an esthetic defect. A case report. *Journal of Periodontology* **50**, 320-322.

Miller, A.J., Brunelle, J.A., Carlos, J.P., Brown, L.J. & Löe, H. (1987). Oral health of United States adults. NIH Publication No. 87-2868, National Institute of Dental Research, Bethesda, Maryland.

Miller, P.D. (1982). Root coverage using a free soft tissue autograft following citric acid application. I. Technique. *International Journal of Periodontics and Restorative Dentistry* **2** (1), 65-70.

Miller, P.D. (1985a). A classification of marginal tissue recession. *International Journal of Periodontics and Restorative Dentistry* **5** (2), 9-13.

Miller, P.D. (1985b). Root coverage using a free soft tissue autograft following citric acid application. III. A successful and predictable procedure in areas of deep-wide recession. *International Journal of Periodontics and Restorative Dentistry* **5** (2), 15-37.

Miller, P.D. Jr. (1986). Ridge augmentation under existing fixed prosthesis. Simplified technique. *Journal of Periodontology* **57**, 742-745.

Miller, P.D. (1987). Root coverage with free gingival graft. Factors associated with incomplete coverage. *Journal of Periodontology* **58**, 674-681.

Miller, P.D. (1993). Root coverage grafting for regeneration and aesthetics. *Periodontology 2000* **1**, 118-127.

Modéer, T. & Odenrick, L. (1980). Post-treatment periodontal status of labially erupted maxillary canines. *Acta Odontologica Scandianvica* **38**, 253-256.

Miyasato, M., Crigger, M. & Egelberg, J. (1977). Gingival condition in areas of minimal and appreciable width of keratinized gingiva. *Journal of Clinical Periodontology* **4**, 200-209.

Murtomaa, H., Meurman, J.H., Rytömaa, I. & Turtola, L. (1987). Periodontal status in university students. *Journal of Clinical Periodontology* **14**, 462-465.

Müller, H.P., Eger, T. & Schorb, A. (1998). Gingival dimensions after root coverage with free connective tissue grafts. *Journal of Clinical Periodontology* **25**, 424-430.

Nabers, C.L. (1954). Repositioning the attached gingiva. *Journal of Periodontology* **25**, 38-39.

Nabers, C.L. (1966). Free gingival grafts. *Periodontics* **4**, 243-245.

Nelson, S.W. (1987). The subpedicle connective tissue graft. A bilaminar reconstructive procedure for the coverage of denuded root surfaces. *Journal of Periodontology* **58**, 95-102.

Nevins, M. (1986). Attached gingiva – mucogingival therapy and restorative dentistry. *International Journal of Periodontics and Restorative Dentistry* **6** (4), 9-27.

Nevins, M. & Mellonig, J.T. (1998). *Periodontal therapy: clinical approaches and evidence of success*. Chicago: Quintessence Publishing Co. Inc.

Nobuto, T., Imai, H. & Yamaoka, A. (1988). Microvascularization of the free gingival autograft. *Journal of Periodontology* **59**, 639-646.

Nordland, W.P. & Tarnow, D.P. (1998). A classification system for loss of papillary height. *Journal of Periodontology* **69**, 1124-1126.

Nyman, S., Karring, T. & Bergenholtz, G. (1982). Bone regeneration in alveolar bone dehiscences produced by jiggling forces. *Journal of Periodontal Research* **17**, 316-322.

Ochsenbein, C. (1960). Newer concept of mucogingival surgery. *Journal of Periodontology* **31**, 175-185.

Okamoto, H., Yoneyama, T., Lindhe, J., Haffajee, A.D. & Socransky, S.S. (1988). Methods of evaluating periodontal disease data in epidemiological research. *Journal of Clinical Periodontology* **15**, 430-439.

Oles, R.D., Ibbott, C.G. & Laverty, W.H. (1985). Effects of citric acid treatment on pedicle flap coverage of localized recession. *Journal of Periodontology* **56**, 259-261.

Oliver, R.G., Löe, H. & Karring, T. (1968). Microscopic evaluation of the healing and re-vascularization of free gingival grafts. *Journal of Periodontal Research* **3**, 84-95.

Orban, B.J. (1957). *Oral Histology and Embryology*, 4th edn. St. Louis: C.V. Mosby Company, pp. 221-264.

Parma-Benfenati, S., Fugazzato, P.A. & Ruben, M.P. (1985). The effect of restorative margins on the postsurgical development and nature of the periodontium. *International Journal of Periodontics and Restorative Dentistry* **5** (6), 31-51.

Pasquinelli, K.L. (1995). The histology of new attachment utilizing a thick autogenous soft tissue graft in an area of deep recession: A case report. *International Journal of Periodontics and Restorative Dentistry* **15**, 248-257.

Patur, B. (1977). The rotation flap for covering denuded root surfaces. A closed wound technique. *Journal of Periodontology* **48**, 41-44.

Pearson, L.E. (1968). Gingival height of lower central incisors orthodontically treated and untreated. *Angle Orthodontist* **38**, 337-339.

Pennel, B.M., Higgison, J.D., Towner, T.D., King, K.O., Fritz, B.D. & Salder, J.F. (1965). Oblique rotated flap. *Journal of Periodontology* **36**, 305-309.

Pfeifer, J. & Heller, R. (1971). Histologic evaluation of full and partial thickness lateral repositioned flaps. A pilot study. *Journal of Periodontology* **42**, 331-333.

Pfeifer, J.S. (1963). The growth of gingival tissue over denuded bone. *Journal of Periodontology* **34**, 10-16.

Pfeifer, J.S. (1965). The reaction of alveolar bone to flap procedures in man. *Periodontics* **3**, 135-140.

Pini Prato, G.P., Baccetti, T., Giorgetti, R., Agudio, G. & Cortellini, P. (2000c). Mucogingival interceptive surgery of buccally-erupted premolars in patients scheduled for orthodontic treatment. II. Surgically treated versus nonsurgically treated cases. *Journal of Periodontology* **71**, 182-187.

Pini Prato, G.P., Baccetti, T., Magnani, C., Agudio, G. & Cortellini, P. (2000b). Mucogingival interceptive surgery of buccally-erupted premolars in patients scheduled for orthodontic treatment. I. A seven-year longitudinal study. *Journal of Periodontology* **71**, 172-181.

Pini Prato, G., Baldi C., Pagliaro U., Nieri M., Saletta D., Rotundo R. & Cortellini P. (1999). Coronally advanced flap procedure for root coverage. Treatment of root surface: root planing versus polishing. *Journal of Periodontology* **70**, 1064-1076.

Pini Prato, G.P., Clauser, C., Cortellini, P., Tinti, C., Vincenzi, G. & Pagliaro, U. (1996). Guided tissue regeneration versus mucogingival surgery in the treatment of human buccal recessions. A 4-year follow-up. *Journal of Periodontology* **67**, 1216-1223.

Pini Prato, G., Pagliaro, U., Baldi, C., Nieri, M., Saletta, D., Cairo, F. & Cortellini, P. (2000a). Coronally advanced flap procedure for root coverage. Flap with tension versus flap without tension: a randomized controlled clinical study. *Journal of Periodontology* **71**, 188-201

Pini Prato, G.P., Tinti, C., Vincenzi, G., Magnani, C, Cortellini, P. & Clauser, C. (1992). Guided tissue regeneration versus mucogingival surgery in the treatment of human buccal gingival recession. *Journal of Periodontology* **63**, 919-928.

Pontoriero, R. & Carnevale, G. (2001). Surgical crown lengthening: a 12-month clinical wound healing study. *Journal of Periodontology* **72**, 841-848.

Pontoriero, R., Celenza, F. Jr., Ricci, G. & Carnevale, M. (1987). Rapid extrusion with fiber resection: a combined orthodontic-periodontic treatment modality. *International Journal of Periodontics and Restorative Dentistry* **5**, 30-43.

Potashnick, S.R. & Rosenberg, E.S. (1982). Forced eruption: principles in periodontics and restorative dentistry. *Journal of Prosthetic Dentistry* **48**, 141-148.

Proceedings of 1st European Workshop on Clinical Periodontology (1994). Lang, N.P. & Karring, T., eds. Consensus report of session II. London: Quintessence Publ. Co Ltd, pp. 210-214.

Proceedings of the World Workshop on Periodontics (1996). Consensus report on mucogingival therapy. *Annals of Periodontology* **1**, 702-706.

Raetzke, P.B. (1985). Covering localized areas of root exposure employing the "envelope" technique. *Journal of Periodontology* **56**, 397-402.

Rateitschak, K.H., Herzog-Specht, F. & Hotz, R. (1968). Reaktion und Regeneration des Parodonts auf Behandlung mit festsitzenden Apparaten und abnehmbaren Platten. *Fortschritte der Kieferorthopädie* **29**, 415-435.

Reitan, K. (1967). Clinical and histologic observations on tooth movement during and after orthodontic treatment. *American Journal of Orthodontics* **53**, 721-745.

Roccuzzo, M., Lungo, M., Corrente, G., et al. (1996). Comparative study of a bioresorbable and a non-resorbable membrane in the treatment of human buccal gingival recessions. *Journal of Periodontology* **67**, 7-14.

Romanos, G.E., Bernimoulin, J.P. & Marggraf, E. (1993). The double lateral bridging flap for coverage of denuded root surface: longitudinal study and clinical evaluation after 5 to 8 years. *Journal of Periodontology* **64**, 683-688.

Rosenberg, N.M. (1960). Vestibular alterations in periodontics. *Journal of Periodontology* **31**, 231-237.

Ruben, M.P. (1979). A biological rationale for gingival reconstruction by grafting procedures. *Quintessence International* **10**, 47-55.

Saletta, D., Pini Prato, G.P., Pagliaro, U., Baldi, C., Mauri, M. & Nieri M. (2001). Coronally advanced flap procedure: is the interdental papilla a prognostic factor for root coverage? *Journal of Periodontology* **72**, 760-766.

Salkin, L.M., Freedman, A.L., Stein, M.D. & Bassiouny, M.A. (1987). A longitudinal study of untreated mucogingival defects. *Journal of Periodontology* **58**, 164-166.

Sangnes, G. (1976). Traumatization of teeth and gingiva related to habitual tooth cleaning procedures. *Journal of Clinical Periodontology* **3**, 94-103.

Sangnes, G. & Gjermo, P. (1976). Prevalence of oral soft and hard tissue lesions related to mechanical tooth cleaning procedures. *Community Dentistry and Oral Epidemiology* **4**, 77-83.

Sbordone, L., Ramaglia, L., Spagnuolo, G. & De Luca, M. (1988). A comparative study of free gingival and subepithelial connective tissue grafts. Periodontal case reports. *Northeastern Society of Periodontology* **10**, 8-12.

Schoo, W.H. & van der Velden, U. (1985). Marginal soft tissue recessions with and without attached gingiva. *Journal of Periodontal Research* **20**, 209-211.

Seibert, J.S. (1983). Reconstruction of deformed, partially edentulous ridges, using full thickness onlay grafts: I. Technique and wound healing. *Compendium of Continuing Education in General Dentistry* **4**, 437-453.

Seibert, J.S. (1991). Ridge augmentation to enhance esthetics in fixed prosthetic treatment. *Compendium of Continuing Education in General Dentistry* **12**, 548-561.

Seibert, J.S. (1993a). Treatment of moderate localized alveolar ridge defects: preventive and reconstructive concepts in therapy. *Dental Clinics of North America* **37**, 265-280.

Seibert, J.S. (1993b). Reconstruction of the partially edentulous ridge: gateway to improved prosthetics and superior esthetics. *Practical Periodontics and Aesthetic Dentistry* **5**, 47-55.

Seibert, J.S. & Louis, J. (1996). Soft tissue ridge augmentation utilizing a combination onlay-interpositional graft procedure: case report. *International Journal of Periodontics and Restorative Dentistry* **16**, 311-321.

Serino, G., Wennström, J.L., Lindhe, J. & Eneroth, L. (1994). The prevalence and distribution of gingival recession in subjects with high standard of oral hygiene. *Journal of Clinical Periodontology* **21**, 57-63.

Staffileno, H. (1964). Management of gingival recession and root exposure problems associated with periodontal disease. *Dental Clinics of North America*, March, 111-120.

Staffileno, H., Levy, S. & Gargiulo, A. (1966). Histologic study of cellular mobilization and repair following a periosteal retention operation via split thickness mucogingival surgery. *Journal of Periodontology* **37**, 117-131.

Staffileno, H., Wentz, F. & Orban, B. (1962). Histologic study of healing of split thickness flap surgery in dogs. *Journal of Periodontology* **33**, 56-69.

Steiner, G.G., Pearson, J.K. & Ainamo, J. (1981). Changes in the marginal periodontium as a result of labial tooth movement in monkeys. *Journal of Periodontology* **52**, 314-320.

Stern, J.B. (1976). Oral mucous membrane. In: Bhaskar, S.N., ed. *Orbans oral histology and embryology*, Chapter 8. St. Louis: C.V. Mosby.

Stetler, K.J. & Bissada, N.B. (1987). Significance of the width of keratinized gingiva on the periodontal status of teeth with submarginal restorations. *Journal of Periodontology* **58**, 696-700.

Stoner, J. & Mazdyasna, S. (1980). Gingival recession in the lower incisor region of 15-year old subjects. *Journal of Periodontology* **51**, 74-76.

Studer, S.P., Lehner, C., Bucher, A. & Schärer, P. (2000). Soft tissue correction of a single-tooth pontic space: a comparative quantitative volume assessment. *Journal of Prosthetic Dentistry* **83**, 402-411.

Studer, S., Naef, R. & Schärer, P. (1997). Adjustment of localized alveolar ridge defects by soft tissue transplantation to improve mucogingival esthetics: a proposal for clinical classification and an evaluation of procedures. *Quintessence International* **28**, 785-805.

Sugarman, E.F. (1969). A clinical and histological study of the attachment of grafted tissue to bone and teeth. *Journal of Periodontology* **40**, 381-387.

Sullivan, H.C. & Atkins, J.H. (1968a). Free autogenous gingival grafts. I. Principles of successful grafting. *Periodontics* **6**, 121-129.

Sullivan, H.C. & Atkins, J.H. (1968b). Free autogenous gingival grafts. III. Utilization of grafts in the treatment of gingival recession. *Periodontics* **6**, 152-160.

Sumner, C.F. (1969). Surgical repair of recession on the maxillary cuspid: incisionally repositioning the gingival tissues. *Journal of Periodontology* **40**, 119-121.

Tarnow, D.P. (1986). Semilunar coronally repositioned flap. *Journal of Clinical Periodontology* **13**, 182-185.

Tarnow, D.P., Magner, A.W. & Fletcher, P. (1992). The effect of the distance from the contact point to the crest of bone on the presence or absence of the interproximal dental papilla. *Journal of Periodontology* **63**, 995-996.

Tenenbaum, H. (1982). A clinical study comparing the width of attached gingiva and the prevalence of gingival recessions. *Journal of Clinical Periodontology* **9**, 86-92.

Tolmie, P.N., Rubins, R.P., Buck, G.S., Vagianos, V. & Lanz, J.C. (1991). The predictability of root coverage by way of free gingival autografts and citric acid application: an evaluation by multiple clinicians. *International Journal of Periodontics and Restorative Dentistry* **11**, 261-271

Trombelli, L. & Scabbia, A. (1997). Healing response of gingival recession defects following guided tissue regeneration procedures in smokers and non-smokers. *Journal of Clinical Periodontology* **24**, 529-533.

Trombelli, L., Schincaglia, G.P., Scapoli, C. & Calura, G. (1995). Healing response of human buccal gingival recessions treated with expanded polytetrafluoroethylene membranes. A retrospective report. *Journal of Periodontology* **66**, 14-22.

Trott, J.R. & Love, B. (1966). An analysis of localized recession in 766 Winnipeg high school students. *Dental Practice* **16**, 209-213.

Valderhaug, J. (1980). Periodontal conditions and caries lesions following the insertion of fixed prostheses: a 10-year follow-up study. *International Dental Journal* **30**, 296-304.

Van der Velden, U. (1982). Regeneration of the interdental soft tissues following denudation procedures. *Journal of Clinical Periodontology* **9**, 455-459.

Van Palenstein Helderman, W.H., Lembariti, B.S., van der Weijden, G.A. & van 't Hof, M.A. (1998). Gingival recession and its association with calculus in subjects deprived of prophylactic dental care. *Journal of Clinical Periodontology* **25**, 106-111.

Vekalahti, M. (1989). Occurrence of gingival recession in adults. *Journal of Periodontology* **60**, 599-603.

Waerhaug, J. (1952). The gingival pocket. Anatomy, pathology, deepening and elimination. *Odontologisk Tidskrift* **60**, Supplement.

Wennström, J.L. (1983). Regeneration of gingiva following surgical excision. A clinical study. *Journal of Clinical Periodontology* **10**, 287-297.

Wennström, J.L. (1987). Lack of association between width of attached gingiva and development of gingival recessions. A 5-year longitudinal study. *Journal of Clinical Periodontology* **14**, 181-184.

Wennström, J.L. (1996) Mucogingival therapy. In: Proceedings of the World Workshop on Periodontics. *Annals of Periodontology* **1**, 671-701.

Wennström, J.L. & Lindhe, J. (1983a). The role of attached gingiva for maintenance of periodontal health. Healing following excisional and grafting procedures in dogs. *Journal of Clinical Periodontology* **10**, 206-221.

Wennström, J.L. & Lindhe, J. (1983b). Plaque-induced gingival inflammation in the absence of attached gingiva in dogs. *Journal of Clinical Periodontology* **10**, 266-276.

Wennström, J.L., Lindhe, J., Sinclair, F. & Thilander, B. (1987). Some periodontal tissue reactions to orthodontic tooth movement in monkeys. *Journal of Clinical Periodontology* **14**, 121-129.

Wennström, J.L. & Zucchelli, G. (1996). Increased gingival dimensions. A significant factor for successful outcome of root coverage procedures? A 2-year prospective clinical study. *Journal of Clinical Periodontology* **23**, 770-777.

Wilderman, M.N. (1963). Repair after a periosteal retention procedure. *Journal of Periodontology* **34**, 484-503.

Wilderman, M.N. (1964). Exposure of bone in periodontal surgery. *Dental Clinics of North America*, March, 23-26.

Wilderman, M.N. & Wentz, F.M. (1965). Repair of a dentogingival defect with a pedicle flap. *Journal of Periodontology* **36**, 218-231.

Wilderman, M.N., Wentz, F.M. & Orban, B.J. (1961). Histogenesis of repair after mucogingival surgery. *Journal of Periodontology* **31**, 283-299.

Yoneyama, T., Okamoto, H., Lindhe, J., Socransky, S.S. & Haffajee, A.D. (1988). Probing depth, attachment loss and gingival recession. Findings from a clinical examination in Ushiku, Japan. *Journal of Clinical Periodontology* **15**, 581-591.

Zabalegui, I., Sicilia, A., Cambra, J. & Gil, J. & Sanz, M. (1999). Treatment of multiple adjacent gingival recessions with the tunnel subepithelial connective tissue graft: a clinical report. *International Journal of Periodontics and Restorative Dentistry* **19**,199-206.

Zucchelli, G., Clauser, C., De Sanctis, M. & Calandriello, M. (2000). Mucogingival versus guided tissue regeneration procedures in the treatment of deep recession type defects. *Journal of Periodontology* **69**, 138-145.

Zucchelli, G. & De Sanctis, M. (2000). Treatment of multiple recession-type defects in patients with esthetic demands. *Journal of Periodontology* **71**, 1506-1514.

CHAPTER 28

Regenerative Periodontal Therapy

THORKILD KARRING, JAN LINDHE AND PIERPAOLO CORTELLINI

INTRODUCTION

At tooth risk assessment in periodontal patients, the presence of sites with a residual pocket depth ≥ 6 mm after active treatment plays a significant role in predicting future periodontal destruction (Haffajee et al. 1991, Grbic & Lamster 1992, Claffey & Egelberg 1995). Thus, an important goal of periodontal therapy is to obtain a reduced pocket depth after treatment in order to arrest further disease progression. Usually, this goal can be accomplished by non-surgical therapy in patients with moderate periodontitis, whereas in advanced cases, particularly in the presence of intrabony defects and furcations, the treatment must be supplemented with periodontal surgery. A fundamental objective of periodontal surgery is to provide access for proper instrumentation and cleaning of the root surface, but in addition, most surgical procedures result in the elimination or the reduction of the soft tissue component of the periodontal pocket. Traditionally, the elimination of deep pockets is achieved by gingivectomy or apical displacement of raised tissue flaps, sometimes associated with bone contouring. In recent years, however, the use of regenerative procedures aimed at restoring the lost periodontal support has become more common.

Indications

Periodontal treatment, either surgical or non-surgical, results in recession of the gingival margin after healing (Isidor et al. 1984). In advanced cases of periodontitis, this may lead to poor esthetics in the front areas of the dentition, in particular when applying surgical procedures including bone contouring for the eradication of bone defects. Treatment of such cases without bone contouring, on the other hand, may result in residual pockets inaccessible to proper cleaning during post-treatment maintenance. These problems can be avoided or reduced by applying regenerative surgical procedures by which the lost periodontal attachment in the bone defects can be restored. Thus, the indication of applying regenerative periodontal therapy is often based on esthetic considerations, besides the fact that the function or long-term prognosis of the treated teeth may be improved.

Localized gingival recession and root exposure may represent an esthetic problem to the patient, and often it is associated with root sensitivity. Such a situation represents an indication to apply regenerative periodontal therapy to obtain root coverage in order to improve esthetics and reduce root sensitivity. Successful root coverage implies regeneration of the attachment apparatus on the exposed root surface including cementum with inserting collagen fibers and alveolar bone as well as an esthetically acceptable restoration of the anatomy of the mucogingival complex.

Another indication for regenerative periodontal therapy is furcation involved teeth. The furcation area is often inaccessible to adequate instrumentation and frequently the roots present concavities and furrows which make proper cleaning of the area after resective surgery impossible. Considering the long-term results and complications reported following treatment of furcation involvements by traditionally resective therapy (Hamp et al. 1975, Bühler 1988), the long-term prognosis of furcation involved teeth can be improved considerably by successful regenerative periodontal therapy.

Case reports also exist demonstrating that "hopeless" teeth with deep vertical defects, increased tooth mobility or through and through furcations can be successfully treated with regenerative periodontal therapy (Gottlow et al. 1986). However, controlled clinical trials or serial case reports presenting a reasonable predictability of treating such advanced cases are not available.

Regenerative surgical procedures

Regenerative periodontal therapy comprises procedures which are specially designed to restore those parts of the tooth-supporting apparatus which have been lost due to periodontitis. Regeneration is defined as a reproduction or reconstruction of a lost or injured part in such a way that the architecture and function of the lost or injured tissues are completely restored (*Glossary of Periodontal Terms* 1992). This means that the attachment of the tooth has been regenerated when new cementum with inserting collagen fibers has formed on the detached root surface, while regeneration of the periodontal supporting apparatus (periodontium) also includes regrowth of the alveolar bone. Procedures aimed at restoring lost periodontal support have also been described as "reattachment" or "new attachment" procedures.

The term "reattachment" was used to describe the regeneration of a fibrous attachment to a root surface surgically or mechanically deprived of its periodontal ligament tissue, whereas the term "new attachment" was preferred in the situation where the fibrous attachment was restored on a root surface deprived of its connective tissue attachment due to the progression of periodontitis. Research findings, however, indicate that there is no difference regarding the possibility of restoring a connective tissue attachment, whether this has been lost because of periodontal disease or mechanically removed (Nyman et al. 1982, Isidor et al. 1985). Therefore, it was suggested that the term "new attachment" should be used to describe the formation of new cementum with inserting collagen fibers on a root surface deprived of its periodontal ligament tissue, whether or not this has occurred because of periodontal disease or by mechanical means, and that the term "reattachment" should be confined to describing the reunion of surrounding soft tissue and a root surface with preserved periodontal ligament tissue (Isidor et al. 1985).

Periodontal regeneration has been reported following a variety of surgical approaches involving root surface biomodification, often combined with coronally advanced flap procedures, the placement of bone grafts or bone substitute implants, or the use of organic or synthetic barrier membranes (guided tissue regeneration). However, many cases that clinically are considered successful, including cases with significant regrowth of alveolar bone, may histologically show an epithelial lining along the treated root surface instead of deposition of new cementum (Listgarten & Rosenberg 1979).

Successful regeneration is assessed by periodontal probing, radiographic analysis, direct measurements of new bone and histology. Although histology remains the ultimative standard in assessing true periodontal regeneration, periodontal probing, direct bone measurements and radiographic measurements of osseous changes are used in the majority of studies of regenerative therapy (Reddy & Jeffcoat 1999).

At the American Academy of Periodontology World Workshop in Periodontics in 1996, the fulfillment of the following criteria was required in order for a periodontal regenerative procedure to be considered as a therapy which can encourage regeneration:

- Human histological specimens demonstrating formation of new cementum, periodontal ligament and bone coronal to a notch indicating the apical extension of the periodontitis affected root surface
- Controlled human clinical trials demonstrating improved clinical probing attachment and bone
- Controlled animal histological studies demonstrating formation of new cementum, periodontal ligament, and bone.

In addition, however, it seems reasonable to require that a regenerative procedure is based on a biological concept which on the basis of current knowledge about periodontal wound healing can explain why the treatment results in periodontal regeneration.

RELIABILITY OF ASSESSMENTS OF PERIODONTAL REGENERATION

In most studies on the effect of regenerative periodontal surgery, the outcomes are evaluated by probing attachment level measurements, radiographic analysis or re-entry operations. However, such methods are not reliable for documentation of a true gain of attachment (i.e. a new connective tissue attachment in an area coronal to the attachment level before treatment).

Periodontal probing

The inability of periodontal probing to determine accurately the coronal level of the connective tissue attachment has been demonstrated by several investigators (Listgarten et al. 1976, Armitage et al. 1977, Van der Velden & de Vries 1978). It is known from these studies that in the inflamed periodontium, the probe does not stop precisely at the coronal level of the connective tissue attachment. Usually it penetrates half a millimeter or more into the connective tissue, surpassing the transition between the apical extension of the dento-gingival epithelium and the coronal level of connective tissue attachment. After therapy, when the inflammatory lesion is resolved, the probe tip tends to stop coronal to the apical termination of the epithelium. Following treatment of intrabony defects, new bone may form so close to the tooth surface that the probe cannot penetrate (Caton & Zander 1976). Thus, a gain of probing attachment level (PAL) following therapy does not necessarily mean that a true gain of connective tissue attachment was accomplished. More likely it is a reflection of improved health of the surrounding soft tissues which offer increased resistance to probe penetration. (For a detailed discussion on errors inherent in clinical probing of periodontal pockets see Chapter 18.)

Radiographic analysis and re-entry operations

Regeneration of bone tissue within intrabony defects following regenerative therapy is often documented by measurements made on radiographs obtained in a standardized and reproducible manner and/or assessed in conjunction with a re-entry operation. Analysis of radiographs before and after therapy and inspection of the treated area during a re-entry operation can certainly provide evidence of new bone formation. However, such "bone fill" does not document formation of new root cementum and a new periodontal ligament. In fact, it was demonstrated by Caton & Zander (1976) and Moscow et al. (1979) that despite the fact that bone regeneration had occurred adjacent to the root in intrabony defects, a junctional epithelium was interposed between the newly formed bone and the curetted root surface. This means that radiographic analysis and assessments of bone formation by re-entry operations are unreliable methods for the documentation of new attachment formation.

Histologic methods

In several studies healing is analyzed in histologic sections of block biopsies obtained after various forms of regenerative periodontal therapy. Histologic analysis is the only valid method to assess the formation of new attachment, but it requires that the location of the attachment level prior to therapy can be assessed with a certain accuracy. In a few studies histologic reference notches were placed in the apical extent of calculus deposits, identified on the root surface at the time of surgery (Cole et al. 1980, Bowers et al. 1989b,c). Usually, however, a reference is obtained by producing a notch in the root surface at the level of the reduced bone height. Although such a notch may not reflect the exact position of the periodontitis-involved root surface prior to treatment, it is considered an adequate landmark for the assessment of new attachment (Isidor et al. 1985).

PERIODONTAL WOUND HEALING

Regeneration of the periodontium must include the formation of new cementum with inserting collagen fibers on the previously periodontitis-involved root surfaces and the regrowth of the alveolar bone. However, whether regrowth of alveolar bone should always be considered a requirement for success following regenerative periodontal surgery is a matter of discussion. The basis for this discussion is that also in a normal non-periodontitis affected dentition in the presence of bone dehiscenses and fenestrations, a fibrous attachment may exist without opposite bone (see Fig. 1-74).

In 1976, Melcher in a review paper suggested that the type of cell which repopulates the root surface after periodontal surgery determines the nature of the attachment that will form. After flap surgery the curetted root surface may be repopulated by four different types of cell (Fig. 28-1):

1. Epithelial cells
2. Cells derived from the gingival connective tissue
3. Cells derived from the bone
4. Cells derived from the periodontal ligament.

Previously, in most attempts to restore lost tooth support, particular attention was directed towards the regeneration of the alveolar bone. In order to examine the relationship between the re-establishment of a

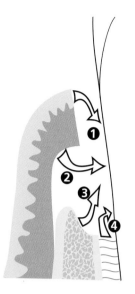

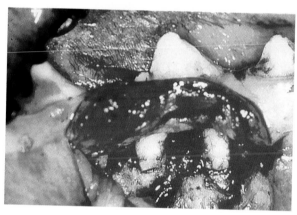

Fig. 28-1. Following flap surgery, the curetted root surface may be repopulated by (1) epithelial cells, (2) gingival connective tissue cells, (3) bone cells, or (4) periodontal ligament cells.

Fig. 28-2. Following flap elevation, the buccal bone, including a part of the interradicular and interproximal alveolar bone, is removed without injuring the connective tissue attachment on the root surface.

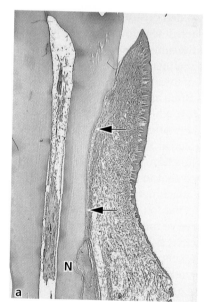

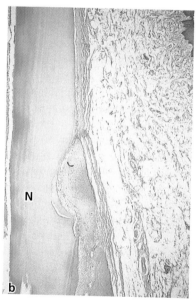

Fig. 28-3. Microphotograph of specimen 8 months following bone removal (a). A connective tissue attachment is re-established (arrows). Bone regeneration is negligible and is confined to the notch (N) in the root surface. (b) Higher magnification of the newly formed bone in the notch area (N).

connective tissue attachment to the root surface and the regrowth of alveolar bone, an investigation was carried out in dogs (Nyman & Karring 1979). After elevation of mucoperiostal flaps, the marginal 5-7 mm of the buccal alveolar bone of each experimental tooth was removed (Fig. 28-2). During this procedure, care was taken to minimize the mechanical injury to the connective tissue attachment on the root surface. A

notch, serving as a landmark for the histologic measurements, was prepared in the root surface at the level of the surgically reduced bone crest. After 8 months of healing, the animals were sacrificed. Histologic analysis demonstrated that although a connective tissue attachment was re-established consistently on the roots, the amount of bone regeneration varied widely. In some roots, bone regrowth was negligible (Fig.

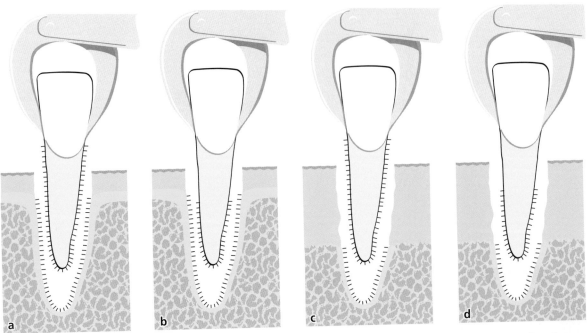

Fig. 28-4. Schematic drawing showing the four experimental conditions (a-d) under which experimental teeth were extracted and reimplanted in their own sockets.

28-3), whereas in others the bone had regenerated to its normal level. These results demonstrated that the amount of bone regrowth is unrelated to the re-establishment of a connective tissue attachment.

Another experiment was carried out in monkeys (Lindhe et al. 1984), in order to examine whether the presence of bone may stimulate the formation of a new connective tissue attachment. Mandibular and maxillary incisors were extracted and reimplanted in their own sockets under the following four experimental conditions (Fig. 28-4):

1. Non-root planed teeth were reimplanted into sockets with normal bone height
2. Teeth, root planed in their coronal portion, were reimplanted into sockets with normal bone height
3. Non-root planed teeth were reimplanted into sockets with a reduced bone height
4. Teeth, root planed in their coronal portion, were reimplanted into sockets with reduced bone height.

Histologic examination after 6 months of healing revealed that a fibrous reunion was established in areas where, at the time of reimplantation, the periodontal connective tissue attachment was retained. However, in areas, where the periodontal ligament tissue was removed, the epithelium had always migrated to the apical extension of root instrumentation (Fig. 28-5). These results of healing occurred irrespective of the presence or absence of bone, indicating that the establishment of a connective tissue attachment is unrelated to the presence of alveolar bone.

Using orthodontic appliances, Karring et al. (1982) tilted maxillary second and third incisors in labial direction in dogs. Subsequently, these teeth were moved back to their original position. During the same time the contralateral incisors were moved to a labially deviated position. The orthodontic appliances were then used to retain the teeth in these positions for a period of 5 months before sacrifice of the animals. Histologic analysis demonstrated that in all experimental teeth, the apical termination of the junctional epithelium was at the cemento-enamel junction. In the teeth which were retained in their labially displaced position, the level of the alveolar bone was reduced to a position about 4.5 mm apical to the cemento-enamel junction (Fig. 28-6a), while in the teeth which were moved back to their original position, the alveolar bone crest was located at a normal level relative to the cemento-enamel junction (Fig. 28-6b). This experiment demonstrated that in the presence of a normal connective tissue attachment, bone may be resorbed or regenerated by orthodontic forces. Thus, the experiments described above indicate that the re-establishment of a connective tissue attachment to the root surface and the regeneration of the alveolar bone are not related to each other.

The use of bone grafts in regenerative periodontal therapy is based on the assumption that the promotion of bone regrowth may also induce cells in the bone to produce a new cementum layer with inserting collagen fibers on previously periodontitis-involved root surfaces. However, histologic studies in both humans and animals have demonstrated that grafting procedures often result in healing with a long junctional epithelium rather than a new connective tissue attachment (Caton & Zander 1976, Listgarten & Rosenberg 1979, Moscow et al. 1979).

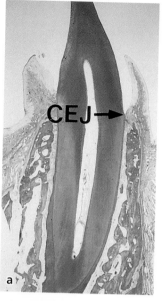

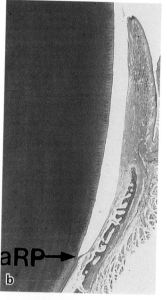

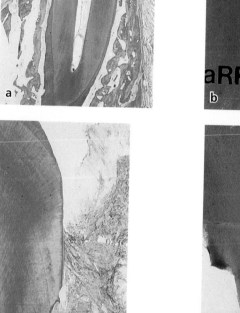

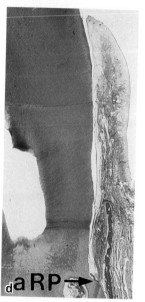

Fig. 28-5. Microphotographs showing the histological features after 6 months of healing, under the four experimental conditions (a-d) illustrated in Fig. 28-4. The teeth in (b) and (d) are those root planed in their coronal portion, and the teeth (a) and (b) are those reimplanted in sockets with normal bone height. A fibrous reunion was established in areas where the connective tissue attachment was retained (a and c) while the epithelium has migrated to the apical extension of root instrumentation (a RP) where the attachment was removed (b and d). CEJ: cementoenamel junction.

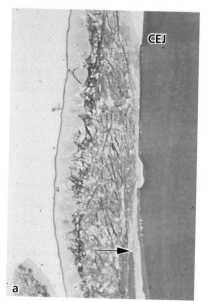

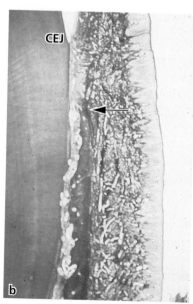

Fig. 28-6. Microphotograph of a tooth retained in its labially displaced position (a) and a tooth (b) moved back to its original position. The level of alveolar bone (arrow) is reduced in (a) while it has regenerated to its normal level (arrow) in (b). The apical termination of the junctional epithelium is at the cemento-enamel junction (CEJ) in both situations.

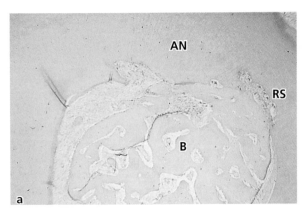

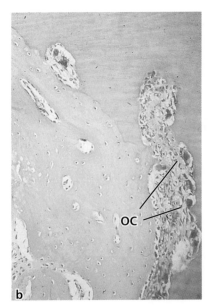

Fig. 28-7. Microphotograph of furcation 6 weeks after grafting with iliac crest marrow (a). The furcation is completely filled with bone (B), but ankylosis (AN) and root resorption (RS) can be seen. (b) Higher magnification of the area in (a) showing ankylosis and resorption. OC: osteoclasts.

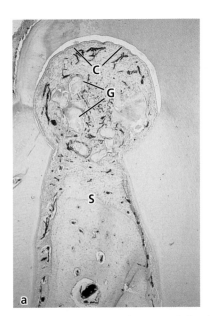

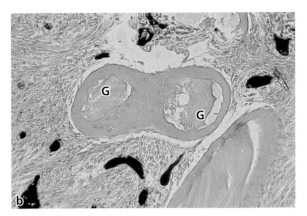

Fig. 28-8. Microphotograph of a healed bifurcation defect following transplantation of non-vital bone grafts (a). The grafts (G) have not been reached by bone formation from the interradicular septum (S), but occur as isolated particles surrounded by "cementum". Cementum (C) and new connective tissue attachment formation have taken place along the entire circumference of the bifurcation. (b) High magnification of isolated bone grafts (G) with newly formed "cementum" on the surface.

Ellegaard et al. (1973, 1974, 1975, 1976) and Nielsen et al. (1980) reported that grafting materials in periodontal bony defects may be:

1. *osteoproliferative* (osteogenetic), which means that new bone is formed by bone forming cells contained in the grafted material
2. *osteoconductive*, which means that the grafted material does not contribute to new bone formation *per se* but serves as scaffold for bone formation originating from adjacent host bone
3. *osteoinductive*, which means that bone formation is

induced in the surrounding soft tissue immediately adjacent to the grafted material.

These studies, where various types of bone graft were placed in intrabony defects or interradicular lesions, revealed that only iliac bone marrow grafts survived transplantation. Transplantation of iliac bone marrow grafts almost consistently resulted in bone fill in the experimental defects, but healing was frequently accompanied by ankylosis and root resorption (Fig. 28-7). The iliac bone marrow grafts exerted an osteogeneic effect, and it was suggested that this was re-

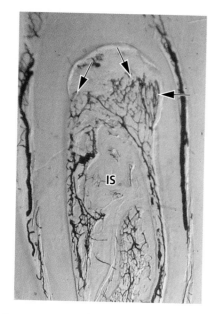

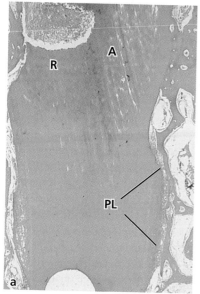

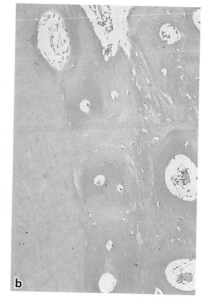

Fig. 28-9. Cleared specimen from a 1-week-old bifurcation defect treated with bone grafts. Judged from the course of the blood vessels, the granulation tissue in the defect has developed mainly from the periodontal ligament (arrows) and only to a minor extent from the interradicular septum (IS).

Fig. 28-10. Microphotograph of a reimplanted root after 3 months of healing (a). A periodontal ligament (PL) has become re-established in the apical portion of the root whereas ankylosis (A) and root resorption (R) is the predominant feature in the coronal portion. (b) High magnification of the ankylosis seen in (a).

sponsible for the induction of root resorption (Ellegaard et al. 1973, 1974). Jaw bone grafts and xenografts did not actively contribute to bone formation but served as a scaffold for bone regeneration (i.e. osteoconductive effect). Often, however, these bone grafts were not reached by the new bone growing out from the host bone, but occurred as isolated particles surrounded by a bone-like or cementum-like substance (Fig. 28-8). It was found that the treated bifurcation defects became filled mainly with granulation tissue derived from the periodontal ligament (Fig. 28-9). The authors (Nielsen et al. 1980) suggested that this ingrowth of ligament tissue inhibited bone formation and that the new cementum on the root surface in the bifurcation defects, including the cementum-like substance observed around the implanted bone particles, were formed by periodontal ligament cells (Fig. 28-8). Thus, it appeared from these studies that the key cells in periodontal regeneration are periodontal ligament cells rather than bone cells.

Regenerative capacity of bone cells

The ability of newly formed tissue originated from bone to produce a new connective tissue attachment was examined in a study by Karring et al. (1980). Roots of periodontitis-affected teeth were extracted and placed in surgically created sockets in edentulous areas of dogs. The implanted roots were covered with tissue flaps (submerged) and the results of healing were examined histologically after 3 months. A periodontal ligament was re-established in the apical portion of the reimplanted roots where, at the time of implantation, remnants of periodontal ligament tissue were preserved. In the coronal portion of the roots which were previously exposed to periodontitis and then scaled and planed, healing had consistently resulted in ankylosis and root resorption (Fig. 28-10). On the basis of this finding, it was concluded that tissue derived from bone lacks cells with the potential to produce a new connective tissue attachment.

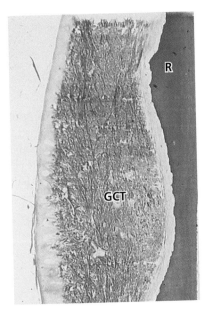

Fig. 28-11. Microphotograph of root (R) which has been reimplanted with its surface facing the gingival connective tissue (GCT). The surface exhibits extensive resorption.

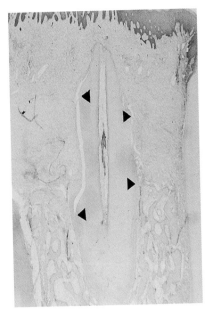

Fig. 28-12. Microphotograph showing new attachment formation (between the arrows) on a submerged root with a non-impaired periodontal ligament. Coronal to the cementum, root resorption is the predominant feature.

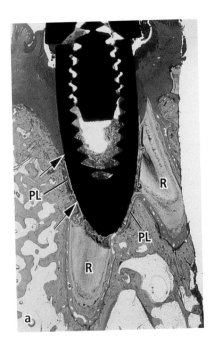

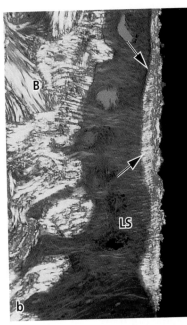

Fig. 28-13. Microphotograph of a titanium implant placed in contact with retained root tips (a). A distinct cementum layer (arrows) and periodontal ligament (PL) in continuity with that on the roots (R) is visible on the implant surface. (b) High magnification in polarized light of the periodontal ligament formed around the implant seen in (a). A cementum layer (arrows) with Sharpey's fibers is present at the implant surface. Principal fibers, oriented perpendicular to the surface, are running across the ligament space (LS) and are inserting in the opposing bone (B) as in natural teeth (see Fig. 1-71).

Regenerative capacity of gingival connective tissue cells

Another experiment (Nyman et al. 1980) was carried out in order to examine the potential of gingival connective tissue to produce a new connective tissue attachment. The teeth were treated as described in the experiment above but were not transplanted into sockets. Instead they were placed in bone concavities prepared on the buccal aspect of the jaw and subsequently covered by tissue flaps. Thus, half the circumference of the roots was in contact with bone while the remaining part was facing the gingival connective tissue at the subsurface of the flaps. Histologic examination after 3 months of healing showed areas with periodontal ligament in the apical portion of the roots where, at the time of implantation, periodontal ligament tissue was preserved. In the coronal, previously exposed part of the roots, no signs of new connective tissue attachment were present. The root portion located in contact with gingival connective tissue demonstrated a connective tissue with fibers oriented parallel to the root surface and without attachment to the root. However, root resorption occurred at the majority of the surfaces (Fig. 28-11). On the basis of this result it was concluded that gingival connective tissue also lacks cells with the potential to produce a new connective tissue attachment.

Regenerative capacity of periodontal ligament cells

In the experiments described above, root resorption was observed occasionally, also in the apical portion of the extracted and reimplanted roots (Karring et al. 1980, Nyman et al. 1980). It was suggested that this occurred because the periodontal ligament tissue retained on this part of the root had become injured during extraction, thereby allowing bone or gingival connective tissue to contact the root surface during healing and induce resorption. It was assumed that this damage of the retained periodontal ligament tissue had also restricted its potential of proliferating in the coronal direction along the root surface. Indeed, in a later study (Karring et al. 1985), where periodontitis-involved roots were retained in their sockets and subsequently submerged, significant amounts of new connective tissue attachment formed on the coronal portion of the roots (Fig. 28-12). The finding of new attachment only on the roots with a non-impaired periodontal ligament, but never on the extracted and reimplanted roots with an impaired ligament, indicates that periodontal ligament tissue contains cells with the potential to form a new connective tissue attachment on a detached root surface.

Active root resorption occurred consistently at the root surfaces above the coronal extension of new attachment. It was suggested that this resorption was induced by gingival connective tissue which had proliferated apically from the covering tissue flap. Thus, only cells in the periodontal ligament seem capable of regenerating lost periodontal attachment.

The final evidence that the progenitor cells for new attachment formation are residing in the periodontal ligament was provided in studies in which titanium dental implants were placed in contact with retained root tips whose periodontal ligament served as a source for cells which could populate the implant surface during healing (Buser et al. 1990a,b, Warrer et al. 1993). Microscopic analysis revealed that a distinct layer of cementum with inserting collagen fibers had formed on the surfaces of the implants (Fig. 28-13a), and that these fibers, often oriented perpendicularly to the surface, were embedded in the opposite bone (Fig. 28-13b). Control implants (Fig. 28-14) placed without contact with retained roots healed with the characteristic features of osseointegration (i.e. direct contact between bone and the implant surface). These results prove that the progenitor cells for periodontal attachment formation reside in the periodontal ligament and not in the alveolar bone as previously assumed (Melcher et al. 1987).

Role of epithelium in periodontal wound healing

Some of the roots in the experiment described above (Karring et al. 1985) penetrated the covering mucosa

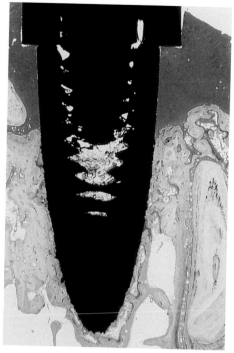

Fig. 28-14. Microphotograph of a titanium implant placed without contact with retained roots (control). This implant has healed with a direct contact between the bone and the implant surface (osseointegration).

at early stages of healing, thereby allowing the epithelium to grow apically along the root surface. The amount of new connective tissue attachment on these roots was considerably smaller than that formed on the roots which remained submerged throughout the study. This finding and those of other investigators (Moscow 1964, Kon et al. 1969, Proye & Polson 1982) indicate that the apical migration of epithelium reduces the coronal gain of attachment, evidently by preventing periodontal ligament cells from repopulating the root surface (Fig. 28-15).

Downgrowth of epithelium into the periodontal lesion has most likely occurred to a varying extent during healing following most flap and grafting procedures applied in regenerative periodontal therapy, which may explain the varying results reported. This view is supported by the results of the monkey study by Caton et al. (1980). These investigators examined healing in ligature-induced periodontal lesions following treatment with four different modalities of regenerative surgical procedures:

1. root planing and soft tissue curettage
2. Widman flap surgery without bone grafting
3. Widman flap surgery with the placement of frozen autogeneous red bone marrow and cancellous bone, or
4. beta tricalcium-phosphate in intrabony defects.

Healing following all treatment modalities resulted in the formation of a long junctional epithelium extending to or close to the same level as before treatment.

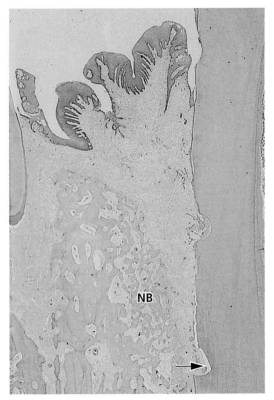

Fig. 28-15. Microphotograph illustrating an intrabony defect after regenerative treatment. New bone (NB) has formed in the defect but epithelium has migrated apically along the root surface to the notch (arrow) in the root surface indicating the bottom of the defect before treatment.

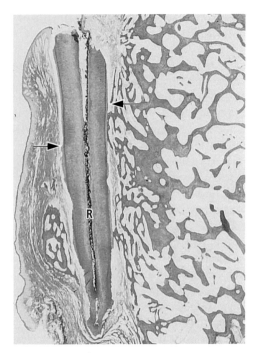

Fig. 28-16. Microphotograph of an implanted root (R) where epithelium was allowed to migrate into the wound after 2 weeks. The epithelium has migrated along the coronal, previously periodontitis-involved root surfaces down to the level indicated by the arrows. In the areas covered by epithelium, there are no signs of resorption. Apical to this level the root surfaces demonstrate root resorption.

Root resorption

In the experimental studies described previously, granulation tissue, derived from gingival connective tissue or bone, produced root resorption when contacting the curetted root surface during healing following surgery (Karring et al. 1980, 1985, Nyman et al. 1980). It should be expected, therefore, that this phenomenon would occur as a frequent complication to regenerative periodontal surgery, particularly following those procedures which include the placement of grafting materials to stimulate bone formation. The reason that root resorption is rarely seen is most likely that postoperatively, the dento-gingival epithelium migrates apically along the root surface, forming a protective barrier towards the root surface (Fig. 28-15). This view is supported by the results of an experimental study in monkeys (Karring et al. 1984) in which roots, which previously had been subjected to ligature-induced periodontitis, were extracted and reimplanted into contact with bone and connective tissue and covered with a tissue flap (submerged). After varying time intervals the submerged roots were exposed to the oral cavity by a second incision (wounding) through the covering mucosa, thereby permitting the epithelium to migrate into the wound. In specimens where the wounding occurred within 2 weeks (Fig. 28-16), the previously diseased part of the roots

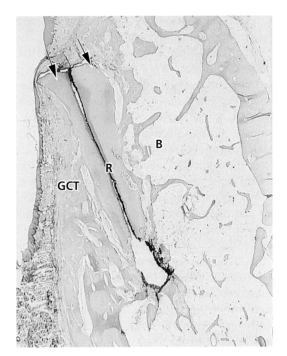

Fig. 28-17. Microphotograph of an implanted root (R) where epithelium was allowed to migrate into the wound after 4 weeks. The epithelium (arrows) covers only the coronal cut root surface. Extensive resorption is seen on the surface facing the gingival connective tissue (GCT) and resorption and ankylosis are seen on the surface facing the bone tissue (B).

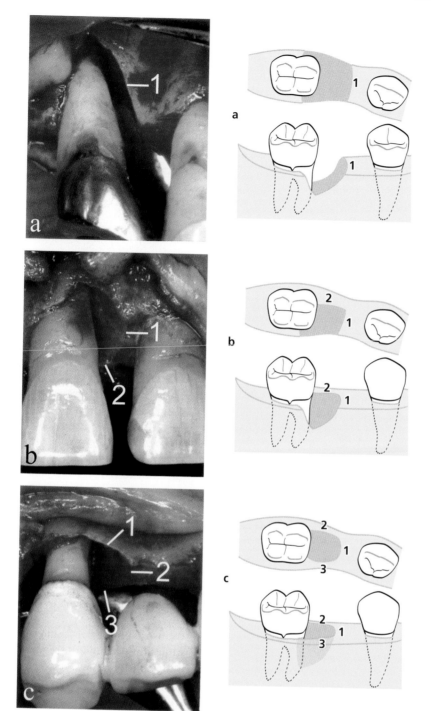

Fig. 28-18. Progression of periodontitis at a different rate on
neighboring tooth surfaces results
in the development of intrabony
defects. Based on the number of
surrounding bone walls such defects are classified as one-wall (a),
two-wall (b) or three-wall (c) defects.

was covered by epithelium and showed no signs of
resorption. With increasing intervals between implantation of the roots and the wounding, a steadily diminishing part of the diseased root surface was covered
by epithelium, and root resorption and ankylosis became progressively pronounced (Fig. 28-17). This observation concurs with results presented by Björn et
al. (1965) who treated 11 periodontally diseased teeth
in seven human volunteers, using the submerging
technique which prevented apical migration of the
dentogingival epithelium. The authors reported that
root resorption was indeed a common complication
following this kind of therapy.

REGENERATIVE PROCEDURES

One of the first methods used in attempts to obtain
new attachment was scaling and root planing combined with soft tissue curettage (i.e. mechanical removal of the diseased root cementum and the pocket
epithelium). Studies in humans (e.g. Younger 1899,
McCall 1926, Orban 1948, Beube 1952, Waerhaug 1952,
Schaffer & Zander 1953, Carranza 1954, 1960) and in
animals (e.g. Beube 1947, Ramfjord 1951, Kon et al.
1969) showed that this type of periodontal therapy
resulted not only in the establishment of gingival
health but also in a reduction of the initially recorded
pocket depth. This decrease in the depth of the peri-

odontal pocket was assumed to be partly the result of shrinkage of the initially inflamed gingiva, but partly also the effect of the formation of a new connective tissue attachment in the apical part of the pocket.

The possibility of obtaining new attachment became widely accepted with the work of Prichard (1957a,b) in which new attachment formation in intrabony periodontal lesions was reported as a predictable outcome of treatment. Seventeen cases were presented out of which four were subjected to a re-entry surgical procedure, revealing that these defects were filled with bone. The technique of Prichard (1957b, 1960) was only used for the treatment of three-wall intrabony defects, and the results obtained suggested that the morphology of the periodontal bony defect was essential for the establishment of a predictable prognosis. Goldman & Cohen (1958) introduced a classification of periodontal intrabony defects which was based on the number of osseous walls surrounding the defect, being either three-wall, two-wall or one-wall defects or a combination of such situations (Fig. 28-18).

The technique of Prichard (1957a,b, 1960) included the elevation of tissue flaps in order to get access to the defect. All granulation tissue in the defect was removed and the root surface was scaled and planed. In order to enhance regeneration of bone, small perforations were made with a bur at several sites of the bone walls. The flaps were sutured to accomplish complete coverage of the defect. Many clinical investigators have claimed that new attachment resulted following this type of treatment but there is little quantitative or qualitative documentation (Patur & Glickmann 1962, Wade 1962, 1966, Ellegaard & Löe 1971, Yukna et al. 1976). Patur & Glickmann (1962) reported a clinical study including 24 intrabony defects treated according to the Prichard technique (1957a,b). The outcome was evaluated by comparing preoperative and postoperative radiographs, measurements of the alveolar bone level adjacent to the root and study casts taken during operation and postoperatively after reflecting buccal and lingual flaps. The authors reported that new attachment had occurred in two-wall and three-wall intrabony defects but not in one-wall defects. Results from a study by Ellegaard & Löe (1971) comprising 191 defects in 24 patients with periodontal disease indicated that complete regeneration, determined radiographically and by periodontal probing, had occurred in around 70% of the three-wall defects, in 40% of the combined two-wall and three-wall defects and in 45% of the two-wall defects.

In a later study by Rosling et al. (1976), 124 intrabony defects in 12 patients were treated by means of the modified Widman flap procedure (Ramfjord & Nissle 1974). Following treatment the patients were recalled twice per month for professional tooth cleaning. Re-examination performed clinically and on radiographs 2 years after therapy demonstrated bone fill in two-wall as well as three-wall defects. The authors suggested that this regrowth of bone was also associ-

ated with the formation of new connective tissue attachment and ascribed the successful healing mainly to the optimal standard of oral hygiene which was maintained in all patients during healing. A clinical study with almost identical results was presented by Polsen & Heijl (1978). The results of several histologic studies in animals and humans, on the other hand, indicate that formation of new periodontal attachment is by no means predictable following subgingival curettage or flap surgery (Listgarten & Rosenberg 1979, Caton & Nyman 1980, Caton et al. 1980, Steiner et el. 1981, Stahl et al. 1983, Bowers et al. 1989a).

Grafting procedures

In a number of clinical trials and animal experiments, the flap approach was combined with the placement of bone grafts or implant materials into the curetted bony defects with the aim of stimulating periodontal regeneration. The various graft and implant materials used so far can be placed into four categories:

1. *Autogenous grafts*: Grafts transferred from one position to another within the same individual. This type of graft comprises (1) cortical bone or (2) cancellous bone and marrow, and is harvested either from intraoral or extraoral donor sites.
2. *Allogeneic grafts*: Grafts transferred between genetically dissimilar members of the same species. (1) Frozen cancellous bone and marrow, and (2) freeze-dried bone have been used.
3. *Xenogeneic grafts*: Grafts taken from a donor of another species.
4. *Alloplastic materials*: Synthetic or inorganic implant materials which are used as substitutes for bone grafts.

The rationale behind the use of bone grafts or alloplastic materials is the assumption that both the regrowth of alveolar bone and the formation of new attachment would be stimulated because these materials may either (1) contain bone forming cells (osteogenesis), or (2) serve as a scaffold for bone formation (osteoconduction), or because (3) the matrix of the bone grafts contains bone-inducing substances (osteoinduction) (Urist 1980, Brunsvold & Mellonig 1993). Such complete regeneration of the periodontal attachment apparatus following grafting procedures would imply that cells derived from bone possess the ability to form new cementum with inserting collagen fibers on a previously periodontitis-involved root surface (Melcher et al. 1987).

The value of using bone grafts or alloplastic materials for periodontal regeneration has mainly been examined in case reports, while histologic evidence of new attachment and controlled clinical studies is limited. The results from such reports vary and the documentation presented usually consists of preoperative and postoperative probing attachment levels, radiographic interpretations or re-entry procedures.

Autogenous grafts

Autogenous grafts (autografts) may retain some cell viability and are considered to promote bone healing mainly through osteogenesis and/or osteoconduction. They are gradually resorbed and replaced by new viable bone. In addition, potential problems of histocompatibility and disease transmission are eliminated with autogenous grafts. Autogenous grafts can be harvested from intraoral or extraoral sites.

Intraoral autogenous grafts

Intraoral autogenous grafts obtained from edentulous areas of the jaw, healing extraction sites, maxillary tuberosities or the mandibular retromolar area were commonly used in periodontal regenerative surgery (Mann 1964, Ellegaard & Löe 1971, Rosenberg 1971a,b, Dragoo & Sullivan 1973a, b, Hiatt & Schallhorn 1973, Froum et al. 1983, Stahl et al. 1983). Generally cancellous bone is preferred as graft material but cortical bone, applied as small chips (Rosenberg et al. 1979), or mixed with blood prior to the placement in the defects (Robinson 1969, Froum et al. 1976), was also reported to be effective in producing regeneration in periodontal intrabony defects.

The effect of intraoral autogenous grafts has been evaluated in both animals and humans. In a study in monkeys, Rivault et al. (1971) observed that intrabony defects filled with intraoral autogenous bone chips mixed with blood (osseous coagulum) healed with new bone formation, but no more bone was found in such experimental defects than was observed in similar control defects treated with surgical curettage. Other studies in monkeys and dogs also failed to demonstrate significant differences in bone formation between grafted and non-grafted intrabony or furcation defects (Ellegaard et al. 1974, Coverly et al. 1975, Nilveus et al. 1978).

In clinical case-series where intraoral autogenous grafts were used for the treatment of intrabony periodontal defects, a mean bone fill ranging from 3.0 mm to 3.5 mm was reported (Nabers & O'Leary 1965, Robinson 1969, Hiatt & Schallhorn 1973, Froum et al. 1975). Hiatt & Schallhorn (1973) treated 166 intrabony lesions with intraoral autogenous cancellous bone. They reported a mean increase in bone height of 3.5 mm, evaluated by clinical measurements. One-wall, two-wall and three-wall defects were included, and the largest bone fill was observed in defects with the highest number of bone walls. A block section obtained from a patient treated in this study presented histologic evidence of new cementum, bone and periodontal ligament formation. In controlled clinical studies, intraoral autogenous grafts were found superior to surgical debridement alone in terms of bone fill (Froum et al. 1976), or probing attachment (PAL) gain (Carraro et al. 1976) in two-wall defects. However, there are controlled studies that demonstrate more modest results regarding bone fill or PAL gain after intraoral grafting when compared to ungrafted controls (Ellegaard & Löe 1971, Renvert et al. 1985).

Ross & Cohen (1968) reported new bone and cementum formation in a human histologic specimen from an intrabony defect retrieved 8 months following debridement and placement of intraoral autogenous grafts. They also found that the grafts were without osteocytes and that the deposition of new alveolar bone had taken place around the grafts. Nabers et al. (1972) observed that new cementum and functionally oriented periodontal ligament fibers were present in half the length of a defect which was biopsied about 4½ years after treatment with intraoral autogenous bone grafts. In other human histologic reports, bone fill and new attachment were observed coronal to reference notches placed on the treated roots at the apical termination of root planing (Hiatt et al. 1978) or at the most apical level of previously existing calculus (Froum et al. 1983, Stahl et al. 1983). Other investigators, however, observed an epithelial lining which occupied a varying portion of the previously diseased part of the root (Hawley & Miller 1975, Listgarten & Rosenberg 1979, Moscow et al. 1979). The results from these studies indicate that the treatment of periodontal osseous defects with intraoral bone grafts may result in periodontal regeneration, but not predictably.

Extraoral autogenous grafts

Schallhorn (1967, 1968) introduced the use of autogeneous hip marrow grafts (iliac crest marrow) in the treatment of furcation and intrabony defects. Later several studies were published demonstrating the osteogenic potentials of this material (Schallhorn et al. 1970, Schallhorn & Hiatt 1972, Patur 1974, Froum et al. 1975), and as much as 3-4 mm gain in crestal bone was reported following the treatment of intrabony defects with hip marrow grafts. The effect of iliac crest marrow and of intraoral cancellous bone grafts in one-wall, two-wall and three-wall bony defects in humans was evaluated by Patur (1974). He reported that bone fill occurred to a varying extent with both types of graft. The amount of bone fill in one-wall bony defects was larger with iliac crest marrow than with cancellous bone or when no grafts were used. Some defects within all three groups showed bone fill, and no difference was observed between the control defects and those treated with intraoral cancellous bone grafts. The author stated that even with fresh iliac crest marrow, bone regeneration is variable and unpredictable.

Healing of interradicular and intrabony lesions following placement of iliac crest marrow was evaluated in monkeys by Ellegaard et al. (1973, 1974). Regeneration occurred more frequently with the use of grafts, but iliac crest marrow frequently resulted in ankylosis and root resorption (Fig. 28-19).

Histologic evidence of periodontal regeneration in humans following the use of iliac crest marrow grafts was provided by Dragoo and Sullivan (1973a,b). At 8 months following therapy a mature periodontal liga-

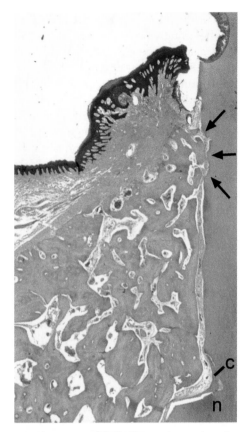

Fig. 28-19. Photomicrograph illustrating an intrabony defect 2 months following grafting with iliac crest marrow. The defect is completely filled with bone, but new cementum (c) is lacking on the root surface except for the most apical part (n) of the defect. Note that anky-losis and root resorption (arrows) are occurring in the coronal part of the defect.

ment was present at the grafted sites and about 2 mm supracrestal new attachment had also formed. Clinical evidence of root resorption was noted in 7 of the 250 grafted sites.

Due to the morbidity associated with the donor site and that root resorption sometimes results, iliac crest marrow grafts are not used in regenerative periodontal therapy today.

Allogeneic grafts
Allogeneic grafts (allografts) were utilized in attempts to stimulate bone formation in intrabony defects in order to avoid the additional surgical insult associated with the use of autogenous grafts. However, the use of allogeneic grafts involves a certain risk regarding antigenicity, although, in order to suppress foreign body reactions, the grafts are usually pretreated by freezing, radiation or chemicals.

The types of allogeneic grafts used are frozen iliac cancellous bone and marrow, mineralized freeze-dried bone grafts (FDBA) and decalcified freeze-dried bone grafts (DFDBA). The need for cross-matching to decrease the likelihood of graft rejection as well as the risk of disease transmission virtually eliminated the use of frozen iliac allogeneic grafts in periodontics.

FDBA is a mineralized bone graft, which through the manufacturing process loses cell viability and, therefore, is supposed to promote bone regeneration through osteoconduction (Goldberg & Stevenson 1987). The freeze drying also markedly reduces the antigenicity of the material (Turner & Mellonig 1981, Quattlebaum et al. 1988). The efficacy of freeze-dried bone allogeneic grafts (FDBA) was evaluated in a study which included 89 clinicians (Mellonig 1991). At re-entry surgery it was found that 67% of the sites treated with FDBA alone and 78% of the sites treated with FDBA plus autogenous bone grafts demon-strated complete or more than 50% bone fill. Thus, FDBA plus autogenous bone appeared more effective than FDBA alone. In split-mouth studies where FDBA was combined with autogenous grafts or tetracycline powder (Sanders et al. 1983, Mabry et al. 1985), a defect fill of 60% and 80% of the initial lesion was reported. In a split-mouth study it was also shown that FDBA implantation had a similar effect on defect reso-lution as that achieved by DFDBA (Rummelhart et al. 1989) or granular porous hydroxyapatite (Barnett et al. 1989). However, the only controlled clinical trial comparing treatment of intrabony defects with FDBA implantation versus flap surgery failed to demon-strate any difference in terms of clinical attachment gain and bone fill between test and control sites at 1 year re-entry examination (Altiere et al. 1979). In ad-dition, human histologic specimens demonstrated that implantation of FDBA in intrabony defects yielded no periodontal regeneration but resulted in a long epithelial attachment on the previously diseased root surface (Dragoo & Kaldahl 1983).

Several animal studies suggested that deminerali-zation of a cortical bone allograft (DFDBA) enhances its osteogenic potential by exposing bone morpho-genic proteins (BMPs) which presumably have the ability to induce host cells to differentiate into osteoblasts (Urist & Strates 1970, Mellonig et al. 1981). Several case reports presented clinical improvements and bone fill after implantation of DFDBA into in-trabony defects (Quintero et al. 1982, Werbitt 1987, Fucini et al. 1993, Francis et al. 1995), and controlled clinical studies documented considerable gain of at-tachment and bone fill in sites treated with DFDBA as compared with non-grafted sites (Pearson et al. 1981, Mellonig 1984, Meadows et al. 1993). However, no statistical differences regarding attachment level changes and bone fill were found when comparing sites treated with FDBA and sites treated with DFDBA (Rummelhart et al. 1989).

Histologic evidence of regeneration following grafting with DFDBA was provided by Bowers et al. (1989b,c). Complete regeneration with new cemen-tum, periodontal ligament and bone amounting to 80% of the original defect depth was reported at sites treated with DFDBA, which was considerably more than that observed in defects treated with surgical debridement alone. However, animal experiments failed to confirm the regenerative potential of DFDBA grafting (Sonis et al. 1985, Caplanis et al. 1998).

The controversial results regarding the effect of DFDBA on the regeneration of periodontal intraosseous defects along with great differences in the osteoinductive potential (ranging from high to no osteoinductive effect) of commercially available DFDBA (Becker et al. 1994, 1995, Shigeyama et al. 1995, Schwartz et al. 1996, Garraway et al. 1998), and the (although minute) risk for disease transmission have raised concern about the clinical applicability of DFDBA. In EU countries, the commercially available DFDBA is not granted a CE mark permitting distribution of the material within the community.

Xenogeneic grafts

The use of xenogeneic bone grafts (xenografts) in regenerative periodontal surgery was examined several years ago. Nielsen et al. (1981) treated 46 intrabony defects with Kielbone® (i.e. defatted and deproteinized ox bone) and another 46 defects with intraoral autogenous bone grafts. The results, which were evaluated by periodontal probing and radiographically, showed no difference between the amount of clinical gain of attachment and bone fill obtained in the two categories of defect. A study in monkeys also demonstrated that the two types of bone graft displayed similar histologic features and were frequently seen in the connective tissue of the healed defects as isolated bone particles surrounded by a cementum-like substance (Nielsen et al. 1980).

Recently, new processing and purification methods have been utilized which make it possible to remove all organic components from a bovine bone source and leave a non-organic bone matrix in an unchanged inorganic form (e.g. Bio-Oss®, Geistlich AG, Wolhusen, Switzerland; Endobone®, Merck Biomaterialen, Darmstadt, Germany; Laddec®, Ost Development, Clermont-Ferrand, France; Bon-Apatite®, Bio-Interfaces Inc., San Diego, US). However, differences in the purification and manipulation methods of the bovine bone exist, leading to commercially available products with different chemical properties and possibly different biological behavior. These materials are available in different particle sizes or as block grafts.

To date, no controlled human study has compared the effect of such graft materials in periodontal defects with flap surgery alone, but a recent clinical study demonstrated that implantation of Bio-Oss® resulted in pocket reduction, gain of attachment and bone fill in periodontal defects to the same extent as that of DFDBA (Richardson et al. 1999). Human histology (Camelo et al. 1998) and animal experiments (Clergeau et al. 1996) have also suggested a beneficial effect of placing bovine bone-derived biomaterials in periodontal bone defects.

The use of coral skeleton as a bone graft substitute was proposed some decades ago (Holmes 1979, Guillemin et al. 1987). Depending on the pre-treatment procedure, the natural coral turns into non-resorbable porous hydroxyapatite (e.g. Interpore 200, Interpore International, Irvine, US) or to a resorbable calcium carbonate (e.g. Biocoral, Inoteb, St Gonnery, France) skeleton (Nasr et al. 1999). Implantation of coralline porous hydroxyapatite in intrabony periodontal defects in humans produced more probing pocket depth reduction, clinical attachment gain and defect fill than non-grafting (Kenney et al. 1985, Krejci et al. 1987, Yukna 1994, Mora & Ouhayoun 1995, Yukna & Yukna 1998), and similar results were found when compared with grafting of FDBA (Barnett et al. 1989). When porous hydroxyapatite was compared with DFDBA for the treatment of intraosseous defects, similar results were also obtained (Bowen et al. 1989), but another study reported clinical results in favor of this material (Oreamuno et al. 1990). However, both animal (West & Brustein 1985, Ettel et al. 1989) and human studies (Carranza et al. 1987, Stahl & Froum 1987) have provided only vague histologic evidence that grafting of natural coral may enhance the formation of true new attachment. In most cases, the graft particles were embedded in connective tissue with minimal bone formation.

Alloplastic materials

Alloplastic materials are synthetic, inorganic, biocompatible and/or bioactive bone graft substitutes which are claimed to promote bone healing through osteoconduction. There are four kinds of alloplastic materials, which are frequently used in regenerative periodontal surgery: hydroxyapatite (HA), beta tricalcium phosphate (β-TCP), polymers, and bio-active glasses (bio-glasses).

Hydroxyapatite (HA)

The HA products used in periodontology are of two forms: a particulate non-resorbable ceramic form (e.g. Periograf®, Miter Inc., Warsaw, IN, US; Calcitite®, Calcitek Inc., San Diego, US) and a particulate, resorbable non-ceramic form (e.g. OsteoGraf/LD®, CeraMed Dental, Lakewood, CO, US). In controlled clinical studies, grafting of intrabony periodontal lesions with HA resulted in a PAL-gain of 1.1-3.3 mm and also in a greater bone defect fill as compared with non-grafted surgically debrided controls (Meffert et al. 1985, Yukna et al. 1985, 1986, 1989, Galgut et al. 1992). In these studies, improvement of clinical parameters (i.e. PPD reduction and PAL gain) was more evident in the grafted sites than in the sites treated only with debridement, especially for initially deep defects. However, animal studies (Barney et al. 1986, Minabe et al. 1988, Wilson & Low 1992), and human histologic data (Froum et al. 1982, Moskow & Lubarr 1983, Ganeles et al. 1986, Sapkos 1986) showed that bone formation was limited and that a true new attachment was not formed consistently after grafting of intrabony periodontal defects with HA. The majority of the HA particles were embedded in connective tissue and new bone was only observed occasionally around particles in close proximity to host bone. A junctional epithelium was lining the major part of the roots.

Beta-tricalcium phosphate (β-TCP)
b-TCP ($Ca_3(PO_4)_2$) (e.g. Synthograft®, Johnson and Johnson, New Brunswick, NJ, US) has been used in a series of case reports for the treatment of periodontal osseous lesions (Nery & Lynch 1978, Strub et al. 1979, Snyder et al. 1984, Baldock et al. 1985). After variable time intervals, a significant gain of bone was observed by means of re-entry or radiographs. However, there is no controlled study comparing the result of β-TCP grafting with that of open flap debridement, and histologic data from animal (Levin et al. 1974, Barney et al. 1986) and human studies (Dragoo & Kaldahl 1983, Baldock et al. 1985, Bowers et al. 1986, Stahl & Froum 1986, Froum & Stahl 1987, Saffar et al. 1990) showed that β-TCP is rapidly resorbed or encapsulated by connective tissue, with minimal bone formation and no periodontal regeneration.

Polymers
There are two polymer materials that have been used as bone graft substitutes in the treatment of periodontal defects: a non-resorbable, calcium hydroxide coated co-polymer of poly-methyl-methacrylate (PMMA) and poly-hydroxylethyl-methacrylate (PHEMA) which is often referred to as HTR (hard tissue replacement) (e.g. HTR™, Bioplant Inc., New York, NY, US), and a resorbable polylactic acid (PLA) polymer (Driloc®, Osmed Corp., Costa Mesa, CA, US).

In controlled clinical studies, implantation of HTR polymer grafts in intrabony defects resulted in a defect fill of approximately 2 mm, representing about 60% of the initial defect depth, but the improved clinical response with grafting was not significantly better than that following solely flap operation (Yukna 1990, Shahmiri et al. 1992). Human histologic data from an experimental study (Plotzke et al. 1993), and from two case reports (Stahl et al. 1990b, Froum 1996) also revealed that grafting of osseous periodontal defects with HTR does not promote periodontal regeneration. The HTR particles were most frequently encapsulated by connective tissue with only scarce evidence of bone formation. Healing resulted in a long junctional epithelium along the root surface, and true new attachment formation was not observed.

When PLA particles were implanted into intrabony defects in humans and compared with DFDBA or surgically debrided controls, it was found that the healing results were less favorable than after flap operation alone, both in terms of clinical parameters (PPD and PAL gain), and in terms of bone fill (Meadows et al. 1993).

Bioactive glasses (Bio-glasses)
Bio-glasses are composed of SiO_2, Na_2O, P_2O_5 and are resorbable or not resorbable depending on the relative proportion of these components. When bio-glasses are exposed to tissue fluids, a double layer of silica gel and calcium phosphate is formed on their surface. Through this layer the material promotes absorption and concentration of proteins used by osteoblasts to form extracellular bone matrix which theoretically may promote bone formation (Hench et al. 1972). Commercially available bio-glasses in particulate form, and theoretically resorbable, have been proposed for periodontal treatment (e.g. PerioGlass®, US Biomaterials Corp., Alachua, FL, US; BioGran®, Orthovita, Malvern, PA, US).

A human case report demonstrated that implantation of bio-glass in periodontal osseous defects resulted in a gain of clinical attachment of 2.0-5.3 mm and a radiographic bone fill of 3.5 mm, and in a controlled study, the treatment with bio-glass in intrabony defects also resulted in greater clinical improvements than surgical debridement alone (Froum et al. 1998). However, other controlled studies (Zamet et al. 1997) and split-mouth studies on grafting of intrabony defects with bio-glass (Ong et al. 1998) failed to demonstrate statistically significant better clinical results than surgery alone or DFDBA grafting (Lovelace et al. 1998). Although experimental studies in monkeys have suggested that bio-glass grafting of periodontal intrabony defects (Karatzas et al. 1999) may favor new cementum formation and inhibit epithelial down-growth, there is no histological evidence in humans that bio-glass may promote true periodontal regeneration. In a histologic evaluation of bio-glass implanted in intrabony defects in humans it was observed that although clinically satisfactory results were produced, healing had most frequently occurred with a junctional epithelium along the previously diseased part of the root, and new cementum with inserting collagen fibers was found in only one out of five treated teeth. Bone formation was limited in all specimens (Nevins et al. 2000).

Evaluation of alloplastic materials
There are no controlled clinical studies demonstrating that grafting with tricalcium phosphate or polymers results in significant clinical improvements beyond that of flap surgery, whereas several reports have indicated that grafting with hydroxyapatite or bio-active glasses may produce more gain of attachment than open flap debridement (Galgut et al. 1992, Zamet et al. 1997, Froum et al. 1998) or a gain similar to that obtained following grafting with DFDBA (Lovelace et al. 1998). Histologic evidence that the use of alloplastic or synthetic graft materials may lead to periodontal regeneration in humans is lacking, and animal experiments have failed to demonstrate regeneration of a functional periodontium following implantation of hydroxyapatite, tricalcium phosphate or polymers in periodontal lesions (Barney et al. 1986, Shahmiri et al. 1992). It was reported, however, that treatment with bio-active glasses in experimental animals produced significantly more bone fill and new attachment compared with that in non-grafted controls (Fetner et al. 1994, Karatzas et al. 1999) or in sites grafted with

hydroxyapatite or tricalcium phosphate (Wilson & Low 1992). Although some bone formation has been reported following the use of alloplastic materials, there is no evidence that these materials may stimulate the formation of new cementum with inserting collagen fibers. At the 1996 American Academy of Periodontology World Workshop, it was concluded that synthetic graft materials function primarily as defect fillers. If regeneration is the desired treatment outcome, other materials are recommended.

Biologic concept of using bone grafts or alloplastic materials

The biologic rationale behind the use of bone grafts or alloplastic materials in periodontal regenerative surgery is the assumption that these materials may either (1) contain bone forming cells (osteogenesis), (2) serve as a scaffold for bone formation (osteoconduction), or that (3) the matrix of the grafting material contains bone inductive substances (osteoinduction). It is believed that the use of such materials may stimulate not only the regrowth of alveolar bone but also the formation of new attachment. However, such complete regeneration of the periodontal attachment apparatus following such grafting procedures would imply that cells derived from bone would possess the ability to form new cementum with inserting collagen fibers on a previously periodontitis-affected root surface. This assumption is in conflict with current knowledge about the biology of periodontal wound healing, that repopulation of the detached root surface with cells from the periodontal ligament is the prerequisite for new attachment formation. This means that all therapeutic procedures involving the placement of bone grafts or bone substitute implants are based on a biologic concept which cannot explain how such treatment should result in regeneration of the periodontium.

Root surface biomodification

Much research has been directed to altering the periodontitis-involved root surface in a manner that will promote the formation of a new connective tissue attachment. Removal of bacterial deposits, calculus and endotoxins in the cementum is generally considered essential for the formation of a new connective tissue attachment (Garrett 1977). However, it was suggested by Stahl et al. (1972) that demineralization of the root surface, exposing the collagen of the dentin, would facilitate the deposition of cementum by inducing mesenchymal cells in the adjacent tissue to differentiate into cementoblasts. The biologic concept is that exposure of collagen fibers of the dentin matrix may facilitate adhesion of the blood clot to the root surface and thereby favor migration of the fibroblasts.

Several studies using various animal models demonstrated an improved healing response histologically following citric acid and tetracycline root surface demineralization (Register & Burdick 1976, Crigger et al. 1978, Polson & Proye 1982, Claffey et al. 1987). However, in a study in dogs where naturally occurring furcations were treated with citric acid, several specimens demonstrated ankylosis and root resorption (Bogle et al. 1981). This finding corroborates that of Magnusson et al. (1985a) in monkeys where citric acid conditioning was evaluated in combination with coronally displaced tissue flaps after 6 months. These investigators found root resorption on 28 out of 40 surfaces examined and 21 of these also presented ankylosis.

New connective tissue attachment following citric acid demineralization of root surfaces has been demonstrated histologically in humans (Cole et al. 1980, Frank et al. 1983, Stahl et al. 1983, Stahl & Froum 1991a). Cole et al. (1980) showed histologic evidence of a new connective tissue attachment and bone formation coronal to reference notches placed in the apical extent of calculus, identified on the root surface at the time of surgery. However, despite histologic evidence of regeneration following root surface biomodification with citric acid, results of controlled clinical trials failed to show any improvements in clinical conditions compared to non-acid treated controls (Moore et al. 1987, Fuentes et al. 1993).

In recent years, biomodification of the root surface with enamel matrix proteins (Emdogain®) during surgery and following demineralization with EDTA has been introduced to encourage periodontal regeneration. The biologic concept is that the application of enamel matrix (amelogenins) proteins may promote periodontal regeneration because it mimics events that took place during the development of the periodontal tissues (Hammarström 1997, Gestrelius et al. 2000). This view is based on the finding that the cells of the Hertwigs epithelial root sheath deposit enamel matrix proteins on the root surface prior to cementum formation and that such proteins are the initiating factor for the formation of cementum. The commercially available product, Emdogain®, a purified acid extract of porcine origin contains enamel matrix derivatives (EMD), supposed to be able to promote periodontal regeneration. In case series reports, 4-4.5 mm gain of clinical attachment, and about 70% bone fill in intrabony defects were reported following treatment with EMD (Heden et al. 1999, Heden 2000).

In a multicenter clinical study involving 33 subjects with 34 paired intrabony defects, application of EMD resulted in larger amounts of PAL-gain (2.2 mm) and statistically significantly more bone gain (2.6 mm) than open flap debridement after 36 months, evaluated clinically and radiographically (Heijl et al. 1997). Similar results were reported in another split-mouth clinical trial (23 patients) published more recently (Froum et al. 2001). In that study a PPD reduction of 4.9 mm, a PAL gain of 4.3, and a bone gain of 3.8 mm (evaluated by re-entry surgery) were observed after EMD application in 53 intrabony defects. These values were statistically significantly larger than those ob-

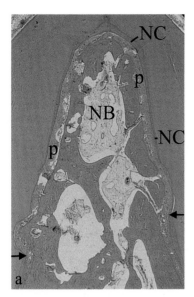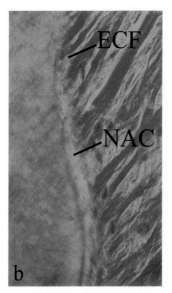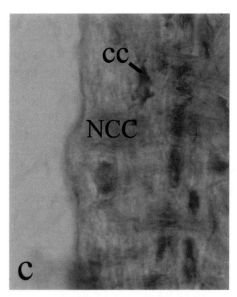

Fig. 28-20. Photomicrograph (a) of a degree III furcation defect in a dog following root surface biomodification with enamel matrix proteins and subsequently covered with a resorbable membrane. The defect has healed completely with bone (NB), a periodontal ligament (p) and new cementum (NC). The arrows indicate the apical extension of the lesion. (b) The cementum (NAC) formed on the root surface in the apical portion of the defect was acellular with inserting extrinsic collagen fibers (ECF) while (c) that (NCC) formed in the coronal portion had a cellular (cc) character.

tained by flap surgery (2.2 mm, 2.7 mm and 1.5 mm, respectively, in 31 defects).

In a more recent prospective multicenter randomized controlled clinical trial, the clinical outcomes of papilla preservation flap surgery (simplified papilla preservation flap, SPPF) with or without the application of enamel matrix proteins, were compared (Tonetti et al. 2002). A total of 83 test and 83 control patients with similar baseline periodontal conditions and defect characteristics were treated with either SPPF and Emdogain® or with SPPF alone. The test defects exhibited significantly more CAL gain than the controls (3.1 ± 1.5 mm and 2.5 ± 1.5 mm, respectively). In addition, this study demonstrated that the treatment outcomes of the test group were significantly affected by the smoking status of the patient and the number of walls of the intrabony defect. Smokers gained less attachment than non-smokers. Defects with very dense cortical or very porous and bleeding walls gained less CAL than normal corticalized defects, and intrabony defects with three walls had a higher predictability in CAL gains than those with one-wall.

Similar results were also reported in other controlled studies (Pontoriero et al. 1999, Silvestri et al. 2000). When application of EMD was compared with GTR treatment, it was found that similar clinical improvements were obtained. In a randomized controlled clinical study, Pontoriero et al. (1999) compared EMD application with GTR with resorbable (two kinds: Guidor and Resolut) and non-resorbable (e-PTFE) membranes in intrabony defects (10 patients per group). After 12 months, there were no significant differences among the groups, and EMD application resulted in a PPD reduction of 4.4 mm and a PAL gain of 2.9 mm, while the corresponding values from the

membrane-treated sites (all GTR groups combined) were 4.5 mm and 3.1 mm, respectively (Pontorierio et al. 1999). Silvestri et al. (2000) reported a PPD reduction of 4.8 mm and a PAL gain of 4.5 mm after EMD application in intrabony defects versus 5.9 mm and 4.8 mm, respectively, after GTR with non-resorbable membranes (randomized controlled study, 10 patients per group). Similar results were reported by Sculean et al. (1999a,b).

Histologic evidence of new cementum formation with inserting collagen fibers on a previously periodontitis-affected root surface and the formation of new alveolar bone in human specimens have been demonstrated following EMD treatment (Mellonig 1999, Sculean et al. 1999b). However, while in the study of Mellonig (1999) healing had occurred with acellular cementum on the root surface, the newly formed cementum in the study of Sculean et al. (1999b) displayed a predominantly cellular character. The ability of EMD to produce regeneration has been confirmed in controlled animal experiments (Fig. 28-20), following the treatment of intrabony, furcation and dehiscence defects (Hammarström et al. 1997, Araújo & Lindhe 1998, Sculean et al. 2000).

Further research is needed to elucidate the function of EMD and the predictability of this regenerative periodontal procedure.

Growth regulatory factors for periodontal regeneration

Growth factor is a general term to denote a class of polypeptide hormones that stimulate a wide variety of cellular events such as proliferation, chemotaxis, differentiation and production of extracellular matrix proteins (Terranova & Wikesjö 1987). Proliferation and migration of periodontal ligament cells and synthesis of extracellular matrix as well as differentiation of cementoblasts and osteoblasts is a prerequisite for obtaining periodontal regeneration. Therefore, it is conceivable that growth factors may represent a potential aid in attempts to regenerate the periodontium. The effects of various growth factors were studied in vitro, and a significant regeneration potential of growth factors was also demonstrated in animal models. Lynch et al. (1989, 1991) examined the effect of placing a combination of platelet derived growth factors (PDGF) and insulin-like growth factors (IGF) in naturally occurring periodontal defects in dogs. The control sites treated without growth factors healed with a long junctional epithelium and no new cementum or bone formation, while regeneration of a periodontal attachment apparatus occurred at the sites treated with growth factors. Similar results were reported by other investigators following application of a combination of PDGF and IGF in experimentally-induced periodontal lesions in monkeys (Rutherford et al. 1992, Giannobile et al. 1994, 1996). One study examined the effect of PDGF and IGF in periodontal intrabony defects and degree II furcations in humans (Howell et al. 1997). At re-entry after 9 months, significantly increased bone fill was only observed at the furcation sites treated with growth factors. It can be concluded that growth factors seem to have a positive effect on periodontal regeneration, but several important questions need to be resolved before this type of regenerative treatment can be used in humans (Graves & Cochran 1994).

Bone morphogenetic proteins (BMPs) are osteoinductive factors that may have the potential to stimulate mesenchymal cells to differentiate into bone-forming cells (Wozney et al. 1988). Sigurdsson et al. (1995) evaluated bone and cementum formation following regenerative periodontal surgery using recombinant human BMP in surgically-created supraalveolar defects in dogs. Following application of BMP the flaps were advanced to submerge the teeth and sutured. Histologic analysis showed significantly more cementum formation and regrowth of alveolar bone on BMP treated sites as compared to the controls. Ripamonti et al. (1994) also reported about the efficacy of bovine BMPs to induce periodontal regeneration in degree II furcations in baboons. On one side BMP was implanted with a collagenous matrix, while at the control sites only the collagen matrix was used. Considerable regeneration of cementum, periodontal ligament and bone was observed in the BMP treated furcations as compared to the control furcations treated without BMP. Further experimentation is needed to evaluate a possible role of BMP in periodontal regeneration.

GUIDED TISSUE REGENERATION (GTR)

The experimental studies (Karring et al. 1980, Nyman et al. 1980, Buser et al. 1990a,b, Warrer et al. 1993) described previously have documented that the progenitor cells for the formation of a new connective tissue attachment are residing in the periodontal ligament. Consequently, it should be expected that a new connective tissue attachment would be predictably achieved if such cells populate the root surface during healing. This view was confirmed in a study in monkeys in which both gingival connective tissue and gingival epithelium were prevented from contacting the root surface during healing by the use of a barrier membrane (Gottlow et al. 1984). After reduction of the supporting tissues around selected experimental teeth, the root surfaces were exposed to plaque accumulation for 6 months. Soft tissue flaps were then raised and the exposed root surfaces were curetted. The crowns of the teeth were resected and the roots were submerged. However, prior to complete closure of the wound, a membrane was placed over the curetted root surfaces on one side of the jaws in order (1) to prevent gingival connective tissue contacting the root surface during healing, and (2) to provide a space for ingrowth of periodontal ligament tissue. No membranes were placed over the contralateral roots. The histologic analysis after 3 months of healing demonstrated that the roots covered with membranes exhibited considerably more new attachment than the non-covered roots (Fig. 28-21). In four of the nine test roots, new cementum covered the entire length of the root. In all control specimens the surface coronal to the newly formed cementum presented multinucleated cells and resorption cavities. In one control specimen virtually half the root was resorbed. Coronal regrowth of alveolar bone had occurred to a varying extent in test and control roots, and no relationship was found between the amount of new cementum formation and the degree of bone regrowth. The results of this study strongly suggested that the exclusion of epithelial and gingival connective tissue cells from the healing area by the use of a physical barrier may allow (guide) periodontal ligament cells to repopulate the detached root surface. This observation provided the basis for the clinical application of the treatment principle termed "guided tissue regeneration" (GTR).

Clinical application of GTR

Clinical application of guided tissue regeneration (GTR) in periodontal therapy involves the placement of a physical barrier to ensure that the previous periodontitis-affected root surface becomes repopulated with cells from the periodontal ligament (Fig. 28-22). Treatment of the first human tooth with GTR was reported by Nyman et al. in 1982. Due to extensive

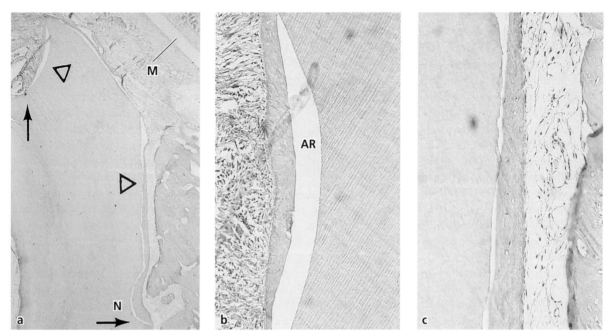

Fig. 28-21. (a) Microphotograph of membrane (M) covered root. Newly formed cementum is visible on the entire length of the buccal root surface coronal to the notch (N) and also on part of the coronal cut surface (arrow). (b, c) Higher magnifications of the areas at the upper and lower triangles in (a), showing that collagen fibers are inserted into the newly formed cementum. AR: artifact.

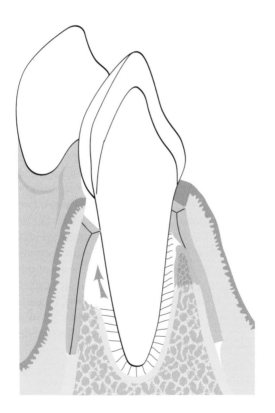

Fig. 28-22. Drawing illustrating the placement of the physical barrier which prevents the epithelium and gingival connective tissue from contacting the root surface during healing. At the same time the membrane allows cells from the periodontal ligament (arrow) to repopulate the previously periodontitis-involved root surface.

periodontal destruction, the tooth was scheduled for extraction. This offered the possibility of obtaining histologic documentation of the result of the treatment. Following elevation of full thickness flaps, scaling of the root surface and removal of all granulation tissue, an 11 mm deep periodontal lesion was ascertained. Prior to flap closure, a membrane was adjusted to cover parts of the detached root surfaces, the osseous defect and parts of the surrounding bone. His-

tologic analysis after 3 months of healing revealed that new cementum with inserting collagen fibers had formed on the previously exposed root surface (Fig. 28-23). In a later study (Gottlow et al. 1986), 12 cases treated with GTR were evaluated clinically, and in five of these cases histologic documentation was also presented. The results showed that considerable but varying amounts of new connective tissue attachment had formed on the treated teeth. Frequently, however,

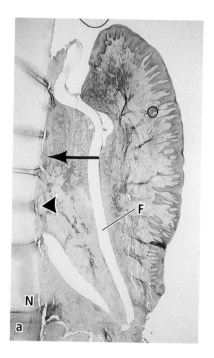
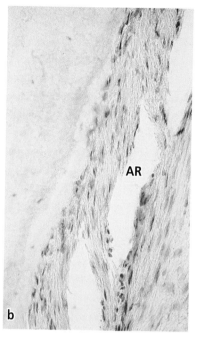

Fig. 28-23. Microphotograph of a human tooth (a) 3 months following GTR treatment using a Millipore filter (F). New cementum with inserting collagen fibers (about 5 mm) has formed from the notch (N) to the level of the arrow. Bone formation underneath the filter is lacking, probably due to the inflammatory infiltrate seen in the tissues adjacent to the filter. (b) Higher magnification of the area indicated by the arrowhead in (a) showing newly formed cementum with inserting collagen fibers. AR: artifact.

bone formation was incomplete. The varying results were ascribed to factors such as the amount of remaining periodontal ligament, the morphology of the treated defect, technical difficulties regarding membrane placement, gingival recession and bacterial contamination of the membrane and the wound during healing.

In the last decades, GTR has been applied in a number of clinical trials for the treatment of various periodontal defects such as intrabony defects (for review see Cortellini & Bowers 1995), furcation involvements (for review see Machtei & Schallhorn 1995, Karring & Cortellini 1999), and localized gingival recession defects (Pini-Prato et al. 1996).

The clinical outcomes of GTR are most frequently evaluated by changes in clinical attachment levels (CAL), bone levels (BL), probing pocket depths (PPD), and the position of the gingival margin. In some of the studies on degree II and III furcations, horizontal changes in clinical attachment, bone level and pocket depth were also measured. As previously pointed out, evidence of true regeneration of periodontal attachment can only be provided by histologic means. However, based on reports about the formation of a new attachment apparatus in histologic specimens from human biopsies harvested following GTR treatment (Nyman et al. 1982, Gottlow et al. 1986, Becker et al. 1987, Stahl et al. 1990a, Cortellini et al. 1993a) and based on the biologic concept of GTR (Karring et al. 1980, 1985, 1993, Nyman et al. 1980, Gottlow et al. 1984), it was suggested that clinical signs of probing attachment gain and bone fill can be accepted as evidence of periodontal regeneration in the evaluation of GTR procedures (Lindhe & Echeverria 1994).

Procedural guidelines

GTR is not a procedure for the treatment of periodontitis, but rather a technique for regenerating defects which have developed as a result of periodontitis. Therefore, appropriate periodontal treatment should always be completed before GTR is initiated.

Surgery is initiated by sulcular or marginal incisions at both the buccal and lingual aspect of the jaw, followed by buccal and vertical releasing incisions. The releasing incisions must be placed a minimum of one tooth anterior and/or posterior to the tooth that is being treated (Fig. 28-24). Care should be taken during this procedure to preserve the interdental papillae. All pocket epithelium is excised so that a fresh connective tissue is left on the full thickness flaps following reflection. After elevation of the tissue flaps, all granulation tissue is removed and thorough debridement of the detached root surfaces is carried out using curettes, burs, etc.

Various types of bioabsorbable and non-bioabsorbable barrier materials are available in a variety of configurations designed for specific applications. The configuration most suitable for covering the defect is selected and additional tailoring of the material is performed. The shaping of the material is carried out in such a way that it is adapting closely to the tooth and is completely covering the defect, extending at least 3 mm on the bone beyond the defect margins after placement (Fig. 28-25). This assures a good stability of the material and protects the underlying blood clot during healing. At placement it is essential to ensure good adaptation of the barrier material to the alveolar bone surrounding the defect and to avoid overlaps or folds of the material.

Although exceptions exist, the barrier materials available are fixed to the tooth with a suture using a

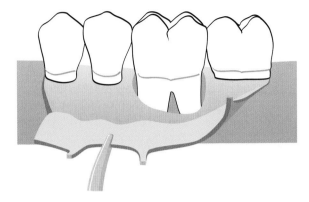

Fig. 28-24. Following marginal incisions and vertical releasing incisions on the buccal aspect of the jaw, buccal and lingual full thickness flaps are elevated.

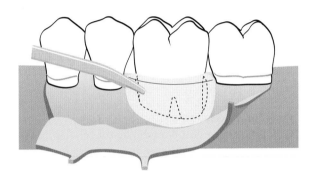

Fig. 28-25. The barrier material is placed in such a way that it completely covers the defect and extends at least 3 mm on the bone beyond the defect margin.

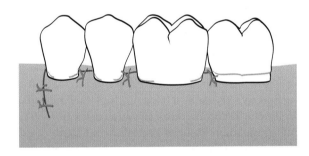

Fig. 28-26. The elevated tissue flaps are coronally displaced and sutured in such a way that the border of the barrier material is at least 2 mm below the flap margin.

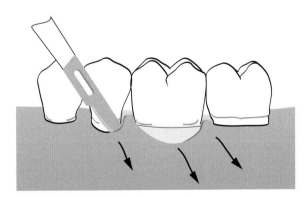

Fig. 28-27. In order to remove the barrier material an incision is made extending one tooth mesially and distally to the border of the barrier. After reflecting the covering tissue flaps, the barrier can be removed without compromising the newly regenerated tissue.

sling technique. For optimal performance, the barrier should be placed with its margin 2-3 mm apically to the flap margin. To maximize coverage of the barrier, a horizontal releasing incision in the periosteum may assist in the coronal displacement of the flap at the suturing of the wound. However, care should be taken not to compromise the blood supply to the flap. The interproximal space near the barrier should be closed first. In order to achieve good closure, a vertical mattress suturing technique is advocated (Fig. 28-26).

To reduce the risk of infection and to assure optimal healing, the patient should be instructed to gently brush the area postoperatively with a soft bristle toothbrush and to rinse with chlorhexidine (0.2%) for a period of 4-6 weeks. In addition, systemic antibiotics are frequently administered immediately prior to surgery and during 1-2 weeks after surgery. When a non-bioabsorbable barrier is used, it should be removed after 4-6 weeks. However, if complications develop it may be necessary to remove it earlier.

Removal of the material requires a minor surgical procedure (Fig. 28-27). To obtain access to the barrier material, a small incision is made extending one tooth mesially and distally of the border of the barrier. The soft tissue flap is gently reflected and the barrier material dissected free from the flap using a sharp blade. During this procedure it is essential not to compromise the newly regenerated tissue. At removal of the barrier material there will usually be some pocket formation on the outer surface of the material. It is important that this epithelium is removed so that fresh connective tissue is in contact with the newly regenerated tissue after wound closure. It is essential that the newly regenerated tissue is completely covered after suturing. The patient is instructed to rinse with chlorhexidine for 2-3 weeks during which period frequent visits for professional tooth cleaning are recommended. After this period, brushing and interproximal cleaning can be resumed, chlorhexidine rinsing discontinued, and the patient enrolled in a regular periodontal maintenance program.

If the flap is excessively traumatized during surgery either part or all of it may slough during healing. Perforations may also occur, particularly in sites with sharp bony ledges. A minor osteoplasty during placement may help to allow the barrier to better follow the contours of the ridge. Abscess formation may also occur in the wound, probably due to severe bacterial contamination of the barrier. Dependent on the severity of such complications, early removal of the barrier may be indicated.

Barrier materials for regenerative surgery
In the first GTR attempts, a bacterial filter produced from cellulose acetate (Millipore®) was used as an occlusive membrane (Nyman et al. 1982, Gottlow et al. 1984, Magnusson et al. 1985b). Although this type of membrane served its purpose, it was not ideal for clinical application. Later studies have utilized membranes of expanded polytetrafluoroethylene (e-PTFE)

especially designed for periodontal regeneration (Gore Tex Periodontal Material®). The basic molecule of this material consists of a carbon-carbon bond with four attached fluorine atoms to form a polymer. It is inert and does not result in any tissue reaction when implanted in the body. This type of membrane persists after healing and must be removed in a second operation. Membranes of e-PTFE have been used successfully in animal experiments and in several clinical studies. It was experienced from such studies that in order for a barrier material to function optimally, it has to meet certain essential design criteria:

1. To allow for good tissue acceptance it is important that the material is biocompatible. The material should not elicit an immune response, sensitization or chronic inflammation which may interfere with healing and present a hazard to the patient. Biocompatibility however, is a relative term since practically no materials are completely inert.
2. The material should act as a barrier to exclude undesirable cell types from entering the secluded space adjacent to the root surface. It is also considered an advantage that the material would allow the passage of nutrients and gases.
3. Tissue integration is another important property of a barrier material. Thus, tissue may grow into the material without penetrating all the way through. The goal of tissue integration is to prevent rapid epithelial downgrowth on the outer surface of the material or encapsulation of the material, and to provide stability to the overlying flap. The importance of tissue integration was demonstrated in a study in monkeys (Warrer et al. 1992) in which bioabsorbable membranes of polylactic acid, a synthetic polymer, were used for treatment of circumferential periodontal defects. Due to the lack of tissue integration, the membranes in this study became surrounded by an epithelial layer and were often encapsulated and exfoliated.
4. It is also essential that the barrier material is capable of creating and maintaining a space adjacent to the root surface. This will allow the ingrowth of tissue from the periodontal ligament. Some materials may be so soft and flexible that they collapse into the defect. Other materials are too stiff and may perforate the overlying tissue.
5. Finally, there are clinical needs in the design of a barrier. It should be provided in configurations which are easy to trim and to place.

Bioabsorbable materials
In recent years, natural or synthetic bioabsorbable barrier materials for GTR have been introduced in order to avoid a second surgery for membrane removal. Barrier materials of collagen from different species and from different anatomical sites have been tested in animals and in humans (Blumenthal 1988, 1993, Pitaru et al. 1988, Tanner et al. 1988, Paul et al. 1992, Wang et al. 1994, Camelo et al. 1998, Mellonig

2000). Often the collagen used is a cross-linked variety of porcine or bovine origin. When a collagen membrane is implanted in the human body it is resorbed by the enzymatic activity of macrophages and polymorphnuclear leucocytes (Tatakis et al. 1999). Successful treatment following the use of such barrier materials has been demonstrated, but the results of the studies vary. Several complications such as early degradation, epithelial downgrowth along the material and premature loss of the material were reported following the use of collagen materials. The varying results are probably due to differences in the properties of the material and the handling of the material at the time of implantation. Although probably very minimal, there is a risk that infectious agents from animal products can be transmitted to humans, and autoimmunization has also been mentioned as a risk.

Barrier materials of polylactic acid or copolymers of polylactic acid and polyglycolic acid were evaluated in animal and human studies and are commonly used (Magnusson et al. 1988, Caffesse et al. 1994, Caton et al. 1994, Gottlow et al. 1994, Laurell et al. 1994, Hugoson et al. 1995, Polson et al. 1995a, Hürzeler et al. 1997, Sculean et al. 1999a). These materials are biocompatible, but by definition they are not inert since some tissue reaction may be expected during degradation. The materials are degradated by hydrolysis and eliminated from the organism through the Krebs cycle as carbon dioxide and water (Tatakis et al. 1999).

The types of barrier materials tested in the studies differ regarding configuration and design. It appears that a number of bioabsorbable materials to a varying extent meet the requirements of a good barrier listed above. Indeed, there are several studies (Hugoson et al. 1995, Cortellini et al. 1996b, Smith et al. 1998, Tonetti et al. 1998, Cortellini & Tonetti 2000a) indicating that similar satisfactory results can be obtained with bioabsorbable barrier materials of polylactic and polyglycolic acid as with non-bioabsorbable materials.

Intrabony defects

Early evidence that GTR treatment of deep intrabony defects may produce clinical improvements in terms of clinical attachment gain was presented in several case reports (Nyman et al. 1982, Gottlow et al. 1986, Becker et al. 1988, Schallhorn & McClain 1988, Cortellini et al. 1990). In recent years, a number of clinical investigations have reported on a total of 1283 intrabony defects treated with GTR (Table 28-1). In these studies, the issue of evaluating the predictability of the clinical outcomes following application of GTR procedures was addressed. The weighted mean of the reported results indicates a mean gain in clinical attachment of 3.8 ± 1.7 mm, with a 95% confidence interval ranging from 3.7 to 4.0 mm (Cortellini & Tonetti 2000a). The reported clinical attachment gains following GTR treatment were significantly larger than the ones obtained from conventional flap surgery. A recent review (Lang 2000) on flap surgery reported a weighted mean of 1.172 defects in 40 studies. CAL gains were 1.8 ± 1.4 mm, with a 95% confidence interval ranging from 1.6 to 1.9 mm.

Different types of non-bioabsorbable (Fig. 28-28) and bioabsorbable (Fig. 28-29) barrier materials were used in the studies summarized in Table 28-1. A subset analysis indicated that cases treated with non-bioabsorbable barrier materials (351 defects) showed a mean gain in clinical attachment of 3.7 ± 1.7 mm which did not differ from that obtained with bioabsorbable barrier materials of 3.6 ± 1.5 mm (592 defects).

Analysis of the results reported in some of the studies in Table 28-1 (i.e. 211 defects in 9 investigations; Proestakis et al. 1992, Cortellini et al. 1993b, 1995c, 1996b, Cortellini & Pini-Prato 1994, Laurell et al. 1994, Mattson et al. 1995, Mellado et al. 1995, Tonetti et al. 1996b) provides important information regarding the predictability of GTR in intrabony defects. Gains of 2-3 mm were observed in 29.2% of the defects, gains of 4-5 mm in 35.4% of the defects, and gains of 6 mm or more in 24.9% of the defects. Only in 10.5% of the treated defects was the gain less than 2 mm, while no change or attachment loss was observed in two cases.

In some of the investigations, changes in bone levels were also reported (Becker et al. 1988, Handelsman et al. 1991, Kersten et al. 1992, Cortellini et al. 1993b,c, Selvig et al. 1993). Bone gains ranged between 1.1 and 4.3 mm and correlated with the reported gains in clinical attachment. In a study by Tonetti et al. (1993b), 1 year after GTR the bone was found to be located 1.5 mm apically to the position of the attained clinical attachment level.

Another important parameter related to the outcome of regenerative procedures is the residual pocket depth. In the studies reported in Table 28-1, shallow pockets were consistently found at 1 year. The weighted mean of residual pocket depth was 3.4 ± 1.2 mm, with a 95% CI ranging from 2.3 to 3.5 mm.

The reported outcomes indicate that GTR procedures predictably result in clinical improvements in intrabony defects beyond that of flap surgery. This was further confirmed in 11 controlled randomized clinical trials in which guided tissue regeneration was compared with conventional flap surgery (Table 28-2). A total of 267 defects were treated with flap surgery and 317 with GTR. In 9 of the 11 investigations, GTR resulted in statistically significantly greater probing attachment level gains when compared to flap surgery. Similar results were also observed for residual pocket depth. It should be emphasized that one of the investigations reporting no significant differences between GTR and flap surgery was carried out in only 9 pairs of defects (18 defects) located on maxillary premolars (Proestakis et al. 1992). In this study the intrabony component of the defects was shallow and 10 of the 18 defects had a furcation involvement. The weighted mean of the results reported in the 11 studies listed in Table 28-2 (Cortellini & Tonetti 2000a) indicated that the gain in clinical attachment in sites

Table 28-1. Clinical outcomes of GTR treatment of deep intrabony defects

Authors	Membranes	N	Gains in CAL ± SD (mm)	Residual PPD ± SD (mm)
Becker et al. 1988	e-PTFE	9	4.5 ± 1.7	3.2 ± 1.0
Chung et al. 1990	collagen	10	0.6 ± 0.6	
Handelsman et al. 1991	e-PTFE	9	4.0 ± 1.4	3.9 ± 1.4
Kersten et al. 1992	e-PTFE	13	1.0 ± 1.1	5.1 ± 0.9
Proestakis et al. 1992	e-PTFE	9	1.2 ± 1.3	3.5 ± 0.9
Quteish & Dolby 1992	collagen	26	3.0 ± 1.5	2.2 ± 0.4
Selvig et al. 1992	e-PTFE	26	0.8 ± 1.3	5.4
Becker & Becker 1993	e-PTFE	32	4.5	3.9 ± 0.3
Cortellini et al. 1993b	e-PTFE	40	4.1 ± 2.5	2.0 ± 0.6
Falk et al. 1993	polylactic acid	25	4.5 ± 1.6	3.0 ± 1.1
Cortellini & Pini-Prato 1994	rubber dam	5	4.0 ± 0.7	2.4 ± 0.5
Laurell et al. 1994	polylactic acid	47	4.9 ± 2.4	3.0 ± 1.4
Al-Arrayed et al. 1995	collagen	19	3.9	2.5
Chen et al. 1995	collagen	10	2.0 ± 0.4	4.2 ± 0.4
Cortellini et al. 1995c	e-PTFE	15	4.1 ± 1.9	2.7 ± 1.0
Cortellini et al. 1995c	e-PTFE+titanium	15	5.3 ± 2.2	2.1 ± 0.5
Cortellini et al. 1995a	e-PTFE+FGG	14	5.0 ± 2.1	2.6 ± 0.9
Cortellini et al. 1995a	e-PTFE	14	3.7 ± 2.1	3.2 ± 1.8
Cortellini et al. 1995b	e-PTFE+fibrin	11	4.5 ± 3.3	1.7
Cortellini et al. 1995b	e-PTFE	11	3.3 ± 1.9	1.9
Mattson et al. 1995	collagen	13	2.5 ± 1.5	3.6 ± 0.6
Mattson et al. 1995	collagen	9	2.4 ± 2.1	4.0 ± 1.1
Mellado et al. 1995	e-PTFE	11	2.0 ± 0.9	
Becker et al. 1996	polylactic acid	30	2.9 ± 2.0	3.6 ± 1.3
Cortellini et al. 1996c	polylactic acid	10	4.5 ± 0.9	3.1 ± 0.7
Cortellini et al. 1996b	e-PTFE	12	5.2 ± 1.4	2.9 ± 0.9
Cortellini et al. 1996b	polylactic acid	12	4.6 ± 1.2	3.3 ± 0.9
Gouldin et al. 1996	e-PTFE	25	2.2 ± 1.4	3.5 ± 1.3
Kim et al. 1996	e-PTFE	19	4.0 ± 2.1	3.2 ± 1.1
Murphy 1996	e-PTFE+ITM	12	4.7 ± 1.4	2.9 ± 0.8
Tonetti et al. 1996b	e-PTFE	23	5.3 ± 1.7	2.7
Benqué et al. 1997	collagen	52	3.6 ± 2.2	3.9 ± 1.7
Caffesse et al. 1997	polylactic acid	6	2.3 ± 2.0	3.8 ± 1.2
Caffesse et al. 1997	e-PTFE	6	3.0 ± 1.2	3.7 ± 1.2
Christgau et al. 1997	e-PTFE	10	4.3 ± 1.2	3.6 ± 1.1
Christgau et al. 1997	polyglactin	10	4.9 ± 1.0	3.9 ± 1.1
Falk et al. 1997	polylactic acid	203	4.8 ± 1.5	3.4 ± 1.6
Kilic et al. 1997	e-PTFE	10	3.7 ± 2.0	3.1 ± 1.4
Cortellini et al. 1998	polylactic acid	23	3.0 ± 1.7	3.0 ± 0.9
Eickholz et al. 1998	polylactic acid	14	3.4 ± 1.6	3.2 ± 0.7
Smith MacDonald et al.1998	e-PTFE	10	4.3 ± 2.1	3.7 ± 0.9
Smith MacDonald et al. 1998	polylactic acid	10	4.6 ± 1.7	3.4 ± 1.2
Parashis et al. 1998	polylactic acid	12	3.8 ± 1.8	3.5 ± 1.4
Tonetti et al. 1998	polylactic acid	69	3.0 ± 1.6	4.3 ± 1.3
Cortellini et al. 1999	polylactic acid	18	4.9 ± 1.8	3.6 ± 1.2
Pontoriero et al. 1999	diff. barriers	30	3.1 ± 1.8	3.3 ± 1.3
Sculean et al. 1999a	polylactic acid	52	3.4 ± 1.4	3.6 ± 1.3

Table 28-1 (*contd*)

Authors	Membranes	N	Gains in CAL ± SD (mm)	Residual PPD ± SD (mm)
Dorfer et al. 2000	polylactic acid	15	4.0 ± 1.2	2.7 ± 0.7
Dorfer et al. 2000	polidiossanon	15	3.4 ± 1.9	3.1 ± 1.1
Eickholz et al. 2000	polylactic acid	30	3.9 ± 1.2	2.6 ± 1.0
Karapataki et al. 2000	polylactic acid	10	4.7 ± 0.7	4.2 ± 1.4
Karapataki et al. 2000	e-PTFE	9	3.6 ± 1.7	4.6 ± 1.3
Ratka-Kruger et al. 2000	polylactic acid	23	3.1 ± 2.3	4.7 ± 1.4
Zybutz et al. 2000	polylactic acid	15	2.4 ± 1.9	
Zubutz et al. 2000	e-PTFE	14	2.4 ± 0.8	
Cortellini & Tonetti 2001	diff. barriers	26	5.4 ± 1.2	3.3 ± 0.6
Cortellini et al. 2001	polylactic acid	55	3.5 ± 2.1	3.8 ± 1.5
Weighted mean		**1283**	**3.8 ± 1.7**	**3.4 ± 1.2**

FGG = Free gingival graft
ITM = Interproximal tissue maintenance

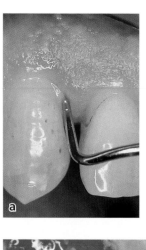
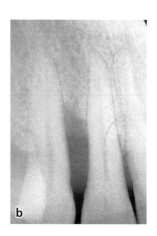
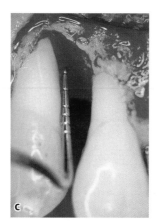
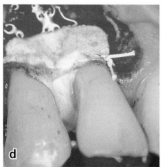
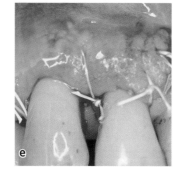
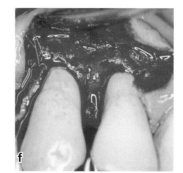
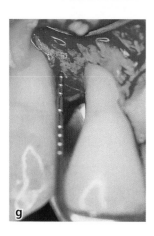
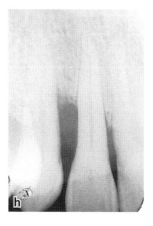

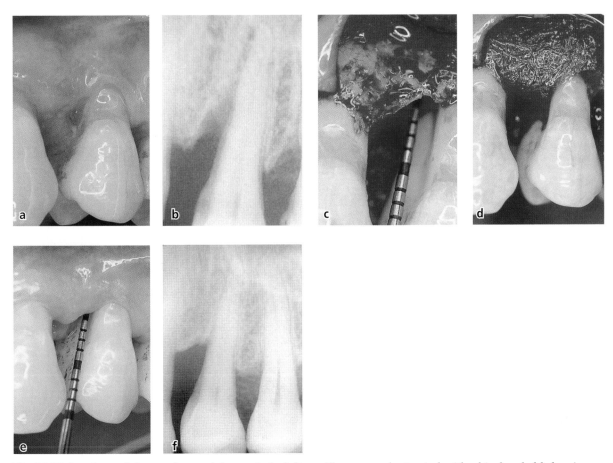

Fig. 28-29. Intrabony defect on the mesial aspect of a left maxillary premolar treated with a bioabsorbable barrier membrane. (a) Clinical attachment loss was 12 mm. (b) Radiograph showing the presence of a deep interproximal intrabony defect approaching the apex of the tooth. (c) A 7 mm interproximal intrabony defect was measured after flap elevation, defect debridement and root planing. (d) A bioabsorbable barrier membrane has been placed and sutured to cover the defect. (e) At 1 year a 4 mm pocket depth and 5 mm clinical gain of attachment were recorded. (f) The 1-year radiograph shows that the intrabony defect is almost resolved.

treated with GTR was 3.3 ± 1.8 mm (95% CI 2.8-3.6 mm), while the flap surgery resulted in a mean gain of 2.1 ± 1.5 mm (95% CI 1.8-2.4 mm). These clinical results strongly indicate that there is an added beneficial effect of placing a barrier material over an intrabony defect in conjunction with surgery.

Factors affecting clinical outcomes of GTR in intrabony defects

The results reported in Table 28-1 indicate that clinical improvements beyond that of flap surgery can be obtained by treating intrabony defects with GTR, but they also suggest a great variability in clinical outcomes among the different studies. In addition, it is apparent from the results that the complete resolution of the intrabony component of the defect is observed in only a minority of sites. A series of factors associated with the clinical outcomes were identified using multivariate approaches (Tonetti et al. 1993a, 1995, 1996a, Cortellini et al. 1994, Machtei et al. 1994). These studies have evaluated three types of factors associated with the observed variability of the results:

1. patient factors
2. defect factors

Fig. 28-28. Intrabony defect on the mesial aspect of a right maxillary canine treated with a non-bioabsorbable barrier membrane. (a) The pocket depth is 9 mm and the loss of clinical attachment 10 mm. (b) Radiograph showing the presence of an interproximal intrabony defect. (c) After full thickness flap elevation, defect debridement, and root planing, a 4 mm intrabony defect is evident. (d) An e-PTFE non-bioabsorbable barrier membrane has been tailored, positioned and tightly sutured around the teeth adjacent to the defect. (e) The flap has been repositioned and sutured to cover the membrane. Optimal preservation of the soft tissues has been accomplished with an intrasulcular incision. (f) After removal of the membrane at 5 weeks, the defect appears to be completely filled with newly formed tissue. (g) The treated site has been surgically re-entered after 1 year. The intrabony defect is completely filled with bone. (h) The 1-year radiograph confirms the complete resolution of the intrabony defect.

Table 28-2. Controlled clinical trials comparing clinical outcomes of GTR procedures with access flap procedures in deep intrabony defects

Authors	Membranes	N	Gains in CAL ± SD (mm)		Residual PPD ± SD (mm)	
			GTR	Access flap	GTR	Access flap
Chung et al. 1990	collagen	10	0.6 ± 0.6		4.0 ± 1.1	
	collagen	9	2.4 ± 2.1			
	control	14		-0.7 ± 0.9		
Proestakis et al. 1992	e-PTFE	9	1.2 ± 1.3		3.5 ± 0.9	
	control	9		0.6 ± 1.0		3.7 ± 3.0
Quteish & Dolby 1992	collagen	26	3.0 ± 1.5		2.2 ± 0.4	
	control	26		1.8 ± 0.9		3.4 ± 0.6
Al-Arrayed et al. 1995	collagen	19	3.9		2.5	
	control	14		2.7		3.5
Cortellini et al. 1995c	e-PTFE	15	4.1 ± 1.9		2.7 ± 1.0	
	e-PTFE+titanium	15	5.3 ± 2.2		2.1 ± 0.5	
	control	15		2.5 ± 0.8		3.7 ± 1.3
Mattson et al. 1995	collagen	13	2.5 ± 1.5		3.6 ± 0.6	
	control	9		0.4 ± 2.1		4.5 ± 1.8
Cortellini et al. 1996b	e-PTFE	12	5.2 ± 1.4		2.9 ± 0.9	
	polylactic acid	12	4.6 ± 1.2		3.3 ± 0.9	
	control	12		2.3 ± 0.8		4.2 ± 0.9
Tonetti et al. 1998	polylactic acid	69	3.0 ± 1.6		4.3 ± 1.3	
	control	67		2.2 ± 1.5		4.2 ± 1.4
Pontoriero et al. 1999	diff. barriers	30	3.1 ± 1.8		3.3 ± 1.3	
	control	30		1.8 ± 1.5		4.0 ± 0.8
Ratka-Kruger et al. 2000	polylactic acid	23	3.1 ± 2.3		4.7 ± 1.4	
	control	21		3.3 ± 2.7		4.9 ± 2.1
Cortellini et al. 2001	polylactic acid	55	3.5 ± 2.1		3.8 ± 1.5	
	control	54		2.6 ± 1.8		4.7 ± 1.4
Weighted mean		**584**	**3.3 ± 1.8**	**2.1 ± 1.5**	**3.5 ± 1.1**	**4.1 ± 1.3**

CAL = Clinical attachment level
PPD = Probing pocket depth
SD = Standard deviation

3. factors associated with the GTR technique and the healing period.

Patient factors
The level of self-performed plaque control had a paramount influence on the outcome of GTR. In fact, better clinical attachment level gains were observed in patients with optimal levels of plaque control as compared with those in patients with poor oral hygiene (Cortellini et al. 1994, Tonetti et al. 1995, 1996a). Patients with plaque on < 10% of the tooth surfaces (full mouth plaque score, FMPS) had a gain of clinical attachment which was 1.89 mm greater than that observed in patients with FMPS > 20% (Tonetti et al. 1995). The authors also demonstrated that cigarette smoking was associated with reduced attachment level gains. The attachment gain in subjects smoking more than 10 cigarettes/day was 2.1 ± 1.2 mm versus 5.2 ± 1.9 mm in non-smokers (Tonetti et al. 1995). Another important variable is the level of residual periodontal infection in the dentition. The higher the level of residual infection, the lower was the attach-

ment gain (Tonetti et al. 1993a, Machtei et al. 1994). It can be concluded that patient selection is critical to the success of GTR therapy (Fig. 28-30).

Defect factors
Defect morphology plays a major role in healing following GTR treatment of intrabony defects. This was demonstrated in studies showing that the depth and width of the intrabony component of the defect influence the amount of clinical attachment and bone gained at 1 year. The deeper the defect, the greater was the amount of clinical improvements, while the wider the defect, the lower were the attachment and bone gains (Garrett et al. 1988, Tonetti et al. 1993a, 1996a).

In a recent controlled study, however, it was demonstrated that deep and shallow defects have the "same potential" for regeneration. In this study, deep defects (deeper than 3 mm) resulted in larger linear amounts of CAL gains than shallow defects (3.7 ± 1.7 mm versus 2.2 ± 1.3 mm), but the percentage of CAL gains as related to baseline defect depth was similar in deep (76.7 ± 27.7%) and in shallow (75.8 ± 45%)

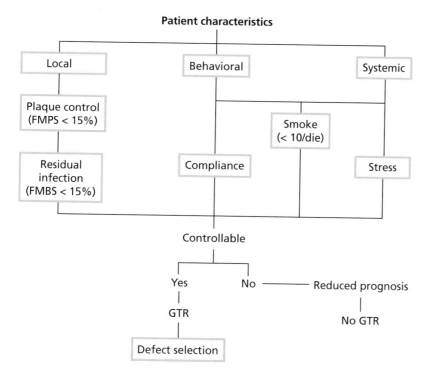

Fig. 28-30. Diagram illustrating patient selection criteria. It can be seen that control of local, behavioral and systemic patient characteristics may improve the treatment outcomes. (Modified from Cortellini & Bowers 1995). FMPS = full mouth plaque score. FMBS = full mouth bleeding score.

defects. The width of the intrabony component of the defects is measured as the angle that the bony wall of the defect forms with the long axis of the tooth. In a recent study on 242 intrabony defects, Cortellini & Tonetti (1999) demonstrated that defects with a radiographic angle of 25° or less gained consistently more attachment (1.6 mm on average) than defects of 37° or more.

It was also shown that the number of residual bony walls was related to the outcomes of various regenerative approaches (Goldman & Cohen 1958, Schallhorn et al. 1970). This issue as related to GTR therapy was addressed in three investigations (Selvig et al. 1993, Tonetti et al. 1993a, 1996a). In one study, the reported 1 year mean clinical attachment level gain was 0.8 ± 1.3 mm. This gain corresponded to the depth of the three-wall intrabony component of the defect (Selvig et al. 1993). In the other two investigations, on the contrary, gains in attachment were not related to the defect configuration in terms of one-wall, two-wall and three-wall subcomponents (Tonetti et al. 1993a, 1996a). A total of 70 defects were examined in these two latter studies, utilizing a multivariate approach. The treatment resulted in mean attachment gains of 4.1 ± 2.5 mm and 5.3 ± 2.2 mm, and it was observed that the most coronal portion of the defects which is most susceptible to negative influences from the oral environment were often incompletely filled with bone.

The endodontic status of the tooth has also been suggested as a potential relevant factor in periodontal therapy. Emerging evidence (see Chapter 14) indicates that root canal treated teeth may respond differently to periodontal therapy. A clinical study on 208 consecutive patients with one intrabony defect each demonstrated that root canal treatment does not negatively affect the healing response and the long-term stability of results of deep intrabony defects treated with GTR (Cortellini & Tonetti 2000b). Finally, a controlled clinical trial demonstrated that severe tooth hypermobility can negatively affect the clinical outcomes of regeneration (Cortellini et al. 2001). Based on these results, it can be concluded that deep and narrow intrabony defects at either vital or endodontically treated teeth are the ones in which the most beneficial outcomes can be achieved by GTR treatment (Fig. 28-31). Severe dental hypermobility may impair the clinical outcomes.

Technical factors
Successful GTR requires careful flap design, correct placement of the material, good closure of the wound and optimal post-operative plaque control.

Membrane exposure is reported to be a major complication with a prevalence in the range of 50 to 100% (Becker et al. 1988, Cortellini et al. 1990, 1993b, Selvig et al. 1992, 1993, Murphy 1995a, DeSanctis et al. 1996a,b, Falk et al. 1997, Trombelli et al. 1997, Mayfield et al. 1998). Cortellini et al. (1995c,d) reported that the prevalence of membrane exposure can be highly reduced with the use of access flaps, specifically designed to preserve the interdental tissues (modified papilla preservation technique) (Fig. 28-32).

Many studies have shown that the exposed membranes are contaminated with bacteria (Selvig et al. 1990, 1992, Grevstad & Leknes 1992, Machtei et al. 1993, Mombelli et al. 1993, Tempro & Nalbandian 1993, Nowzari & Slots 1994, Novaes-Jr et al. 1995, Nowzari et al. 1995, DeSanctis et al. 1996a,b). Contamination of exposed non-bioabsorbable as well as bioabsorbable membranes was associated with lower probing attachment level gains in intrabony defects (Selvig et al. 1992, Nowzari & Slots 1994, Nowzari et al. 1995, DeSanctis et al. 1996a,b). The impaired clini-

Defect anatomy

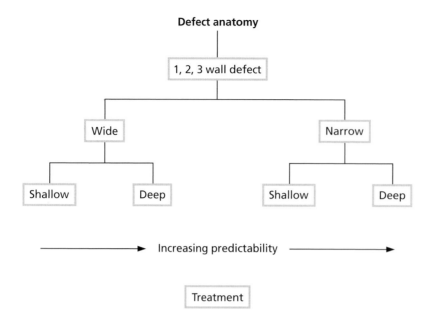

Fig. 28-31. Diagram illustrating defect selection criteria. It can be seen that deep and narrow defects, whether they are one-wall, two-wall or three-wall defects, have the greatest possibility to show gain of attachment after treatment. (Modified from Cortellini & Bowers 1995.)

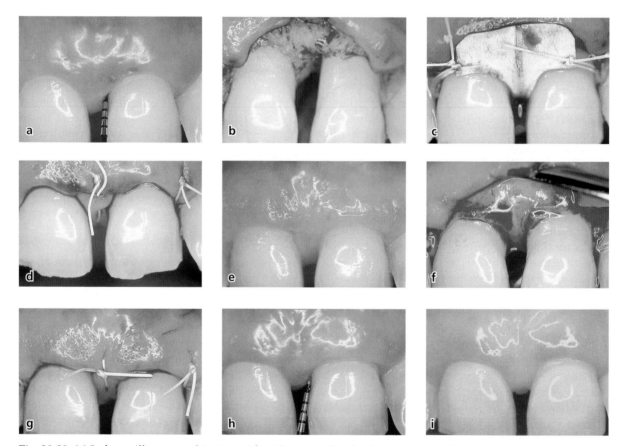

Fig. 28-32. (a) Left maxillary central incisor with a 10 mm pocket depth and 11 mm of clinical attachment loss on the mesial surface. A diastema is present between the two central incisors. (b) Full thickness buccal and palatal flaps have been raised and an intrabony defect can be seen. The interdental papilla has been incised on the buccal aspect and elevated with the palatal flap (modified papilla preservation technique). (c) A titanium-reinforced e-PTFE barrier membrane has been placed and fixed close to the level of the cemento-enamel junction. (d) The membrane is completely covered. This primary closure has been obtained by preserving the interdental papilla and by coronal displacement of the buccal tissue flap. (e) At 6 weeks, the membrane is completely covered with healthy tissue. (f) After membrane removal at 6 weeks, dense newly formed tissue is evident in the defect and in the supracrestal space maintained by the titanium-reinforced membrane. (g) The newly formed tissue is completely covered by the raised and well preserved tissue flaps. (h) The photograph after 1 year shows a 4 mm residual pocket depth. A gain of clinical attachment of 6 mm was recorded, and no recession has occurred compared to baseline. (j) 1 year photograph showing the optimal preservation of the interdental tissues.

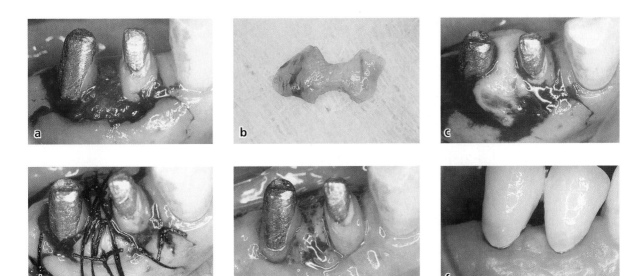

Fig. 28-33. (a) At 5 weeks after treatment of an intrabony defect with a non-resorbable barrier membrane, the covering tissue was largely dehiscent. After membrane removal, the flaps could not properly cover the newly formed tissue. (b) A free gingival graft has been harvested from the palate and saddle shaped to fit the interdental space. (c) The free gingival graft is placed to cover the newly regenerated tissue. (d) The graft is kept in position by interrupted and suspended sutures. (e) Healing after 1 week. (f) Appearance of the treated site after 1 year.

cal results in some studies were associated with high counts of bacteria and with the presence of *P. gingivalis* and *A. actinomycetemcomitans* (Machtei et al. 1994, Nowzari & Slots 1994, Nowzari et al. 1995).

Bacterial contamination of the membrane may occur during surgery, but also during the postoperative healing phase. After placement, bacteria from the oral cavity may colonize the coronal part of the membrane. Frequently, this results in recession of the gingival tissues, which allows colonization of the membrane material further apically. In addition, "pocket" formation may occur on the outer surface of the membrane due to apical migration of the epithelium on the inner surface of the covering gingival tissue. This may allow bacteria from the oral cavity to colonize the subgingival area. The significance of bacterial contamination was addressed in an investigation in monkeys (Sander & Karring 1995). The findings of this study showed that new attachment and bone formation occurred consistently when bacteria were prevented from invading the membrane and the wound during healing.

In order to prevent wound infection, some investigators have administered systemic antibiotics to patients before and during the first weeks after membrane application (Demolon et al. 1993, Nowzari & Slots 1994). However, despite the application of systemic antibiotics, occurrence of postoperative wound infection related to implanted barrier membranes was noticed. This indicates that either the drug administered is not directed against the microorganisms responsible for the wound infection, or that the drug does not reach the infected site at a concentration sufficiently high to inhibit the target microorganisms. An improved effect on periodontal healing after GTR in association with local application of metronidazol was reported by Sander et al. (1994). Twelve patients

with one pair of intrabony defects participated in the study. Metronidazol was placed in the defects and on the membrane prior to wound closure, while the controls were treated with a membrane alone. Six months following membrane removal the medium gain in probing attachment level, presented as a percentage of the initial defect depth, was 92% for test defects versus 50% for the control defects. Other clinical parameters, like plaque index, bleeding on probing, pocket depth reduction or recession of the gingival margin were similar in the test and control sites. Although the use of local or systemic antibiotics may reduce the bacterial load on exposed membranes, it seems ineffective in preventing the formation of a microbial biofilm (Frandsen et al. 1994, Nowzari et al. 1995). Apart from the erythema and swelling related to such infection of the wound, more severe postoperative complications such as suppuration, sloughing or perforation of the flap, membrane exfoliation, and post-operative pain have been reported (Murphy 1995a, b).

Another important issue associated with the clinical results is the coverage of the regenerated tissue after removal of a non-bioabsorbable membrane. Many authors have reported that the frequent occurrence of a gingival dehiscence over the membrane is likely to result in insufficient protection of the interproximal regenerated tissue (Becker et al. 1988, Selvig et al. 1992, Cortellini et al. 1993b, Tonetti et al. 1993a). Exposure of the regenerated tissue to the oral environment entails the risks of mechanical and infectious insults which in turn may prevent complete maturation of the regenerated tissue into a new connective tissue attachment. In fact, incomplete coverage of the regenerated tissue was associated with reduced attachment and bone gain at 1 year (Tonetti et al. 1993a).

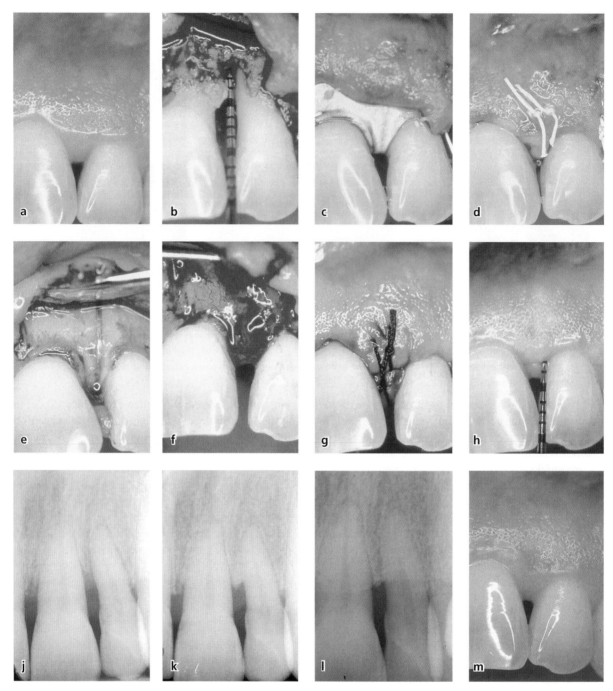

Fig. 28-34. (a,b) Left maxillary lateral incisor with a deep interproximal intrabony defect on the mesial surface. (c) Flaps are raised according to the modified papilla preservation technique, and a titanium reinforced barrier membrane is placed over the defect. (d) By coronal displacement of the flap and preservation of the interdental papilla, the membrane is completely covered. (e,f) After 6 weeks of uneventful postoperative healing the membrane was removed, (g) and the newly formed tissue was completely covered. (h) At 1 year, residual probing pocket depth was 2 mm and no buccal or interdental recession had occurred. (j) The baseline radiograph shows radiolucency approaching the apex of the tooth, but (k) after 1 year the intrabony defect is resolved and some supracrestal bone apposition seems to have occurred (k). The radiograph taken at 6 years confirms the supracrestal bone regeneration (l) and the clinical image shows the integrity of the interdental papilla with optimal preservation of the esthetic appearance (m).

Recently, the positioning of a saddle-shaped free gingival graft over the regenerated interproximal tissue (Fig. 28-33) was suggested (Cortellini et al. 1995a) to offer better coverage and protection than a dehiscent gingival flap. In this randomized controlled study, more gain of attachment was observed in the 14 sites where a free gingival graft was positioned after membrane removal (5.0 ± 2.1 mm), than in the 14 sites where a conventional protection of the regenerated tissue was accomplished (3.7 ± 2.1 mm).

In order to increase the space for regeneration, and in order to achieve and maintain primary closure of the flap in the interdental area, the modified papilla preservation technique (MPPT) was developed (Cortellini et al. 1995c,d). This approach combines special soft tissue management with use of a self-supporting titanium-reinforced membrane capable of maintaining a supra-alveolar space for regeneration. The MPPT allows primary closure of the interdental space, resulting in better protection of the membrane from the oral environment (Cortellini et al. 1995d). The technique involves the elevation of a full thickness palatal flap which includes the entire interdental papilla. The buccal flap is mobilized with vertical and periosteal incisions, coronally positioned to cover the membrane, and sutured to the palatal flap through a horizontal internal crossed mattress suture over the membrane. A second internal mattress suture warrants primary closure between the flap and the interdental papilla. A representative case is shown in Fig. 28-34. In a randomized controlled clinical study on 45 patients (Cortellini et al. 1995c), significantly greater amounts of attachment gain were obtained with the MPPT (5.3 ± 2.2 mm), in comparison with either conventional GTR (4.1 ± 1.9 mm) or flap surgery (2.5 ± 0.8 mm), demonstrating that a modified surgical approach can result in improved clinical outcomes.

In this study 100% of the sites were closed on top of a titanium-reinforced membrane and 73% remained closed for up to 6 weeks, when the barrier membrane was removed. The reported procedure can be successfully applied in sites where the interdental space width is at least 2 mm at the most coronal portion of the papilla. When interdental sites are narrower, the reported technique is difficult to apply. In order to overcome this problem, a different papilla preservation procedure (the simplified papilla preservation flap) has been proposed to apply in narrow interdental spaces (Cortellini et al. 1999). This approach includes an oblique incision across the defect-associated papilla, starting from the buccal angle of the defect associated tooth to reach the mid-interdental part of the papilla at the adjacent tooth under the contact point. In this way, the papilla is cut into two equal parts of which the buccal is elevated with the buccal flap and the lingual with the lingual flap. In the cited study, 100% of the narrow interdental papilla could be closed on top of bioresorbable barriers, and 67% maintained primary closure over time, resulting in 4.9 ± 1.8 mm of clinical attachment level gains. This approach has been successfully applied in different multicenter randomized clinical trials designed to test the generalizability of the added benefits of using barrier membranes on deep intrabony defects (Tonetti et al. 1998, Cortellini et al. 2001).

In the cited studies, GTR therapy of deep intrabony defects performed by different clinicians on various patient populations resulted in both greater amounts and improved predictability of CAL gains than access flap alone. The issue of soft tissue manipulation to obtain a stable protection of the regeneration site has been further explored, applying a microsurgical approach in the regenerative therapy of deep intrabony defects (Fig. 28-35). In a patient cohort study on 26 patients with 26 intrabony defects treated with papilla preservation techniques, primary closure on the barrier was obtained in 100% of the cases and maintained over time in 92.3% of the sites. Treatment resulted in large amounts of CAL gains (5.4 ± 1.2 mm) and minimal gingival recession (0.4 ± 0.7 mm). Thus, the improved vision and better soft tissue handling improved the predictability of periodontal regeneration.

Postoperative morbidity

To date, little consideration has been given to critical elements that could contribute to the patient's assessment of the cost-benefit ratio of GTR procedures. These include postoperative pain, discomfort, complications, and the perceived benefits from the treatment. A parallel group, randomized, multicenter and controlled clinical trial designed to test the efficacy of GTR and flap surgery alone assessed these patient issues (Cortellini et al. 2001). During the procedure, 30.4% of the test and 28.6% of the controls reported moderate pain and subjects estimated the hardship of the procedure as 24 ± 25 units on a visual analog scale (VAS in a scale from 0 to 100) in the test group and to 22 ± 23 VAS in the controls. Test surgery with membranes required longer chair time than flap surgery (on average 20 minutes longer). Among the postoperative complications, edema was most prevalent at week 1 and most frequently associated with the GTR treatment, while postoperative pain was reported by fewer than 50% of both test and control patients. Pain intensity was described as mild and lasted on average 14.1 ± 15.6 hours in the test patients and 24.7 ± 39.1 hours in the controls. Postoperative morbidity was limited to a minority of subjects: 35.7% of the test and 32.1% of the controls reported that the procedures interfered with daily activities for an average of 2.7 ± 2.3 days in the test group and 2.4 ± 1.3 days in the control group. These data indicate that GTR adds almost 30 minutes to a flap procedure and is followed by a greater prevalence of post surgical edema, while no difference could be observed between GTR and flap surgery alone in terms of postoperative pain, discomfort and interference with daily activities.

Furcation involvements

The invasion of the furcation area of multirooted teeth by periodontitis represents a serious complication in periodontal therapy. The furcation area is often inaccessible to adequate instrumentation, and frequently the roots present concavities and furrows which make proper cleaning of the area impossible (see Chapter 29). As long as the pathologic process is extending only a minor distance (< 5 mm; degree I and II involvements) into the furcation area, further progress of the disease can usually be prevented by scaling and root planing, provided a proper oral hygiene program is established after treatment. In more advanced cases (5-6 mm; degree II involvements), the initial cause-re-

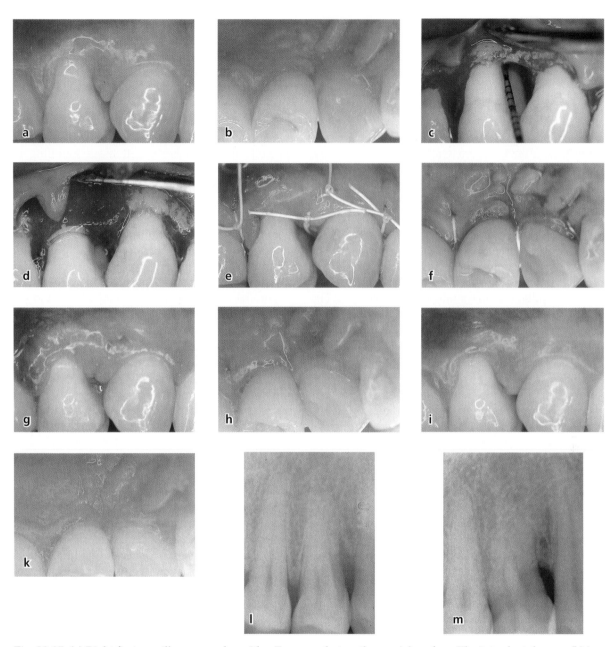

Fig. 28-35. (a) Right first maxillary premolar with a 7 mm pocket on the mesial surface. The interdental space (b) is very narrow (> 2 mm), and is accessed with a simplified papilla preservation flap. The 5 mm deep intrabony defect (c) is covered with a bioresorbable barrier membrane (d). Primary closure of the flap over the membrane (e,f) is maintained over time (g,h). After 1 year the interdental papilla is completely preserved and the residual pocket depth is 3 mm (j,k). The radiograph taken at baseline (l) compared with that taken 1 year after treatment (m) shows that the intrabony defect has healed completely.

lated treatment is frequently supplemented with surgery involving contouring of the interradicular bone (osteoplasty) or reduction of the tooth prominence at the furcation entrance by grinding (odontoplasty), in order to reduce the horizontal extension of the furcation involvement. In cases where the involvement is extending deeper into the furcation area (> 5 mm; degree II involvements), or a through and through defect (degree III involvements) has developed, tunnel preparation or root resection has been advocated as the choice of treatment. However, both of these latter treatments involve a risk of complications on a long-term basis. Following tunnel preparation, caries

frequently develops in the furcation area and root resected teeth often present complications of non-periodontal nature, although controversial reports exist regarding the long-term results of these treatment modalities (Hamp et al. 1975, Langer et al. 1981, Erpenstein 1983, Bühler 1988, Little et al. 1995).

Considering the complexity of current techniques for the treatment of furcation problems, and in view of the long-term results and complications reported following treatment of advanced furcation involvements by traditionally resective therapy, predictable regeneration of the periodontium at furcation-in-

Table 28-3. Clinical outcomes and weighted mean of GTR treatment of mandibular degree II furcations

Authors	Type of Study	Treatment	N	Defect Depth (mm)	H-CAL Gain (mm)	H-OPAL Gain (mm)	N of Furca closed
Pontoriero et al. 1988	Controlled clinical trial	e-PTFE	21	4.4 ± 1.2	3.8 ± 1.2	NA	14 (67%)
Becker et al. 1988	Case cohort	e-PTFE	6	8.3 ± 2.3	NA	1.8 ± 1.5	0
Schallhorn & McClain 1988	Case cohort	e-PTFE	16	NA	NA	3.1 ± 1.7	5 (31%)
Lekovic et al. 1989	Controlled clinical trial	e-PTFE	6	NA	NA	0.2 ± 0.5	NA
Lekovic et al. 1990	Controlled clinical trial	e-PTFE	15	4.2 ± 0.2	NA	0.1 ± 0.1	NA
Caffesse et al. 1990	Controlled clinical trial	e-PTFE	9	4.8 ± ?	0.8 ± ?	NA	NA
Anderegg et al. 1991	Controlled clinical trial	e-PTFE	15	4.2 ± 2.2	NA	1.0 ± 0.8	NA
Yukna 1992	Controlled clinical trial	e-PTFE	11	3.0 ± ?	NA	1.0 ± ?	0
		FDDMA	11	4.0 ± ?	NA	2.0 ± ?	0
Blumenthal 1993	Controlled clinical trial	e-PTFE	12	4.4 ± 0.9	1.8 ± 1	1.7 ± 0.5	4 (33%)
		Collagen	12	4.5 ± 0.9	2.5 ± 0.8	2.5 ± 0.7	1 (8%)
Bouchard et al. 1993	Controlled clinical trial	e-PTFE	12	NA	2.8 ± 1.3	2.2 ± 1.4	4 (33%)
		Conn. Graft	12	NA	1.5 ± 1.5	1.5 ± 1.1	2 (17%)
Machtei et al. 1993	Controlled clinical trial	e-PTFE	18	NA	2.3 ± 1.7	NA	NA
Parashis & Mitsis 1993	Controlled clinical trial	e-PTFE	9	5.7 ± 0.7	4.7 ± 1.5	NA	4 (44%)
Van Swol et al. 1993	Controlled clinical trial	Collagen	28	5.1 ± 1.4	2.3 ± 1	1.7 ± ?	NA
Wallace et al. 1994	Controlled clinical trial	e-PTFE	7	NA	NA	2.3 ± ?	NA
Black et al. 1994	Controlled clinical trial	e-PTFE	13	4.3 ± 2	0.8 ± 2.2	NA	NA
		Collagen	13	4.4 ± 1.5	1.5 ± 2	NA	NA
Laurell et al. 1994	Case cohort	Polylactic Acid	19	NA	3.3 ± 1.4	NA	9 (47%)
Machtei et al. 1994	Controlled clinical trial	e-PTFE	30	7.7 ± 1.8	2.6 ± 1.7	NA	NA
Mellonig et al. 1994	Controlled clinical trial	e-PTFE	11	8.4 ± 1.2	NA	4.5 ± 1.6	1 (9%)
Wang et al. 1994	Controlled clinical trial	Collagen	12	6.0 ± 2.7	2.0 ± 0.4	2.5 ± ?	NA
Hugoson et al. 1995	Controlled clinical trial	e-PTFE	38	5.9 ± 1.3	1.4 ± 2.2	NA	4 (11%)
		Polylactic Acid	38	5.6 ± 1.4	2.2 ± 2	NA	13 (34%)
Polson et al. 1995	Case cohort*	Polylactic Acid	29	5.4 ± 0.2	2.5 ± 0.1	NA	0
Weighted Mean			**423**	**5.4 ± 1.3 ‡**	**2.3 ± 1.4$**	**1.9 ± 1 ^**	

H-CAL = Horizontal Clinical Attachment. H-OPAL = Horizontal Open Probing Attachment. NA = data not available. e-PTFE = expanded Polytetrafluoroethylene. FDDMA = Freeze Dried Dura Mater Allograft. Conn. Graft = Connective Tissue Graft. ‡ N = Mean (340) ± S.D. (302); $ N = Mean (325) ± S.D. (316); ^N = Mean (186) ± S.D. (177). * Mandibular and maxillary molars.

volved sites would represent a considerable progress in periodontics.

Mandibular degree II furcations
Pontoriero et al. (1988) reported a controlled randomized clinical trial in which significantly greater amounts of horizontal clinical attachment (H-CAL) gain (3.8 ± 1.2 mm) were obtained in 21 mandibular degree II furcations treated with e-PTFE membranes as compared to that in a control group treated with open flap debridement alone (H-CAL gains of 2.0 ± 1.2 mm). Complete closure of the furcation was observed in 67% of the test sites and in only 10% of the control sites. Other studies, however, have failed to confirm these promising results to the same extent (Becker et al. 1988, Lekovic et al. 1989, Caffesse et al. 1990). Analysis of a series of studies published between 1988 and 1996 demonstrates a great variability in the clinical outcomes (Figs. 28-36 and 28-37). Table 28-3 summarizes the outcomes of 21 clinical trials in which a total of 423 mandibular degree II furcations were treated with different types of non-bioabsorbable and bioabsorbable barrier membranes. The weighted mean of the reported results shows a H-CAL gain of 2.3 ± 1.4 mm with a 95% confidence interval ranging from 2.0 to 2.5 mm in defects with a baseline horizontal probing depth of 5.4 ± 1.3 mm. The reported number of complete furcation closures after GTR range from 0 to 67%. In three studies none of the treated furcations were closed (Becker et al. 1988, Yukna 1992,

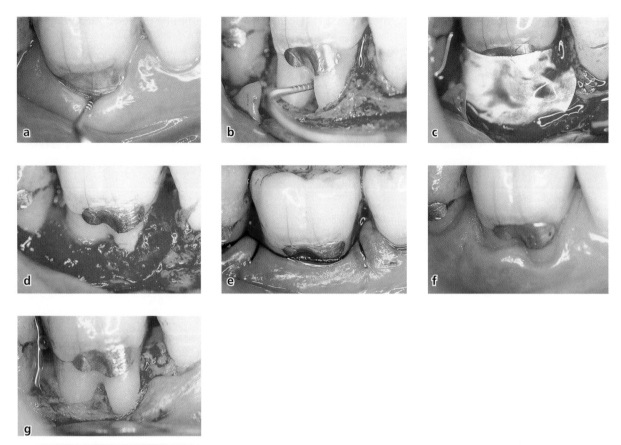

Fig. 28-36. (a) Right mandibular first molar presenting with a degree II furcation involvement. (b) Full thickness buccal flaps have been raised, the defect debrided and the root carefully planed. (c) A non-bioabsorbable barrier membrane has been placed to cover the defect. (d) After membrane removal, newly formed tissue appears to fill the furcation completely. (e) The regenerated tissue is covered with the flap. (f) Clinical appearance and surgery entry (g) after 1 year shows that the degree II furcation is almost completely resolved.

Polson et al. 1995b), in seven studies fewer than 50% were closed (Schallhorn & McClain 1988, Blumenthal 1993, Bouchard et al. 1993, Parashis & Mitsis 1993, Laurell et al. 1994, Mellonig et al. 1994, Hugoson et al. 1995), and in only one study were more than 50% of the treated furcations completely resolved (Pontoriero et al. 1988).

A subset analysis of the studies reported in Table 28-3 indicated that furcations treated with non-bioabsorbable barrier membranes (287) showed a gain in horizontal clinical attachment of 1.8 ± 1.4 mm (95% CI 1.5-2.1 mm) as compared with 2.3 ± 1.2 mm H-CAL gain (95% CI 2-2.6 mm) in 174 defects treated with bioabsorbable barrier membranes. Five controlled clinical trials compared treatment with non-resorbable e-PTFE membranes and treatment with different types of bioabsorbable membranes (Table 28-4). In particular, one investigation reported significantly greater H-CAL gain in the non-bioabsorbable group (Bouchard et al. 1993), while another one (Hugoson et al. 1995) showed a significantly greater H-CAL gain in the bioabsorbable group. The remaining three investigations failed to detect any significant differences between the outcomes of treatment with bioabsorbable or non-bioabsorbable membranes. Generally the results indicate that the predictability of GTR in

the treatment of mandibular degree II furcations is questionable, if the treatment objective is the complete resolution of the furcation involvement.

Significant gain in vertical attachment level (V-CAL) and reduction in pocket depth (PPD) was also reported by several investigators following treatment of mandibular degree II furcation defects (Pontoriero et al. 1988, Lekovic et al. 1989, 1990, Blumenthal 1993, Machtei et al. 1993, 1994, Black et al. 1994, Laurell et al. 1994, Mellonig et al. 1994, Wang et al. 1994, Hugoson et al. 1995, Polson et al. 1995b). The reported mean values ranged from 0.1 mm to 3.5 mm for V-CAL gain and from 1 mm to 4 mm for PPD reduction.

The effect of using barrier membranes for the treatment of mandibular degree II furcations was investigated in six controlled randomized clinical trials in which GTR procedures were directly compared to flap surgery (Table 28-5). Sixty-six furcations treated with flap surgery and 87 treated with GTR were included. Three of the four studies reporting H-CAL gains concluded that GTR resulted in statistically significantly greater horizontal attachment level gains than flap surgery (Pontoriero et al. 1988, Van Swol et al. 1993, Wang et al. 1994). The weighted mean of the results reported in Table 28-5 indicated that the H-CAL in furcations treated with GTR was 2.5 ± 1 mm (95% CI

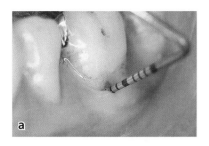
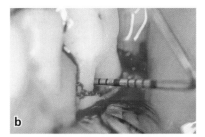
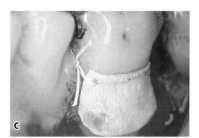
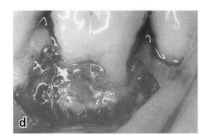
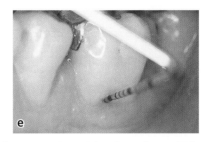

Fig. 28-37. (a) Left mandibular first molar presenting with a deep degree II furcation involvement. (b) Horizontal loss of tooth support of 7 mm was probed. (c) An e-PTFE barrier membrane has been trimmed and sutured to cover the furcation. (d) At membrane removal after 5 weeks, newly formed tissue fills the furcation completely. (e) At 1 year, a 3 mm gain of tooth support was measured, but a residual 4 mm degree II furcation involvement was still present.

Table 28-4. Controlled clinical trials comparing clinical outcomes of GTR procedures with e-PTFE non- bioabsorbable barrier membranes with different types of bioabsorbable barrier membranes in mandibular degree II furcations

Authors	Design & Treatment (GTR C/GTR T)	N C/T	Defect Depth (mm)		H-CAL Gain (mm)		H-OPAL Gain (mm)	
			GTR C	GTR T	GTR C	GTR T	GTR C	GTR T
Yukna 1992	Intraindividual (e-PTFE/FDDMA)	11/11	3.0 ± ?	4.0 ± ?	NA	NA	1.0 ± ?	2.0 ± ?
Blumenthal 1993	Intraindividual (e-PTFE/Collagen)	12/12	4.4 ± 0.9	4.5 ± 0.9	1.8 ± 1	2.5 ± 0.8	1.7 ± 0.5	2.5 ± 0.7
Bouchard et al. 1993	Intraindividual (e-PTFE/Conn. Graft)	12/12	NA	NA	2.8 ± 1.3*	1.5 ± 2	2.2 ± 1.4	1.5 ± 1.1
Black et al. 1994	Intraindividual (e-PTFE/Collagen)	13/13	4.3 ± 2	4.4 ± 1.5	0.8 ± 2.2	1.5 ± 2	NA	NA
Hugoson et al. 1995	Intraindividual (e-PTFE/Polytetra-fluoroethylene)	38/38	5.9 ± 1.3	5.6 ± 1.4	1.4 ± 2.2*	2.2 ± 2.0*	NA	NA
Weighted Mean		86/86	4.9 ± 1.4 §	5 ± 1.3 §	1.6 ± 1.9 ‡	2 ± 1.7 ‡	1.3 ± 1 #	1.4 ± 0.9 #

GTR C = Guided Tissue Regeneration Control Treatment. GTR T = Guided Tissue Regeneration Test Treatment.
N C/T = Number of defects in the Control (C) and in the Test (T) treatment arm.
H-CAL = Horizontal Clinical Attachment. H-OPAL = Horizontal Open Probing Attachment. NA = data not available.
e-PTFE = expanded Polytetrafluoroethylene. FDDMA = Freeze Dried Dura Mater Allograft. Conn. Graft = Connective Tissue Graft.
* = Difference between treatments statistically significant.   § N = Mean (74) ± S.D. (63); ‡ N = Mean (75) ± S.D. (75); # N = Mean (35) ± S.D. (24).

2.1-2.9 mm) while the flap surgery resulted in a mean H-CAL gain of 1.3 ± 1 mm (95% CI.0.8-1.8 mm). These results indicate an added benefit from GTR in the treatment of mandibular degree II furcations.

Maxillary degree II furcations
Results reported in three controlled studies (Metzeler et al. 1991, Mellonig et al. 1994, Pontoriero & Lindhe 1995a) comparing GTR treatment of maxillary degree II furcations with non-bioabsorbable e-PTFE membranes and with open flap debridement, indicate that GTR treatment of such defects is generally unpredictable. Metzeler et al. (1991) in a study including 17 pairs of degree II furcations measured CAL gains of

Table 28-5. Controlled clinical trials comparing clinical outcomes of GTR procedures with access flap procedures in mandibular degree II furcations

Authors	Design (GTR Treatment)	N C/T	Defect Depth (mm)		H-CAL Gain (mm)		H-OPAL Gain (mm)	
			Access Flap	GTR	Access Flap	GTR	Access Flap	GTR
Pontoriero et al. 1988	Intraindividual (e-PTFE)	21/21	4.0 ± 0.8	4.4 ± 1.2	2.0 ± 1.2*	3.8 ± 1.2*	NA	NA
Lekovic et al. 1989	Intraindividual (e-PTFE)	6/6	NA	NA	NA	NA	-0.1 ± 0.3	0.2 ± 0.5
Caffesse et al. 1990	Parallel (e-PTFE)	6/9	5.3 ± ?	4.8 ± ?	0.3 ± ?	0.8 ± ?	NA	NA
Van Swol et al. 1993	Parallel (Collagen)	10/28	5.7 ± 2.5	5.1 ± 1.4	0.7 ± 1.2*	2.3 ± 1*	0.8 ± ?	1.7 ± ?
Mellonig et al. 1994	Intraindividual (e-PTFE)	6/6	7.5 ± 2.3	8.4 ± 1.2	NA	NA	1.1 ± 1.3*	4.5 ± 1.6*
Wang et al. 1994	Intraindividual (Collagen)	12/12	5.6 ± 2.7	6.0 ± 2.7	1.1 ± 0.6*	2.0 ± 0.4*	1.5 ± ?	2.5 ± ?
Weighted Mean		66/87	**5.4 ± 1.8 §**	**5.5 ± 1.5 $**	**1.3 ± 1^**	**2.5 ± 1 #**	**1 ± 1 °**	**2.3 ± 1.2 ‡**

N C/T = Number of defects in the Control (C) and in the Test (T) treatment arm.
H-CAL = Horizontal Clinical Attachment. H-OPAL = Horizontal Open Probing Attachment. NA = data not available.
e-PTFE = expanded Polytetrafluorethylene. * = Difference between treatments statistically significant.
§ N = Mean (60) ± S.D. (54); $ N = Mean (81) ± S.D. (72); ^N = Mean (49) ± S.D. (43); # N = Mean (70) ± S.D. (61); °N = Mean (39) ± S.D. (17);
‡ N = Mean (57) ± S.D. (17).

1.0 ± 0.9 mm in the GTR treated sites versus 0.2 ± 0.6 mm in the control sites. Following re-entry, horizontal probing attachment gains (H-OPAL) of 0.9 ± 0.4 mm and 0.3 ± 0.6 mm were detected in the GTR and flap treated furcations, respectively. No differences were found and none of the furcations of the two groups were completely resolved. Similarly, Mellonig et al. (1994) treated eight pairs of maxillary degree II furcations which resulted in H-OPAL gains of 1.0 mm (GTR sites) and 0.3 mm (flap treated sites). No differences were found and none of the treated furcations were completely closed. Pontoriero & Lindhe (1995a), on the other hand, in a study on 28 maxillary degree II furcations found a significant gain in CAL (1.5 mm) and horizontal bone (1.1 mm) in buccal degree II furcations.

Although these three investigations show a slight clinical improvement following treatment of degree II maxillary furcations with GTR, the results are generally inconsistent.

Degree III furcations

Four investigations on the treatment of mandibular degree III furcations (Becker et al. 1988, Pontoriero et al. 1989, Cortellini et al. 1990, Pontoriero & Lindhe 1995b) indicate that the treatment of such defects with GTR is unpredictable. A controlled study of Pontoriero et al. (1989) showed that only 8 out of 21 "through and through" mandibular furcations treated with non-bioabsorbable barrier membranes healed with complete closure of the defect. Another ten defects were partially filled, and three remained open. In the control group, treated with open flap debridement, 10 were partially filled and 11 remained open. Similar results were reported by Cortellini et al. (1990) who, in a case cohort of 15 degree III mandibular furcations, found that 33% of the defects had healed completely,

33% were partially closed, and 33% were still through and through following treatment. Becker et al (1988) did not observe complete closure of any of 11 treated degree III mandibular furcations. Similarly, in a controlled clinical trial of Pontoriero & Lindhe (1995b) on 11 pairs of maxillary degree III furcations randomly assigned to GTR or flap surgery, none of the furcation defects were closed.

Factors affecting the clinical outcomes of GTR in furcations

The studies considered above have demonstrated that treatment of maxillary degree II furcations and maxillary and mandibular degree III furcation involvements with GTR is unpredictable, while clinical improvements can be expected treating mandibular degree II furcations. The great variability in clinical outcomes, following treatment of mandibular degree II furcations with GTR, is probably related to the factors discussed relative to intrabony defects.

Regarding defect factors, it was shown that first and second mandibular molars and buccal and lingual furcations respond equally well to GTR treatment (Pontoriero et al. 1988, Machtei et al. 1994). It was also demonstrated that the preoperative horizontal pocket depth is directly correlated with the magnitude of attachment gain and bone formation in the furcation area (Machtei et al. 1993, 1994). The deeper the baseline horizontal pocket, the greater was the H-CAL and bone gain. The anatomy of the furcations in terms of height, width, depth and volume, however, did not correlate with the clinical outcome (Machtei et al. 1994). Anderegg et al. (1995) demonstrated that sites with a gingival thickness of > 1 mm exhibited less gingival recession post surgery than sites with a gingival thickness of < 1 mm. The authors concluded that the thickness of the gingival tissue covering a barrier

Table 28-6. Summary of controlled clinical trials evaluating the combined effects of decalcified freeze-dried bone allografts (DFDBA) and barrier membranes in deep intrabony defects

Authors	Design (GTR Treatment)	N*	Gains in CAL (mm)		Significance	Residual PD (mm)		Significance
			GTR	GTR + DFDBA		GTR	GTR + DFDBA	
Chen et al. 1995	Intraindividual (Collagen)	8	2.0 ± 0.4	2.3 ± 0.5	P > 0.05,NS	4.2 ± 0.4	4.2 ± 0.5	P > 0.05,NS
Mellado et al. 1995	Intraindividual (e-PTFE)	11	2.0 ± 0.9	2.0 ± 1.4	P = 0.86,NS	NA	NA	NA
Gouldin et al. 1996	Intraindividual (e-PTFE)	26	2.2 ± 1.4	2.4 ± 1.6	NS	3.7 ± 1.6	3.7 ± 1.8	NS
Weighted Mean		**45**	**2.1 ± 1.1**	**2.3 ± 1.4**		**3.8 ± 1.3 §**	**3.8 ± 1.5 §**	

* = Defects per treatment arm. CAL = Clinical Attachment Level. PD = Pocket Depth. e-PTFE = expanded Polytetrafluoroethylene. DFDBA = Decalcified Freeze Dried Bone Allograft.
NS = not significant. NA = Data not available. § N = Mean (34) ± S.D. (34).

material must be considered if post-treatment recession is to be minimized or avoided.

Based on present evidence, it seems that mandibular degree II furcations in the first or second molars, either buccal or lingual, with deep pockets at baseline and a gingival thickness of > 1 mm, may benefit from GTR treatment.

GTR combined with other regenerative procedures
Compromised results after GTR may be obtained in cases where the membrane collapses/falls (partially or totally) into the defect and/or towards the root surface, thereby reducing the space available for invasion of new tissue capable of forming periodontal ligament and bone in particular. Reduced amounts of regenerated bone due to membrane collapse were noticed in early studies of GTR. In the study of Gottlow et al. (1984), it was observed that collapse of the membrane towards the root surface resulted in new cementum formation on the entire exposed root surfaces, whereas bone regeneration was minimal. Although the authors reported that the degree of coronal regrowth of bone was unrelated to the amount of new cementum formation, they did not comment on what effect membrane collapse might have had. Recent experimental studies, however, recognized the negative effect of membrane collapse on periodontal regeneration generally and on bone formation in particular (Caton et al. 1992, Haney et al. 1993, Sigurdsson et al. 1994, Sallum et al. 1998). Haney et al. (1993) observed a highly significant correlation between the space provided by the membrane and the amount of regenerated alveolar bone using a supra-alveolar defect model in dogs. This finding corroborates that of Cortellini et al. (1995c) who reported that clinical application of self-supporting (reinforced with titanium) e-PTFE membranes, which could be positioned more coronally than ordinary e-PTFE membranes, yielded statistically significantly more PAL-gain in intrabony defects. A particular risk for membrane collapse exists

in cases where the configuration of the defect is incapable of supporting/preserving the membrane at the position where it was originally placed.

As already discussed, membrane materials must possess certain characteristics in order to be efficient. Among those it is important that the membrane is capable of keeping its shape and integral features, thereby maintaining the space created adjacent to the root surface. The e-PTFE membranes reinforced with titanium are the closest in meeting these requirements but they have the disadvantage that they are non-resorbable. At present there are no resorbable membranes available that fulfill this requirement sufficiently, which means that the placement of a resorbable membrane on, for instance, a wide one-wall defect involves the risk of membrane collapse. The collapse may be prevented by means of implantation of a biomaterial into the defect to support the membrane so that it preserves its original position. However, the biomaterial to be used for this purpose must not interfere with the process of periodontal regeneration and ideally it may also promote bone regeneration.

As previously described, periodontal regeneration has been attempted with a variety of grafting materials, among which demineralized freeze-dried bone allografts (DFDBA) apparently facilitated regeneration in humans (Ouhayoun 1996). Schallhorn and McClain (1988) reported on improved clinical results in intrabony defects and degree II furcations, following a combination therapy including barrier membranes plus DFDBA and citric acid root conditioning.

In three controlled clinical trials, the treatment of a total of 45 pairs of intrabony defects with DFDBA grafting and GTR were compared to GTR alone (Table 28-6). The weighted mean of the results of the reported investigations showed similar gain in CAL in the GTR group (2.1 ± 1.1 mm, 95% CI 1.6-2.6 mm) and in the GTR plus DFDBA group (2.3 ± 1.4 mm, 95% CI 1.7-2.9 mm). The differences between the two treatments did

Table 28-7. Controlled clinical trials comparing clinical outcomes of GTR procedures with e-PTFE non- bioabsorbable barrier membranes with or without the adjunctive use of grafts in mandibular degree II furcations

Authors	Design & Treatment (GTR C/GTR T)	N C/T	Defect Depth (mm)		H-OPAL Gain (mm)	
			GTR C	GTR T	GTR C	GTR T
Lekovic et al. 1990	Intraindividual (e-PTFE/e-PTFE + HA)	15/15	4.2 ± 0.2	4.3 ± 0.2	0.1 ± 0.1	1.6 ± 0.2
Anderegg et al. 1991	Intraindividual (e-PTFE/e-PTFE + DFDBA)	15/15	4.2 ± 2.2	5.3 ± 2.6	1.0 ± 0.8*	2.4 ± 1.5*
Wallace et al. 1994	Parallel (e-PTFE/e-PTFE + DFDBA)	7/10	6.0 ± ?	6.5 ± ?	2.3 ± ?	2.4 ± ?
Weighted Mean		**37/40**	**4.5 ± 1.2 §**	**5.2 ± 1.4 ‡**	**0.9 ± 0.5 §**	**2.1 ± 0.9 #**

GTR C = Guided Tissue Regeneration Control Treatment. GTR T = Guided Tissue Regeneration Test Treatment. N C/T = Number of defects in the Control (C) and in the Test (T) treatment arm. H-OPAL = Horizontal Open Probing Attachment.
e-PTFE = expanded Polytetrafluoroethylene. HA = Hydroxylapatite. DFDBA = Decalcified Freeze Dried Bone Allograft.
* = Difference between treatments statistically significant. § N = Mean (37) ± S.D. (30); ‡ N = Mean (40) ± S.D. (30)
# N = Mean (35) ± S.D. (24).

not reach statistical significance, thus indicating no added effect of combining DFDBA with barrier materials in the treatment of intrabony defects. Guillemin et al. (1993), on the other hand, compared the effect of DFDBA alone with a combination of barrier materials and DFDBA in 15 pairs of intrabony defects. Both treatments resulted in significant amounts of CAL gains and bone fill at 6 months, but no difference was found between the treatments.

In three studies on mandibular degree II furcations, GTR treatment alone was compared with GTR treatment combined with hydroxylapatite or DFDBA (Table 28-7). In one of these investigations, a statistically significant improvement was found in terms of horizontal open probing attachment levels (H-OPAL) in the group of furcations treated with the combination therapy (Anderegg et al. 1991). In another of these three studies the difference between the two treatments was not statistically significant, but the combination therapy resulted in a greater extent of furcation fill (Lekovic et al. 1990). In the third investigation (Wallace et al. 1994), the two treatments were equivalent in terms of H-OPAL gains. The weighted mean of the cited studies showed greater H-OPAL gains in the cases treated with the combination therapy (2.1 ± 0.9 mm, 95% CI 1.6-2.6 mm) when compared to GTR treatment alone (0.9 ± 0.5 mm, 95% CI 0.6-1.1 mm), indicating a possible added benefit from the use of grafting materials in combination with non-bioabsorbable barrier membranes for the treatment of mandibular degree II furcations.

Promising clinical results with a PAL-gain of 1.0-5.5 mm were obtained in human case reports, in which the GTR technique was combined with grafting of Bio-Oss® for the treatment of intrabony periodontal defects (Lundgren & Slotte 1999, Mellonig 2000, Paolantonio et al. 2001). The combined Bio-Oss® and GTR treatment resulted in greater PPD reduction, PAL gain and defect fill than the mere implantation of Bio-Oss® in case series (Camelo et al. 1998, Hutchens 1999) and

than flap surgery alone in a split-mouth study (Camargo et al. 2000).

In a recent randomized controlled clinical study including 60 patients (Stavropoulos et al. 2002), Bio-Oss® alone or impregnated with gentamicin was used as an adjunct to GTR in the treatment of one-wall or two-wall intrabony defects, and the outcomes were compared to those obtained following GTR alone or flap surgery. Treatment with a membrane alone (Fig. 28-38) resulted in a mean PAL gain of 2.9 mm, while it was 3.8 and 2.5 mm, respectively, when Bio-Oss® grafts with or without gentamicin were placed in the defects prior to membrane coverage (Fig. 28-39). The control defects treated with flap surgery demonstrated a gain of PAL of only 1.5 mm. The clinical improvements in defects treated with GTR alone or in combination with Bio-Oss® grafting were significantly better than those obtained with flap surgery, whereas the differences between the groups treated with membranes were not statistically significant.

In a controlled study (Pietruska 2001), similar clinical improvements were obtained when Bio-Oss® combined with GTR was compared with biomodification of the root surface with enamel matrix protein (Emdogain®).

Camelo et al. (1998) and Mellonig (2000) presented histologic data indicating that the use of Bio-Oss® under a membrane may result in partial regeneration of the periodontal apparatus, but in all the cases, most of the defect was still occupied by deproteinized bone particles. Bone was not observed near the root, and the connective tissue fibers of the "new" periodontal ligament were mostly oriented parallel to the root surface. These results corroborate findings reported by Paolantonio et al. (2001), who observed only limited bone formation in the vicinity of the pre-existing bone in a biopsy, taken from a site treated 8 months earlier with Bio-Oss® and a collagen membrane. Most of the space in the defect was occupied by Bio-Oss® particles embedded in connective tissue. However, in a case report,

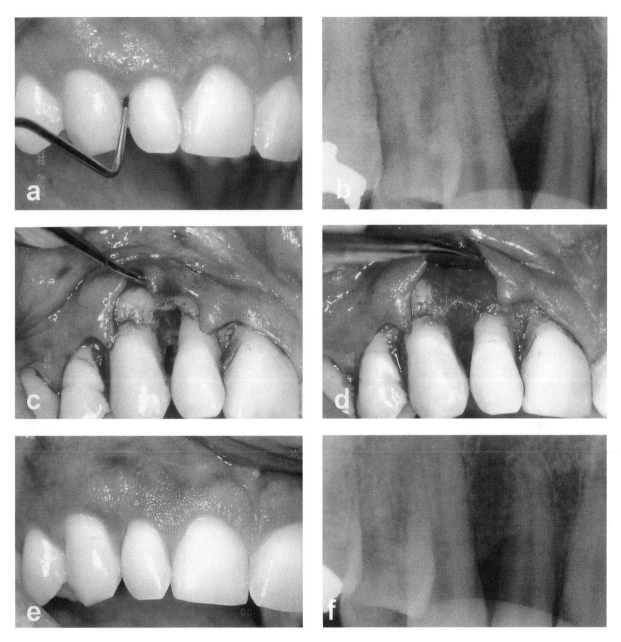

Fig. 28-38. Right lateral maxillary incisor with an 8 mm deep pocket associated with an intrabony defect on the distal aspect (a), as seen on the radiograph (b). Full thickness buccal and palatal flaps have been raised and the defect has been debrided (c). A bioabsorbable membrane has been adopted over the defect (d). The level of the interdental gingiva is maintained after 1 year (e) and the intrabony defect (f) is resolved.

where intrabony defects were treated with Bio-Oss® combined with intraoral autogenous bone and GTR, new attachment formation had occurred consistently, but a major portion of the regenerated osseous tissue consisted of deproteinized bone particles (Camelo et al. 2001). The effect of combining citric acid root biomodification with GTR treatment was evaluated in two randomized controlled clinical trials in intrabony defects. The first investigation (Handelsman et al. 1991) demonstrated significant amounts of CAL gains in both the test (e-PTFE membranes and citric acid; CAL gain 3.5 ± 1.6 mm) and control sites (e-PTFE membranes alone; CAL gain 4.0 ± 1.4 mm). Less favorable results following these two treatment modalities were reported by Kersten et al. (1992) who found CAL gains of 1.0 ± 1.1 mm in the test group, and CAL gains of 0.7 ± 1.5 mm in the control group. Both studies, however, failed to demonstrate any added effect of the use of citric acid in combination with non-bioabsorbable barrier membranes.

Root surface biomodification with tetracycline alone and in combination with GTR was evaluated in two controlled studies on degree II furcations (Machtei et al. 1993, Parashis & Mitsis 1993). Both investigations failed to show significant differences between sites treated with non-bioabsorbable barrier membranes alone or in combination with tetracycline root surface biomodification. Similarly, the use of other surface active chemicals like EDTA also failed to

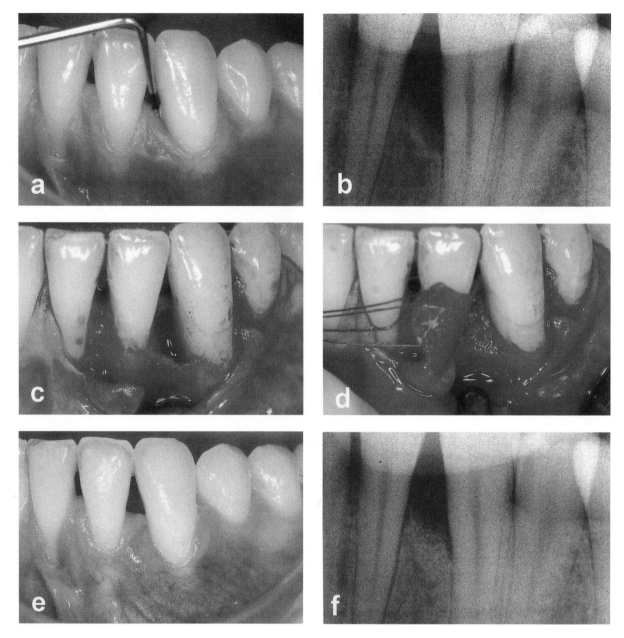

Fig. 28-39. Left mandibular canine with an 8 mm deep pocket (a) associated with an intrabony defect on its mesial aspect (b). The defect is debrided after flap elevation (c) and Bio-Oss® particles are placed in the defect (d) prior to placement of a bioabsorbable membrane. After 1 year (e) no gingival recession has occurred and the intrabony defect is almost resolved (f).

provide a significant added effect to GTR treatment in humans (Lindhe & Cortellini 1996).

Evaluation of GTR

Several reports, case series and controlled clinical trials have demonstrated successful results following GTR treatment of a variety of periodontal defects (for review see Cortellini & Tonetti 2000a, Sanz & Giovannoli 2000, Trombelli 1999). These results have been confirmed in animal experiments involving GTR treatment of intrabony defects (Caffesse et al. 1988, Caton et al. 1992), furcation defects (Niedermann et al. 1989, Caffesse et al. 1990, Araújo et al. 1996) and recession defects (Gottlow et al. 1990, Cortellini et al. 1991). The effect of placing non-bioabsorbable or

bioabsorbable membranes on degree II and III furcation defects as compared to that in control defects treated without membranes was evaluated in dogs (Claffey et al. 1989, Caffesse et al. 1990, Pontoriero et al. 1992, Lindhe et al. 1995). In both degree II and III furcation defects, GTR treatment resulted in significantly more gain of connective tissue attachment and regrowth of alveolar bone than control therapy.

In the studies of Pontoriero et al. (1992) and Lindhe et al. (1995), complete closure of through and through furcation defects with the formation of a periodontal ligament and regrowth of the alveolar bone was achieved (Fig. 28-40). It was suggested that the size of the furcation defects as well as the shape of the surrounding alveolar bone were determining for the out-

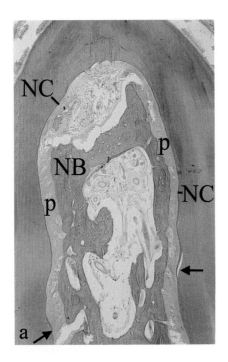
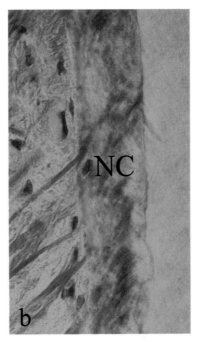

Fig. 28-40. (a) Photomicrograph of a degree III furcation in a dog 5 months after GTR treatment in combination with coronally displaced flaps. The defect has become filled with new bone (NB), and a periodontal ligament (p) and new cementum (NC) can be seen along the entire surface of the furcation defect. The arrows indicate the apical level of the original defect. (b) A high magnification of the cementum formed on the root surface in a healed bifurcation defect. Note the cellular nature of the new cementum (NC).

come of GTR treatment. The treatment failures were consistently associated with recession of the covering tissue flaps, which resulted in exposure of the furcation defect. Provided this was prevented, even comparatively large furcation defects were successfully regenerated by GTR therapy. The results also demonstrated that bioabsorbable membranes provided a barrier which was equally as effective as that of non-bioabsorbable Teflon membranes.

Histologic evidence in humans that regeneration of the attachment apparatus on previously periodontitis affected roots can be attained by means of the GTR technique was provided in several reports (Nyman et al. 1982, Gottlow et al. 1986, Becker et al. 1987, Stahl et al. 1990a, Stahl & Froum 1991b, Cortellini et al. 1993a, Parodi et al. 1997, Vincenzi et al. 1998, Sculean et al. 1999a). New cementum, periodontal ligament and variable amounts of new bone formation were observed in these studies, also above notches placed in the root surface at the apical extent of calculus. Thus, the GTR technique is fulfilling the criteria set by the American Academy of Periodontology at the World Workshop in Periodontics in 1996, and is also based on a biologic concept that, according to the current knowledge about periodontal wound healing, can explain why this method leads to periodontal regeneration.

Long-term evaluation

A pertinent question with respect to regenerative treatment is whether the achieved attachment gain can be maintained over an extended period of time. In a study in monkeys (Kostopoulos & Karring 1994), periodontal breakdown was produced by the placement and retention of orthodontic elastics on experimental teeth until 50% bone loss was recorded. The experimental teeth were endodontically treated and subjected to a flap operation and all granulation tissue

was removed. The crowns of the teeth were resected at the level of the cemento-enamel junction and a barrier membrane was placed to cover the roots before they were submerged. Following 4 weeks of healing, the membranes were removed. At the same time the contralateral teeth which served as controls were endodontically treated and subjected to a sham operation during which the crowns were resected at the level of the cemento-enamel junction. Artificial composite crowns were then placed on both the experimental and the control roots. The sites were allowed to heal for 3 months during which period careful plaque control was performed. At the end of this period cotton-floss ligatures were placed on both experimental and control teeth to induce periodontal tissue breakdown. After another 6 months, the animals were sacrificed. With respect to attachment level, bone level, pocket depth and gingival recession, similar results were recorded in histologic specimens of experimental (Fig. 28-41) and control (Fig. 28-42) teeth. This indicates that the new connective tissue attachment formed with GTR is not more susceptible to periodontitis than the naturally existing periodontium.

In a long-term follow-up study, Gottlow et al. (1992) assessed the stability of new attachment gained through GTR procedures. Eighty sites in 39 patients, which 6 months after surgery exhibited a gain of clinical attachment of ≥ 2 mm (2-7 mm), were monitored during additional periods of 1 to 5 years. Of the 80 sites, 65 were monitored for 2 years, 40 for 3 years, 17 for 4 years and 9 sites for 5 years. The results of this study and those of other trials indicate that attachment gain obtained following GTR treatment can be maintained on a long-term basis (Becker & Becker 1993, McClain & Schallhorn 1993).

An investigation on intrabony defects demonstrated that the stability of sites treated with GTR was

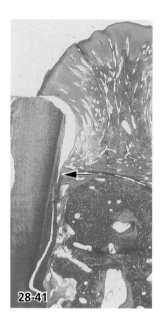
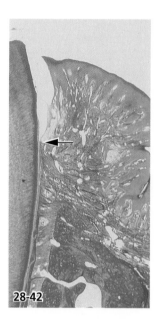

Fig. 28-41. Microphotograph of test specimen with a reformed connective tissue attachment. After 6 months of ligature induced periodontitis, loss of attachment has occurred from the coronal cut root surface to the level indicated by the arrow.

Fig. 28-42. Microphotograph of control specimen with a naturally existing periodontium. After 6 months of ligature induced periodontitis, loss of attachment has occurred from the coronal cut tooth surface to the level indicated by the arrow.

dependent on participation of the patients into a recall program, and on the absence of bacterial plaque, bleeding on probing and re-infection of the treated sites with periodontal pathogens (Cortellini et al. 1994). In addition, the susceptibility to disease recurrence at sites treated with non-bioabsorbable barrier membranes was compared to that at sites treated with root planing in a controlled clinical trial (Cortellini et al. 1996a). The results indicated that patient factors such as compliance with oral hygiene, smoking habits, and susceptibility to disease progression rather than the employed treatment modality, were the major determinants of stability of the treated sites.

A few studies have evaluated the long-term prognosis for furcation defects treated with regenerative therapy. Sixteen mandibular degree II furcation defects, following coronal flap positioning and citric acid root biomodification with and without implantation of demineralized freeze-dried bone allografts (DFDBA), were determined as completely resolved with bone fill assessed by re-entry surgery. They were re-evaluated after 4-5 years (Haney et al. 1997), when 12 of the 16 sites exhibited recurrent degree II furcations and all 16 sites demonstrated probable buccal furcation defects. The investigators concluded that these findings question the long-term stability of bone regeneration in furcations following coronally advanced flap procedures.

The long-term stability of mandibular furcation defects regenerated following GTR alone or in combination with root surface biomodification with citric acid and bone grafting, was also evaluated by McClain & Schallhorn (1993). Out of the 57% of the furcation defects which were assessed as completely filled at 6 and 12 months, only 29% were completely filled after 4 to 6 years. However, 74% of the furcations treated with GTR in combination with the placement of

DFDBA were completely filled at both the short and long-term evaluation, suggesting that the results obtained with the combined procedure were more stable over time. Long-term results of GTR treatment of mandibular degree II furcations with e-PTFE membranes were also reported by Machtei et al. (1996). The teeth were followed up to 4 years and compared with non-furcated molars. Improvements assessed in vertical (V-CAL) and horizontal (H-CAL) clinical attachment levels after treatment were maintained also after 4 years, suggesting that changes obtained in degree II furcation defects by GTR are stable. Only 9% of the treated defects were unstable, which was similar to that observed for non-furcated molars. Good oral hygiene as reflected in low plaque scores and elimination of periodontal pathogens were closely related to the long-term stability. On the basis of these results, it was concluded that furcation defects treated with membrane barriers can be maintained in health for at least 4 years, provided good oral hygiene and frequent recall visits are established.

CONCLUSIONS

GTR represents the most well-documented regenerative procedure for obtaining periodontal regeneration in intrabony defects and in degree II furcations. GTR has demonstrated significant clinical improvements beyond that achieved with only debridement in such defects. Regarding degree II maxillary furcations, the results following GTR treatment are inconsistent, and the treatment of degree III furcation defects is unpredictable. An added benefit may be obtained by the use of grafting materials in combination with GTR in some situations.

Differences between individuals and studies regarding the results of treating intrabony defects and class II furcations are related to patient compliance, maintenance procedures, selection of defects, surgical management, etc.

Periodontal regeneration obtained following GTR is stable on a long-term basis, provided good oral hygiene is maintained and a proper recall program is established.

REFERENCES

Al-Arrayed, F., Adam, S., Moran, J. & Dowell, P. (1995). Clinical trial of cross-linked human type I collagen as a barrier material in surgical periodontal treatment. *Journal of Clinical Periodontology* **22**, 371-379.

Altiere, E., Reeve, C. & Sheridan, P. (1979). Lyophilized bone allografts in periodontal osseous defects. *Journal of Periodontology* **50**, 510-519.

Anderegg, C., Martin, S., Gray, J., Mellonig, J. & Gher, M. (1991). Clinical evaluation of the use of decalcified freeze-dried bone allograft with guided tissue regeneration in the treatment of molar furcation invasions. *Journal of Periodontology* **62**, 264-268.

Anderegg, C., Metzeler, D. & Nicoll, B. (1995). Gingival thickness in guided tissue regeneration and associated recession at facial furcation defects. *Journal of Periodontology* **66**, 397-402.

Araùjo, M., Berglundh, T. & Lindhe, J. (1996). The periodontal tissues in healed degree III furcation defects. An experimental study in dogs. *Journal of Clinical Periodontology* **23**, 532-541.

Araùjo, M. & Lindhe, J. (2001). GTR treatment of degree III furcation defects following application of enamel matrix proteins. An experimental study in dogs. *Journal of Clinical Periodontology* **27** (in press).

Armitage G.C., Svanberg, G.K. & Löe, H. (1977). Microscopic evaluation of clinical measurements of connective tissue attachment levels. *Journal of Clinical Periodontology* **4**, 173-190.

Baldock, W.T., Hutchens, L.H. Jr., McFall, W.T. Jr. & Simpson, D.M. (1985). An evaluation of tricalcium phosphate implants in human periodontal osseous defects of two patients. *Journal of Periodontology* **56**, 1-7.

Barnett, J.D., Mellonig, J.T., Gray, J.L. & Towle, H.J. (1989). Comparison of freeze-dried bone allograft and porous hydroxyapatite in human periodontal defects. *Journal of Periodontology* **60**, 231-237.

Barney, V.C., Levin, M.P. & Adams, D.F. (1986). Bioceramical implants in surgical periodontal defects. A comparison study. *Journal of Periodontology* **57**, 764-770.

Becker, W. & Becker, B. (1993). Treatment of mandibular three-wall intrabony defects by flap debridement and expanded polytetrafluoroethylene barrier membranes. Long term evaluation of 32 treated patients. *Journal of Periodontology* **64**, 1138-1144.

Becker, W., Becker, B. E., Berg, L., Pritchard, J., Caffesse, R. & Rosenberg, E. (1988). New attachment after treatment with root isolation procedures: Report for treated class III and class II furcations and vertical osseous defects. *International Journal of Periodontics and Restorative Dentistry* **8**, 2-16.

Becker W., Becker, B.E. & Caffesse, R. (1994). A comparison of demineralized freeze-dried bone and autologous bone to induce bone formation in human extraction sockets. *Journal of Periodontology* **65**, 1128-1133.

Becker, W., Becker, B.E., Mellonig, J. Caffesse, R.G., Warrer, K., Caton, J.G. & Reid, T. (1996). A prospective multicenter study evaluating periodontal regeneration for class II furcation invasions and intrabony defects after treatment with a biosorbable barrier membrane: 1 year results. *Journal of Periodontology* **67**, 641-649.

Becker, W., Becker, B.E., Prichard, J.F., Caffesse, R., Rosenberg, E. & Gian-Grasso, J. (1987). Root isolation for new attachment procedures. A surgical and suturing method: three case reports. *Journal of Periodontology* **58**, 819-825.

Becker, W., Urist, M.R., Tucker, L.M., Becker, B.E. & Ochsenbein, C. (1995). Human demineralized freeze-dried bone: inadequate induced bone formation in athymic mice. A preliminary report. *Journal of Periodontology* **66**, 822-828.

Benqué, E., Zahedi, S., Brocard, D., Oscaby, F., Justumus, P. & Brunel, G. (1997). Guided tissue regeneration using a collagen membrane in chronic adult and rapidly progressive periodontitis patients in the treatment of 3-wall intrabony defects. *Journal of Clinical Periodontology* **24**, 544-549.

Beube, F.E. (1947). A study of reattachment of the supporting structures of teeth. *Journal of Periodontology* **18**, 55-56.

Beube, F.E. (1952). A radiograhic and histologic study on reattachment. *Journal of Periodontology* **23**, 158-164.

Björn H., Hollender, L. & Lindhe, J. (1965). Tissue regeneration in patients with periodontal disease. *Odontologisk Revy* **16**, 317-326.

Black, S., Gher, M., Sandifer, J., Fucini, S. & Richardson, C. (1994). Comparative study of collagen and expanded polytetrafluoroethylene membranes in the treatment of human class II furcation defects. *Journal of Periodontology* **65**, 598-604.

Blumenthal, N.M. (1988). The use of collagen membranes to guide regeneration of new connective tissue attachment in dogs. *Journal of Periodontology* **59**, 830-836.

Blumenthal, N.M. (1993). A clinical comparison of collagen membranes with e-PTFE membranes in the treatment of human mandibular Class II furcation defects. *Journal of Periodontology* **64**, 925-933.

Bogle, G., Adams, D., Crigger, M., Klinge, B. & Egelberg, J. (1981). New attachment after surgical treatment and acid conditioning of roots in naturally occurring periodontal disease in dogs. *Journal of Periodontal Research* **16**, 130-133.

Bouchard, P., Ouhayoun, J. & Nilveus, R. (1993). Expanded polytetrafluorethylene membranes and connective tissue grafts support bone regeneration for closing mandibular class II furcations. *Journal of Periodontology* **64**, 1193-1198.

Bowen, J.A., Mellonig, J.T., Gray, J.L. & Towle, H.T. (1989). Comparison of decalcified freeze-dried bone allograft and porous particulate hydroxyapatite in human periodontal osseous defects. *Journal of Periodontology* **60**, 647-654.

Bowers, G.M., Chadroff, B., Carnevale, R., Mellonig, J., Corio, R., Emerson, J., Stevens, M. & Romberg, E. (1989a). Histologic evaluation of new attachment apparatus formation in humans. Part I. *Journal of Periodontology* **60**, 664-674.

Bowers, G.M., Chadroff, B., Carnevale, R., Mellonig, J., Corio, R., Emerson, J., Stevens, M. & Romberg, E. (1989b). Histologic evaluation of new human attachment apparatus formation in humans. Part II. *Journal of Periodontology* **60**, 675-682.

Bowers, G.M., Chadroff, B., Carnevale, R., Mellonig, J., Corio, R., Emerson, J., Stevens, M. & Romberg, E. (1989c). Histologic evaluation of a new attachment apparatus formation in humans. Part III. *Journal of Periodontology* **60**, 683-693.

Bowers, G.M., Vargo, J.W., Lerg, B., Emerson, J.R. & Bergquist, J.J. (1986). Histologic observations following the placement of tricalcium phosphate implants in human intrabony defects. *Journal of Regeneration* **57**, 286-287.

Brunsvold, M.A. & Mellonig, J. (1993). Bone grafts and periodontal regeneration. *Periodontology 2000* **1**, 80-91.

Buser, D., Warrer, K. & Karring, T. (1990a). Formation of a periodontal ligament around titanium implants. *Journal of Periodontology* **61**, 597-601.

Buser, D., Warrer, K., Karring, T. & Stich, H. (1990b). Titanium implants with a true periodontal ligament. An alternative to osseointegrated implants. *International Journal of Oral and Maxillofacial Implants* **5**, 113-116.

Bühler, H. (1988). Evaluation of root-resected teeth. Results after 10 years. *Journal of Periodontology* **59**, 805-810.

Caffesse, R., Mota, L., Quinones, C. & Morrison, E.C. (1997). Clinical comparison of resorbable and non-resorbable barriers for guided tissue regeneration. *Journal of Clinical Periodontology* **24**, 747-752.

Caffesse, R.G., Nasjleti, C.E., Morrison, E.C. & Sanchez, R. (1994). Guided tissue regeneration: comparison of bioabsorbable and non-bioabsorbable membranes. Histologic and histometric study in dogs. *Journal of Periodontology* **65**, 583-591.

Caffesse, R.G., Smith, B.A., Castelli, W.A. & Nasjleti, C.E. (1988). New attachment achieved by guided tissue regeneration in beagle dogs. *Journal of Periodontology* **59**, 589-594.

Caffesse, R., Smith, B., Duff, B., Morrison, E., Merril, D. & Becker, W. (1990). Class II furcations treated by guided tissue regeneration in humans: case reports. *Journal of Periodontology* **61**, 510-514.

Camargo, P.M., Lekovic, V., Weinlander, M., Nedic, M., Vasilic, N., Wolinsky, L.E. & Kenney, E.B. (2000). A controlled re-entry study on the effectiveness of bovine porous bone mineral used in combination with a collagen membrane of porcine origin in the treatment of intrabony defects in humans. *Journal of Clinical Periodontology* **27**, 889-986.

Camelo, M., Nevins, M.L., Lynch, S.E., Schenck, R.K., Simion, M. & Nevins, M. (2001). Periodontal regeneration with an autogenous bone-Bio-Oss composite graft and a Bio-Gide membrane. *International Journal of Periodontics and Restorative Dentistry* **21**, 109-119.

Camelo, M., Nevins, M., Schenk, R., Simion, M., Rasperini, C., Lynch, S. & Nevins, M. (1998). Clinical radiographic, and histologic evaluation of human periodontal defects treated with Bio-Oss® and Bio-Gide. *International Journal of Periodontics and Restorative Dentistry* **18**, 321-331.

Caplanis, N., Lee, M.B., Zimmerman, G.J., Selvig, K.A. & Wikesjö, U.M. (1998). Effect of allogeneic freeze-dried demineralized bone matrix on regeneration of alveolar bone and periodontal attachment in dogs. *Journal of Clinical Periodontology* **25**, 801-806.

Carranza, F.A. (1954). A technique for reattachment. *Journal of Periodontology* **25**, 272-277.

Carranza, F.A. (1960). A technique for treating infrabony pockets so as to obtain reattachment. *Dental Clinics of North America* **5**, 75-83.

Carranza, F.A., Kenney, E.B., Lekovic, V., Talamante, E., Valencia, J. & Dimitrijevic, B. (1987). Histologic study of healing of human periodontal defects after placement of porous hydrozylapatite implants. *Journal of Periodontology* **58**, 682-688.

Carraro, J.J., Sznajder, N. & Alonso, C.A. (1976). Intraoral cancellous bone autografts in the treatment of infrabony pockets. *Journal of Clinical Periodontology* **3**, 104-109.

Caton, J., Greenstein, G. & Zappa, U. (1994). Synthetic bioabsorbable barrier for regeneration in human periodontal defects. *Journal of Periodontology* **65**, 1037-1045.

Caton J. & Nyman, S. (1980). Histometric evaluation of periodontal surgery. I. The modified Widman flap procedure. *Journal of Clinical Periodontology* **7**, 212-223.

Caton, J., Nyman, S. & Zander, H. (1980). Histometric evaluation of periodontal surgery. II. Connective tissue attachment levels after four regenerative procedures. *Journal of Clinical Periodontology* **7**, 224-231.

Caton, J., Wagener, C., Polson, A., Nyman, S., Frantz, B., Bouwsma, O. & Blieden, T. (1992). Guided tissue regeneration in interproximal defects in the monkey. *International Journal of Periodontics and Restorative Dentistry* **12**, 266-277.

Caton, J. & Zander, H.A. (1976). Osseous repair of an infrabony pocket without new attachment of connective tissue. *Journal of Clinical Periodontology* **3**, 54-58.

Chen, C., Wang, H., Smith, F., Glickman, G., Shyr, Y. & O'Neal, R. (1995). Evaluation of a collagen membrane with and without bone grafts in treating periodontal intrabony defects. *Journal of Periodontology* **66**, 838-847.

Christgau, M., Schamlz, G., Wenzel, A. & Hiller, K.A. (1997). Periodontal regeneration of intrabony defects with resorbable and non-resorbable membranes: 30 month results. *Journal of Clinical Periodontology* **24**, 17-27.

Chung, K.M., Salkin, L.M., Stein, M.D. & Freedman, A.L. (1990). Clinical evaluation of a biodegradable collagen membrane in guided tissue regeneration. *Journal of Periodontology* **61**, 732-736.

Claffey, N., Bogle, G., Bjoruatn, K., Selvig, K. & Egelberg, J. (1987). Topical application of tetracycline in regenerative periodontal surgery in beagles. *Acta Odontologica Scandinavica* **45**, 141-146.

Claffey, N. & Egelberg, J. (1995). Clinical indicators of probing attachment loss following initial periodontal treatment in advanced periodontitis patients. *Journal of Clinical Periodontology* **22**, 690-696.

Claffey, N., Motsinger, S., Ambruster, J. & Egelberg, J. (1989). Placement of a porous membrane underneath the mucoperiosteal flap and its effect on periodontal wound healing in dogs. *Journal of Clinical Periodontology* **16**, 12-16.

Clergeau, L.P., Danan, M., Clergeau-Guerithault, S. & Brion, M. (1996). Healing response to anorganic bone implantation in periodontal intrabony defects in dogs. Part I. Bone regeneration. A microradiographic study. *Journal of Periodontology* **67**, 140-149.

Cole, R.T., Crigger, M., Bogle, G., Egelberg, J. & Selvig, K.A. (1980). Connective tissue regeneration to periodontally diseased teeth. A histological study. *Journal of Periodontal Research* **15**, 1-9.

Cortellini, P. & Bowers, G. (1995). Periodontal regeneration of intrabony defects: an evidence based treatment approach. *International Journal of Periodontics and Restorative Dentistry* **15**, 129-145.

Cortellini, P., Carnevale, G., Sanz, M. & Tonetti, M.S. (1998). Treatment of deep and shallow intrabony defects. A multicenter randomized controlled clinical trial. *Journal of Clinical Periodontology* **25**, 981-987.

Cortellini, P., Clauser, C. & Pini Prato, G. (1993a). Histologic assessment of new attachment following the treatment of a human buccal recession by means of a guided tissue regeneration procedure. *Journal of Periodontology* **64**, 387-391.

Cortellini, P., De Sanctis, M., Pini, P.G., Baldi, C. & Clauser, C. (1991). Guided tissue regeneration procedure using a fibrin-fibronectin system in surgically induced recession in dogs. *International Journal of Periodontics and Restorative Dentistry* **11**, 150-163.

Cortellini, P. & Pini-Prato, G. (1994). Guided tissue regeneration with a rubber dam; A five case report. *International Journal of Periodontics and Restorative Dentistry* **14**, 9-15.

Cortellini, P., Pini-Prato, G., Baldi, C. & Clauser, C. (1990). Guided tissue regeneration with different materials. *International Journal of Periodontics and Restorative Dentistry* **10**, 137-151.

Cortellini, P., Pini-Prato, G. & Tonetti, M. (1993b). Periodontal regeneration of human infrabony defects. I. Clinical Measures. *Journal of Periodontology* **64**, 254-260.

Cortellini, P., Pini-Prato, G. & Tonetti, M. (1993c). Periodontal regeneration of human infrabony defects. II. Re-entry procedures and bone measures. *Journal of Periodontology* **64**, 261-268.

Cortellini, P., Pini-Prato, G. & Tonetti, M. (1994). Periodontal regeneration of human infrabony defects. V. Effect of oral hygiene on long term stability. *Journal of Clinical Periodontology* **21**, 606-610.

Cortellini, P., Pini-Prato, G. & Tonetti, M. (1995a). Interproximal free gingival grafts after membrane removal in GTR treatment of infrabony defects. A controlled clinical trial indicating improved outcomes. *Journal of Periodontology* **66**, 488-493.

Cortellini, P., Pini-Prato, G. & Tonetti, M. (1995b). No detrimental effect of fibrin glue on the regeneration of infrabony defects. A controlled clinical trial. *Journal of Clinical Periodontology* **22**, 697-702.

Cortellini, P., Pini-Prato, G. & Tonetti, M. (1995c). Periodontal regeneration of human infrabony defects with titanium reinforced membranes. A controlled clinical trial. *Journal of Periodontology* **66**, 797-803.

Cortellini, P., Pini-Prato, G. & Tonetti, M. (1995d). The modified papilla preservation technique. A new surgical approach for interproximal regenerative procedures. *Journal of Periodontology* **66**, 261-266.

Cortellini, P., Pini-Prato, G. & Tonetti, M. (1996a). Long term stability of clinical attachment following guided tissue regeneration and conventional therapy. *Journal of Clinical Periodontology* **23**, 106-111.

Cortellini, P., Pini-Prato, G. & Tonetti, M. (1996b). Periodontal regeneration of human intrabony defects with bioresorbable membranes. A controlled clinical trial. *Journal of Periodontology* **67**, 217-223.

Cortellini, P., Pini-Prato, G. & Tonetti, M. (1996c). The modified papilla preservation technique with bioresorbable barrier membranes in the treatment of intrabony defects. Case reports. *International Journal of Periodontics and Restorative Dentistry* **14**, 8-15.

Cortellini, P., Prato, G.P. & Tonetti, M.S. (1999). The simplified papilla preservation flap. A novel surgical approach for the management of soft tissues in regenerative procedures. *International Journal of Periodontics and Restorative Dentistry* **19**, 589-599.

Cortellini, P. & Tonetti, M. (1999). Radiographic defect angle influences the outcome of GTR therapy in intrabony defects. *Journal of Dental Research* **78**, 381 (abstract).

Cortellini, P. & Tonetti, M.S. (2000a). Focus on intrabony defects: guided tissue regeneration (GTR). *Periodontology 2000* **22**, 104-132.

Cortellini, P. & Tonetti, M. (2000b). Evaluation of the effect of tooth vitality on regenerative outcomes in intrabony defects. *Journal of Clinical Periodontology* **28**, 672-679.

Cortellini, P. & Tonetti, M.S. (2001). Microsurgical approach to periodontal regeneration. Initial evaluation in a case cohort. *Journal of Periodontology* **72**, 559-569.

Cortellini, P., Tonetti, M.S., Lang, N.P., Suvan, J.E., Zucchelli, G., Vangsted, T., Silvestri, M., Rossi, R., McClain, P., Fonzar, A., Dubravec, D. & Adriaens, P. (2001). The simplified papilla preservation flap in the regenerative treatment of deep intrabony defects: clinical outcomes and postoperative morbidity. *Journal of Periodontology* **72**, 1701-1712.

Coverly, L., Toto, P.D. & Gargiulo, A.W. (1975). Osseous coagulum. A histologic evaluation. *Journal of Periodontology* **46**, 596-606.

Crigger, M., Bogle, G., Nilveus, R., Egelberg, J. & Selvig, K.A. (1978). The effect of topical citric acid application on the healing of experimental furcation defects in dogs. *Journal of Periodontal Research* **13**, 538-549.

Demolon, I.A., Persson, G.R., Johnson, R.H. & Ammons, W.F. (1993). Effect of antibiotic treatment of clinical conditions and bacterial growth with guided tissue regeneration. *Journal of Periodontology* **64**, 609-616.

DeSanctis, M., Clauser, C. & Zucchelli, G. (1996b). Bacterial colonization of barrier material and periodontal regeneration. *Journal of Clinical Periodontology* **23**, 1039-1046.

DeSanctis, M., Zucchelli, G. & Clauser, C. (1996a). Bacterial colonization of bioabsorbable barrier material and periodontal regeneration. *Journal of Periodontology* **67**, 1193-1200.

Dorfer, C.E., Kim, T.S., Steinbrenner, H., Holle, R. & Eickholz, P. (2000). Regenerative periodontal surgery in interproximal intrabony defects with biodegradable barriers. *Journal of Clinical Periodontology* **27**, 162-168.

Dragoo, M.R. & Kaldahl, W.B. (1983). Clinical and histological evaluation of alloplasts and allografts in regenerative periodontal surgery in humans. *International Journal of Periodontics and Restorative Dentistry* **3**, 8-29.

Dragoo, M.R. & Sullivan, H.C. (1973a). A clinical and histological evaluation of autogenous iliac bone grafts in humans. I. Wound healing 2 to 8 months. *Journal of Periodontology* **44**, 599-613.

Dragoo, M.R. & Sullivan H.C. (1973b). A clinical and histological evaluation of autogenous iliac bone grafts in humans. II. External root resorption. *Journal of Periodontology* **44**, 614-625.

Eickholz, P., Kim, T.S., Steinbrenner, H., Dorfer, C. & Holle, R. (2000). Guided tissue regeneration with bioabsorbable barriers: intrabony defects and class II furcations. *Journal of Periodontology* **71**, 999-1008.

Eickholz, P., Lenhard, M., Benn, D.K. & Staehle, H.J. (1998). Periodontal surgery of vertical bony defects with or without synthetic bioabsorbable barriers. 12-month results. *Journal of Periodontology* **69**, 1210-1217.

Ellegaard, B., Karring, T., Davies, R. & Löe, H. (1974). New attachment after treatment of intrabony defects in monkeys. *Journal of Periodontology* **45**, 368-377.

Ellegaard, B., Karring, T., Listgarten, M. & Löe, H. (1973). New attachment after treatment of interradicular lesions. *Journal of Periodontology* **44**, 209-217.

Ellegaard, B., Karring, T. & Löe, H. (1975). The fate of vital and devitalized bone grafts on the healing of interradicular lesion. *Journal of Periodontal Research* **10**, 88-97.

Ellegaard, B. & Löe, H. (1971). New attachment of periodontal tissues after treatment of intrabony lesions. *Journal of Periodontology* **42**, 648-652.

Ellegaard, B., Nielsen, I.M. & Karring, T. (1976). Composite jaw and iliac cancellous bone grafts in intrabony defects in monkeys. *Journal of Periodontal Research* **11**, 299-310.

Erpenstein, H. (1983). A three year study of hemisected molars. *Journal of Clinical Periodontology* **10**, 1-10.

Ettel, R.G., Schaffer, E.M., Holpuch, R.C. & Brandt, C.L. (1989). Porous hydroxyapatite grafts in chronic subcrestal periodontal defects in rhesus monkeys: a histological investigation. *Journal of Periodontology* **60**, 342-351.

Falk, H., Fornell, J. & Teiwik, A. (1993). Periodontal regeneration using a bioresorbable GTR device. *Journal of the Swedish Dental Association* **85**, 673-681.

Falk, H., Laurell, L., Ravald, N., Teiwik, A. & Persson, R. (1997). Guided tissue regeneration therapy of 203 consecutively treated intrabony defects using a bioabsorbable matrix barrier. Clinical and radiographic findings. *Journal of Periodontology* **68**, 571-581.

Fetner, A.E., Hartigan, M.S. & Low, S.B. (1994). Periodontal repair using PerioGlas in non-human primates: clinical and histologic observations. *Compendium* **15**, 932-935.

Francis, J.R., Brunsvold, M.A., Prewett, A.B. & Mellonig, J.T. (1995). Clinical evaluation of an allogenic bone matrix in the treatment of periodontal osseous defects. *Journal of Periodontology* **66**, 1074-1079.

Frandsen, E., Sander, L., Arnbjerg, D. & Theilade, E. (1994). Effect of local metronidazole application on periodontal healing following guided tissue regeneration. Microbiological findings. *Journal of Periodontology* **65**, 921-928.

Frank, R.M., Fiore-Donno, G. & Cimasoni, G. (1983). Cementogenesis and soft tissue attachment after citric acid treatment in a human. An electron microscopic study. *Journal of Periodontology* **54**, 389-401.

Froum, S. (1996). Human histologic evaluation of HTR polymer and freeze-dried bone allografts. A case report. *Journal of Clinical Periodontology* **23**, 615-620.

Froum, S.J., Kushnek, L., Scopp, I.W. & Stahl, S.S. (1982). Human clinical and histologic responses to durapatite in intraosseous lesions. Case reports. *Journal of Periodontology* **53**, 719-729.

Froum, S.J., Kushnek, L., Scopp, I.W. & Stahl, S.S. (1983). Healing responses of human intraosseous lesions following the use of debridement, grafting and citric acid root treatment. I. Clinical and histologic observations six months postsurgery. *Journal of Periodontology* **54**, 67-76.

Froum, S.J., Ortiz, M., Witkin, R.T., Thaler, R., Scopp, I.W. & Stahl, S.S. (1976). Osseous autografts. III. Comparison of osseous coagulum-bone blend implant with open curettage. *Journal of Periodontology* **47**, 287-294.

Froum, S. & Stahl, S.S. (1987). Human intraosseous healing responses to the placement of tricalcium phosphate ceramic implants. II. 13 to 18 months. *Journal of Periodontology* **58**, 103-109.

Froum, S.J., Thaler, R., Scopp, I.W. & Stahl, S.S. (1975). Osseous autografts. I. Clinical responses to bone blend or hip marrow grafts. *Journal of Periodontology* **46**, 515-521.

Froum, S.J., Weinberg, M.A., Rosenberg, E. & Tarnow, D. (2001). A comparative study utilizing open flap debridement with and without enamel matrix derivate in the treatment of periodontal intrabony defects: a 12 month re-entry study. *Journal of Periodontology* **72**, 25-34.

Froum, S.J., Weinberg, M.A. & Tarnov, D. (1998). Comparison of bioactive glass, synthetic bone graft particles and open debridement in the treatment of human periodontal defects. A clinical study. *Journal of Periodontology* **69,** 698-709.

Fucini, S.E., Quintero, G., Gher, M.E., Black, B.S. & Richardson, A.C. (1993). Small versus large particles of demineralized freeze-dried bone allografts in human intrabony periodontal defects. *Journal of Periodontology* **64**, 844-847.

Fuentes, P., Garrett, S., Nilveus, R. & Egelberg, J. (1993). Treatment of periodontal furcation defects. Coronally positioned flaps with or without citric acid root conditioning in Class II defects. *Journal of Clinical Periodontology* **20**, 425-430.

Galgut, P.N., Waite, I.M., Brookshaw, J.D. & Kingston, C.P. (1992). A 4-year controlled clinical study into the use of a ceramic hydroxyapatite implant material for the treatment of periodontal bone defects. *Journal of Clinical Periodontology* **19,** 570-577.

Ganeles, J., Listgarten, M.A. & Evian, C. I. (1986). Ultrastructure of durapatite periodontal tissue interface in human intrabony defects. *Journal of Periodontology* **57**, 133-140.

Garraway, R., Young, W.G., Daley, T., Harbrow, D. & Bartold, P.M. (1998). An assessment of the osteoinductive potential of commercial demineralized freeze-dried bone in the murine thigh muscle implantation model. *Journal of Periodontology* **69**, 1325-1336.

Garrett, S. (1977). Root planing: a perspective. *Journal of Periodontology* **48**, 553-557.

Garrett, S., Loos, B., Chamberlain, D. & Egelberg, J. (1988). Treatment of intraosseous periodontal defects with a combined therapy of citric acid conditioning, bone grafting and placement of collagenous membranes. *Journal of Clinical Periodontology* **15**, 383-389.

Gestrelius, S., Lyngstadaas, S.P. & Hammarström, L. (2000). Emdogain – periodontal regeneration based on biomimicry. *Clinical Oral Investigations* **2**, 120-125.

Giannobile, W.V., Finkelman, R.D. & Lynch, S.E. (1994). Comparison of canine and non-human primate animal models for periodontal regenerative therapy: results following a single administration of PDGF/IGF-I. *Journal of Periodontology* **65**, 1158-1168.

Giannobile, W.V., Hernandez, R.A., Finkelman, R.D., Ryan, S., Kinitsy, C.P., D'Andrea, M. & Lynch, S.E. (1996). Comparative effects of platelet-derived growth factor-BB and insulin-like growth factor-I, individually and in combination, on periodontal regeneration in Macaca fascicularis. *Journal of Periodontal Research* **31**, 301-312.

Glossary of Periodontal Terms (1992). 3rd edn. Chicago: The American Academy of Periodontology.

Goldberg, V.M. & Stevenson, S. (1987). The natural history of autografts and allografts. *Clinical Orthopaedics* **225**, 7-16.

Goldman, H. & Cohen, W. (1958). The infrabony pocket: classification and treatment. *Journal of Periodontology* **29**, 272-291.

Gottlow, J., Karring, T. & Nyman, S. (1990). Guided tissue regeneration following treatment of recession-type defects in the monkey. *Journal of Periodontology* **61**, 680-685.

Gottlow, J., Laurell, L., Lundgren, D., Mathiesen, T., Nyman, S., Rylander, H. & Bogentoft, C. (1994). Periodontal tissue response to a new bioresorbable guided tissue regeneration device. A longitudinal study in monkeys. *International Journal of Periodontics and Restorative Dentistry* **14**, 437-449.

Gottlow, J., Nyman, S. & Karring, T. (1992). Maintenance of new attachment gained through guided tissue regeneration. *Journal of Clinical Periodontology* **19**, 315-317.

Gottlow, J., Nyman, S., Karring, T. & Lindhe, J. (1984). New attachment formation as the result of controlled tissue regeneration. *Journal of Clinical Periodontology* **11**, 494-503.

Gottlow, J., Nyman, S., Lindhe, J., Karring, T. & Wennström, J. (1986). New attachment formation in the human periodontium by guided tissue regeneration. *Journal of Clinical Periodontology* **13**, 604-616.

Gouldin, A., Fayad, S. & Mellonig, J. (1996). Evaluation of guided tissue regeneration in interproximal defects. II. Membrane and bone versus membrane alone. *Journal of Clinical Periodontology* **23**, 485-491.

Graves, D.T. & Cochran, D.L. (1994). Periodontal regeneration with polypeptide growth factors. In: Williams, R.C., Yukna, R.A. & Newman, M.G., eds. *Current Opinion in Periodontology*. Philadelphia: Current Science, pp. 178-186.

Grbic, J.T. & Lamster, I.B. (1992). Risk indicators for future clinical attachment loss in adult periodontitis. Tooth and site variables. *Journal of Periodontology* **63**, 262-269.

Grevstad, H. & Leknes, K.N. (1992). Epithelial adherence to polytetrafluoroethylene (PTFE) material. *Scandinavian Journal of Dental Research* **100**, 236-239.

Guillemin, M., Mellonig, J. & Brunswold, M. (1993). Healing in periodontal defects treated by decalcified freeze-dried bone allografts in combination with e-PTFE membranes. (I) Clinical and scanning electron microscope analysis. *Journal of Clinical Periodontology* **20**, 528-536.

Guillemin, G., Patat, J.L., Fournie, J. & Chetail, M. (1987). The use of coral as a bone graft substitute. *Journal of Biomedical Material Research* **21**, 557-567.

Haffajee, A.D., Socransky, S.S., Lindhe, J., Kent, R.L., Okamoto, H. & Yoneyama, T. (1991). Clinical risk indicators for periodontal attachment loss. *Journal of Clinical Periodontology* **18**, 117-125.

Hammarström, L. (1997). Enamel matrix, cementum development and regeneration. *Journal of Clinical Periodontology* **24**, 658-668.

Hammarström, L., Heijl, L. & Gestrelius, S. (1997). Periodontal regeneration in a buccal dehiscence model in monkeys after application of enamel matrix proteins. *Journal of Clinical Periodontology* **24**, 669-677.

Hamp, S.E., Nyman, S. & Lindhe, J. (1975). Periodontal treatment of multirooted teeth after 5 years. *Journal of Clinical Periodontology* **2**, 126-135.

Handelsman, M., Davarpanah, M. & Celletti, R. (1991). Guided tissue regeneration with and without citric acid treatment in vertical osseous defects. *International Journal of Periodontics and Restorative Dentistry* **11**, 351-363.

Haney, J.M., Leknes, K.N. & Wikesjö, U.M.E. (1997). Recurrence of mandibular molar furcation defects following citric acid root treatment and coronally advanced flap procedures. *International Journal of Periodontics and Restorative Dentistry* **17**, 3-10.

Haney, J.M., Nilveus, R.E., McMillan, P.J. & Wikesjö, U.M.E. (1993). Periodontal repair in dogs: expanded polytetraflouroethylene barrier membranes support wound stabilization and enhance bone regeneration. *Journal of Periodontology* **64**, 883-890.

Hawley, C.E. & Miller, J. (1975). A histologic examination of a free osseous autograft. *Journal of Periodontology* **46**, 289-293.

Heden, G. (2000). A case report study of 72 consecutive Emdogain-treated intrabony periodontal defects: clinical and radiographic findings after 1 year. *International Journal of Periodontics and Restorative Dentistry* **20**, 127-139.

Heden, G., Wennström, J. & Lindhe, J. (1999). Periodontal tissue alterations following Emdogain treatment of periodontal sites with angular bone defects. A series of case reports. *Journal of Clinical Periodontology* **26**, 855-860.

Heijl, L., Heden, G., Svärdström, C. & Ostgren, A. (1997). Enamel matrix derivate (EMDOGAIN®) in the treatment of intrabony periodontal defects. *Journal of Clinical Periodontology* 24, 705-714.

Hench, L.L., Splinter, R.J., Allen, W.C. & Greenlee, T.K. (1972). Bonding mechanism at the interface of ceramic prosthetic materials. *Journal of Biomedical Materials Research* 2, 117-141.

Hiatt, W.H. & Schallhorn, R.G. (1973). Intraoral transplants of cancellous bone and marrow in periodontal lesions. *Journal of Periodontology* 44, 194-208.

Hiatt, W.H., Schallhorn, R.G. & Aaronian, A.J. (1978). The induction of new bone and cementum formation. IV. Microscopic examination of the periodontium following human bone and marrow allograft, autograft and non-graft periodontal regenerative procedures. *Journal of Periodontology* 49, 495-512.

Holmes, R.E. (1979). Bone regeneration within a corraline hydroxyapatite implant. *Journal of Plastic and Reconstructive Surgery* 63, 626-633.

Howell, T.H., Fiorellini, J.P., Paquette, D.W., Offenbacher, S., Giannobile, W.V. & Lynch, S. (1997). A phase I/II clinical trial to evaluate a combination of recombinant human platelet-derived growth factor-BB and recombinant human insulin-like growth factor-I in patients with periodontal disease. *Journal of Periodontology* 68, 1186-1193.

Hugoson, A., Ravald, N., Fornell, J., Johard, G., Teiwik, A. & Gottlow, J. (1995). Treatment of class II furcation involvements in humans with bioresorbable and nonresorbable guided tissue regeneration barriers. A randomized multicenter study. *Journal of Periodontology* 66, 624-634.

Hutchens, L.H. Jr. (1999). The use of a bovine bone mineral in periodontal osseous defects: case reports. *Compendium of Continuing Education in Dentistry* 20, 365-376.

Hürzeler, M.B., Quinones, C.R., Caffesse, R.G., Schupback, P. & Morrison, E.C. (1997). Guided periodontal tissue regeneration in interproximal intrabony defects following treatment with a synthetic bioabsorbable barrier. *Journal of Periodontology* 68, 489-497.

Isidor, F., Karring, T. & Attström, R. (1984). The effect of root planing as compared to that of surgical treatment. *Journal of Clinical Periodontology* 11, 669-681.

Isidor, F., Karring, T., Nyman, S. & Lindhe, J. (1985). New attachment-reattachment following reconstructive periodontal surgery. *Journal of Clinical Periodontology* 12, 728-735.

Karapataki, S., Hugoson, A., Falk, H., Laurell, L. & Kugelberg, C.F. (2000). Healing following GTR treatment of intrabony defects distal to mandibular second molars using resorbable and non-resorbable barriers. *Journal of Clinical Periodontology* 27, 333-340.

Karatzas, S., Zavras, A., Greenspan, D. & Amar, S. (1999). Histologic observations of periodontal wound healing after treatment with PerioGlass in non-human primates. *International Journal of Periodontics and Restorative Dentistry* 19, 489-499.

Karring, T. & Cortellini, P. (1999). Regenerative therapy: furcation defects. *Periodontology 2000* 19, 115-137.

Karring, T., Isidor, F., Nyman, S. & Lindhe, J. (1985). New attachment formation on teeth with a reduced but healthy periodontal ligament. *Journal of Clinical Periodontology* 12, 51-60.

Karring, T., Nyman, S., Gottlow, J. & Laurell, L. (1993). Development of the biological concept of guided tissue regeneration – animal and human studies. *Periodontology 2000* 1, 26-35.

Karring, T., Nyman, S. & Lindhe, J. (1980). Healing following implantation of periodontitis affected roots into bone tissue. *Journal of Clinical Periodontology* 7, 96-105.

Karring, T., Nyman, S., Lindhe, J. & Sirirat, M. (1984). Potentials for root resorption during periodontal healing. *Journal of Clinical Periodontology* 11, 41-52.

Karring, T., Nyman, S., Thilander, B. & Magnusson, I. (1982). Bone regeneration in orthodontically produced alveolar bone dehiscences. *Journal of Periodontal Research* 17, 309-315.

Kenney, E.B., Lekovic, V., Han, T., Carranza, F.A. & Demitrijevic, B. (1985). The use of porous hydroxylapatite implant in periodontal defects. I. Clinical results after six months. *Journal of Periodontology* 56, 82-88.

Kersten, B., Chamberlain, A., Khorsandl, S., Wikesjö, U.M.E., Selvig, K. & Nilveus, R. (1992). Healing of the intrabony periodontal lesion following root conditioning with citric acid and wound closure including an expanded PTFE membrane. *Journal of Periodontology* 63, 876-882.

Kilic, A., Efeoglu, E. & Yilmaz, S. (1997). Guided tissue regeneration in conjunction with hydroxyapatite-collagen grafts for intrabony defects. A clinical and radiological evaluation. *Journal of Clinical Periodontology* 24, 372-383.

Kim, C., Choi, E., Chai, J.K. & Wikesjö, U.M. (1996). Periodontal repair in intrabony defects treated with a calcium carbonate implant and guided tissue regeneration. *Journal of Periodontology* 67, 1301-1306.

Kon, S., Novaes, A.B., Ruben, M.P. & Goldman, H.M. (1969). Visualization of microvascularization of the healing periodontal wound II. Curettage. *Journal of Periodontology* 40, 96-105.

Kostopoulos, L. & Karring, T. (1994). Resistance of new attachment to ligature induced periodontal breakdown. An experiment in monkeys. *Journal of Dental Research* 73, 963 (abstract).

Krejci, C.B., Bissada, N.F., Farah, C. & Greenwell, H. (1987). Clinical evaluation of porous and nonporous hydroxyapatite in the treatment of human periodontal bony defects. *Journal of Periodontology* 58, 521-528.

Lang, N.P. (2000). Focus on intrabony defects – conservative therapy. *Periodontology 2000* 22, 51-58.

Langer, B., Stein, S.D. & Wagenberg, B. (1981). An evaluation of root resection. A ten year study. *Journal of Periodontology* 52, 719-722.

Laurell, L., Falk, H., Fornell, J., Johard, G. & Gottlow, J. (1994). Clinical use of a bioresorbable matrix barrier in guided tissue regeneration therapy. Case series. *Journal of Periodontology* 65, 967-975.

Lekovic, V., Kenney, E.B., Carranza, F.A. & Danilovic, V. (1990). Treatment of class II furcation defects using porous hydroxylapatite in conjunction with a polytetrafluoroethylene membrane. *Journal of Periodontology* 61, 575-578.

Lekovic, V., Kenney, E., Kovacevic, K. & Carranza, F. (1989). Evaluation of guided tissue regeneration in class II furcation defects. A clinical re-entry study. *Journal of Periodontology* 60, 694-698.

Levin, M.P., Getter, L., Adrian, J. & Cutright, D.E. (1974). Healing of periodontal defects with ceramic implants. *Journal of Clinical Periodontology* 1, 197-205.

Lindhe, J. & Cortellini, P. (1996). Consensus report of session 4. In: Lang, N.P., Karring, T. & Lindhe, J., eds. *Proceedings of the 2nd European Workshop on Periodontology.* London: Quintessence Publishing Co. Ltd, pp. 359-360.

Lindhe, J. & Echeverria, J. (1994). Consensus report of session II. In: Lang, N.P. & Karring, T., eds. *Proceedings of the 1st European Workshop on Periodontology.* London: Quintessence Publishing Co. Ltd, pp. 210-214.

Lindhe, J., Nyman, S. & Karring, T. (1984). Connective tissue attachment as related to presence or absence of alveolar bone. *Journal of Clinical Periodontology* 11, 33-40.

Lindhe, J., Pontoriero, R., Berglundh, T. & Araújo, M. (1995). The effect of flap management and bioresorbable occlusive devices in GTR treatment of degree III furcation defects. An experimental study in dogs. *Journal of Clinical Periodontology* 22, 276-283.

Listgarten, M.A., Moa, R. & Robinson, P.J. (1976). Periodontal probing and the relationship of the probe to the periodontal tissues. *Journal of Periodontology* 47, 511-513.

Listgarten, M.A. & Rosenberg, M.M. (1979). Histological study of repair following new attachment procedures in human periodontal lesions. *Journal of Periodontology* 50, 333-344.

Little, L.A., Beck, F.M., Bugci, B. & Horton, J.E. (1995). Lack of furcal bone loss following the tunneling procedure. *Journal of Clinical Periodontology* 22, 637-641.

Lovelace, T.B., Mellonig, J.T., Meffert, R.M., Jones, A.A., Nummikoski, P.V. & Cochran, D.L. (1998). Clinical evaluation of bioactive glass in the treatment of periodontal osseous defects in humans. *Journal of Periodontology* **69**, 1027-1035.

Lundgren, D. & Slotte, C. (1999). Reconstruction of anatomically complicated periodontal defects using a bioresorbable GTR barrier supported by bone mineral. A 6-months follow-up study of 6 cases. *Journal of Clinical Periodontology* **26**, 56-62.

Lynch, S.E., deCustilla, G.R., Williams, R.C., Kinitsy, C.P., Howell, H., Reddy, M.S. & Antoniades, H.N. (1991). The effects of short-term application of a combination of platelet derived and insulin like growth factors on periodontal wound healing. *Journal of Periodontology* **62**, 458-467.

Lynch, S.E., Williams, R.C., Polson, A.M., Howell, T.H., Reddy, M.S., Zappa, U.E. & Antoniades, H.N. (1989). A combination of platelet derived and insulin like growth factors enhances periodontal regeneration. *Journal of Clinical Periodontology* **16**, 545-548.

Mabry, T.W., Yukna, R.A. & Sepe, W.W. (1985). Freeze-dried bone allografts combined with tetracycline in the treatment of juvenile periodontitis. *Journal of Periodontology* **56**, 74-81.

Machtei, E., Cho, M., Dunford, R., Norderyd, J., Zambon, J. & Genco, R. (1994). Clinical, microbiological, and histological factors which influence the success of regenerative periodontal therapy. *Journal of Periodontology* **65**, 154-161.

Machtei, E., Dunford, R., Norderyd, J., Zambon, J. & Genco, R. (1993). Guided tissue regeneration and anti-infective therapy in the treatment of class II furcation defects. *Journal of Periodontology* **64**, 968-973.

Machtei, E., Grossi, S., Dunford, R., Zambon, J. & Genco, R. (1996). Long-term stability of class II furcation defects treated with barrier membranes. *Journal of Periodontology* **67**, 523-527.

Machtei, E. & Schallhorn, R.G. (1995). Successful regeneration of mandibular class II furcation defects. An evidence-based treatment approach. *International Journal of Periodontics and Restorative Dentistry* **15**, 146-167.

Magnusson, I., Batich, C. & Collins, B.R. (1988). New attachment formation following controlled tissue regeneration using biodegradable membranes. *Journal of Periodontology* **59**, 1-6.

Magnusson, I., Claffey, N., Bogle, S., Garrett, S. & Egelberg, J. (1985a). Root resorption following periodontal flap procedures in monkeys. *Journal of Periodontal Research* **20**, 79-85.

Magnusson, I., Nyman, S., Karring, T. & Egelberg, J. (1985b). Connective tissue attachment formation following exclusion of gingival connective tissue and epithelium during healing. *Journal of Periodontal Research* **20**, 201-208.

Mann, W. (1964). Autogenous transplant in the treatment of an infrabony pocket. *Periodontics* **2**, 205-208.

Mattson, J., McLey, L. & Jabro, M. (1995). Treatment of intrabony defects with collagen membrane barriers. Case reports. *Journal of Periodontology* **66**, 635-645.

Mayfield, L., Söderholm, G., Hallström, H., Kullendorff, B., Edwardsson, S., Bratthall, G., Brägger, U. & Attström, R. (1998). Guided tissue regeneration for the treatment of intraosseous defects using a bioabsorbable membrane. A controlled clinical study. *Journal of Clinical Periodontology* **25**, 585-595.

McCall, J.O. (1926). An improved method of inducing reattachment of the gingival tissue in periodontoclasia. *Dental Items of Interest* **48**, 342-358.

McClain, P. & Schallhorn, R.G. (1993). Long term assessment of combined osseous composite grafting, root conditioning and guided tissue regeneration. *International Journal of Periodontics and Restorative Dentistry* **13**, 9-27.

Meadows, C.L., Gher, M.E., Quintero, G. & Lafferty, T.A. (1993). A comparison of polylactic acid granules and decalcified freeze-dried bone allograft in human periodontal osseous defects. *Journal of Periodontology* **64**, 103-109.

Meffert, R.M., Thomas, J.R., Hamilton, K.M. & Brownstein, C.R. (1985). Hydroxylapatite as an alloplastic graft in the treatment of human periodontal osseous defects. *Journal of Periodontology* **56**, 63-73.

Melcher, A.H. (1976). On the repair potential of periodontal tissues. *Journal of Periodontology* **47**, 256-260.

Melcher, A.H., McCulloch, C.A.G., Cheong, T., Nemeth, E. & Shiga, A. (1987). Cells from bone synthesize cementum like and bone like tissue in vitro and may migrate into periodontal ligament in vivo. *Journal of Periodontal Research* **22**, 246-247.

Mellado, J., Salkin, L., Freedman, A. & Stein, M. (1995). A comparative study of e-PTFE periodontal membranes with and without decalcified freeze-dried bone allografts for the regeneration of interproximal intraosseous defects. *Journal of Periodontology* **66**, 751-755.

Mellonig, J.T. (1984). Decalcified freeze-dried bone allografts as an implant material in human periodontal defects. *International Journal of Periodontics and Restorative Dentistry* **4**, 41-55.

Mellonig, J.T. (1991). Freeze-dried bone allografts in periodontal reconstructive surgery. *Dental Clinics of North America* **35**, 505-520.

Mellonig, J.T. (1999). Enamel matrix derivate for periodontal reconstructive surgery: Technique and clinical and histologic case report. *International Journal of Periodontics and Restorative Dentistry* **19**, 9-19.

Mellonig, J.T. (2000). Human histologic evaluation of a bovine-derived bone xenograft in the treatment of periodontal osseous defects. *International Journal of Periodontics and Restorative Dentistry* **20**, 18-29.

Mellonig, J.T., Bowers, G. & Bully, R. (1981). Comparison of bone graft materials. I. New bone formation with autografts and allografts determined by strontium-85. *Journal of Periodontology* **52**, 291-296.

Mellonig, J.T., Semons, B., Gray, J. & Towle, H. (1994). Clinical evaluation of guided tissue regeneration in the treatment of grade II molar furcation invasion. *International Journal of Periodontics and Restorative Dentistry* **14**, 255-271.

Metzeler, D.G., Seamons, B.C., Mellonig, J.T., Gher, M.E. & Gray, J.L. (1991). Clinical evalution of guided tissue regeneration in the treatment of maxillary class II molar furcation invasions. *Journal of Periodontology* **62**, 353-360.

Minabe, M., Sugaya, A., Satou, H., Tamara, T., Ogawa, Y., Huri, T. & Watanabe, Y. (1988). Histologic study of the hydroxyapatite-collagen complex implants in periodontal osseous defects in dogs. *Journal of Periodontology* **59**, 671-678.

Mombelli, A., Lang, N. & Nyman, S. (1993). Isolation of periodontal species after guided tissue regeneration. *Journal of Periodontology* **64**, 1171-1175.

Moore, J.A., Ashley, F.P. & Watermann, C.A. (1987). The effect on healing of the application of citric acid during replaced flap surgery. *Journal of Clinical Periodontology* **14**, 130-135.

Mora, F. & Ouhayoun, J.P. (1995). Clinical evaluation of natural coral and porous hydroxyapatite implants in periodontal bone lesions: results of a 1-year follow-up. *Journal of Clinical Periodontology* **22**, 877-884.

Moscow, B.S. (1964). The response of the gingival sulcus to instrumentation: A histological investigation. *Journal of Periodontology* **35**, 112-126.

Moscow, B.S., Karsh, F. & Stein, S.D. (1979). Histological assessment of autogenous bone graft. A case report and critical evaluation. *Journal of Periodontology* **6**, 291-300.

Moscow, B.S. & Lubarr, A. (1983). Histological assessment of human periodontal defects after durapatite ceramic implant. *Journal of Periodontology* **51**, 455-464.

Murphy, K. (1995a). Post-operative healing complications associated with Gore-tex periodontal material. Part 1. Incidence and characterization. *International Journal of Periodontics and Restorative Dentistry* **15**, 363-375.

Murphy, K. (1995b). Post-operative healing complications associated with Gore-tex periodontal material. Part 2. Effect of complications on regeneration. *International Journal of Periodontics and Restorative Dentistry* **15**, 549-561.

Murphy, K. (1996). Interproximal tissue maintenance in GTR procedures: description of a surgical technique and 1 year reentry results. *International Journal of Periodontics and Restorative Dentistry* **16**, 463-477.

Nabers, C.L. & O'Leary, T.J. (1965). Autogenous bone transplant in the treatment of osseous defects. *Journal of Periodontology* **36**, 5-14.

Nabers, C.L., Reed, O.M. & Hamner, J.E. (1972). Gross and histologic evaluation of an autogenous bone graft 57 months postoperatively. *Journal of Periodontology* **43**, 702-704.

Nasr, H.F., Aichelmann-Reidy, M.E. & Yukna, R.A. (1999). Bone and bone substitutes. *Periodontology 2000* **19**, 74-86.

Nery, E.B. & Lynch, K.L. (1978). Preliminary clinical studies of bioceramic in periodontal osseous defects. *Journal of Periodontology* **49**, 523-527.

Nery, E.M., Lynch, K.L. Hirthe, W.M. & Mueller, B.H. (1975). Bioceramic implants in surgically produced infrabony defects. *Journal of Periodontology* **46**, 328-347.

Nevins, M.L., Camelo, M., Nevins, M., King, C.J., Oringer, R.J., Schenk, R.K. & Fiorellini, J.P. (2000). Human histologic evaluation of bioactive ceramic in the treatment of periodontal osseous defects. *International Journal of Periodontics and Restorative Dentistry* **20**, 458-467.

Niederman, R., Savitt, E.D., Heeley, J.D. & Duckworth, J.E. (1989). Regeneration of furca bone using Gore-Tex periodontal material. *International Journal of Periodontics and Restorative Dentistry* **9**, 468-480.

Nielsen, I.M., Ellegaard, B. & Karring, T. (1980). Kielbone® in healing interradicular lesions in monkeys. *Journal of Periodontal Research* **15**, 328-337.

Nielsen, I.M., Ellegaard, B. & Karring, T. (1981). Kielbone® in new attachment attempts in humans. *Journal of Periodontology* **52**, 723-728.

Nilveus, R., Johansson, O. & Egelberg, J. (1978). The effect of autogenous cancellous bone grafts on healing of experimental furcation defects in dogs. *Journal of Periodontal Research* **13**, 532-537.

Novaes-Jr, A., Gutierrez, F., Francischetto, I. & Novaes, A. (1995). Bacterial colonization of the external and internal sulci and of cellulose membranes at times of retrieval. *Journal of Periodontology* **66**, 864-869.

Nowzari, H., Matian, F. & Slots, J. (1995). Periodontal pathogens on polytetrafluoroethylene membrane for guided tissue regeneration inhibit healing. *Journal of Clinical Periodontology* **22**, 469-474.

Nowzari, H. & Slots, J. (1994). Microorganisms in polytetrafluoroethylene barrier membranes for guided tissue regeneration. *Journal of Clinical Periodontology* **21**, 203-210.

Nyman, S. & Karring, T. (1979). Regeneration of surgically removed buccal alveolar bone in dogs. *Journal of Periodontal Research* **14**, 86-92.

Nyman, S., Karring, T., Lindhe, J. & Planten, S. (1980). Healing following implantation of periodontitis-affected roots into gingival connective tissue. *Journal of Clinical Periodontology* **7**, 394-401.

Nyman, S., Lindhe, J., Karring, T. & Rylander, H. (1982). New attachment following surgical treatment of human periodontal disease. *Journal of Clinical Periodontology* **9**, 290-296.

Ong, M.M., Eber, R.M., Korsnes, M.I., MacNeil, R.L., Glickman, G.R., Shyr, Y. & Wang, H.L. (1998). Evaluation of bioactive glass alloplast in treating periodontal intrabony defects. *Journal of Periodontology* **69**, 1346-1354.

Orban, B. (1948). Pocket elimination or reattachment? *New York Dental Journal* **14**, 227-232.

Oreamuno, S., Lekovic, V., Kenney, E.B., Carranza, F.A. Jr., Takei, H.H. & Prokic, B. (1990). Comparative clinical study of porous hydroxyapatite and decalcified freeze-dried bone in human periodontal defects. *Journal of Periodontology* **61**, 399-404.

Ouhayoun, J. (1996). Biomaterials used as bone graft substitutes. In: Lang, N.P., Karring, T. & Lindhe, J., eds. *Proceedings of the 2nd European Workshop on Periodontology.* London: Quintessence Publishing Co. Ltd, pp. 313-358.

Paolantonio, M., Scarano, A., DiPlacido, G., Tumini, V., D'Archivio, D. & Piattelli, A. (2001). Periodontal healing in humans using anorganic bovine bone and bovine peritoneum-derived collagen membrane: a clinical and histologic case report.

International Journal of Periodontics and Restorative Dentistry **21**, 505-515.

Parashis, A., Andronikaki-Faldami, A. & Tsiklakis, K. (1998). Comparison of two regenerative procedures – guided tissue regeneration and demineralized freeze-dried bone allograft – in the treatment of intrabony defects: a clinical and radiographic study. *Journal of Periodontology* **69**, 751-758.

Parashis, A. & Mitsis, F. (1993). Clinical evaluation of the effect of tetracycline root preparation on guided tissue regeneration in the treatment of class II furcation defects. *Journal of Periodontology* **64**, 133-136.

Parodi, R., Carusi, G., Santarelli, G., Nanni, F., Pingitore, R. & Brunel, G. (1997). Guided tissue regeneration employing a collagen membrane in a human periodontal bone defect: a histologic evaluation. *International Journal of Periodontics and Restorative Dentistry* **17**, 282-291.

Patur, B. (1974). Osseous defects. Evaluation, diagnostic and treatment methods. *Journal of Periodontology* **45**, 523-541.

Patur, B. & Glickman, I. (1962). Clinical and roentgenographic evaluation of the post-treatment healing of infrabony pockets. *Journal of Periodontology* **33**, 164-171.

Paul, B.F., Mellonig, J.T., Towle, H.J. & Gray, J.L. (1992). The use of a collagen barrier to enhance healing in human periodontal furcation defects. *International Journal of Periodontics and Restorative Dentistry* **12**, 123-131.

Pearson, G.E., Rosen, S. & Deporter, D.A. (1981). Preliminary observations on the usefulness of decalcified freeze-dried cancellous bone allograft material in periodontal surgery. *Journal of Periodontology* **52**, 55-59.

Pietruska, M.D. (2001). A comparative study on the use of Bio-Oss and enamel matrix derivative (Emdogain) in the treatment of periodontal bone defects. *European Journal of Oral Science* **109**, 178-181.

Pini-Prato, G., Clauser, C., Tonetti, M.S. & Cortellini, P. (1996). Guided tissue regeneration in gingival recessions. *Periodontology 2000* **11**, 49-57.

Pitaru, S., Tal, H., Soldinger, M., Grosskopf, A. & Noff, M. (1988). Partial regeneration of periodontal tissues using collagen barriers. Initial observations in the canine. *Journal of Periodontology* **59**, 380-386.

Plotzke, A.E., Barbosa, S., Nasjleti, C.E., Morrison, E.C. & Caffesse, R.G. (1993). Histologic and histometric responses to polymeric composite grafts. *Journal of Periodontology* **64**, 343-348.

Polson, A.M, Garrett, S., Stoller, N.H., Greenstein, G., Polson, A., Harrold, C. & Laster, L. (1995b). Guided tissue regeneration in human furcation defects after using a biodegradable barrier: a multi-center feasibility study. *Journal of Periodontology* **66**, 377-385.

Polson, A. M. & Heijl, L. (1978). Osseous repair in infrabony defects. *Journal of Clinical Periodontology* **5**, 13-23.

Polson, A.M. & Proye, M.P. (1982). Effect of root surface alterations on periodontal healing. II. Citric acid treatment of the denuded root. *Journal of Clinical Periodontology* **9**, 441-454.

Polson, A.M., Southard, G.L., Dunn, R.L., Polson, A.P., Yewey, G.L., Swanbom, D.D., Fulfs, J.C. & Rodgers, P.W. (1995a). Periodontal healing after guided tissue regeneration with Atrisorb barriers in beagle dogs. *International Journal of Periodontics and Restorative Dentistry* **15**, 574-589.

Pontoriero, R. (1996) *Studies on regenerative therapy in furcation defects.* Thesis. Department of Periodontology, Faculty of Odontology, University of Gothenburg, p. 44.

Pontoriero, R. & Lindhe, J. (1995a). Guided tissue regeneration in the treatment of degree II furcations in maxillary molars. *Journal of Clinical Periodontology* **22**, 756-763.

Pontoriero, R. & Lindhe, J. (1995b). Guided tissue regeneration in the treatment of degree III furcations in maxillary molars. Short communication. *Journal of Clinical Periodontology* **22**, 810-812.

Pontoriero, R., Lindhe, J., Nyman, S., Karring, T., Rosenberg, E. & Sanavi, F. (1988). Guided tissue regeneration in degree II furcation-involved mandibular molars. A clinical study. *Journal of Clinical Periodontology* **15**, 247-254.

Pontoriero, R., Lindhe, J., Nyman, S., Karring, T., Rosenberg, E. & Sanavi, F. (1989). Guided tissue regeneration in the treatment of furcation defects in mandibular molars. A clinical study of degree III involvements. *Journal of Clinical Periodontology* **16**, 170-174.

Pontoriero, R., Nyman, S., Ericsson, I. & Lindhe, J. (1992). Guided tissue regeneration in surgically produced furcation defects. An experimental study in the beagle dog. *Journal of Clinical Periodontology* **19**, 159-163.

Pontoriero, R., Wennström, J. & Lindhe, J. (1999). The use of barrier membranes and enamel matrix proteins in the treatment of angular bone defects. A prospective controlled clinical study. *Journal of Clinical Periodontology* **26**, 833-840.

Prichard, J. (1957a). Regeneration of bone following periodontal therapy. *Oral Surgery* **10**, 247-252.

Prichard, J. (1957b). The infrabony technique as a predictable procedure. *Journal of Periodontology* **28**, 202-216.

Prichard, J. (1960). A technique for treating infrabony pockets based on alveolar process morphology. *Dental Clinics of North America* **4**, 85-105.

Proestakis, G., Bratthal, G., Söderholm, G., Kullendorff, B., Gröndahl, K., Rohlin, M. & Attström, R. (1992). Guided tissue regeneration in the treatment of infrabony defects on maxillary premolars. A pilot study. *Journal of Clinical Periodontology* **19**, 766-773.

Proye, M. & Polson, A.M. (1982). Effect of root surface alterations on periodontal healing. I. Surgical denudation. *Journal of Clinical Periodontology* **9**, 428-440.

Quattlebaum, J.B., Mellonig, J.T. & Hensel, N.F. (1988). Antigenicity of freeze-dried cortical bone allograft in human periodontal osseous defects. *Journal of Periodontology* **59**, 394-397.

Quintero, G., Mellonig, J.T., Gambill, V.M. & Pelleu, G.B. Jr. (1982). A six-month clinical evaluation of decalcified freeze-dried bone allografts in periodontal osseous defects. *Journal of Periodontology* **53**, 726-730.

Quteish, D. & Dolby, A. (1992). The use of irradiated-crosslinked human collagen membrane in guided tissue regeneration. *Journal of Clinical Periodontology* **19**, 476-484.

Ramfjord, S.P. (1951). Experimental periodontal reattachment in Rhesus monkeys. *Journal of Periodontology* **22**, 67-77.

Ramfjord, S.P. & Nissle, R.R. (1974). The modified Widman flap. *Journal of Periodontology* **45**, 601-607.

Ratka-Kruger, P., Neukranz, E. & Raetzke, P. (2000). Guided tissue regeneration procedure with bioresorbable membranes versus conventional flap surgery in the treatment of infrabony periodontal defects. *Journal of Clinical Periodontology* **27**, 120-127.

Reddy, M.S. & Jeffcoat, H.K. (1999). Methods of assessing periodontal regeneration. *Periodontology 2000* **19**, 87-103.

Register, A.A. & Burdick, F.A. (1976). Accelerated reattachment with cementogenesis to dentin, demineralized in situ. II. Defect repair. *Journal of Periodontology* **47**, 497-505.

Renvert, S., Garrett, S., Schallhorn, R.G. & Egelberg, J. (1985). Healing after treatment of periodontal intraosseous defects. III. Effect of osseous grafting and citric acid conditioning. *Journal of Clinical Periodontology* **12**, 441-455.

Richardson, C.R., Mellonig, J.T., Brunsvold, M.A., McDonnell, H.T. & Cochran, D.L. (1999). Clinical evaluation of Bio-Oss: a bovine-derived xenograft for the treatment of periodontal osseous defects in humans. *Journal of Clinical Periodontology* **26**, 421-428.

Ripamonti, U., Heliotis, M., van der Heerer, B. & Reddi, A.H. (1994). Bone morphogenetic proteins induce periodontal regeneration in the baboon (papio ursinus). *Journal of Periodontal Research* **29**, 439-445.

Rivault, A.F., Toto, P.D., Levy, S. & Gargiulo, A.W. (1971). Autogenous bone grafts: osseous coagulum and osseous retrograde procedures in primates. *Journal of Periodontology* **42**, 787-788.

Robinson, R.E. (1969). Osseous coagulum for bone induction. *Journal of Periodontology* **40**, 503-510.

Rosenberg, M.M. (1971a). Free osseous tissue autografts as a predictable procedure. *Journal of Periodontology* **42**, 195-209.

Rosenberg, M.M. (1971b). Re-entry of an osseous defect treated by a bone implant after a long duration. *Journal of Periodontology* **42**, 360-363.

Rosenberg, E.S., Garber, D.A. & Abrams, B. (1979). Repair of bony defects using an intraoral exostosis as a donor site. A case report. *Journal of Periodontology* **50**, 476-478.

Rosling, B., Nyman, S. & Lindhe, J. (1976). The effect of systematic plaque control on bone regeneration in infrabony pockets. *Journal of Clinical Periodontology* **3**, 38-53.

Ross, S. & Cohen, W. (1968). The fate of an osseous tissue autograft. A clinical and histologic case report. *Periodontics* **6**, 145-151.

Rummelhart, J.M., Mellonig, J.T., Gray, J.L. & Towle, H.J. (1989). A comparison of freeze-dried bone allograft and demineralized freeze-dried bone allograft in human periodontal osseous defects. *Journal of Periodontology* **60**, 655-663.

Rutherford, R.B., Niekrash, C.E., Kennedy, J.E. & Charette, M.F. (1992). Platelet-derived and insulin-like growth factors stimulate regeneration of periodontal attachment in monkeys. *Journal of Periodontal Research* **27**, 285-290.

Saffar, J.L., Colombier, M.L. & Detienville, R. (1990). Bone formation in tricalcium phosphate-filled periodontal intrabony lesions. Histological observations in humans. *Journal of Periodontology* **61**, 209-216.

Sallum, E.A., Sallum, A.W., Nociti, F.H. Jr., Marcantonio, R.A. & de Toledo, S. (1998). New attachment achieved by guided tissue regeneration using a bioresorbable polylactic acid membrane in dogs. *International Journal of Periodontics and Restorative Dentistry* **18**, 502-510.

Sander, L., Frandsen, E.V.G., Arnbjerg, D., Warrer, K. & Karring, T. (1994). Effect of local metronidazol application on periodontal healing following guided tissue regeneration. Clinical findings. *Journal of Periodontology* **65**, 914-920.

Sander, L. & Karring, T. (1995). New attachment and bone formation in periodontal defects following treatment of submerged roots with guided tissue regeneration. *Journal of Clinical Periodontology* **22**, 295-299.

Sanders, J.J., Sepe, W.W., Bowers, G.M., Koch, R.W., Williams, J.E., Lekas, J.S., Mellonig, J.T., Pelleu, G.B. Jr. & Gambill, V. (1983). Clinical evaluation of freeze-dried bone allografts in periodontal osseous defects. Part III. Composite freeze-dried bone allografts with and without autogenous bone grafts. *Journal of Periodontology* **54**, 1-8.

Sanz, M. & Giovannoli, J.L. (2000). Focus on furcation defects: guided tissue regeneration. *Periodontology 2000* **22**, 169-189.

Sapkos, S.W. (1986). The use of periograft in periodontal defects. Histologic findings. *Journal of Periodontology* **57**, 7-13.

Schaffer, E.M. & Zander, H.A. (1953). Histological evidence of reattachment of periodontal pockets. *Parodontologie* **7**, 101-107.

Schallhorn, R.G. (1967). Eradication of bifurcation defects utilizing frozen autogenous hip marrow implants. *Periodontal Abstracts* **15**, 101-105.

Schallhorn, R.G. (1968). The use of autogenous hip marrow biopsy implants for bony crater defects. *Journal of Periodontology* **39**, 145-147.

Schallhorn, R.G. & Hiatt, W.H. (1972). Human allografts of iliac cancellous bone and marrow in periodontal osseous defects. II. Clinical observations. *Journal of Periodontology* **43**, 67-81.

Schallhorn, R.G., Hiatt, W.H, & Boyce, W. (1970). Iliac transplants in periodontal therapy. *Journal of Periodontology* **41**, 566-580.

Schallhorn, R. G. & McClain, P. K. (1988). Combined osseous composite grafting, root conditioning, and guided tissue regeneration. *International Journal of Periodontics and Restorative Dentistry* **4**, 9-31.

Schwartz, Z., Mellonig, J.T., Carnes, D.L. Jr., de la Fontaine, J., Cochran, D.L., Dean, D.D. & Boyan, B.D. (1996). Ability of commercial demineralized freeze-dried bone allograft to induce new bone formation. *Journal of Periodontology* **67**, 918-926.

Sculean, A., Donos, N., Brecx, M., Reich, E. & Karring, T. (2000). Treatment of intrabony defects with guided tissue regeneration and enamel-matrix proteins. An experimental study in monkeys. *Journal of Clinical Periodontology* **27**, 466-472.

Sculean, A., Donos, N., Chiantella, G.C., Windisch, P., Reich, E. & Brecx, M. (1999a). GTR with bioresorbable membranes in the treatment of intrabony defects: a clinical and histologic study. *International Journal of Periodontics and Restorative Dentistry* **19**, 501-509.

Sculean, A., Donos, N., Windisch, P. Brecx, M., Gera, I., Reich, E. & Karring, T. (1999b). Healing of human intrabony defects following treatment with enamel matrix proteins or guided tissue regeneration. *Journal of Periodontal Research* **34**, 310-322.

Selvig, K., Kersten, B., Chamberlain, A., Wikesjo, U.M.E. & Nilveus, R. (1992). Regenerative surgery of intrabony periodontal defects using e-PTFE barrier membranes. Scanning electron microscopic evaluation of retrieved membranes vs. clinical healing. *Journal of Periodontology* **63**, 974-978.

Selvig, K., Kersten, B. & Wikesjö, U.M.E. (1993). Surgical treatment of intrabony periodontal defects using expanded polytetrafluoroethylene barrier membranes: influence of defect configuration on healing response. *Journal of Periodontology* **64**, 730-733.

Selvig, K. A., Nilveus, R. E., Fitzmorris, L., Kersten, B. & Thorsandi, S. S. (1990). Scanning electron microscopic observations of cell population and bacterial contamination of membranes used for guided periodontal tissue regeneration in humans. *Journal of Periodontology* **61**, 515-520.

Shahmiri, S., Singh, I.J. & Stahl, S.S. (1992). Clinical response to the use of the HTR polymer implant in human intrabony lesions. *International Journal of Periodontics and Restorative Dentistry* **12**, 294-299.

Shigeyama, Y., D'Errico, J.A., Stone, R. & Somerman, M.J. (1995). Commercially-prepared allograft material has biological activity in vitro. *Journal of Periodontology* **66**, 478-487.

Sigurdsson, J.T., Hardwick, R., Bogle, G.C. & Wikesjö, U.M.E. (1994). Periodontal repair in dogs: space provision by reinforced e-PTFE membranes enhances bone and cementum regeneration in large supraalveolar defects. *Journal of Periodontology* **65**, 350-356.

Sigurdsson, T.J., Lee, M.B., Kubota, K., Turek, T.J., Wazney, J.M. & Wikesjö, U.M.E. (1995). Periodontal repair in dogs: Recombinant human bone morphogenetic protein-2 significantly enhances periodontal regeneration. *Journal of Periodontology* **66**, 131-138.

Silvestri, M., Ricci, G., Rasperini, G., Sartori, S. & Cattaneo, V. (2000). Comparison of treatments of infrabony defects with enamel matrix derivate, guided tissue regeneration with a nonresorbable membrane and Widman modified flap. A pilot study. *Journal of Clinical Periodontology* **27**, 603-610.

Smith, M.E., Nowzari, H., Contreras, A., Flynn, J., Morrison, J. & Slots, J. (1998). Clinical and microbiological evaluation of a bioabsorbable and a nonresorbable barrier membrane in the treatment of periodontal intraosseous lesions. *Journal of Periodontology* **69**, 445-453.

Smith MacDonald, E., Nowzari, H., Contreras, A., Flynn, J., Morrison, J. & Slots, J. (1998). Clinical evaluation of a bioabsorbable and a nonresorbable membrane in the treatment of periodontal intraosseous lesions. *Journal of Periodontology* **69**, 445-453.

Snyder, A.J., Levin, M.P. & Cutright, D.E. (1984). Alloplastic implants of tricalcium phosphate ceramic in human periodontal osseous defects. *Journal of Periodontology* **55**, 273-277.

Sonis, S.T., Williams, R.C., Jeffcoat, M.K., Black, R. & Shklar, G. (1985). Healing of spontaneous periodontal defects in dogs treated with xenogeneic demineralized bone. *Journal of Periodontology* **56**, 470-479.

Stahl, S. & Froum, S. (1986). Histologic evaluation of human intraosseous healing responses to the placement of tricalcium phosphate ceramic implants. I. Three to eight months. *Journal of Periodontology* **57**, 211-217.

Stahl, S. & Froum, S. (1987). Histologic and clinical responses to porous hydroxylapatite implants in human periodontal defects. Three to twelve months postimplantation. *Journal of Periodontology* **58**, 689-695.

Stahl, S. & Froum, S. (1991a). Human suprabony healing responses following root demineralization and coronal flap anchorage. Histologic responses in seven sites. *Journal of Clinical Periodontology* **18**, 685-689.

Stahl, S. & Froum, S. (1991b). Healing of human suprabony lesions treated with guided tissue regeneration and coronally anchored flaps. Case reports. *Journal of Clinical Periodontology* **18**, 69-74.

Stahl, S., Froum, S. & Kushner, L. (1983). Healing responses of human teeth following the use of debridement grafting and citric acid root conditioning. II. Clinical and histologic observations: One year post-surgery. *Journal of Periodontology* **54**, 325-338.

Stahl, S., Froum, S. & Tarnow, D. (1990a). Human histologic responses to the placement of guided tissue regenerative techniques in intrabony lesions. Case reports on nine sites. *Journal of Clinical Periodontology* **17**, 191-198.

Stahl, S., Froum, S. & Tarnow, D. (1990b). Human clinical and histologic responses to the placement of HTR polymer particles in 11 intrabony lesions. *Journal of Periodontology* **61**, 269-274.

Stahl, S., Slavkin, H.C., Yamada, L. & Levine, S. (1972). Speculations about gingival repair. *Journal of Periodontology* **43**, 395-402.

Stavropoulos, A., Karring, E.S., Kostopoulos, L. & Karring, T. (2002). Deproteinized bovine bone and gentamicin as an adjunct to GTR in the treatment of intrabony defects. A randomized controlled clinical study. *Journal of Clinical Periodontology* (in press).

Steiner, S.S., Crigger, M. & Egelberg, J. (1981). Connective tissue regeneration to periodontal diseased teeth. II. Histologic observation of cases following replaced flap surgery. *Journal of Periodontal Research* **16**, 109-116.

Strub, J.R., Gaberthüel, T.W. & Firestone A.R. (1979). Comparison of tricalcium phosphate and frozen allogenic bone implants in man. *Journal of Periodontology* **50**, 624-629.

Tanner, M.G., Solt, C.W. & Vuddhakanok, S. (1988). An evaluation of new attachment formation using a microfibrillar collagen barrier. *Journal of Periodontology* **59**, 524-530.

Tatakis, D.N., Promsudthi, A. & Wikesjö, U.M.E. (1999). Devices for periodontal regeneration. *Periodontology 2000* **19**, 59-73.

Tempro, P. & Nalbandian, J. (1993). Colonization of retrieved polytetrafluoroethylene membranes: morphological and microbiological observations. *Journal of Periodontology* **64**, 162-168.

Terranova, V. & Wikesjö, U.M.E. (1987). Extracellular matrices and polypeptide growth factors as mediators of functions of cells of the periodontium. *Journal of Periodontology* **58**, 371-380.

Tonetti, M., Cortellini, P., Suvan, J.E., Adriaens, P., Baldi, C., Dubravec, D., Fonzar, A., Fourmosis, I., Magnani, C., Muller-Campanile, V., Patroni, S., Sanz, M., Vangsted, T., Zabalegui, I., Pini Prato, G. & Lang, N.P. (1998). Generalizability of the added benefits of guided tissue regeneration in the treatment of deep intrabony defects. Evaluation in a multi-center randomized controlled clinical trial. *Journal of Periodontology* **69**, 1183-1192.

Tonetti, M., Lang, N.P., Cortellini, P. et al. (2002). Enamel matrix proteins in the regenerative therapy of deep intrabony defects. A multicenter randomized controlled clinical trial. *Journal of Clinical Periodontology* **28** (in press).

Tonetti, M., Pini-Prato, G. & Cortellini, P. (1993a). Periodontal regeneration of human infrabony defects. IV. Determinants of the healing response. *Journal of Periodontology* **64**, 934-940.

Tonetti, M., Pini-Prato, G. & Cortellini, P. (1995). Effect of cigarette smoking on periodontal healing following GTR in infrabony defects. A preliminary retrospective study. *Journal of Clinical Periodontology* **22**, 229-234.

Tonetti, M., Pini-Prato, G. & Cortellini, P. (1996a). Factors affecting the healing response of intrabony defects following guided tissue regeneration and access flap surgery. *Journal of Clinical Periodontology* **23**, 548-556.

Tonetti, M., Pini-Prato, G. & Cortellini, P. (1996b). Guided tissue regeneration of deep intrabony defects in strategically important prosthetic abutments. *International Journal of Periodontics and Restorative Dentistry* **16**, 378-387.

Tonetti, M. S., Pini-Prato, G. P., Williams, R. C. & Cortellini, P. (1993b). Periodontal regeneration of human infrabony defects. III. Diagnostic strategies to detect bone gain. *Journal of Periodontology* **64**, 269-277.

Trombelli, L. (1999). Periodontal regeneration in gingival recession defects. *Periodontology 2000* **19**, 138-150.

Trombelli, L., Kim, C.K., Zimmerman, G.J. & Wikesjö, U.M.E. (1997). Retrospective analysis of factors related to clinical outcome of guided tissue regeneration procedures in intrabony defects. *Journal of Clinical Periodontology* **24**, 366-371.

Turner, D.W. & Mellonig, J.T. (1981). Antigenicity of freeze-dried bone allograft in periodontal osseous defects. *Journal of Periodontal Research* **16**, 89-99.

Urist, M.R. (1980) *Fundamental and Clinical Bone Physiology*. Philadelphia: J.B. Lippincott Co. pp. 348-353.

Urist, M.R. & Strates, B. (1970). Bone formation in implants of partially and wholly demineralized bone matrix. *Journal of Clinical Orthopedics* **71**, 271-278.

Van der Velden, U. & de Vries, J.H. (1978). Introduction of a new periodontal probe: the pressure probe. *Journal of Clinical Periodontology* **5**, 188-197.

Van Swol, R., Ellinger, R., Pfeifer, J., Barton, N. & Blumenthal, N. (1993). Collagen membrane barrier therapy to guide regeneration in class II furcations in humans. *Journal of Periodontology* **64**, 622-629.

Vincenzi, D., De Chiesa, A. & Trisi, P. (1998). Guided tissue regeneration using a resorbable membrane in gingival recession-type defects: a histologic case report in humans. *International Journal of Periodontics and Restorative Dentistry* **18**, 24-33.

Wade, A.B. (1962). An assessment of the flap operation. *Dental Practitioner and Dental Records* **13**, 11-20.

Wade, A.B. (1966). The flap operation. *Journal of Periodontology* **37**, 95-99.

Waerhaug, J. (1952). The gingival pocket. *Odontologisk Tidsskrift* **60**, Supplement 1.

Wallace, S., Gellin, R., Miller, C. & Miskin, D. (1994). Guided tissue regeneration with and without decalcified freeze-dried bone in mandibular class II furcation invasions. *Journal of Periodontology* **65**, 244-254.

Wang, H., O'Neal, R., Thomas, C., Shyr, Y. & MacNeil, R. (1994). Evaluation of an absorbable collagen membrane in treating Class II furcation defects. *Journal of Periodontology* **65**, 1029-1036.

Warrer, K., Karring, T. & Gotfredsen, K. (1993). Periodontal ligament formation around different types of dental titanium implants. I. The selftapping screw type implant system. *Journal of Periodontology* **64**, 29-34.

Warrer, K., Karring, T., Nyman, S. & Gogolewski, S. (1992). Guided tissue regeneration using biodegradable membranes of polylactic acid or polyurethane. *Journal of Clinical Periodontology* **19**, 633-640.

Werbitt, M. (1987). Decalcified freeze-dried bone allografts: a successful procedure in the reduction of intrabony defects. *International Journal of Periodontics and Restorative Dentistry* **7**, 56-63.

West, T.L. & Brustein, D.D. (1985). Freeze-dried bone and coralline implants compared in the dog. *Journal of Periodontology* **56**, 348-351.

Wilson, J. & Low, S.B. (1992). Bioactive ceramics for periodontal treatment: comparative studies in the Patus monkey. *Journal of Applied Biomaterials* **3**, 123-129.

World Workshop in Periodontology (1996). The American Academy of Periodontology. *Annals of Periodontology* **1**, 618-670.

Wozney, J.M., Rosen, V.B., Celeste, A.J., Mitsock, L.M., Whitters, M.J., Kriz, R.W., Hewick, R.M. & Wang, E.M. (1988). Novel regulators of bone formation: molecular clones and activities. *Science* **243**, 1528-1534.

Younger, W.J. (1970). Pyorrhea alveolaris from a bacteriological standpoint with a report of some investigations and remarks on the treatment. *International Dental Journal* **20**, 413-423.

Yukna, R. (1990). HTR polymer grafts in human periodontal osseous defects. I. 6-month clinical results. *Journal of Periodontology* **61**, 633-642.

Yukna, R. (1992). Clinical human comparison of expanded polytetrafluoroethylene barrier membrane and freeze dried dura mater allografts for guided tissue regeneration of lost periodontal support. *Journal of Periodontology* **63**, 431-442.

Yukna, R. (1994). Clinical evaluation of coralline calcium carbonate as a bone replacement graft material in human periodontal osseous defects. *Journal of Periodontology* **65**, 177-185.

Yukna, R., Bowers, G.M., Lawrence, J.J. & Fedi, P.F. (1976). A clinical study of healing in humans following the excisional new attachment procedure. *Journal of Periodontology* **47**, 696-700.

Yukna, R., Cassingham, R.J., Caudill, R.F., Evans, G.F., Miller, S., Mayer, E.T. & Simon, J.F. (1986). Six month evaluation of Calcitite (hydroxyapatite ceramics) in periodontal osseous defects. *International Journal of Periodontics and Restorative Dentistry* **6**, 34-45.

Yukna, R., Harrison, B.G., Caudill, R.F., Evans, G.H., Mayer, E.T. & Miller, S. (1985). Evaluation of durapatite as an alloplastic implant in periodontal osseous defects. II. Twelve month re-entry results. *Journal of Periodontology* **56**, 540-547.

Yukna, R., Mayer, E.T. & Amos, S.M. (1989). 5-year evaluation of durapatite ceramic alloplastic implants in periodontal osseous defects. *Journal of Periodontology* **60**, 544-551.

Yukna, R. & Yukna, C.N. (1998). A 5-year follow-up of 16 patients treated with coralline calcium carbonate (BIOCORAL) bone replacement grafts in infrabony defects. *Journal of Clinical Periodontology* **25**, 1036-1040.

Zamet, J.S., Darbar, U.R., Griffiths, G.S., Bulman, J.S., Brägger, U., Burgin, W. & Newman, H.N. (1997). Particulate bioglass as a grafting material in the treatment of periodontal intrabony defects. *Journal of Clinical Periodontology* **24**, 410-418.

Zybutz, M.D., Laurell, L., Rapoport, D.A. & Persson, G.R. (2000). Treatment of intrabony defects with resorbable materials, non-resorbable materials and flap debridement. *Journal of Clinical Periodontology* **27**, 167-178.

CHAPTER 29

Treatment of Furcation-Involved Teeth

GIANFRANCO CARNEVALE, ROBERTO PONTORIERO AND JAN LINDHE

Terminology

Anatomy

Diagnosis

Differential diagnosis

Therapy
  Scaling and root planing
  Furcation plasty
  Tunnel preparation
  Root separation and resection (RSR)
  Regeneration of furcation defects
  Extraction

Prognosis

Detailed knowledge of the morphology of the multi-rooted teeth and their position in the dental arch is a fundamental prerequisite for a proper understanding of problems which may occur when such teeth become involved in destructive periodontal disease. The first part of this chapter therefore includes a brief description of some important anatomic features of the root complexes and related structures of premolars and molars.

TERMINOLOGY

Root complex is the portion of a tooth that is located apical of the cemento-enamel junction (CEJ), i.e. the portion that normally is covered with a root cementum. The root complex may be divided into two parts: the *root trunk* and the *root cone(s)* (Fig. 29-1).

The *root trunk* represents the *undivided region* of the root. The height of the root trunk is defined as the distance between the CEJ and the separation line (furcation) between two root cones (roots). Depending on the position of the separation line the height of the root trunk may vary from one surface to the next in one given molar or premolar.

The *root cone* is included in the *divided region* of the root complex. The root cone (root) may vary in size and position and may at certain levels be connected to or separated from other root cones. Two or more root

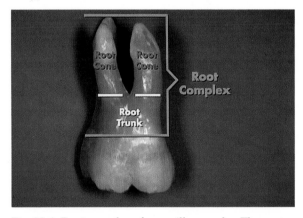

Fig. 29-1. Root complex of a maxillary molar. The root complex is separated into one undivided region: the root trunk, and one divided region: the (3) root cones.

cones make up the *furcated region* of the root complex (Fig. 29-2a).

The *furcation* is the area located between individual root cones.

Furcation entrance: the transitional area between the undivided and the divided part of the root (Fig. 29-2a,b).

Furcation fornix: the roof of the furcation (Fig. 29-2b).

Degree of separation: the angle of separation between two roots (cones) (Fig. 29-3a).

Divergence is the distance between two roots; this distance normally increases in apical direction (Fig. 29-3a).

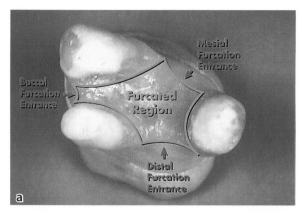
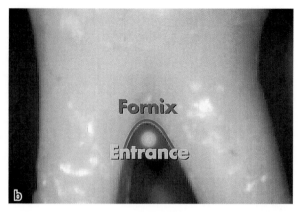

Fig. 29-2. Apical-occlusal view of a maxillary molar where the three root cones make up the furcated region and the three furcation entrances (a). A buccal view of the furcation entrance and of its roof (b).

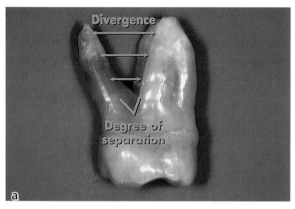
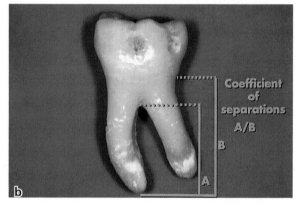

Fig. 29-3. Photographs illustrating the angle (degree) of separation and the divergence between the mesiobuccal and the palatal roots of a maxillary molar (a). The coefficient of separation (A/B) of the illustrated mandibular molar is 0.8 (A = 8 mm; B = 10 mm).

Coefficient of separation: the length of the root cones in relation to the length of the root complex (Fig. 29-3b).

Fusion between divergent root cones may occur. The fusion may be complete or incomplete. In the case of an incomplete fusion, the root cones may be fused in the area close to the CEJ but separated in a more apical region of the root complex.

ANATOMY

Maxillary molars

As a general rule the maxillary first molar, in all respects – crown and individual roots – is larger than the second molar, which in turn is larger than the third molar.

The first and second molars most often have three roots; one mesiobuccal, one distobuccal and one palatal. The mesiobuccal root is normally vertically positioned while the distobuccal and the palatal roots are inclined. The distobuccal root projects distally and the palatal root projects in palatal direction (Fig. 29-4a-c). The cross-sections of the distobuccal and the palatal roots are generally circular. The palatal root is gener-

ally wider in mesiodistal than in buccopalatal direction. The distal surface of the mesiobuccal root has a concavity which is about 0.3 mm deep (Bower 1979a,b). This concavity gives the cross-section of the mesiobuccal root an "hour-glass" configuration (Fig. 29-5).

The three furcation entrances of the maxillary first and second molars vary in width and are positioned at varying distances apical of the CEJ. As a rule, the first molar has a shorter root trunk than the second molar. In the first molar the mesial furcation entrance is located about 3 mm from the CEJ, while the buccal is 3.5 mm and the distal entrance about 5 mm apical of CEJ (Abrams & Trachtenberg 1974, Rosenberg 1988). This implies that the furcation fornix is inclined; in the mesiodistal plane the fornix is comparatively close to CEJ at the mesial but closer to apex at the distal surface. The buccal furcation entrance is narrower than its distal and mesial counterparts.

The degree of separation between the roots and their divergence decreases from the first to the second, and from the second to the third maxillary molar.

The mesiobuccal root of the first molar is frequently located more buccally in the arch than the distobuccal root. If the buccal bone plate is thin, the mesiobuccal root frequently projects through the outer surface of

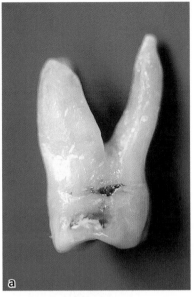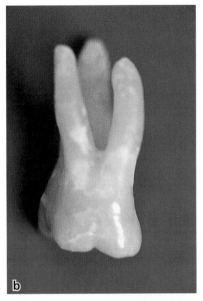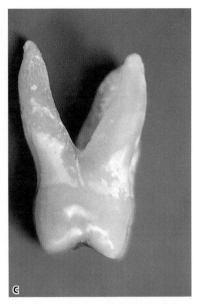

Fig. 29-4. Furcation entrances (a, mesial; b, buccal; c, distal) and the position of the roots of a maxillary first molar.

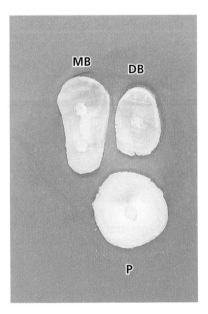

Fig. 29-5. Root-shape of a maxillary first molar in a horizontal cut at the level of the coronal third of the cones. Note the circular shape of the palatal root in comparison with the mesiodistally compressed shape of the mesiobuccal root, which also exhibits a concavity in the distal aspect.

the alveolar bone and bone fenestrations and/or dehiscences may occur.

Maxillary premolars

In about 40% of cases the maxillary first premolars have two root cones – one buccal and one palatal, and hence a mesiodistal furcation. A concavity (about 0.5 mm deep) is often present in the furcation aspect of the buccal root. The furcation is in many cases located in the middle or in the apical third of the root complex (Fig. 29-6). The mean distance between CEJ and the furcation entrance is about 8 mm. The width of the furcation entrance is about 0.7 mm.

Mandibular molars

The mandibular first molar is larger than the second molar, which in turn is larger than the third molar. In the first and second molars the root complex almost always includes two root cones, one mesial and one distal. The mesial root is larger than the distal. The mesial root has a position which is mainly vertical while the distal root projects distally. The mesial root is wider in the buccolingual direction and has a larger cross-section area than the distal root. The cross-section of distal root is circular while the mesial root has an "hour-glass" shape. In addition, on the distal surface of the mesial root, furrows and concavities often occur (Fig. 29-7). The distal concavity of the mesial root is more pronounced than that of the distal root (Bower 1979a,b, Svärdström & Wennström 1988).

The root trunk of the first molar is often shorter than the trunk of the second molar. The furcation entrances of the mandibular first molar, similar to those of the maxillary first molar, are located at different distances from the CEJ. Thus, the lingual entrance is frequently found more apical of CEJ (> 4 mm) than the buccal

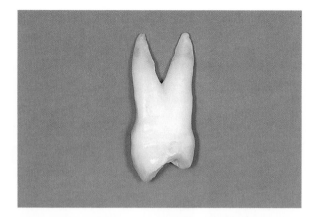

Fig. 29-6. A maxillary first premolar with the furcation located in the apical third of the root complex.

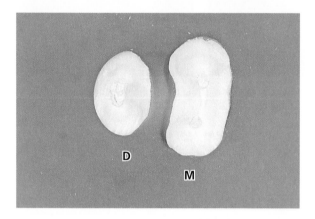

Fig. 29-7. "Hour-glass" shape of the mesial root – with a concavity in the distal aspect – and the circular shape of the distal root (horizontal section at the level of the coronal third of the cones).

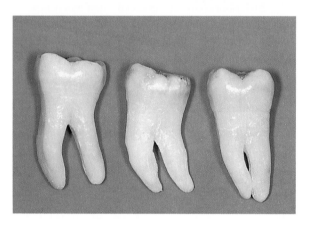

Fig. 29-8. From left to right, differences in degree of separation and in divergence between the root cones from the first to the mandibular third molar.

entrance (> 3 mm). Thus, the furcation fornix is inclined in the buccolingual direction. The buccal furcation entrance is often < 0.75 mm wide while the lingual entrance is > 0.75 mm in most cases (Bower 1979a,b).

The degree of separation and divergence between the roots decreases from the first to the third molar (Fig. 29-8).

It should also be observed that the buccal bone plate is thinner outside the roots of the first than of the second molar. Bone fenestrations and dehiscences are, as a consequence, more frequent in the first than in the second molar region.

Other teeth

Furcations may be present also in teeth which normally have only one root. In fact, two-rooted incisors (Fig. 29-9a), canines (Fig. 29-9b) and mandibular premolars may exist. Occasionally three-rooted maxillary premolars (Fig. 29-10a) and three-rooted mandibular molars can be found (Fig. 29-10b).

DIAGNOSIS

The presence of furcation-involved teeth in a periodontal patient will influence the treatment plan (see Chapter 19). The selection of procedures to be used in the treatment of periodontal disease at multirooted teeth can first be made when the presence and depth of furcation lesions have been assessed. In this examination traditional measures of periodontal disease are used (see Chapter 18) but special attention is paid to

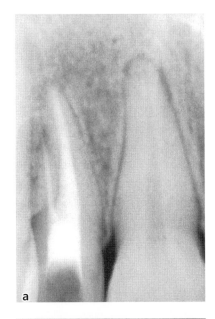

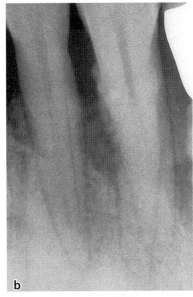

Fig. 29-9. Radiographs illustrating morphologic variations represented by two-rooted (a) maxillary lateral incisor and (b) mandibular canine.

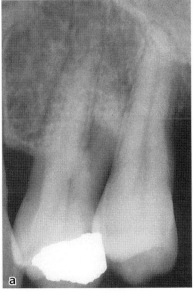

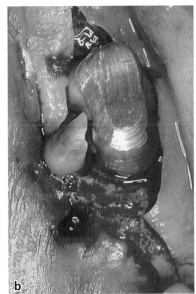

Fig. 29-10. Anatomic variation represented in a radiograph of a three-rooted mandibular first premolar (a). Clinical photograph illustrating, during surgery, the separation – before extraction – of an "abnormal" second mesial root of a mandibular molar (b).

findings from clinical *probing* and analysis of *radiographs* from the premolar-molar regions.

The classification description of the involved furcation is based on the amount of periodontal tissue destruction that has occurred in the interradicular area, i.e. degree of "horizontal root exposure" or attachment loss that exists within the root complex. Hamp et al. (1975) has suggested the following classification of the involved furcation:

- Degree I: Horizontal loss of periodontal support not exceeding ⅓ of the width of the tooth (Fig. 29-11a).
- Degree II: Horizontal loss of periodontal support exceeding ⅓ of the width of the tooth, but not encompassing the total width of the furcation area (Fig. 29-11b).
- Degree III: Horizontal "through and through" destruction of the periodontal tissues in the furcation area (Fig. 29-11c).

It is important to understand that each furcation en-

trance must be examined and each entrance must be classified according to the above criteria.

Probing

The buccal furcation entrance of the *maxillary molars* and the buccal and lingual furcation entrances of the *mandibular molars* are normally accessible for examination using a curved graduated periodontal probe (Fig. 29-12a,b), an explorer or a small curette. The examination of approximal furcations is more difficult, in particular when neighboring teeth are present. Large contact areas between the teeth further impair access to approximal furcation entrances.

In maxillary molars the mesial furcation entrance is located much closer to the palatal than to the buccal tooth surface. Thus, the mesial furcation should be probed from the palatal aspect of the tooth (Fig. 29-13). The distal furcation entrance of a *maxillary molar* is generally located midway between the buccal and palatal surfaces and, as a consequence, this furcation

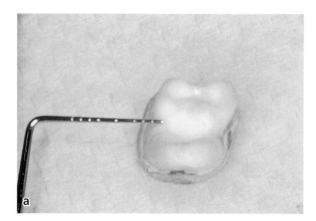

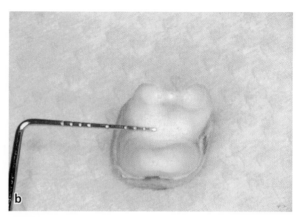

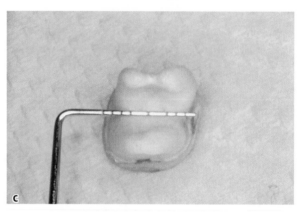

Fig. 29-11. Different degrees of furcation involvement in relation to the probe (penetration/superimposition) in the interradicular space of a mandibular molar. (a) degree I; (b) degree II; (c) degree III.

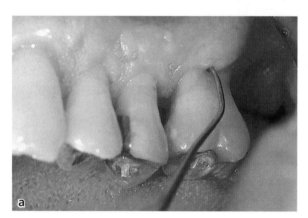

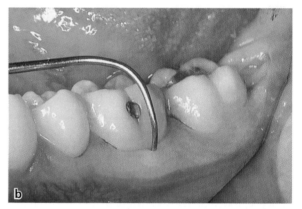

Fig. 29-12. Easily accessible vestibular furcation entrances for probing of a (a) maxillary molar and (b) mandibular molar.

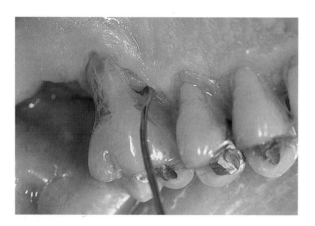

Fig. 29-13. Common access for probing of a mesial furcation entrance of a maxillary molar. The mesial furcation entrance is generally located at the palatal aspect of the tooth, while the distal entrance is located midway between the buccal and the palatal surface.

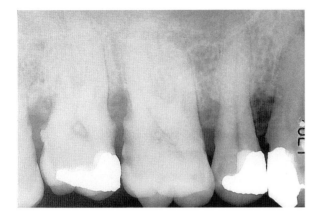

Fig. 29-14. Radiograph showing the location of the interdental bone level in relation to the furcation entrances of the maxillary first and second molar.

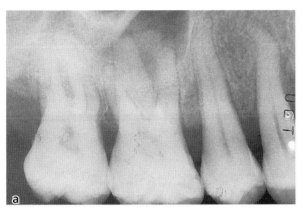

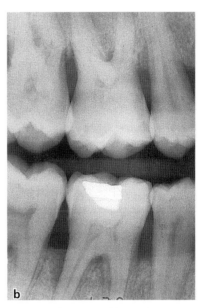

Fig. 29-15. Radiographs of the right maxillary molar region where, with a normal bisecting projection, the furcation defect of the first molar is not evident (a). It is, however, easily identified in a bitewing radiograph (b).

could be probed from either the buccal or the palatal aspect of the tooth.

In *maxillary premolars* the root anatomy often varies considerably. The roots may also harbor irregularities such as longitudinal furrows, invaginations or true furcations, which may open at varying distances from the CEJ. Due to the above variations and due to the limited access, the clinical assessment of a furcation involvement in maxillary premolars is often difficult. In some patients, a furcation involvement may, in such teeth, first be identified after the elevation of a soft tissue flap.

Radiographs

Radiographs must always be obtained to confirm findings made during probing of a furcation-involved tooth. The radiographic examination should include both paralleling "periapical" and vertical "bite-wing" radiographs. In the radiographs the location of the interdental bone as well as the bone level within the root complex should be examined (Fig. 29-14). Situations may occur when findings from clinical probing

and from the radiographs are inconsistent. Thus, the localized but extensive attachment loss which may be detected within the root complex of a maxillary molar with the use of a probe, will not always appear in the radiograph. This may be due to the superimposition in the radiograph of the palatal root and of remaining bone structures (Fig. 29-15a). In such a case, additional radiographs with different angles of orientation of the central beam should be used to identify bone loss within the root complex (Fig. 29-15b).

DIFFERENTIAL DIAGNOSIS

A lesion in the interradicular space of a multirooted tooth may be associated with problems originating from the root canal or be the result of occlusal overload. The treatment of a furcation-involved tooth, therefore, should not be initiated until a proper differential diagnosis of the lesion has been made.

Pulpal pathosis may sometimes cause a lesion in the periodontal tissues of the furcation (see Chapter 14). The radiographic appearance of such a defect may

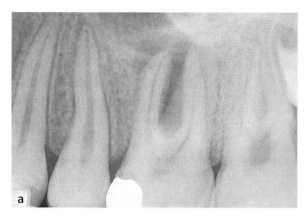 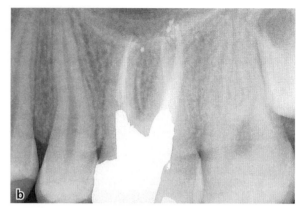

Fig. 29-16. Radiographs demonstrating a destruction of interradicular bone and the presence of periapical defects at the mesial and distal roots of a maxillary first molar (a). Radiographic appearance of complete healing of the interradicular and periapical lesions after endodontic treatment (b).

have some features in common with a plaque-associated furcation lesion. In order to differentiate between the two lesions the vitality of the affected tooth must *always* be tested. If the tooth is vital, a plaque-associated lesion should be suspected. If the tooth is non-vital, the furcation involvement may have an endodontic origin. In such a case, proper endodontic treatment must *always* precede periodontal therapy. In fact, endodontic therapy may resolve the inflammatory lesion, soft and hard tissue healing occur and the furcation defect disappear (Fig. 29-16a,b). If signs of healing of a furcation defect fail to appear within 2 months following endodontic treatment, the furcation involvement is probably associated with marginal periodontitis.

Trauma from occlusion

Forces elicited by occlusal interferences, e.g. bruxers and clenchers (see Chapters 15, 30), may cause inflammation and tissue destruction or adaptation within the interradicular area of a multirooted tooth. In such a tooth a radiolucency may be seen in the radiograph of the root complex. The tooth may exhibit increased mobility. Probing, however, fails to detect an involvement of the furcation. In this particular situation, occlusal adjustment must always precede periodontal therapy. If the defects seen within the root complex are of "occlusal" origin, the tooth will become stabilized and the defects disappear within weeks following correction of the occlusal overload (Fig. 29-17a,b).

THERAPY

Treatment of a defect in the furcation region of a multi-rooted tooth is intended to meet two objectives:

1. the elimination of the microbial plaque from the exposed surfaces of the root complex
2. the establishment of an anatomy of the affected

surfaces that facilitates proper self-performed plaque control.

Different methods of therapy are recommended:

Furcation involvement degree I

Recommended therapy: Scaling and root planing. Furcation plasty.

Furcation involvement degree II

Recommended therapy: Furcation plasty. Tunnel preparation. Root resection. Tooth extraction. Guided tissue regeneration at mandibular molars.

Furcation involvement degree III

Recommended therapy: Tunnel preparation. Root resection. Tooth extraction.

Scaling and root planing

Scaling and planing of the root surfaces in the furcation entrance of a degree I involvement in most situations result in the resolution of the inflammatory lesion in the gingiva. Healing will re-establish a normal gingival anatomy with the soft tissue properly adapted to the hard tissue walls of the furcation entrance (Fig. 29-18a,b).

Furcation plasty

Furcation plasty (Fig 29-19a-f) is a resective treatment modality which should lead to the elimination of the interradicular defect. Tooth substance is removed (odontoplasty) and the alveolar bone crest is remodeled (osteoplasty) at the level of the furcation entrance.

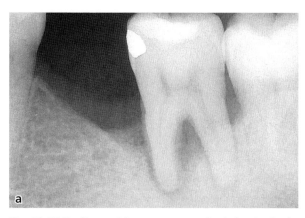
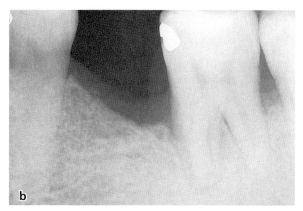

Fig. 29-17. Radiographic appearance of a defect in the furcation area caused by occlusal overload (a). After occlusal adjustment the interradicular defect spontaneously healed, as documented 6 months after therapy in a radiograph (courtesy of M. Cattabriga).

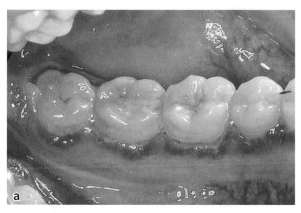
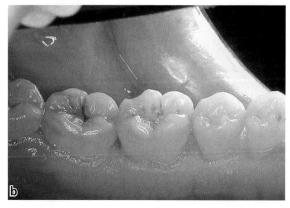

Fig. 29-18. Resolution of inflammatory lesions in the gingiva achieved by scaling, root planing and the re-establishment of a correct tissue morphology in the interradicular area of degree I furcation involved mandibular molars. (a) Before therapy, (b) 6 months after therapy.

Furcation plasty is used mainly at buccal and lingual furcations. At approximal surfaces access is often too limited for this treatment.

Furcation plasty involves the following procedures:

- The dissection and reflection of a soft tissue flap to obtain access to the interradicular area and the surrounding bone structures.
- The removal of the inflammatory soft tissue from the furcation area followed by careful scaling and root planing of the exposed root surfaces.
- The removal of crown and root substance in the furcation area (odontoplasty) to eliminate or reduce the horizontal component of the defect and to widen the furcation entrance.
- The recontouring of the alveolar bone crest in order to reduce the buccal-lingual dimension of a bone defect in the furcation area.
- The positioning and the suturing of the mucosal flaps at the level of the alveolar crest in order to cover the furcation entrance with soft tissue. Following healing a "papilla"-like tissue should close the entrance of the furcation.

Care must be exercised when odontoplasty is per-

formed on vital teeth. Excessive removal of tooth structure will enhance the risk for increased root sensitivity.

Tunnel preparation

Tunnel preparation is a technique used to treat deep degree II and degree III furcation defects in mandibular molars. This type of resective therapy can be offered at mandibular molars which have a short root trunk, a wide separation angle and long divergence between the mesial and distal root. The procedure includes the surgical exposure and management of the entire furcation area of the affected molar.

Following the reflection of buccal and lingual mucosal flaps, the granulation tissue in the defect is removed and the root surfaces are scaled and planed. The furcation area is widened by the removal of some of the interradicular bone. The alveolar bone crest is recontoured and to obtain a flat outline of the bone, some of the interdental bone, mesial and distal to the tooth in the region, is also removed. Following hard tissue resection enough space has been established in the furcation region to allow access for cleaning devices to be used during self-performed plaque control

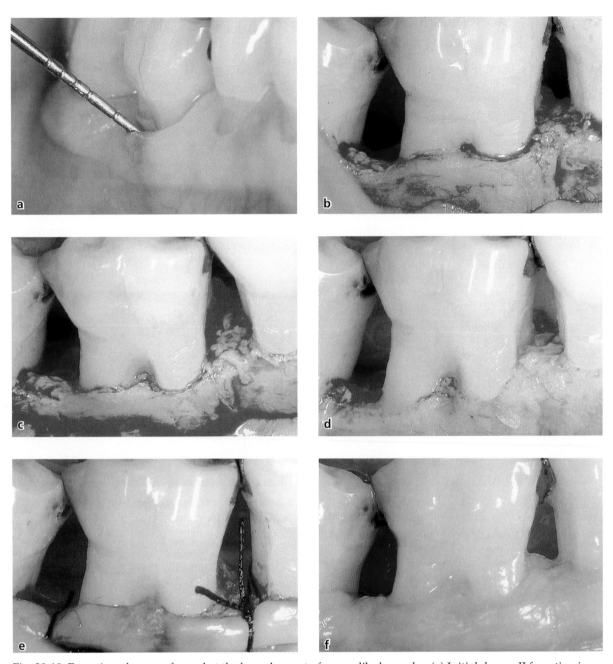

Fig. 29-19. Furcation plasty performed at the buccal aspect of a mandibular molar. (a) Initial degree II furcation involvement. (b) After flap elevation, removal of the granulation tissue and scaling of the exposed root surfaces. (c) After odontoplasty. (d) After osteoplasty. (e) Apical position of the flap managed by periosteal sutures. (f) Healing resulting in the elimination of the furcation defect and in the establishment of a proper soft tissue morphology.

measures (Fig. 29-20a,b). The flaps are apically positioned to the surgically established interradicular and interproximal bone level.

During maintenance the exposed root surfaces should be treated by topical application of chlorhexidine digluconate and fluoride varnish. This surgical procedure should be used with caution, because there is a pronounced risk for root sensitivity and for carious lesions developing on the denuded root surfaces within artificially prepared tunnels (Hamp et al. 1975).

Root separation and resection (RSR)

Root separation involves the sectioning of the root complex and the maintenance of all roots. *Root resection* involves the sectioning and the removal of one or two roots of a multirooted tooth.

RSR is frequently used in cases of deep degree II and degree III furcation involved molars.

Before RSR is performed the following factors must be considered:

The length of the root trunk
In a patient with progressive periodontal disease a tooth with a *short* root trunk may have an early involvement of the furcation (Larato 1975, Gher & Vern-

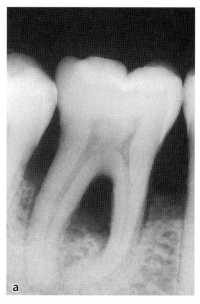
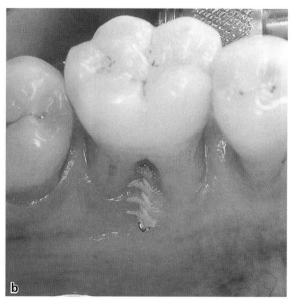

Fig. 29-20. Tunnel preparation of a degree III-involved mandibular molar. Radiograph (a) and photograph (b) showing a wide interradicular space where self-performed plaque control can be obtained by the use of an interproximal brush.

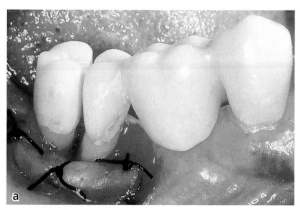
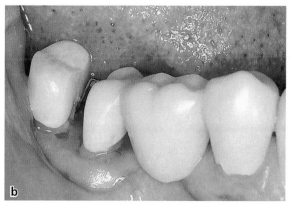

Fig. 29-21. Effect of orthodontic treatment of a separated mandibular molar with a small root divergence. (a) After root separation. (b) 3 months after completion of orthodontic therapy.

ino 1980). A tooth with a short root trunk is a good candidate for RSR; the amount of remaining periodontal tissue support following separation and resection is often sufficient to ensure the stability of the remaining root cone. If the root trunk is *long*, the furcation involvement occurs later in the disease process, but once established the amount of periodontal tissue support left apical of the furcation may be insufficient to allow RSR.

The divergence between the root cones
The distance between the root cones must be considered. Roots with a short divergence are technically more difficult to separate than roots which are wide apart. In addition, the smaller the divergence is, the smaller also is the interradicular (furcation) space. In cases where the divergence between two roots is small, the possibility of increasing the interradicular distance with an orthodontic root movement may be considered (Fig. 29-21a,b).

The furcation space may also be increased by odontoplasty performed during surgery. Fig. 29-22a-c illustrates that *odontoplasty* was performed on (1) the distal part of the mesial root and (2) the mesial part of the distal root and deep finishing lines prepared for the subsequent restoration (Di Febo et al. 1985).

The length and the shape of the root cones
Short and small root cones (Fig. 29-23) following separation tend to exhibit an increased mobility. Such roots, in addition, have narrow root canals which are difficult to ream. Short and small roots consequently should be regarded as poor abutments for prosthetic restorations.

Fusion between root cones
When a decision has been made to perform RSR, it is important that the clinician first determines that the cones within the root complex are not fused. This is generally an uncomplicated diagnostic problem for

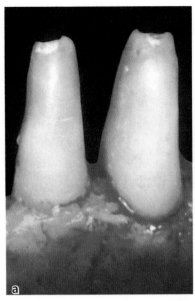
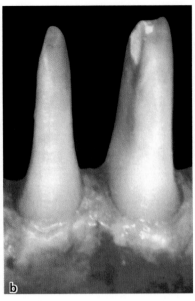
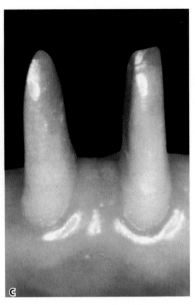

Fig. 29-22. Odontoplasty of a separated mandibular molar performed during surgery to increase the furcation space. After flap elevation and exposure of the alveolar bone, it is evident that the distance between the two roots is small (a). By preparing the interradicular surfaces during surgery (b) the furcation space is increased and is sufficient for self-performed plaque control measures (c).

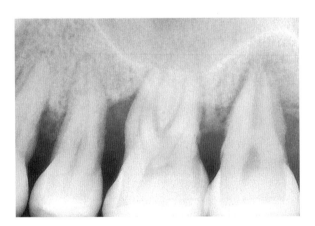

Fig. 29-23. Radiograph showing maxillary molars with thin, short and conical roots.

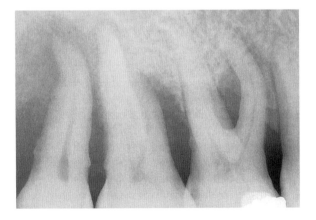

Fig. 29-24. Radiograph indicating the presence of a degree III involvement of the buccal furcation of the maxillary first molar. This tooth is a candidate for root resection.

mandibular molars or for the buccal furcation of maxillary molars (Fig. 29-24). At such teeth the separation area between the roots can easily be identified both with the probe and in a radiograph. It is more difficult to identify a separation line between mesiobuccal (or distobuccal) and palatal roots of a maxillary molar or maxillary first premolar with a narrow root complex. In such situations, a soft tissue flap must often be raised to allow the operator to get proper access to the approximal tooth surfaces. The mesial (or distal) entrance of the furcation must be probed to a depth of 3-5 mm to ascertain that a fusion does NOT exist between the roots scheduled for RSR.

Table 29-1. Root resective treatment possibilities in molars with furcation involvement

Furcation involvement	Root resection	Root resection plus separation of the remaining roots
1 Buccal	Mesiobuccal, Distobuccal	
Mesial	Mesiobuccal, Palatal	
Distal	Distobuccal, Palatal	
2 Buccal & Distal	Distobuccal, Mesiobuccal & Palatal	Palatal
Buccal & Mesial	Mesiobuccal, Distobuccal & Palatal	Palatal, Distobuccal
Mesial & Distal	Palatal, Mesial & Distobuccal	Distobuccal
3 Buccal, Distal & Mesial	Distobuccal & Palatal, Mesiobuccal & Palatal, Mesio & Distobuccal	Palatal, Distobuccal

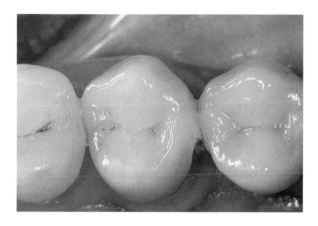

Fig. 29-25. Occlusal view of a restoration using the mesial root of a maxillary first molar as abutment. Note the alignment of the mesial root and the adjacent premolars.

Amount of remaining support around individual roots

This should be determined by probing the entire circumference of the separated roots. It should be observed that a localized deep attachment loss at one surface of one particular root (e.g. on the buccal surface of the palatal root, or the distal surface of the mesiobuccal root of a maxillary molar) may compromise the long-term prognosis for an otherwise ideal root.

Stability of individual roots

Must be examined following root separation. Rule of thumb: the more mobile the root cone is, the less periodontal tissue support remains.

Access for oral hygiene devices

The site must after completion of therapy have an anatomy which facilitates proper self-performed toothcleaning.

Maxillary molars

General example

Several decisions must be made when RSR is planned for a furcation-involved maxillary molar. Since such teeth have three root cones, one or two cones may be retained after separation. Different treatment alternatives exist. They are listed in Table 29-1.

Prior to RSR, the morphology of the individual roots as well as the surface area of each root must be carefully analyzed.

The *distobuccal root* of a maxillary molar (1) is the shortest of the three roots; (2) the root trunk is comparatively long. Thus, the distal root has a small quantity of bone support and once separated, the cone may exhibit increased mobility. The distobuccal root is, therefore, often removed as part of RSR (Rosenberg 1978, Ross & Thompson 1980).

The *mesiobuccal root* has (1) a wide buccopalatal dimension, (2) an hour-glass cross section, and therefore a large root surface area. In fact, the mesiobuccal cone often has a total root surface area that is equal to or greater than that of the palatal root cone. The mesiobuccal root (1) is located centrally in the alveolar process, (2) is properly aligned with the maxillary premolars and is in an ideal position to function as a separate unit (Fig. 29-25). For these reasons, the mesiobuccal root may be preferred for retention when the clinician is selecting between the mesiobuccal or palatal root. It should be remembered, however, that the root canals of the mesiobuccal root are narrow and more difficult to treat than the single and wide canal of the palatal root.

The tissue destruction in the furcation area often causes deep attachment and bone loss at the distal-

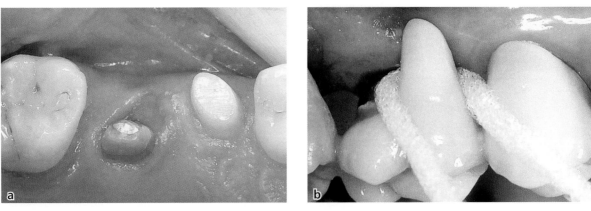

Fig. 29-26. Palatal root of a root-resected maxillary molar serving as a single abutment for a crown restoration (a). A mesiobuccal root was included in the restoration for esthetic reasons (b).

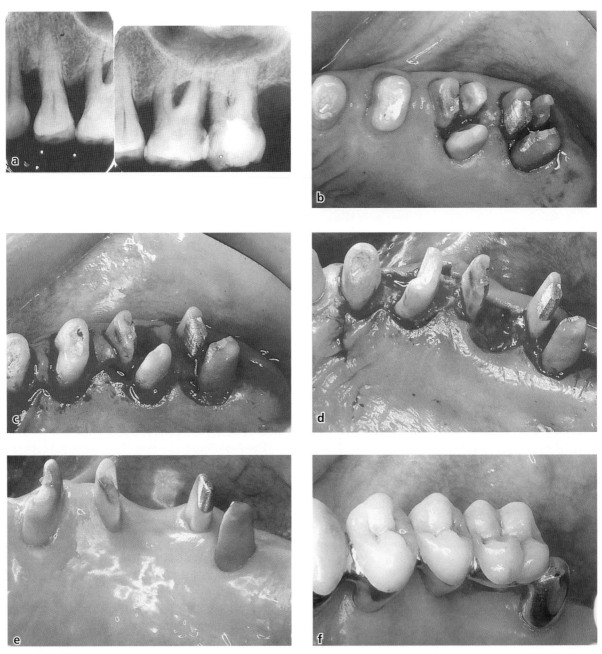

Fig. 29-27. The sequential stages of root resection of two maxillary molars with degree III involvement. Radiograph showing the pre RSR situation (a). The roots were separated before flap elevation (b). The distal roots of both molars and the palatal root of the first molar were extracted and the teeth prepared (c,d). After 3 months of healing (e). The final prosthetic restoration of the site (f).

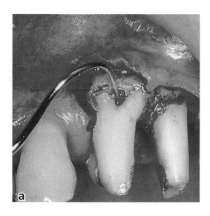
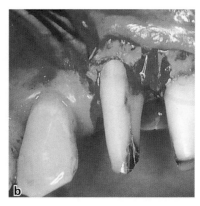

Fig. 29-28. Resection of the distobuccal root of a three-rooted maxillary first premolar.

palatal surface of the mesiobuccal root. In such situations the palatal root remains as the only candidate for retention (Fig. 29-26a,b).

The series of illustrations presented in Fig. 29-27 demonstrates two left maxillary molars (teeth 26 and 27) with degree III involvement of all six furcation entrances. Both teeth were, following a detailed examination and diagnosis, scheduled for treatment with RSR. Note that in this case the second premolar was missing. In cases of advanced periodontal disease at maxillary molars, it is often necessary to separate all three roots of the individual tooth to obtain access to the interradicular area for assessment of the height of the remaining bone at (1) the buccal surface of the palatal root and (2) the palatal surfaces of the buccal roots. Fig. 29-27b illustrates the two maxillary molars with all six roots separated. Because of anatomic considerations and increased mobility, the distobuccal roots of 26 and 27 were extracted (Fig. 29-27c). The palatal root of the first molar had a deep area of localized attachment loss on its buccal surface, was considered to be a poor candidate for a bridge abutment and was extracted. The mesiobuccal root of the first molar as well as the mesiobuccal and palatal roots of the second molar (27) were stable and exhibited moderate probing depth. It was anticipated that at all three roots the anatomy following healing after treatment would allow proper plaque control. The three roots were maintained (Fig. 29-27d). Fig. 29-27e shows the area after 3 months' healing and Fig. 29-27f illustrates the segment properly restored. Since in this segment one premolar was missing, the mesiobuccal root of the first molar was used as second premolar in the prosthetic reconstruction and the two roots of the second molar served as abutments for a crown restoration in the position of a molar.

Maxillary premolars

Root resection of maxillary first premolars is possible only in rare instances due to the anatomy of the root complex (Joseph et al. 1996) (Fig. 29-28a,b). The furcation of this premolar is often located at such an apical level that the maintenance of one root serves no meaningful purpose. In most cases, therefore, the presence

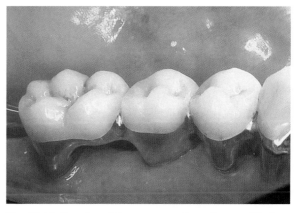

Fig. 29-29. Results of the root resection of a mandibular first molar of which the distal root was retained.

of a deep furcation involvement of degree II or degree III in a maxillary first premolar calls for tooth extraction.

Mandibular molars

If RSR must be applied in a furcation-involved mandibular molar, three treatment alternatives exist:

1. separate the two roots, but maintain both roots (premolarization)
2. separate and extract the mesial root
3. separate and extract the distal root

In some situations, both roots may be maintained following separation.

If one root is to be removed, the following facts must be considered:

The *mesial* root has a significantly greater root surface area than the distal root. The mesial root, however, has an hour-glass-shaped cross section which may be difficult to manage (1) in the self-performed plaque control and (2) in the restorative procedure. In addition, the mesial root frequently has two narrow root canals. The root canals are often close to the external root surface. This may complicate root preparation during the subsequent restorative treatment.

The *distal* root has an oval cross section and, as a rule, only one, wide root canal. The distal root (1) is

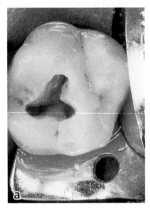
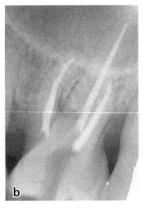
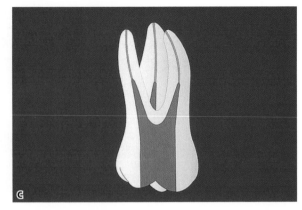

Fig. 29-30. Combined photograph and radiograph showing the "conservative" approach both regarding the access to the pulp chamber (a) and the shaping and filling of the root canal system (b). Schematic illustration showing the temporary restoration of the endodontically treated tooth (c).

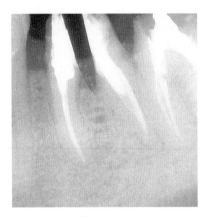

Fig. 29-31. Radiograph illustrating the damage which occurred to the interradicular septum during root separation.

comparatively large, providing a greater mass of dentin to resist root fracture (Langer et al. 1981); (2) is a good candidate for pin or post placement. Further, when the resected mandibular molar is a terminal abutment for a bridge, the retention of the distal root will result in a longer dental arch than would be the case had the mesial root been retained (Fig. 29-29).

Sequence of treatment at RSR

Once anatomic and pathologic characteristics of the root complex (es) of multirooted teeth have been documented, treatment should follow a logical plan (see also Chapter 19).

Endodontic treatment
If the tooth to be resected is vital or if an improper root canal filling was placed in a non-vital tooth, RSR starts with endodontic therapy. Rubber dam can be placed, and optimal conditions thus be established for the important management (cleaning and shaping) of the root canal. The structural integrity of the root must be maintained and minimal amounts of root dentin should be removed (Fig. 29-30a,b). Direct filling with amalgam or chemically cured composite of the endo-

dontically treated tooth should be performed before RSR (Fig. 29-30c). Each root should have individual retention for a restoration which should not break or detach during RSR, removal and relining of the provisional restorations, impressions and prosthetic trys-in. Endocanal posts or endodontic screws are used only if natural retention needs improvement.

Occasionally, a furcation involvement may first be identified during periodontal surgery. In this emergency situation RSR may be completed but the root canal entrance(s) of the remaining root(s) must be properly sealed. Definitive root canal therapy must be completed within two weeks (Smukler & Tagger 1976).

Provisional restoration
Alginate impressions of the area to be treated are taken and sent to the laboratory together with a wax record of the intercuspal position. A provisional restoration is prepared.

RSR
Root separation and root resection may be performed as part of the preparation of the segment for prosthetic rehabilitation ("prosthetic preparation"), i.e. prior to periodontal surgery (Carnevale et al. 1981). During the prosthetic preparation it is important to *avoid*

- exposing the interradicular bone to undue mechanical trauma (Fig. 29-31)
- leaving behind parts of the furcation fornix (Fig. 29-32a-d)
- perforating the root canals
- preparing the vertical surfaces of the remaining roots with sharp angles (Fig. 29-33).

Situation 1: mandibular molar
Following separation, both roots are maintained. The distal surface of the distal root and the mesial surface of the mesial root must be prepared parallel with each other to increase the retention for a subsequent restoration. The mesial surface of the distal root and the distal surface of the mesial root should be prepared

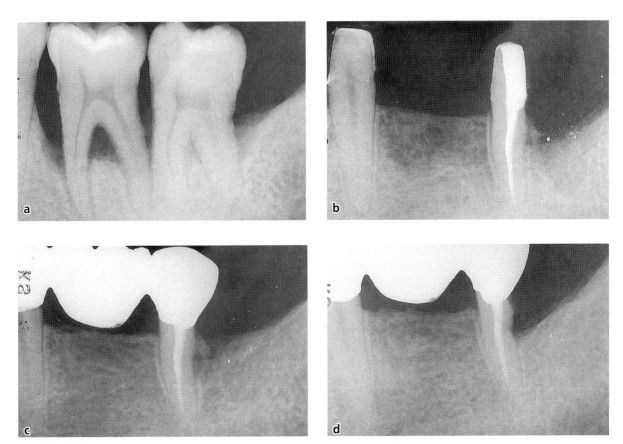

Fig. 29-32. Radiographs of a mandibular first molar to be extracted and of a second molar to be root resected (a). During hemisection an overhang is left behind as a result of an oblique sectioning of the tooth distal to the furcation (b). In a radiograph obtained 2 years later, the presence of an angular bony defect can be seen adjacent to the "overhang" (c). The lesion was resolved and the angular defect disappeared following removal of the "overhang". Radiograph after 2 years (d).

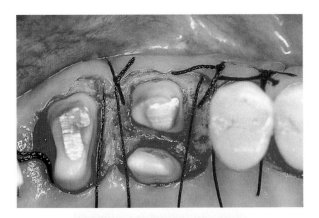

Fig. 29-33. Maintenance of the two fused buccal roots of a maxillary first molar. The buccal roots were separated from the palatal root. Note the rounded line angles and the wide space created between the separated roots.

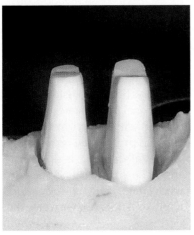

Fig. 29-34. Mandibular molar after root separation. Note the diverging angle of preparation performed to increase the interradicular space between the mesial and distal roots and the parallel approximal surfaces.

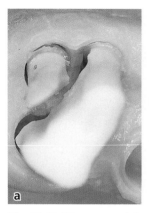
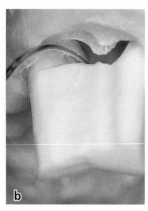
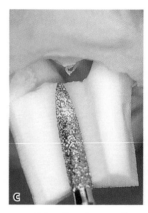
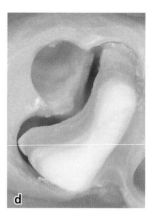

Fig. 29-35. The sequential stages of root resection and extraction of the distal root of a maxillary molar. In order to minimize the concave outline of the cut surfaces, the sectioning should be performed with a straight line cut (a,b). After extraction of the distal root, the furcation area of the remaining roots must be re-prepared to eliminate undercuts (c, d).

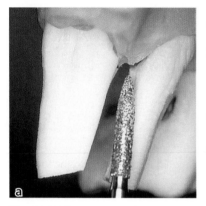
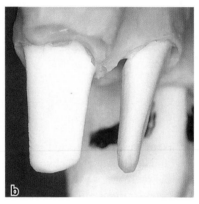
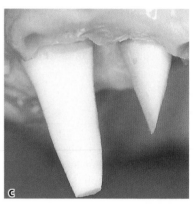

Fig. 29-36. Preparation, during separation, of the mesiobuccal and palatal roots after the distobuccal root of a maxillary molar had been extracted. The internal (furcation) surfaces of the two roots should be prepared with diverging angles to increase the interradicular space, while the external surfaces of the two roots should be prepared parallel to each other to increase the subsequent retention of the restoration (a,b). When the palatal surface of the palatal root is not prepared parallel to the buccal surface (c), the palatal abutment will become shortened and not self-retentive.

with diverging angles to increase the space available between the separated roots (Fig. 29-34).

Situation 2: maxillary molar
Following separation, the distobuccal root was extracted. The distal surface of the crown is prepared with a bevel cut and in such a way that the concave curvature (in apicocoronal direction) is eliminated (Fig. 29-35a-d).

If the mesiobuccal and the palatal roots of this molar must be separated but maintained, it is important that the buccal surface of the mesiobuccal root and the palatal surface of the palatal root are prepared parallel with each other. This will enhance the retention of the subsequent restoration. The palatal surface of the mesiobuccal root and the buccal surface of the palatal root must be prepared at diverging angles to increase the space available between the separated roots (Fig. 29-36a-c).

The provisional restoration is at this stage relined with cold cured acrylic and cemented after RSR.

Periodontal surgery
Following flap elevation, osseous resective techniques are used to eliminate angular bone defects that may exist around the maintained roots. Bone resection may also be performed to reduce the buccolingual dimension of the alveolar process of the extraction site. The remaining root(s) may be prepared with a bevel cut to the level of the supporting bone (Levine 1972, Ramfjord & Nissle 1974, Carnevale et al. 1983). This additional preparation may serve the purpose of (1) eliminating residual soft and hard deposits and (2) eliminating existing undercuts to facilitate the final impression (Fig. 29-37a-f). The provisional restoration is relined. The margins of the provisional restoration must end ≥ 3 mm coronal of the bone crest. The soft tissue flaps are secured with sutures at the level of the bone crest. The relined provisional restoration is cemented and a periodontal dressing is applied to cover the surgical area. The dressing and the sutures are removed 1 week later. The roots are debrided and a new dressing applied. After another week, the dressing is

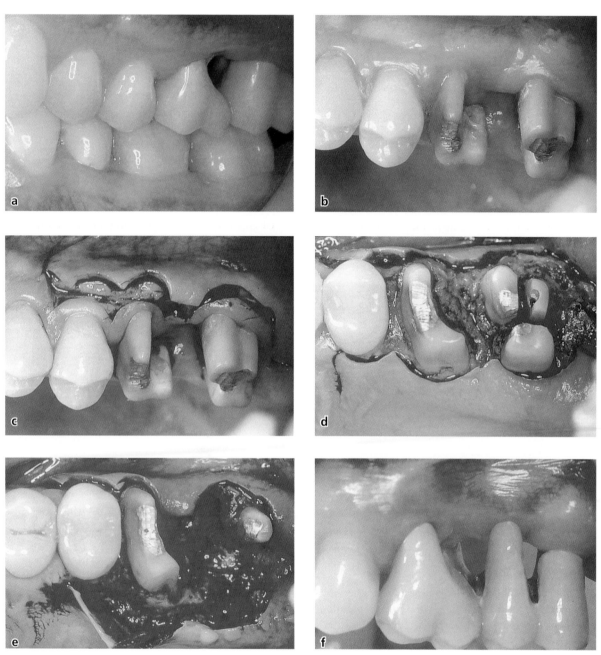

Fig. 29-37. Sequential stages of root resection at maxillary first and second molars. The extraction of the distal root of the first molar was performed during tooth preparation and prior to the insertion of the provisional restoration (a,b). During the surgical procedure, after flap elevation, the furcation-involved second molar was separated, the mesial and palatal roots were extracted and the osseous defects were eliminated (c, d, e). Healing with the definitive prosthetic restoration in place (f).

finally removed and the patient instructed in proper plaque control techniques.

Final prosthetic restoration

Since the prosthetic preparation of the roots was completed during surgery, the clinician concerns him/herself with only minor adjustments. The preparation margins are located supragingivally, which improves the precision of the definitive crown restoration. The framework of the restoration must be rigid to compensate for the compromised abutments (roots) with a compromised periodontal tissue support. The occlusion should be designed to minimize the infliction of lateral deflective forces (see Chapter 30) (Fig. 29-38a,b).

Regeneration of furcation defects

The possibility of regenerating and closing a furcation defect has been investigated (see Chapter 28).

Following an early case report publication (Gottlow et al. 1986), where histologic documentation of new attachment formation in human furcation de-

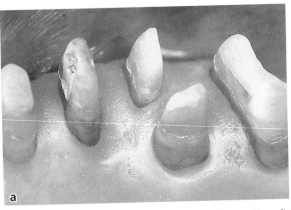
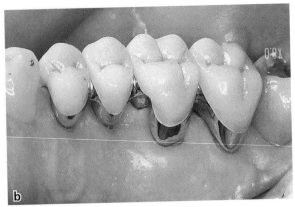

Fig. 29-38. Soft tissue healing at a separated maxillary first molar and at a root-resected second molar (a). The final prosthetic restoration in place with the occlusion designed to minimize the lateral stresses on the roots left as abutments (b).

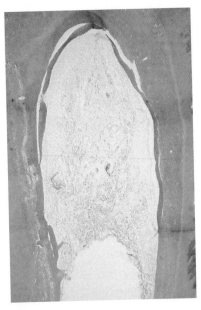

Fig. 29-39. Histologic mesiodistal section of a previous degree II furcation involvement of a human mandibular molar, treated with GTR. The section demonstrates that the newly formed cementum covers the entire circumference of the furcation defect.

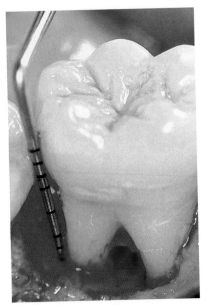

Fig. 29-40. Position of the furcation fornix in relation to the level of the supporting bone and attachment apparatus in a lingual degree II furcation-involved mandibular molar.

fects (Fig. 29-39) treated by "guided tissue regeneration" (GTR) therapy was provided, the results of several investigations on this form of treatment in furcation-involved teeth have been presented. In these reports, a reasonably predictable outcome of GTR therapy was demonstrated only in degree II furcation-involved mandibular molars, where a clinical soft tissue closure or a decreased probing depth of the furcation defect was recorded (Pontoriero et al. 1988, Lekovic et al. 1989, Caffesse et al. 1990).

Less favorable results have been reported when GTR therapy was used in other types of furcation defects such as degree III furcation-involved mandibular and maxillary molars (Pontoriero et al. 1989, Pontoriero & Lindhe 1995a) and degree II furcations in maxillary molars (Metzeler et al. 1991, Pontoriero & Lindhe 1995b).

The reason for the limited predictability of GTR

therapy in furcation-involved teeth may be related to several factors:

- The morphology of the periodontal defect, which in the root complex often has the character of a "horizontal lesion". New attachment formation is hence dependent on coronal upgrowth of periodontal ligament tissue (Fig. 29-40).
- The anatomy of the furcation, with its complex internal morphology, may prevent proper instrumentation and debridement of the exposed root surface (Fig. 29-41).
- The varying and changing location of the soft tissue margins during the early phase of healing with a possible recession of the flap margin and early exposure of both the membrane material and the fornix of the furcation (Fig. 29-42).

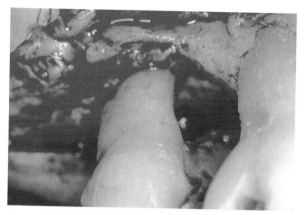

Fig. 29-41. Internal morphology of the furcation of a maxillary molar. Note the invagination of the palatal root.

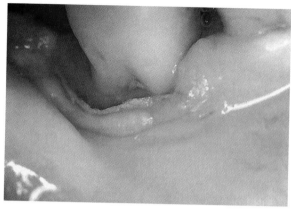

Fig. 29-42. Exposure of the membrane and of the furcation entrance as a consequence of recession of the flap margin. The photograph is taken at 3 weeks of healing after GTR treatment of a degree II buccal furcation of a mandibular molar.

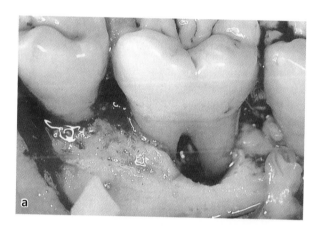

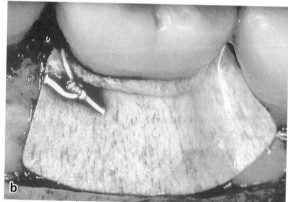

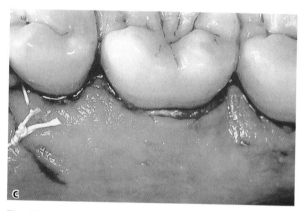

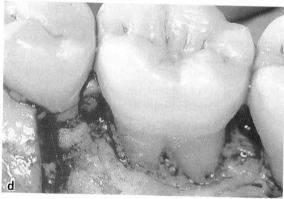

Fig. 29-43. Aspect of a lingual degree II furcation involvement in a mandibular first molar. Note the infrabony component of the defect and the level of the approximal supporting bone in relation to the furcation fornix (a). The Teflon membrane sutured in position and supported by the interproximal alveolar bone (b). The flap positioned and sutured over the membrane (c). At re-entry, after 6 months of healing, the previously exposed furcation defect was closed and filled with bone tissue (d).

GTR treatment could be considered in dentitions with isolated degree II furcation defects in mandibular molars. The predictability of this treatment outcome improves following GTR therapy if:

- The *interproximal* bone is located at a level which is close to the CEJ of the approximal surface. This "key-hole" type of degree II involvement allows for

an effective retention of the membrane material and retention also of the position of the coronally placed flap margins (Fig. 29-43a-d).

- The debridement of the exposed root surfaces in the furcation area is comprehensive. Since the width of the furcation entrance and the internal morphology of the interradicular area may limit the access of the curettes for proper debridement, the removal of

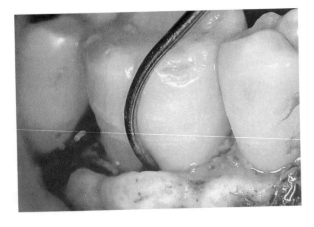

Fig. 29-44. Phase of debridment of a buccal degree II furcation defect by the use of an "extra-fine" ultrasonic tip.

hard and soft bacterial deposits from the root surfaces must frequently be made with ultrasonic instruments, rotating, flame-shaped fine diamond burs and endodontic files (Fig. 29-44).

- The membrane material is properly placed and a "space" between the tooth and the material established. A "primary" wound closure is hereby obtained, blood-clot protection will occur and recession of the soft tissue margin during the early phase of healing will be minimized (Fig. 29-45a-h).
- A plaque control program is put in place. This should include daily rinsing with a chlorhexidine solution and professional toothcleaning once a week for the first month, and once every 2-3 weeks for at least another 6 months of healing following the surgical procedure.

The outcome of the regenerative procedures at furcation-involved molars should result in the complete elimination of the defect within the interradicular space in order to establish anatomic conditions which facilitate optimal self-performed plaque control measures. In fact, partial gain of clinical attachment levels within the furcation defect, although statistically significant, will not necessarily improve the site's accessibility for plaque control measures.

Extraction

The extraction of a furcation-involved tooth must be considered when the attachment loss is so extensive that no root can be maintained or when the treatment will not result in a tooth/gingival anatomy which allows proper self-performed plaque control measures.

Moreover, extraction can be considered as an alternative form of therapy when the maintenance of the affected tooth will not improve the overall treatment plan or when, due to endodontic or caries-related lesions, the preservation of the tooth will represent a risk factor for the long-term prognosis of the overall treatment.

The possibility of substituting a furcation-involved tooth with an osseointegrated implant should be considered with extreme caution and only if implant therapy will improve the prognosis of the overall treatment (see Chapter 31). In fact, the implant alternative has obvious anatomic limitations in the maxillary and mandibular molar regions.

PROGNOSIS

Several studies have evaluated the long-term prognosis of multirooted teeth with furcation involvement that were treated in accordance with the principles described in this chapter (Table 29-2). In a 5-year study, Hamp et al. (1975) observed the outcome of treatment of 175 teeth with various degrees of furcation involvement in 100 patients. Of the 175 teeth, 32 (18%) were treated by scaling and root planing alone, 49 (28%) were subjected, in addition to scaling and root planing, to furcation plasty which included odonto and/or osteoplasty. In 87 teeth (50%) root resection had been carried out and in seven teeth (4%) a tunnel had been prepared. At the completion of the active phase of therapy the patients were enrolled in a maintenance program which included a recall visit every 3-6 months. The plaque and gingivitis scores assessed immediately after treatment and once a year during maintenance indicated that the patients' oral hygiene was of high quality. None of the teeth treated was lost during the 5 years of study. Only 16 furcation sites exhibited probing depths exceeding 3 mm. During the observation period carious lesions were detected in 12 surfaces of the 32 teeth which had been treated by scaling and root planing, in three surfaces of the 49 teeth subjected to furcation plasty, in five surfaces of the 78 root-resected teeth and in four surfaces of the seven teeth where a tunnel was prepared. The results of this study were basically confirmed in a more recent investigation (Hamp et al. 1992). In this 7-year study, the authors followed 100 patients with 182 furcation-involved teeth. Out of the 182 furcation-involved teeth, 57 had been treated by scaling and root planing only, 101 were treated by furcation plasty and 24 were subjected to root resection or hemisection. No tunnel preparation was performed. After the active phase of therapy, the patients were enrolled in a meticulous

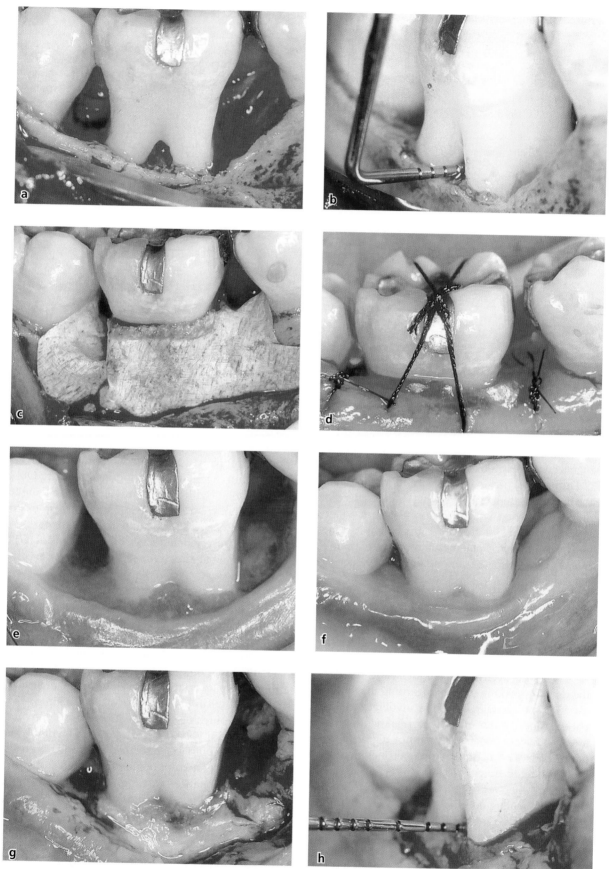

Fig. 29-45a-f. The sequential stages of GTR treatment of a buccal degree II furcation-involved mandibular first molar. The clinical appearance and the horizontal probing of the defect (a, b). Membrane placement and retention (c, d). The clinical aspect of the soft tissue at 4 weeks after membrane removal (e). The clinical aspect after 6 months of healing (f). During the re-entry procedure the furcation defect appeared completely closed (g) and was not probeable (h).

Table 29-2. Long-term clinical studies on root resection therapy in molars with furcation involvement

Author	Observation period	No. of teeth examined	% teeth lost	Causes of tooth loss				
				% root/ tooth fracture	% perio-dontal	% endo-dontic	% caries or decemen-tation	% strategic
Bergenholtz (1972)	21 teeth / 2-5 yrs 17 teeth / 5-10 yrs	45	6		4	2		
Klavan (1975)	3 yrs	34	3		3			
Hamp et al. (1975)	5 yrs	87	0					
Langer et al. (1981)	10 yrs	100	38	18	10	7	3	
Erpenstein (1983)	4-7 yrs	34	9		3	6		
Bühler (1988)	10 yrs	28	32	3.6	7.1	17.7	3.6	
Carnevale et al. (1991)	303 teeth / 3-6 yrs 185 teeth / 7-11 yrs	488	4	1.8	0.4	0.9	0.9	
Basten et al. (1996)	2-23 yrs	49	8			2	4	2
Carnevale et al. (1998)	10 yrs	175	7	1.1	1.8	2.3	1.8	

maintenance-care program including recall appointments once every 3-6 months.

During the course of the study, more than 85% of the furcations treated with scaling root planing alone, or in conjunction with furcation plasty, maintained stable conditions or showed signs of improvement. Only one tooth and one mesial root of a mandibular molar were extracted among the root-resected or hemisected teeth.

Carnevale et al. (1998), in a 10-year prospective controlled clinical trial, demonstrated a 93% survival rate of root resected furcation-involved teeth and a 99% survival rate of non-furcation involved teeth.

More recently, Svärdström (2001) presented the results of a retrospective analysis on factors influencing the decision-making process regarding the treatment for 1313 molars with furcation involvement in 222 patients and the outcome of the treatment decisions after 8-12 years (mean 9.5 years) of regular maintenance care. The treatment options included were: tooth extraction, root separation/resection and maintenance of the tooth with non-surgically/surgically performed scaling and root-planing with or without furcation plasty. Of the 1313 furcation-involved molars, 366 (28%) were extracted during the active phase of therapy. The decision for tooth extraction was primarily influenced by factors such as tooth mobility, tooth position, absence of occulusal antagonism, the degree of furcation involvement, probing depth and the amount of remaining periodontal support. Out of the 685 molars with furcation involvement and the 160 patients that were available for the follow-up examination 8-12 years after treatment, 47 teeth were root separated/resected and 638 teeth were considered to be maintainable after a non-surgical or conservative surgical therapy.

The factor found to have the strongest influence for the decision to perform root separation/resection was the degree of furcation involvement (class II and III). Tooth position, probing depth and tooth mobility were also factors of statistical significance. The author explained that other factors such as endodontic conditions, root anatomy and overall treatment strategy may also have influenced the choice of treatment. The long-term outcome of the treatment decisions made for furcation-involved molars showed a favorable survival rate for both root resective (89%) and non-resective (96%) therapy options in patients included in a proper maintenance care program.

Of the 47 root separated/resected teeth, only 5 (11%) were lost during the 9.5 years of follow-up. Of the 638 molars initially considered to be maintainable by a non-resective treatment, 21 teeth (3.5%) were extracted and 3 teeth were root resected.

Table 29-3. Factors to consider in treatment of furcation-involved molars

Tooth-related factors
Degree of furcation involvement
Amount of remaining periodontal support
Probing depth
Tooth mobility
Endodontic conditions and root/root-canal anatomy
Available sound tooth-substance
Tooth position and occlusal antagonisms

Patient-related factors
Strategic value of the tooth in relation to the overall plan
Patient's functional and esthetic demands
Patient's age and health conditions
Oral hygiene capacity

Conclusion

When it comes to treatment decisions for furcation-involved molars, it must be realized that there is no scientific evidence that a given treatment modality is superior to the others (Table 29-3).

REFERENCES

Abrams, L. & Trachtenberg, D.I. (1974). Hemisection-technique and restoration. *Dental Clinics of North America* **18**, 415-444.

Basten, C.H.J., Ammons, W.F.J. & Persson, R. (1996). Long-term evaluation of root-resected molars: a retrospective study. *International Journal of Periodontics and Restorative Dentistry* **16**, 207-219.

Bergenholtz, G. (1972). Radectomy of multi-rooted teeth. *Journal of American Dental Association* **85**, 870-875.

Bower, R.C. (1979a). Furcation morphology relative to periodontal treatment. Furcation entrance architecture. *Journal of Periodontology* **50**, 23-27.

Bower, R.C. (1979b). Furcation morphology relative to periodontal treatment. Furcation root surface anatomy. *Journal of Periodontology* **50**, 366-374.

Bühler, H. (1988). Evaluation of root resected teeth. Results after ten years. *Journal of Periodontology* **59**, 805-810.

Caffesse, R., Smith, B., Duff, B., Morrison, E., Merril, D. & Becker, W. (1990). Class II Furcations treated by guided tissue regeneration in humans: case reports. *Journal of Periodontology* **61**, 510-514.

Carnevale, G., Di Febo, G. & Trebbi, L. (1981). A patient presentation: planning a difficult case. *International Journal of Periodontics and Restorative Dentistry* **6**, 51-63.

Carnevale, G., Di Febo, G., Tonelli, M.P., Marin, C. & Fuzzi, M. (1991). A retrospective analysis of the periodontal-prosthetic treatment of molars with interradicular lesions. *International Journal of Periodontics and Restorative Dentistry* **11**, 189-205.

Carnevale, G., Freni Sterrantino, S. & Di Febo, G. (1983). Soft and hard tissue wound healing following tooth preparation to the alveolar crest. *International Journal of Periodontics and Restorative Dentistry* **3**, 36-53.

Carnevale, G., Pontoriero, R. & Di Febo, G. (1998). Long-term effects of root-resective therapy in furcation-involved molars. A 10-year longitudinal study. *Journal of Clinical Periodontology* **25**, 209-214.

Di Febo, G., Carnevale, G. & Sterrantino, S.F. (1985). Treatment of a case of advanced periodontitis: clinical procedures utilizing the "combined preparation" technique. *International Journal of Periodontics and Restorative Dentistry* **1**, 52-63.

Erpenstein, H. (1983). A 3 year longitudinal study of hemisectioned molars. *Journal of Clinical Peridontology* **10**, 1-10.

Gher, M.E. & Vernino, A.R. (1980). Root morphology-clinical significance in pathogenesis and treatment of periodontal disease. *Journal of American Dental Association* **101**, 627-633.

Gottlow, J., Nyman, S., Lindhe, J., Karring, T. & Wennström, J. (1986). New attachment formation in the human periodontium by guided tissue regeneration. Case reports. *Journal of Clinical Periodontology* **13**, 604-616.

Hamp, S.E., Nyman, S. & Lindhe, J. (1975). Periodontal treatment of multirooted teeth. Results after 5 years. *Journal of Clinical Periodontology* **2**, 126-135.

Hamp, S.E., Ravald, N., Tewik, A. & Lundström, A. (1992). Perspective a long terme des modalités de traitement des lesions inter-radiculaires. *Journal de Parodontologie* **11**, 11-23.

Joseph, I., Varma, B.R.R. & Bhat, K.M. (1996). Clinical significance of furcation anatomy of the maxillary first premolar: a biometric study on extracted teeth. *Journal of Periodontology* **67**, 386-389.

Klavan, B. (1975). Clinical observation following root amputation in maxillary molar teeth. *Journal of Periodontology* **46**, 1-5.

Langer, B., Stein, S.D. & Wagenberg, B. (1981). An evaluation of root resection. A ten years study. *Journal of Periodontology* **52**, 719-722.

Larato, D.C. (1975). Some anatomical factors related to furcation involvements. *Journal of Periodontology* **46**, 608-609.

Lekovic, V., Kenney, E.B., Kovacevic, K. & Carranza, F.A. Jr. (1989). Evaluation of guided tissue regeneration in class II furcation defects. A clinical re-entry study. *Journal of Periodontology* **60**, 694-698.

Levine, H.L. (1972). Periodontal flap surgery with gingival fiber retention. *Journal of Periodontology* **43**, 91-98.

Metzeler, D., Seamons, B.C., Mellonig, J.T., Marlin, G.E. & Gray, J.L. (1991). Clinical evaluation of guided tissue regeneration in the treatment of maxillary class II molar furcation invasion. *Journal of Periodontology* **62**, 353-360.

Pontoriero, R. & Lindhe, J. (1995a). Guided tissue regeneration in the treatment of degree III furcations defects in maxillary molars. *Journal of Clinical Periodontology* **22**, 810-812.

Pontoriero, R. & Lindhe, J. (1995b). Guided tissue regeneration in the treatment of degree II furcations in maxillary molars. *Journal of Clinical Periodontology* **22**, 756-763.

Pontoriero, R., Lindhe, J., Nyman, S., Karring, T., Rosenberg, E. & Sanavi, F. (1988). Guided tissue regeneration in degree II furcation involved mandibular molars. A clinical study. *Journal of Clinical Periodontology* **15**, 247-254.

Pontoriero, R., Lindhe, J., Nyman, S., Karring, T., Rosenberg, E. & Sanavi, F. (1989). Guided tissue regeneration in the treatment of furcation defects in mandibular molars. A clinical study of degree III involvements. *Journal of Clinical Periodontology* **16**, 170-174.

Ramfjord, S.P., Nissle, L.L. (1974). The modified Widman flap. *Journal of Periodontology* **45**, 601-607.

Rosenberg, M.M. (1978). Management of osseous defects. *Clinical Dentistry* **3**, 103.

Rosenberg, M.M. (1988). Furcation involvement: periodontic, endodontic and restorative interrelationships. In: Rosenberg, M.M., Kay, H.B., Keough, B.E. & Holt, R.L., eds. *Periodontal and prosthetic management for advanced cases* Chichago: Quintessence, pp. 249-251.

Ross, I.F. & Thompson, R.H. (1980). Furcation involvement in maxillary and mandibular molars. *Journal of Periodontology* **51**, 450-454.

Smukler, H. & Tagger, M. (1976). Vital root amputation. A clinical and histologic study. *Journal of Periodontology* **47**, 324-330.

Svärdström, G. (2001). *Furcation involvements in periodontitis patients. Prevalence and treatment decisions.* Thesis. Department of Peridontology, Faculty of Odontology, Göteborg University, pp. 31.

Svärdström, G. & Wennström, J. (1988). Furcation topography of the maxillary and mandibular first molars. *Journal of Clinical Periodontology* **15**, 271-275.

CHAPTER 30

Occlusal Therapy

JAN LINDHE AND STURE NYMAN

Clinical symptoms of trauma from occlusion
  Angular bony defect
  Increased tooth mobility
  Progressive tooth mobility

Tooth mobility
  Initial and secondary tooth mobility
  Clinical assessment of tooth mobility

Treatment of increased tooth mobility

CLINICAL SYMPTOMS OF TRAUMA FROM OCCLUSION

Angular bony defect

It has been claimed that *angular bony defects* and *increased tooth mobility* are important symptoms of trauma from occlusion (Glickman 1965, 1967). The validity of this suggestion has, however, been questioned (see Chapter 15). Thus, angular bony defects have been found at teeth affected by *trauma from occlusion* as well as at teeth with normal occlusal function (Waerhaug 1979). *This means that the presence of angular bony defects cannot* per se *be regarded as an exclusive symptom of trauma from occlusion.*

Increased tooth mobility

Increased tooth mobility, determined clinically, is expressed in terms of amplitude of displacement of the crown of the tooth. Increased tooth mobility can, indeed, be observed in conjunction with *trauma from occlusion*. It may, however, also be the result of a reduction of the height of the alveolar bone with or without an accompanying angular bony defect caused by plaque-associated periodontal disease (see Chapter 5). Increased tooth mobility resulting from occlusal interferences may further indicate that the periodontal structures have become adapted to an altered functional demand, i.e. a widened periodontal ligament with a normal tissue composition has become the end result of a previous phase of progressive tooth mobility (see Chapter 15) associated with trauma from occlusion.

Progressive (increasing) tooth mobility

In Chapter 15, it was concluded that the diagnosis trauma from occlusion should be used solely in situations where a progressive mobility could be observed. Progressive tooth mobility can be identified only through a series of repeated tooth mobility measurements carried out over a period of several days or weeks.

TOOTH MOBILITY CROWN EXCURSION / ROOT DISPLACEMENT

Initial and secondary tooth mobility

A tooth which is surrounded by a normal periodontium may be moved (displaced) in horizontal and vertical directions and may in addition be forced to perform limited rotational movements. Clinically, tooth mobility is usually assessed by exposing the crown of the tooth to a certain force and determining the distance the crown can be displaced in buccal and/or lingual direction. The mobility (= movability) of a tooth in a horizontal direction is closely dependent on the height of the surrounding supporting bone, the width of the periodontal ligament as well as the shape and number of roots present (Fig. 30-1).

The mechanism of tooth mobility was studied in detail by Mühlemann (1954, 1960) who described a standardized method for measuring even minor tooth displacements. By means of the "Periodontometer" a small force (~100 pounds) is applied to the crown of a tooth (Fig. 30-2). The crown starts to tip in the direction of the force. The resistance of the tooth-supporting

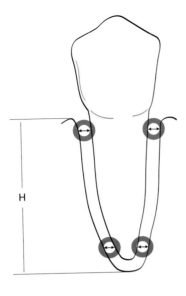

Fig. 30-1. The mobility of a tooth in horizontal direction is dependent on the height of the alveolar bone (H), the width of the periodontal ligament (encircled arrows) and the shape and number of roots.

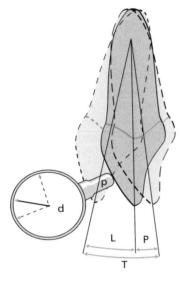

Fig. 30-2. Tooth mobility measurements by means of the Periodontometer. d: dial indicator. p: pointer. L: labial excursion of the crown. P: palatal excursion of the crown, T = L+P: total excursion of the crown.

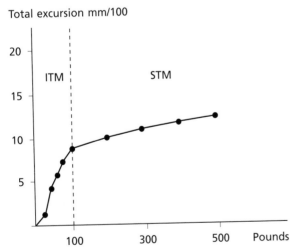

Fig. 30-3. Initial tooth mobility (ITM) means the excursion of the crown of a tooth when a force of 100 pounds is applied to the crown. Secondary tooth mobility (STM) means the excursion of the crown of the tooth when a force of 500 pounds is applied.

structures against displacement of the root is low in the initial phase of force application and the crown is

moved only 5/100-10/100 mm. This movement of the tooth was called "initial tooth mobility-ITM" by Mühlemann (1954) and is the result of an intraalveolar displacement of the root (Fig. 30-3). In the pressure zone (see Chapter 15) there is a 10% reduction in the width of the periodontal ligament and in the tension zone there is a corresponding increase. Mühlemann & Zander (1954) stated that "there are good reasons to assume that the initial displacement of the root (initial-TM) corresponds to a reorientation of the periodontal membrane fibers into a position of functional readiness towards tensile strength". The magnitude of the "initial-TM" varies from individual to individual, from tooth to tooth, and is mainly dependent on the structure and organization of the periodontal ligament. The "initial-TM" value of ankylosed teeth is therefore zero.

When a larger force (~ 500 pounds) is applied to the crown, the fiber bundles on the tension side cannot offer sufficient resistance to further root displacement. The additional displacement of the crown that is observed in "secondary tooth mobility-secondary-TM" (Fig. 30-3) is allowed by distortion and compression of the periodontium in the pressure side. According to

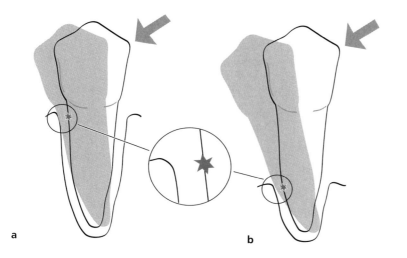

Fig. 30-4. (a) The normal "physiologic" mobility of a tooth with normal height of the alveolar bone and normal width of the periodontal ligament. (b) The mobility of a tooth with reduced height of the alveolar bone. The distance of the horizontal displacement of the reference point (*) on the roots is the same in the two situations (a,b).

Mühlemann (1960) the magnitude of *"secondary-TM"*, i.e. the excursion of the crown of the tooth when a force of 500 pounds is applied, (1) varies between different types of teeth (e.g. incisors 10-12/100 mm, canines 5-9/100 mm, premolars 8-10/100 mm and molars 4-8/100 mm), (2) is larger in children than in adults, and (3) is larger in females than males and increases during, for example, pregnancy. Furthermore, tooth mobility seems to vary during the course of the day; the lowest value is found in the evening and the largest in the morning.

A new method for determining tooth mobility was presented by Schulte and co-workers (Schulte 1987, Schulte et al. 1992) when the Periotest® (SiemensAG, Bensheim, Germany) system was introduced. The Periotest device measures the reaction of the periodontium to a defined percussion force which is applied to the tooth and delivered by a tapping instrument. A metal rod is accelerated to a speed of 0.2 m/s with the device and maintained at a constant velocity. Upon impact the tooth is deflected and the rod decelerated. The contact time between the tapping head and the tooth varies between 0.3 and 2 milliseconds and is shorter for stable than mobile teeth. The Periotest scale (the Periotest values) ranges from − 8 to + 50 and the following ranges should be considered:

- − 8 to +9: clinically firm teeth
- 10 to 19: first distinguishable sign of movement
- 20 to 29: crown deviates within 1 mm of its normal position
- 30 to 50: mobility is readily observed.

The Periotest values correlate well with (1) tooth mobility assessed with a metric system, and (2) degree of periodontal disease and alveolar bone loss. There are reasons to suggest that the simple Periotest device in the future will be used in both the clinic and in research settings.

Clinical assessment of tooth mobility (physiologic and pathologic tooth mobility)

If, in the traditional clinical measurement of tooth mobility, a comparatively large force is exerted on the crown of a tooth which is surrounded by a normal periodontium, the tooth will tip within its alveolus until a closer contact has been established between the root and the marginal (or apical) bone tissue. The magnitude of this tipping movement, which is normally assessed using the tip of the crown as a reference point, is referred to as the *"physiologic"* tooth mobility. The term *"physiologic"* implies that *"pathologic"* tooth mobility may also occur.

What, then, is "pathologic" tooth mobility?
1. If a similar force is applied to a tooth which is surrounded by a periodontal ligament with an increased width, the excursion of the crown in horizontal direction will become increased; the clinical measurement consequently demonstrates that the tooth has an increased mobility. Should this increased mobility be regarded as *"pathologic"*?
2. An increased tooth mobility, i.e. an increased displacement of the crown of the tooth after force application, can also be found in situations where the height of the alveolar bone has been reduced but the remaining periodontal ligament has a normal width. At sites where this type of bone loss is extensive, the degree of tooth mobility (i.e. excursion of the crown) may be pronounced. Should this increased tooth mobility be regarded as "pathologic"?

Fig. 30-4b illustrates a tooth which is surrounded by alveolar bone of reduced height. The width of the remaining periodontal ligament, however, is within normal limits. A horizontally directed force applied to the crown of the tooth will in this case result in a larger excursion of the crown than if a similar force is applied to a tooth with normal height of the alveolar bone and normal width of the periodontal ligament (Fig. 30-4a). There are reasons to suggest that the *so-called increased mobility* meas-

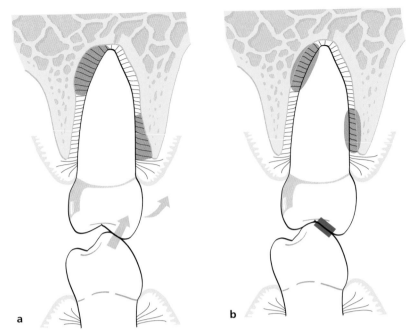

Fig. 30-5. (a) Contact relationship between a mandibular and a maxillary premolar in occlusion. The maxillary premolar is fitted with an artificial restoration with an improperly designed occlusal surface. Occlusion results in horizontally directed forces (arrows) which may produce an undue stress concentration within the "brown" areas of the periodontium of the maxillary tooth. Resorption of the alveolar bone occurs in these areas. A widening of the periodontal ligament can be detected as well as increased mobility of the tooth. Following adjustment of the occlusion, the horizontal forces are reduced. This results in bone apposition ("red areas") and a normalization of the tooth mobility (b).

ured in the case of Fig. 30-4b is, indeed, *"physiologic"*. The validity of this statement can easily be demonstrated if the displacement of the two teeth is assessed not from the crown but from a point on the root at the level of the bone crest. If a horizontal force is directed to the teeth as indicated in Fig. 30-4a,b, the reference points (*) on the root surfaces will be displaced a similar distance in both instances. *Obviously, it is not the length of the excursive movement of the crown that is important from a biologic point of view, but the displacement of the root within its remaining periodontal ligament.*

In plaque-associated periodontal disease, bone loss is a prominent feature. Another so-called classical symptom of periodontitis is "increased tooth mobility". It is important to realize, however, that in many situations with even or "horizontal" bone loss patterns, the increased crown displacement (tooth mobility) which is assessed in clinical measurements should, according to the above discussion, also be regarded as physiologic; the movement of the root within the space of its remaining "normal" periodontal ligament is normal.

3. Increased crown displacement (tooth mobility) may also be detected in a clinical measurement where a "horizontal" force is applied to teeth with angular bony defects and/or increased width of the periodontal ligament. If this mobility is not gradually increasing – from one observation interval to the next – the root is surrounded by a periodontal ligament of increased width but normal composi-

tion. This mobility should also be considered *"physiologic"* since the movement is a function of the height of the alveolar bone and the width of the periodontal ligament.

4. Only *progressively increasing tooth mobility* which may occur in conjunction with trauma from occlusion and which is characterized by active bone resorption (see Chapter 15) and which indicates the presence of inflammatory alterations within the periodontal ligament tissue, may be considered *"pathologic"*.

TREATMENT OF INCREASED TOOTH MOBILITY

A number of situations will be described below which may call for treatment aimed at reducing an increased tooth mobility .

Situation I

Increased mobility of a tooth with increased width of the periodontal ligament but normal height of the alveolar bone

If a tooth (for instance a maxillary premolar) is fitted with an improper filling or crown restoration, occlusal interferences develop and the surrounding periodontal tissues become the seat of inflammatory reactions,

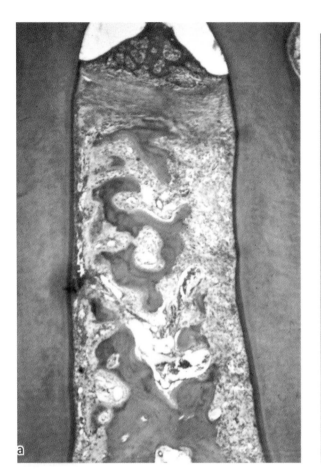
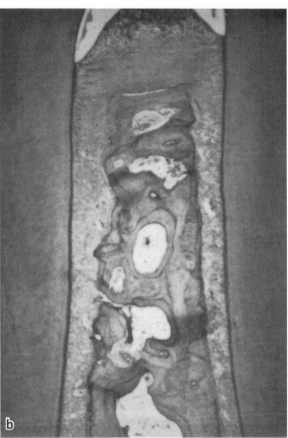

Figs. 30-6. Photomicrograph illustrating the interdental area between two mandibular premolars in the monkey. In (a) the two premolars are exposed to jiggling forces. Note the reduction of alveolar bone in the area and the location of the bone crest. Ten weeks after the elimination of the jiggling forces (b) a considerable regeneration of bone has occurred. Note the increase of the height of the interdental bone and the normalization of the width of the periodontal ligaments. The apical end of the junctional epithelium is located at the cemento-enamel junction. Courtesy of Dr Polson; from Polson et al. (1976a).

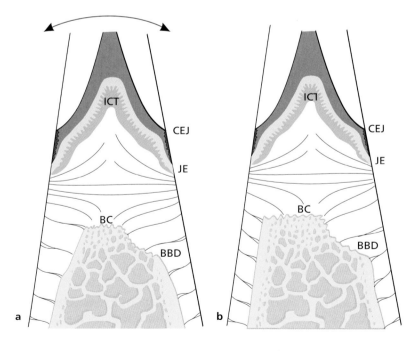

Figs. 30-7. In the presence of an existing marginal inflammation, alveolar bone, lost by jiggling trauma (a), will not always regenerate following elimination of the traumatic forces (b). ICT: infiltrated connective tissue. CEJ: cemento-enamel junction. JE: apical end of junctional epithelium. BC: alveolar bone crest. BBD: bottom of angular bony defect. From Polson et al. (1976b).

i.e. trauma from occlusion (Fig. 30-5). If the restoration is so designed that the crown of the tooth in occlusion is subjected to undue forces directed in a buccal direc-

tion, bone resorption phenomena develop in the buccal-marginal and lingual-apical pressure zones with a resulting increase of the width of the periodontal liga-

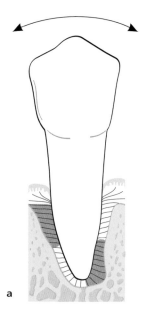
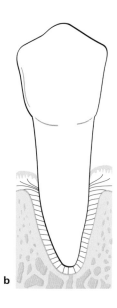

a   b

Figs. 30-8. If a tooth with reduced periodontal tissue support (a) has been exposed to excessive horizontal forces, a widened periodontal ligament space ("brown" areas) and increased mobility (arrow) result. Following reduction or elimination of such forces, bone apposition will occur and the tooth will become stabilized (b).

ment in these zones. The tooth becomes hypermobile or moves away from the "traumatizing" position. Since such traumatizing forces in teeth with normal periodontium or overt gingivitis cannot result in pocket formation or loss of connective tissue attachment, the resulting increased mobility of the tooth should be regarded as a physiologic adaptation of the periodontal tissues to the altered functional demands. A proper correction of the anatomy of the occlusal surface of such a tooth, i.e. occlusal adjustment, will normalize the relationship between the antagonizing teeth in occlusion, thereby eliminating the excessive forces. As a result, apposition of bone will occur in the zones previously exposed to resorption, the width of the periodontal ligament will become normalized and the tooth stabilized, i.e. it reassumes its normal mobility (Fig. 30-5). In other words, resorption of alveolar bone which is caused by trauma from occlusion is a reversible process which can be treated by the elimination of occlusal interferences.

The capacity for bone regeneration after resorption following trauma from occlusion has been documented in a number of animal experiments (Waerhaug & Randers-Hansen 1966, Polson et al. 1976a, Karring et al. 1982, Nyman et al. 1982). In such experiments, the induced bone resorption not only involved the bone within the alveolus but also the alveolar bone crest. When the traumatizing forces were removed, bone tissue was deposited not only in the walls of the alveolus, thereby normalizing the width of the periodontal ligament, but also on the bone crest area, whereby the height of the alveolar bone was normalized (Fig. 30-6; Polson et al. 1976a). In the presence of an untreated, plaque-associated lesion in the soft tissue, however, substantial bone regrowth did not always occur (Fig. 30-7; Polson et al. 1976b) .

Situation II

Increased mobility of a tooth with increased width of the periodontal ligament and reduced height of the alveolar bone

When a dentition has been properly treated for moderate to advanced periodontal disease, gingival health is established in areas of the dentition where teeth are surrounded by periodontal structures of reduced height. If a tooth with a reduced periodontal tissue support is exposed to excessive horizontal forces (trauma from occlusion), inflammatory reactions develop in the pressure zones of the periodontal ligament with accompanying bone resorption. These alterations are similar to those which occur around a tooth with normal height of the supporting structures; the alveolar bone is resorbed, the width of the periodontal ligament is increased in the pressure/tension zones and the tooth becomes hypermobile (Fig. 30-8a). If the excessive forces are reduced or eliminated by occlusal adjustment, bone apposition to the "pre-trauma" level will occur, the periodontal ligament will regain its normal width and the tooth will become stabilized (Fig. 30-8b).

Conclusion: Situations I and II

Occlusal adjustment is an effective therapy against increased tooth mobility when such mobility is caused by an *increased width* of the periodontal ligament.

Situation III

Increased mobility of a tooth with reduced height of the alveolar bone and normal width of the periodontal ligament

The increased tooth mobility which is the result of a reduction in height of the alveolar bone without a concomitant increase in width of the periodontal membrane cannot be reduced or eliminated by oc-

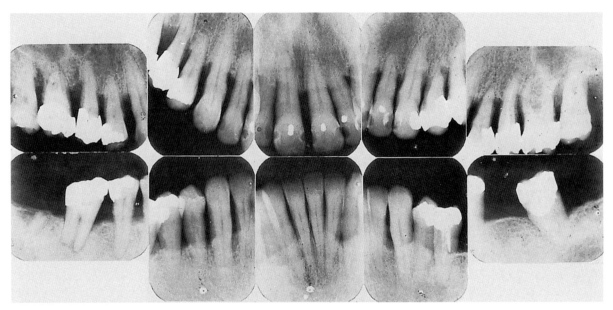

Fig. 30-9. Case A, 64-year-old male. Periodontal status and radiographs prior to therapy.

clusal adjustment. In teeth with normal width of the periodontal ligament, no further bone apposition on the walls of the alveoli can occur. If such an increased tooth mobility does not interfere with the patient's chewing function or comfort, no treatment is required. If the patient experiences the tooth mobility as disturbing, however, the mobility can in this situation be reduced only by splinting, i.e. by joining the mobile tooth/teeth together with other teeth in the jaw into a fixed unit – a SPLINT.

A SPLINT, according to the Glossary of Periodontic Terms (1986) is "an appliance designed to stabilize mobile teeth". A splint can be fabricated in the form of joined composite fillings, fixed bridges, removable partial prostheses, etc.

Example: Case A, 64-year-old male

The periodontal condition of this patient is illustrated by the probing depth, furcation involvement and tooth mobility data as well as the radiographs from the initial examination in Fig. 30-9. Periodontal disease has progressed to a level where, around the maxillary teeth, only the apical third or less of the roots is invested in supporting alveolar bone. The following discussion is related to the treatment of the maxillary dentition.

In the treatment planning of this case it was decided that the first premolars (teeth 14 and 24) had to be extracted due to advanced periodontal disease and furcation involvement of degree III. For the same reasons, teeth 17 and 27 were scheduled for extraction. Teeth 16 and 26 were also found to have advanced loss of periodontal tissue support in combination with deep furcation involvements. The most likely *definitive* treatment should include periodontal and adjunctive therapy in the following parts of the dentition: 15 and 25, and 13, 12, 11, 21, 22, 23. For functional and esthetic reasons, 14 and 24 obviously had to be replaced. The question now arose as to whether these

two premolars should be replaced by two separate unilateral bridges, using 13, 15 and 23, 25 as abutment teeth, or if the increased mobility of these teeth and

Periodontal chart

Tooth	Pocket depth M B D L	Furcation involvement	Tooth mobility
18			
17	6 6 8 8	b2, m2, d1	
16	6 6 8 8	m1, d2	2
15	8 8 6 7		2
14	7 7 7 4	3	2
13	8 4 8 4		2
12	8 4 8 4		2
11	6 4 7 4		1
21	6 4 6 4		1
22	6 5 7		2
23	6 6 4		2
24	7 8	3	2
25	6 8 8 4		2
26	8 6	b2, m2, d2	
27	6 6 10 8	b2, d2	1
28			
48			
47			
46	8 6 6 7	b1, l2	
45	6 7 4		1
44	6 6 4		
43	7 7 6 4		
42	4 4 4		1
41	6 4		1
31	6		1
32	4 6 4		1
33	6 6 6		2
34	4 7 4		
35	7 4 6		2
36			
37	8 5 6 4	b2, l2	3
38			

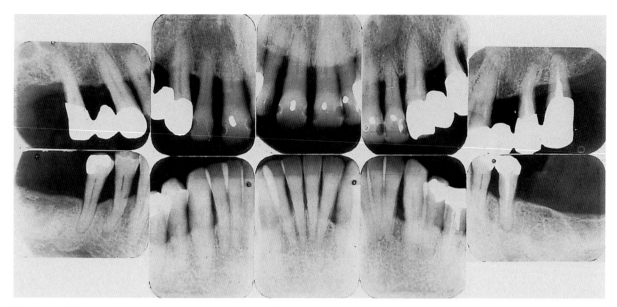

Fig. 30-10. Case A. Radiographs obtained 10 years after periodontal therapy and installation of two unilateral bridges in the maxilla.

also of the anterior teeth (12, 11, 21, 22; Fig. 30-9) called for a bridge of cross-arch design, with the extension 15-25, to obtain a splinting effect. If 14 and 24 are replaced by two unilateral bridges, each one of these 3-unit bridges will exhibit the same degree of mobility in buccolingual direction as the individual abutment teeth (degree II: Fig. 30-9), since a unilateral straight bridge will not have a stabilizing effect on the abutment teeth in this force direction.

From the radiographs it can be seen that the increased mobility observed in the maxillary teeth of this patient is associated mainly with reduced height of the alveolar bone and not with increased width of the periodontal ligaments. This means that the mobility of the individual teeth should be regarded as normal or "physiologic" for teeth with such a reduced height of the supporting tissues. This in turn implies that the increased tooth mobility in the present case does not call for treatment unless it interferes with the chewing comfort or jeopardizes the position of the front teeth. This particular patient had not recognized any functional problems related to the increased mobility of his maxillary teeth. Consequently, there was no reason to install a cross-arch bridge in order to splint the teeth, i.e. to reduce tooth mobility.

Following proper treatment of the plaque-associated periodontal lesions, two separate provisional bridges of unilateral design were produced (15, 14, 13; 23, 24, 25, 26 palatal root). The provisional acrylic bridges were used for 6 months during which the occlusion, the mobility of the two bridges and the position of the front teeth were all carefully monitored. When, after 6 months, no change of position of the lateral and central incisors had occurred and no increase of the mobility of the two provisional bridges had been noted, the definitive restorative therapy was performed.

Fig. 30-10 presents radiographs obtained 10 years

after initial therapy. The position of the front teeth and the mobility of the incisors and the two bridges have not changed during the course of the maintenance period. There has been no further loss of periodontal tissue support during the 10 years of observation, no further spread of the front teeth and no widening of the periodontal ligaments around the individual teeth, including the abutment teeth for the bridgework.

Conclusion: Situation III
Increased tooth mobility (or bridge mobility) as a result of reduced height of the alveolar bone can be accepted and splinting avoided, provided the occlusion is stable (no further migration or further increasing mobility of individual teeth), and provided the degree of existing mobility does not disturb the patient's chewing ability or comfort. Consequently, splinting is indicated when the mobility of a tooth or a group of teeth is so increased that chewing ability and/or comfort are disturbed.

Situation IV

Progressive (increasing) mobility of a tooth (teeth) as a result of gradually increasing width of the reduced periodontal ligament
Often in cases of advanced periodontal disease the tissue destruction may have reached a level where extraction of one or several teeth cannot be avoided. Teeth which in such a dentition are still available for periodontal treatment may, after therapy, exhibit such a high degree of mobility – or even signs of progressively increasing mobility – that there is an obvious risk that the forces elicited during function may mechanically disrupt the remaining periodontal ligament components and cause extraction of the teeth.

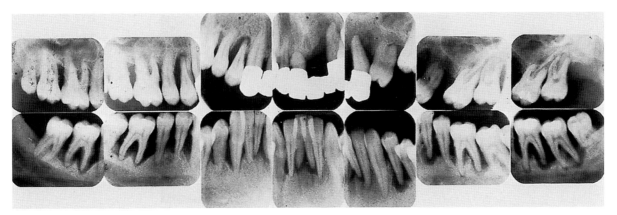

Fig. 30-11. Case B, 26-year-old male. Radiographs illustrating the periodontal conditions prior to therapy.

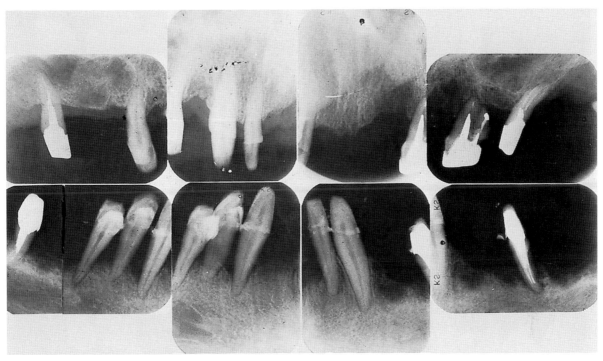

Fig. 30-12. Case B. Radiographs obtained after periodontal treatment and preparation of the abutment teeth for two fixed splints.

Only by means of a splint will it be possible to maintain such teeth. In such cases a fixed splint has two objectives: (1) to stabilize hypermobile teeth and (2) to replace missing teeth.

Example: Case B, 26-year-old male
Fig. 30-11 presents radiographs taken prior to therapy and Fig. 30-12 those obtained after periodontal treatment and preparation of the remaining teeth as abutments for two fixed splints. All teeth except 13, 12 and 33 have lost around 75% or more of the alveolar bone and widened periodontal ligaments are a frequent finding. The four distal abutments for the two splints are root-separated molars, the maintained roots being the following: the palatal root of 17, the mesiobuccal root of 26 and the mesial roots of 36 and 47. It should be observed that tooth 24 is root-separated and the palatal root maintained with only minute amounts of periodontium left. Immediately prior to insertion of the two splints, all teeth except 13, 12 and 33 displayed a mobility varying between degrees 1 and 3. From the radiographs in Fig. 30-12 it can be noted that there is an obvious risk of extraction of a number of teeth such as 24, 26, 47, 45, 44, 43 and 36 if the patient is allowed to bite with a normal chewing force without the splints in position.

Despite the high degree of mobility of the individual teeth, the splints were, after insertion, entirely stable and have maintained their stability during a maintenance period of more than 12 years. Fig. 30-13 describes the clinical status and Fig. 30-14 presents the radiographs obtained 10 years after therapy. From these radiographs it can be observed (compare with Fig. 30-12) that during the maintenance period there has been no further loss of alveolar bone or widening of the various periodontal ligament spaces.

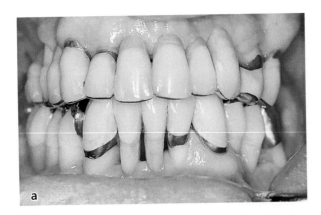

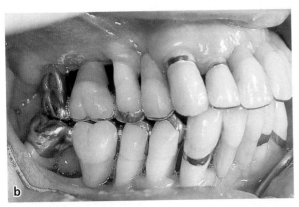

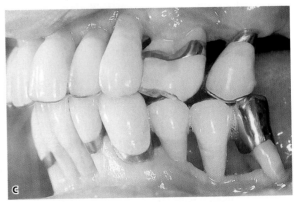

Fig. 30-13. Case B. Clinical status 9 years after therapy.

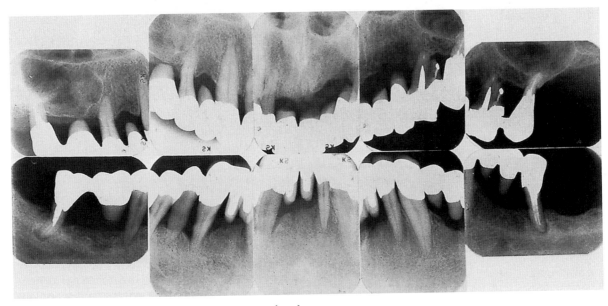

Fig. 30-14. Case B. Radiographs obtained 10 years after therapy.

Conclusion: Situation IV

Splinting is indicated when the periodontal support is so reduced that the mobility of the teeth is progressively increasing, i.e. when a tooth or a group of teeth during function are exposed to extraction forces.

Situation V

Increased bridge mobility despite splinting

In patients with advanced periodontal disease it can often be observed that the destruction of the periodontium has progressed to varying levels around different teeth and tooth surfaces in the dentition. Proper treatment of the plaque-associated lesions often includes multiple extractions. The remaining teeth may display an extreme reduction of the supporting tissues concomitant with increased or progressive tooth mobility. They may also be distributed in the jaw in such a way as to make it difficult, or impossible, to obtain a proper splinting effect even by means of a cross-arch bridge.

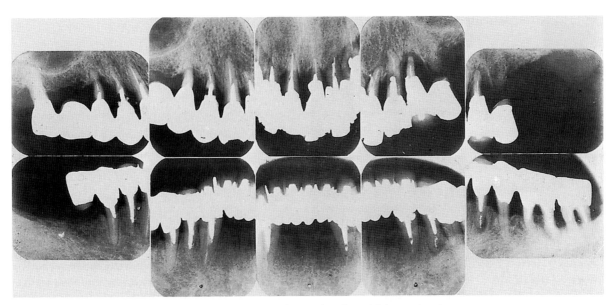

Fig. 30-15. Case C, 52-year-old female. Radiographs obtained at the initial examination.

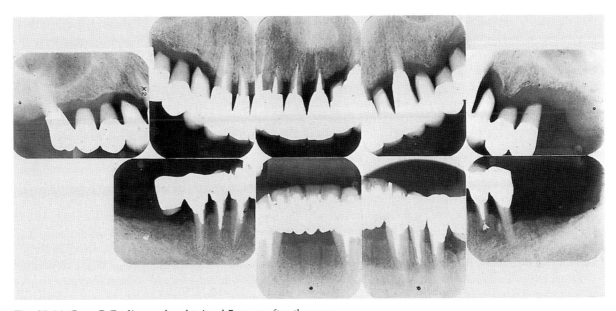

Fig. 30-16. Case C. Radiographs obtained 5 years after therapy.

The entire bridge/splint may exhibit mobility in frontal and or lateral directions.

It was stated above (Situation III) that a certain mobility of a tooth or a bridge of unilateral design can be accepted provided this mobility does not interfere with the patient's chewing ability or comfort. This is also valid for a cross-arch bridge/splint. From a biologic point of view there is no difference between increased tooth mobility on the one hand and increased bridge mobility on the other. However, neither progressive tooth mobility nor progressive bridge mobility can be accepted. In cases of extremely advanced periodontal disease, a cross-arch splint with an increased mobility may be regarded as an acceptable result of rehabilitation. The maintenance of status quo of the bridge/splint mobility and the prevention of tipping or orthodontic displacement of the total splint, however, requires particular attention regarding the design of the occlusion. Below, a case is reported which may serve as an interesting illustration of this particular clinical problem.

Example: Case C, 52-year-old female

Fig. 30-15 shows radiographs obtained at the initial examination. A 12-unit maxillary bridge was installed 10-15 years prior to the present examination using 18, 15, 14, 13, 12, 11, 21, 22, 23 and 24 as abutments. After a detailed clinical examination it was obvious that 15, 14, 22 and 24 could not be maintained because of severe symptoms of caries and periodontal disease. The remaining teeth were subjected to periodontal therapy and maintained as abutments for a new bridge/splint in the maxilla extending from tooth 18 to the region of 26, i.e. a cross-arch splint was installed which carried three cantilever units, namely 24, 25 and 26. The mobility of the individual abutment teeth immediately prior to insertion of the splint was the following: degree 1 (tooth 18), degree 0 (tooth 13),

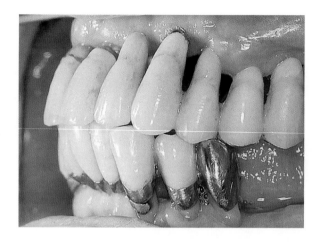

Fig. 30-17. Case C. The cantilever section including teeth 24, 25 and 26.

degree 2 (teeth 12 and 11), degree 3 (tooth 21) and degree 2 (tooth 23).

Radiographs obtained 5 years after therapy are shown in Fig. 30-16. The bridge/splint had a mobility of degree 1 immediately after its insertion and this mobility was unchanged 5 years later. The radiographs demonstrate that no further widening of the periodontal ligament occurred around the individual teeth during the maintenance period.

When a cross-arch bridge/splint exhibits increased mobility, the center (fulcrum) of the movement must be identified. In order to prevent further increase of the mobility and/or to prevent displacement of the bridge, it is essential to design the occlusion in such a way that the bridge/splint, when in contact with the teeth of the opposing jaw, is subjected to a balanced load, i.e. equal force on each side of the fulcrum. If this can be achieved, the force to which the bridge is exposed in occlusion can be used to retain the fixed prosthesis in proper balance (further increase of the mobility being thereby prevented).

Balanced loading of a mobile bridge/splint has to be established not only in the intercuspal position (IP) and centric occlusion (CP) but also in frontal and lateral excursive movements of the mandible if the bridge shows mobility or a tendency for tipping in the direction of such movements. In other words, a force which tends to displace the bridge in a certain direction has to be counteracted by the introduction of a balancing force on the opposite side of the fulcrum of the movement. If, for instance, a cross-arch splint in the maxilla exhibits mobility in frontal direction in conjunction with protrusive movements of the mandible, the load applied to the bridge in the frontal region has to be counterbalanced by a load in the distal portions of the splint; this means that there must be a simultaneous and equal contact relationship between the occluding teeth in both the frontal and the posterior regions of the splint. If the splint is mobile in a lateral direction, the force acting on the working side of the jaw must be counteracted by a force established by the introduction of balancing contacts in the non-working side of the jaw. The principle for establishing stability of a *mobile* cross-arch splint is consequently

the same as that used to obtain stability in a complete denture. In situations where distal abutment teeth are missing in a cross-arch bridge/splint with increased mobility, balance and functional stability may be obtained by means of cantilever units. It is important in this context to point out that balancing contacts on the non-working side should not be introduced in a bridge/splint in which no increased mobility can be observed.

The maxillary splint in the patient described in Figs. 30-13 to 30-16 exhibited increased mobility in frontal direction. Considering the small amount of periodontal support left around the anterior teeth, it is obvious that there would have been a risk of frontal displacement of the total bridge had the bridge terminated at the last abutment tooth (23) on the left side of the jaw. The installation of cantilever units in the 24 and 25 region prevented such a displacement of the bridge/splint by the introduction of a force counteracting frontally directed forces during protrusive movements of the mandible (Fig. 30-17). In addition, the cantilever units provide bilateral contact relationship towards the mandibular teeth in the intercuspal position, i.e. bilateral stability of the bridge.

In cases similar to the one described above, cantilever units can thus be used to prevent increasing mobility or displacement of a bridge/splint. It should, however, be pointed out that the insertion of cantilever units increases the risk of failures of a technical and biophysical character (fracture of the metal frame, fracture of abutment teeth, loss of retention, etc).

In cases of severely advanced periodontal disease it is often impossible to anticipate in the planning phase whether a bridge/splint after insertion will show signs of instability and increasing (progressive) mobility. In such cases, a provisional splint should always be inserted. Any alterations of the mobility of the bridge/splint can be observed over a prolonged period of time and the occlusion continuously adjusted until, after 4-6 months, it is known whether stability (i.e. no further increase of the mobility) can be achieved. The design of the occlusion of the provisional acrylic bridge is then reproduced in the permanent bridge construction. If, on the other hand, stability cannot be obtained, the rehabilitation of the case cannot be achieved with a fixed splint. The alternative treatment then is a complete denture or an implant supported restoration.

Conclusion: Situation V

An increased mobility of a cross-arch bridge/splint can be accepted provided the mobility does not disturb chewing ability or comfort and the mobility of the splint is not progressively increasing.

References

Glickman, I. (1965). Clinical significance of trauma from occlusion. *Journal of the American Dental Association* **70**, 607-618.

Glickman, I. (1967). Occlusion and periodontium. *Journal of Dental Research* **46**, Supplement, 53.

Glossary of Periodontic Terms (1986). *Journal of Periodontology*. Supplement.

Karring, T., Nyman, S., Thilander, B. & Magnusson, I. (1982). Bone-regeneration in orthodontically produced alveolar bone dehiscences. *Journal of Periodontal Research* **17**, 309-315.

Mühlemann, H.R. (1954). Tooth mobility. The measuring method. Initial and secondary tooth mobility. *Journal of Periodontology* **25**, 22-29.

Mühlemann, H.R. (1960). Ten years of tooth mobility measurements. *Journal of Periodontology* **31**, 110-122.

Mühlemann, H.R. & Zander, H.A. (1954). Tooth mobility, III. The mechanism of tooth mobility. *Journal of Periodontology* **25**, 128.

Nyman, S., Karring, T., & Bergenholtz, G. (1982). Bone regeneration in alveolar bone dehiscences produced by jiggling forces. *Journal of Periodontal Research* **17**, 316-322.

Polson, A.M., Meitner, S.W. & Zander, H.A. (1976a). Trauma and progression of marginal periodontitis in squirrel monkeys. III. Adaptation of interproximal alveolar bone to repetitive injury. *Journal of Periodontal Research* **11**, 279-289.

Polson, A.M., Meitner, S.W. & Zander, H.A. (1976b). Trauma and progression of marginal periodontitis in squirrel monkeys. IV. Reversibility of bone loss due to trauma alone and trauma superimposed upon periodontitis. *Journal of Periodontal Research* **11**, 290-298.

Schulte, W. (1987). Der Periotest-Parodontalstatus. *Zahnärztliche Mitteilung* **76**, 1409-1414.

Schulte, W., Hoedt, B., Lukas, D., Maunz, M. & Steppeler, M. (1992). Periotest for measuring periodontal characteristics – Correlation with periodontal bone loss. *Journal of Periodontal Research* **27**, 184-190.

Waerhaug, J. (1979). The infrabony pocket and its relationship to trauma from occlusion and subgingival plaque. *Journal of Periodontology* **50**, 355-365.

Waerhaug, J. & Randers-Hansen, E. (1966). Periodontal changes incident to prolonged occlusal overload in monkeys. *Acta Odontologica Scandinavica* **24**, 91-105.

CHAPTER 31

Orthodontics and Periodontics

BJÖRN U. ZACHRISSON

Orthodontic treatment may be adjunctive to periodontal therapy. The loss of periodontal support or teeth may result in elongation, spacing and proclination of incisors, rotation and tipping of premolars and molars with collapse of the posterior occlusion, and decreasing vertical dimension. But orthodontic tooth movement can also facilitate the management of several restorative and esthetic problems in adults. Such difficulties may be related to subgingivally fractured or lost teeth, tipped abutment teeth, excess spacing, inadequate implant or pontic space, supra-erupted teeth, narrow alveolar ridges that prevent implant placement, and other conditions (Ong et al. 1998). The purpose of this chapter is to discuss how recent basic and clinical information may be used to improve treatment planning, clinical management, and retention for patients in whom different malocclusions are caused or complicated by moderate to advanced periodontal destruction.

ORTHODONTIC TOOTH MOVEMENT IN ADULTS WITH PERIODONTAL TISSUE BREAKDOWN

Poorly executed orthodontic treatment in periodontal patients can certainly contribute to further periodontal tissue breakdown. In particular, the combination of inflammation, orthodontic forces and occlusal trauma

Fig. 31-1. Adult male patient with advanced periodontitis and marked pathologic migration of the anterior teeth before (left column) and after (right column) periodontal and orthodontic fixed-appliance treatment for 2 years. Clinical appearance of the face and dentition are dramatically improved after the combined periodontic/orthodontic treatment. The dental result is maintained by means of bonded lingual retainer wires. A maxillary two-unit and a mandibular three-unit bridge were constructed. Some interdental recession was unavoidable in the mandibular anterior region (d), but it does not show much clinically (b).

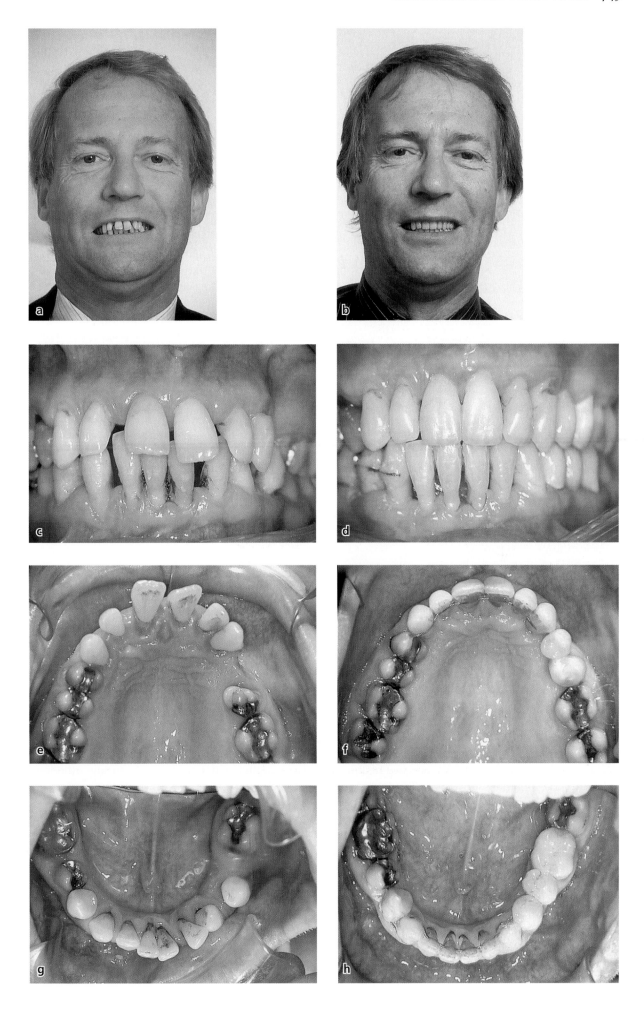

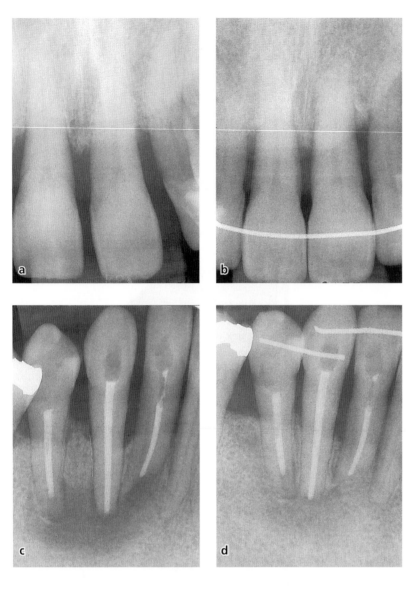

Fig. 31-2. Long-term radiographic follow-up of the same patient as in Fig. 31-1. Radiographs of maxillary and mandibular anterior regions 7 years after the completion of orthodontic therapy (b,d) show reduced but healthy periodontium, with no progression of periodontal tissue destruction compared with the initial situation (a,c).

may produce a more rapid destruction than would occur with inflammation alone (Kessler 1976). However, with properly performed treatment, extensive orthodontic tooth movement can be made in adults with a reduced but healthy periodontium without further periodontal deterioration. Figs. 31-1 to 31-6 show the pretreatment and post-treatment conditions in four different adult orthodontic patients with advanced periodontitis. The findings of no significant further periodontal tissue breakdown in these patients was the result of carefully controlled treatment planning considerations.

Only a few well-controlled studies have been published on groups of adults with advanced periodontitis, who have received comprehensive orthodontic fixed-appliance treatment. Boyd et al. (1989) described 10 adults with generalized periodontitis who received preorthodontic periodontal treatment including surgery, and then regular maintenance at 3-month intervals during a 2-year orthodontic treatment period. They were compared with 10 control adults who had normal periodontal tissues, and 20 adolescent orthodontic patients. The results demonstrated that:

- Adults were more effective than adolescents in removing plaque, especially late in the orthodontic treatment period
- Tooth movement in adults with reduced, but healthy, periodontium did not result in significant further loss of attachment (none of the adults had additional mean loss of attachment of more than 0.3 mm)
- Adults with teeth that did *not* have healthy periodontal tissues may experience further breakdown and tooth loss due to abscesses during orthodontic treatment.

In another study by Årtun & Urbye (1988) 24 patients with advanced loss of marginal bone and pathologic tooth migration received active appliance therapy for an average of 7 months, following periodontal treatment. Bone level measurements on radiographs indicated that the majority of sites showed little or no additional loss of bone support. However, a few sites demonstrated pronounced additional bone loss.

More recent studies on much larger groups (350-400 patients) of consecutively treated adult patients from different practices (Nelson & Årtun 1997, Re et al.

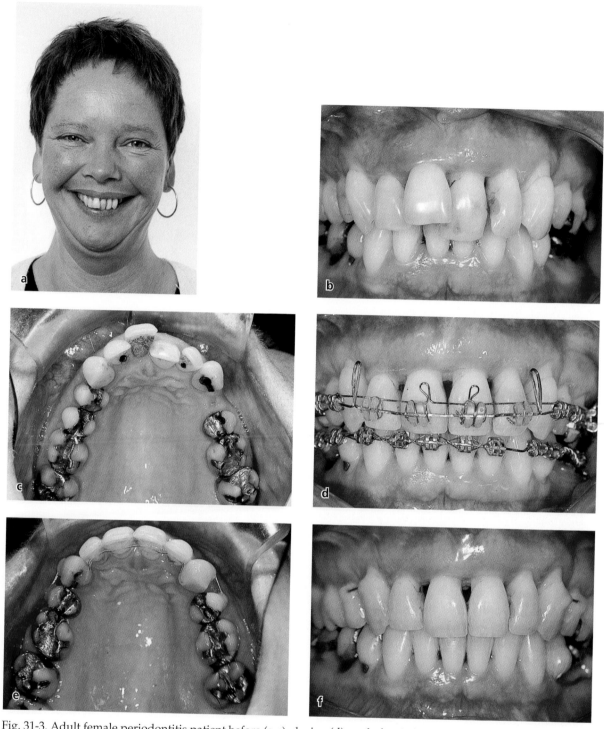

Fig. 31-3. Adult female periodontitis patient before (a-c), during (d), and after (e,f) periodontal and orthodontic treatment. The initial extensive destruction of bone around the maxillary incisors had resulted in pathologic migration (b,c), and the loss of the left first premolar. The right first premolar was extracted as part of the treatment plan. The treatment result is retained with a gold-coated maxillary retainer bonded lingually from canine to canine, and two short labial retainers in the closed extraction sites (e,f). The esthetic result is much improved, even in the presence of some interdental gingival recession post-treatment (f). No apparent further progression of the periodontal tissue breakdown occurred during the orthodontic space closure and levelling of the teeth.

2000) have confirmed that (1) pretreatment evidence of periodontal tissue destruction is no contraindication for orthodontics, (2) orthodontic therapy improves the possibilities of saving and restoring a deteriorated dentition, and (3) the risk of recurrence of an active disease process is not increased during appliance therapy. However, these larger samples have

indicated that adult orthodontic patients are at a somewhat higher risk than adolescents for tissue breakdown. The mean bone loss on radiographs of the six anterior teeth in the study of Nelson & Årtun (1997) was 0.54 mm (SD 0.62). Only 2.5% of the patients had average bone loss of 2 mm or more, but as many as

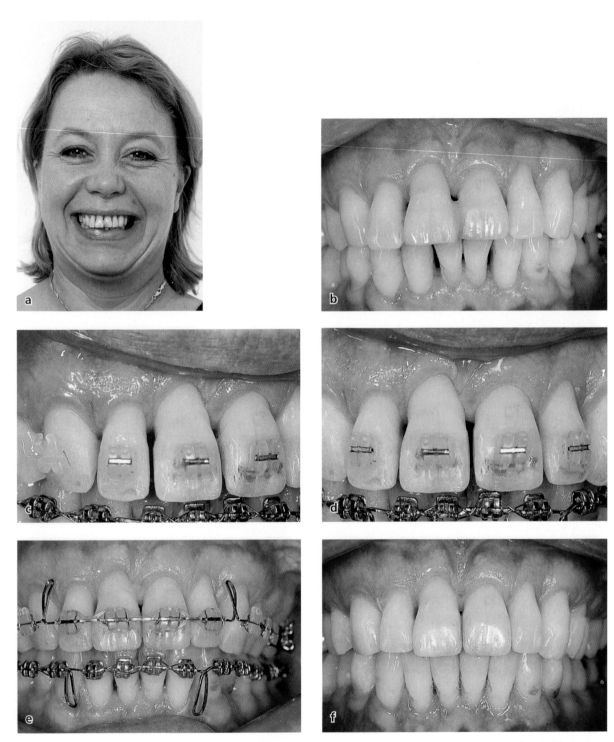

Fig. 31-4. Adult female periodontitis patient with pathologic migration of the maxillary incisors before (a,b), during (c-e) and after (f) periodontal and orthodontic treatment. An attempt had been made by the periodontist to grind and splint the overextruded right central incisor with composite resin (b) before orthodontic treatment was started. Due to extensive mesial and distal recontouring of the incisors (stripping) during the treatment (c,d), it was possible to obtain an esthetic final result with almost intact gingival papillae between the incisors in both the maxilla and in the mandible (f).

36% of these patients had one or more surfaces with bone loss exceeding 2 mm.

Orthodontic treatment considerations

The key element in the orthodontic management of adult patients with periodontal disease is to eliminate, or reduce, plaque accumulation and gingival inflammation. This implies much emphasis on oral hygiene instruction, appliance construction, and periodical check-ups throughout treatment (Zachrisson 1996).

The most appropriate method for tooth movement must be determined in each particular case. Although minor or partial orthodontic treatment with sectional or removable appliances may be possible in some

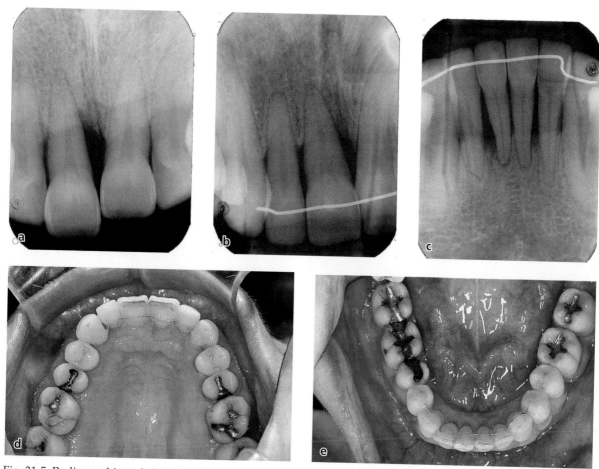

Fig. 31-5. Radiographic and clinical occlusal appearance of the same patient as in Fig. 31-4. No noticeable progression of the periodontal tissue destruction has occurred (compare a and b), and although markedly reduced the periodontium is healthy after the orthodontic therapy (b,c). The treatment result is maintained by means of gold-coated lingual retainers over six maxillary and eight mandibular anterior teeth (d,e). These bonded retainers act as effective orthodontic retainers as well as neat and hygienic periodontal splints.

instances, in the majority of cases a fully controlled technique with fixed appliances in both dental arches is preferred in order to carefully control the movement of teeth in three planes.

The orthodontic appliance has to be properly designed. It must provide stable anchorage without causing tissue irritation, and must be esthetically acceptable. For psychologic reasons bonded ceramic brackets are preferred in the most visible regions (Figs. 31-3 to 31-6), generally for the maxillary teeth, whereas stainless steel or gold-coated attachments are commonly used elsewhere in the mouth (Figs. 31-3, 31-4).

To counteract the tendency of orthodontic appliances to increase the accumulation of plaque on the teeth, attempts should be made to keep the appliances and mechanics simple, and avoid hooks, elastomeric rings and excess bonding resin outside the bracket bases. The use of steel ligatures is recommended on all brackets (Figs. 31-3, 31-4, 31-6), since elastomeric rings have been shown to be significantly more plaque attractive than steel ties (Forsberg et al. 1991). Bonds are preferrable to bands (Boyd & Baumrind 1992). Bonded molars show less plaque accumulation, gingivitis and loss of attachment interproximally than banded molars during orthodontic treatment of adults. However, bonding is more complicated in adult patients than in adolescents. Many adults have amalgam restorations and crown-and-bridge restorations made of porcelain or precious metals. Thanks to the introduction of new techniques and materials, it is feasible to bond orthodontic brackets, buccal tubes and retainer wires to artificial surfaces. Clinical experience with bonding to different artificial tooth surfaces, except gold, is excellent (Zachrisson 2000a,b).

Renewed oral hygiene instruction and motivation is made after the placement of the orthodontic appliances. During the treatment period professional tooth cleaning by dental hygienist or periodontist may be performed at 3 month intervals (Boyd et al. 1989, Boyd & Baumrind 1992), or after regular examination updates at 6 and 12 month intervals, depending on the situation. The re-examinations should include recordings of probing depths, mobility, bleeding on probing, suppuration, gingival recessions, bone levels, etc. Professional scaling may be indicated during *active intrusion* of elongated maxillary incisors, since orthodontic intrusion may shift supragingival plaque to a subgingival location (Ericsson et al. 1977, 1978). If efforts at maintaining excellent-to-good oral hygiene are un-

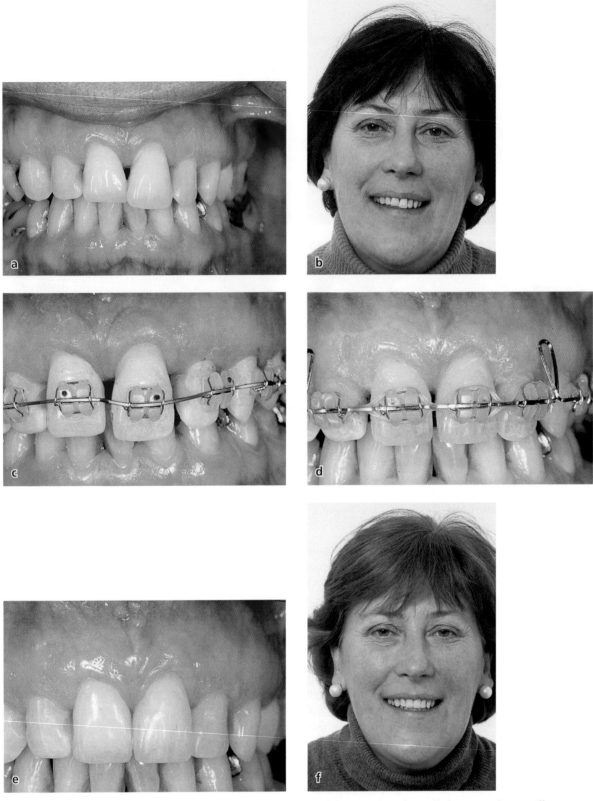

Fig. 31-6. Adult female periodontitis patient with marked loss of the interdental papilla between the maxillary central incisors (a,b). This gap is caused by the "fan-shaped" morphology of the central incisors, which places the interproximal contact too near the incisal edge. To eliminate the unesthetic soft tissue gap, the mesial surfaces of the central incisors were reshaped (c) to lengthen their connector area and move the contact point gingivally (d). After continued orthodontic space closure, a more esthetic final result was achieved (e,f).

successful, orthodontic treatment should be terminated (Machen 1990).

After appliance removal, reinstruction in oral hygiene measures should be given. Otherwise, subsequent labial gingival recession may be risked due to overzealous toothbrushing, since cleaning is now easier to perform.

Esthetic finishing of treatment results

Adults with a reduced periodontium represent different challenges for orthodontists than adolescents. Worn or abraded teeth, missing papillae and uneven crown lengths are common problems, and it is therefore more difficult to obtain an esthetically optimal appearance of the teeth and gingiva after bracket removal.

Most incisor teeth in adults with malocclusions have more or less worn incisal edges, which represent an adaptation to the functional demands. When the axial inclinations and rotations of such incisors are corrected, there is frequently need for incisal grinding towards a more normal contour. Such grinding can be performed safely as long as the wear is limited, the overbite is adequate, and the patients display enough tooth material in conversation and on smiling. When the abrasion is more significant, however, co-operation with a restorative dentist is generally indicated.

The presence of papillae between the maxillary incisors is a key esthetic factor after orthodontic treatment. Normally, when a long-standing crowding with incisor overlap is corrected orthodontically in adults, it is generally not possible to have an intact papilla. This is because the contact point becomes located too far incisally on the triangular crowns that have not had a normal interdental wear pattern. Similarly, in patients with advanced periodontal disease and destruction of the crestal bone between the incisors, the papillae may be absent. This produces unesthetic gaps between the teeth after orthodontics. The best method of correcting this problem is to recontour the mesiodistal surfaces of the incisors during the orthodontic finishing stage (Tuverson 1980). When the diastemata thus created are closed, the roots of the teeth can come closer together. The contact point is lengthened and moved apically, and the papilla can fill out the interdental space more easily (Figs. 31-4, 31-6).

In patients with high or normal smile lines, the relationship of the gingival margins of the maxillary anterior teeth may be another important factor in the esthetic appearance of the crowns (Kokich 1996a,b). When adult patients have gingival margin discrepancies between adjacent teeth, the orthodontist must determine the proper solution for the problem: orthodontic movement to reposition the gingival margin (Fig. 31-17) or surgical correction (gingivectomy) to increase the crown length of single or several teeth (Figs. 31-29, 31-30).

Retention – problems and solutions; long-term follow-up

Due to the anatomic and biologic differences in tissue reaction between adults and children (Melsen 1991), adults undergoing extensive orthodontic treatment will generally need, at least, a longer period of retention than would an adolescent patient. Also, growth and development no longer take place and cannot aid in changing occlusal levels or in space closure by the eruption of posterior teeth with mesial drift. The space reopening tendency of closed extraction sites in adults can be mitigated by use of labially bonded retainers (Figs. 31-1, 31-3).

The migration of teeth associated with periodontal tissue breakdown around the incisors in adults is usually blamed on inflammatory swelling or the tongue thrust. However, according to Proffit (1978), two major primary factors are involved in the equilibrium which determines the final position of teeth. These are the resting pressures of lip or cheek and tongue, and forces produced by metabolic activity within the periodontal membrane. With an intact periodontium, unbalanced tongue-lip forces are normally counteracted by forces from the periodontal membrane. However, when the periodontium breaks down, its stabilizing function no longer exists and the incisors begin to move. A consequence of this concept would be that persons with advanced periodontal disease and tooth migration would need permanent retention after the orthodontic correction. For patients with minimum-to-moderate loss of periodontal tissue support, more "normal" retention periods may be sufficient.

The optimal long-term retainer for adults with reduced periodontium is the flexible spiral wire (FSW) retainer bonded lingually on each tooth in a segment. The bonded retainer in the anterior region is generally used together with a maxillary removable plate. The fabrication and long-term evaluation of bonded retainers is described by Dahl and Zachrisson (1991). Figs. 31-1, 31-3, and 31-5 demonstrate different designs of FSW retainers in the maxilla and the mandible in several patients. At the same time as the FSW retainer works as a reliable, invisible orthodontic retainer, it concomitantly acts as a periodontal splint, which allows the individual teeth within the splint to exert physiological mobility. As long as the retainer remains intact, small spaces might open up distal to, but not within, the retainer.

Splinting may not be needed for most teeth with increased mobility after periodontal therapy (Ramfjord 1984). However, reduced mobility of teeth after combined periodontal and orthodontic treatment by using a bonded retainer would seem to be of considerable benefit. If a bonded retainer is not used, and instead a removable plate or spring retainer is used at night on a long-term basis, there is a risk for ongoing jiggling of the teeth because of the relapse tendency during the day. Experimental studies in animals indicate that jiggling forces may facilitate the progress of attachment loss in periodontitis, or at least result in more bone resorption. Also, more connective tissue reattachment and bone regeneration may occur around non-jiggled teeth. Monkey experiments have shown that when experimental jiggling of teeth was stopped, a significant gain of alveolar bone occurred (Nyman et al. 1982). Similarly, Burgett et al. (1992) demonstrated that the healing following periodontal therapy may be more advantageous in patients who received occlusal adjustment than in non-adjusted patients.

Long-term follow-up of patients who have received combined periodontal and orthodontic treatment, and have used bonded retainers for several years, demonstrates excellent stability and apparently unchanged, or even improved, periodontal condition (Figs. 31-7, 31-8). It should be pointed out, however, that a bonded maxillary retainer must be placed out of occlusion with the mandibular incisors, because biting on a retainer wire will lead to unacceptably high bond failure rates (Årtun & Urbye 1988).

Possibilities and limitations; legal aspects

Adult orthodontic patients with marked periodontal destruction may represent potential problems even when optimal treatment is provided. There are, however, no definite metric limits in terms of probing depths or loss of attachment when orthodontic tooth movement can no longer be performed (Diedrich 1999). Each individual treatment plan may depend on a variety of factors and can be limited by biomechanical considerations (force systems, limited anchorage), by periodontal risk factors (tooth/alveolar bone topography, sinus recesses, activity and prognosis of the periodontitis), and by limited patient motivation and poor oral hygiene co-operation.

Single case reports have documented successful periodontal-orthodontic treatment with localized juvenile periodontitis (LJP) after conventional periodontal therapy (Harpenau & Boyd 2000), or with continous antiseptic and short-term systemic (Folio et al. 1985) or local (Hoerman et al. 1985) antibiotic applications, and microbiologic testing during the orthodontic treatment period to reduce the risk of recurrent disease. However, until more evidence is accumulated, it may seem wise to avoid orthodontic treatment in patients with particularly aggressive forms of periodontal disease. Similarly, multirooted teeth with questionable prognosis should be moved orthodontically only in exceptional situations.

"Hopeless teeth": According to old concepts, the retention of teeth diagnosed as periodontally "hopeless" would accelerate the destruction of the adjacent interproximal periodontium. Such teeth were therefore frequently extracted in the past. However, the theoretic rationale for such extractions would seem unsupported, and recent follow-up studies have demonstrated that retained periodontally "hopeless" teeth do not significantly affect the interproximal periodontium of adjacent teeth following periodontal therapy (Chace & Low 1993). The clinical implication is that these teeth can be useful for orthodontic anchorage, if the periodontal inflammation can be controlled (Fig. 31-9). Occasionally, the hopeless tooth may be so improved after orthodontic treatment that it is retained (Mathews & Kokich 1997). Alternatively, a hopeless molar may be hemisectioned after the orthodontic treatment, and the best root may be used as a bridge abutment (Fig. 31-10). Most of the time, however, the hopeless tooth will be extracted, especially if other restorations are planned in the segment.

For improved patient care, stress reduction, and reduction or elimination of law-suits, careful examination protocols, documentation and correspondence techniques, and regular progress evaluations are important. The legal implications of orthodontic risk management concepts may be that it is preferable to terminate treatment for patients who fail to improve oral hygiene care, despite the orthodontist's efforts. In the long term, this will be better for both patient and orthodontist, since termination, if properly handled, will be more easily defended than permitting the condition to worsen (Machen 1990). However, if proper procedures are followed, termination of orthodontic care for periodontal patients will very rarely be needed.

SPECIFIC FACTORS ASSOCIATED WITH ORTHODONTIC TOOTH MOVEMENT IN ADULTS

Tooth movement into infrabony pockets

Orthodontic forces *per se* are unlikely to convert gingivitis into destructive periodontitis. The plaque-induced lesion in gingivitis is confined to the supra-alveolar connective tissue, whereas tissue reactions to orthodontic forces occur in the connective tissue between the root and the alveolar bone. However, infrabony pockets, i.e. angular bony defects with inflamed connective tissue and epithelium apical to the bone crest, may develop as a result of destructive periodontitis. Infrabony pockets may also be created by orthodontic tipping and/or intruding movements of teeth harboring plaque (Ericsson et al. 1977). The effect of bodily tooth movement into infrabony defects has been evaluated experimentally in monkeys (Polson et al. 1984) and in dogs (Wennström et al. 1993). Provided elimination of the subgingival infection was performed before the orthodontic tooth movement was started, no detrimental effects on the attachment level were observed. The angular bony defect was eliminated by the orthodontic treatment, but no coronal gain of attachment was found and a thin epithelial

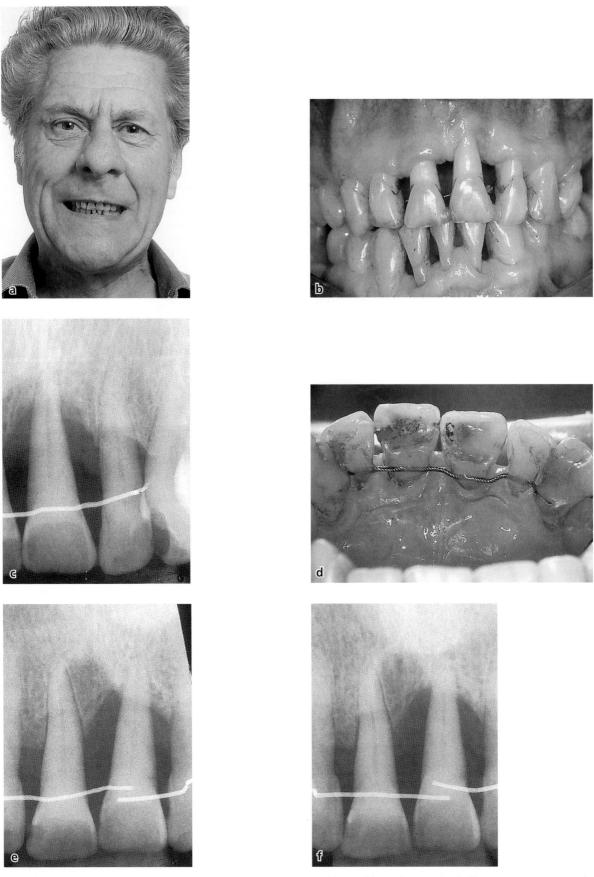

Fig. 31-7. Adult male periodontitis patient after periodontal and orthodontic therapy (a-d). The patient was treated with generalized gingivectomies according to concepts aiming at pocket elimination. The orthodontic result is maintained with a six-unit lingually bonded retainer (d). The bonded wire will act both as an orthodontic retainer and as a periodontal splint, which would appear advantageous in cases where the tissue destruction is as advanced as in this patient. (e) and (f) show the radiographic appearances 7 and 9 years, respectively, after removal of the orthodontic appliances. The left central incisor had so little bone support that if the bonded retainer had not been used, the tooth would probably had been lost over time (see also Fig. 31-8).

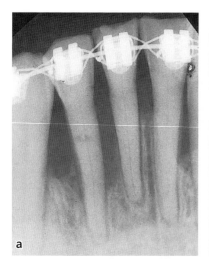
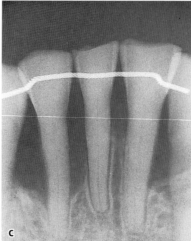
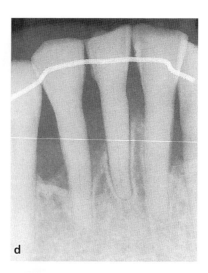
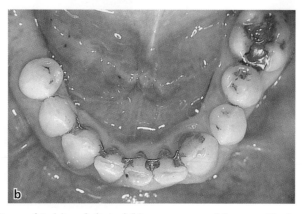

Fig. 31-8. Post-treatment radiographic (a) and clinical (b) appearance of the mandibular dentition in the same patient as in Fig. 31-7 after periodontal and orthodontic treatment. The mandibular six-unit retainer bonded lingual retainer (b) concomitantly acts as a periodontal splint. Note signs of improvement of periodontal condition 7 and 9 years, respectively, after the orthodontic treatment (c,d), with marked crestal lamina dura contours.

lining covered the root surface corresponding to its pretreatment position (Fig. 31-11). It was therefore concluded that orthodontic tooth movement into infrabony periodontal defects had no favorable effects on the level of connective tissue attachment. However, it was possible to move teeth with reduced *healthy* periodontium without additional attachment loss. If, on the other hand, the orthodontic treatment involved movement of teeth into and through a site with inflammation and angular bone loss, an enhanced rate of periodontal destruction was noted.

Conclusion

Since orthodontic movement of teeth into inflamed infrabony pockets may create a high risk for additional periodontal destruction, and because infrabony pockets are frequently found at teeth that have been tipped and/or elongated as a result of periodontal disease, it is clinically essential that periodontal treatment with elimination of the plaque-induced lesion is performed before orthodontic therapy is begun. It is equally important that excellent oral hygiene is maintained throughout the course of the orthodontic treatment. Following these principles, clinical and radiographic observations confirm that orthodontic treat-

ment can be successfully performed in patients with infrabony pockets resulting from periodontal disease.

Tooth movement into compromised bone areas

Orthodontic tooth movement may sometimes be performed in adults with partially edentulous dentitions (due to agenesis or previous extractions of teeth) and such patients may have a more or less compromised alveolar process. Experimental reports (Lindskog-Stokland et al. 1993) and clinical studies (Stepovich 1979, Hom & Turley 1984, Goldberg & Turley 1989, Thilander 1996) have shown that a reduction in vertical bone height is not a contraindication for orthodontic tooth movement towards, or into, the constricted area. Mandibular second molars can be moved mesially through remodeled edentulous first molar areas in adults (Fig. 31-12), with only a limited reduction in vertical bone height, averaging –1.3 mm (Hom & Turley 1984). Space closure is possible also in edentulous maxillary first molar areas, although vertical bone loss and some space re-opening can be a complication.

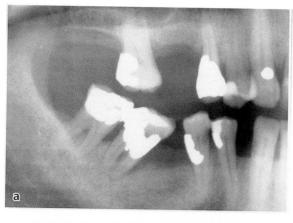
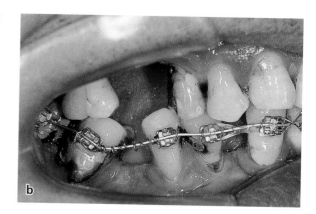
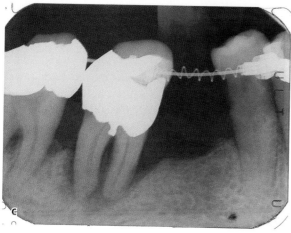
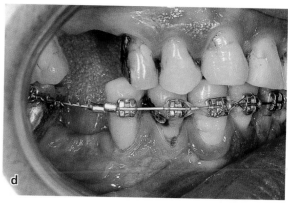

Fig. 31-9. "Hopeless" mandibular right first molar (a) can be used as part of anchorage to move the premolars mesially and upright the second molar (b-d). The first molar may be kept, or extracted, after the orthodontic treatment period.

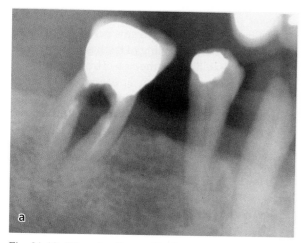
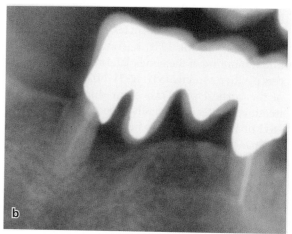

Fig. 31-10. "Hopeless" mandibular right first molar (a) was used as anchorage during orthodontic treatment to close spaces anteriorly, before it was hemisectioned and the distal root employed as a bridge abutment (b).

Histologic observations in animal experiments have confirmed that when light forces were applied to move teeth bodily into an area with reduced bone height, a thin bone plate was recreated ahead of the moving tooth (Fig. 31-13) (Lindskog-Stokland et al. 1993). The key to moving teeth with bone is direct resorption in the direction of tooth movement, and avoiding hyalinization. Teeth can be moved with bone into the maxillary sinus also (Melsen 1991).

Conclusion

Although the results of clinical experiments and follow-ups are encouraging, provided light forces are used and excellent oral hygiene is maintained, it is probably wise not to stretch the indications for tooth movement into constricted bone areas too far. Marked gingival invaginations are sometimes seen in such areas (Fig. 31-12), and computer tomography analysis and human histological findings indicate that buccal

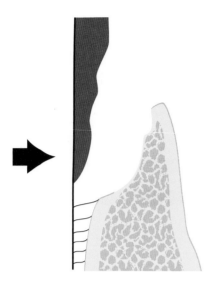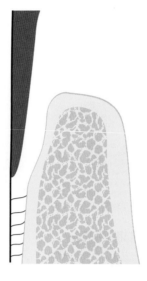

Fig. 31-11. Schematic illustration of persisting junctional epithelium subsequent to orthodontic tooth movement (direction of arrow) into an infrabony pocket.

or lingual bone dehiscences may occur (Diedrich 1996). Such defects are not revealed by conventional radiography. The clinical significance of the gingival clefts and bone dehiscences with regard to relapse tendency and periodontal status is not known. For orthodontic tooth movement into markedly atrophied alveolar ridges, the possibility to acquire new bone by, for example, GBR procedures (see Chapter 38) should be considered.

Tooth movement through cortical bone

Experimental studies in animals have demonstrated that when a tooth is moved bodily in a labial direction towards and through the cortical plate of the alveolar bone, no bone formation will take place in front of the tooth (Steiner et al. 1981, Karring et al. 1982). After initial thinning of the bone plate, a labial bone dehiscence is therefore created (Fig. 31-14). Such perforation of the cortical plate can occur during orthodontic treatment either accidentally or because it was considered unavoidable. It may happen for example (1) in the mandibular anterior region due to frontal expansion of incisors (Wehrbein et al. 1994), (2) in the maxillary posterior region during lateral expansion of cross-bites (Greenbaum & Zachrisson 1982), (3) lingually in the maxilla associated with retraction and lingual root torque of maxillary incisors in patients with large overjets (Ten Hoeve & Mulie 1976), and (4) by pronounced traumatic jiggling of teeth (Nyman et al. 1982). The soft tissue reactions accompanying such tooth movements are discussed later in this chapter and in Chapter 30.

Interestingly, however, there is potential for repair when malpositioned teeth are moved back toward their original positions, and bone apposition may take place (Fig. 31-14). Evidently, the soft tissue facial to an orthodontically produced bone dehiscence may contain soft tissue components (vital osteogenic cells) with a capacity for forming bone following repositioning of the tooth into the alveolar process (Nyman et al. 1982).

Conclusion

The clinical implication of these observations is encouraging. Bone dehiscences which may occur due to uncontrolled expansion of teeth through the cortical plate may be repaired when the teeth are brought back, or relapse, towards a proper position within the alveolar process, even if this occurs several months later. Similar repair mechanisms may be expected to occur when marked jiggling of teeth is brought under control and stabilized. In the case of buccal cross-bites, the initial discrepancy can apparently be overcorrected with both slow and rapid expansion treatment approaches without causing permanent periodontal injury to the settled occlusion.

Extrusion and intrusion of single teeth – effects on periodontium, clinical crown length and esthetics

Extrusion

Orthodontic extrusion of teeth, or so-called "forced eruption", may be indicated for (1) shallowing out intraosseous defects and (2) for increasing clinical crown length of single teeth. The forced eruption technique was originally described by Ingber (1974) for

Fig. 31-12. Orthodontic tooth movements into edentulous areas with reduced bone height in compromised mandible of adult female patient. During the orthodontic treatment (c-g), the teeth were moved to close three areas of marked alveolar bone constriction (a,b), most notably in the right first molar area. Note that the impacted third molar erupted spontaneously as the second molar was moved mesially (g). (h) shows final result with bonded six-unit lingual and two-unit labial retainers.

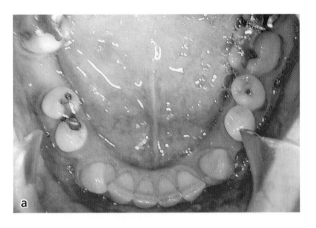

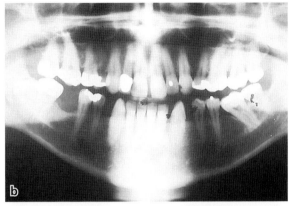

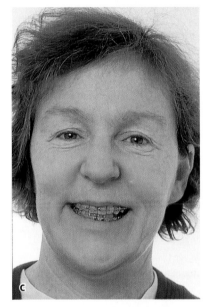

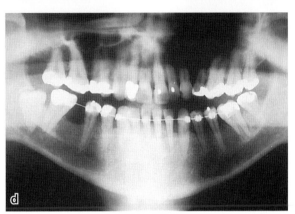

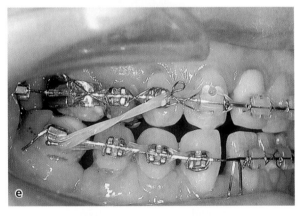

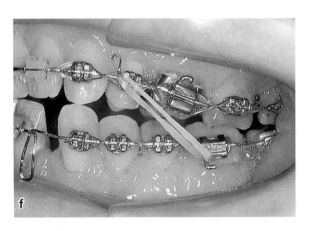

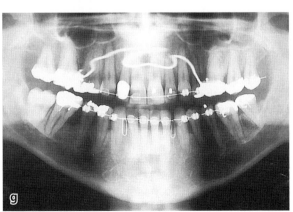

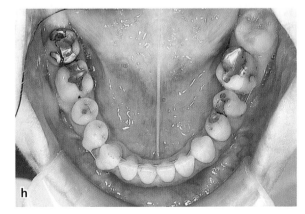

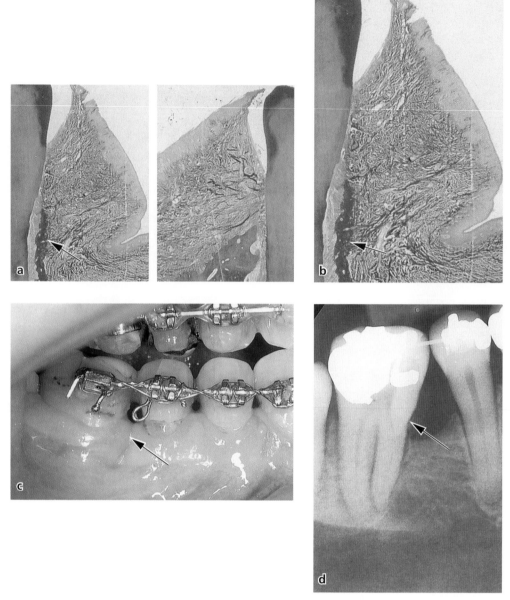

Fig. 31-13. (a) and (b) show histologic specimens from experimental orthodontic tooth movement into edentulous areas in dogs. The thin bone spicule along the pressure side of the test tooth (b) indicates tooth movement with, and not through, bone. (c) and (d) show the same patient as in Fig. 31-12. Note radiographic visualization of the thin bone spicule on the mesial side of the second molar (arrow in d). Although the molar is moved to contact the second premolar, a marked gingival invagination is present in the area (arrow in c). (a) and (b) from Lindskog-Stokland et al. (1993).

treatment of one-wall and two-wall bony pockets that were difficult to handle by conventional therapy alone. The extrusive tooth movement leads to a coronal positioning of intact connective tissue attachment, and the bony defect is shallowed out. This was confirmed in animal experiments (van Venroy & Yukna 1985) and clinical trials. Because of the orthodontic extrusion, the tooth will be in supraocclusion. Hence, the crown of the tooth will need to be shortened, in some cases followed by endodontic treatment.

During the elimination of an intraosseous pocket by means of orthodontic extrusion, the relationship between the CEJ and the bone crest is maintained. This means that the bone follows the tooth during the extrusive movement. This may or may not be benefi-

cial depending on the clinical situation. In other words, it is sometimes desirable to have the periodontium follow the tooth and in other situations it is desirable to move a tooth out of the periodontal support. This is further discussed under slow versus rapid eruption of teeth in Chapter 30.

Extrusion with periodontium

Orthodontic extrusion of a single tooth that needs to be extracted is an excellent method for improvement of the marginal bone level before the surgical placement of single implants (Figs. 31-15, 31-21). Not only the bone, but also the soft supporting tissues will move vertically with the teeth during orthodontic extrusion. Using tattoo marks in monkeys to indicate

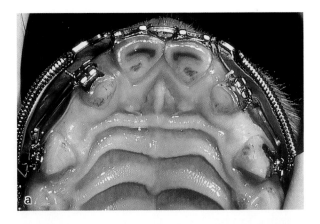
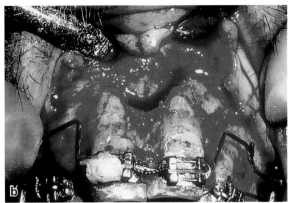
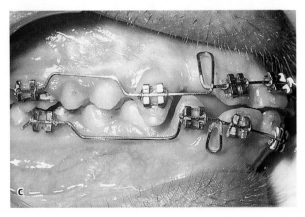
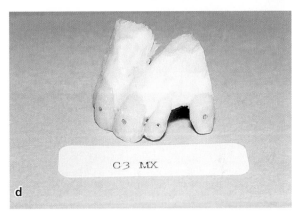

Fig. 31-14. Techniques used by Steiner et al. (1981) to bodily advance incisors through the labial bone plate in monkeys (a,b) and by Engelking & Zachrisson (1982) to retract the incisors to their original position (after the teeth had remained in extreme labioversion for 8 months) in a study of periodontal regeneration to such tooth movement. Tissue blocks after tooth repositioning (d) show evident bone regeneration.

the mucogingival junction and clinical sulcus bottom, Kajiyama et al. (1993) made a metric evaluation of the gingival movement associated with vertical extrusion of incisors. The results indicated that the free gingiva moved about 90% and the attached gingiva about 80% of the extruded distance. The width of the attached gingiva and the clinical crown length increased significantly, whereas the position of the mucogingival junction was unchanged. Orthodontic extrusion of a "hopeless" incisor is therefore a useful method also for esthetic improvement of the marginal gingival level associated with the placement of implants (Fig. 31-15).

Extrusion out of periodontium
In teeth with crown-root fracture, or other subgingival fractures, the goal of treatment may be to extrude the root out of the periodontium (Fig. 31-16), and then provide it with an artificial crown. When an increased distance between the CEJ and the alveolar bone crest is aimed at, the forced eruption should be combined with gingival fiberotomy (Pontoriero et al. 1987, Kozlowsky et al. 1988). Berglundh et al. (1991) showed in animal experiments that when the fiberotomy (i.e. excision of the coronal portion of the fiber attachment around the tooth) was performed frequently (every 2 weeks), the tooth was virtually moved out of the bony periodontium, without affecting the bone heights or

level of the marginal gingiva of the neighboring teeth. This procedure is illustrated in Fig. 31-16.

Intrusion
Similar to the indications for extrusion, the orthodontic intrusion of teeth has been recommended (1) for teeth with horizontal bone loss or infrabony pockets, and (2) for increasing the clinical crown length of single teeth. However, the benefits of intrusion for improvement of the periodontal condition around teeth are controversial.

As mentioned, the intrusion of plaque-infected teeth may lead to the formation of angular bony defects and increased loss of attachment. When oral hygiene is inadequate, tipping and intrusion of the teeth may shift supragingivally located plaque into a subgingival position, resulting in periodontal destruction (Ericsson et al. 1977, 1978). This explains why professional subgingival scaling is particularly important during the phase of active intrusion of elongated, tipped and migrated maxillary incisors commonly occurring in association with advanced periodontal disease. Even in a healthy periodontal environment the question remains as to whether the orthodontic tooth movement intrudes a long epithelial attachment beneath the margin of the alveolar bone or whether the alveolar crest is continuously resorbed in front of the intruding tooth.

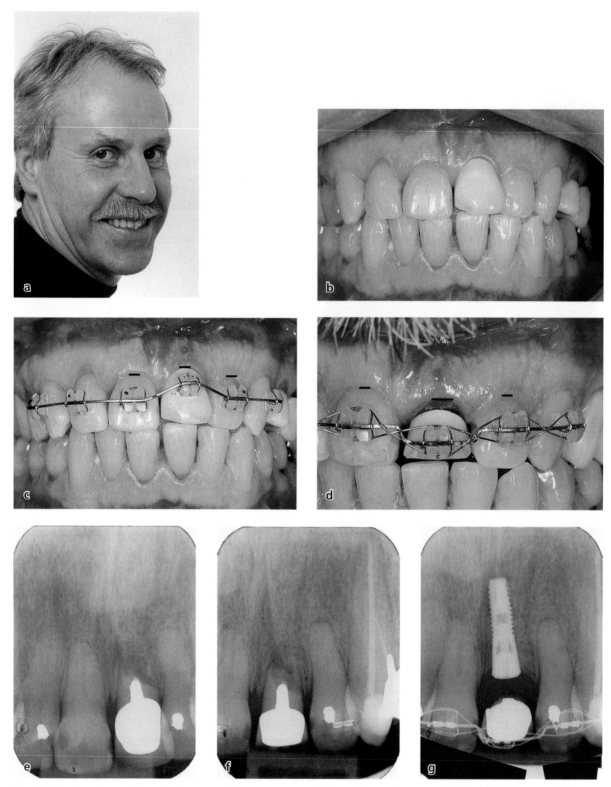

Fig. 31-15. Extrusion with periodontium. Selective extrusion of maxillary left central incisor to improve periodontal soft and hard tissues before placement of single implant. As shown in (b) to (d), it is necessary to extensively grind the extruding incisor crown to avoid jiggling with the mandibular teeth. Note evident differences in marginal gingival levels (lines) on the left central incisor during its extrusion (b-d). (e) to (g) show radiographic appearance at start, after 4 months and after 10 months, respectively.

Histologic (Melsen 1986, Melsen et al. 1988) and clinical (Melsen et al. 1989) studies indicate that new attachment is possible associated with orthodontic intrusion of teeth. In monkey experiments, periodontal tissue breakdown was induced and intrusion along the axis of the incisors with light forces was initiated following flap surgery. Histologic analysis showed new cementum formation and connective tissue attachment on the intruded teeth, by an average of 1.5 mm, provided a healthy gingival environment was

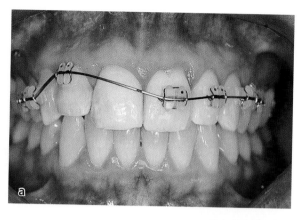
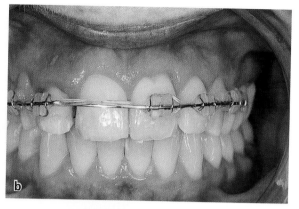

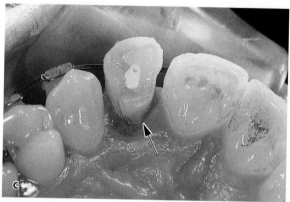

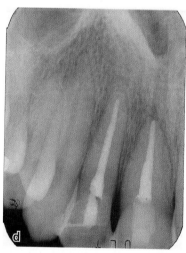
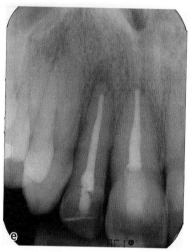

Fig. 31-16. Extrusion out of periodontium. Due to subgingival crown-root fracture on the maxillary right lateral incisor (a,d), this tooth was extruded out of the periodontium with a continous force (a-b) and fiberotomy was made with two-week intervals. The amount of extrusion is evident by comparison of the relationship between lateral and central incisor root ends in (d) and (e). Having moved the fracture line to a supragingival position (arrow in c), the tooth can now be safely restored.

maintained throughout the tooth movement. The increased activity of periodontal ligament cells and the approximation of formative cells to the tooth surface was suggested to contribute to the new attachment. In the clinical study, the periodontal condition was evaluated following the intrusion of extruded and spaced incisors in patients who had advanced periodontal disease. Judging from clinical probing depths and radiography, there was despite a large individual variation a beneficial effect on clinical crown lengths and marginal bone levels in many cases.

However, the reported clinical and histologic find-

ings associated with a combined orthodontic-periodontal approach must be assessed with great caution, and these findings have not been confirmed by others. Furthermore, new techniques like the GTR and other regenerative procedures (see below) would appear to be more promising when it comes to creation of new attachment.

Similar to the case with extrusion, metric and histologic studies have been made after experimental intrusion of teeth in monkeys. According to Murakami et al. (1989), the gingiva moved only about 60% of the distance when the teeth were intruded with a

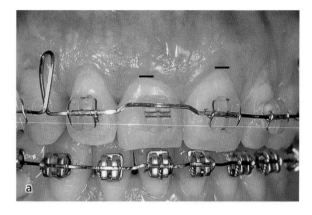
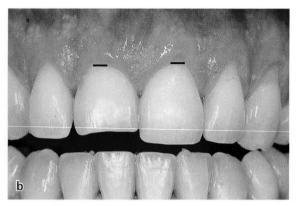
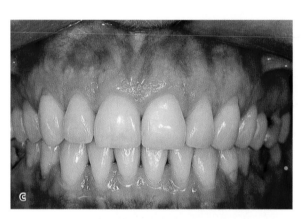
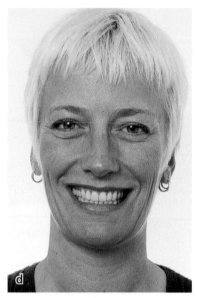

Fig. 31-17. Adult female patient in whom the clinical crown length of the maxillary right central incisor was shorter than that of the left central incisor (a). Because the sulcular depths were normal, the crown lengths were corrected by orthodontic intrusion of the right central incisor (b) and restoring the incisal edge (b) with enamel-bonded ultrathin porcelain laminate veneer (c,d). The alignment and correction of the crown length discrepancy has improved the esthetic appearance of the dentition. Restoration courtesy of Dr S. Toreskog.

continuous force of 80-100 g. However, Kokich et al. (1984) recommended an interrupted, continuous force for levelling of gingival margins on supra-erupted teeth (Fig. 31-17).

The key to understanding why intrusion can be used to increase clinical crown length is related to the subsequent restorative treatment. When orthodontic intrusion is used for levelling of the gingival margins to desired heights, such teeth must then be provided with porcelain laminate veneers or crowns (Fig. 31-17).

Regenerative procedures and orthodontic tooth movement

The development of barrier membranes to prevent cells of the epithelium and gingival connective tissue from colonizing the decontaminated root surface, as well as the use of Emdogain, would appear to provide a distinct improvement in orthodontic therapy in the periodontally compromised patient. New supracre-

stal and periodontal ligament collagen fibers may be gained on the tension side, which can transfer the orthodontic force stimulus to the alveolar bone (Diedrich 1996). In theory, the regenerative techniques would be advantageous associated with both extrusion and intrusion of teeth with infrabony defects, and for uprighting of tipped molars with mesial angular lesions. Moreover, if the epithelium can be prevented from proliferating apically, a bodily tooth movement into or through an intraosseous defect could eliminate the bony pocket more effectively than in the past (Fig. 31-11).

So far, however, relatively little clinical information is available about the use of different regenerative procedures in connection with orthodontic treatment. Diedrich (1996) reported an experiment in dogs in which orthodontic intrusion with flap surgery and GTR were compared with flap surgery only on periodontally affected teeth. In the presence of minimal or no round cell infiltration, the marking notch was located beneath the alveolar margin indicating that new attachment had formed. The potential of the intru-

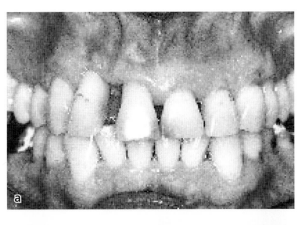
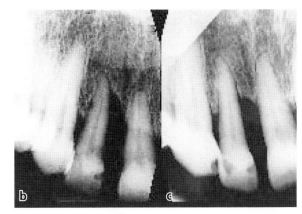
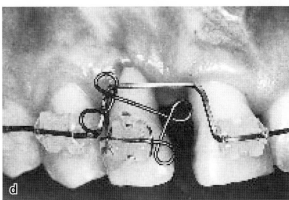
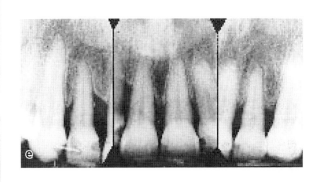

Fig. 31-18. Pathologic tooth migration as a result of an advanced periodontal lesion in adult female patient (a). Severe intraosseous defect between the right central and lateral incisors (b). Three months after GTR treatment (GoreTex membrane) partial reossification is evident (c), possibly with new attachment. Orthodontic leveling (d) with controlled space closure and intrusion of the lateral incisor. Result 6 months after orthodontic tooth movements shows no root resorption and a consolidated alveolar crest (e). From Diedrich (1996).

sive/regenerative mechanism was most impressive within the interradicular area. Some clinical observations (Nemcovsky et al. 1996, Stelzel & Flores-de-Jacoby 1998, Rabie et al. 2001) confirm that different regenerative procedures may enrich the therapeutic spectrum in combined periodontal/orthodontic approaches (Fig. 31-18). The combined regenerative and periodontal surgical treatments used together with orthodontic tooth movements create new perspectives and should be an interesting field for further experiments on adults with severe loss of periodontal tissues.

However, other clinical trials have demonstrated that treatment results with barrier membranes in the GTR technique may vary between different patients and that the method is operator and technique-sensitive (Leknes 1995). The patient's oral hygiene during the healing phase is critical, and inflammation around the membrane, particularly if it becomes exposed and contaminated, may lead to discouraging clinical results with marked gingival retraction (Fig. 31-19).

Since the membrane is covered in the GBR technique, the risk for inflammation is reduced. The possibility for orthodontic movement of teeth into alveolar processes with deficient bone volume may thus be improved (Basdra et al. 1995). Preorthodontic GBR of markedly constricted alveolar ridges also has the ad-

vantage that tooth movement through cancellous bone is easier, and the formation of interfering gingival invaginations can be reduced.

Traumatic occlusion (jiggling) and orthodontic treatment

As discussed in Chapter 15, the role of occlusal trauma in periodontal treatment has not been determined. From an orthodontic perspective, it is of interest that several studies indicate that traumatic occlusion forces (1) do not produce gingival inflammation or loss of attachment in teeth with healthy periodontium, (2) do not aggravate and cause spread of gingivitis or cause loss of attachment in teeth with established gingivitis, (3) may aggravate an active periodontitis lesion, i.e. be a co-destructive factor in an ongoing process of periodontal tissue breakdown (in one way or another favor the apical proliferation of plaque-induced destruction), and (4) may lead to less gain of attachment after periodontal treatment – non-surgical or surgical.

A major problem in this regard is the lack of established and reliable criteria to identify and quantitate different degrees of traumatic occlusion. Various clinical and radiographic indications, such as unfavorable

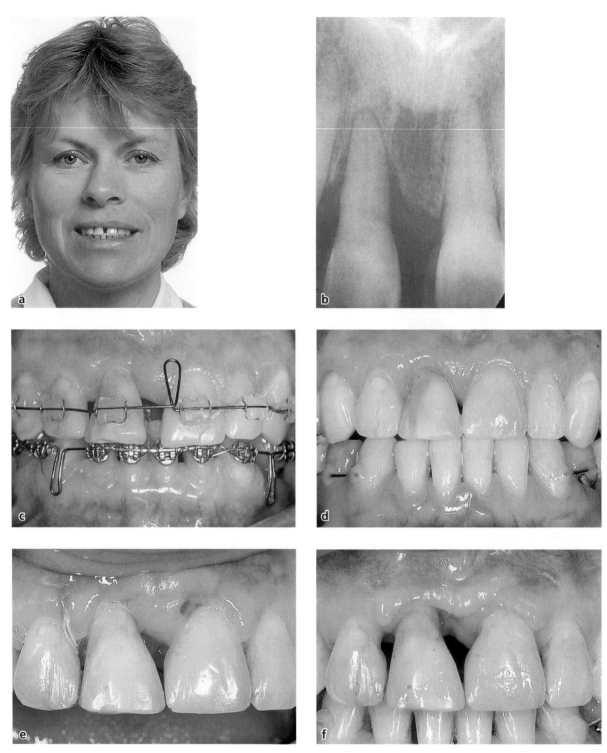

Fig. 31-19. Adult female periodontitis patient with marked vertical bone loss around the maxillary right central incisor before (a,b), during (c) and after (d) orthodontic treatment. Attempt to improve the periodontal situation by means of GTR treatment failed. Due to infection around the GoreTex membrane (e) marked gingival retraction occurred (f).

crown/root ratio, increased tooth mobility, widened periodontal ligament space, angular bone loss, alterations in root morphology, etc. are uncertain and insufficient in diagnosis of occlusal trauma, and there have been few scientific clinical reports to evaluate these signs (Jin & Cao 1992).

The extent to which it is necessary to avoid, or reduce, occlusal trauma during orthodontic treatment is controversial and unsupported by scientific evidence. Some orthodontists use bite-planes in virtually every periodontal case with bone deformities, to reduce occlusal trauma and for the purpose of shallowing the bony defects, as teeth supra-erupt. However, independent studies have shown that surgical pocket elimination including bone sculpturing offers no advantage compared with more conservative periodontal treatment (Ramfjord 1984), and apparently there is little need to shallow or eliminate bony deformities. It

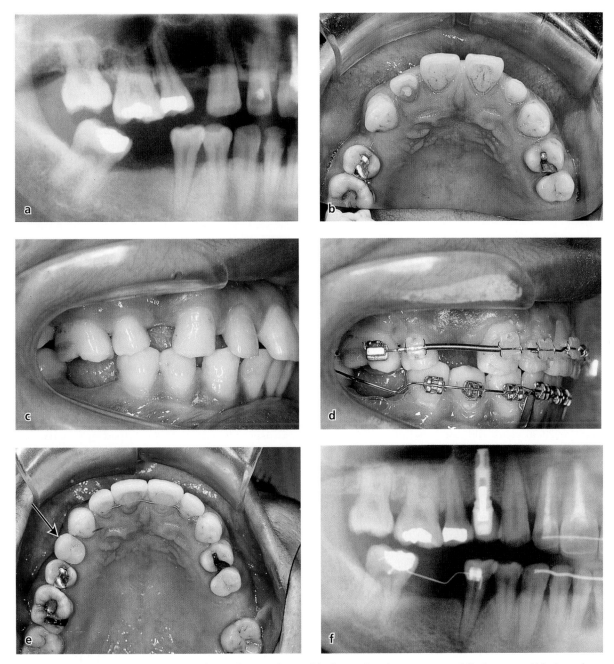

Fig. 31-20. Uprighting and leveling of maxillary and mandibular molars (compare a and f) plus consolidation of multiple small spaces into one area before placing single-tooth implant for missing maxillary right first premolar (arrow) in adult female patient.

would still appear sensible to avoid gross interferences, like raising the bite when a maxillary incisor in lingual inversion is moved over the mandibular teeth, and to mitigate evident occlusal interferences on single teeth with markedly increased mobility. However, it may be a futile exercise to try and eliminate all occlusal trauma during active tooth movement and a more practical solution is to concentrate on controlling the inflammation. After appliance removal, however, occlusal adjustment by selective grinding may be required. Even though good occlusal function is part of the orthodontic treatment goal, correct cusp-fossa relationships cannot always be achieved in adults with orthodontic therapy alone. In general terms, the adjustment should be directed toward obtaining even

and stable tooth contacts in centric relation, a straight forward slide from centric relation to centric occlusion without any side shifts or lateral deviation, freedom in centric, smooth gliding contacts in centric and eccentric mandibular motion, and elimination of balancing side interferences (Burgett et al. 1992).

The importance of reducing jiggling of teeth *after* orthodontic treatment of patients with moderate to advanced periodontitis may be significant: (1) tooth mobility generally increases with loss of support for the teeth, (2) animal experiments have shown that bone dehiscences produced by jiggling forces will regenerate after elimination of the jiggling trauma, and (3) occlusal adjustment may be a factor in the healing of periodontal defects, especially bony defects, after periodontal treatment. Therefore, the bonded orthodontic retainers, which stabilize the teeth, may secure optimal conditions for improved periodontal healing and bone regeneration after the orthodontic treatment period (Fig. 31-5). In fact, long-term follow-ups of orthodontic patients with advanced periodontal tissue breakdown may demonstrate better periodontal conditions, with marked crestal lamina dura contours, many years after appliance removal than at the end of the orthodontic treatment (Figs. 31-7, 31-8). If bonded retainers had not been used in many such cases, the most affected teeth would probably have been lost with time.

Molar uprighting, furcation involvement

The problem of mesially tipped mandibular molars because of non-replacement of missing first molars has been the subject of many anecdotal reports over the past 30 years. Tipped molars have been considered a causative or at least an aggravating factor for future periodontal tissue breakdown. However, Lundgren et al. (1992) recently observed that 73 molars that had remained in a markedly tipped position for at least 10 years, with most molars having been tipped for as long as 20-30 years, did not constitute an increased risk for initiation or aggravation of moderate periodontal disease at their mesial surface. The study did not consider the potential risk for aggravation of already established advanced periodontitis lesions. This lack of correlation may not exclude other indications for molar uprighting, such as functionally disturbing interferences, paralleling or space problems associated with prosthetic rehabilitation (Fig. 31-20), or traumatic occlusion.

In this context it must be emphasized that the apparent angular bone loss along the mesial surface of tipped molars may be illusive and solely represent an anatomic variation, since lines drawn from the adjacent cemento-enamel junctions appear to parallel the alveolar crest (Ritchey & Orban 1954). While uprighting such a tooth appears to cause a shallowing-out of the angular defect, with new bone forming at the mesial alveolar crest, it may merely reflect the inclination of the molar relative to the alveolar bone, and the attachment level remains unchanged. When there is a definite osseous defect caused by periodontitis on the mesial surface of the inclined molar, uprighting the tooth and tipping it distally will widen the osseous defect. Any coronal position of bone may be due to the extrusion component of the mechanotherapy.

Furcation defects generally remain the same or get worse during orthodontic treatment. For example, if tipped molars have furcation involvement before orthodontic uprighting, simultaneous extrusion may increase the severity of the furcation defects, especially in the presence of inflammation (Burch et al. 1992). Hence, initial periodontal therapy and maintenance is essential. The mandibular molar can be split into two roots, one or both of which may be kept and moved orthodontically into new positions. However, this is difficult treatment (Müller et al. 1995).

In a thorough study of periodontal condition around tipped mandibular molars before prosthetic replacement, Lang (1977) reported that after completion of the hygiene phase, significant pocket reduction (mean 1.0 mm) was noted on all surfaces. In addition, a further significant reduction in pocket depth (mean 0.6 mm), associated with a gain of clinical attachment (mean 0.4 mm), was found on the mesial and lingual aspects of the molars as a result of the orthodontic uprighting. He concluded that uprighting of tipped molars is a simple and predictable procedure, provided excellent plaque control is maintained.

Kessler (1976), on the other hand, stated that uprighting of mesially inclined molars is not a panacea, and showed some cases in which evident bone loss and furcation involvement developed during the orthodontic uprighting procedure. Because of the furcation involvement and increased mobility, these teeth were no longer considered suitable as abutments, although they were properly uprighted. Radiographic indications that furcation involvement may develop between the roots at the end of orthodontic molar uprighting is evident also in other studies, even when extrusive movement of the tipped molars has been avoided (Diedrich 1989). However, it is not unlikely that this radiolucent area reflects immature bone.

Conclusion

As risks may be involved in orthodontic uprighting of mesially tipped molars in cases with periodontal lesions along their mesial surface, or with furcation involvement, the indications for molar uprighting must be apparent. Excellent oral hygiene is required during the orthodontic treatment, with careful consideration of the force distribution, and avoiding extrusion as much as possible. The developments of regenerative techniques may make it possible in the future to obtain better outcomes in orthodontic therapy of periodontally compromised patients.

Tooth movement and implant esthetics

Osseointegrated implants may be used (1) to provide anchorage for orthodontic tooth movement and later serve as abutments for restorative treatment, and (2) to replace single missing teeth. The use of implants as anchors for orthodontic treatment is discussed in Chapter 43, and will not be dealt with here.

It is difficult to achieve esthetically satisfactory results with artificial crowns on single-tooth implants, and the orthodontist may play a role in the interdisciplinary treatment planning team of specialists. There are at least three areas where orthodontics may be considered:

• redistribution of the available space in the dental

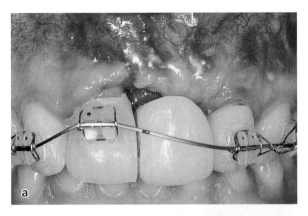
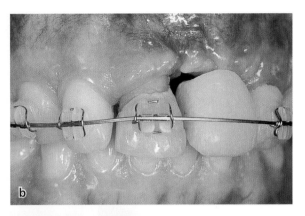

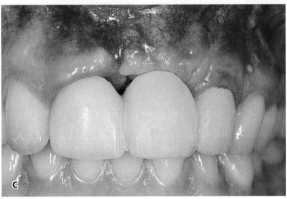

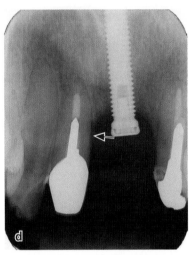
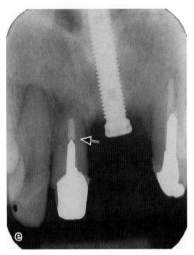

Fig. 31-21. Orthodontic improvement of periodontal soft and hard tissues associated with implant placement and a large anterior defect in young adult female patient. As in Fig. 31-15 the periodontal tissues will follow the selectively extruded incisor incisally (a-c), and thus improve the possibilities for a successful connective tissue graft from the palate when the gingival papillae is reconstructed. Note the more incisal relationship of bone level relative to the implant in the radiographs before and after treatment (arrows in d,e).

arch when tooth positions for implant placement are not optimal
• orthodontic ridge augmentation by vertical tooth movement
• orthodontic ridge augmentation by horizontal tooth movement.

Redistribution of space
Orthodontic movement of neighboring teeth to optimal positions is often required in association with placement of implants substituting missing maxillary central or lateral incisors (Spear et al. 1997). Another

common indication is a lack of adequate space for the implant. Fig. 31-20 illustrates a typical case with multiple small spaces between the teeth and not enough room to place an implant in the maxillary first premolar region.

Ridge augmentation – vertical movement
During selective orthodontic extrusion of one single tooth, both the alveolar bone and the soft periodontal tissues will follow the extruded tooth in an incisal direction, as discussed under forced eruption earlier in this chapter. By this means, it is possible to signifi-

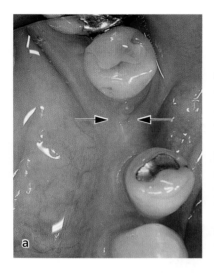
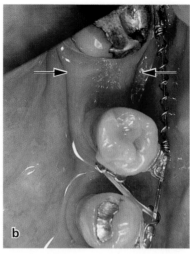

Fig. 31-22. Orthodontic ridge augmentation before implant placement. Since the buccolingual width of the alveolar bone on the left side of the mandible was too narrow for an implant, the second premolar was orthodontically rotated and moved mesially. Note that the bone volume on the tension side of the mesially moved premolar is markedly greater than that on the pressure side (arrows). It will now be possible to place the implant in the position previously occupied by the second premolar.

cantly improve the periodontal tissue esthetics associated with fabrication of prosthetic crowns on single implants (Fig. 31-21). The technique of "orthodontic extraction" of a hopeless incisor or molar may be useful to improve the results for single-tooth implants in patients in whom one or more teeth are to be extracted. Following progressive grinding of the extruded tooth to prevent it from jiggling, new periodontal tissues are generated that provide improved conditions for the implant, after extraction of the extruded tooth (Fig. 31-15).

Ridge augmentation – horizontal movement

If an implant cannot be placed because of reduced buccolingual ridge thickness after a previous extraction, one option is to move a premolar into the edentulous space and to place the implant in the position previously occupied by the premolar (Spear et al. 1997). The buccolingual volume of the new bone on the tension side will be markedly greater than that on the pressure side (Fig. 31-22). This is an alternative to surgical ridge augmentation (GBR or bone graft). Fig. 31-22 shows a case in which the mesial movement and uprighting of a mandibular first premolar provided new bone of adequate width for implant placement in a previously atrophied alveolar bone area. Similar generation of bone can be obtained in patients who have no molars by moving a terminal premolar distally in the dental arch.

GINGIVAL RECESSION

Labial recession

"Normal" age changes

Gingival recession, with exposure of cementum on facial surfaces of teeth, may occur on single or multiple teeth. Many factors have been implicated in the etiology, including plaque, position of the tooth in the arch, faulty toothbrushing, traumatic occlusion, high frenum or muscle attachments, lack in dimension of gingiva, lip pressure, etc. (Baker & Seymor 1976). It is difficult to see a single cause of, or a solitary mechanism in the development of, labial gingival recession. Two basic types of recession may occur, one related to periodontal disease, or to factors associated with periodontal disease, and the other relating to mechanical factors, including toothbrushing.

Labial gingival recessions are always accompanied by alveolar bone dehiscences, and there is a direct correlation between the millimetric extension of labial bone dehiscences and the corresponding gingival recessions (Bernimoulin & Curilovic 1977). It has been postulated that a root dehiscence may establish an environment which, for one reason or another, may predispose to gingival recession (Wennström 1990). The position in which a tooth erupts through the alveolar process has a profound influence on the amount of gingiva that will be established around the tooth. When a tooth erupts close to the mucogingival line, only a minimal width, or complete lack, of gingiva may be observed labially, and localized gingival recessions may occur in patients at a young age. Thus the "normal" age changes that will then take place are important. Longitudinal monitoring of labial gingival dimensions during the development of the dentition has shown that provided adequate plaque control is established and maintained, a significant increase of the gingival height will generally occur. Spontaneous improvement of localized mandibular labial recessions is the rule rather than the exception, and in some teeth the recessions were totally eliminated during a 3-year observation period (Andlin-Sobocki et al. 1991). Also, spontaneous changes of tooth positions in a buccolingual direction will affect the gingival dimension. These alterations in gingival dimensions are similar to, albeit less pronounced than, those observed during orthodontic treatment (see below).

Favorable tooth movements, and tissue factors

Alterations of mucogingival dimensions may occur

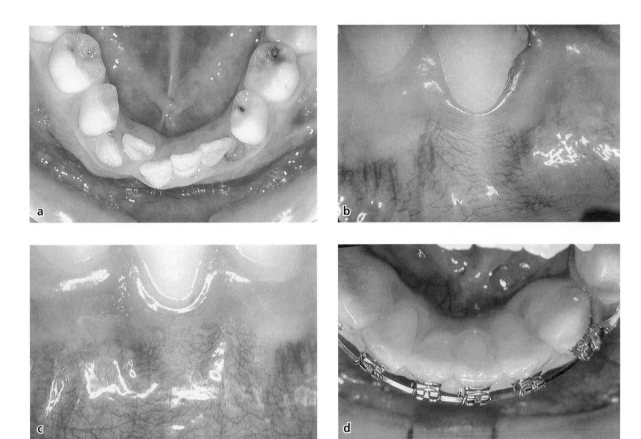

Fig. 31-23. Thin labial gingiva on prominent mandibular right central incisor (a,b) spontaneously became thicker when the incisor was orthodontically moved lingually and aligned (c) after premolar extractions. (d) shows condition after appliance removal.

during orthodontic treatment. Contrary to beliefs in the past, these changes are independent of the apico-coronal width of the keratinized and attached gingiva. Wennström et al. (1987) found no relationship between the initial width of keratinized gingiva and the tendency for development of gingival recession during orthodontic tooth movements in monkeys. Instead, it is the buccolingual thickness (volume), which may be the determining factor for the development of gingival recession and attachment loss at sites with gingivitis during orthodontic treatment.

A tooth that is facially positioned within the alveolar process may show an alveolar bone dehiscence with a thin covering soft tissue. When such a tooth is moved lingually during orthodontic treatment, the gingival dimensions on the labial aspects will increase in thickness (Figs. 31-23, 31-24). Furthermore, because the mucogingival junction is a stable anatomical landmark and the gingiva is anchored to the supracrestal portion of the root, it will follow the tooth during the movement lingually and will consequently get an increase in gingival height (decreased clinical crown height).

Conclusion

It follows that in cases with a thin (delicate) gingiva caused by a prominent position of the teeth, there is no need for a preorthodontic gingival augmentation procedure. Neither in the case of labial gingival reces-

sions should a mucogingival surgical procedure be performed before orthodontic therapy, when the position of the tooth is improved by the treatment. The recession, as well as the bone dehiscence, will decrease as a consequence of the lingual movement of the tooth into a more proper position within the alveolar bone. If still indicated at the end of orthodontic therapy, the surgical procedure will have a higher predictability of success than if it had been performed before the tooth movement (Wennström 1996).

Unfavorable tooth movements, and tissue factors

Orthodontic movements of teeth *away* from the genetically determined envelope of the alveolar process are risk movements for development of mucogingival problems, particularly in thin bone and gingival tissues. During frontal and lateral expansion of teeth, tension may develop in the marginal tissues due to the forces applied to the teeth. This stretching may result in thinning of the soft tissues. However, recession-type defects will not develop as long as the tooth is moved within the alveolar bone. If, however, the expansion results in the establishment of a bone dehiscence, the volume (thickness) of the covering soft tissue must be considered as a factor that may influence the development of soft tissue recessions. This may be true both during and after the active orthodontic treatment period. The labial orthodontic tooth movement *per se* will not cause soft tissue recession.

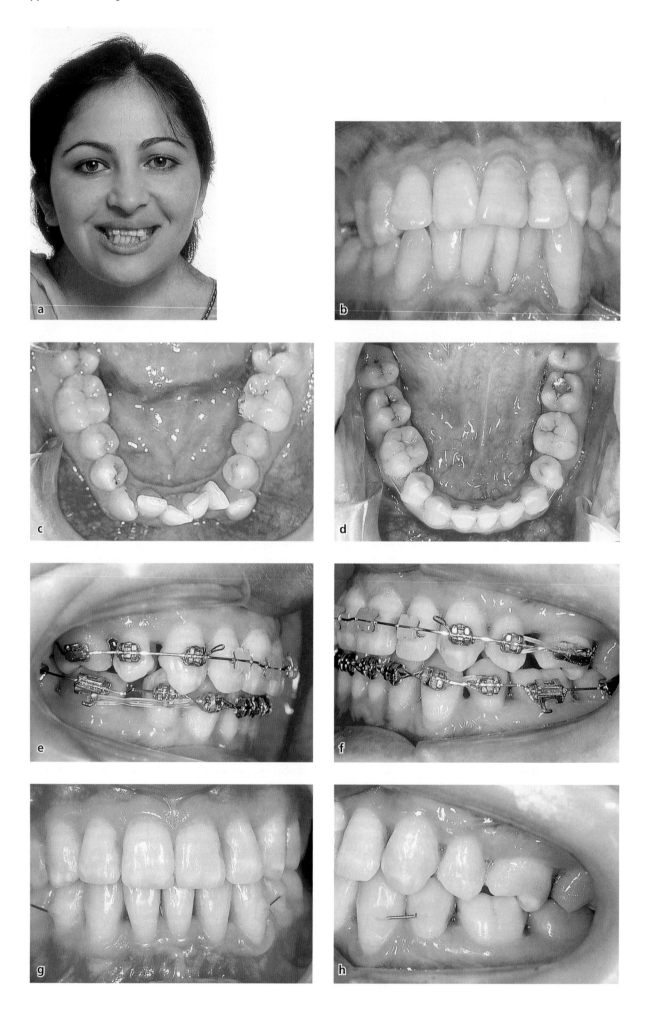

However, the thin gingiva that will be the consequence of such movement may serve as a locus minoris resistentia to developing soft tissue defects in the presence of bacterial plaque and/or mechanical trauma caused by improper toothbrushing techniques, or orthodontic correction of marked rotations of the incisors.

For stability reasons as well, expansion in the mandibular arch should normally be avoided, if possible. If frontal expansion is still performed in association with orthodontic therapy, the buccolingual thickness of the hard and soft tissues should be evaluated. If surgical intervention is considered necessary in order to reduce the risk for development of soft tissue recessions, this should aim at increasing the thickness of the covering tissue (e.g. grafts), and not the apicocoronal width of the gingiva.

Conclusion

Before any kind of orthodontic therapy is started, it is important to check the buccolingual thickness of the bone and soft tissues on the pressure side of all teeth, which are to be moved. When tissues are delicate and thin, careful instructions in adequate plaque control measures should be provided, and controlled before and during treatment as well as after removal of the fixed appliances, in order to reduce the risk for development of labial gingival recession.

Interdental recession

Esthetic considerations with regard to defect papillae

Until recently, most clinical emphasis with regard to gingival recession was given to the labial defects. If left untreated, most labial gingival recessions will not progress significantly with time, at least if oral hygiene is good, and the main indication for treatment is the esthetic implications for the patient. From an esthetic point of view, however, it would appear that interdental recession, manifest as more or less pronounced empty spaces ("dark triangles") between the teeth, would be equally or more important. Compared with a labial recession, in most patients the loss of interdental papillae would be more visible, both in normal conversation and upon smiling.

Since quality of life (esthetics and lack of pain) has become increasingly more important in recent years in selection of periodontal therapies, disfigurement of the gingival papillae during orthodontic treatment of periodontal patients must be avoided, if possible. The development of interdental recession during orthodontic treatment in adults may be caused by one of three factors: (1) advanced periodontal disease, by the

tissue destruction or due to pocket elimination by surgery, (2) triangular tooth shape due to abnormal interproximal wear of teeth in crowded positions before the orthodontic treatment, and (3) diverging roots of teeth due to improper bracket placement. To begin with, there is an obvious difference in dental esthetics between patients with advanced periodontitis who have been treated according to "old" and "new" concepts for periodontal therapy. In the past, pocket elimination by gingivectomies frequently resulted in advanced root exposure and complete loss of interdental papillae (Fig. 31-7). However, even with careful nonsurgical periodontal therapy in the preparation of patients with advanced periodontal disease for orthodontic treatment, the clinical outcome of the interdisciplinary treatment will normally result in marked interdental recessions, if special precautions are not taken (see below).

Clinical options for treatment

There are only a few options available for the treatment of interdental gingival recession associated with orthodontic treatment in the periodontal patient:

1. mucogingival surgery, using coronally positioned flaps and GTR techniques (Pini Prato et al. 1992)
2. the provision of a gingival prosthesis
3. orthodontic paralleling of the roots of neighboring teeth
4. mesio-distal enamel reduction ("stripping").

Of these techniques, the mucogingival surgery aspects are discussed in Chapter 27, and will not be commented on here. The gingival prosthesis may be useful in cases of markedly compromised dentitions, where the psychological implications of having pronounced retractions are serious. It may be regarded as a last resort. In contrast, the mesio-distal contouring of teeth is a very useful technique to routinely improve the esthetic results achieved by orthodontic treatment in most adult and adolescent patients (Figs. 31-3, 31-4, 31-6, 31-25).

Benefits of mesiodistal enamel reduction ("stripping")

Introduced by Tuverson in 1980, mesio-distal recontouring of teeth has now become a routine procedure in orthodontics. It is generally performed on three indications: (1) treatment of slight-to-moderate crowding without arch expansion, (2) correction of width discrepancies (so-called TSD = tooth size discrepancies) between maxillary and mandibular teeth, and (3) to prevent interdental recession from developing during orthodontic treatment. The principle in-

---

Fig. 31-24. Marked labial gingival recession on prominent left mandibular canine in female young adult patient (a-c). After extraction of two premolars and the left central incisor (sic!), the mandibular arch was leveled orthodontically (d). (e) and (f) show the clinical condition towards end of orthodontic therapy, and (g-h) at follow-up 1 year after appliance removal. Note spontaneous improvement of gingival recession (f-h).

volved in stripping is to recontour those teeth which for one reason or another have abnormal morphology, towards an ideal anatomical shape (Figs. 31-6, 31-25). In doing so, a good occlusion with optimal tooth contact point relationships and normal interdental gingival papillary contours will be achievable (Figs. 31-5, 31-6, 31-25).

In many adult patients with malocclusion, particularly in cases with crowded and overlapping incisors, the crowns of the incisors are much wider at their incisal edges than at the cervical region. As the crowding is unraveled by orthodontic levelling in these instances, the contact point between the incisors will become located in the incisal 1 mm, and a more or less evident space develops above the interproximal contacts of the incisors. Similar, or even more pronounced, loss of the interdental papillae between the maxillary and mandibular incisors, is commonly seen after orthodontic treatment in patients with advanced periodontal destruction.

Short-term (Zachrisson & Mjör 1975) and long-term (> 10 years)(Thordarson et al. 1991) follow-up studies after extensive grinding of teeth have demonstrated that no harmful side-effects are observed subsequent to the procedure, provided adequate cooling is used during the grinding and the prepared surfaces are made smooth and self-cleansing. After the diastema is created, the space between the teeth is closed orthodontically. As this occurs, the roots of neighboring teeth come closer together, the contact area is lengthened, and the reduced papilla can fill out the small space between the teeth (Tarnow et al. 1992). In patients with advanced periodontal disease, it is not always possible to restitute all papillae in the dentition. Even if it is not possible to eliminate the interdental recession completely after the orthodontic treatment, the esthetic appearance is in most patients substantially improved by stripping (Figs. 31-3, 31-4).

MINOR SURGERY ASSOCIATED WITH ORTHODONTIC THERAPY

Several forms of minor periodontal surgery may be used to improve or stabilize the results achieved by orthodontic treatment of malocclusion. More than 30 years ago, Edwards (1970) described clinical techniques to help prevent rotational relapse, re-opening of closed extraction spaces (Edwards 1971), and a simple yet effective technique for frenotomy (Edwards 1977). At about the same time, a gingivectomy technique to increase clinical crown length for esthetic improvement of orthodontic results in specific situations was reported (Monefeldt & Zachrisson 1977). Removal of gingival invaginations in extraction sites following orthodontic space closure has also been a subject of considerable interest to orthodontists.

Fiberotomy

The problem of relapse of orthodontically treated teeth in general, and rotated teeth in particular, has been well recognized for years. Methods to reduce the occurrence of rotational relapse may include (1) complete correction, or overcorrection, of rotated teeth, (2) long-term retention with bonded lingual retainers, and (3) the use of fiberotomy.

Two soft-tissue periodontal entities may influence the stability: the principal fibers of the periodontal ligament, and the supra-alveolar fibers. Whereas the fibers of the periodontal ligament and transseptal groups remodel efficiently and histologically completely in only 2 to 3 months after orthodontic rotation of teeth, the supra-alveolar fibers are apparently more stable, with a slow turnover. Since the gingival soft tissues are composed primarily of non-elastic collagenous fibers, the exact mechanism by which the gingival soft tissues may apply a force capable of moving the teeth is as yet unknown. From a practical and clinical point of view, however, the supracrestal gingival tissues seemingly do contribute to rotational relapse, as evidenced by the effect of the circumferential supracrestal fiberotomy (CSF) technique.

Basically this technique consists of inserting a scalpel into the gingival sulcus and severing the epithelial attachment surrounding the involved teeth. The blade also transects the transseptal fibers by interdentally entering the periodontal ligament space. Various modifications of the original CSF technique have been described, in which the scalpel is inserted below the gingival margin, or the cut is reduced to interdental vertical incisions buccally and lingually (Fig. 31-26). In neither case are surgical dressings indicated, and clinical healing is usually complete in 7-10 days.The fiberotomy procedure is not recommended during active tooth movement, or in the presence of gingival inflammation. When performed in healthy tissues after orthodontic therapy, there is negligible loss of attachment (Edwards 1988).

The long-term effectiveness of fiberotomy was evaluated in a prospective follow-up study over a period of 15 years by Edwards (1988). The degree of crowding was examined for CSF and control cases at 4-6 years and at 12-14 years after treatment. A significant effect of the fiberotomy was observed at both time intervals. The surgical procedure was more successful in the maxillary than in the mandibular anterior region; more effective in alleviating rotational than labiolingual relapse; and more useful in reducing relapse in cases with severe rather than mild irregularity of teeth. There was no clinically significant increase in sulcus depth, nor signs of gingival labial recession.

Frenotomy

The contribution of the maxillary labial frenum to the etiology of a persisting midline diastema, and to re-

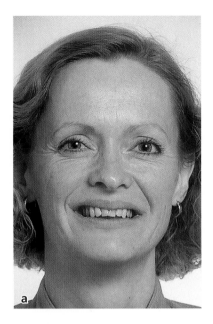

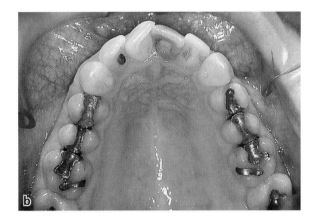

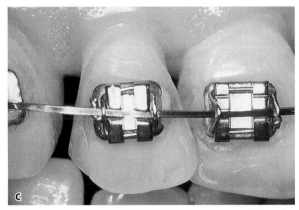

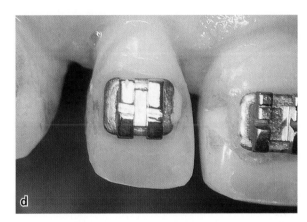

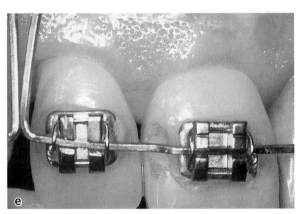

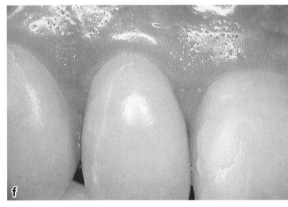

Fig. 31-25. Adult female patient with maxillary crowding and large overjet (a,b). After premolar extractions, orthodontic distalization of canines resulted in the development of marked interdental recessions in the anterior region (c). Marked triangular incisor morphology and uneven incisal edges necessitated extensive recontouring (c,d) to allow gingival fill-in after treatment (e,f).

opening of diastemas after orthodontic closure, is controversial. The probability for diastema closure in the long run is the same whether or not frenectomy is performed. However, very hyperplastic types of frenum, with a fan-like attachment, may obstruct diastema closure and should be relocated.

In the past, the most common surgical procedure was *frenectomy*, an excision-type operation, which was often carried over to the palatal aspects. However, a frequently observed complication may be an undesirable loss of the interdental papilla between the maxillary central incisors. For this reason, the *frenotomy* (Fig. 31-27), which represents a more gentle operation, will produce esthetically preferable results. With frenotomy, the attachment of the frenum to gingiva and periosteum is severed, and the insertion of the frenum

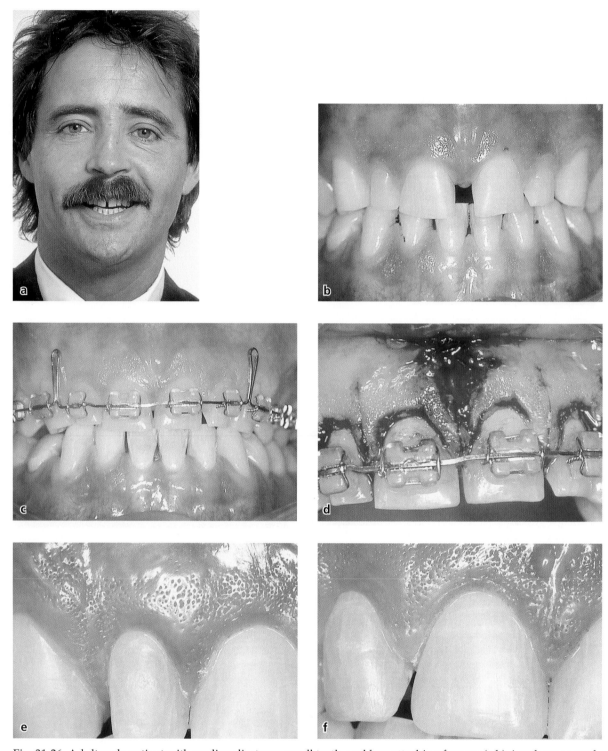

Fig. 31-26. Adult male patient with median diastema, small teeth, and low attaching frenum (a,b), in whom several different types of minor surgeries were performed (d) in order to improve and stabilize the orthodontic treatment result (c). Gingivectomy over four incisors increased crown length. Note healing with intact stippling 2 months later (e,f). The surgical procedure also comprised frenotomy and fiberotomies with interdental vertical cuts (d).

is relocated several millimeters up onto the alveolar mucosa. If a marked sutural bone cleft is observed in the pretreatment radiographs, the cut is extended to sever the fibers within the coronal part of the mid-palatal suture. Tissue healing after a frenotomy procedure is usually uneventful (Fig. 31-27). To further reduce the relapse tendency and/or increase clinical crown height of single or several teeth, the frenotomy may be combined with fiberotomy and gingivectomy (Fig. 31-26).

Removal of gingival invaginations (clefts)

Incomplete adaptation of supporting structures during orthodontic closure of extraction spaces in adults

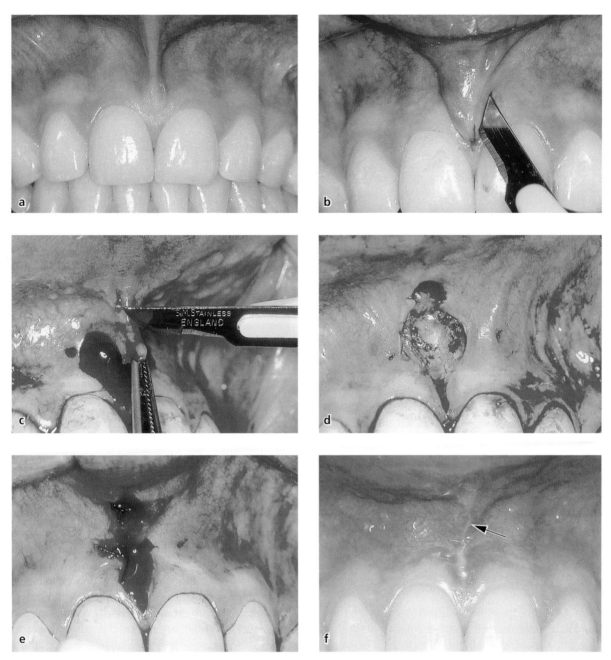

Fig. 31-27. Clinical illustration of Edwards' frenotomy procedure. The surgery includes a V-incision (b), removal of the frenum tip (c), some vertical and horizontal cuts into periosteum (d), and, optionally, one or two sutures (e). One month later (f), some slight scarring may be observed below the relocated frenum attachment (arrow), but there is predictably no loss of the interdental gingival papilla.

may result in infolding or invagination of the gingiva (Fig. 31-28). The clinical appearance of such invaginations may range from a minor one-surface crease to deep clefts that extend across the interdental papilla from the buccal to the lingual gingivae. Although gingival invaginations are quite common, the precise cause of the infolding as teeth are moved through an extraction area remains unclear. Since approximated teeth appear to displace the gingival tissue more than move through it, a "piling-up" of gingival tissue is conceivable. There is some resolution of these defects with time, but many invaginations persist for 5 years or more after completion of orthodontic therapy.

Several authors have suggested that compression of transseptal fibers and alterations of gingival tissue will contribute to extraction-space reopening, but no correlation was found between space reopening and presence and severity of invaginations by Rivera Circuns and Tulloch (1983). They still felt the damage to the gingiva was severe enough to warrant the surgical removal of these defects in selected patients (Fig. 31-28). Edwards (1971) suggested that simple removal of only the excess gingiva in the buccal and lingual area of approximated teeth would be sufficient to alleviate the tendency for the teeth to separate after orthodontic movement. The removal of the gingival papillae in closure sites may enhance the restitution of a more normal connective tissue, although the epithelial hy-

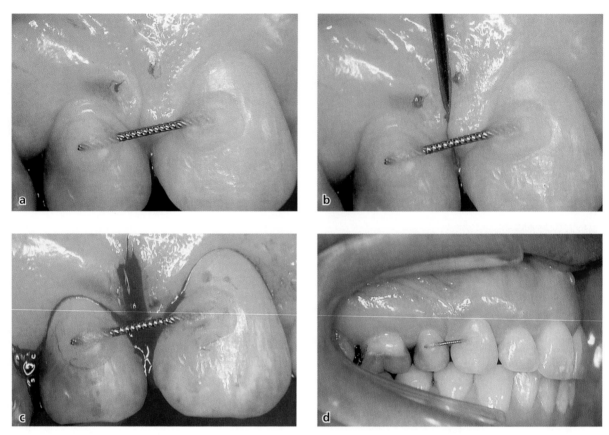

Fig. 31-28. Surgical removal of gingival invagination after first premolar extraction and orthodontic space closure in adult female patient (a,b). A mesiodistally narrow but deep excision of tissue (c) was made to avoid loss of the interdental papilla. (d) shows condition 2 years later.

perplasia, invaginations, and loss of collagen in the underlying gingiva are surprisingly long-standing.

Gingivectomy

The relationship of the gingival margins of the six maxillary anterior teeth plays an important role in the esthetic appearance of the crowns (Kokich 1996a,b). In some instances, it may be necessary to increase clinical crown length of one or several teeth during or after orthodontic treatment. If a gingival margin discrepancy is present, but the patient's lip does not move upward to expose the discrepancy upon smiling, it does not require correction. If the gingival discrepancy is apparent, however, one of four different techniques may be used:

1. gingivectomy
2. intrusion + incisal restoration or porcelain laminate veneer (Fig. 31-17)
3. extrusion + fiberotomy + porcelain crown (Fig. 31-16)
4. surgical crown lengthening, by flap procedure and ostectomy/ostoplasty of bone (Brägger et al. 1992).

Each of these techniques has its specific indications, and whenever gingival margin discrepancies are present, the clinician must determine the proper solution

(see also Chapter 27). For example, gingivectomy is not indicated when there is a risk for root exposure, such as when one single incisor has supra-erupted (Fig. 31-17).

The gingivectomy technique has proven to be useful in improving orthodontic results, particularly in difficult cases with missing maxillary central or lateral incisors (Fig. 31-29); after premolar autotransplantation to the anterior region; and in some "gummy" smiles (Fig. 31-30). Clinical and histologic examination demonstrated that it was possible to permanently increase clinical crown length after orthodontic treatment by making a labial gingivectomy to the bottom of the clinical pocket. The healing and regeneration of the gingiva was uneventful, provided excellent oral hygiene was maintained in the wound area for 2 months. The result may be explained by one or more of three factors: (1) the effect of the gingivectomy itself, (2) elimination of accumulated hyperplastic gingiva often seen associated with fixed appliance therapy (Fig. 31-29), and (3) elimination of a normally occurring deep pocket. Whatever the reason, the net gain in crown length was close to half the probing depth in all instances (Monefeldt & Zachrisson 1977). The increase in crown length of 1-2 mm may be important to improve the clinical outcome, as shown in Figs. 31-29 and 31-30. Similar long-term results on the position of the marginal soft tissue following periodontal surgery have been reported by others (Lindhe & Nyman 1980).

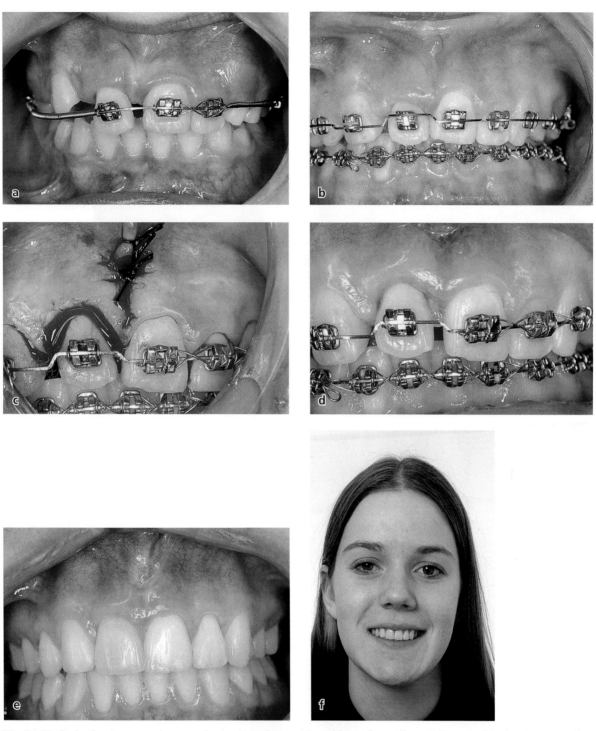

Fig. 31-29. Orthodontic space closure substitution after accidental loss of maxillary right central incisor in young female patient (a). The marginal gingival level on the "new" central incisor was corrected by selective intrusion bends in the archwire (b-d) and local gingivectomy and frenotomy (c-d). Local gingivectomies were also performed on the right first premolar in the canine position, and on the left lateral incisor (e). Enamel-bonded ultrathin porcelain veneer on lateral incisor, and vital bleaching of right canine courtesy of Dr S. Toreskog. By these means, it was possible to obtain an optimally esthetic result (e,f).

Interestingly, Wennström (1983) demonstrated that even if the gingivectomy is extended into the alveolar mucosa, the regenerated tissue will still be normal gingiva with keratinized epithelium. Thus the human periodontal membrane tissue has the capacity to form a granulation tissue which will prevent the alveolar mucosa from becoming the border-tissue against the tooth. When local labial gingivectomies are made in adults, the cut is reduced mesiodistally in order to eliminate the risk for developing interdental recession. Then the incision should not follow the gingival contour all the way, but should be limited by two small vertical cuts towards the interdental papillae (Fig. 31-26, 31-30).

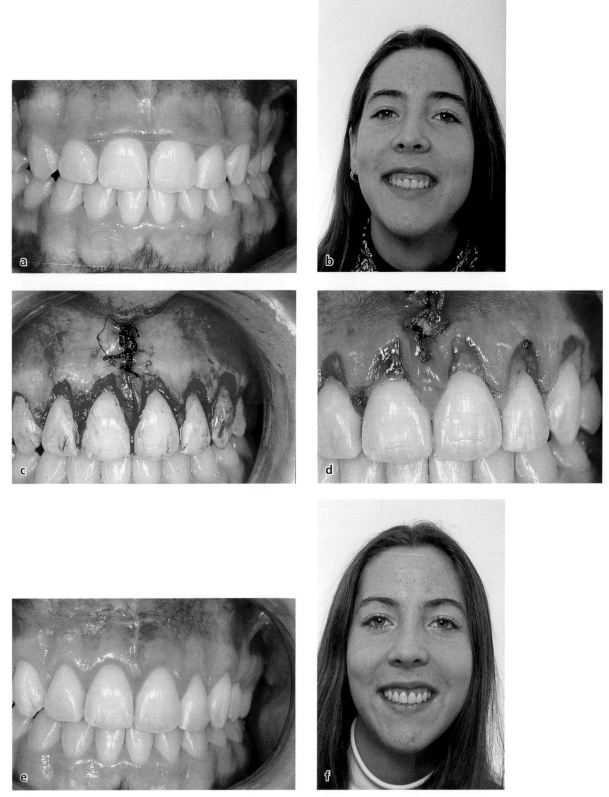

Fig. 31-30. Young female with long face and pronounced "gummy" smile remaining after active maxillary incisor intrusion (a,b). Labial gingivectomies over six anterior teeth, using "adult" excisions, with frenum relocated and sutured (c). Healing of gingiva after one week (d) and four months (e) resulted in acceptable tooth display and smile (f). Further improvement can be expected with normal aging.

REFERENCES

Andlin-Sobocki, A., Marcusson, A. & Persson, M. (1991). 3-year observation on gingival recession in mandibular incisors in children. *Journal of Clinical Periodontology* **18**, 155-159.

Årtun, J. & Urbye, K.S. (1988). The effect of orthodontic treatment on periodontal bone support in patients with advanced loss of marginal periodontium. *American Journal of Orthodontics* **93**, 143-148.

Baker, D.L. & Seymor, G.J. (1976). The possible pathogenesis of gingival recession. *Journal of Clinical Periodontology* **3**, 208-219.

Basdra, E.K., Mayer, T. & Komposch, G. (1995). Guided tissue regeneration precedes tooth movement and crossbite correction. *The Angle Orthodontist* **65**, 307-310.

Berglundh, T., Marinello, C.P., Lindhe, J., Thilander, B. & Liljenberg, B. (1991). Periodontal tissue reactions to orthodontic extrusion. An experimental study in the dog. *Journal of Clinical Periodontology* **18**, 330-336.

Bernimoulin, J.P. & Curilovic, Z. (1977). Gingival recession and tooth mobility. *Journal of Clinical Periodontology* **4**, 107-114.

Boyd, R.L. & Baumrind, S. (1992). Periodontal considerations in the use of bonds or bands on molars in adolescents and adults. *The Angle Orthodontist* **62**, 117-126.

Boyd, R.L., Leggott, P.J., Quinn, R.S., Eakle, W.S. & Chambers, D. (1989). Periodontal implications of orthodontic treatment in adults with reduced or normal periodontal tissues versus those of adolescents. *American Journal of Orthodontics and Dentofacial Orthopedics* **96**, 191-199.

Brägger, U., Lauchenauer, D. & Lang, N.P. (1992). Surgical lengthening of the clinical crown. *Journal of Clinical Periodontology* **19**, 58-63.

Burch, J.G., Bagci, B., Sabulski, D. & Landrum, C. (1992). Periodontal changes in furcations resulting from orthodontic uprighting of mandibular molars. *Quintessence International* **23**, 509-513.

Burgett, F.G., Ramfjord, S.P., Nissle, R.R., Morrison, E.C., Charbeneau, T.D. & Caffesse, R.G. (1992). A randomized trial of occlusal adjustment in the treatment of periodontitis patients. *Journal of Clinical Periodontology* **19**, 381-387.

Chace, R. & Low, S.B. (1993). Survival characteristics of periodontally-involved teeth: A 40-year study. *Journal of Periodontology* **64**, 701-705.

Dahl, E.H. & Zachrisson, B.U. (1991). Long-term experiences with direct-bonded lingual retainers. *Journal of Clinical Orthodontics* **25**, 619-630.

Diedrich, P. (1989). Wechselbeziehungen zwischen Kieferorthopädie und Parodontologie. *Fortschritte der Kieferorthopädie* **50**, 347-364.

Diedrich, P. (1996). Guided tissue regeneration associated with orthodontic therapy. *Seminars in Orthodontics* **2**, 39-45.

Diedrich, P. (1999). The eleventh hour or where are our orthodontic limits? *Journal of Orofacial Orthopedics/Fortschritte der Kieferorthopädie* **60**, 60-65.

Edwards, J.G. (1970). A surgical procedure to eliminate rotational relapse. *American Journal of Orthodontics* **57**, 33-46.

Edwards, J.G. (1971). The reduction of relapse in extraction cases. *American Journal of Orthodontics* **60**, 128-141.

Edwards, J.G. (1977). The diastema, the frenum, the frenectomy: A clinical study. *American Journal of Orthodontics* **71**, 489-508.

Edwards, J.G. (1988). A long-term prospective evaluation of the circumferential supracrestal fiberotomy in alleviating orthodontic relapse. *American Journal of Orthodontics and Dentofacial Orthopedics* **93**, 380-387.

Engelking, G. & Zachrisson, B.U. (1982). Effects of incisor repositioning on monkey periodontium after expansion through the cortical plate. *American Journal of Orthodontics* **83**, 23-32.

Ericsson, I., Thilander, B. & Lindhe, J. (1978). Periodontal condition after orthodontic tooth movements in the dog. *The Angle Orthodontist* **48**, 210-218.

Ericsson, I., Thilander, B., Lindhe, J. & Okamoto, H. (1977). The effect of orthodontic tilting movements on the periodontal tissues of infected and non-infected dentitions in the dog. *Journal of Clinical Periodontology* **4**, 78-293.

Folio, J., Rams, T.E. & Keyes, P.H. (1985). Orthodontic therapy in patients with juvenile periodontitis. Clinical and microbiologic effects. *American Journal of Orthodontics* **87**, 421-431.

Forsberg, C.M., Brattstrom, V., Malmberg, E. & Nord, C.E. (1991). Ligature wires and elastomeric rings: Two methods of ligation, and their association with microbial colonization of *Streptococcus mutans* and lactobacilli. *European Journal of Orthodontics* **13**, 416-420.

Goldberg, D. & Turley, P. (1989). Orthodontic space closure of edentulous maxillary first molar area in adults. *International Journal of Orthodontics and Orthognathic Surgery* **4**, 255-266.

Greenbaum, K.R. & Zachrisson, B.U. (1982). The effect of palatal expansion therapy on the periodontal supporting tissues. *American Journal of Orthodontics* **81**, 12-21.

Harpenau, L.A. & Boyd, R.L. (2000). Long-term follow-up of successful orthodontic-periodontal treatment of localized aggressive periodontitis: a case report. *Clinical Orthodontics and Research* **3**, 220-229.

Hoerman, K.C., Lang, R.L., Klapper, L., & Beery, J. (1985). Local tetracycline therapy of the periodontium during orthodontic treatment. *Quintessence International* **16**, 161-166.

Hom, B.M. & Turley, P.K. (1984). The effects of space closure on the mandibular first molar area in adults. *American Journal of Orthodontics* **85**, 457-469.

Ingber, J. (1974). Forced eruption. Part I. A method of treating isolated one and two wall infrabony osseous defects – rationale and case report. *Journal of Periodontology* **45**, 199-206.

Jin, L.J. & Cao, C.F. (1992). Clinical diagnosis of trauma from occlusion and its relation with severity of periodontitis. *Journal of Clinical Periodontology* **19**, 92-97.

Kajiyama, K., Murakami, T. & Yokota, S. (1993). Gingival reactions after experimentally induced extrusion of the upper incisors in monkeys. *American Journal of Orthodontics and Dentofacial Orthopedics* **104**, 36-47.

Karring, T., Nyman, S., Thilander, B. & Magnusson, B. (1982). Bone regeneration in orthodontically produced alveolar bone dehiscences. *Journal of Periodontal Research* **17**, 309-315.

Kessler, M. (1976). Interrelationships between orthodontics and periodontics. *American Journal of Orthodontics* **70**, 154-172.

Kokich, V. (1996a). Managing complex orthodontic problems: the use of implants for anchorage. *Seminars in Orthodontics* **2**, 153-160.

Kokich, V. (1996b). Esthetics: the ortho-perio restorative connection. *Seminars in Orthodontics* **2**, 21-30.

Kokich, V., Nappen, D. & Shapiro, P. (1984). Gingival contour and clinical crown length: their effect on the esthetic appearance of maxillary anterior teeth. *American Journal of Orthodontics* **86**, 89-94.

Kozlowsky, A., Tal, H. & Lieberman, M. (1988). Forced eruption combined with gingival fiberotomy. A technique for clinical crown lengthening. *Journal of Clinical Periodontology* **15**, 534-538.

Lang, N.P. (1977). Das präprotetische Aufrichten von gekippten unteren Molaren im Hinblick auf den parodontalen Zustand. *Schweizerische Monatsschrift für Zahnheilkunde* **87**, 560-569.

Leknes, K.N. (1995). Membrane surgery – possibilities and limitations. *Den Norske Tannlegeforenings Tidende* **105**, 352-359.

Lindhe, J. & Nyman, S. (1980). Alterations of the position of the marginal soft tissue following periodontal surgery. *Journal of Clinical Periodontology* **7**, 525-530.

Lindskog-Stokland, B., Wennström, J.L., Nyman, S. & Thilander, B. (1993). Orthodontic tooth movement into edentulous areas with reduced bone height. An experimental study in the dog. *European Journal of Orthodontics* **15**, 89-96.

Lundgren, D., Kurol, J., Thorstensson, B. & Hugoson, A. (1992).

Periodontal conditions around tipped and upright molars in adults. An intra-individual retrospective study. *European Journal of Orthodontics* **14**, 449-455.

Machen, D.E. (1990). Periodontal evaluation and updates: don't abdicate your duty to diagnose and supervise. *American Journal of Orthodontics and Dentofacial Orthopedics* **98**, 84-85.

Mathews, D.P. & Kokich, V.G. (1997). Managing treatment for the orthodontic patient with periodontal problems. *Seminars in Orthodontics* **3**, 21-38.

Melsen, B. (1986). Tissue reaction following application of extrusive and intrusive forces to teeth in adult monkeys. *American Journal of Orthodontics* **89**, 469-475.

Melsen, B. (1991). Limitations in adult orthodontics. In: Melsen, B., ed. *Current Controversies in Orthodontics*. Chicago: Quintessence, pp. 147-180.

Melsen, B., Agerbæk, N., Eriksen, J. & Terp, S. (1988) New attachment through periodontal treatment and orthodontic intrusion. *American Journal of Orthodontics and Dentofacial Orthopedics* **94**,104-116.

Melsen, B., Agerbæk, N. & Markenstam, G. (1989). Intrusion of incisors in adult patients with marginal bone loss. *American Journal of Orthodontics and Dentifacial Orthopedics* **96**, 232-241.

Monefeldt, I. & Zachrisson, B.U. (1977). Adjustment of clinical crown height by gingivectomy following orthodontic space closure. *The Angle Orthodontist* **47**, 256-264.

Müller, H-P, Eger, T. & Lange, D.E. (1995). Management of furcation-involved teeth. A retrospective analysis. *Journal of Clinical Periodontology* **22**, 911-917.

Murakami, T., Yokota, S., & Takahama, Y. (1989). Periodontal changes after experimentally induced intrusion of the upper incisors in Macaca fuscata monkeys. *American Journal of Orthodontics and Dentofacial Orthopedics* **95**, 115-126.

Nelson, P.A. & Årtun, J. (1997). Alveolar bone loss of maxillary anterior teeth in adult orthodontic patients. *American Journal of Orthodontics and Dentofacial Orthopedics* **111**, 328-334.

Nemcovsky, C.E., Zubery, Y., Artzi, Z. & Lieberman, M.A. (1996). Orthodontic tooth movement following guided tissue regeneration: report of three cases. *International Journal of Adult Orthodontics and Orthognathic Surgery* **11**, 347-355.

Nyman, S., Karring, T. & Bergenholz, G. (1982). Bone regeneration in alveolar bone dehiscences produced by jiggling forces. *Journal of Periodontal Research* **17**, 316-322.

Ong, M.A., Wang, H-L. & Smith, F.N. (1998). Interrelationship between periodontics and adult orthodontics. *Journal of Clinical Periodontology* **25**, 271-277.

Pini Prato, G., Tenti, C., Vincenzi, G., Magnani, C., Cortellini, P. & Clauser, C. (1992). Guided tissue regeneration versus mucogingival surgery in the treatment of human buccal gingival recession. *Journal of Periodontology* **63**, 919-928.

Polson, A., Caton, J., Polson, A.P., Nyman, S., Novak, J. & Reed, B. (1984). Periodontal response after tooth movement into intrabony defects. *Journal of Periodontology* **55**, 197-202.

Pontoriero, R., Celenza, F., Ricci, G. & Carnevale, G. (1987). Rapid extrusion with fiber resection: a combined orthodontic-periodontic treatment modality. *International Journal of Periodontics and Restorative Dentistry* **7**, 31-43.

Proffit, W.R. (1978). Equilibrium theory revisited: Factors influencing position of the teeth. *The Angle Orthodontist* **48**, 175-186.

Rabie, A.B.M.,Gildenhuys, R. & Boisson, M. (2001). Management of patients with severe bone loss: bone induction and orthodontics. *World Journal of Orthodontics* **2**, 142-153.

Ramfjord, S.P. (1984). Changing concepts in periodontics. *Journal of Prosthetic Dentistry* **52**, 781-785.

Re, S., Corrente, G., Abundo, R. & Cardaropoli, D. (2000). Orthodontic treatment in periodontally compromised patients: 12-year report. *International Journal of Periodontics and Restorative Dentistry* **20**, 31-39.

Ritchey, B. & Orban, B. (1954). Crests of the interdental alveola septa. *Dental Radiography and Photography* **27**, 37-56.

Rivera Circuns, A.L. & Tulloch, J.F.C. (1983). Gingival invagination in extraction sites of orthodontic patients: Their incidence, effects on periodontal health, and orthodontic treatment. *American Journal of Orthodontics* **83**, 469-476.

Spear, F.M., Mathews, D.M. & Kokich, V.G. (1997). Interdisciplinary management of single-tooth implants. *Seminars in Orthodontics* **3**, 45-72.

Steiner, G.G., Pearson, J.K. & Ainamo, J. (1981). Changes of the marginal periodontium as a result of labial tooth movement in monkeys. *Journal of Periodontology* **52**, 314-320.

Stelzel, M.J. & Flores-de-Jacoby, L. (1998). Guided tissue regeneration in a combined periodontal and orthodontic treatment: a case report. *International Journal of Periodontics and Restorative Dentistry* **18**, 189-195.

Stepovich, M.L. (1979). A clinical study on closing edentulous spaces in the mandible. *The Angle Orthodontist* **49**, 227-233.

Tarnow, D.P., Magner, A.W. & Fletcher, P. (1992). The effect of the distance from the contact point to the crest of bone on the presence or absence of the interproximal papilla. *Journal of Periodontology* **63**, 995-996.

Ten Hoeve, A. & Mulie, R.M. (1976). The effect of anteroposterior incisor repositioning on the palatal cortex as studied with laminography. *Journal of Clinical Orthodontics* **6**, 804-822.

Thilander, B. (1996). Infrabony pockets and reduced alveolar bone height in relation to orthodontic therapy. *Seminars in Orthodontics* **2**, 55-61.

Thilander, B., Nyman, S., Karring, T. & Magnusson, I. (1983). Bone regeneration in alveolar bone dehiscences related to orthodontic tooth movements. *European Journal of Orthodontics* **5**, 105-114.

Thordarson, A., Zachrisson, B.U. & Mjör, I.A. (1991). Remodeling of canines to the shape of lateral incisors by grinding: a long-term clinical and radiographic evaluation. *American Journal of Orthodontics and Dentofacial Orthopedics* **100**, 123-132.

Tuverson, D.L. (1980). Anterior interocclusal relations. *American Journal of Orthodontics* **78**, 361-393.

van Venroy, J.R. & Yukna, R.A. (1985). Orthodontic extrusion of single-rooted teeth affected with advanced periodontal disease. *American Journal of Orthodontics* **87**, 67-73.

Wehrbein, H., Fuhrmann, R.A.W. & Diedrich, P.R. (1994). Periodontal conditions after facial root tipping and palatal root torque of incisors. *American Journal of Orthodontics and Dentofacial Orthopedics* **106**, 455-462.

Wennström, J.L. (1983). Regeneration of gingiva following surgical excision. A clinical study. *Journal of Clinical Periodontology* **10**, 287-297.

Wennström, J.L. (1990). The significance of the width and thickness of the gingiva in orthodontic treatment. *Deutsche Zahnärztliche Zeitschrift* **45**, 136-141.

Wennström, J.L. (1996). Mucogingival considerations in orthodontic treatment. *Seminars in Orthodontics* **2**, 46-54.

Wennström, J.L., Lindhe, J., Sinclair, F. & Thilander, B. (1987). Some periodontal tissue reactions to orthodontic tooth movement in monkeys. *Journal of Clinical Periodontology* **14**, 121-129.

Wennström, J.L., Lindskog Stokland, B., Nyman, S. & Thilander, B. (1993). Periodontal tissue response to orthodontic movement of teeth with infrabony pockets. *American Journal of Orthodontics and Dentofacial Orthopedics* **103**, 313-319.

Zachrisson, B.U. (1996). Clinical implications of recent orthodontic-periodontic research findings. *Seminars in Orthodontics* **2**, 4-12.

Zachrisson, B.U. (2000a). Bonding in Orthodontics. In: Graber, T.M. & Vanarsdall, R.L., eds. *Orthodontics. Current Principles and Techniques*, 3rd edn, St. Louis: Mosby, Inc., pp. 557-645.

Zachrisson, B.U. (2000b). Orthodontic bonding to artificial tooth surfaces: clinical versus laboratory findings. *American Journal of Orthodontics and Dentofacial Orthopedics* **117**, 592-594.

Zachrisson, B.U. & Mjör, I.A. (1975). Remodelling of teeth by grinding. *American Journal of Orthodontics* **68**, 545-553.

CHAPTER 32

Supportive Periodontal Therapy (SPT)

Niklaus P. Lang, Urs Brägger, Giovanni Salvi and Maurizio S. Tonetti

Clinical trials on the long-term effects of treatment of periodontitis have clearly demonstrated that post-therapeutic professional maintenance care is an integral part of the treatment. This also constitutes the only means of assuring the maintenance of long-term beneficial therapeutic effects. Mainly through the rigid surveillance of patients involving professional visits at regular intervals could reinfection be prevented or kept to a minimal incidence in most patients. However, the maintenance systems presented in various studies do not allow the presentation of a clear concept with general validity for the frequency of professional maintenance visits and the mode of maintenance therapy. A danger for supervised neglect of reinfection and recurrent disease in some patients coexists with a tendency for overtreatment in others.

Objective criteria for assessing the patient's individual risk for recurrent disease have been the focus of attention of recent years. However, the evaluation of the patient's individual risk still has to be based on a probability estimation based on the analysis of patient, tooth or tooth site risk assessments.

The purpose of this chapter is to discuss the basics of continuous patient monitoring following active periodontal therapy in order to prevent reinfection and the continued progression of periodontal disease following therapy. Also, the mode and extent of interceptive therapeutic measures needed to achieve this goal will be evaluated.

DEFINITIONS

Periodontal treatment includes:

1. systemic evaluation of the patient's health
2. a cause-related therapeutic phase with, in some cases,
3. a corrective phase involving periodontal surgical procedures
4. *maintenance phase*

The 3rd World Workshop of the American Academy of Periodontology (1989) has renamed this treatment phase "supportive periodontal therapy" (SPT). This term expresses the essential need for therapeutic measures to support the patient's own efforts to control the periodontal infections and to avoid reinfection. Regular visits to the therapist should serve as a positive feedback mechanism between the patient and the therapist with the purpose of ensuring that the patients have the opportunity to maintain their dentitions in a healthy status for the longest possible time. An integral part of SPT is the continuous diagnostic monitoring of the patient in order to intercept with adequate therapy and to optimize the therapeutic interventions tailored to the patient's needs.

BASIC PARADIGMS FOR THE PREVENTION OF PERIODONTAL DISEASE

Periodontal maintenance care, or SPT, follows the paradigms of the etiology and pathogenesis of periodontal disease and – at the present time – must consider the fact that these diseases are coping with the result of the host defense on an opportunistic infection.

Almost 40 years ago, a cause-effect relationship between the accumulation of bacterial plaque on teeth and the development of gingivitis was proven (Löe et al. 1965). This relationship was also documented by the restoration of gingival health following plaque removal. Ten years later, a corresponding relationship between plaque accumulation and the development of periodontal disease, characterized by loss of connective tissue attachment and resorption of alveolar bone, was shown in laboratory animals (Lindhe et al. 1975). Since some of these animals did not develop periodontal disease despite a persistent plaque accumulation for 48 months, it must be considered that the composition of the microbiota or the host's defense mechanisms or susceptibility for disease may vary from individual to individual. Nevertheless, in the study mentioned, the initiation of periodontal disease was always preceded by obvious signs of gingivitis. Hence, it seems reasonable to predict that the elimination of gingival inflammation and the maintenance of healthy gingival tissues will result in the prevention of both the initiation and the recurrence of periodontal disease. In fact, already in 1746, Fauchard stated that "little or no care as to the cleaning of teeth is ordinarily the cause of all diseases that destroy them" (Fauchard 1746).

From the clinical point of view, the above-mentioned results must be translated into the necessity for proper and regular personal plaque elimination, at least in patients treated for or susceptible to periodontal disease. This simple principle may be difficult to implement in all patients; however, interceptive professional supportive therapy at regular intervals may, to a certain extent, compensate for the lack of personal compliance with regard to oral hygiene standards.

These aspects have been imitated in a beagle dog model with naturally occurring periodontal disease (Morrison et al. 1979). Two groups of animals were used. The test group was subjected to initial scaling and root planing and, subsequently, plaque was eliminated by daily toothbrushing and biweekly polishing with rubber cups for a period of 3 years. In the control group, no initial scaling and no oral hygiene practices were performed during the same period of time. Every 6 months, however, the teeth in two diagonally opposed jaw quadrants in both test and control animals were scaled and root planed. The results showed that the reduction of probing depth and the gain of probing attachment, obtained after the initial scaling and root planing in the test animals, were maintained throughout the entire course of the study irrespective of whether or not repeated scaling and root planing had been performed. The control animals, on the other hand, continued to show increasing probing depths and loss of attachment in all quadrants irrespective of whether or not repeated scaling and root planing had been performed. However, in the jaw quadrants where the teeth were repeatedly instrumented every 6 months, the progression of periodontal destruction was significantly less pronounced (Fig. 32-1a,b). These results indicate that professional supportive therapy, performed at regular intervals, may, at least to a certain extent, compensate for a "suboptimal" personal oral hygiene standard. In this respect, it has been demonstrated that following root instrumentation, the subgingival microbiota is significantly altered in quantity and quality (Listgarten et al. 1978), and that the re-establishment of a disease-associated, subgingival microbiota may require several months (Listgarten et al. 1978, Slots et al. 1979, Mousquès et al. 1980, Caton et al. 1982, Magnusson et al. 1984.)

In a number of longitudinal, clinical studies on the outcome of periodontal therapy, the crucial role of SPT in maintaining successful results has been documented (Ramfjord et al. 1968, 1975, Lindhe & Nyman 1975, 1984, Rosling et al. 1976, Nyman et al. 1977, Knowles et al. 1979, 1980, Badersten et al. 1981, 1987, Hill et al. 1981, Lindhe et al. 1982a,b, Pihlström et al. 1983, Westfelt et al. 1983, 1985, Isidor & Karring 1986, Kaldahl et al. 1988). In all these studies, probing depths and clinical attachment levels were maintained as a result of a well-organized professional maintenance care program (recall intervals varying between 3 and 6 months) irrespective of the initial treatment modality performed. In one of the studies (Nyman et al. 1977) an alarming result was that patients treated for advanced periodontal disease involving surgical techniques, but not incorporated in a supervised maintenance care program, exhibited recurrent periodontitis including loss of attachment at a rate three to five times higher than documented for natural progression of periodontal disease in population groups with high disease susceptibility (Löe et al. 1978, 1986). Within this area, the effect of negligence in providing adequate supportive maintenance care following periodontal treatment has been studied over a 6-year period by Axelsson & Lindhe (1981a). Following presurgical root instrumentation and instruction in oral hygiene practices, all study patients were subjected to modified Widman flap procedures. During a 2-month healing period, professional toothcleaning was performed every 2 weeks. Following this time period, baseline clinical data were obtained and one out of every third patient was dismissed from the clinic, while the two others were incorporated in a professionally conducted maintenance program with a recall once every 3 months. These patients maintained excellent oral hygiene and consequently

Reduction (+) or Increase (-) in Pocket Depth

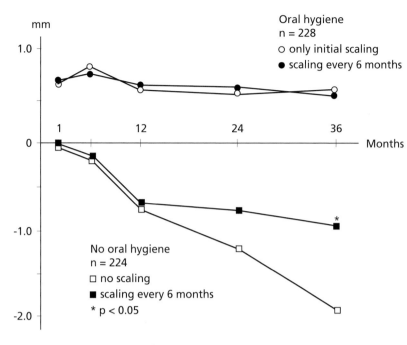

Fig. 32-1a. Mean probing depth reduction (+) or increase in probing depth (-) in millimeters with or without repeated scaling and root planing in experimental (oral hygiene) and control (no oral hygiene) animals relative to baseline means.

Gain (+) or Loss (-) of Attachment

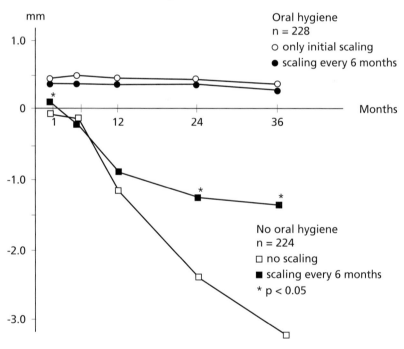

Fig. 32-1b. Mean gain (+) or loss (-) of probing attachment with or without repeated scaling and root planing in experimental (oral hygiene) and control (no oral hygiene) animals relative to baseline means. (Data from Morrison et al. 1979).

yielded a very low frequency of bleeding sites. In addition, probing depths and probing attachment levels were maintained unchanged over the 6-year period. In contrast, the non-recalled patients demonstrated obvious signs of recurrent periodontitis at the 3-year and 6-year re-examinations. Further evidence for the likelihood of recurrent disease in patients not subjected to professional maintenance care was presented by Kerr (1981). Five years after successful treatment, 45% of the patients presented with periodontal conditions similar to their status before treatment. Supportive therapy had only been provided at intervals varying between 9 and 18 months.

Similar results have been described for private practice patients who decided not to participate in an organized maintenance care program following active periodontal therapy (Becker et al. 1984). Subsequent examinations revealed clear signs of recurrent periodontal disease including increased probing depths and involvements of furcations of multirooted teeth concomitant with tooth loss. Also, loss of alveolar bone observed in radiographs and tooth loss have been reported for a group of patients in whom posttherapeutic supportive maintenance care was provided less frequently than once every 12 months (De Vore et al. 1986). From all these studies it is evident that periodontal treatment is ineffective in maintaining periodontal health if supportive maintenance care is neglected, denied or omitted.

Even though the number of well-controlled longitudinal clinical trials is rather limited for patients who, in addition to periodontal treatment, have undergone extensive reconstructive therapy, it should be realized that the concept of professional maintenance care has unrestricted validity. In a longitudinal study of combined periodontal and prosthetic treatment of patients with advanced periodontal disease, periodontal health could be maintained over a study period of 5-8 years with regular recall appointments scheduled every 3-6 months (Nyman & Lindhe 1979). Similar results have been presented by Valderhaug & Birkeland (1976) and by Valderhaug (1980) for periods of up to 15 years. Another study of 36 patients who received extensive poly-unit cantilevered bridgework following periodontal therapy, confirmed the maintenance of periodontal health over 5-12 years (Laurell et al. 1991). More recent studies on the long-term maintenance over 10 and 11 years of periodontal patients who, following successful treatment of chronic periodontitis, were reconstructed with extensive fixed reconstructions revealed that regularly performed SPT resulted in periodontal stability. Only 1.3% (Hämmerle et al. 2000) and 2.0% (Moser et al. 2002) of the abutments showed some minor attachment loss during these long periods of observation. In contrast, a report of insurance cases who were not regularly maintained by SPT yielded a recurrence rate for periodontitis of almost 10% after an observation of 6.5 years (Randow et al. 1986).

Summary

The etiology of gingivitis and periodontitis is fairly well understood. However, the causative factors, i.e. the microbial challenge which induces and maintains the inflammatory response, may not be completely eliminated from the dento-gingival environment for any length of time. This requires the professional removal of all microbial deposits in the supragingival and subgingival areas at regular intervals, since recolonization will occur following the debridement procedures, leading to a reinfection of the ecologic niche and hence, giving rise to further progression of the disease process. Numerous well-controlled clinical trials, however, have documented that such a development can be prevented over very long periods of time only by the regular interference with the subgingival environment which aims at the removal of the subgingival bacteria.

PATIENTS AT RISK FOR PERIODONTITIS WITHOUT SPT

The effect of an omission of SPT in patients with periodontitis may best be studied either in untreated populations or patient groups with poor compliance.

One of the few studies documenting untreated periodontitis-susceptible patients reported on the continuous loss of periodontal attachment as well as teeth in Sri Lankan tea plantation workers receiving no dental therapy (Löe et al. 1986). In such a – for the western world – rather unique model situation an average loss of 0.3 mm per tooth surface and year was encountered. Also, the laborers lost between 0.1 and 0.3 teeth per year as a result of periodontitis. In another untreated group in the United States, 0.61 teeth had been lost per year during an observation period of 4 years (Becker et al. 1979). This is in dramatic contrast to reports on tooth loss in well-maintained patients treated for periodontitis (e.g. Hirschfeld & Wasserman 1978, McFall 1982, Becker et al. 1984, Wilson et al. 1987). Such patients were either completely stable and lost no teeth during maintenance periods ranging up to 22 years or lost only very little periodontal attachment and only 0.03 teeth (Hirschfeld & Wasserman 1978) or 0.06 teeth (Wilson et al. 1987), respectively.

Non-complying, but periodontitis-susceptible patients receiving no SPT following periodontal surgical interventions continued to lose periodontal attachment at a rate of approximately 1 mm per year regardless of the type of surgery chosen (Nyman et al. 1977). This is almost three times more than would have to be expected as a result of the "natural" course of periodontal disease progression (Löe et al. 1978, 1986).

In a British study of a private practice situation (Kerr 1981) where the patients were referred back to the general dentist after periodontal therapy, 45% of the patients showed a complete reinfection after 5 years.

Probably the most impressive documentation of the lack of SPT in disease-susceptible individuals arises from a clinical trial in which one third of the patients had been sent back to the referring general practitioner for maintenance, while two thirds of the patients received SPT in a well-organized maintenance system (Axelsson & Lindhe 1981a). The 77 patients were examined before treatment, 2 months after the last surgical procedure and 3 and 6 years later. The 52 patients on the carefully designed SPT system visited the program every 2 months for the first 2 years and every 3 months for the remaining 4 years of the observation period. The results obtained from the second examination (2 months after the last surgery) showed that the effect of the initial treatment was good in both groups. Subsequently, the recall patients were able to maintain proper oral hygiene and unaltered attachment levels. In the non-recall group, plaque scores increased markedly from the baseline values, as did the number of inflamed gingival units (Fig. 32-2a). Concomitantly, there were obvious signs of recurrent periodontitis. The mean values for pocket depth and attachment levels at the 3-year and 6-year examinations were higher than at baseline (Fig. 32-2b). In the recall group, approximately 99% of the tooth surfaces showed either improvement, no change or less than 1 mm loss of attachment, compared to 45% in the non-

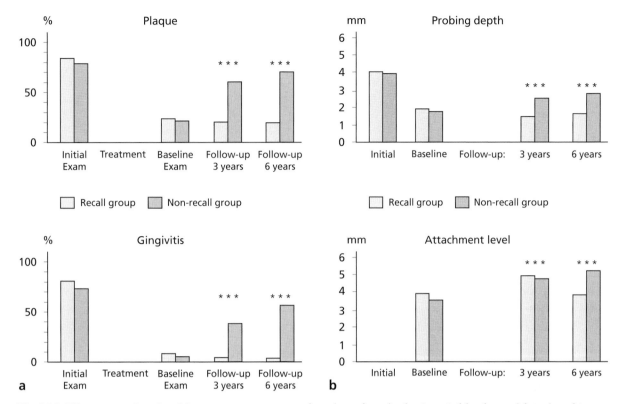

Fig. 32-2. Histograms showing (a) average percentages of tooth surfaces harboring visible plaque (above) and inflamed gingival units (bleeding on probing) (below), and (b) average probing depth (above) and probing attachment levels (below), at initial, baseline and follow-up examinations. (Data from Axelsson & Lindhe 1981b.)

recall group (Table 32-1). In the latter patients, 55% of the sites showed a 2-5 mm further loss of attachment at the 6-year examination, and 20% of the pockets were 4 mm deep or more (Tables 32-1 & 32-2).

Summary
Patients susceptible to periodontal disease are at high risk for reinfection and progression of periodontal lesions without meticulously organized and performed SPT. Since all patients who were treated for periodontal diseases belong to this risk category by virtue of their past history, an adequate maintenance care program is of utmost importance for a beneficial long-term treatment outcome. SPT has to be aimed at the regular removal of the subgingival microbiota and must be supplemented by the patient's efforts for optimal supragingival plaque control.

Table 32-1. Percentage of sites showing various changes in probing attachment level between baseline examination, 2 months after completion of active periodontal therapy and follow-up examination 6 years later. (Adapted from Axelsson & Lindhe 1981b)

Change in attachment level	Percentage of surfaces showing change	
	Recall	Non-recall
Attachment level improved	17	1
No change	72	10
Attachment level worse by		
≥ 1 mm	10	34
2 to 5 mm	1	55

Table 32-2. Percentage of various probing depths in recall and non-recall patients at the initial examination, 2 months after active periodontal treatment and at 3 and 6-year follow-up visits. (Adapted from Axelsson & Lindhe 1981b)

Examinations	Percentage of pockets of various depths					
	≤ 3 mm		4-6 mm		≥ 7 mm	
	Recall	Non-recall	Recall	Non-recall	Recall	Non-recall
Initial	35	50	58	38	8	12
Baseline	99	99	1	1	0	0
3 years	99	91	1	9	0	0
6 years	99	80	1	19	0	1

SPT FOR PATIENTS WITH GINGIVITIS

Several studies – predominantly in children – have documented that periodic professional prophylactic visits in conjunction with reinforcement of personal oral hygiene are effective in controlling gingivitis (Badersten et al. 1975, Poulsen et al. 1976, Axelsson & Lindhe 1981a,b, Bellini et al. 1981). This, however, does not imply that maintenance visits in childhood preclude the development of more severe disease later in life. It is obvious that SPT, therefore, must be a lifelong commitment of both the patient and the profession.

Adults whose effective oral hygiene was combined with periodic professional prophylaxes clearly were healthier periodontally than patients who did not participate in such programs (Lövdal et al. 1961, Suomi et al. 1971). One particular study of historic significance was performed on 1428 adults from an industrial company in Oslo, Norway (Lövdal et al. 1961). Over a 5-year observation period, the subjects were recalled 2-4 times per year for instruction in oral hygiene and supragingival and subgingival scaling. Gingival conditions improved by approximately 60% and tooth loss was reduced by about 50% of what would be expected without these efforts.

In another study (Suomi et al. 1971) loss of periodontal tissue support in young individuals with gingivitis or only loss of small amounts of attachment was followed over 3 years. An experimental group receiving scaling and instruction in oral hygiene every 3 months yielded significantly less plaque and gingival inflammation than the control group in which no special efforts had been made. The mean loss of probing attachment was only 0.08 mm per surface in the experimental as opposed to 0.3 mm in the control group.

When adult patients with gingivitis were treated with scaling and root planing, but did not improve their oral hygiene procedures, the gingival condition did not improve compared with individuals receiving prophylaxes at 6-month intervals (Listgarten & Schifter 1982).

Summary
The available information indicates that the prevention of gingival inflammation and early loss of attachment in patients with gingivitis depends primarily on the level of personal plaque control, but also on further measures to reduce the accumulation of supragingival and subgingival plaque.

SPT FOR PATIENTS WITH PERIODONTITIS

As mentioned previously, a series of longitudinal studies on periodontal therapeutic modalities was performed in the past 25 years, first at the University of Michigan, later at the University of Gothenburg, Sweden, and also at the Universities of Minnesota, Nebraska and Loma Linda. These studies always incorporated the patients into a well-organized maintenance care system with recall visits at regular intervals (generally 3-4 months). Although the patients performed plaque control with various degrees of efficacy, the SPT resulted in excellent maintenance of postoperative attachment levels in most patients (Knowles 1973, Ramfjord et al. 1982).

On average, excellent treatment results with maintained reduced probing depths and maintained gains of probing attachment were documented for most of the patients in the longitudinal studies irrespective of the treatment modality chosen (Ramfjord et al. 1975, Lindhe & Nyman 1975, Rosling et al. 1976, Nyman et al. 1977, Knowles et al. 1979, 1980, Badersten et al. 1981, 1987, Hill et al. 1981, Lindhe et al. 1982a, Pihlström et al. 1983b, Westfelt et al. 1983a,b, 1985, Isidor & Karring 1986).

In a study on 75 patients with extremely advanced periodontitis, who had been successfully treated for the disease, a result of cause-related therapy and modified Widman flap procedures (Lindhe & Nyman 1984), recurrent infection occurred in only very few sites during a 14-year period of effective SPT. However, it has to be realized that recurrent periodontitis was noticed at completely unpredictable time intervals, but was concentrated in about 25% of the patient population (15 out of 61). This suggests that, in a periodontitis-susceptible risk population, the majority of patients can be "cured" provided an optimally organized SPT is performed, while a relatively small proportion of patients (20-25%) will suffer from occasional episodes of recurrent periodontal reinfection. It is obviously a challenge for the diagnostician to identify such patients with very high disease susceptibility and to monitor the dentitions for recurrent periodontitis on a long-term basis.

As opposed to the study by Lindhe & Nyman (1984) which involved exclusively patients with advanced periodontitis, another study on 52 patients with generalized mild to moderate adult periodontitis addressed the efficacy of SPT 8 years following completion of cause-related periodontal therapy (Brägger et al. 1992). Full mouth intraoral radiographs were used to assess changes in the radiographic alveolar bone height as a percentage of the total tooth length. As a result of cause-related therapy, a gain in probing attachment followed by a loss of 0.5-0.8 mm over the following 8 years was observed. The radiographic loss of alveolar bone height in the same time period was less than 2% and thus clinically insignificant. In this patient group initially presenting with mild to moderate periodontitis, the frequency of SPT rendered per year did not affect the rate of progression of periodontal desease. However, patients seeking SPT less than once per year over 8 years lost further periodontal attachment during the period of observation. From these studies it is evident that patients having experienced periodontitis need some kind of SPT. Obviously, the frequency of SPT visits has to be adapted to the risk of susceptibility for the disease. Patients with advanced periodontitis may need SPT at a regular and rather short time interval (3-4 months), while for mild to moderate forms of periodontitis, one annual visit may be enough to prevent further loss of attachment.

Summary

SPT is an absolute prerequisite to guarantee beneficial treatment outcomes with maintained levels of clinical attachment over long periods of time. While the maintenance of treatment results for the majority of patients has been documented up to 14 years, it has to be realized that a small proportion of patients will experience recurrent infections with progression of periodontal lesions in a few sites in a completely unpredictable mode. The continuous risk assessment at subject, tooth and tooth site levels, therefore, represents a challenge for the SPT concept.

Continuous multilevel risk assessment

As opposed to an initial periodontal diagnosis which considers the sequelae of the disease process, i.e. documents the net loss of periodontal attachment and the concomitant formation of periodontal pockets and the existence of inflammation, clinical diagnosis during SPT has to be based on the variations of the health status obtained following successful active periodontal treatment. This, in turn, means that a new baseline will have to be established once the treatment goals of active periodontal therapy (i.e. phases 1-3) are reached and periodontal health is restored (Claffey 1991). This baseline includes the level of clinical attachment achieved while the inflammatory parameters are supposed to be under control. Under optimal circumstances, supportive periodontal care would maintain clinical attachment levels obtained after active therapy for the years to come. The relevant question would, therefore, be which clinical parameters may serve as early indicators for a new onset or recurrence of the periodontal disease process, i.e. reinfection and progression of periodontal breakdown of a previously treated periodontal site.

From a clinical point of view the stability of periodontal conditions reflects a dynamic equilibrium between bacterial aggression and effective host response. As such, this homeostasis is prone to sudden changes whenever one of the two factors prevails.

Hence, it is evident that the diagnostic process must be based on a continuous monitoring of the multilevel risk profile. The intervals between diagnostic assessments must also be chosen based on the overall risk profile and the expected benefit. To schedule patients for supportive periodontal therapy on the basis of an individual risk evaluation for recurrence of disease has been demonstrated to be cost-effective (Axelsson & Lindhe 1981a,b, Axelsson et al. 1991).

By virtue of their previous disease predisposition, all patients under a periodontal maintenance program represent a population with a moderate to high risk for recurrent periodontal infection. As opposed to the general population without such a history, periodontal patients need to participate in a well-organized recall system which should provide both continuous risk assessment and adequate supportive care. Without this, the patients are likely to experience progressive loss of periodontal attachment (Axelsson & Lindhe 1981a, Kerr 1981, Becker et al. 1984, Cortellini et al. 1994, 1996). On the other hand, it is important to determine the level of risk for progression in each individual patient in order to be able to determine the frequency and extent of professional support necessary to maintain the attachment levels obtained following active therapy. The determination of such risk level would thus prevent undertreatment, and also excessive overtreatment, during SPT (Brägger et al. 1992).

Subject risk assessment

The patient's risk assessment for recurrence of periodontitis may be evaluated on the basis of a number of clinical conditions whereby no single parameter displays a more paramount role. The entire spectrum of risk factors and risk indicators ought to be evaluated simultaneously. For this purpose, a functional diagram has been constructed (Fig. 32-3) (Lang & Tonetti 2003) including the following aspects:

1. Percentage of bleeding on probing
2. Prevalence of residual pockets greater than 4 mm
3. Loss of teeth from a total of 28 teeth
4. Loss of periodontal support in relation to the patient's age
5. Systemic and genetic conditions
6. Environmental factors such as cigarette smoking.

Each parameter has its own scale for minor, moderate and high risk profiles. A comprehensive evaluation, the functional diagram will provide an individualized total risk profile and determine the frequency and complexity of SPT visits. Modifications may be made to the functional diagram if additional factors become important from future evidence.

Compliance with recall system

Several investigations have indicated that only a mi-

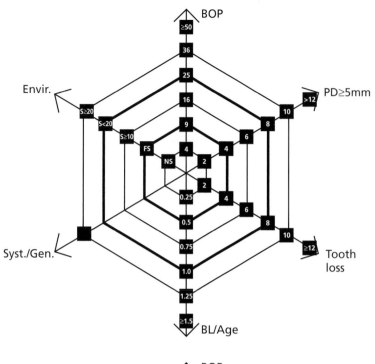

Fig. 32-3a. Functional diagram to evaluate the patient's risk for recurrence of periodontitis. Each vector represents one risk factor or indicator with an area of relatively low risk, an area of moderate risk and an area of high risk for disease progression. All factors have to be evaluated together and hence the area of relatively low risk is found within the center circle of the polygon, while the area of high risk is found outside the periphery of the second ring in bold. Between the two rings in bold, there is the area of moderate risk.

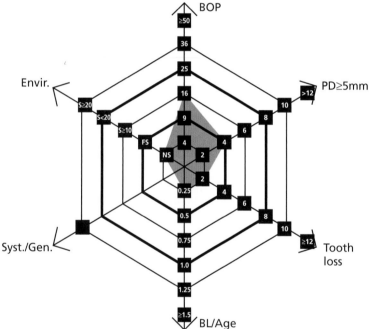

Fig. 32-3b. Functional diagram of a low risk maintenance patient. BOP is 15%, four residual pockets ≥ 5 mm are diagnosed, two teeth have been lost, the bone factor in relation to the age is 0.25, no systemic factor is known and the patient is a non-smoker.

nority of periodontal patients comply with the prescribed supportive periodontal care (Wilson et al. 1984, Mendoza et al. 1991, Checchi et al. 1994, Demetriou et al. 1995). Since it has been clearly established that treated periodontal patients who comply with regular periodontal maintenance appointments have a better prognosis than patients who do not comply (Axelsson & Lindhe 1981a, Kent 1981, Becker et al. 1984, Cortellini et al. 1994, 1996), non-compliant or poorly compliant patients should be considered at higher risk for periodontal disease progression. A report that investigated the personality differences of patients participating in a regular recall program as compared to patients who did not, revealed that patients who did not take part in a maintenance program

following periodontal therapy had higher incidences of stressful life events and less stable personal relationships in their lives (Becker et al. 1988).

Oral hygiene
Since bacterial plaque is by far the most important etiologic agent for the occurrence of periodontal diseases (for review see Kornman & Löe 1993), it is evident that the full mouth assessment of the bacterial load must have a pivotal impact in the determination of the risk for disease recurrence. It has to be realized, however, that regular interference with the microbial ecosystem during periodontal maintenance will eventually obscure such obvious associations. In patients treated with various surgical and non-surgical mo-

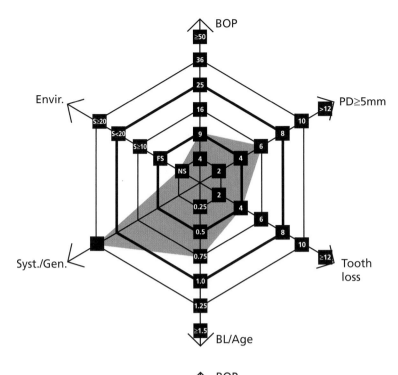

Fig. 32-3c. Functional diagram of a medium risk maintenance patient. BOP is 9%, 6 residual pockets ≥ 5 mm are diagnosed, four teeth have been lost, the bone factor in relation to the age is 0.75, the patient is a Type I diabetic, but a non-smoker.

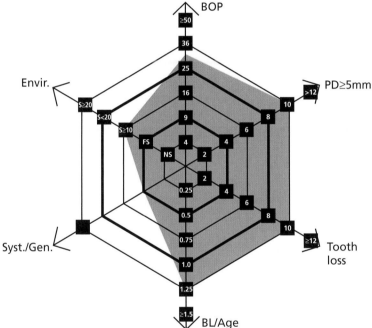

Fig. 32-3d. Functional diagram of a high risk maintenance patient. BOP is 32%, ten residual pockets ≥ 5 mm are diagnosed, ten teeth had been lost, the bone factor in relation to the age is 1.25, no systemic factor is known and the patient is a occasional smoker.

dalities, it has been clearly established that plaque-infected dentitions will yield recurrence of periodontal disease in multiple locations, while dentitions under plaque control and regular supportive care maintain periodontal stability for many years (Rosling et al. 1976, Axelsson & Lindhe 1981a,b). Studies have thus far not identified a level of plaque infection compatible with maintenance of periodontal health. However, in a clinical set-up, a plaque control record of 20-40% might be tolerable by most patients. It is important to realize that the full mouth plaque score has to be related to the host response of the patient, i.e. compared to inflammatory parameters.

Percentage of sites with bleeding on probing
Bleeding on gentle probing represents an objective inflammatory parameter which has been incorporated into index systems for the evaluation of periodontal conditions (Löe & Silness 1963, Mühlemann & Son 1971) and is also used as a parameter by itself. In a patient's risk assessment for recurrence of periodontitis, BOP reflects, at least in part, the patient's compliance and standards of oral hygiene performance. Although there is no established acceptable level of prevalence of bleeding on probing in the dentition above which a higher risk for disease recurrence has been established, a BOP prevalence of 25% has been the cut-off point between patients with maintained periodontal stability for 4 years and patients with

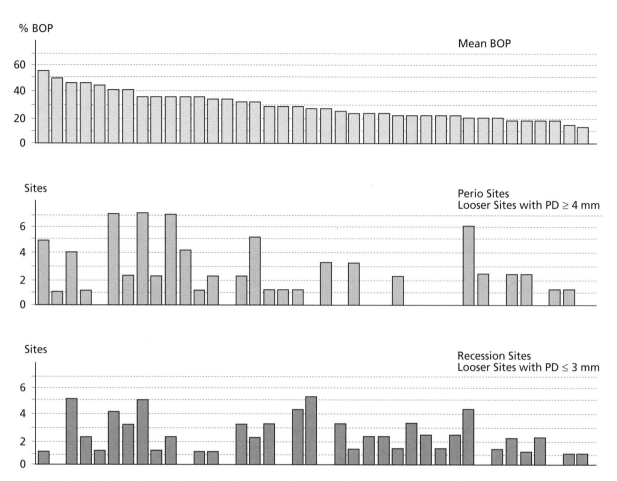

Fig. 32-4. Distribution of "looser" sites (probing depth PD ≥ 4 mm) due to periodontal disease progression with or without concomitant recession, dependent on the mean bleeding on probing percentage (BOP) during an observation period of 4 years. Patients are sorted by decreasing mean BOP percentages. Patients with < 20% BOP have a significantly lower risk for disease recurrence. (Data from Joss et al. 1994.)

recurrent disease in the same time frame in a prospective study in a private practice (Joss et al. 1994) (Fig. 32-4). Further evidence of BOP percentages between 20% and 30% determining a higher risk for disease progression originates from studies of Claffey et al. (1990) and Badersten et al. (1990).

In assessing the patient's risk for disease progression, BOP percentages reflect a summary of the patient's ability to perform proper plaque control, the patient's host response to the bacterial challenge and the patient's compliance. The percentage of BOP, therefore, is used as the first risk factor in the functional diagram of risk assessment (Fig. 32-3). The scale runs in a quadratic mode with 4, 9, 16, 25, 36 and > 49% being the divisions on the vector.

Individuals with low mean BOP percentages (< 10% of the surfaces) may be regarded as patients with a low risk for recurrent disease (Lang et al. 1990), while patients with mean BOP percentages > 25% should be considered to be at high risk for reinfection.

Prevalence of residual pockets greater than 4 mm
The enumeration of the residual pockets with probing depths greater than 4 mm represents – to a certain extent – the degree of success of periodontal treatment rendered. Although this figure *per se* does not make

much sense when considered as a sole parameter, the evaluation in conjunction with other parameters such as bleeding on probing and/or suppuration will reflect existing ecologic niches from and in which reinfection might occur. It is, therefore, conceivable that periodontal stability in a dentition would be reflected in a minimal number of residual pockets. Presence of high frequencies of deep residual pockets and deepening of pockets during supportive periodontal care has, in fact, been associated with high risk for disease progression (Badersten et al. 1990, Claffey et al. 1990). On the other hand, it has to be realized that an increased number of residual pockets does not necessarily imply an increased risk for re-infection or disease progression, since a number of longitudinal studies have established the fact that, depending on the individual supportive therapy provided, even deeper pockets may be stable without further disease progression for years (e.g. Knowles et al. 1979, Lindhe & Nyman 1984).

Nevertheless, in assessing the patient's risk for disease progression, the number of residual pockets with a probing depth of ≥ 5 mm is assessed as the second risk indicator for recurrent disease in the functional diagram of risk assessment (Fig. 32-3). The scale runs in a linear mode with 2, 4, 6, 8, 10 and ≥ 12% being the divisions on the vector.

Individuals with up to four residual pockets may be regarded as patients with a relatively low risk, while patients with more than eight residual pockets may be regarded as individuals with high risk for recurrent disease.

Loss of teeth from a total of 28 teeth

Although the reason for tooth loss may not be known, the number of remaining teeth in a dentition reflects the functionality of the dentition. Mandibular stability and individual optimal function may be assured even with a shortened dental arch of premolar to premolar occlusion, i.e. 20 teeth. The shortened dental arch does not seem to predispose the individual to mandibular dysfunction (Witter et al. 1990, 1994). However, if more than eight teeth from a total of 28 teeth are lost, oral function is usually impaired (Käyser 1981, 1994, 1996). Since tooth loss also represents a true end-point outcome variable reflecting the patient's history of oral diseases and trauma, it is logical to incorporate this risk indicator as the third parameter in the functional diagram of risk assessment (Fig. 32-3). The number of teeth lost from the dentition without the third molars (28 teeth) is counted, irrespective of their replacement. The scale runs also in a linear mode with 2, 4, 6, 8, 10 and ≥ 12% being the divisions on the vector.

Individuals with up to four teeth lost may be regarded as patients in low risk, while patients with more than eight teeth lost may be considered as being in high risk.

Loss of periodontal support in relation to the patient's age

The extent and prevalence of periodontal attachment loss (i.e. previous disease experience and susceptibility), as evaluated by the height of the alveolar bone on radiographs, may represent the most obvious indicator of subject risk when related to the patient's age. In light of the present understanding of periodontal disease progression, and the evidence that both onset and rate of progression of periodontitis might vary among individuals and during different time frames (van der Velden 1991), it has to be realized that previous attachment loss in relation to the patient's age does not rule out the possibility of rapidly progressing lesions. Therefore, the actual risk for further disease progression in a given individual may occasionally be underestimated. Hopefully, the rate of progression of disease has been positively affected by the treatment rendered and, hence, previous attachment loss in relation to patient's age may be a more accurate indicator during SPT than before active periodontal treatment. Given the hypothesis that a dentition may be functional for the most likely life expectancy of the subject in the presence of a reduced height of periodontal support (i.e. 25-50% of the root length), the risk assessment in treated periodontal patients may represent a reliable prognostic indicator for the stability of the overall treatment goal of keeping a functional dentition for a lifetime (Papapanou et al. 1988).

The estimation of the loss of alveolar bone is performed in the posterior region on either periapical radiographs, in which the worst site affected is estimated gross as a percentage of the root length, or on bite-wing radiographs in which the worst site affected is estimated in mm. One mm is equated with 10% bone loss. The percentage is then divided by the patient's age. This results in a factor. As an example, a 40-year-old patient with 20% of bone loss at the worst posterior site affected would be scored BL/Age = 0.5. Another 40-year-old patient with 50% bone loss at the worst posterior site scores BL/Age = 1.25.

In assessing the patient's risk for disease progression, the extent of alveolar bone loss in relation to the patient's age is estimated as the fourth risk indicator for recurrent disease in the functional diagram of risk assessment (Fig. 32-3). The scale runs in increments of 0.25 of the factor BL/Age, with 0.5 being the division between low and moderate risk and 1.0 being the division between moderate and high risk for disease progression. This, in turn, means that a patient who has lost a higher percentage of posterior alveolar bone than his/her own age is at high risk regarding this vector in a multifactorial assessment of risk.

Systemic conditions

The most substantiated evidence for modification of disease susceptibility and/or progression of periodontal disease arises from studies on Type I and Type II (insulin-dependent and non-insulin-dependent) diabetes mellitus populations (Gusberti et al. 1983, Emrich et al. 1991, Genco & Löe 1993).

It has to be realized that the impact of diabetes on periodontal diseases has been documented in patients with untreated periodontal disease, while, as of today, no clear evidence is available for treated patients. It is reasonable, however, to assume that the influence of the systemic conditions may also affect recurrence of disease.

In recent years, genetic markers have become available to determine various genotypes of patients regarding their susceptibility for periodontal diseases. Research on the interleukin-1 (IL-1) polymorphisms has indicated that IL-1 genotype positive patients show more advanced periodontitis lesions than IL-1 genotype negative patients of the same age group (Kornman et al. 1997). Also, there is a trend to higher tooth loss in the IL-1 genotype positive subjects (McGuire & Nunn 1999). In a retrospective analysis of over 300 well-maintained periodontal patients, the IL-1 genotype positive patients showed significantly higher BOP percentages and a higher proportion of patients which yielded higher BOP percentages during a 1-year recall period than the IL-1 genotype negative control patients (Lang et al. 2000). Also, the latter group had twice as many patients with improved BOP percentages during the same maintenance period, indicating that IL-1 genotype positive subjects do indeed represent a group of hyper-reactive subjects even if they are regularly maintained by effective SPT (Lang et al. 2000). In a prospective study over 5 years on Australian white collar and blue collar workers on a University campus, the IL-1 genotype positive age group above 50 years showed significantly deeper probing depth than their IL-1 genotype negative counterparts, especially when they were non-smokers.

In assessing the patient's risk for disease progression, systemic factors are only considered, if known, as the fifth risk indicator for recurrent disease in the functional diagram of risk assessment (Fig. 32-3). In this case, the area of high risk is marked for this vector. If not known or absent, systemic factors are not taken into account for the overall evaluation of risk.

Research on the association and/or modifying influence in susceptibility and progression of periodontitis of physical or psychologic stress is sparse (Cohen-Cole et al. 1981, Green et al. 1986, Freeman & Goss 1993). The hormonal changes associated with this condition, however, are well documented (Selye 1950).

Cigarette smoking
Consumption of *tobacco*, predominantly in the form of smoking or chewing, affects the susceptibility and the treatment outcome of patients with adult periodontitis. Classical explanations for these observations have included the association between smoking habits and poor oral hygiene as well as unawareness of general health issues (Pindborg 1949, Rivera-Hidalgo 1986). More recent evidence, however, has established that smoking *per se* represents not only a risk marker, but probably a true risk factor for periodontitis (Ismail et al. 1983, Bergström 1989, Bergström et al. 1991, Haber et al. 1993). In a young population (19-30 years of age), 51-56% of periodontitis was associated with cigarette smoking (Haber et al. 1993). The association of smoking and periodontitis has been shown to be dose-dependent (Haber et al. 1993). It has also been shown that smoking will affect the treatment outcome after scaling and root planing (Preber & Bergström 1985), modified Widman flap surgery (Preber & Bergström 1990), and regenerative periodontal therapy (Tonetti et al. 1995). Furthermore, a high proportion of so-called refractory patients has been identified as consisting of smokers (Bergström & Blomlöf 1992). The impact of cigarette smoking on the long-term effects of periodontal therapy in a population undergoing supportive periodontal care has been reported. Smokers displayed less favorable healing responses both at re-evaluation and during a 6-year period of supportive periodontal care (Baumert-Ah et al. 1994). In spite of the paucity of evidence relating cigarette smoking to impaired outcomes during supportive periodontal care, it seems reasonable to incorporate heavy smokers (> 20 cigarettes/day) in a higher risk group during maintenance.

In assessing the patient's risk for disease progression, environmental factors such as smoking must be considered as the sixth risk factor for recurrent disease

in the functional diagram of risk assessment (Fig. 32-3). While non-smokers (NS) and former smokers (FS) (more than 5 years since cessation) have a relatively low risk for recurrence of periodontitis, the heavy smokers (HS), as defined by smoking more than one pack per day, are definitely at high risk. Occasional (OS; < 10 cigarettes a day) and moderate smokers (MS) may be considered in moderate risk for disease progression.

Calculating the patient's individual periodontal risk assessment (PRA)
Based on the six parameters specified above, a multi-functional diagram is constructed for the PRA. In this diagram, the vectors have been constructed on the basis of the scientific evidence available. It is obvious that ongoing validation may result in slight modifications.

A low PR patient has all parameters within the low risk categories or at the most one parameter in the moderate risk category (Fig. 32-3b).
A moderate PR patient has at least two parameters in the moderate category, but at most one parameter in the high risk category (Fig. 32-3c).
A high PR patient has at least two parameters in the high risk category (Fig. 32-3d).

Summary
The subject risk assessment may estimate the risk for susceptibility for progression of periodontal disease. It consists of an assessment of the level of infection (full mouth bleeding scores), the prevalence of residual periodontal pockets, tooth loss, an estimation of the loss of periodontal support in relation to the patient's age, an evaluation of the systemic conditions of the patient, and finally, an evaluation of environmental and behavioral factors such as smoking and stress. All these factors should be contemplated and evaluated together. A functional diagram (Fig. 32-3) may help the clinician in determining the risk for disease progression on the subject level. This may be useful in customizing the frequency and content of SPT visits.

Tooth risk assessment

Tooth position within the dental arch
Early clinical surveys have associated the prevalence and severity of periodontal diseases with malocclusion and irregularities of tooth position (Ditto & Hall 1954, Bilimoria 1963). However, many subsequent studies using clinical evaluation methods could not confirm these conclusions (Beagrie & James 1962, Geiger 1962, Gould & Picton 1966). Although a relationship between crowding and increased plaque retention and gingival inflammation has been established (Ingervall et al. 1977, Buckley 1980, Griffith & Addy 1981, Hörup et al. 1987), no significant correlation

between anterior overjet and overbite (Geiger et al. 1973), crowding and spacing (Geiger et al. 1974) or axial inclinations and tooth drifts (Geiger & Wasserman 1980) and periodontal destruction, i.e. attachment loss subsequent to gingival inflammation, could be established. It is evident from the literature mentioned that crowding of teeth might eventually affect the amount of plaque mass formed in dentitions with irregular oral hygiene practices, thus contributing to the development of chronic gingivitis, but, as of today, it remains to be demonstrated whether tooth malposition within the dental arch will lead to an increased risk for periodontal attachment loss.

Furcation involvement

It is evident that multirooted teeth with periodontal lesions extending into the furcation area have been the subject of intensive therapeutic studies for many years (Kalkwarf & Reinhardt 1988). Retrospective analyses of large patient populations in private periodontal practices of periodontal specialists (Hirschfeld & Wasserman 1978, McFall 1982) have clearly established that multirooted teeth appear to be at high risk for tooth loss during the maintenance phase. The most impressive long-term documentation maintained 600 patients for an average duration of 22 years, and 10% of these patients were even maintained for more than 30 years (Hirschfeld & Wasserman 1978). While 83% of the patients could be considered "well maintained" and had lost only 0-3 teeth during the observation period, a patient group of 4% (25) was identified with an extreme risk for disease progression and had lost between 10 and 23 teeth during a regularly scheduled maintenance program. Irrespective of the patient group of low, moderate, and high risk for disease progression during maintenance, the majority of the teeth lost were furcation-involved molars (Hirschfeld & Wasserman 1978). Similar results were obtained in a study on 100 treated periodontal patients maintained for 15 years or longer (McFall 1982).

Prospective studies on periodontal therapy in multirooted teeth have also revealed significant differences between non-molar sites and molar flat surfaces on the one hand and molar furcation sites on the other, when looking at the treatment outcomes evaluated as bleeding frequency, probing depth reductions and levels of attachment (Nordland et al. 1987). Again, teeth with furcation involvement and original probing depths > 6 mm had reduced treatment outcomes.

The assumption that the prognosis for single rooted teeth and non-furcation-involved multirooted teeth is better than the prognosis for furcation-involved multirooted teeth has also been confirmed by Ramfjord et al. (1987) in a prospective study over 5 years. It has to be realized, however, that these results are not intended to imply that furcation-involved teeth should be extracted, since all the prospective studies have documented a rather good overall prognosis for such teeth if regular supportive care is provided by a well-organized maintenance program.

Iatrogenic factors

Overhanging restorations and ill-fitting crown margins certainly represent an area for plaque retention, and there is an abundance of association studies documenting increased prevalence of periodontal lesions in the presence of iatrogenic factors (for review see Leon 1977). Depending on the supragingival or subgingival location of such factors, their influence on the risk for disease progression has to be considered. It has been established that slightly subgingivally located overhanging restorations will, indeed, change the ecologic niche, providing more favorable conditions for the establishment of a Gram-negative anaerobic microbiota (Lang et al. 1983). There is no doubt that shifts in the subgingival microflora towards a more periodontopathic microbiota, if unaffected by treatment, represent an increased risk for periodontal breakdown.

Residual periodontal support

Although many clinicians believe that teeth with reduced periodontal support are unable to function alone and should be extracted or splinted, there is clear evidence from longitudinal studies that teeth with severely reduced, but healthy, periodontal support can function either individually or as abutments for many years without any further loss of attachment (Nyman & Lindhe 1979, Nyman & Ericsson 1982, Brägger et al. 1990). Hence, successfully periodontally treated teeth can be maintained over decades and function as abutments in fixed bridgework or as individual chewing units irrespective of the amount of residual periodontal support, provided that physiologic masticatory forces do not subject such teeth to a progressive trauma which may lead to spontaneous extraction. Obviously, by virtue of the already reduced support, should disease progression occur in severely compromised teeth, this may lead to spontaneous tooth exfoliation.

Mobility

In light of the discussion of abutment teeth with severely reduced but healthy periodontal support, tooth mobility may be an indicator for progressive traumatic lesions, provided that the mobility is increasing continuously (Nyman & Lang 1994). When assessing tooth mobility, it has to be realized that two factors may contribute to hypermobility: (1) a widening of the periodontal ligament as a result of unidirectional or multidirectional forces to the crown, high and frequent enough to induce resorption of the alveolar bone walls; and (2) the height of the periodontal supporting tissues. If this is reduced due to prior periodontal disease, but the width of the periodontal ligament is unchanged, the amplitude of root mobility within the remaining periodontium is the same as in a tooth with normal height, but the leverage on the tooth following application of forces to the crown is changed. Therefore, it has to be realized that all teeth that have lost periodontal support have increased tooth mobility as defined by crown displacement upon application of a given force. Nevertheless, this hypermobility should be regarded as physiologic (Nyman & Lindhe 1976).

Since tooth mobility is probably more frequently affected by reduced periodontal height rather than unidirectional or multidirectional application of forces onto the tooth, its significance for the evaluation of the periodontal conditions has to be questioned. Several studies have indicated that tooth mobility varies greatly before, during and after periodontal therapy (Persson 1980, 1981a,b). From these studies it can be concluded that periodontally involved teeth show a decrease in mobility following non-surgical and/or surgical periodontal procedures. However, following surgical procedures, tooth mobility may temporarily increase during the healing phase and may resume decreased values later on. Provisional splinting as an adjunct to non-surgical or surgical therapy does not seem to affect the final result of tooth mobility.

Summary

The tooth risk assessment encompasses an estimation of the residual periodontal support, an evaluation of tooth positioning, furcation involvements, presence of iatrogenic factors and a determination of tooth mobility to evaluate functional stability. A risk assessment on the tooth level may be useful in evaluating the prognosis and function of an individual tooth and may indicate the need for specific therapeutic measures during SPT visits.

Site risk assessment

Bleeding on probing

Absence of bleeding on probing is a reliable parameter to indicate periodontal stability if the test procedure for assessing bleeding on probing has been standardized (Lang et al. 1990). Presence of bleeding upon standardized probing will indicate presence of gingival inflammation. Whether or not repeated bleeding on probing over time will predict the progression of a lesion is, however, questionable (Lang et al. 1986, 1990, Vanooteghem et al. 1987). Nevertheless, a 30% probability for attachment loss to occur in the future may be predicted for sites repeatedly positive for bleeding on probing (Fig. 32-5) (Badersten et al. 1985, 1990, Lang et al. 1986, Vanooteghem et al. 1987, 1990, Claffey et al. 1990).

Obviously, bleeding on probing is rather sensitive to different forces applied to the tissues. An almost linear relationship (R = 0.87) existed between the probing force applied and the percentage of bleeding sites in a study on healthy young adults (Fig. 32-6) (Lang et al. 1991). If the probing force exceeded 0.25 N (25 g), the tissues were traumatized and bleeding was provoked as a result of trauma, rather than as a result of tissue alterations due to inflammation. To assess the

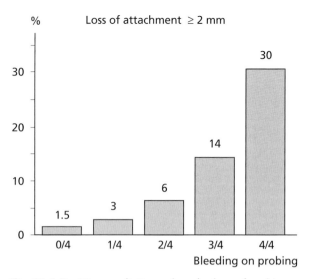

Fig. 32-5. Positive predictive values for loss of probing attachment of ≥ 2 mm in 2 years in sites which bled on probing 0, 1, 2, 3 or 4 times out of four SPT visits in a total of 48 patients following active periodontal therapy. (Data from Lang et al. 1986.)

"true" percentage of bleeding sites due to inflammation, a probing force of 0.25 N or less should be applied, which clinically means a light probing force. This has also been confirmed for patients who have experienced loss of attachment, i.e. with successfully treated advanced periodontitis (Fig. 32-7) (Karayiannis et al. 1991, Lang et al. 1991).

Since absence of bleeding on probing at 0.25 N indicated periodontal stability with a negative predictive value of 98-99% (Lang et al. 1990), this clinical parameter is the most reliable for monitoring patients over time in daily practice. Non-bleeding sites may be considered periodontally stable. On the other hand, bleeding sites seem to have an increased risk for progression of periodontitis, especially when the same site is bleeding at repeated evaluations over time (Lang et al. 1986, Claffey et al. 1990).

It is, therefore, advisable to register the sites which bleed on probing (BOP) in a dichotomous way using a constant force of 0.25 N. This allows the calculation of the mean BOP for the patient, and yields also the topographic location of the bleeding site. Repeated scores during maintenance will yield the surfaces at higher risk for loss of attachment.

Probing depth and loss of attachment

Clinical probing is the most commonly used parameter both to document loss of attachment and to establish a diagnosis of periodontitis. There are, however, some sources of error inherent in this method which contribute to the variability in the measurements. Among these are (1) the dimension of the periodontal probe; (2) the placement of the probe and obtaining a reference point; (3) the crudeness of the measurement scale; (4) the probing force; and (5) the gingival tissue conditions.

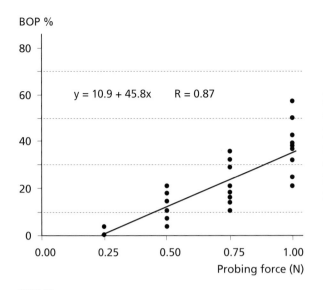

Fig. 32-6. Regression analysis between mean bleeding on probing (BOP) percentage and probing forces applied in young dental hygiene students with a healthy gingiva and normal anatomy. A very high correlation coefficient (R = 0.87) and an almost linear correlation between probing force and BOP% was found. (Data from Lang et al. 1991.)

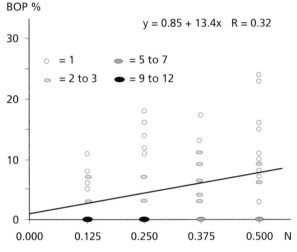

Fig. 32-7. Regression analysis between mean bleeding on probing (BOP) percentage and probing forces applied in subjects with successfully treated periodontitis: a reduced, but healthy, periodontium. (Data from Karayiannis et al. 1991.)

Clinical probing

In spite of the recognized method errors inherent in clinical probing, this diagnostic procedure has not only been the most commonly used but is also the most reliable parameter for the evaluation of the periodontal tissues. It has to be realized that increased probing depth and loss of probing attachment are parameters which reflect the history of periodontitis rather than its current state of activity. In order to obtain a more realistic assessment of the disease progression or, more commonly, the healing following therapy, multiple evaluations should be performed. Obviously, the first evaluation prior to therapy will yield results confounded by greater measurement error than evaluations following therapy. The reference point (cemento-enamel junction) may be obstructed by calculus or by dental restorations, and the condition of the gingival tissues may allow an easy penetration of the periodontal probe into the tissues, even though the probe position and force applied are standardized. These biologic variables (tissue conditions and calculus) may be minimized following initial periodontal therapy, and hence, repeated periodontal evaluations using probing will improve the metric assessment. Therefore, the first periodontal evaluation after healing following initial periodontal ther-

apy should be taken as the baseline for long-term clinical monitoring (Claffey 1994).

Suppuration

In a proportion of periodontal lesions pus will develop and may drain through the orifice of a pocket. This criterion of suppuration may be recognized while clinically probing the lesion, or preferably, by using a ball burnisher (Singh et al. 1977). Several longitudinal studies on the results of periodontal therapy have evaluated clinical parameters, including suppuration, for the prediction of future loss of attachment (Badersten et al. 1985, 1990, Claffey et al. 1990). In all these studies, the presence of suppuration increased the positive predictive value for disease progression in combination with other clinical parameters such as bleeding on probing and increased probing depth. Hence, following therapy a suppurating lesion may provide evidence that the periodontitis site is undergoing a period of exacerbation (Kaldahl et al. 1990).

Summary

The tooth site risk assessment includes the registration of bleeding on probing, probing depth, loss of attachment, and suppuration. A risk assessment on the site level may be useful in evaluating periodontal disease

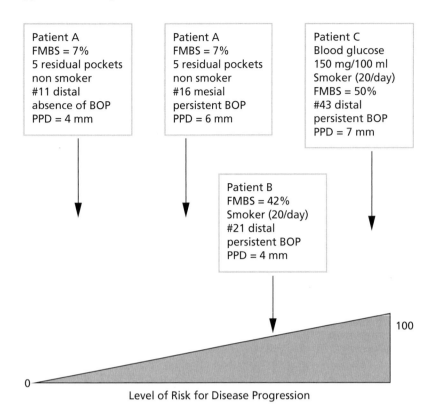

Patient A
FMBS = 7%
5 residual pockets
non smoker
#11 distal
absence of BOP
PPD = 4 mm

Patient A
FMBS = 7%
5 residual pockets
non smoker
#16 mesial
persistent BOP
PPD = 6 mm

Patient C
Blood glucose
150 mg/100 ml
Smoker (20/day)
FMBS = 50%
#43 distal
persistent BOP
PPD = 7 mm

Patient B
FMBS = 42%
Smoker (20/day)
#21 distal
persistent BOP
PPD = 4 mm

100

0

Level of Risk for Disease Progression

Fig. 32-8. Continuous multiple level risk assessment. Subject, tooth and site parameters are combined to establish the clinical risk for disease progression. Note that different sites in the same patient may have a different level of risk. Subject-based risk factors are used to put the tooth and/or site risk assessment in perspective.

activity and determining periodontal stability or ongoing inflammation. The site risk assessment is essential for the identification of the sites to be instrumented during SPT.

Radiographic evaluation of periodontal disease progression

As a consequence of the clinical risk assessments the decision may be made to gather radiographic information on the periodontal conditions as well (Hirschmann et al. 1994). The task may be related to a generalized pattern of disease progression or a localized monitoring. Not only periodontal aspects, but a comprehensive approach, should influence the choice of the radiographic technique (Rohlin & Akerblom 1992). Periodic radiographic surveys not based on clinical signs and symptoms should not be scheduled simply to confirm health.

Radiographic perception of periodontal changes is characterized by a high specificity, but a low sensitivity, with underestimation of the severity of a periodontal defect (Hämmerle et al. 1990, Åkesson et al. 1992). Undetectability of minute changes at the alveolar crest is related to overprojections and variations in projection geometry when taking repeated radiographs (Lang & Hill 1977, Goodson et al. 1984, Jenkins et al. 1992). This may result in mimicked variations in the alveolar bone height, obscured furcation status, etc. In addition, film processing variations may result in unreliable assessments of alveolar bone density changes (Rams et al. 1994).

The standard procedure for periodontal evaluations is based on a filmholder system with an align-

ment for long-cone paralleling technique (Rushton & Horner 1994). With the addition of simple pins to the filmholders as a repositioning reference, the methodologic error was impressively reduced (Carpio et al. 1994).

It is a fact that, in general, the standards in oral radiology related to agreement in the choice of a technique, the quality of film processing and the agreement in the diagnosis need to be improved (Brägger 1996).

Clinical implementation

The *three levels* of risk assessment presented represent a logic sequence of clinical evaluation to be performed prior to rendering treatment during maintenance. The information gathered from a stepwise evaluation should not impinge on, but rather improve, the efficacy of secondary prophylactic periodontal care and treatment. A logic sequence of checks and examinations may be easily obtained in a short period of time and at no extra cost for laboratory tests. The information obtained from clinical monitoring and multilevel risk assessment facilitates an immediate appreciation of the periodontal health status of an individual and the possible risk for further infection and/or disease progression.

Most longitudinal studies published to date have been based on single level, i.e. site or tooth, risk assessment, rather than accounting for the most evident factor in risk assessment: the patient. Ample evidence indicates that a minority of patients will continue to present problems and hence, differ completely from the maintenance pattern visualized in the majority of the patients. Even in the studies where this fact has been explicitly addressed (Hirschfeld & Wasserman 1978), the factors which determined whether or not a patient belonged to a well-maintained group or to a group with continuous loss of periodontal attachment have not been identified.

Summary
It is suggested that patients be evaluated on the *three different levels* mentioned. At the patient level, loss of support in relation to patient age, full mouth plaque and/or bleeding scores and prevalence of residual pockets are evaluated together with the presence of systemic conditions or environmental factors, such as smoking, which can influence the prognosis. The clinical utility of this first level of risk assessment influences primarily the determination of the recall frequency and time requirements. It should also provide a perspective for the evaluation of risk assessment conducted at the tooth and site levels.

At the tooth and tooth site levels, residual periodontal support, inflammatory parameters and their persistence, presence of ecologic niches with difficult access such as furcations, and presence of iatrogenic factors have to be put into perspective with the patient overall risk profile (Fig. 32-8). The clinical utility of tooth and site risk assessment relates to rational allocation of the recall time available for therapeutic intervention to the sites with higher risk, and possibly to the selection of different forms of therapeutic intervention.

OBJECTIVES FOR SPT

The objective of maintenance care must be the continued preservation of gingival and periodontal health, obtained as a result of the active periodontal treatment. Irrespective of whether or not additional treatment such as prosthetic reconstructions or placement of implants has been rendered, the regular and adequate removal of supragingival plaque by the patient is, therefore, a prerequisite for a good long-term prognosis. In order to reach these goals, regular clinical re-evaluations with appropriate interceptive treatment, continued psychologic support and encouragement of the patient and a lifelong commitment by the therapists are required.

General rules regarding frequency of maintenance care visits are difficult to define. However, there are a few aspects to consider in this respect: the patient's individual oral hygiene standard, the prevalence of sites exhibiting bleeding on probing, and the pretherapeutic attachment level and alevolar bone height. This in turn means that patients with suboptimal plaque control and/or concomitant high prevalence of bleeding sites should be recalled more frequently than patients exhibiting excellent plaque control and healthy gingival tissues. Nevertheless, pa-

tients with healthy gingival conditions, but with a severely reduced height of periodontal support, should also be recalled with short time intervals (not exceeding 3-4 months) in order to exclude or at least reduce the risk of additional tooth loss. In most of the longitudinal studies referred to above, positive treatment results were maintained with regular maintenance care provided at 3-6-month intervals. It seems reasonable to commence post-therapeutic maintenance with recall visits once every 3-4 months and then shorten or prolong these intervals in accordance with the aspects discussed above.

Since clinical attachment levels are usually stable 6 months following active periodontal therapy, it has been suggested that the first 6 months after completion of therapy be considered a healing phase (Westfelt et al. 1983b) during which frequent professional tooth-cleaning has been recommended. Following this healing phase, it is generally agreed to recall patients treated for periodontal disease at intervals of 3-4 months in a well-organized system of SPT. It has to be realized that tissue contours may be subjected to re-modeling processes despite stable clinical attachment levels and, hence, morphologic changes may still improve the accessibility of all tooth surfaces to oral hygiene practices for months and years. Proper oral hygiene practices appear to be the most important patient factor to guarantee long-term stability of treatment results (Knowles et al. 1979, Ramfjord et al. 1982, 1987, Lindhe & Nyman 1984). This, in turn, necessitates optimization of the patient's skills and continuous motivation and reinforcement to perform adequate mechanical oral hygiene practices, although chemical agents such as the potent antiseptic chlorhexidine may substitute and later complement the patient's efforts during the healing phase, when mechanical practices are difficult (Westfelt et al. 1983a). It is obvious that regular recall visits for SPT should be scheduled soon after completion of cause-related therapy, even if periodontal surgical procedures are still to be performed following a careful re-evaluation of the tissue response. To postpone the organization of a maintenance care program until corrective procedures such as surgery, endodontic, implant, operative or reconstructive therapy have been performed may reinforce a possible misconception of the patient that the professional visits to a therapist or hygienist guarantee positive treatment outcomes and optimal long-term prognosis rather than the patient's own regular performance of individually optimal and adequate oral hygiene practices.

SPT IN DAILY PRACTICE

The recall hour should be planned to meet the patient's individual needs. It basically consists of four different sections which may require various amounts of time during a regularly scheduled visit:

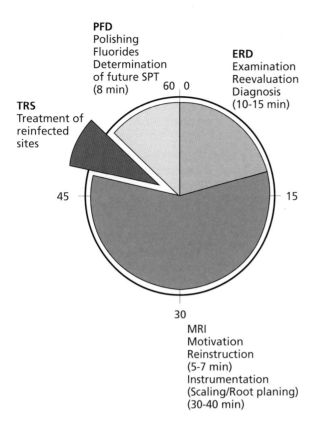

PFD
Polishing
Fluorides
Determination
of future SPT
(8 min)

ERD
Examination
Reevaluation
Diagnosis
(10-15 min)

TRS
Treatment of
reinfected
sites

60   0

45

15

30

MRI
Motivation
Reinstruction
(5-7 min)
Instrumentation
(Scaling/Root planing)
(30-40 min)

Fig. 32-9. The SPT recall hour is divided into four sections: 1. Examination, re-evaluation and diagnosis (ERD) providing information on stable and inflamed sites. This segment uses 10-15 min. 2. Motivation, reinstruction of oral hygiene where indicated and instrumentation (MRI) will use the bulk of the recall hour (30-40 min). Sites which were diagnosed as not stable are instrumented. 3. Treatment of reinfected sites (TRS) may require a second appointment. 4. Polishing all tooth surfaces, application of fluorides and determination of the future recall interval (PFD) conclude the recall hour (5-10 min).

1. Examination, Re-evaluation and Diagnosis (ERD)
2. Motivation, Reinstruction and Instrumentation (MRI)
3. Treatment of Reinfected Sites (TRS)
4. Polishing of the entire dentition, application of Fluorides and Determination of future SPT (PFD)

The SPT recall hour (Fig. 32-9) is generally composed of 10-15 min of diagnostic procedures (ERD) followed by 30-40 min of motivation, reinstruction and instrumentation (MRI) during which time the instrumentation is concentrated on the sites diagnosed with persistent inflammation. Treatment of reinfected sites (TRS) may include small surgical corrections, applications of local drug delivery devices or just intensive instrumentation under local anesthesia. Hence, such procedures, if judged necessary, may require an additional appointment. The recall hour is normally concluded with polishing of the entire dentition, application of fluorides and another assessment of the situation including the determination of future SPT visits (PFD). Approximately 5-10 min have to be reserved for this section.

Examination, Re-evaluation and Diagnosis (ERD)

Since patients on SPT may experience significant changes in their health status and the use of medications, an update of the information on general health issues is appropriate. Changes in health status and medications should be noted. Especially in the middle-aged to elderly patients, these aspects might influence the future management of the patient. An extraoral and intraoral soft tissue examination should be performed at any SPT visit to detect any abnormalities and to act as a screening for oral cancer. Especially the lateral borders of the tongue and the floor of the mouth should be inspected. An evaluation of the patient's risk factors will also influence the choice of future SPT and the determination of the recall interval at the end of the maintenance visit. Following the assessment of the subject's risk factors, the tooth site-related risk factors are evaluated. As indicated above, the diagnostic procedure usually includes an assessment of the following:

1. the oral hygiene and plaque situation
2. the determination of sites with bleeding on probing, indicating persistent inflammation
3. the scoring of clinical probing depths and clinical attachment levels. The latter is quite time-consuming and requires the assessment of the location of the cemento-enamel junction as a reference mark on all (six) sites of each root. Therefore, an SPT evaluation usually only includes scoring of clinical probing depths
4. the inspection of reinfected sites with pus formation
5. the evaluation of existing reconstructions, including vitality checks for abutment teeth
6. the exploration for carious lesions.

All these evaluations are performed for both teeth and oral implants. Occasionally, conventional dental radiographs should be obtained at SPT visits. Especially for devitalized teeth, abutment teeth and oral im-

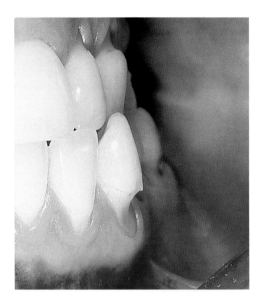

Fig. 32-10. Wedge-shaped defects apical to the cemento-enamel junction following recession of the gingival tissues resulting from overzealous or faulty toothbrushing.

plants, single periapical films exposed with a parallel and preferably standardized technique are of great value. Bite-wing radiographs are of special interest for caries diagnostic purposes. They also reveal plaque retentive areas such as overhanging fillings and ill-fitting crown margins. Since only approximately 10-15 min are available for this section, these assessments have to be performed in a well-organized fashion. It is preferable to have a dental assistant available to note all the results of the diagnostic tests unless a voice-activating computer-assisted recording system is used.

Motivation, Reinstruction and Instrumentation (MRI)

This aspect uses most of the available time of the SPT visit. When informed about the results of the diagnostic procedures, e.g. the total percentage of the bleeding on probing (BOP) score or the number of pockets exceeding 4 mm, the patient may be motivated either in a confirmatory way in case of low scores or in a challenging fashion in case of high scores. Since encouragement usually has a greater impact on future positive developments than negative criticism, every effort should be made to acknowledge the patient's performance.

Patients who have experienced a relapse in their adequate oral hygiene practices need to be further motivated. Especially if the personal life situation has influenced the performance, positive encouragement is appropriate. Standard "lecturing" should be replaced by an individual approach.

Occasionally, patients present with hard tissue lesions (wedge-shaped dental defects) which suggest overzealous and/or faulty mechanical toothcleaning (Fig. 32-10). Such habits should be broken and the patient reinstructed in toothbrushing techniques which emphasize vibratory rather than scrubbing movements.

Since it appears impossible to instrument 168 tooth sites in a complete dentition in the time allocated, only

those sites will be reinstrumented during SPT visits which exhibit signs of inflammation and/or active disease progression. Hence, all the BOP positive sites and all pockets with a probing depth exceeding 5 mm are carefully rescaled and root planed. Repeated instrumentation of healthy sites will inevitably result in mechanically caused continued loss of attachment (Lindhe et al. 1982a).

Similar observations were made in clinical studies by Claffey et al. (1988) where loss of clinical attachment levels immediately following instrumentation was observed in 24% of the sites. Also, it is known from regression analyses of several longitudinal studies (e.g. Lindhe et al. 1982b) that probing attachment may be lost following instrumentation of pockets below a "critical probing depth" of approximately 2.9 mm. Instrumentation of shallow sulci is, therefore, not recommended. As it has been shown in several studies that non-bleeding on probing sites represent stable sites (Lang et al. 1986, 1990, Joss et al. 1994), it appears reasonable to leave non-bleeding sites for polishing only and concentrate on periodontal sites with a positive BOP test or probing depths exceeding 5 mm. To protect the hard tissues, root planing should be performed with great caution. The deliberate removal of "contaminated" cementum during SPT is no longer justified (Nyman et al. 1986, 1988, Mombelli et al. 1995). Especially during SPT visits, root surface instrumentation should be aimed at the removal of subgingival plaque rather than "diseased" cementum. This may require a more differentiated approach than hitherto recommended. In this respect, the use of ultrasonics may have to be re-evaluated.

Treatment of Reinfected Sites (TRS)

Single sites, especially furcation sites or sites with difficult access, may occasionally be reinfected and demonstrate suppuration. Such sites require a thorough instrumentation under anesthesia, the local application of antibiotics in controlled release devices or

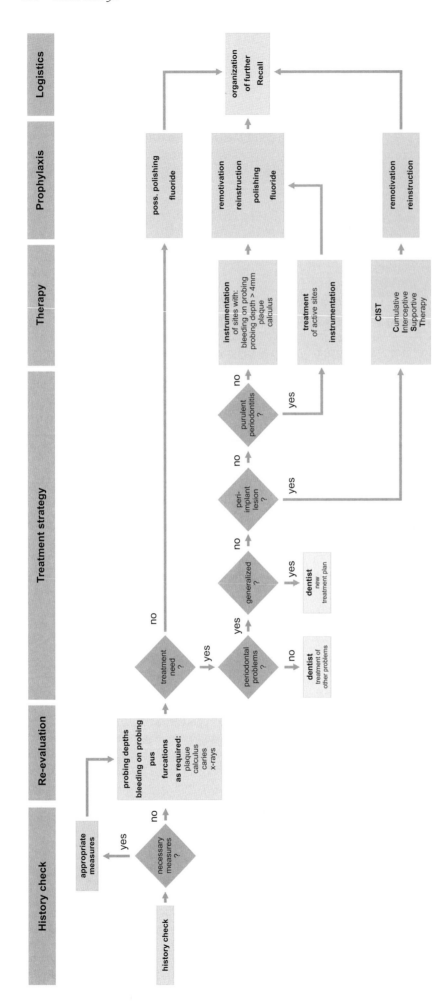

Fig. 32-11. Flow sheet of supportive periodontal therapy (SPT) with strategic decision tree for the recall visit.

even open debridement with surgical access. It is evident that such therapeutic procedures may be too time-consuming to be performed during the routine recall hour, and hence, it may be necessary to reschedule the patient for another appointment. Omission of thoroughly retreating such sites or only performing incomplete root instrumentation during SPT may result in continued loss of probing attachment (Kaldahl et al. 1988, Kalkwarf et al. 1989).

Treatment choices for reinfected sites should be based on an analysis of the causes most likely responsible for the reinfection.

Generalized reinfections are usually the result of inadequate SPT. Although not all sites positive for bleeding on probing may further progress and lose attachment, high BOP percentages call for more intensive care and more frequent SPT visits. Sometimes, a second visit 2-3 weeks after the recall may be indicated to check the patient's performance in oral home care. It is particularly important to supervise patients closely for advanced periodontitis if they have a high subject risk assessment (Westfelt et al. 1983b, Ramfjord 1987).

Local reinfections may either be the result of inadequate plaque control in a local area or the formation of ecologic niches conducive to periodontal pathogens. The risk assessment on the tooth level may identify such niches which are inaccessible for regular oral hygiene practices. Furcation involvements often represent special periodontal risk factors which may require additional therapy to be performed following diagnosis in the regular SPT visit.

Polishing, Fluorides, Determination of recall interval (PFD)

The recall hour is concluded with polishing the entire dentition to remove all remaining soft deposits and stains. This may provide freshness to the patient and facilitates the diagnosis of early carious lesions. Following polishing, fluorides should be applied in high concentration in order to replace the fluorides which might have been removed by instrumentation from the superficial layers of the teeth. Fluoride or chlorhexidine varnishes may also be applied to prevent root surface caries, especially in areas with gingival recessions. The determination of future SPT visits must be based on the patient's risk assessment.

Summary

Fig. 32-11 provides a flow sheet for SPT. The SPT recall hour is divided into four sections. While the first 10-15 min are reserved for Examination, Re-evaluation and Diagnosis, the second and most time-consuming section of 30-40 min is devoted to reinstruction and instrumentation of sites at risk identified in the diagnostic process. Some reinfected sites may require futher treatment, and hence, the patient may have to be rescheduled for an additional appointment. The recall hour is concluded by polishing the dentition, applying fluorides and determining the frequency of future SPT visits.

REFERENCES

Åkesson, L., Håkonsson, J. & Rohlin, M. (1992). Comparison of panoramic and intraoral radiography and pocket probing for the measurement of alveolar bone. *Journal of Clinical Periodontology* **19**, 326-332.

Axelsson, P. & Lindhe, J. (1981a). Effect of controlled oral hygiene procedures on caries and periodontal disease in adults. Results after 6 years. *Journal of Clinical Periodontology* **8**, 239-248.

Axelsson, P. & Lindhe, J. (1981b). The significance of maintenance care in the treatment of periodontal disease. *Journal of Clinical Periodontology* **8**, 281-294.

Axelsson, P., Lindhe, J., & Nyström, B. (1991). On the prevention of caries and periodontal disease. Results of a 15-year longitudinal study in adults. *Journal of Clinical Periodontology* **18**, 182-189.

Badersten, A., Egelberg, J. & Koch, G. (1975). Effects of monthly prophylaxis on caries and gingivitis in school children. *Community Dentistry and Oral Epidemiology* **3**, 1-4.

Badersten, A., Nilvéus, R. & Egelberg, J. (1981). Effect of non-surgical periodontal therapy. I. Moderately advanced periodontitis. *Journal of Clinical Periodontology* **8**, 57-72.

Badersten, A., Nilvéus, R. & Egelberg, J. (1985). Effect of non-surgical periodontal therapy. (VII) Bleeding, suppuration and probing depths in sites with probing attachment loss. *Journal of Clinical Periodontology* **12**, 432-440.

Badersten, A., Nilvéus, R. & Egelberg, J. (1987). Effect of non-surgical periodontal therapy. (VIII) Probing attachment changes related to clinical characteristics. *Journal of Clinical Periodontology* **14**, 425-437.

Badersten, A., Nilvéus, R. & Egelberg, J. (1990). Scores of plaque, bleeding, suppuration and probing depth to predict probing attachment loss. *Journal of Clinical Periodontology* **17**, 102-107.

Baumert-Ah, M., Johnson, G., Kaldahl, W., Patil, K. & Kalkwarf, K. (1994). The effect of smoking on the response to periodontal therapy. *Journal of Clinical Periodontology* **21**, 91-97.

Beagrie, G. & James, G. (1962). The association of posterior tooth irregularities and periodontal disease. *British Dental Journal* **113**, 239-243.

Becker, B., Karp, C., Becker, W. & Berg, L. (1988). Personality differences and stressful life events. Differences between treated periodontal patients with and without maintenance. *Journal of Clinical Periodontology* **15**, 49-52.

Becker, W., Becker, B.E. & Berg, L.E. (1984). Periodontal treatment without maintenance. A retrospective study in 44 patients. *Journal of Periodontology* **55**, 505-509.

Becker, W., Berg, L.E. & Becker, B.E. (1979). Untreated periodontal disease: A longitudinal study. *Journal of Periodontology* **50**, 234-244.

Bellini, H., Campi, R. & Denardi, J. (1981). Four years of monthly professional tooth cleaning and topical fluoride application in Brazilian school children. *Journal of Clinical Periodontology* **8**, 231-238.

Bergström, J. (1989). Cigarette smoking as a risk factor in chronic periodontal disease. *Journal of Clinical Periodontology* **17**, 245-247.

Bergström, J. & Blomlöf, L. (1992). Tobacco smoking a major risk factor associated with refractory periodontal disease. *Journal of Dental Research* 71(spec issue), 297 #1530 (IADR Abstr).

Bergström, J., Eliasson, S. & Preber, H. (1991). Cigarette smoking and periodontal bone loss. *Journal of Periodontology* **62**, 242-246.

Bilimoria, K. (1963). Malocclusion – Its role in the causation of periodontal disease. *Journal of the All-India Dental Association* **35**, 293-300.

Brägger, U. (1996). Radiographic diagnosis of periodontal disease progression. *Current Opinions in Dentistry* **3**, 59-67.

Brägger, U., Håkanson, D. & Lang, N.P. (1992). Progression of periodontal disease in patients with mild to moderate adult periodontitis. *Journal of Clinical Periodontology* **19**, 659-666.

Brägger, U., Nyman, S., Lang, N.P., von Wyttenbach, T., Salvi, G. & Schürch, Jr. E. (1990). The significance of alveolar bone in periodontal disease. A long-term observation in patients with cleft lip, alveolus and palate. *Journal of Clinical Periodontology* **17**, 379-384.

Buckley, L. (1980). The relationship between irregular teeth, plaque, calculus and gingival disease. A study of 300 subjects. *British Dental Journal* **148**, 67-69.

Carpio, L.C., Hausmann, E., Dunford, R.G., Allen, R.M., Christensson, L.A. (1994). Evaluation of a simple modified radiographic alignment system for routine use. *Journal of Periodontology* **65**, 62-67.

Caton, J.G., Proye, M. & Polson, A.M. (1982). Maintenance of healed periodontal pockets after a single episode of root planing. *Journal of Periodontology* **53**, 420-424.

Checchi, L., Pellicioni, G., Gatto, M. & Kelescian, L. (1994). Patient compliance with maintenance therapy in an Italian periodontal practice. *Journal of Clinical Periodontology* **21**, 309-312.

Claffey, N. (1991). Decision making in periodontal therapy. The re-evaluation. *Journal of Clinical Periodontology* **18**, 384-389.

Claffey, N. (1994). Gold Standard clinical and radiographical assessment of disease activity. In: Lang, N. & Karring, T., eds. *Proceedings of the 1st European Workshop on Periodontology.* London: Quintessence, pp. 42-53.

Claffey, N., Loos, B., Gantes, B., Martin, M., Heins, P. & Egelberg, J. (1988). The relative effects of therapy and periodontal disease on loss of probing attachment after root debridement. *Journal of Clinical Periodontology* **15**, 163-169.

Claffey, N., Nylund, K., Kiger, R., Garrett, S. & Egelberg, J. (1990). Diagnostic predictability of scores of plaque, bleeding, suppuration, and probing pocket depths for probing attachment loss. 3½ years of observation following initial therapy. *Journal of Clinical Periodontology* **17**, 108-114.

Cohen-Cole, S., Cogen, R., Stevens, A., Kirk, K., Gaitan, E., Hain, J. & Freeman, A. (1981). Psychosocial, endocrine and immune factors in acute necrotizing ulcerative gingivitis. *Psychosomatic Medicine* **43**, 91.

Cortellini, P., Pini Prato, G. & Tonetti, M. (1994). Periodontal regeneration of human infrabony defects. V. Effect of oral hygiene on long term stability. *Journal of Clinical Periodontology* **21**, 606-610.

Cortellini, P., Pini Prato, G. & Tonetti, M. (1996). Long term stability of clinical attachment following guided tissue regeneration and conventional therapy. *Journal of Clinical Periodontology* **23**, 106-111.

Cullinan, M.P., Westermann, B., Hamlet, S.P., Palmer J.E., Faddy, M.J., Lang, N.P. & Seymour, G.J. (2001). A longitudinal study of interleukin-1 gene polymorphisms and periodontal disease in a general adult population. *Journal of Clinical Periodontology* **28**, 1137-1144.

Demetriou, N., Tsami-Pandi, A. & Parashis, A. (1995). Compliance with supportive periodontal treatment in private periodontal practice. A 14-year retrospective study. *Journal of Periodontology* **66**, 145-149.

De Vore, C.H., Duckworth, J.E., Beck, F.M., Hicks, M.J., Brumfield, F.W. & Horton, J.E. (1986). Bone loss following periodontal therapy in subjects without frequent periodontal maintenance. *Journal of Periodontology* **57**, 354-359.

Ditto, W. & Hall, D. (1954). A survey of 143 periodontal cases in terms of age and malocclusion. *American Journal of Orthodontics* **40**, 234-243.

Emrich, L., Schlossman, M. & Genco, R. (1991). Periodontal disease in non-insulin dependent diabetes mellitus. *Journal of Periodontology* **62**, 123-130.

Fauchard, P. (1746). *Le Chirurgien Dentiste, au Traité des Dents.* Chap. XI. Paris: P-J Mariette, pp. 177-182.

Freeman, R. & Goss, S. (1993). Stress measures as predictors of periodontal disease – a preliminary communication. *Community Dentistry and Oral Epidemiology* **21**, 176-177.

Geiger, A. (1962). Occlusal studies in 188 consecutive cases of periodontal disease. *American Journal of Orthodontics* **48**, 330-360.

Geiger, A. & Wassermann, B. (1980). Relationship of occlusion and periodontal disease. Part XI. Relation of axial inclination (mesial-distal) and tooth drift to periodontal status. *Journal of Periodontology* **51**, 283-290.

Geiger, A., Wasserman, B. & Turgeon, L. (1973). Relationship of occlusion and periodontal disease. Part VI. Relation of anterior overjet and overbite to periodontal destruction and gingival inflammation. *Journal of Periodontology* **44**, 150-157.

Geiger, A., Wassermann, B. & Turgeon, L. (1974). Relationship of occlusion and gingival inflammation. *Journal of Periodontology* **45**, 43-49.

Genco, R. & Löe, H. (1993). The role of systemic conditions and disorders in periodontal disease. *Periodontology 2000* **2**, 98-116.

Goodson, J.M., Haffajee, A.D. & Socransky, S.S. (1984). The relationship between attachment level loss and alveolar bone loss. *Journal of Clinical Periodontology* **11**, 348-359.

Gould, M. & Picton, D. (1966). The relation between irregularities of teeth and periodontal disease. *British Dental Journal* **121**, 20-23.

Green, L., Tryon, W., Marks, B. & Huryn, J. (1986). Periodontal disease as a function of life events stress. *Journal of Human Stress* **12**, 32-36.

Griffith, G. & Addy, M. (1981). Effects of malalignment of teeth in the anterior segments on plaque accumulation. *Journal of Clinical Periodontology* **8**, 481-490.

Gusberti, F.A., Syed, S.A, Bacon, G., Grossman, N. & Loesche, W.J. (1983). Puberty gingivitis in insulin-dependent diabetic children. I. Cross-sectional observations. *Journal of Periodontology* **54**, 714-720.

Haber, J., Wattles, J., Crowley, M., Mandell, R., Joshipura, K. & Kent, R. (1993). Evidence for cigarette smoking as a major risk factor for periodontitis. *Journal of Periodontology* **64**, 16-23.

Hämmerle, C.H.F., Ingold, H-P. & Lang, N.P. (1990). Evaluation of clinical and radiographic scoring methods before and after initial periodontal therapy. *Journal of Clinical Periodontology* **17**, 255-263.

Hämmerle, C.H.F., Ungerer, M.C., Fantoni, P.C., Brägger, U., Bürgin, W. & Lang, N.P. (2000). Long-term analysis of biological and technical aspects of fixed partial dentures with cantilevers. *International Journal of Prosthodontics* **13**, 409-415.

Hill, R.W., Ramfjord, S.P., Morrison, E.C., Appleberry, E.A., Caffesse, R.G., Kerry, G.J. & Nissle, R.R. (1981). Four types of periodontal treatment compared over two years. *Journal of Periodontology* **52**, 655-677.

Hirschfeld, L. & Wasserman, B. (1978). A long-term survey of tooth loss in 600 treated periodontal patients. *Journal of Periodontology* **49**, 225-237.

Hirschmann, P.N., Horner, K. & Rushton, V.E. (1994). Selection criteria for periodontal radiography. *Journal of Clinical Periodontology* **176**, 324-325.

Hörup, N., Melsen, B. & Terp, S. (1987). Relationship between malocclusion and maintenance of teeth. *Community Dentistry and Oral Epidemiology* **15**, 74-78.

Ingervall, B., Jacobsson, U. & Nyman, S. (1977). A clinical study of the relationship between crowding of teeth, plaque and gingival conditions. *Journal of Clinical Periodontology* **4**, 214-222.

Isidor, F. & Karring, T. (1986). Long-term effect of surgical and non-surgical periodontal treatment. A 5-year clinical study. *Journal of Periodontal Research* **21**, 462-472.

Ismail, A.L., Burt, B.A. & Eklund, S.A. (1983). Epidemiologic patterns of smoking and periodontal disease in the United States. *Journal of the Alabama Dental Association* **106**, 617-621.

Jenkins, S.M., Dammer, P.M. & Addy, M. (1992). Radiographic evaluation of early periodontal bone loss in adolescents. An overview. *Journal of Clinical Periodontology* **19**, 363-366.

Joss, A., Adler, R. & Lang, N.P. (1994). Bleeding on probing. A parameter for monitoring periodontal conditions in clinical practice. *Journal of Clinical Periodontology.* **21**, 402-408.

Kaldahl, W.B., Kalkwarf, K.L., Patil, K.D., Dyer, J.K. & Bates, R.E. (1988). Evaluation of four modalities of periodontal therapy. Mean probing depth, probing attachment level and recession changes. *Journal of Periodontology* **59**, 783-793.

Kaldahl, W., Kalkwarf, K., Patil, K. D. & Molvar, M. (1990). Evaluation of gingival suppuration and supragingival plaque following 4 modalities of periodontal therapy. *Journal of Clinical Periodontology* **17**, 642-649.

Kalkwarf, K.L., Kaldahl, W.B., Patil, K.D. & Molvar M.P. (1989). Evaluation of gingival bleeding following 4 types of periodontal therapy. *Journal of Clinical Periodontology* **16**, 601-608.

Kalkwarf, K. & Reinhardt, R. (1988). The furcation problem: current controversies and future directions. *Dental Clinics of North America* **22**, 243-266.

Karayiannis, A., Lang, N.P., Joss, A. & Nyman, S. (1991). Bleeding on probing as it relates to probing pressures and gingival health in patients with a reduced but healthy periodontium. A clinical study. *Journal of Clinical Periodontology* **19**, 471-475.

Käyser, A.F. (1981). Shortened dental arches and oral function. *Journal of Oral Rehabilitation* **8**, 457-462.

Käyser, A.F. (1994). Limited treatment goals – shortened dental arches. *Periodontology 2000* **4,** 7-14.

Käyser, A.F. (1996). Teeth, tooth loss and prosthetic appliances. In: Øwall, B., Käyser, A.F. & Carlsson, G.E., eds. *Prosthodontics: Principles and Management Strategies*. London: Mosby-Wolfe, pp. 35-48.

Kerr, N.W. (1981). Treatment of chronic periodontitis. 45% failure rate. *British Dental Journal* **150**, 222-224.

Knowles, J.W. (1973). Oral hygiene related to long-term effects of periodontal therapy. *Journal of the Michigan State Dental Association* **55**, 147-150.

Knowles, J.W., Burgett, F.G., Morrison, E.C., Nissle, R.R. & Ramfjord, S.P. (1980). Comparison of results following three modalities of periodontal therapy related to tooth type and initial pocket depth. *Journal of Clinical Periodontology* **7**, 32-47.

Knowles, J.W., Burgett, F.G., Nissle, R.R., Shick, R.A., Morrison, E.C. & Ramfjord, S.P. (1979). Results of periodontal treatment related to pocket depth and attachment level. Eight years. *Journal of Periodontology* **50**, 225-233.

Kornman, K. & Löe, H. (1993). The role of local factors in the etiology of periodontal dieases. *Periodontology 2000* **2**, 83-97.

Kornman, K.S., Crane, A., Wang, H.Y., di Giovine, F.S., Newman, M.G., Pirk, F.W., Wilson, T.G. Jr., Higginbottom, F.L. & Duff, G.W. (1997). The interleukin-1 genotype as a severity factor in adult periodontal disease. *Journal of Clinical Periodontology* **24,** 72-77.

Lang, N.P., Adler, R., Joss, A. & Nyman, S. (1990). Absence of bleeding on probing. An indicator of periodontal stability. *Journal of Clinical Periodontology* **17**, 714-721.

Lang, N.P. & Hill, R.W. (1977). Radiographs in periodontics. *Journal of Clinical Periodontology* **4**, 16-28.

Lang, N.P., Joss, A., Orsanic, T., Gusberti, F.A. & Siegrist, B.E. (1986). Bleeding on probing. A predictor for the progression of periodontal disease? *Journal of Clinical Periodontology* **13**, 590-596.

Lang, N.P., Kiel, R. & Anderhalden, K. (1983). Clinical and microbiological effects of subgingival restorations with overhanging or clinically perfect margins. *Journal of Clinical Periodontology* **10**, 563-578.

Lang, N.P., Nyman, S., Senn, C. & Joss, A. (1991). Bleeding on probing as it relates to probing pressure and gingival health. *Journal of Clinical Periodontology* **18**, 257-261.

Lang, N.P. & Tonetti, M.S. (2003). Periodontal risk assessment for patients in supportive periodontal therapy (SPT). *Oral Health and Preventive Dentistry* **1** (in press).

Lang, N.P., Tonetti, M.S., Suter, J., Duff, G.W. & Kornmann, K.S. (2000). Effect of interleukin-1 gene polymorphisms on gingival inflammation assessed by bleeding on probing in a periodontal maintenance population. *Journal for Periodontal Research* **35**, 102-107.

Langer, B., Stein, S.D. & Wagenberg, B. (1981). An evaluation of root resections: A ten-year study. *Journal of Periodontology* **52**, 719-722.

Laurell, K., Lundgren, D., Falk, H. & Hugoson, A. (1991). Long-term prognosis of extensive poly-unit cantilevered fixed partial dentures. *Journal of Prosthetic Dentistry* **66**, 545-552.

Leon, A. (1977). The periodontium and restorative procedures. A critical review. *Journal of Oral Rehabilitation* **21**, 105-117.

Lindhe, J., Hamp, S-E. & Löe, H. (1975). Plaque induced periodontal disease in beagle dogs. A 4-year clinical, roentgenographical and histometric study. *Journal of Periodontal Research* **10**, 243-253.

Lindhe, J. & Nyman, S. (1975). The effect of plaque control and surgical pocket elimination on the establishment and maintenance of periodontal health. A longitudinal study of periodontal therapy in cases of advanced disease. *Journal of Clinical Periodontology* **2**, 67-79.

Lindhe, J. & Nyman, S. (1984). Long-term maintenance of patients treated for advanced periodontal disease. *Journal of Clinical Periodontology* **11**, 504-514.

Lindhe, J., Nyman, S. & Karring, T. (1982a). Scaling and root planing in shallow pockets. *Journal of Clinical Periodontology* **9**, 415-418.

Lindhe, J., Socransky, S.S., Nyman, S., Haffajee, A. & Westfelt, E. (1982b). "Critical probing depths" in periodontal therapy. *Journal of Clinical Periodontology* **9**, 323-336.

Lindhe, J., Westfelt, E., Nyman, S., Socransky, S.S., Heijl, L. & Bratthall, G. (1982c). Healing following surgical/non-surgical treatment of periodontol disease. A clinical study. *Journal of Clinical Periodontology* **9**, 115-128.

Listgarten, M.A. & Helldén, L. (1978). Relative distribution of bacteria at clinically healthy and periodontally diseased sites in humans. *Journal of Clinical Periodontology* **5**, 115-132.

Listgarten, M.A. & Levin, S. (1981). Positive correlation between the proportions of subgingival spirochetes and motile bacteria and susceptibility of human subjects to periodontal deterioration. *Journal of Clinical Periodontology* **8**, 122-138.

Listgarten, M.A., Lindhe, J. & Helldén, L. (1978). Effect of tetracycline and/or scaling on human periodontal disease. Clinical, microbiological and histological observations. *Journal of Clinical Periodontology* **5**, 246-271.

Listgarten, M.A. & Schifter, C. (1982). Differential darkfield microscopy of subgingival bacteria as an aid in selecting recall intervals: Results after 18 months. *Journal of Clinical Periodontology* **9**, 305-316.

Löe, H, Ånerud, Å., Boysen, H. & Smith, M. (1978). The natural history of periodontal disease in man. The role of periodontal destruction before 40 years. *Journal of Periodontal Research* **49**, 607-620.

Löe, H., Ånerud, Å., Boysen, H. & Morrison, E.C. (1986). Natural history of periodontal disease in man. Rapid, moderate and no loss of attachment in Sri Lankan laborers 14-46 years of age. *Journal of Clinical Periodontology* **13**, 431-440.

Löe, H. & Silness, J. (1963). Periodontal disease in pregnancy. I.

Prevalence and severity. *Acta Odontologica Scandinavia* **21**, 533-551.

Löe, H., Theilade, E. & Jensen, S.B. (1965). Experimental gingivitis in man. *Journal of Periodontology* **36**, 177-187.

Lövdal, A., Arnö, A., Schei, O. & Waerhaug, J. (1961). Combined effect of subgingival scaling and controlled oral hygiene on the incidence of gingivitis. *Acta Odontologica Scandinavia* **19**, 537-553.

Magnusson, I., Lindhe, J., Yoneyama, T. & Liljenberg, B. (1984). Recolonization of a subgingival microbiota following scaling in deep pockets. *Journal of Clinical Periodontology* **11**, 193-207.

McFall, W.T. (1982). Tooth loss in 100 treated patients with periodontal disease in a long-term study. *Journal of Periodontology* **53**, 539-549.

McGuire, M.K. & Nunn, M.E. (1999). Prognosis versus actual outcome. IV. The effectiveness of clinical parameters and IL-1 genotype in accurately predicting prognoses and tooth survival. *Journal of Periodontology* **70**, 49-56.

Mendoza, A., Newcomb, G. & Nixon, K. (1991). Compliance with supportive periodontal therapy. *Journal of Periodontology* **62**, 731-736.

Mombelli, A., Nyman, S., Brägger, U., Wennström, J. & Lang, N.P. (1995). Clinical and microbiological changes associated with an altered subgingival environment induced by periodontal pocket reduction. *Journal of Clinical Periodontology* **22**, 780-787.

Morrison, E.C., Lang, N.P., Löe, H. & Ramfjord, S.P. (1979). Effects of repeated scaling and root planing and/or controlled oral hygiene on the periodontal attachment level and pocket depth in beagle dogs. I. Clinical findings. *Journal of Periodontal Research* **14**, 428-437.

Moser, P., Hämmerle, C.H.F., Lang, N.P., Schlegel-Bregenzer, B. & Persson, R.G. (2002). Maintenance of periodontal attachment levels in prosthetically treated patients with gingivitis or moderate chronic periodontitis 5-17 years post therapy. *Journal of Clinical Periodontology* **29** (in press).

Mousquès, T., Listgarten, M.A. & Phillips, R.W. (1980). Effect of scaling and root planing on the composition of the human subgingival microbial flora. *Journal of Periodontal Research* **15**, 144-151.

Mühlemann, H.R. & Son, S. (1971). Gingival sulcus bleeding – a leading symptom in initial gingivitis. *Helvetica Odontologica Acta* **15**, 107-113.

Nordland, P., Garret, S., Kiger, R., Vanooteghem, R., Hutchens, L. H. & Egelberg, J. (1987). The effect of plaque control and root debridement in molar teeth. *Journal of Clinical Periodontology* **14**, 231-236.

Nyman, S. & Ericsson, I. (1982). The capacity of reduced periodontal tissues to support fixed bridgework. *Journal of Clinical Periodontology* **9**, 409-414.

Nyman, S. & Lang, N.P. (1994). Tooth mobility and biological rationale for splinting teeth. *Periodontology 2000* **4**, 15-22.

Nyman, S. & Lindhe, J. (1976). Persistent tooth hypermobility following completion of periodontal treatment. *Journal of Clinical Periodontology* **3**, 81-93.

Nyman, S. & Lindhe, J. (1979). A longitudinal study of combined periodontal and prosthetic treatment of patients with advanced periodontal disease. *Journal of Periodontology* **50**, 163-169.

Nyman, S., Lindhe, J. & Rosling, B. (1977). Periodontal surgery in plaque-infected dentitions. *Journal of Clinical Periodontology* **4**, 240-249.

Nyman, S., Rosling, B. & Lindhe, J. (1975). Effect of professional tooth cleaning on healing after periodontal surgery. *Journal of Clinical Periodontology* **2**, 80-86.

Nyman, S., Sarhed, G., Ericsson, I., Gottlow, J. & Karring, T. (1986). The role of "diseased" root cementum for healing following treatment of periodontal disease. *Journal of Periodontal Research* **21**, 496-503.

Nyman, S., Westfelt, E., Sarhed, G. & Karring, T. (1988). Role of "diseased" root cementum in healing following treatment of periodontal disease. A clinical study. *Journal of Clinical Periodontology* **15**, 464-468.

Papapanou, P., Wennström, J. & Gröndahl, K. (1988). Periodontal status in relation to age and tooth type. A cross-sectional radiographic study. *Journal of Clinical Periodontology* **15**, 469-478.

Persson, R. (1980). Assessment of tooth mobility using small loads. II. Effect of oral hygiene procedures. *Journal of Clinical Periodontology* **7**, 506-515.

Persson, R. (1981a). Assessment of tooth mobility using small loads. III. Effect of periodontal treatment including a gingivectomy procedure. *Journal of Clinical Periodontology* **8**, 4-11.

Persson, R. (1981b). Assessment of tooth mobility using small loads. IV. The effect of periodontal treatment including gingivectomy and flap procedures. *Journal of Clinical Periodontology* **8**, 88-97.

Pihlström, B.L., McHugh, R.B., Oliphant, T.H. & Ortiz-Campos, C. (1983). Comparison of surgical and non-surgical treatment of periodontal disease. A review of current studies and additional results after 6 ½ years. *Journal of Clinical Periodontology* **10**, 524-541.

Pindborg, J. (1949). Correlation between consumption of tobacco, ulcero-membraneous gingivitis and calculus. *Journal of Dental Research* **28**, 461-463.

Poulsen, S., Agerbaek, N., Melsen, B., Korts, D., Glavind, L. & Rölla, G. (1976). The effect of professional tooth cleaning on gingivitis and dental caries in children after 1 year. *Community Dentistry and Oral Epidemiology* **4**, 195-199.

Preber, H. & Bergström, J. (1985). The effect of non-surgical treatment on periodontal pockets in smokers and nonsmokers. *Journal of Clinical Periodontology* **13**, 319-323.

Preber, H. & Bergström, J. (1990). Effect of cigarette smoking on periodontal healing following surgical therapy. *Journal of Clinical Periodontology* **17**, 324-328.

Ramfjord, S.P. (1987). Maintenance care for treated periodontitis patients. *Journal of Clinical Periodontology* **14**, 433-437.

Ramfjord, S.P., Caffesse, R.G., Morrison, E. C., Hill, R., Kerry, G. J., Appleberry, E., Nissle, R. R. & Stults, J. (1987). Four modalities of periodontal treatment compared over 5 years. *Journal of Clinical Periodontology* **14**, 445-452.

Ramfjord, S.P., Knowles, J.W., Nissle, R.R., Shick, R.A. & Burgett, F.G. (1975). Results following three modalities of periodontal therapy. *Journal of Periodontology* **46**, 522-526.

Ramfjord, S.P., Morrison, E.C., Burgett, F.G., Nissle, R.R., Shick, R.A., Zann, G.J. & Knowles, J.W. (1982). Oral hygiene and maintenance of periodontal support. *Journal of Periodontology* **53**, 26-30.

Ramfjord, S.P., Nissle, R.R., Shick, R.A. Cooper, H. (1968). Subgingival curettage versus surgical elimination of periodontal pockets. *Journal of Periodontology* **39**, 167-175.

Rams, T.E., Listgarten, M.A. & Slots, J. (1994). Utility of radiographic crestal lamina dura for predicting periodontal disease activity. *Journal of Clinical Periodontology* **21**, 571-576.

Randow, K., Glantz, P-O. & Zöger, B. (1986). Technical failures and some related clinical complications in extensive fixed prosthodontics. *Acta Odontontilogica Scandinavia* **44**, 241-255.

Rivera-Hidalgo, F. (1986). Smoking and periodontal disease. *Journal of Periodontology* **57**, 617-624.

Rohlin, M. & Akerblom, A. (1992). Individualized periapical radiography determined by clinical and panoramic examination. *Dental and Maxillofacial Radiology* **21**, 135-141.

Rosling, B., Nyman, S., Lindhe, J. & Jern, B. (1976). The healing potential of the periodontal tissues following different techniques of periodontal surgery in plaque-free dentitions. *Journal of Clinical Periodontology* **3**, 233-250.

Rushton, V.E. & Horner, K. (1994). A comparative study of radiographic quality with five periapical techniques in general dental practice. *Dental and Maxillofacial Radiology* **23**, 37-45.

Selye, H. (1950). *The physiology and pathology of stress: a treatise based on the concepts of the general-adaptation-syndrome and the diseases of adaptation*. Montreal: Acta Medical Publishers, pp. 203.

Singh, S., Cianciola, L. & Genco, R. (1977). The suppurative index: an indicator of active periodontal disease. *Journal of Dental Research* **56**, 200 #593.

Slots, J., Mashimo, P., Levine, M.J. & Genco, R.J. (1979). Periodontal therapy in humans. I. Microbiological and clinical effects of a single course of periodontal scaling and root planing, and of adjunctive tetracycline therapy. *Journal of Periodontology* **50**, 495-509.

Suomi, J.D., Greene, J.C., Vermillion, J.R., Doyle Chang, J.J. & Leatherwood, E.C. (1971). The effect of controlled oral hygiene procedures on the progression of periodontal disease in adults: Results after third and final year. *Journal of Periodontology* **42**, 152-160.

Tonetti, M., Pini Prato, G. & Cortellini, P. (1995). Effect of cigarette smoking on periodontal healing following GTR in infrabony defects. A preliminary retrospective study. *Journal of Clinical Periodontology* **22**, 229-234.

Valderhaug, J. (1980). Periodontal conditions and carious lesions following the insertion of fixed prostheses: a 10-year follow-up study. *International Dental Journal* **30**, 296-304.

Valderhaug, J. & Birkeland, J.M. (1976). Periodontal conditions in patients 5 years following insertion of fixed prostheses. *Journal of Oral Rehabilitation* **3**, 237-243.

Vanooteghem, R., Hutchens, L. H., Bowers, G., Kramer, G., Schallhorn, R., Kiger, R., Crigger, M. & Egelberg, J. (1990). Subjective criteria and probing attachment loss to evaluate the effects of plaque control and root debridement. *Journal of Clinical Periodontology* **17**, 580-587.

Vanooteghem, R., Hutchens, L.H., Garrett, S., Kiger, R. & Egelberg, J. (1987). Bleeding on probing and probing depth as indicators of the response to plaque control and root debridement. *Journal of Clinical Periodontology* **14**, 226-230.

van der Velden, U. (1991). The onset age of periodontal destruction. *Journal of Clinical Periodontology* **18**, 380-383.

Westfelt, E., Bragd, L., Socransky, S.S., Haffajee, A.D., Nyman, S. & Lindhe, J. (1985). Improved periodontal conditions following therapy. *Journal of Clinical Periodontology* **12**, 283-293.

Westfelt, E., Nyman, S., Lindhe, J. & Socransky, S.S. (1983a). Use of chlorhexidine as a plaque control measure following surgical treatment of periodontal disease. *Journal of Clinical Periodontology* **10**, 22-36.

Westfelt, E., Nyman, S., Socransky, S.S. & Lindhe, J. (1983b). Significance of frequency of professional tooth cleaning for healing following periodontal surgery. *Journal of Clinical Periodontology* **10**, 148-156.

Wilson, T.G., Glover, M.E., Malik, A.K., Schoen, J.A. & Dorsett, D. (1987). Tooth loss in maintenance patients in a private periodontal practice. *Journal of Periodontology* **58**, 231-235.

Wilson, T., Glover, M., Schoen, J., Baus, C. & Jacobs, T. (1984). Compliance with maintenance therapy in a private periodontal practice. *Journal of Periodontology* **55**, 468-473.

Witter, D.J., Cramwinckel, A.B., van Rossum, G.M. & Käyser, A.F. (1990). Shortened dental arches and masticatory ability. *Journal of Dentistry* **18**, 185-189.

Witter, D.J., De Haan, A.F.J., Käyser, A.F. & van Rossum, G.M. (1994). A 6-year follow-up study of oral function in shortened dental arches. *Journal of Oral Rehabiltation* **21**, 113-125.

Implant Concepts

CHAPTER 33

Osseointegration: Historic Background and Current Concepts

TOMAS ALBREKTSSON, TORD BERGLUNDH AND JAN LINDHE

Development of the osseointegrated implant

Early tissue response to osseointegrated implants

Osseointegration from a mechanical and biologic viewpoint

Osseointegration in the clinical reality

Future of osseointegrated oral implants

DEVELOPMENT OF THE OSSEOINTEGRATED IMPLANT

In the early 1960s, Brånemark and co-workers at the University of Göteborg started developing a novel implant that for clinical function depended on direct bone anchorage – termed osseointegration. Osseointegration was certainly not an accepted phenomenon at the time. Instead, the notion was that an oral implant was embedded in soft tissue whether one liked it or not. Therefore, the implanted device was never as strongly anchored in the host tissues as immediately after its insertion. Animal experiments performed at Brånemark's laboratory clearly indicated that it was possible to establish a direct bone anchorage, provided that a number of defined guidelines were followed (Brånemark et al. 1969). This was further documented in the first clinical report published a few years later (Brånemark et al. 1977).

Even though Brånemark's team was the first to suggest a direct bone anchorage and the potential clinical advantages of such osseointegration, the scientific community remained unconvinced of osseointegration and its potentials. The reason for this reluctance to accept the new ideas was partly a methodological shortcoming: in the 1970s there were no methods available to section intact bone to metal specimens. Therefore, the histologic evidence of osseointegration remained indirect (Fig. 33-1). Only after re-

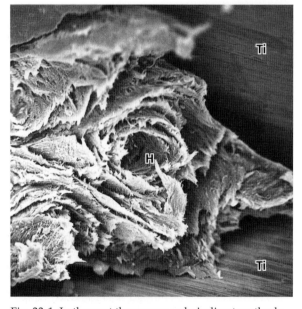

Fig. 33-1. In the past there were only indirect methods for verifying osseointegration. In this formalin-fixed and thereby slightly shrunk specimen, one sees bone tissue with a Haversian (H) system in close relation to the titanium (Ti) threaded implant.

moval of the implant with potential simultaneous removal of some soft interfacial tissues was it possible to inspect and analyze the interface. The first investigator to clearly demonstrate osseointegration was Schroeder from Switzerland. Schroeder worked from the mid 1970s, quite independently from Brånemark, with research on direct bone anchored implants. Schroeder's team used newly developed techniques to cut through undecalcified bone and implant without previous separation of the anchorage. In, for their time, excellent illustrations, a direct bone to implant contact was proved beyond doubt (Schroeder et al. 1976, 1978, 1981). Other pioneering work on osseointegration was conducted at roughly the same time by the German clinical scientist Schulte (1978).

Albrektsson et al. (1981) presented information on a series of background factors that needed control in order for a reliable osseointegration of an implant to ensue. These factors involved (1) the biocompatibility, (2) design and (3) surface conditions of the implant, (4) the status of the host bed, (5) the surgical technique at insertion, and (6) the loading conditions applied afterwards. All these factors needed more or less simultaneous control in order to result in osseointegration of the implanted device. Albrektssons laboratory has since been devoted to learning more about these various background factors. Twenty-eight PhD theses on these topics have been published at the laboratory.

Ossseointegration, once looked upon with scepticism, is now even regarded by some investigators as a frequently occurring, primitive foreign body reaction to an implanted material. A biomechanical factor alone is thought to determine whether a fibrous encapsulation or a bone covering will develop around an implanted device. Indeed, the authors behind these statements have demonstrated that even amalgam compounds will be embedded in bone (Donath et al. 1992). However, opposed to this view of osseointegration as simply a foreign body reaction is the documented evidence of the bone response being quantitatively different depending on the type of biomaterial and its surface roughness (Johansson 1991, Gottlander 1994, Wennerberg 1996).

EARLY TISSUE RESPONSE TO OSSEOINTEGRATED IMPLANTS

The site in the edentulous alveolar ridge that is selected for implant insertion is lined with a mucosa, in most situations a keratinized mucosa, which guards the hard tissue compartment. The surface of the bony part of the ridge – the compact bone – is lined with the periosteum, below which a layer of cortical bone can be found. The cortical bone serves as an envelope for the spongious or trabecular bone and the bone marrow that are included in the central portion of the ridge (Fig. 33-2)

In order to acquire proper conditions for healing, the implant following installation must exhibit good mechanical stability. It has been assumed that proper stability can be achieved when the marginal and/or "apical" portion of the site harbors sufficient amounts of compact bone and/or when the spongious (cancel-

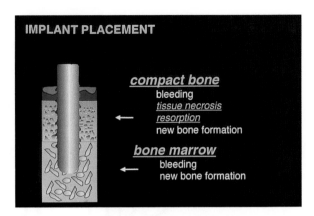

Fig. 33-2.

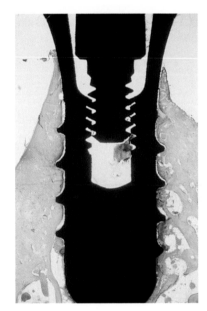

Fig. 33-3.

lous) bone contributes with sufficient amounts of trabeculae.

The various steps used in the surgical procedure – e.g. the incision in the mucosa, the elevation of the mucoperiosteal flaps, the careful preparation of a canal in the cortical and spongy bone, and finally the insertion of the titanium device – bring to bear a series of mechanical insults which result in injury to both the mucosa and the bone tissue. To the above described injury must be added the adverse effects obtained by the so called "press fit", namely the collapse of the vasculature which occurs in the cortical portion of the bone wall when the slightly wider implant is inserted in the canal prepared in the hard tissue.

The damage to the soft and hard tissue initiates the process of wound healing which ultimately allows (1) the implant to become "anchylotic" with the bone, i.e. osseointegrated, and (2) the establishment of a delicate mucosal attachment or barrier to the titanium device, which serves as a seal that prevents products from the oral cavity reaching the anchoring bone tissue.

The healing of the severed bone tissue is a complicated process and apparently involves different steps

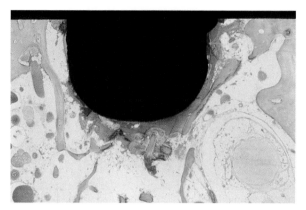

Fig. 33-4.

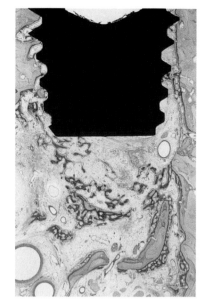

Fig. 33-5.

in the cortical and spongious parts of the surgical site. In the cortical bone region resorption of mineralized, avascular necrotic tissue must occur before new bone can form on the implant surface. In the spongious region of the site, on the other hand, woven bone formation and osseointegration occur early in the process of healing.

Some important features of the early wound, that occur in the bone at the recipient site, can be observed in Fig. 33-3 (ITI solid screw), which illustrates an implant with surrounding tissues 24 hours after installation surgery. The implant has proper mechanical stability, achieved by the "press-fit", i.e. the minute lateral displacement of bone tissue and the tight contact that was established following installation between the metal screw and the avascular cortical bone in the marginal two-thirds of the site. This zone of "press-fit" has been calculated to be about 1 mm wide. During site preparation and fitting of the implant, bone trabeculae were in the apical portion of the site, dislocated into the marrow space, blood vessels were severed and bleeding occurred (Fig. 33-4) (ITI implant, apical part). In Fig. 33-3 blood clot formation can also be observed between the implant body and the host bone. During the course of the following days, the blood clot will mature and become substituted with a granulation tissue, rich in neutrophils and macrophages. The leucocytes will start to decontaminate the wound, and from the marrow spaces of the peripheral vital bone, vascular structures will proliferate into the newly formed granulation tissue.

Reparative macrophages and undifferentiated mesenchymal cells will about one week after implant insertion start to produce and release growth factors, which stimulate *fibroplasias* through which an undifferentiated *provisional connective tissue* forms in (1) the apical, trabecular regions of the implant site, and (2) the "furcation sites" (F) of a screw-shaped implant. A "furcation site" (F) may be defined as the inner parts of the threaded regions of the implant which, following insertion, are without contact with the surrounding bone.

Osteoclasts will at this stage start to appear in the bone marrow spaces more remote from the implant surface, and the necrotic bone will gradually be resor-

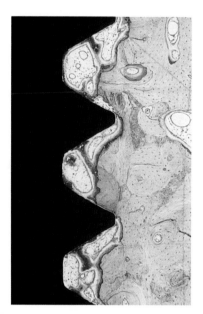

Fig. 33-6.

bed. The provisional connective tissue is rich in (1) newly formed vessels, (2) fibroblasts, and (3) undifferentiated mesenchymal cells and will gradually mature into an osteoid from which (4) *woven bone* (primary osteons) will form to fill the void with bone tissue. This phase of wound healing and early bone formation is called *modeling*.

Fig. 33-5 (Astra implant) illustrates an implant site 2 weeks after installation surgery. Note that woven bone with primary osteons has formed at the base of the surgical site and that newly formed bone has been laid down not only in the apical part of the implant, but also in the "furcation sites" of the implant surface (Fig. 33-6, enlargement of Fig. 33-5).

A further examination of the bone tissue next to the implant documents the presence of so called reversal lines (Fig. 33-7) (enlargement of a 3I implant), which indicate the level, lateral to the titanium screw, to

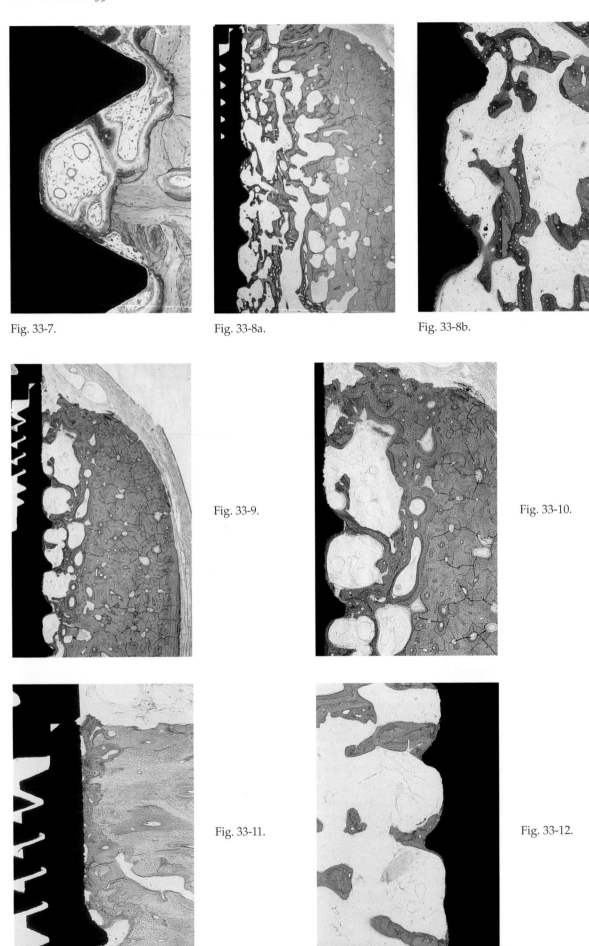

Fig. 33-7.

Fig. 33-8a.

Fig. 33-8b.

Fig. 33-9.

Fig. 33-10.

Fig. 33-11.

Fig. 33-12.

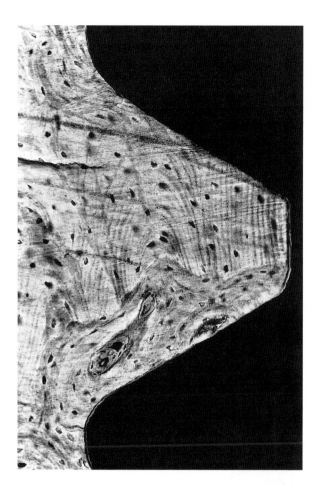

Fig. 33-13. Osseointegration represents a direct bone to implant contact at the resolution level of the light microscope, but is still best defined based on maintained stability of the implant. Retrieved clinical specimen showing a high degree of bone to implant direct contact.

which resorption of the necrotic tissue has occurred. In the "furcation sites" of the implant, new bone formation – osseointegration – is at this stage of healing the dominating feature, while at the peaks of the threads of the screw-type implant, discrete areas of bone resorption can be seen, since the newly-formed woven bone has poor loading capacity – implant stability is at this interval still maintained through the "press-fit" upheld in the necrotic part of the cortical bone.

Fig. 33-8 (ITI solid screw) presents an implant site after 4 weeks of wound healing. In this particular implant the distance between the threads is about 1 mm. The bone tissue within a zone – about 1 mm wide – lateral to the implant contains remnants of old bone that have been partly replaced by newly formed woven bone. The non-mineralized part of the bone tissue (primary bone marrow) contains at this stage no adipocytes. Note the presence of newly formed woven bone that lines most parts of the implant surface. This newly formed bone represents the first phase of true osseointegration.

The phase of modeling is followed by a phase of *remodeling* during which the woven bone is substituted with lamellar bone with a good potential to take up and distribute load. The woven bone is through a process of osteoclastic activity gradually removed and replaced by lamellar bone and bone marrow. Figs. 33-9 and 33-10 (ITI screw; different enlargements) illustrate an implant site 8 weeks after the insertion of the titanium screw. The titanium surface is lined with a thin rim of lamellar bone, lateral of which a bone marrow rich in adipocytes can be observed. Typical secondary osteons with concentric lamellae and a central Haversian canal can be observed in the lamellar bone within the zone of "press-fit", and in the adjacent bone tissue.

As healing continues, all portions of the original bone become replaced with new bone. Fig. 33-11 (ITI solid screw) illustrates a site 4 months after implant installation. The newly formed lamellar bone, next to the implant, is continuous with the more lightly-stained old bone tissue. In the apical, bone marrow part of the site (Fig. 33-12), a thin rim of lamellar bone can be seen in contact with the implant surface.

OSSEOINTEGRATION FROM A MECHANICAL AND BIOLOGIC VIEWPOINT

Osseointegration represents a direct connection between bone and implant without interposed soft tissue layers (Fig. 33-13). However, 100% bone connection to the implant does not occur. Problems in identifying the exact degree of bone attachment for the implant to be termed osseointegrated have led to a definition of osseointegration based on stability instead of on histologic criteria: "A process whereby clinically asymptomatic rigid fixation of alloplastic

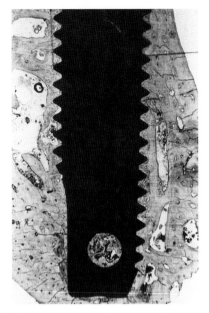

Fig. 33-14. Post mortem specimen of a titanium screw implant showing a high degree of bone to implant contact after 4 years of clinical loading.

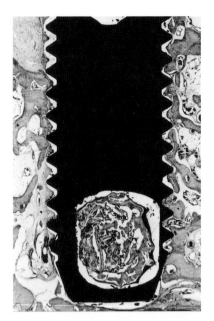

Fig. 33-15. Post mortem specimen of a maxillary implant inserted together with a bone graft, immediately prior to planned second stage surgery. Note the poor bone to implant contact percentage in this specimen that was basically similar to five other implants from the same maxilla.

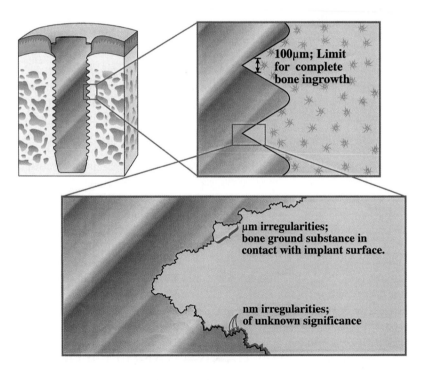

100μm; Limit for complete bone ingrowth

μm irregularities; bone ground substance in contact with implant surface.

nm irregularities; of unknown significance

Fig. 33-16. Even if complete bone tissue with cells and ground substance requires a minimum of 100 μm thickness for ingrowth, ground substance alone may invade pores of much smaller sizes, leading to the establishment of biomechanical bonds typical for properly osseointegrated implants. Bone ground substance invasion of nm-sized irregularities is only hypothetical and without any proven significance for implant stabilization.

materials is achieved, and maintained, in bone during functional loading" (Zarb & Albrektsson 1991). From different retrieval studies of implants removed from human jaws, despite maintained stability some information regarding bone to metal contact percentage has become available. Investigating more than 100 retrieved Nobelpharma type implants we have experienced more than 60% bone to implant contact for implants loaded between 1 and 18 years (Fig. 33-14). With increasing time of loading, there is a clear tendency for there to be more bone in contact with

mandibular implants than with maxillary ones (Albrektsson et al. 1993). In some grafted cases we found a very sparse amount of bone to implant contact, despite the implants being clinically stable (Fig. 33-15) (Nyström et al. 1993).

It has been suggested that the nature of the osseointegrated bond is related to physical and chemical forces acting over the interface (Albrektsson et al. 1983). However, even if such forces may act over the bone to c.p. titanium interface, there is no evidence that they play any dominant role in the strength of the

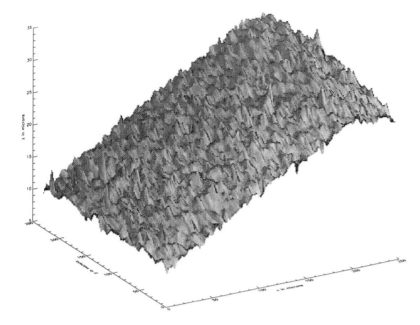

Fig. 33-17. The optimal surface roughness in experimental studies is of an s_a of about 1.4. s_a represents the arithmetic mean of the absolute values of the surface departures (i.e. peaks and valleys) from the mean plane within the sampling area.

osseointegrated bond. The bond is in all probability predominantly biomechanical. Having said this, surface modified titanium implants may indeed show bioactive properties. NaOH/heat-treated titanium plates have been found to resist much higher failure loads than non-treated controls (Yan et al 1997, Skripitz & Aspenberg 1998, Nishiguchi et al 1999). Sul (2002) has presented some evidence that titanium implants oxidized in a calcium hydroxide solution likewise become bioactive.

It is known that complete bone ingrowth does not occur in spaces much smaller than 100 microns (Albrektsson 1979). However, bone ground substance will adapt to surface irregularities in the 1-100 microns range, explaining why changing the surface topography at this level will result in a profound impact on the holding power of the implant (Wennerberg 1996). There is no scientific evidence that irregularities even in the nm range will affect the bone response, though this has been suggested by some investigators (Fig. 33-16). Commercially available oral implants have average surface irregularity values (s_a) beween 0.5 and 2.5 microns. In animal experiments there is a significantly stronger bone response to surfaces with s_a-values of 1.0-1.5 microns (Fig. 33-17). Surface irregularities in the 2.0 microns range or greater will show a diminished bone response, possibly because of increasing ionic leakage from these relatively rough surfaces.

Osseointegration is a time-related phenomenon. Johansson & Albrektsson (1987) demonstrated that during the first few weeks after implant insertion there were no signs of proper osseointegration. Three months after implant insertion there was a relatively high proportion of bone to implant direct contact (Fig. 33-18) and a clearly increased resistance to torque removal. The amount of bone and resistance to torque increased further, in the rabbit model used, at 6 and 12 months of follow-up. Yamanaka et al. (1992) investi-

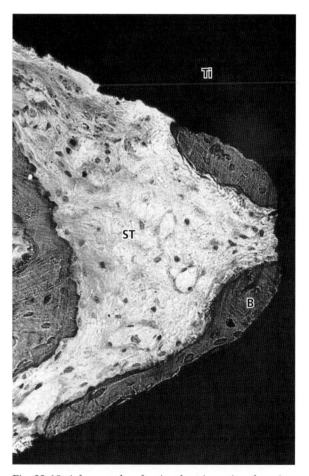

Fig. 33-18. A few weeks after implant insertion there is very sparse bone to implant contact. The bone tissue (B) contact with the implant (Ti) increases with time, represented by this rabbit tibial implant at three months after insertion. ST= Soft tissue.

gated the holding power of temporal bone implants in humans and found a gradually increasing removal torque up to 3 years after implant insertion. Taken together these results imply that c.p. titanium im-

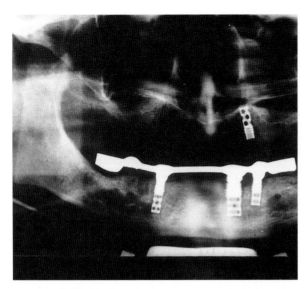

Fig. 33-19. A hollow basket implant made from Ti-6Al-4V that was demonstrated to fail clinically in many cases due to ongoing bone saucerization. This implant was launched without any published clinical long-term follow-up results, yet was at one time the most frequently used oral implant in the USA. Stricter attitudes from authorities and more critical analyses from dentists will, hopefully, prevent human experimentation with untested products in the future.

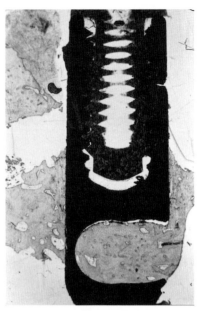

Fig. 33-20. A solid cylinder implant removed because of pain 3 years after its insertion. There is not one single study documenting steady state bone levels around solid cylindrical implants without special retention elements such as threads. Since numerous studies of this design have documented an ongoing gradual loss of anchoring bone tissue, responsible dentists should avoid working with cylindrical implant designs.

plants are not very stable in bone during the first weeks after their insertion. Despite this observation primary loading of implants seems possible at least in the mandible, mainly dependent on the previously described "press-fit" (for review see Albrektsson & Sennerby 2000). This does not prevent the possibility that there may a slightly increased failure rate for early loading even in mandibular sites. Furthermore, since the implants are dependent on "press-fit" for maintained stability, the surgical technique must be carefully controlled. In the maxilla, there is as yet sparse information about early loading. These data point to the importance of diagnosing the stability of implants which may differ considerably, e.g. in mandibles between the mental foraminae compared to in maxillae of poor bone quantity and quality.

Previous attempts to measure implant stability and thereby assess its degree of osseointegration have included Periotest measurements (Schulte & Lukas 1993). The Periotest uses a metal probe accelerated by an electromagnet. The contact duration of the probe on the implant is measured by an accelerometer. Contact time is then related to implant mobility. Despite being frequently used, the Periotest approach results in widely different data, and individual measurements have failed to reveal whether an implant is osseointegrated or not. The device cannot be recommended for clinical decisions on implant stability. Meredith and co-workers (1994, 1996) have described a different approach to assess bone formation around an implant, measuring the resonance frequency of a small transducer attached to an implant fixture. In a

clinical application of this new so-called RFA technique (Resonance Frequency Analysis), Meredith et al. (1996) investigated one group of nine patients with 56 Brånemark implants during their first year of insertion. They found the resonance frequency to rise from an average of 7473 Hz at implant placement to an average of 7915 Hz, 8 months later. In contrast, two implants that failed to integrate showed clearly lowered frequency data. Furthermore, the authors collected data obtained with 52 other Brånemark implants in nine patients examined 5 years after implant placement and compared those with radiograms with special reference to the exposed threads and the length of each abutment. The findings indicated a clear correlation ($r = -0.78$) between the length of the non-osseointegrated part of the implant pillar and resonance frequency. Resonance frequency of an implant/transducer system was found to be related to the height of the implant not surrounded by bone and the stability of the implant/tissue interface. The innovative work by Meredith has resulted in clearly improved ways of measuring implant stability in clinical routine.

Once established, the osseointegrated interface is relatively resistant but certainly not immune to various types of outer stimuli. Whereas the healing bed around an implant is highly sensitive to irradiation or heat injuries, once osseointegration has occurred, the same trauma levels will seemingly not affect the bond (Eriksson 1984, Jacobsson 1985). However, prolonged adverse conditions may result in breakage of osseointegration and subsequent implant failure (Fig.

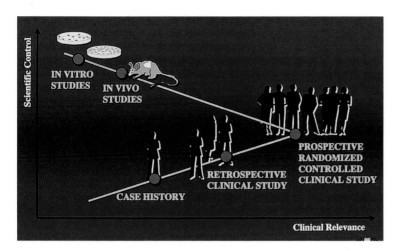

Fig. 33-21. *In vitro* studies are scientifically very controlled, but simultaneously of very low clinical relevance. The clinical case report is of lower scientific but higher clinical relevance than *in vitro* and *in vivo* studies. The prospective, randomized, controlled clinical study is at an intermediate level of scientific but a high level of clinical relevance.

33-19). A good example is overload. Overload is detrimental to osseointegration during the first few months after implant insertion, because interfacial movements will stimulate soft tissue formation in the interface, but once osseointegrated, the interface is capable of carrying occasional strong loads. Continuous, dynamic overloading of osseointegrated implants, however, will lead to micromovements and subsequent bone resorption. If the conditions are not altered in time (precise time/load relations are unknown), continuing bone resorption will result in increasing micromovements, eventually leading to implant failure (Hoshaw et al. 1994, Isidor 1996, 1997). This sequence of events is, in fact, typical for cylindrical oral implants without any macroscopic retention elements in the form of threads (Fig. 33-20) (Albrektsson 1993). Another documented secondary failure load of oral implants is peri-implantitis, defined as a combination of inflammation and bone loss (Lindhe et al 1992, Berglundh 1993). It is not known which of these two secondary implant failure modes is clinically most common.

OSSEOINTEGRATION IN THE CLINICAL REALITY

Although there are a great number of scientific investigations behind osseointegrated implants, a high proportion of the hardware and software preferences are based on empirical data only. We have simply learnt to follow a certain protocol that, if used in combination with a well-investigated oral implant, will result in a predictable outcome under defined conditions. It is indeed reasonable to challenge the osseointegrated protocol, provided this is done in a scientifically controlled manner. Obviously, more basic science is needed to learn more about optimal biomaterials, designs and surfaces of oral implants. However, one must interpret such data with some caution. *In vitro* findings may be of some scientific interest, but the glass disk represents a highly artificial environment devoid of blood flow, hormonal or loading influences. It is not uncommon for *in vivo* studies to produce

results opposite to those of the test tube. *In vivo* studies in animals over short and long follow-up times do provide interesting data. Such studies should be mandatory before the clinical trial is initiated. Yet, even those generally referred to as long-term animal studies span a follow-up time limited to about 1 year. Therefore, when the animal studies have been completed, we are not even halfway to collecting data necessary for widespread clinical introduction. There is now the need for controlled, preferably prospective, clinical studies that should be carried out under the guidance of a university ethical committee, with every patient consenting to treatment with a changed clinical routine or an untested product, spanning a minimum of 5 years. Only when the new clinical routine or novel implant has passed all these hurdles would a widespread clinical usage seem reasonable (Fig. 33-21). However, this is indeed a wish for the future, since the oral implant community of today does not seem to ask for anything but some animal pre-studies.

Lamentably, the high standards of clinical reporting set by Adell et al. (1981) were not followed in later times. Instead, osseointegration was regarded as equivalent to long-term implant success. New oral implant systems appeared and were marketed based only on sketchy short-term animal data with evidence of direct bone to implant contact. Well-known examples of such untested products that achieved great popularity despite lack of clinical documentation were a threaded, hollow cylinder device and a solid cylindrical implant with or without hydroxyapatite. These different types of implants had two things in common: they were supported by experimental evidence of osseointegration but, unknown to the treating dentist, they were prone to lose their bone anchorage with time due to progressive bone saucerization, which often resulted in subsequent implant failure (Albrektsson 1993). Furthermore, many types of screw design implants were introduced claiming that documentation was unnecessary since they allegedly resembled the original, well-documented Swedish c.p. titanium implant. This reasoning was based on the opinion that oral implants represent generic products – a misconceived notion at this stage. The various look-alike implants differ from one another with re-

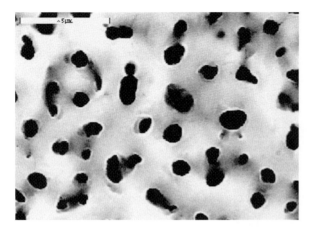

Fig. 33-22. Calcium incorporated, oxidized titanium implants are probably anchored to bone through ionic bonding. These implants have a unique porous surface and differ from non-oxidized c.p. titanium implants in other aspects such as crystallinity and presence of interfacial calcium ions.

spect to titanium composition, thread configuration and surface topography (Wennerberg et al. 1993). Indeed, the observed differences in surface topography alone are such that they will clearly influence the results in experimental studies (Wennerberg 1996). At present, there is insufficient knowledge about what governs the incorporation of an oral implant and we lack a great deal of information about optimal composition of the biomaterial, the design and the surface finish of an implant. Therefore, every oral implant must be supported by clinical documentation of the specific product without reference to any other implant of assumed similarity.

Unfortunately, the progress with respect to clinical reporting has been quite slow. When papers claiming high success rates of oral implants for 5 years are scrutinized, all too often there are numerous shortcomings, making the true results difficult to interpret. Common errors in most reports of the clinical outcome of oral implants are a failure to account for patients who dropped out, misinterpretation of survival and success, forgetting to report on bone height levels and claiming a 5-year outcome when implants have been followed only for up to 5 years. When critically analyzed, by far the best documented oral implant is the original Brånemark screw (Albrektsson et al. 1986, Albrektsson & Sennerby 1991, Lang & Karring 1994). However, there is no long-term clinical documentation of the novel, oxidized TiUnite implant from the same company. The turned version of the Astra Tech implant has been documented with positive results for 5 years (Arvidsson et al. 1998), whereas the newer Tioblast design has been reported for long term only in clinical materials, most limited in size (Palmer et al. 2000, Norton 2001). The original ITI solid screw implant has been positively documented for survival for more than 5 years, but the lack of reported bone height data makes any evaluation of implant success uncertain. Newer ITI designs, such as the Osseotite implant, lack proper long-term documentation. The same is true for the 3I implant. Another implant that has been positively documented for a full 5 years, at least in the mandible, is the Endopore (Deporter et al 1999).

FUTURE OF OSSEOINTEGRATED ORAL IMPLANTS

New developments of oral implants have, generally, been focused on changes in the hardware of the implant, i.e. new materials, designs or surfaces have been introduced with simultaneous claims of these being superior to those used in the past. Albeit of some relevance for biomaterials research, this approach has not been without pitfalls. Hydroxyapatite-coated implants have not been documented with good clinical results for 5 years or more, despite these implants being originally launched in the mid 1980s (Albrektsson 1998). The clinical results of intermediary roughened implants have not been as positive as once postulated, since the only three controlled clinical studies as yet published have failed to find any clear advantages of such implants in comparison to smoother controls (Lindhe 1997, Karlsson et al. 1998, Åstrand et al. 1999). The only published, long-term clinical study of oxidized implants (Graf et al. 2001) is of a quality that does not seem to allow for any reliable conclusions with respect to the outcome of the implants. Naturally, this does not prevent oxidized implants being of interest for the future, particularly since there is some evidence (Sul 2002) of the establishment of a bioactive implant surface, at least with certain types of anodized implants (Fig. 33-22).

However, if we base our look at the future on what is known today, there are obvious ways to improve clinical results. Although the main focus in the past has been on the three hardware parameters, the present authors foresee a substantial development in the realization of the importance of software parameters such as surgery and prosthodontics. Improvements of the surgical technique seem to be a reliable way of increasing oral implant success (Albrektsson 2002). The future of osseointegrated implants will mean a greater understanding of the important contributions by the responsible surgeon and prosthodontist (Bryant 2001).

REFERENCES

Adell, R., Lekholm, U., Rockler, B. & Brånemark, P-I. (1981). A 15-year study of osseointegrated implants in the treatment of the edentulous jaw. *International Journal of Oral Surgery* **6**, 387-399.

Albrektsson, T., (1979). *Healing of bone grafts. In vivo studies of tissue reactions at autografting of bone in the rabbit tibia.* PhD thesis. Göteborg: Biomaterials Group, University of Göteborg.

Albrektsson, T. (1993). On long term maintenance of the osseointegrated response. *Australian Prosthetic Journal* **7**, suppl., 15-24.

Albrektsson, T. (1998). Hydroxyapatite-coated implants. A case against their use. *Journal Oral Maxillofacial Surgery* **56**, 1312-1326.

Albrektsson, T. (2002). Is surgical skill more important for clinical success than changes in implant hardware? Editorial. *Clinical Implant Dentistry and Related Research* **3**, 174-175.

Albrektsson, T., Brånemark, P.I., Hansson, H.A., Kasemo, B., Larsson, K., Lundsström, I., McQueen, D. & Skalak, R. (1983). The interface zone of inorganic implants *in vivo*: Titanium implants in bone. *Annals of Biomedical Engineering* **11**, 1-27.

Albrektsson, T., Brånemark, P-I., Hansson, H-A. & Lindström, J. (1981). Osseointegrated titanium implants. Requirements for ensuring a long-lasting, direct bone anchorage in man. *Acta Orthopaedica Scandinavica* **52**, 155-170.

Albrektsson, T., Eriksson, A.R., Friberg, B., Lekholm, U., Lindahl, I., Nevins, M., Oikarinen, V., Roos, J., Sennerby, L. & Åstrand, P. (1993). Histologic investigations on 33 retrieved Nobelpharma implants. *Clinical Materials* **12**, 1-9.

Albrektsson, T. & Sennerby, L. (1991). State of the art in oral implants. *Journal of Clinical Periodontology* **18**, 474-481.

Albrektsson, T. & Sennerby, L. (2000). Einphasiges Implantatverfahren und Sofortbelastung von Implantaten. *Implantologie* **2**, 145-160.

Albrektsson, T., Zarb, G., Worthington, P. & Eriksson, R.A. (1986). The long-term efficacy of currently used dental implants: a review and proposed criteria of success. *International Journal of Oral and Maxillofacial Implants* **1**, 11-25.

Arvidsson K., Bystedt, H., Frykholm, A., von Konow, L. & Lothigius, E. (1998). Five year prospective follow up report of the Astra tech dental implant system in the treatment of edentulous mandibles. *Clinical Oral Implants Research* **9**, 225-234.

Åstrand, P., Engquist, B., Dahlgrens, S., Engquist, E., Feldmann, H. & Gröndahl, K. (1999). Astra tech and Brånemark system implants. A prospective 5-year comparative study. Results after one year. *Clinical Implant Dentistry and Related Research* **1**, 17-26.

Berglundh, T. (1993). *Studies on gingival and periimplant mucosa in the dog.* PhD thesis. Göteborg: University of Göteborg.

Bodine, R., Yanase, R. & Bodine, A. (1996). Forty years of experience with subperiosteal implant dentures in 41 edentulous patients. *Journal of Prosthetic Dentistry* **75**, 33-44.

Brånemark, P.I., Adell, R., Breine, U., Hansson, B.O., Lindström, J. & Ohlsson, Å. (1969). Intra-osseous anchorage of dental prostheses I. Experimental studies. *Scandinavian Journal of Plastic Reconstructive Surgery* **3**, 81-100.

Brånemark, P.I., Hansson, B.O., Adell, R., Breine, U., Lindström, J., Hallén, O. & Öhman, A. (1977). Osseointegrated implants in the treatment of the edentulous jaw. Experience from a 10-year period. *Scandinavian Journal of Plastic Reconstructive Surgery* **16**, (suppl).

Bryant, S.R. (2001). *Oral implant outcomes predicted by age- and site specific aspects of bone condition.* PhD thesis. Toronto: University of Toronto.

Buser, D., Merickse-Stern R., Bernard, J.P., Behneke, A., Behneke, N. & Hirt, H.P. (1997) Long-term evaluation of non-submerged ITI-implants. Part 1: 8-year life table analysis of a prospective multicenter study with 2359 implants. *Clinical Oral Implants Research* **8**, 161-172.

Deporter, D.A., Watson, P.A., Pharoah, M., Levy, D. & Todescan, R. (1999). Five-to six year results of aprospective clinical trial using the Endopore dental implant and mandibular overdenture. *Clinical Oral Implants Research* **10**, 95-102.

Donath, K., Laass, M. & Günzl, H.J. (1992). The histopathology of different foreign-body reactions in oral soft tissue and bone tissue. *Virchows Archiv. A: Pathological Anatomy and Histopathology* (Berlin) **420**, 131-137.

Eriksson, R.A. (1984). *Heat induced bone tissue injury.* PhD thesis. Göteborg: Biomaterials Group, University of Göteborg.

Gottlander, M. (1994). *On hard tissue reactions to hydroxyapatite-coated titanium implants.* PhD thesis. Göteborg: Biomaterials/Handicap Research, University of Göteborg.

Graf, H.L., Geu, B., Knöfler, W. & Hemprich, A. (2001). Klinisches verhalten des ZL-Duraplant-Implantatsystems mit Ticer-Oberfläche. *Zeitschrift Zahnärtzliche Implantologie* **17**, 124-131.

Hoshaw, S.J., Brunski, J.B. & Cochran, G.V.B. (1994). Mechanical loading of Brånemark implants affects interfacial bone modeling and remodeling. *Journal Oral Maxillofacial Surgery* **9**, 345-360.

Isidor, F. (1996). Loss of osseointegration caused by occlusal load of oral implants. A clinical and radiographic study in monkeys. *Clinical Oral Implants Research* **7**, 143-152.

Isidor F. (1997). Histological evaluation of peri-implant bone at implants subjected to occlusal overload or plaque accumulation. *Clinical Oral Implants Research* **8**, 1-9.

Johansson, C. (1991). *On tissue reactions to metal implants.* PhD thesis. Göteborg: Biomaterials/Handicap Research, University of Göteborg.

Johansson, C. & Albrektsson, T. (1987). Integration of screw implants in the rabbit. A 1-year follow-up of removal of titanium implants. *International Journal of Oral and Maxillofacial Implants* **2**, 69-75.

Kapur, K.K. (1989). Veterans Administration cooperative dental implant study – comparisons between fixed partial dentures supported by blade vent implants and removable part dentures. Part II. Comparisons of success rates and periodontal health between two treatment modalities. *Journal of Prosthetic Dentistry* **62**, 685-703.

Karlsson, U., Gotfredsen, K. & Olsson, C. (1998). A 2-year report on maxillary and mandibular fixed partial dentures supported by Astra Tech dental implants. A comparison of two implants with different surface textures. *Clinical Oral Implants Research* **9**, 235-242.

Lang, N. & Karring, T. (1994). *Proceedings of the 1st European Workshop on Periodontology.* Berlin: Quintessence.

Lindhe, J. (1997). Prospective clinical trials on implant therapy in the partially edentulous dentition using the Astra tech dental implant system. In: *Proceedings of 13th European conference on Biomaterials.* European Society for Biomaterials, transactions of workshops, p. 9.

Lindhe, J., Berglundh, T., Ericsson, I., Liljenberg, B. & Marinello, C.P. (1992). Experimental breakdown of periimplant and periodonotal tissues. A study in the beagle dog. *Clinical Oral Implants Research* **3**, 9-16.

Meredith, N., Alleyne, D. & Cawley, P. (1996). Quantitative determination of the stability of the implant-tissue interface using resonance frequency analysis. *Clinical Oral Implants Research* **7**, 261-267.

Meredith, N., Book, K., Friberg, B., Jemt, T. & Sennerby, L. (1997). Resonance frequency measurements of implant stability *in vivo*. *Clinical Oral Implants Research* **8**, 226-233.

Meredith, N., Cawley, P. & Alleyne, D. (1994). The application of modal vibration analysis to study bone healing *in vivo*. *Journal of Dental Research* **73**, 793.

Nishiguchi, S., Nakamura, T., Kobayashi, M., Kim, H.Y., Miyajji,

F. & Kokubo, T. (1999). The effect of heat treatment on bone-bonding ability of alkali-treated titanium. *Biomaterials* **20**,491-500.

Norton, M.R. (2001). Biologic and mechanical stability of single-tooth implants: 4-7 year follow-up. *Clinical Implant Dentistry and Related Research* **3**, 214-220.

Nyström, E., Kahnberg, K.E. & Albrektsson, T. (1993). Treatment of the severely resorbed maxillae with bone graft and titanium implants. Histologic review of autopsy specimens. *International Journal of Maxillofacial Implants* **8**, 167-172.

Palmer, R.M., Palmer, P.J. & Smith, B.J. (2000). A 5-year prospective study of Astra single tooth implants. *Clinical Oral Implants Research* **11**, 179-182.

Schroeder, A., Pohler, O. & Sutter, F. (1976). Gewebsreaktion auf ein Titan-Hohlzylinderimplantat mit Titan-Spritzschicht-oberfläche. *Schweizerisches Monatsschrift für Zahnheilkunde* **86**, 713-727.

Schroeder, A., Stich, H., Straumann, F. & Sutter, F. (1978). Über die Anlagerung von Osteozement an einen belasteten Implantatkörper. *Schweizerisches Monatsschrift für Zahnheilkunde* **88**, 1051-1058.

Schroeder, A., van der Zypen, E., Stich, H. & Sutter, F. (1981). The reactions of bone, connective tissue, and epithelium to endosteal implants with titanium-sprayed surfaces. *Journal of Maxillofacial Surgery* **9**, 15-25.

Schulte, W. (1978). Das Tübingen Implantat aus Frialit – Fünfjährige Erfahrungen. *Deutsche Zahnärztliche Zeitung* **33**, 326-331

Schulte, W. & Lukas, D. (1993). Periotest to monitor osseointegration and to check the occlusion in oral implantology. *Journal of Oral Implantology* **XIX**, 23-32.

Sennerby, L. (1991). *On the bone tissue response to titanium implants.* PhD thesis. Göteborg: Biomaterials/Handicap Research, University of Göteborg.

Skripitz, R. & Aspenberg, P. (1998). Tensile bond between bone and titanium. *Acta Orthopaedica Scandinavica* **69**, 2-6.

Spiekermann, H. (1980). Clinical and animal experiences with endosseous metal implants. In: Heimke, G., ed. *Dental Implants, Materials and Systems.* Vienna: Hanser Verlag, pp. 49-54.

Sul, Y.T. (2002). *On the bone tissue response to oxidized titanium implants.* PhD thesis, Göteborg: Department of Biomaterials, University of Göteborg.

Wennerberg, A., Albrektsson, T. & Andersson, B. (1993). Design and surface characteristics of 13 commercially available oral implant systems. *International Journal of Oral and Maxillofacial Implants* **8**, 622-633.

Wennerberg, A. (1996). *On surface roughness and implant incorporation.* PhD thesis. Göteborg: Biomaterials/Handicap Research, Göteborg University.

Yamanaka, E., Tjellström, A., Jacobsson, M. & Albrektsson, T. (1992). Long-term observations on removal torque of directly bone-anchored implants. In: *Transplants and Implants in Otology,* II. Ingelheim: Kugler.

Yan, W.Q., Nakamura, T., Kobayashi, M., Kim, H.M., Miyaji, F. & Kokubo, T. (1997). Bonding of chemically treated titanium implants to bone. *Journal Biomedical Materials Research* **37**, 267-275.

Zarb, G.A. & Albrektsson, T. (1991). Osseointegration – A requiem for the periodontal ligament? Editorial. *International Journal of Periodontology and Restorative Dentistry* **11**, 88-91.

Zarb, G. & Symington, J. (1983). Osseointegrated dental implants: preliminary report on a replication study. *Journal of Prosthetic Dentistry* **50**, 271-279.

CHAPTER 34

Surface Topography of Titanium Implants

ANN WENNERBERG, TOMAS ALBREKTSSON AND JAN LINDHE

Implant surface/osseointegration

Measurement of surface topography
  Instruments
  Procedure

Implant surface roughness
  Experimental studies
  Surface roughness of some commercially available implants

IMPLANT SURFACE/OSSEOINTEGRATION

Dental implants supplied with a turned surface configuration have been used for more than 30 years and have been shown to have great long-term success when used for the rehabilitation of the partially dentate and fully edentulous patient (Albrektsson & Sennerby 1991, Eckert et al. 1997, Roos et al. 1997, Arvidsson et al. 1998). Based mainly on results from experimental studies, however, several manufacturers of dental implants have gradually substituted the "old-fashioned" turned implant with implants designed with enlarged surfaces. It was suggested that implants with such modified surfaces can be loaded at an earlier time following installation than was generally recommended for implants with a turned surface. Thus, arguments used in the promotion of surface modified implants were that they (1) provided a better mechanical stability between bone and implant immediately following installation – established by a greater contact area, (2) provided a surface configuration that properly retained the blood clot, and (3) stimulated the bone healing process. Indeed, findings from experimental studies documented that a firmer bone fixation (osseointegration) was established to implants with a roughened surface than to implants with a turned surface (Carlsson et al. 1988, Feighan et al. 1995, Gotfredsen et al. 2000, Ivanoff et al. 2001).

Examples of methods that are used to alter the surface topography of commercially available dental implants include *grit blasting, titanium plasma spraying, etching* and/or *coating*. Such surface conditioning methods will result in *irregularities* of *height, wavelength* and *spatial dimension*. It is currently not known whether it is variation in height of the irregularities of a given surface or their wavelength or a combination of the two factors, that will promote the rate of incorporation of the implant in bone tissue.

It is reasonable to assume that new surface modifications of dental implants will be introduced and claims will be made that this or that particular surface will most ideally promote osseointegration. Thus, it will become important for the student of dentistry to understand how a surface is changed, how this surface is characterized and how it may indeed enhance bone healing and osseointegration.

The characterization of a surface requires not only the use of an appropriate measuring device but also knowledge regarding how the results of the measurements should be interpreted.

MEASUREMENT OF SURFACE TOPOGRAPHY

Instruments

The surface topography describes (1) the degree of *roughness* that the surface exhibits as well as (2) the *orientation* of the irregularities on the surface. Surface roughness occurs in two principal planes: one perpendicular to the surface and one in the plane of the surface (Thomas 1999). The orientation of the irregularities may be either isotropic or anisotropic.

For a proper topographical characterization of a surface, instruments and methods must be used that

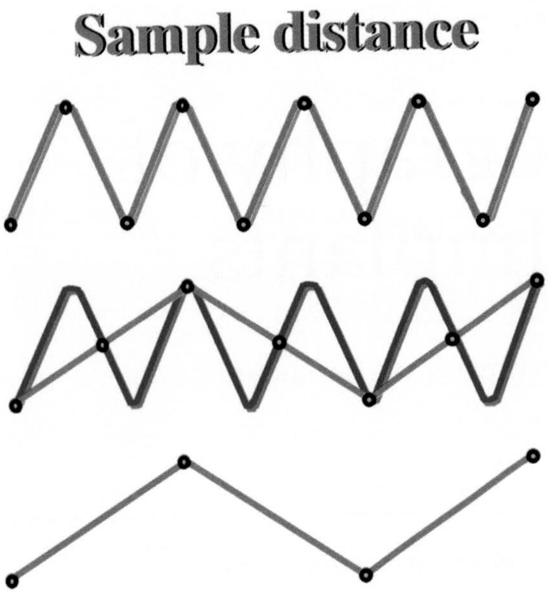

Sample distance

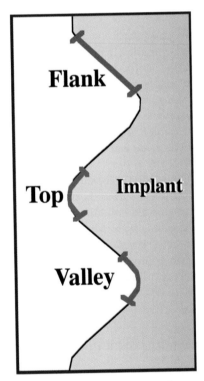

Fig. 34-1. Too large a distance between the measuring points will result in a loss of information and an artificial increase of wavelength.

Fig. 34-2. A drawing that demonstrates the measuring areas – top, flank and valley – of a threaded oral implant.

provide both numerical and visual data. Currently three groups of instruments are available that may provide such information:

1. mechanical contact stylus instruments
2. optical instruments
3. scanning probe microscopes (SPM).

Each of the above instruments has its own area of application. However, in studying the surface characteristics of screw-type oral implants only optical instruments may provide proper information (Wennerberg & Albrektsson 2000). Among the optical instruments that are available, confocal laser scanning profilometers and interferometers are preferred. It must be realized that the horizontal resolution in such an optical instrument is dependent on the wavelength of the light used and cannot be much better that 0.3 µm, while the vertical resolution may approach values close to 0.05 nm. The size of the area of the implant surface to be analyzed is about 1 mm² and the vertical range for the optical instruments is about 100 µm. It is also important to define a proper sampling distance, i.e. the interval or distance between the points to be measured along the profile of the surface. If this distance is too long, important surface features will be lost and the surface (profile) may appear to be smoother than is actually the case (Fig.34-1).

Measuring and evaluating procedure

The threaded portion of a screw-shaped implant has three typical regions: the top, the flank and the valley region (Fig.34-2). Of the three different sites, the top region generally has the roughest surface (Wennerberg & Albrektsson 2000). If we assume that all parts of an implant are equally important with respect to osseointegration, a proper characterization of the implant surface must include measurements made in all three regions. The number of measurements required for the characterization depends on the homogeneity of the surface structure within the three regions (Bennett & Mattson 1989). Findings from an analysis of dental implants reported by Wennerberg (1996) indicated that for threaded implants nine measurements are sufficient for a comprehensive surface characterization – three from the top, three from the flank and three from the valley regions. Further, three-dimensional (3D) measurements are more reliable than two-dimensional (2D) determinations due to the increased amount of data obtained in the 3D assessment.

The topography of a surface is defined in terms of *form, waviness* and *roughness* (Fig.34-3). Waviness and roughness are often presented together under the term *texture* (Thomas 1999). Undercuts present in the surface are not possible to measure (Fig.34-4).

In the analysis, data describing form and waviness are first determined, after which the roughness is assessed. As can be seen in Fig. 34-3, the roughness describes the smallest irregularities in the surface, while form relates to the largest structure (profile). Surface roughness is further described in terms of *amplitude, spatial distribution* (spacing) and *hybrid* parameters. For the proper characterization of dental implants at least one parameter from each of the three groups – amplitude, spacing and hybrid – must be included in the topographical evaluation of the top,

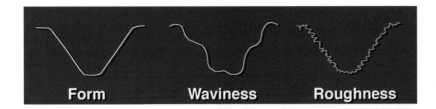

Fig. 34-3. A schematic drawing of an implant, which demonstrates the terms form, waviness and roughness.

the flank and the valley regions (Wennerberg & Albrektsson 2000).

Amplitude parameters describe the vertical height of the irregularities and are determined in both 2D and 3D measurements (for example correspond the 2D parameters Ra, Rq, Rz with the 3D Sa, Sq, Sz) (Fig.34-5).

Spacing parameters describe the space between the irregularities and are also determined in both 2D and 3D measurements. Sm (2D) and Scx (3D) report the average length between profile peaks (Fig.34-6).

Hybrid parameters (Sdq and Sdr) include information regarding both amplitude and spacing.

These parameters describe whether the irregularities have rounded or pointed curvatures (Fig.34-7).

IMPLANT SURFACE ROUGHNESS

Surface structures without a dominating direction are called *isotropic*. Techniques to produce such surfaces include abrasive blasting, plasma spraying, etching and oxidizing. Other processes such as turning or milling result in a surface that has a distinct and regular pattern. Such a surface structure is denoted *anisotropic*.

Experimental studies investigating surface roughness and osseointegration

Several studies including *in vivo* experiments have reported that a better bone fixation (osseointegration) will be achieved with implants with an enlarged, isotropic surface as compared to implants with a turned, anisotropic surface structure (e.g. Wennerberg 1996, Ivanoff et al. 2001). In some studies, by for example Hahn & Palich 1970, Roberson et al. 1976, Carlsson et al. 1988, Gotfredsen et al. 2000, a positive correlation was found between increasing surface roughness and degree of implant incorporation (osseointegration), while in other studies no such direct correlation was observed (Vercaigne et al. 1998).

Wennerberg and co-workers (Wennerberg et al 1995a,b, 1996a,b,c, 1997) performed a series of investigations in an attempt to identify the surface structure of the "optimal" implant. Threaded (screw-type) implants made of commercially pure titanium were

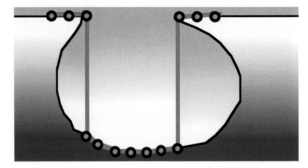

Fig. 34-4. Undercuts cannot be measured; a loss of spatial information will occur.

used. They all had a diameter of 3.75 mm and a pitch-height of 0.6 mm. Implants with a turned surface were used as negative controls. The surface structure of the test implants was altered by exposing the implants to different blasting materials and of different particle size. The blasting materials used were either TiO_2 or Al_2O_3 and the particles used for blasting were 25 µm, 75 µm or 250 µm large. Following the surface modification procedure, the implants were cleaned in an ultrasonic bath and their surface topography characterized with the use of an optical confocal profilometer.

The implants were subsequently implanted in the tibia of rabbits and allowed to heal for 4, 12 or 52 weeks. The degree of bone fixation (osseointegration) was determined by mechanical (torque removal force) and histologic (amount of bone to implant contact) means. The analysis of the findings from these *in vivo* experiments revealed that implants designed with a surface characterized by the following exhibited the most ideal degree of osseointegration:

- S_a value (amplitude 3D) of 1.45 µm
- S_{cx} value (spacing 3D) of 11 µm
- S_{dr} ratio (hybrid 3D) of 1.5

In a second study, the research protocol was slightly amended in that each individual, screw-shaped implant was prepared with two different surfaces with different roughness. The implant was thus acting as its own control. The same blasting technique, materials and particle size were used to modify the surface as in the previous study. The implants were inserted, allowed to heal and were exposed to the same determinations as in the experiments described above. The mechanical and histologic measurements performed revealed again that a surface with a S_a value of 1.45 µm, a S_{cx} value of 11 µm and a S_{dr} value of 1.5 provided

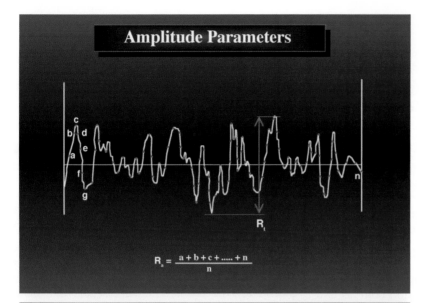

Fig. 34-5. A profile demonstrating how 2D height amplitude descriptive parameters are calculated.

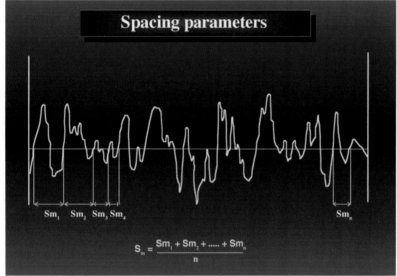

Fig. 34-6. A profile demonstrating how 2D spatial descriptive parameters are calculated.

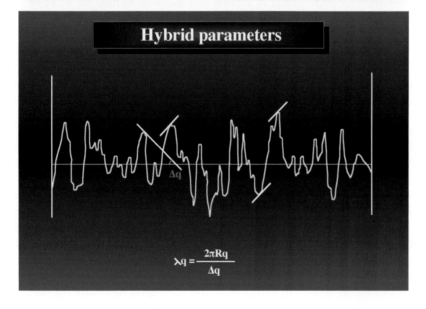

Fig. 34-7. A profile demonstrating how 2D hybrid parameters are calculated.

the most ideal conditions for bone fixation and osseointegration (Wennerberg et al. 1998).

In a third study (Ivanoff et al. 2001) "micro-sized" screw type implants with either a turned or a TiO_2 blasted surface were installed in human volunteers. The implants were allowed to heal for 4 months (mandible) and 6 months (maxilla) and were subsequently removed in a biopsy and prepared for a histological examination. It was observed that significantly larger amounts of bone-to-implant contact had been establ-

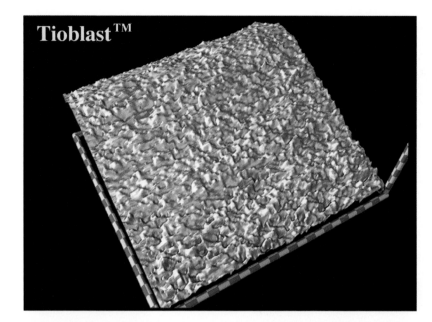

Fig. 34-8. A blasted surface, Tioblast™, a flank area showing an isotropic surface with fine irregularities. Each section of the red and white bars represents a length of 10 μm.

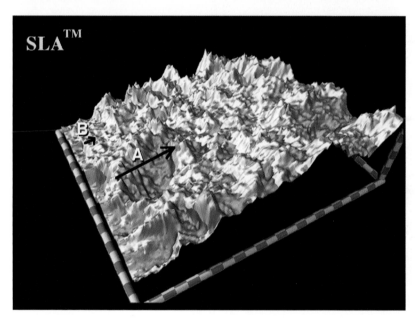

Fig. 34-9. A blasted and etched surface, SLA™, a flank area demonstrating two dominating surface features, pronounced pits (A) and high frequency irregularities (B). Each section of the red and white bars represents a length of 10 μm.

ished to the implants that were prepared with a rough surface than to the control device. The study further documented that the S_a value used to characterize a surface may be of lesser importance than the S_{cx} value and the S_{dr} ratio in discriminating between surfaces that may promote osseointegration.

The findings from the studies by Wennerberg and co-workers, discussed above, were confirmed in a thesis by Hallgren Höstner (2001). In this series of studies it was observed that implants with blasted isotropic surfaces were superior to implants with anisotropic or chequered surface patterns in terms of bone fixation and osseointegration.

Surface roughness of some commercially available implants

All values presented below are from measurements made with a confocal laser scanning profilometer (TopScan 3D, Heidelberg, Germany). The diameter of the helium-neon laser beam used in this instrument is approximately 1 μm. All measurement areas had a size of 250 × 250 μm. Nine measurements were taken from each implant (three top regions, three valley regions and three flank regions) and three implants from each manufacturer were included in the assessments. A Gaussian filter, sized 50 × 50 μm, was used to separate roughness from errors of form and waviness.

Blasted surface

(Tioblast™, AstraTech AB, Mölndal, Sweden.) A surface blasted with TiO_2 particles. The blasting procedure resulted in an isotropic surface; no topographical remnants from the underlying machining process were visible. The implants had an average height deviation (S_a) of 1.07 μm, an average wavelength (S_{cx}) of 10.11 μm and an increased surface area (S_{dr}) of 29% (Fig.34-8).

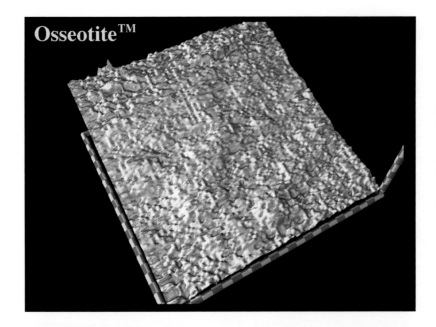

Osseotite™

Fig. 34-10. An etched surface, Osseotite™, with a flank area with fine irregularities and a pronounced isotropy. A smoother surface compared to the Tioblast surface in Fig. 34-8. Each section of the red and white bars represents a length of 10 μm.

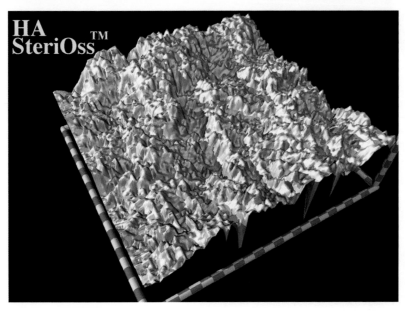

HA SteriOss™

Fig. 34-11. An implant surface coated with hydroxyapatite, SteriOss™. This surface has a rather increased average height deviation and short average wavelength resulting in an intermediately increased surface area. Each section of the red and white bars represents a length of 10 μm.

Blasted + etched surface

(SLA™, Institute Straumann AG, Waldenburg, Switzerland.) The surface is blasted followed by acid etching. The measurements disclosed a surface that included high frequency wavelength and medium frequency wavelength. The implant surface had an average height deviation of 1.42 μm (S_a), an average wavelength of 16.60 μm (S_{cx}) and an increased surface area of 33% (S_{dr}) (Fig.34-9).

Etched surface

(Osseotite™, 3i, Implant innovations, Palm Beach, Florida, US.) The surface is etched in a two-step procedure. The surface examination disclosed an isotropic surface with high frequency irregularities visible (Fig.34-10). The measured implants had an average height deviation of 0.94 μm (S_a), an average wavelength of 11.68 μm (S_{cx}) and an increased surface area of 20% (S_{dr}).

Hydroxyapatite coated surface

(SteriOss™, Replace system, Nobel Biocare, US.) With the coating procedure used not only the surface chemistry but also the topography will be altered. In general this procedure gives a rather rough and isotropic surface. The surface of the SteriOss HA coated implants were found to have an average height deviation of 1.68 μm (S_a), an average wavelength of 13.74 μm (S_{cx}) and an increased surface area of 55% (S_{dr}) (Fig.34-11).

Oxidized surfaces

(TiUnite™, Nobel Biocare AB, Göteborg, Sweden.) The surface is oxidized in a manner that progressively increases the thickness of the oxidized layer in "apical" direction. The process results in an isotropic surface that is characterized by the presence of craterous structures. The implant surface was found to have an average height deviation of 1.08 μm (S_a), an average wavelength of 10.98 μm (S_{cx}) and an increased surface area of 37% (S_{dr}) (Fig.34-12).

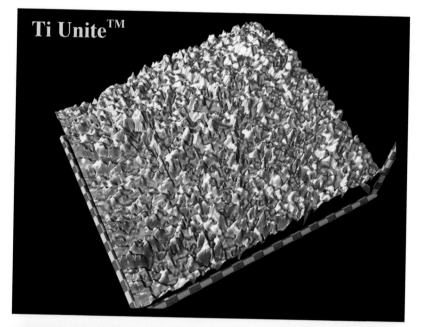

Ti Unite™

Fig. 34-12. A TiUnite™ flank, where the oxidation process has resulted in a lot of pores. The porous structure will increase the surface area more than other surfaces with similar average height deviation. Each section of the red and white bars represents a length of 10 μm.

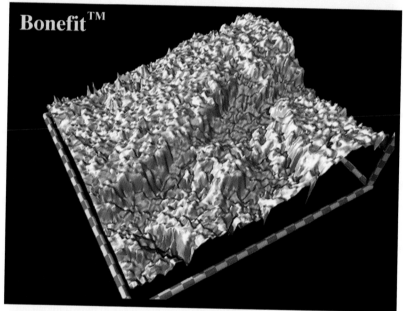

Bonefit™

Fig. 34-13. Bonefit™, a titanium plasma sprayed surface with a rough structure. Some parts of this area are rather smooth, others very rough. Each section of the red and white bars represents a length of 10 μm.

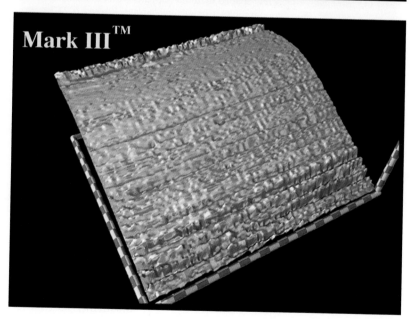

Mark III™

Fig. 34-14. A turned implant flank with marks from the cutting procedure clearly visible. Each section of the red and white bars represents a length of 10 μm.

Titanium plasma sprayed surface

(Bonefit™, Institute Straumann AG, Waldenburg, Switzerland.) Plasma spraying results in a rough but still isotropic surface. The surface of the implants was found to have an average height deviation of 2.35 μm (S_a), an average wavelength of 13.15 μm (S_{cx}) and an increased surface area of 87% (S_{dr}). (Fig.34-13).

(SteriOss™, Replace system, Nobel Biocare, US.) This was the roughest implant surface among those measured. The implant surface was found to have an average height deviation of 3.86 μm (S_a), an average wavelength of 19.55 μm (S_{cx}) and an increased surface area of 134% (S_{dr}).

Turned surface

(MKIII™, Nobel Biocare, Göteborg, Sweden.) Cutting marks from the machining process result in an oriented anisotropic surface. The surface of the implants had an average height deviation of 0.71 μm (S_a), an average wavelength of 9.84 μm (S_{cx}) and an increased surface area of 19% (S_{dr}) (Fig.34-14).

The MK III implants had a rougher surface compared to the turned "coronal part" of the Osseotite™ implant. The average height deviation was for Osseotite "coronal part", 0.53 μm, and the average wavelength and developed surface area was 8.6 μm and 15%, respectively.

REFERENCES

Albrektsson, T. & Sennerby, L. (1991). State of the art in oral implants. *Journal of Clinical Parodontology* **18**, 474-481.

Arvidsson, K., Bystedt, H., Frykholm, A., von Konow, L. & Lothigius, E. (1998). Five-year prospective follow-up report of the AstraTech dental implant system in the treatment of edentulous mandibles. *Clinical Oral Implants Reseach* **9**, 225-234.

Bennett, J.M. & Mattsson, L. (1989). *Introduction to Surface Roughness and Scattering*, 1st edn. Washington DC: Optical Society of America.

Carlsson, L., Röstlund, T., Albrektsson, B. & Albrektsson, T. (1988). Removal torques for polished and rough titanium implants. *International Journal of Oral and Maxillofacial Implants* **3**, 21-24.

Eckert, S.E., Parein, A., Myshin, H.L. & Padilla, J.L. (1997). Validation of dental implant systems through a review of the literature supplied by system manufacturers. *Journal of Prosthetic Dentistry* **77**, 271-279.

Feighan, J.E., Goldberg, V.M., Davy, D., Parr, J.A. & Stevensson, S. (1995). The influence of surface blasting on the incorporation of titanium-alloy implants in a rabbit intramedullary model. *Journal of Bone and Joint Surgery* **77-A**, 1380-1395.

Gotfredsen, K., Berglundh, T. & Lindhe, J. (2000). Anchorage of titanium implants with different surface characteristics: an experimental study in rabbits. *Clinical Implant Dentistry and Related Research* **2**(3), 120-128.

Hahn, H. & Palich, W. (1970). Preliminary evaluation of porous metal surfaced titanium for orthopedic implants. *Journal of Biomedical Material Research* **14**, 571-577.

Hallgren Höstner, C. (2001). *On the bone response to different implant textures. A 3D analysis of roughness, wavelength and surface pattern of experimental implants.* PhD thesis. Göteborg: Dept Biomaterials/Handicap Research, Göteborg University.

Ivanoff, C.J, Widmark, G., Hallgren, C., Sennerby, L. & Wennerberg, A. (2001). Histologic evaluation of the bone integration of TiO2 blasted and turned titanium microimplants in humans. *Clinical Oral Implants Research* **12**, 128-134.

Roberson, D.M., St Pierre, L. & Chahal, R. (1976). Preliminary oberservations of bone ingrowth into porous materials. *Journal of Biomedical Material Research* **10**, 335-344.

Roos, J., Sennerby, L. & Albrektsson, T. (1997). An update on the clinical documentation on currently used bone-anchored endosseous implants. *Clinical Update* **24**, 194-200.

Thomas, T. (1999). *Rough Surfaces*, 2nd edn. London: Imperial Collage Press.

Vercaigne, S., Wolke, J,G,, Naert, I. & Jansen, J.A. (1998). Bone healing capacity of titanium plasma-sprayed and hydroxylapatite-coated oral implants. *Clinical Oral Implants Research* **9**, 261-271.

Wennerberg, A. (1996). *On surface roughness and implant incorporation.* PhD thesis. Göteborg: Dept Biomaterials/Handicap Research, Göteborg University.

Wennerberg, A. & Albrektsson, T. (2000). Suggested guidelines for the topographic evaluation of implant surfaces. *International Journal of Oral and Maxillofacial Implants* **15**, 331-344.

Wennerberg, A., Albrektsson, T. & Andersson, B. (1995b). An animal study of c.p. titanium screws with different surface topographies. *Journal of Materials Science: Materials in Medicine* **6**, 302-309.

Wennerberg, A., Albrektsson, T. & Andersson, B. (1996b). Bone tissue response to commercially pure titanium implants blasted with fine and coarse particles of aluminum oxide. *International Journal of Oral and Maxillofacial Implants* **11**, 38-45.

Wennerberg, A., Albrektsson, T., Andersson, B. & Krol, J.J. (1995a). A histomorphometric and removal torque study of screw-shaped titanium implants with three different surface topographies. *Clinical Oral Implants Research* **6**, 24-30.

Wennerberg, A., Albrektsson, T., Johansson, C. & Andersson, B. 1996a). Experimental study of turned and grit-blasted screw-shaped implants with special emphasis on effects of blasting material and surface topography. *Biomaterials* **17**, 15-22.

Wennerberg, A., Albrektsson, T. & Lausmaa, J.(1996c). Torque and histomorphometric evaluation of c.p. titanium screws blasted with 25- and 75-microns-sized particles of Al2O3. *Journal of Biomedical Material Research* **30**, 251-260.

Wennerberg, A., Ektessabi, A., Albrektsson, T., Johansson, C. & Andersson, B. (1997). A 1-year follow-up of implants of differing surface roughness placed in rabbit bone. *International Journal of Oral and Maxillofacial Implants* **12**, 486-494.

Wennerberg, A., Hallgren, C., Johansson, C. & Danelli, S. (1998). A histomorphometric evaluation of screw-shaped implants each prepared with two surface roughnesses. *Clinical Oral Implants Research* **9**, 11-19.

CHAPTER 35

The Transmucosal Attachment

JAN LINDHE AND TORD BERGLUNDH

Normal peri-implant mucosa
   Dimensions
   Composition
   Vascular supply

Probing gingiva and peri-implant mucosa

The wound healing that occurs following the closure of mucoperiosteal flaps during implant surgery results in the establishment of a mucosal attachment (transmucosal attachment) to the implant. The transmucosal attachment serves as a seal that prevents products from the oral cavity reaching the bone tissue that anchors the implant.

NORMAL PERI-IMPLANT MUCOSA

Dimensions

The structure and function of the mucosa that surrounds implants made of commercially pure (c.p.) titanium has been examined in man and several animal models (for review see Berglundh 1999). In an early study in the dog, Berglundh et al. (1991) compared some anatomical features of the gingiva (at teeth) and the mucosa at implants. Since the research protocol from this study was used in subsequent experiments that will be described in this chapter, details regarding the protocol are briefly outlined here.

The mandibular premolars in one side of the mandible were extracted, leaving the teeth in the contralateral jaw quadrant. After 3 months of healing following tooth extraction (Fig. 35-1) implants (i.e. the fixture part; Fig. 35-2; Brånemark System®, Nobel Biocare, Gothenburg, Sweden) made of c.p. titanium were installed according to the guidelines given in the manual for the system. Another 3 months later, abutment connection was performed (Fig. 35-3) in a second-stage procedure and the animals were placed in a careful plaque control program. This called for tooth and implant cleaning five times a week. Four months

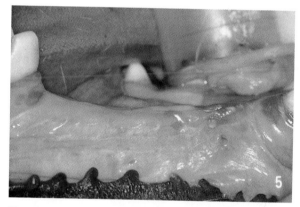

Fig. 35-1. The edentulous mandibular right premolar region 3 months following tooth extraction (from Berglundh et al. 1991).

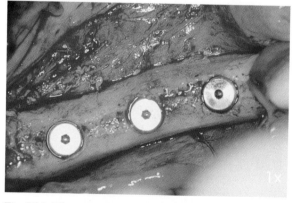

Fig. 35-2. Three titanium implants (i.e. the fixture part and cover screw; Brånemark System®) are installed.

subsequent to abutment connection, the dogs were exposed to a clinical examination following which biopsies of several tooth and all implant sites were harvested.

The clinically healthy gingiva and peri-implant

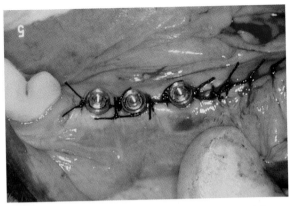

Fig. 35-3. Abutment connection is performed and the mucosa sutured with interrupted sutures.

mucosa had a pink color and a firm consistency (Figs. 35-4a,b). In radiographs obtained from the tooth sites it was observed that the alveolar bone crest was located about 1 mm apical of a line connecting the cemento-enamel junction of neighboring premolars (Fig. 35-5a). The radiographs from the implant sites disclosed that the marginal termination of the bone crest was close to the junction between the abutment and fixture part of the implant system (Fig. 35-5b).

The histologic examination of the sections (prepared in a buccal-lingual direction) revealed that the two soft tissue units, the gingiva and the peri-implant mucosa, have several features in common. The oral epithelium of the gingiva is well keratinized and is continuous with a smooth junctional epithelium that faces the crown of the tooth and ends at the cemento-enamel junction (arrow) (Fig. 35-6). The supra-alveolar connective tissue is about 1 mm high (arrows) and the periodontal ligament about 0.2-0.3 mm wide. The principal fibers extend from the root cementum in a fan-shaped pattern into the soft and hard tissues of the marginal periodontium (arrows; Fig. 35-7).

The outer surface of the peri-implant mucosa is also covered by a well-keratinized oral epithelium, which in the marginal border (arrow) connects with a barrier epithelium that is facing the abutment part of the implant (Fig. 35-8). This barrier epithelium has several features in common with the junctional epithelium found on the tooth site. The barrier epithelium is only a few cell layers thick (Fig. 35-9) and terminates about 2 mm apical of the soft tissue margin (arrows; Fig. 35-8). In a zone that is about 1-1.5 mm high, between the apical level of the barrier epithelium and the alveolar bone crest, the connective tissue appears to be in direct contact with the TiO_2 layer of the implant (Figs. 35-8, 35-10). The collagen fibers seem to originate from the periosteum of the bone crest and extend towards the margin of the soft tissue in directions parallel to the surface of the abutment.

The observation that the barrier epithelium – dur-

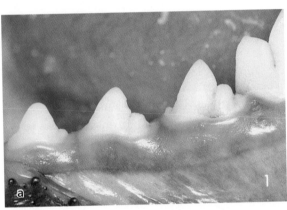

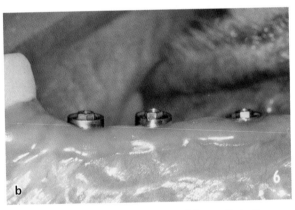

Fig. 35-4. After 4 months of careful plaque control the gingiva (a) and the peri-implant mucosa (b) are clinically healthy.

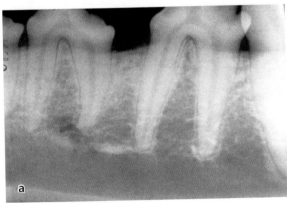

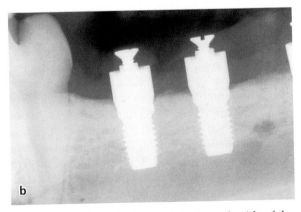

Fig. 35-5. Radiographs obtained from the premolars in the left side (a) and from the implants in the right side of the mandible (b).

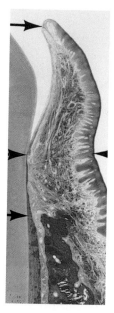

Fig. 35-6. Microphotograph of a cross-section of the buccal and coronal part of the periodontium of a mandibular premolar. Note the position of the soft tissue margin (top arrow), the apical cells of the junctional epithelium (center arrow) and the crest of the alveolar bone (bottom arrow). The junctional epithelium is about 2 mm long and the supracrestal connective tissue portion about 1 mm high.

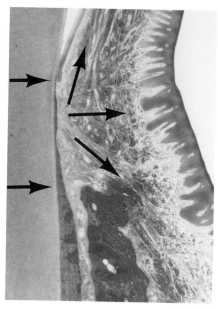

Fig. 35-7. Higher magnification of the supracresta connective tissue portion seen in Fig. 35-6. Note the direction of the principal fibers (arrows).

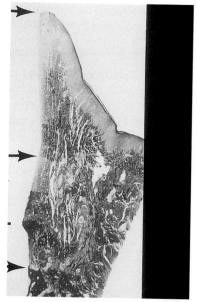

Fig. 35-8. Microphotograph of a buccal/lingual section of the peri-implant mucosa. Note the position of the soft tissue margin (top arrow), the apical cells of the junctional epithelium (center arrow) and the crest of the marginal bone (bottom arrow). The junctional epithelium is about 2 mm long and the implant/connective tissue interface about 1.5 mm high.

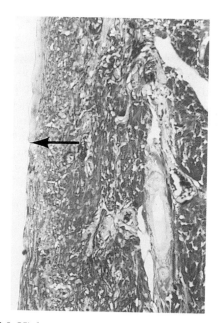

Fig. 35-9. Higher magnification of the apical portion of the barrier epithelium (arrow) in Fig. 35-8.

ing healing following the abutment connection procedure – consistently ends at a certain distance from the bone is important. During the surgical procedure an incision is made in the ridge mucosa, the marginal portion of the fixture is identified and the abutment is connected. The severed connective tissue parts of the mucosa are placed in contact with the abutment. The process of healing starts and in the "apical" parts of the abutment an interaction must occur between the connective tissue and the TiO_2 layer of the metal de-

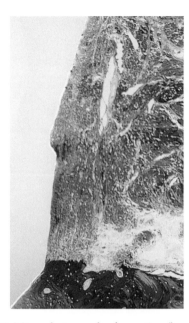

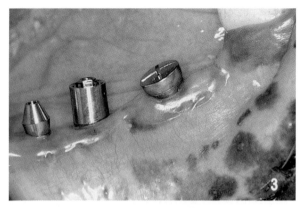

Fig. 35-11. Implants of three systems installed in the mandible of a beagle dog. Astra Tech Implants® Dental System (left), Brånemark System® (center) and ITI® Dental Implant System (right).

Fig. 35-10. Microphotograph of a section (buccal/lingual) of the implant/connective tissue interface of the peri-implant mucosa. The collagen fibers invest in the periosteum of the bone and project in directions parallel to the implant surface towards the margin of the soft tissue.

vice. This zone of interaction is apparently not recognized as a wound and therefore does not call for an epithelial lining.

Summary
The junctional and barrier epithelia are about 2 mm long and the zones of supra-alveolar connective tissue are between 1 and 1.5 mm high. Both epithelia are via hemi-desmosomes attached to the tooth/implant surface (Gould et al. 1984). The main attachment fibers (the principal fibers) invest in the root cementum of the tooth, but at the implant site the corresponding

fibers apparently originate from the periosteum of the adjacent bone crest.

In further dog experiments of similar design (Abrahamsson et al. 1996, 2001) it was observed that identical transmucosal attachment features occurred when different types of implant systems were used (e.g. Astra Tech Implants®, Dental system, Mölndal, Sweden; Brånemark System®, Nobel Biocare, Gothenburg, Sweden; ITI® Dental Implant System, Straumann AG, Waldenburg, Switzerland; 3i® Implant System, Implant Innovation Inc., West Palm Beach, FL, US) and also independent of whether the implant was initially submerged.

The clinical characteristics of the peri-implant mucosa that occurred with three different implant systems (Astra Tech, Brånemark and ITI systems) are presented in Fig. 35-11. The Astra Tech and the Brånemark implants were initially submerged and abutments installed in a second surgical procedure, while

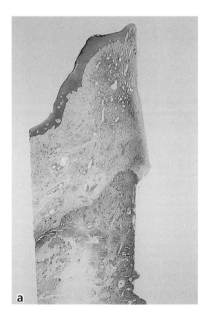

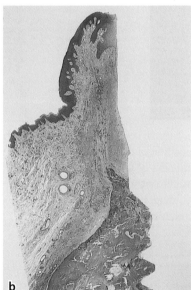

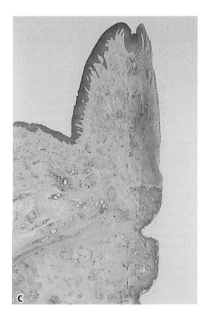

Fig. 35-12. Microphotographs illustrating the mucosa (buccal/lingual view) facing the three implant systems: (a) Astra, (b) Brånemark and (c) ITI.

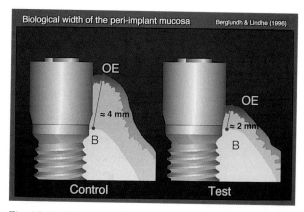
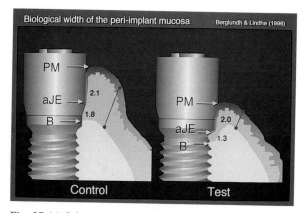

Fig. 35-13. Schematic drawing illustrating that the mucosa at the test site was reduced to about 2 mm.

Fig. 35-14. Schematic drawing illustrating that the peri-implant mucosa at both control and test sites contained a 2 mm long barrier epithelium and a zone of connective tissue that was about 1.3-1.8 mm high. Bone resorption occurred in order to accommodate the soft tissue attachment at sites with a thin mucosa.

the ITI implant was placed in a one-stage procedure. The geometry of the transmucosal part of the implants varied considerably from one system to the next. Fig. 35-12 presents microphotographs documenting the transmucosal soft tissue attachment of the three implant systems. Note that in all three sites examined:

- the profile of the implant is recorded in the adjacent tissue
- the transmucosal attachment is comprised of one barrier epithelium (about 2 mm) and one zone of connective tissue attachment (about 1-1.5 mm high).

In another study using the same model (Abrahamsson et al. 1996), it was demonstrated that the material used in the abutment part of the implant was of decisive importance for the quality of the attachment that occurred between the abutment and the surrounding mucosa. Thus, abutments made of aluminum-based sintered ceramic (Al_2O_3) allowed for the establishment of a mucosal attachment similar to that which occurred at titanium implants. Abutments made of gold alloy or dental porcelain provided inferior mucosal healing. Thus, to abutments made of such materials a zone of connective tissue attachment failed to develop. The mucosal attachment occurred instead in a more apical location, i.e. at the fixture level. Thus, during healing following abutment connection some resorption of the marginal bone must occur to "open" the titanium portion (i.e. the fixture) of the implant for the formation of a connective tissue attachment.

The biological height of the transmucosal attachment was further examined in a dog experiment by Berglundh & Lindhe (1996). All mandibular premolars were first removed and the extraction sites allowed to heal for several months after which implants (fixtures) of the Brånemark System® were installed and submerged. After 3 months of healing, abutment connection was performed. In the left side of the mandible the volume of the ridge mucosa was maintained while in the right jaw the vertical dimension of the mucosa was reduced to ≤2 mm (Fig. 35-13). In biopsies obtained after 6 months of careful plaque control, it

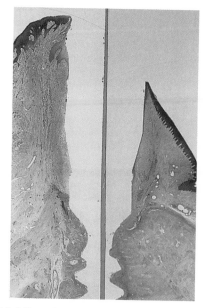

Fig. 35-15. Microphotograph illustrating the peri-implant mucosa of a normal dimension (left) and reduced dimension (right). Note the angular bone loss that had occurred at the site with the thin mucosa.

was observed that the transmucosal attachment at all implants included one barrier epithelium that was 2 mm long and one zone of connective tissue attachment that was 1-1.5 mm high.

A further examination of the peri-implant tissues at sites where the mucosa prior to abutment connection was made thin (≤2 mm), disclosed that wound healing consistently had included marginal bone resorption to establish a mucosa that was ≥ 3 mm high. In this context it must be realized that the connective tissue attachment at such sites occurred not at the abutment but at the fixture level (Figs. 35-14, 35-15).

Conclusion

The transmucosal attachment that occurs at implants made of c.p. titanium is comprised of two parts: one

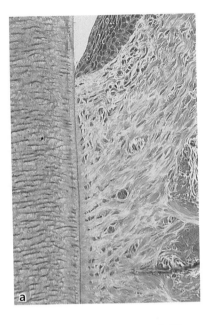
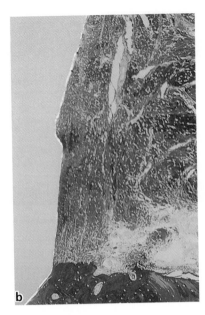

Fig. 35-16. (a) Microphotograph of a tooth with marginal periodontal tissues (buccal/lingual section). Note on the tooth side the presence of an acellular root cementum with inserting collagen fibers. The fibers are orientated more or less perpendicular to the root surface. (b) Microphotograph of the peri-implant mucosa and the bone at the tissue/titanium interface. Note that the orientation of the collagen fibers is more or less parallel (not perpendicular) to the titanium surface.

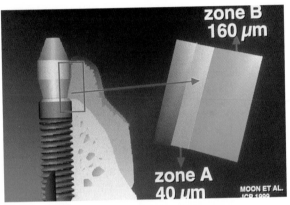

Fig. 35-17. Schematic drawing illustrating the two zones in the implant/connective tissue interface. Zone A (40 μm wide) is located next to the implant surface, while zone B (160 μm wide) resides lateral to zone A.

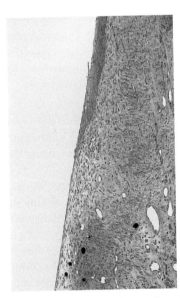

Fig. 35-18. Microphotograph of the implant/connective tissue interface of the peri-implant mucosa. A large number of fibroblasts reside in the tissue next to the implant.

barrier epithelium that has features in common with a junctional epithelium and is about 2 mm long. This barrier epithelium is continuous with one zone of connective tissue, about 1-1.5 mm high, that attaches ("integrates") to the implant and contains collagen fiber bundles, some of which invest in the periosteum of the bone crest and run a course parallel with the surface of the implant.

Composition

The quality, i.e. the composition, of the connective tissue in the supra-alveolar compartments at teeth and implants was examined by Berglundh et al. (1991). The authors stated that the main difference between the mesenchymal tissue present at a tooth and at an implant site is the occurrence of a cementum (acellular or cellular) on the root surface. From this, often-acellular extrinsic fiber cementum (Fig. 35-16a), coarse dento-gingival and dento-alveolar collagen fiber bundles project in lateral, coronal and apical directions (Fig. 35-7).

At the implant site, the collagen fiber bundles are orientated in a completely different manner. Thus, the fibers invest in the periosteum at the bone crest and either project in directions parallel with the implant surface (Fig. 35-16b), or aligned as coarse bundles which – in areas distant from the implant – run a course more or less perpendicular to the implant surface. These "horizontal fibers" appear to bend in a "vertical" direction, i.e. become parallel with the implant surface, in compartments close to the implant (Buser et al. 1992).

The connective tissue in the attachment zone at implants contains more collagen, but fewer fibroblasts and vascular structures, than the tissue in the corresponding location at teeth. A more detailed analysis of the composition of the connective tissue in the attachment zone at implants (made of c.p. titanium)

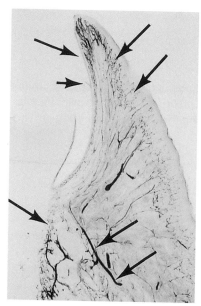 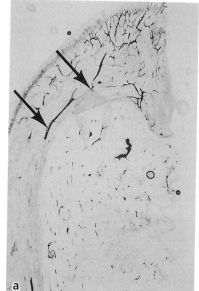 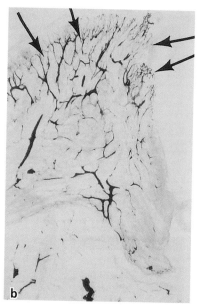

Fig. 35-19. A buccal/lingual section of a beagle dog gingiva. Cleared section. The vessels have been filled with carbon. Note the presence of a supraperiosteal vessel on the outside the alveolar bone, the presence of a plexus of vessels within the periodontal ligament, as well as vascular structures in the very marginal portion of the gingiva.

Fig. 35-20. (a) A buccal/lingual cleared section of a beagle dog mucosa facing an implant (the implant was positioned to the right). Note the presence of a supraperiosteal vessel on the outside of the alveolar bone, but also that there is no vasculature that corresponds to the periodontal ligament plexus. (b) Higher magnification (of a) of the peri-implant soft tissue and the bone implant interface. Note the presence of a vascular plexus lateral to the junctional epithelium, but the absence of vessels in the more apical portions of the soft tissue facing the implant and the bone.

was made by Moon et al. (1999) in a dog experiment. They reported that this border tissue could be divided into two zones: zone A and zone B (Fig. 35-17). Zone A is about 40 μm wide and resides next to the implant surface. In this zone there are virtually no blood vessels but a large number of fibroblasts that are orientated with their long axes parallel with the implant surface (Fig. 35-18) (collagen 67%, vascular structures 0.3% and fibroblasts 32%). In zone B – that in lateral direction is continuous with zone A and is 160 μm wide – there are fewer fibroblasts but more collagen fibers and more vascular structures (collagen 85%, vascular structures 3% and fibroblasts 11%). Abrahamsson et al. (2002) analyzed the connective tissue attachment at implant abutments with different surface roughness in dogs. It was reported (1) that the composition of the connective tissue facing the different surfaces was virtually similar, and (2) that the cell-rich interface portion was comprised of round and flat-shaped fibroblasts. From these findings it may be concluded that the attachment between the TiO_2 layer on the titanium surface and the connective tissue is maintained, and if damaged is repaired, by cellular (fibroblast) activity.

Vascular supply

The vascular supply to the gingiva comes from two different sources (Fig. 35-19). The first source is the large *supraperiosteal blood vessels*, which put forth branches to form (1) the capillaries of the connective tissue papillae under the oral epithelium and (2) the vascular plexus lateral to the junctional epithelium. The second source is the *vascular plexus of the periodontal ligament*, from which branches run in a coronal direction, pass the alveolar bone crest and terminate in the supra-alveolar portion of the free gingiva. It is, thus, important to realize that the blood supply to the zone of connective tissue attachment in the periodontium is derived from two apparently independent sources (see also Chapter 1).

Berglundh et al. (1994) observed that the vascular system of the peri-implant mucosa of dogs (Fig. 35-20a,b) originated *solely* from the large *supraperiosteal blood vessel* on the outside of the alveolar ridge. This vessel gives off branches to the supra-alveolar mucosa and forms (1) the capillaries beneath the oral epithelium and (2) a vascular plexus located immediately lateral to the barrier epithelium. Further, the implant site lacks a periodontal ligament, and consequently the site also lacks a vascular plexus in the interface between the bone and the titanium surface. As a consequence, the connective tissue part of the transmucosal attachment to titanium implants contains only a few vessels, all of which are terminal branches of the *supraperiosteal blood vessels*.

Conclusion

The gingiva at teeth and the mucosa at implants made

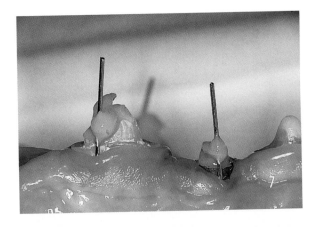

Fig. 35-21. Clinical photograph illustrating the position of the periodontal probes which via a cementing substance were attached to the tooth and the implant surface.

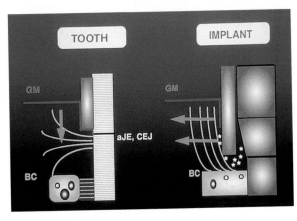

Fig. 35-22. Schematic drawing illustrating the probe in position at the tooth site and at the implant site. Note that at the tooth site the probe fails to reach the apical cells of the junctional epithelium, and that the gingiva becomes compressed in apical direction. On the implant site, the probe passes beyond the apical cells of the junctional epithelium. Note also that the peri-implant mucosa during probing is displaced mainly in the lateral direction.

of titanium have some characteristics in common, but differ in the composition of the connective tissue, the alignment of the collagen fiber bundles and the distribution of vascular structures in the compartment apical of the barrier epithelium.

PROBING GINGIVA AND PERI-IMPLANT MUCOSA

It has been demonstrated in several studies (see Chapter 18) that the tip of a periodontal probe in a "pocket depth" measurement at a *tooth site* seldom identifies the apical termination of the dentogingival epithelium. Thus, the junctional epithelium offers no resistance to the probe. If an inflammatory lesion – rich in leukocytes and poor in collagen – is present in the gingival connective tissue, the probe may penetrate beyond the apical termination of the epithelium and reach the apical-lateral border of the infiltrate. In the absence of an inflammatory lesion, e.g. following successful therapy, however, the probe frequently fails to reach the apical part of the junctional epithelium.

The outcome of probing depth measurements at *implant sites* was examined in the beagle dog model by Ericsson & Lindhe (1993) and Lang et al. (1994) and in monkeys (*Macaca fascicularis*) by Schou et al (2002).

Ericsson & Lindhe (1993) used the model by Berglundh et al. (1991) referred to above and, hence, had both teeth and implants available for examination. The gingiva at mandibular premolars and the mucosa

at correspondingly positioned implants (Brånemark System®) were, after extended periods of plaque control, considered clinically healthy. A probe with a tip diameter of 0.5 mm was inserted into the buccal "pocket" using a standardized force of 0.5 N (Fig. 35-21). The probe was anchored to the tooth or to the implant and biopsies from the various sites were harvested. The histologic examination of the biopsy material revealed that probing the dento-gingival interface had resulted in a slight compression of the gingival tissue. The resulting "histologic" probing depth was 0.7 mm. The tip of the probe was located coronal to the apical cells of the junctional epithelium (Fig. 35-22). At the implant sites, probing caused both compression and a lateral dislocation of the peri-implant mucosa, and the average "histologic" probing depth was markedly deeper than at the tooth site, namely 2.0 mm. The tip of the probe was consistently positioned deep in the connective tissue/abutment interface and apical of the barrier epithelium. The distance between the probe tip and the bone crest at the tooth sites was about 1.2 mm. The corresponding distance at the implant site was 0.2 mm. This means that at the implant sites, the probe almost made contact with the bone crest. From these observations, it may be concluded that the attachment between the implant surface and the mucosa was weaker than the corresponding attachment between the tooth and the gingiva, and that care must be exercised when data from probing depth measurements from tooth and implant sites are compared.

Lang et al. (1994) used five beagle dogs and prepared the implant (ITI® Dental Implant System) sites in such a way that at the probing experiment some regions were healthy, a few sites exhibited signs of mucositis and some sites exhibited more advanced peri-implantitis. Probes with different geometry were inserted into the pockets using a standardized probing procedure and a small force of only 0.2 N. The probes were anchored and block biopsies were harvested. The probe locations were studied in histologic ground sections. The authors reported that the mean "histologic" probing depth at healthy sites was 1.75 mm, i.e. similar to the depth (about 2 mm) recorded by Ericsson & Lindhe (1993). The corresponding depth at sites with mucositis and peri-implantitis was 1.62 mm and 3.8 mm respectively. Lang et al. (1994) further stated that at healthy and mucositis sites, the probe tip identified "the connective tissue adhesion level" (i.e. the base of the barrier epithelium) while at peri-implantitis sites, the probe exceeded the base of the ulcerated pocket epithelium by a mean distance of 0.5 mm. At such peri-implantitis sites the probe reached the base of the inflammatory cell infiltrate.

Schou et al. (2002) compared probing measurements at implants and teeth in eight cynomolgus monkeys. Ground sections were produced from tooth and implant sites that were (1) clinically healthy, (2) slightly inflamed (mucositis/gingivitis), and (3) severely inflamed (peri-implantitis/peridodontitis) and in which probes had been inserted. An electronic probe (Peri-Probe®) with a tip diameter of 0.5 mm and a standardized probing force of 0.3-0.4 N was used. It was demonstrated that the probe tip was located at a similar distance from the bone in healthy tooth sites and implant sites. On the other hand, at implants exhibiting mucositis and peri-implantitis, the probe tip was consistently identified at a more apical position than at corresponding sites at teeth (gingivitis and periodontitis). The authors concluded that (1) probing depth measurements at implant and teeth yielded different information, and (2) small alterations in probing depth at implants may reflect changes in soft tissue inflammation rather than loss of supporting tissues.

By comparing the findings from the studies reported above, it becomes apparent that meaningful – in comparison to tooth sites – probing depth and probing attachment level measurements at implant sites can be obtained only if the force used during probing is light, i.e. about 0.2–0.3 N. If a greater force is utilized, the attachment between the mucosa and the implant surface may be mechanically compromised; the mucosa becomes dislocated in lateral, "apical", direction and the probe tip is allowed to end close to the bone level. In this context it should be realized that the probing force used by different professionals varies between 0.5 and 1.3 N (Freed et al. 1983). Further, in the presence of inflammation in the peri-implant mucosa, the probe penetrates to a more "apical" position than at inflamed sites at teeth.

REFERENCES

Abrahamsson, I., Berglundh, T., Glantz, P.O. & Lindhe, J. (1998). The mucosal attachment at different abutments. An experimental study in dogs. *Journal of Clinical Periodontology* **25**, 721-727.

Abrahamsson, I., Berglundh, T., Wennström, J. & Lindhe, J. (1996). The peri-implant hard and soft tissues at different implant systems. A comparative study in the dog. *Clinical Oral Implants Research* **7**, 212-219.

Abrahamsson, I., Zitzmann, N.U., Berglundh, T., Linder, E., Wennerberg, A. & Lindhe, J. (2002) The mucosal attachment to titanium implants with different surface characteristics. An experimental study in dogs. *Journal of Clinical Periodontology* (in press).

Abrahamsson, I., Zitzmann, N.U., Berglundh, T., Wennerberg, A. & Lindhe, J. (2001). Bone and soft tissue integration to titanium implants with different surface topography. An experimental study in the dog. *Journal of Maxillofacial Implants* **16**, 323-332.

Berglundh, T. (1999). Soft tissue interface and response to microbial challenge. In: Lang, N.P., Lindhe, J. & Karring, T., eds. *Implant dentistry. Proceedings from 3rd European Workshop on Periodontology.* Berlin: Quintessence, pp. 153-174.

Berglundh, T. & Lindhe, J. (1996). Dimensions of the peri-implant mucosa. Biological width revisited. *Journal of Clinical Periodontology* **23**, 971-973.

Berglundh, T., Lindhe, J., Ericsson, I, Marinello, C.P., Liljenberg, B. & Thomsen, P. (1991). The soft tissue barrier at implants and teeth. *Clinical Oral Implants Research* **2**, 81-90.

Berglundh, T., Lindhe, J., Jonsson, K. & Ericsson, I. (1994). The topography of the vascular systems in the periodontal and peri-implant tissues dog. *Journal of Clinical Periodontology* **21**, 189-193.

Buser, D., Weber, H.P., Donath, K., Fiorellini, J.P., Paquette, D.W. & Williams, R.C. (1992). Soft tissue reactions to non-submerged unloaded titanium implants in beagle dogs. *Journal of Periodontology* **63**, 226-236.

Ericsson, I. & Lindhe, J. (1993). Probing depth at implants and teeth. *Journal of Clinical Periodontology* **20**, 623-627.

Freed, H.K, Gapper, R.L, & Kalkwarf, K.L. (1983). Evaluation of periodontal probing forces. *Journal of Periodontology* **54**, 488-492.

Gould, T.R.L., Westbury, L. & Brunette, D.M. (1984). Ultrastructural study of the attachment of human gingiva to titanium in vivo. *Journal of Prosthetic Dentistry* **52**, 418-420.

Lang, N.P, Wetzel, A.C., Stich, H. & Caffesse, R.G. (1994). Histologic probe penetration in healthy and inflamed peri-implant tissues. *Clinical Oral Implants Research* **5**, 191-201.

Moon, I-S, Berglundh, T., Abrahamsson, I., Linder, E. & Lindhe, J. (1999). The barrier between the keratinized mucosa and the dental implant. An experimental study in the dog. *Journal of Clinical Periodontology* **26**, 658-663.

Schou, S., Holmstrup, P., Stolze, K., Hjørting-Hansen, E., Fien, N.E. & Skovgaard, L.T. (2002). Probing around implants and teeth with healthy or inflamed marginal tissues. A histologic comparison in cynomolgus monkeys (*Macaca fascicularis*). *Clinical Oral Implants Research* **13**, 113-126.

CHAPTER 36

Radiographic Examination

HANS-GÖRAN GRÖNDAHL

BASIC RADIOLOGIC PRINCIPLES

Whenever radiographic methods are used to acquire information in a clinical context it is of great importance that one makes sure that the benefit of using them exceeds the costs involved. When radiographic methods are employed, the costs are not only of a monetary nature. Not least important are those which comprise radiation risks. With the growing number of subjects for whom implant treatment is considered, there is a risk that the population dose will increase. This is because both preoperatively and postoperatively, more radiographs are often required when implant treatment is performed than when conventional prosthetic treatment is done. In addition, radiographic methods which deliver higher radiation doses to the patient than do conventional methods are sometimes used.

It must thus be remembered that radiography should be based on a comprehensive clinical examination from which is determined the clinically indispensable information that can only be obtained through radiographic methods. Furthermore, the required information should be obtained with techniques yielding the smallest possible radiation dose.

SPECIAL REQUIREMENTS IN THE PERIODONTALLY COMPROMISED PATIENT

The placement of implants in the partially dentate patient and, particularly, in the periodontally compromised patient, requires careful attention to both the remaining teeth and the potential implant sites. The state of the remaining teeth in a patient in whom implant treatment is contemplated must be thoroughly evaluated to enable necessary treatment to be performed and a long-term prognosis to be made before the implant treatment is initiated. Failures to diagnose and treat pathologic conditions in and around remaining teeth can seriously compromise the results of implant therapy in both the short-term and the long-term perspective. Hence, the partially dentate patient must be subjected to a detailed clinical and radiographic examination of the teeth and surrounding alveolar bone. The examination should include the potential implant sites to determine the presence of pathologic conditions, root remnants, foreign bodies and other factors which may require surgical intervention and a subsequent healing period before a decision to insert implants can be made.

RADIOGRAPHIC TECHNIQUES FOR PRIMARY PREOPERATIVE EVALUATIONS

Intraoral and panoramic radiography

The radiographic technique of choice is the intraoral paralleling technique (Fig. 36-1) with projections perpendicular to the tangent of the dental arch in the areas of interest. The bisecting-angle technique should be avoided because this distorts vertical dimensions. To decrease doses as much as possible, fast (E or F speed) films should be used in combination with narrowly collimated X-ray beams. When applied also to the edentate regions the intraoral technique provides

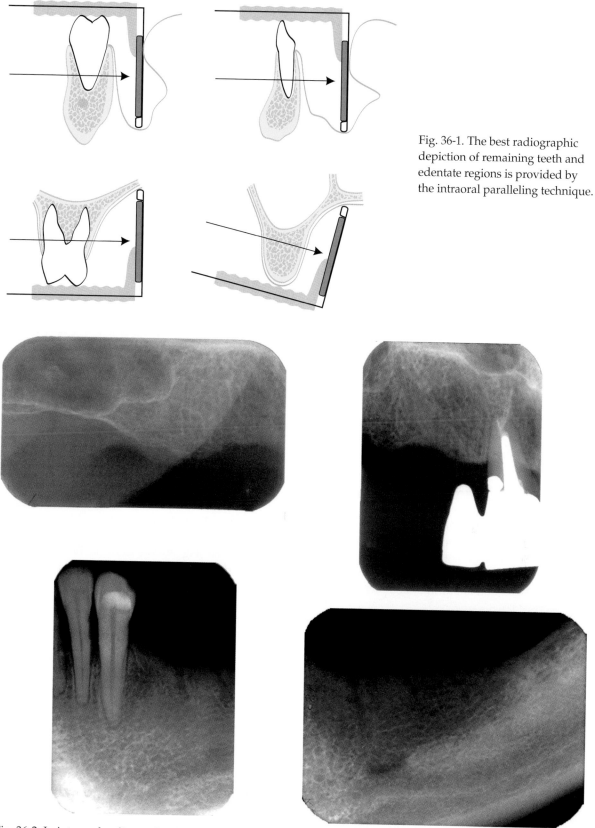

Fig. 36-1. The best radiographic depiction of remaining teeth and edentate regions is provided by the intraoral paralleling technique.

Fig. 36-2. In intraoral radiographs the mesiodistal dimension of the intended implant site can be evaluated. The number of implants that can be inserted can thus be assessed. Intraoral radiographs also provide a preliminary estimate of the vertical bone dimension.

valuable information concerning the mesiodistal dimension of the region in which implants are considered and, thus, about the number of implants that can be inserted. The radiographs also provide information about the potentially available bone height relative to, for example, the mandibular canal and the maxillary sinus (Fig. 36-2). From the intraoral radiographs it can therefore be determined in which cases implant treat-

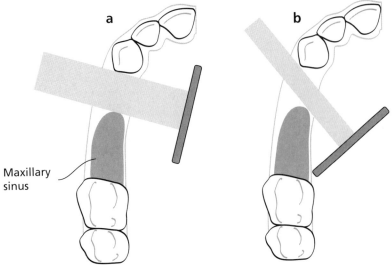

Fig. 36-3. To be able to correctly estimate horizontal distances in the region of interest, radiographs must be taken with the incident beam perpendicular to the tangent of the alveolar process (a). An incorrect beam angulation can make the mesiodistal dimension appear smaller than it is (b).

Maxillary sinus

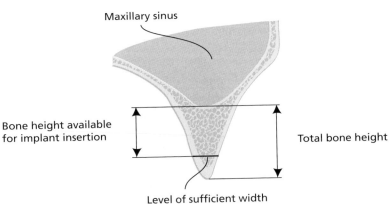

Maxillary sinus

Bone height available for implant insertion

Total bone height

Level of sufficient width

Fig. 36-4. Ideally, the implant should be surrounded by bone in its entire length. The bone height available for implant insertion therefore corresponds to the distance from a bone level, where the bone width is sufficient, to a limiting anatomic structure. Bone width is most accurately measured in tomograms. A measure of the total bone height can be used as a reference during surgery.

ment cannot be performed due to lack of available bone volume unless bone augmentation procedures are performed. It cannot, however, be determined whether implant treatment can be made because of the lack of information about the buccolingual bone dimensions.

While panoramic radiography can provide some of the information that is necessary to determine whether implant treatment may be contemplated, its lack of detail often prohibits a sufficiently accurate diagnosis of tooth-related diseases. Furthermore, in panoramic radiographs distortions are frequently found, above all concerning horizontal dimensions (Tronje 1982). This makes panoramic images less well suited for accurate estimates of the amount of bone available in the mesiodistal direction, particularly in the anterior parts of the jaws. However, when the anatomic conditions make it impossible to place intraoral films parallel to the vertical axis of the alveolar process, a better estimate of the bone height can be made in panoramic radiographs. It is important that due account is taken of the magnification in panoramic radiographs, as this can vary between panoramic units.

When implants are to be inserted between teeth, between a tooth and the mental foramen, or between a tooth and the anterior border of the maxillary sinus, supplementary intraoral radiographs should always

be obtained. They should be taken with a direction of the X-ray beam perpendicular to the tangent of the alveolar arch (Fig. 36-3). Inaccurate horizontal angulation of the X-ray beam can easily make the distances of interest appear too small or, less frequently, too large (Gröndahl et al. 1996).

RADIOGRAPHIC TECHNIQUES FOR SECONDARY PREOPERATIVE EVALUATIONS

An important objective of the preoperative radiographic evaluation of the implant patient is to determine the height and width of the bone available for implant insertion. Ideally, the bone width should allow complete coverage of all implant threads on both the buccal and the lingual sides. The available bone height must therefore be estimated from that part of the alveolar bone in which a sufficient bone width is found to a site specific anatomic border in the vertical direction, e.g. the lower border of the nasal cavity, the lower border of the maxillary sinus or the upper border of the mandibular canal. Sufficiently accurate estimations of bone width and height cannot be obtained without cross-sectional tomography. To obtain

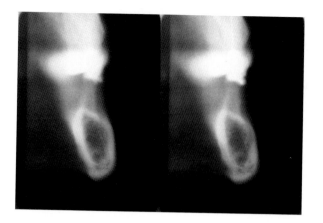

Fig. 36-5. Cross-sectional tomography of the mandible provides information about the position of the mandibular canal relative to the marginal bone crest and about the width of the mandible.

a reference measurement that can be used during surgery in order to determine to what depth the drilling can be performed, measures should also be taken from the marginal border of the alveolar crest to the anatomic structure that limits the depth to which the preparation can be made (Fig. 36-4).

To achieve ideal conditions for a successful integration of the implant with the surrounding bone it is important that good stability of the implant can be obtained during the healing period (Sennerby et al. 1992, Ivanoff et al. 1996). The most important factor in this respect is the presence of a sufficient amount of compact bone in which the implant can be anchored. The compact bone at the marginal bone crest can provide stability of the marginal part of the implant. Stability of its "apical" part can, in the anterior part of the mandible, be obtained by anchoring the implant in a layer of cortical bone at the base of the mandible. In the maxilla the lower border of the nasal cavity or the maxillary sinus can provide the necessary "apical" stability. If neither of these possibilities are at hand, stability of the "apical" part can sometimes be achieved by placing it in a layer of buccal or, more often, lingual bone cortex. When an apically located cortical layer cannot be used for anchoring the implant, a relatively narrow width of the jaw bone in combination with a thick, cortical marginal border may provide proper conditions for immediate implant stability. On the other hand, a wide alveolar bone with a thin layer of compact bone at the alveolar crest often provides less than optimal conditions for implant treatment. However, the presence of thick trabeculae in the spongious bone can provide the necessary conditions for good primary stability. Adequate information about bone width and bone content consequently is of importance in the planning of where and how to place implants. While bone width can be determined by tomography, the number and size of bone trabeculae can be difficult to evaluate. The best information is provided by the intraoral radiographs (Lindh et al. 1996a) but it must be remembered that the trabecular pattern seen in these images primarily reflects the conditions in the junctional area between compact and trabecular bone (van der Stelt 1979, Lindh et al. 1996b). Thus, the presence in the radiograph of a trabecular pattern is no guarantee that bone

trabeculae will be found in the interior parts of the jaw bone. On the other hand, the absence of such a pattern strongly indicates a definite absence of bone trabeculae. In such cases, nutrient canals are frequently seen. Absence of bone trabeculae and presence of nutrient canals are also a frequent finding in alveolar processes of a narrow buccolingual dimension.

An accurate estimate of the distance between the marginal bone crest and the lower border of the nasal cavity or the maxillary sinus is necessary in order to select implants of appropriate lengths for placement in the maxilla. Rather than choosing an implant that does not reach the border, an implant should be used that just penetrates the cortical border to obtain the necessary anchorage.

In the mandible, the distance between the marginal bone crest and the upper border of the mandibular canal must be determined with great accuracy so that the insertion of implants, or the preparation preceding the insertion of an implant, does not interfere with the infra-alveolar neurovascular bundle. If it does, permanent paresthesia may follow. Since this is a serious complication, the risk for it must be minimized. Only cross-sectional tomography can provide a good enough depiction of the mandibular canal and provide a basis for the necessary measurements (Fig. 36-5). In contrast to the maxilla, one must rather choose an implant that is a little too short than too long. Radiographic measurements are neither so accurate nor so precise that they can be completely trusted (Gröndahl et al. 1991, Ekestubbe & Gröndahl 1993, Lindh et al. 1995). One must therefore decrease the calculated distances by 1-2 mm. Due account must also be taken of the fact that the drilling procedure which precedes the implant insertion goes deeper than the implant itself. One must also take into account that the upper part of the implant cannot always be placed at the level of the marginal bone crest, e.g. in cases when an implant has to be placed buccal or lingual to the upper bone margin or when a narrow width of the marginal bone makes reduction of the bone height necessary (Fig. 36-6). Hence, the need for a reference measurement between the marginal bone crest and the upper border of the mandibular canal is obvious.

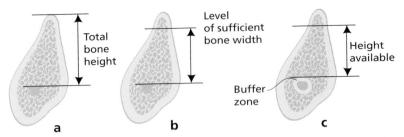

Fig. 36-6. The total height between the upper border of the mandibular canal and the marginal bone crest can be used as a reference during surgery (a). The total bone height may have to be reduced due to too narrow a marginal bone width (b). To decrease the risk for nerve damage, the bone height measurements should be further reduced (c).

Conclusion

A comprehensive clinical examination must precede the radiographic examination. The latter should be done with techniques yielding the lowest possible doses, yet all clinically necessary information.

Failure to diagnose and treat pathologic conditions in and around remaining teeth can seriously compromise the results of implant therapy.

The intra-oral paralleling technique is recommended for an estimate of horizontal dimensions of the intended implant site, and for a preliminary estimate of its vertical dimensions.

When panoramic techniques are used, supplementary intraoral radiographs should always be obtained when horizontal distances are critical.

For the best estimate of height and width of the implant site, cross-sectional tomography should be carried out.

To avoid damages of the infra-alveolar neurovascular bundle, a safety margin should be applied to the calculated distances between the marginal bone crest and the upper border of the mandibular canal.

Requirements for cross-sectional tomography

In cross-sectional tomography with conventional tomographic techniques (motion tomography) one must take into account the curvature of the jaws. For each intended implant site, the placement of the tomographic layers must be individualized. This is possible with some computer-operated tomographic units because of special software. Other units require that the patient is moved and his/her head rotated in the horizontal plane to achieve the appropriate position. A correct position of the tomographic layer implies that it is perpendicular to the tangent of the jaw curvature and to a horizontal reference plane (Fig. 36-7). In the maxilla the reference plane is the hard palate, in the mandible the mandibular canal, which in the premolar to first molar region often runs parallell to the base of the mandible. To obtain correct positions of the tomographic layer relative to one of these horizontal reference planes the patient's head may have to be slightly tilted forwards or backwards. The latter is the case for a tomographic examination in the mandibular premolar and molar regions. Incorrect angulation of the tomographic layer decreases the visibility of the cortical bone plates and the mandibu-

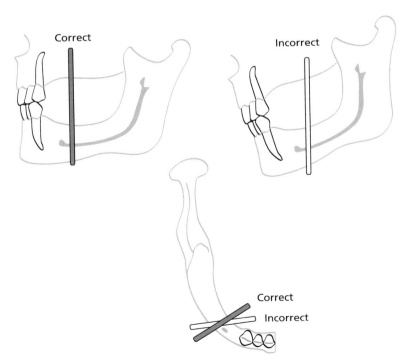

Fig. 36-7. In cross-sectional tomography a proper placement of the tomographic layers is essential for correct estimates of bone height and width.

lar canal and can lead to incorrect estimates of both bone height and width (Gröndahl et al. 1996).

Implants in the premolar and molar regions

In the maxillary premolar and molar regions, the extension of the maxillary sinus limits the amount of bone available for implant placement both in the horizontal and the vertical direction. In cases where teeth remain in the anterior part of the jaw, but are missing posteriorly, one must be able to determine the number of implants that can be inserted between the most posteriorly positioned tooth and the anterior border of the maxillary antrum. An estimate of the horizontal dimension of the potential implant site can be made from panoramic or intraoral radiographs. If the implant site is within a curved part of the jaw, measurements from panoramic radiographs can be inaccurate. Orthoradially obtained radiographs are therefore to be preferred. These can also be used for a preliminary estimate of the available bone height between the marginal bone crest and the lower border of the maxillary sinus. When the film cannot be placed parallel to the vertical axis of the alveolar process, the vertical measurements are best made in the panoramic image.

The bone height actually available for implant insertion also depends upon the width of the alveolar process. For example, when the bone width is too narrow in the marginal part of the alveolar process, the bone height has to be surgically reduced until a level is reached where the bone width is sufficient for implant placement. To determine the height of the bone in areas with proper width, supplementary tomography is often needed. This can also establish whether bone of sufficient width is present lingual to the maxillary sinus (Fig. 36-8), which neither intraoral nor panoramic radiographs can reveal (Gröndahl et al. 1996). To be able to give as accurate information as possible about the height and width of the jaw bone, the tomographic layers must be perpendicular to the hard palate and to the tangent of the jaw curvature. Because of the shape of the dental arch, each side and region must be examined with individual adjustments of the direction of the X-ray beam (Eckerdal & Kvint

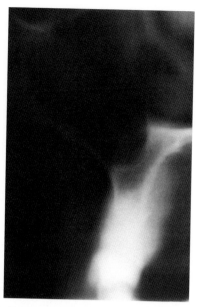

Fig. 36-8. Tomography can reveal whether bone of sufficient width for implant placement is present on the lingual side of the maxillary sinus.

1986). To obtain the best possible image quality the amount of scatter radiation should be small. This is achieved by narrowly collimated X-ray beams that also reduce the radiation dose to the patient.

In the premolar and molar regions of the mandible, the position of the mental foramen and the mandibular canal must be identified. If there is a certain minimum distance between a tooth and the anterior border of the mental foramen, it may be possible to insert an implant between the tooth and the foramen. Because the mental foramen on the one hand and the root of an anteriorly positioned tooth on the other are at different distances from the X-ray source, the horizontal distance between the tooth and the foramen can be misinterpreted. In images taken from a mesio-oblique direction the distance can appear too long, while it can appear too short in images taken from a disto-oblique direction. Therefore, the X-ray beam must be perpendicular to the tangent of the dental arch in the area between the foramen and the anteriorly positioned tooth (Fig. 36-9).

The mandibular canal often makes a more or less

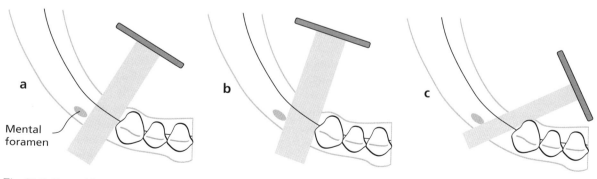

Mental foramen

Fig. 36-9. To enable a correct estimate of the distance between the mental foramen and an anteriorly positioned tooth, a correct horizontal angulation of the X-ray beam (a) is essential. Incorrect angulations can make the distance appear too large (b) or too small (c).

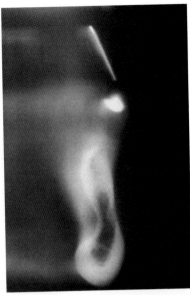

Fig. 36-10. Cross-sectional tomography of a mandibular molar region revealing a deep lingual concavity.

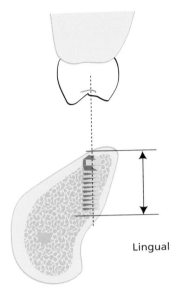

Lingual

Fig. 36-11. Cross-sectional tomography of the posterior parts of the mandible can reveal a lingual inclination of the alveolar process and the presence of a lingual fossa. It can also be used to determine proper implant placement for good primary stability as well as optimal placement and inclination relative to teeth in the maxilla.

anteriorly convex loop before it reaches the mental foramen. To avoid damaging the nerve, the distance between the anterior border of the mental foramen and the tooth must allow for some safety margin between the foramen and an implant.

The insertion of implants above the mandibular canal should be preceded by a radiographic evaluation which provides information not only on the width of the jaw bone and the distance between the upper border of the mandibular canal and the marginal bone crest, but also of the cross-sectional shape of the jaw. Not infrequently, the width of the jaw is limited by lingual concavities, most notably the submandibular gland fossa within which a branch from the facial artery can be found. Failure to take account of this cavity can lead to a lingual perforation of the mandible during surgery and damage to the artery. The subsequent bleeding can be life threatening (Bruggenkate et al. 1993). Failure to observe the sometimes pronounced lingual inclination of the posterior part of the alveolar process can also lead to unintentional perforation of the lingual border of the mandible. The necessary information about lingual concavities or a marked lingual inclination of the posterior part of the mandible can only be obtained through cross-sectional tomography (Fig. 36-10). This not only prevents serious complications, it also provides information about where sufficient amount of bone can be found in which the apical part of the implant can be anchored (Fig. 36-11). Tomographic images which include the crowns of the teeth in the maxilla also provide guidance for an appropriate buccolingual placement and inclination of the mandibular implant.

Regardless of technique used, the tomographic lay-

ers should be placed as perpendicular as possible to the mandibular canal and to the tangent of the jaw curvature. This provides the most distinct images of the canal and the borders of the mandible while offering the best possibilities for reliable measurements.

Although it is true that the mandibular canal occasionally can be difficult to perceive even in high quality tomograms (Lindh et al. 1992) the combination of intraoral, panoramic and tomographic images usually provides a solid radiographic foundation for subsequent treatment decisions.

Conclusion

The horizontal dimension of an intended implant site can be determined from intraoral or panoramic radiographs. In curved parts of the dental arch, measurements in panoramic radiographs can be inaccurate due to distortions.

Preliminary estimates of the bone height can be made in intraoral radiographs, provided that a paralleling technique has been used, or in panoramic radiographs.

Determination of the bone height actually available is best made in cross-sectional tomograms in which the width of the jaw bone also can be determined.

Cross-sectional tomography should be done perpendicular to the tangent of the dental arch and perpendicular to a horizontal reference plane, the hard palate for maxillary examinations and the base of the mandible for mandibular examinations.

To determine the distance between the mental foramen and an anteriorly positioned tooth, intraoral radiographs should be obtained with an X-ray beam

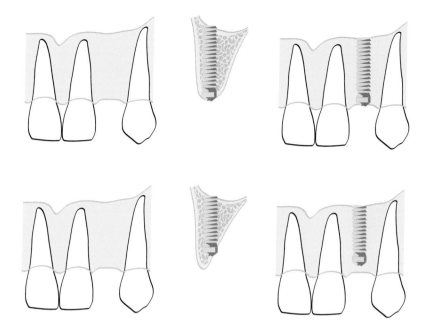

Fig. 36-12. The eventual position of the marginal part of an implant depends on the width of the marginal bone. Tomography can reveal where sufficient bone width is located and, thus, where the marginal part of the fixture will become placed once the necessary bone reduction has been made.

direction perpendicular to the tangent of the dental arch.

Cross-sectional tomography in the mandible is needed to determine the distance between the marginal bone crest and the upper border of the mandibular canal as well as the presence of lingual concavities and the inclination of the alveolar process.

Conventional versus computed tomography

Conventional tomography is to be preferred for implant treatment in the partially dentate patient not least because computed tomography delivers considerably larger radiation doses (Clark et al. 1990, Ekestubbe et al. 1993, Fredriksen et al. 1995). For conventional tomography, equipment with which multidirectional tomography – hypocycloidal or spiral – can be performed provides the best image quality due to less disturbing ghost shadows from surrounding structures (Curry et al. 1990). When computed tomography has to be done, because of lack of conventional tomographic equipment, lower doses can be achieved through a lowering of the X-ray tube current (Ekestubbe et al. 1996). If possible, so-called direct computed tomography should be done instead of axial tomography, which requires subsequent reformatting to obtain cross-sectional images. Direct computed tomography, in which the scan planes are positioned as in conventional tomography, requires a careful, individual positioning of the patient relative to each region of interest, to obtain high quality images (Lindh et al. 1995, Gröndahl et al. 1996). In many patients this can be difficult to achieve. In addition, the presence of metal components within the scan plane can cause disturbing artifacts.

Conclusion
Conventional tomography delivers lower doses than computed tomography and is therefore to be preferred.

Multidirectional tomography provides the best image quality due to a smaller amount of ghost shadows from surrounding structures.

Lower doses in computed tomography can be achieved by a lowering of the X-ray tube current.

In computed tomography, direct techniques provide better image quality than techniques requiring image reformatting. However, direct techniques can be difficult to use clinically.

The single implant case

When an implant is to be inserted between neighboring teeth, the distance between the opposing root surfaces must be determined to make sure that the implant does not become placed too close to either tooth. It has been shown that marginal bone loss can occur at the approximal bone surfaces facing the implant and that this bone loss becomes more pronounced, the closer to the tooth the implant is placed (Esposito et al. 1993, Andersson et al. 1995). Another factor which can affect the marginal bone at adjacent teeth is the vertical position at which the most marginal part of the implant is positioned relative to the neighboring teeth. A long vertical distance between the level of the marginal part of the implant and the bone level at adjacent root surfaces is unfavorable and the more so, the smaller the horizontal distance between the implant and the root surface. In a region with a narrow marginal width of the alveolar bone, and therefore a need to reduce its height to reach a bone level of sufficient width, the eventual vertical position of the marginal part of the implant can be best predicted through a preceding tomographic examination (Fig. 36-12).

The most accurate estimation of the distance be-

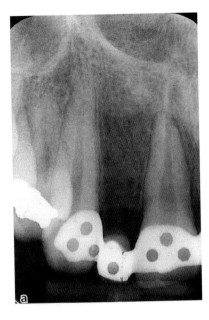

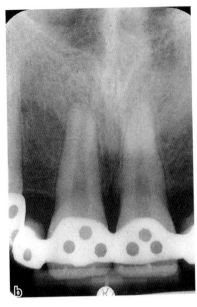

Fig. 36-13. The most correct information about the distance between opposing root surfaces is obtained from an orthoradially obtained radiograph relative to the region of implant placement (a). A mesio-oblique beam direction can make the distance appear too small (b).

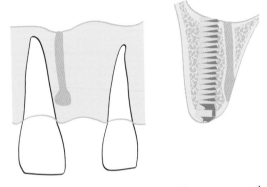

Fig. 36-14. If the horizontal distance between a tooth and the incisive canal appears too small for implant placement, tomography may reveal sufficient bone width anterior to the incisive canal.

tween neighboring root surfaces is made from orthoradially obtained intraoral radiographs (Fig. 36-13). Panoramic radiographs can easily depict such a distance incorrectly and make it either too large or too small. This is especially the case in the anterior regions of the jaws and depends on incorrect patient positioning in the panoramic machine (Gröndahl et al. 1996). In the anterior part of the maxilla, one must also take the proximity of the incisive canal into account. In cases where the mesiodistal distance between the canal and the intended implant site appears too small in an intraoral radiograph, tomography can be used to determine whether sufficient amount of bone is present buccal to the canal (Figs. 36-14, 36-15).

Tomography within a small region surrounded by teeth can lead to disturbing ghost shadows from the

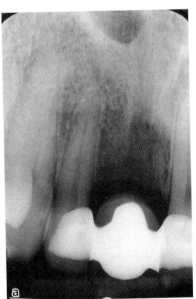

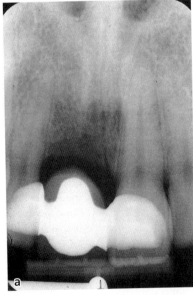

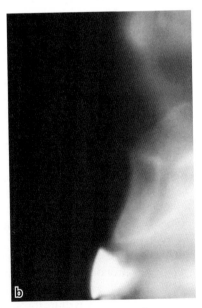

Fig. 36-15. Intraoral radiographs (a) in which the distance between the lateral incisor and the incisive canal appears too small for implant placement. A tomographic examination (b) reveals sufficient bone width anterior to the canal.

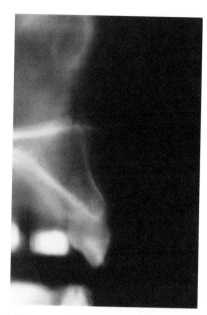

Fig. 36-16. When a tomographic technique is used with which thin tomographic layers can be produced, ghost shadows from surrounding teeth are minimized.

surrounding teeth, particularly if metal crowns or fillings are present. A technique yielding thin (≤ 2 mm) tomographic layers (Fig. 36-16) should be used (Gröndahl et al. 1996).

In many single implant cases, sufficient information about the width and height of available bone volume can be obtained from a clinical examination supplemented by intraoral radiography. Tomography is recommended when patient history, the clinical examination and intraoral radiographs lead to a suspicion of a narrow width of the jaw bone. Tomography is also recommended when a single implant is to be placed above the mandibular canal.

Conclusion

The distance between opposing root surfaces is preferably measured in intraoral radiographs. Slight variations in patient positioning can make such a distance appear too small or too large in panoramic images.

If tomography is considered necessary, thin tomographic layers should be used to avoid disturbing ghost shadows.

Tomography is recommended when a single implant is to be placed above the mandibular canal.

POSTOPERATIVE RADIOGRAPHY

At abutment connection

For some implant systems such as the Brånemark System® it is necessary to control the fit between the abutment and the implant pillar once the abutment has been seated. Even a small intermediary gap means that forces from the suprastructure will not be opti-

mally transferred to the implant pillar. Later, this can cause a fracture of the abutment screw or of the implant pillar itself. To be able to radiographically disclose a small misfit, intraoral radiographs should be used because of their high geometric resolution. The irradiation geometry has to be such that the X-ray beam is directed at a right angle to the longitudinal axis of the implant. Even small deviations from a direction of the incident radiation parallel to the upper surface of the implant and the opposing surface of the abutment can make a clinically significant gap invisible. Because of less geometric resolution and difficulties in individual adjustment of the radiation beam direction, panoramic images cannot be recommended for abutment controls.

Following crown-bridge installation

Immediately following the connection of the crowns or the bridgework, radiographs should be taken both to provide necessary information at this point in time and to serve as reference images for subsequent follow-up radiographs. The information to be obtained at this time again concerns the fit between implant and abutment, but also that between abutment and the suprastructure. In addition, the level of the marginal bone must be determined and the conditions of the bone that surrounds the implant evaluated.

High demands on image quality

To be meaningful, images obtained in conjunction with crown or bridge installation as well as at subsequent follow-ups must be of the best possible quality as regards density and contrast as well as radiation geometry. Most problems concerning density and contrast depend on suboptimal film developing. Consequently, a strict program for quality maintenance of the dark-room procedure must be followed. Throughout the follow-up period the exposure factors (tube current, tube voltage and focus-to-film distance) must be kept constant. As regards radiation geometry it is of the utmost importance that images are taken with the film placed parallel to the implant and that the radiation beam is directed perpendicular to the longitudinal axis of the implant (Fig. 36-17). Only then can a correct estimate of the marginal bone level relative to some reference point on the implant be obtained. Furthermore, the bone-implant interface zone cannot be evaluated in its entirety if the bone, reaching into the inner parts of the threads, is not visualized. Because of the high demands made in terms of irradiation geometry and resolution, intraoral radiographs are to be preferred for all follow-up examinations. In some cases it is not possible to display the implant in its entire length when a strict paralleling technique is used. In the absence of clinical signs and symptoms this is acceptable, because the significant changes that

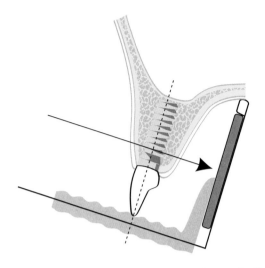

Fig. 36-17. For postoperative control radiographs the incident X-ray beam should be perpendicular to the longitudinal axis of the implant and the film.

may occur are most often found around the marginal part of the implant. In the presence of clinical signs and symptoms, such as pain, suppuration and implant mobility, radiographs obtained with the paralleling technique can be supplemented with radiographs obtained with a radiation beam angulation which visualizes the "apical" part of the implant.

Analysis of postoperative radiographs

In the postoperative radiographs the marginal bone level is compared with that in radiographs obtained immediately following crown and bridge installation (Brägger 1994). Therefore, the demands on radiographs similar in irradiation geometry, density and contrast are high (Fig. 36-18). When threaded implants are used, optimal projections in the vertical plan are at hand when the threads on both sides of the implant are clearly seen. Due to the spiral right-turned path of

the threads it is possible to determine how to adjust the angulation of the X-ray beam if the threads are not clearly seen on either side. Diffuse threads on the right side of the implant indicate a direction of the X-ray beam too much from above while diffuse threads on the left side indicate a beam direction too much from below. Corrections of the irradiation geometry are necessary to make it possible to correctly ascertain any changes in the marginal bone level over time. Even relatively moderate variations in irradiation geometry between radiographs to be compared can lead to differences in the bone level estimates. Because the marginal bone often can be relatively thin in the buccolingual direction, or less well mineralized in the early stages of the postoperative phase, a high density of the radiographs can make it less visible. This can also lead to erroneous conclusions about bone level changes.

An important aim of the postoperative controls is to determine lack of osseointegration. Because it would be both too costly and inconvenient to detach the bridgework at all postoperative clinical controls, radiography is the most feasible tool to use. Radiographically, lack of osseointegration and thus lack of clinical stability of the implant is indicated by a radiolucent line along the implant surface (Fig. 36-19). However, false-negative diagnoses can be made when the soft tissue layer surrounding the implant is not wide enough to overcome the resolution of the radiographic system, including that of the observer. On the other hand, false-positive diagnoses can be made, above all due to the presence of a so-called Mach band effect. This causes a thin area adjacent to an area of a lower radiographic density, in this case the implant, to look darker than it is in reality. Although radiography is not a perfect tool to reveal lack of osseointegration, it has been demonstrated that it performs as well in this respect as it does for approximal caries diagnosis (Sundén et al. 1995). However, an important prerequisite is radiographs of high quality.

At the postoperative follow-ups the state of the implant components should also be controlled. Al-

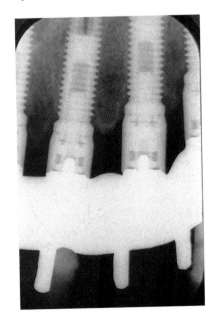

Fig. 36-18. When proper projections are used, the threads on both sides of the implant are clearly seen. The marginal bone level can be evaluated relative to a reference point on the implant.

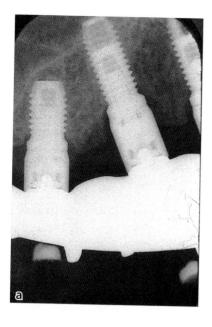
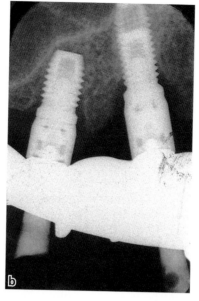

Fig. 36-19. Postoperative radiograph taken in connection with bridge installation (a) with no signs of failure. In a radiograph taken 2 years later (b) the most posterior implant is surrounded by a radiolucent zone indicating lack of osseointegration.

though infrequently, fractures of the abutment screw (Fig. 36-20) or the implant pillar itself (Fig. 36-21) occur. An indirect sign of a fracture of the abutment screw is the appearance of a gap between abutment and the implant pillar. An indirect sign of a fracture of the implant pillar itself is a pronounced, localized reduction in the marginal bone level. To be able to directly detect fractures of the implant components, the density of the radiographs has to be relatively high. Hence, there are conflicting demands on the density of the postoperative radiographs.

Subsequent follow-up examinations

Most clinically significant changes occur during the first year of function. Control radiographs 6-12 months after crown or bridge installation can therefore be recommended. When using systems for which high success rates have been reported, the application of rigid protocols for subsequent, frequent radiographic examinations can be questioned, once a clinician has established that his/her success rate is similar to that reported from multi-center studies. However, for a clinician to determine that he/she has reached a similar, high success rate, control radiography can be recommended at intervals of 2-3 years. The same is the case when systems are used for which long-term results are still lacking. Naturally, any clinical signs and symptoms which cannot be explained without radiography make this justified at any point in time.

Since pathologic conditions in and around remaining teeth can have a negative effect on the fate of the implants, control radiographs covering the teeth should also be considered. When and how often these should be obtained depends on the results of the clinical examination. However, for conditions for which the clinical examination gives little guidance, e.g. periapical lesions, annual radiography can be

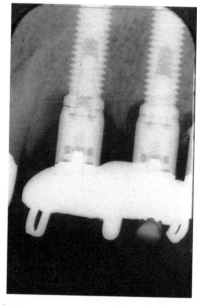

Fig. 36-20. Fracture of the abutment screw (left implant). Notice dislocation of fragments and small gap between abutment and implant pillar.

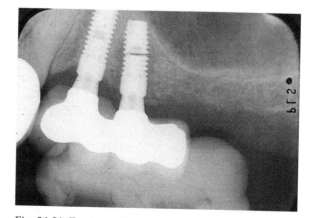

Fig. 36-21. Fracture of the implant pillar. Also notice lack of osseo-integration.

recommended until it is clear that healing is well under way.

Conclusion

For abutment controls and all follow-up examinations, intraoral radiography should be used.

Reference images should be taken immediately following crown/bridge installation.

The film should be placed parallel to the implant and the radiation beam be directed perpendicular to its longitudinal axis. Small deviations from optimal projections can make small misfits between abutment and implant or between implant and suprastructure invisible. They can also cause significant variability in bone level estimates.

The visibility of the threads can be used to determine whether proper projections have been used or not.

A quality assurance protocol should be used to maintain optimal image quality over time in terms of density and contrast.

Variations in film density and contrast can lead to erroneous conclusions regarding bone level changes over time.

Provided there is proper image quality, lack of osseointegration can be determined with a reasonably high accuracy.

A gap between the implant pillar and the abutment may be an indirect sign of abutment screw fracture.

A pronounced, localized loss of marginal bone may indicate fracture of the implant pillar.

Most clinically significant changes occur during the first year of function. Control radiographs should therefore be taken 6-12 months after crown/bridge installation.

Subsequent radiographs in asymptomatic patients should be obtained with intervals of 2-3 years dependent on system used and success rates obtained, otherwise when clinically needed.

Remaining teeth should be regularly controlled!

DIGITAL INTRAORAL RADIOGRAPHY

To avoid problems pertaining to the darkroom procedures it seems tempting to use a digital system for intraoral radiography. These could also contribute to a lowering of the radiation doses, since all digital systems require considerably lower exposures than film (Wenzel & Gröndahl 1995, Borg & Gröndahl 1996). Because implant radiography requires that rather thin and thus quite radiolucent structures – the marginal bone – should be visualized at the same time as more radiopaque structures – the implant and its components – a system with a wide dynamic range can be recommended. Among the systems so far tested, the image plate systems seem to have the widest dynamic range. They can thus show structures with a small mass density with the same exposure with which they can show structures with a considerably larger mass density. A wide dynamic range also means that exposure variations exert a limited influence on image quality (Borg & Gröndahl 1996).

Digital radiographs can be subjected to image processing with which the images can be altered to achieve task specific image characteristics. For example, density and contrast can be lowered for evaluations of the marginal bone and increased for evaluations of the implant components. It is also conceivable that the influence of the Mach band effect can be reduced through image processing. The possibilities of pseudo-coloring, that is, to assign different colors to different gray-level values, have been suggested to be of value in evaluating the bone surrounding the implant. So has the possibility to graphically display the variations in gray-level values over a distance, e.g. one that covers the implant-bone interface.

Little scientific evidence of the value of these types of image processing procedures in implant evaluation has been presented. However, subtraction of serially taken radiographs in combination with pseudo-coloring has been able to demonstrate changes between radiographs not readily apparent by unaided visual observations (Brägger & Pasquali 1989, Brägger et al. 1991). It has also been shown that edge enhancement can be of value to detect a distance between implant and surrounding bone that may be undetected in conventional radiographs (Borg et al. 2000).

REFERENCES

Andersson, B., Ödman, P., Lindvall, A-M. & Lithner, B. (1995). Single-tooth restorations on osseointegrated implants. Results and experiences from a prospective study after 2-3 years. *International Journal of Oral and Maxillofacial Implants* 10, 702-711.

Borg, E. & Gröndahl, H-G. (1996). On the dynamic range of different X-ray photon detectors in intra-oral radiography. A comparison of image quality in film, charge-coupled device and storage phosphor systems. *Dentomaxillofacial Radiology* 25, 82-88.

Borg, E., Gröndahl, K., Persson, L.G. & Gröndahl, H-G. (2000). Marginal bone level around implants assessed in digital and film radiographs: *in vivo* study in the dog. *Clinical Implant Dentistry and Related Research* 2, 10-17.

Brägger, U. (1994). Radiographic parameters for the evaluation of peri-implant tissues. *Periodontology 2000* 4, 87-97.

Brägger, U., Bürgin, W., Lang, N.P. & Buser, D. (1991). Digital subtraction radiography for the assessment of changes in peri-implant bone density. *International Journal of Oral and Maxillofacial Implants* **6**, 160-166.

Brägger, U. & Pasquali, L. (1989). Color conversion of alveolar bone density changes in digital subtraction images. *Journal of Clinical Periodontology* **16**, 209-214.

Bruggenkate, C.M., Krekeler, G., Kraaijenhagen, H.A., Foizik, C., Nat, P. & Oosterbeek, H.S. (1993). Hemorrhage of the floor of the mouth resulting from lingual perforation during implant placement: a clinical report. *International Journal of Oral and Maxillofacial Implants* **8**, 329-334.

Clark, D.E., Danforth, R.A., Barnes, R.W. & Burtch, M.L. (1990). Radiation absorbed from dental implant radiography: A comparison of linear tomography, CT scan and panoramic and intra-oral techniques. *Journal of Oral Implants* **16**, 156-164.

Curry, T., Dowdey, J. & Murry, R. (1990). *Christensen's introduction to the physics of radiology*. Philadelphia: Lea and Febiger.

Eckerdal, O. & Kvint, S. (1986). Presurgical planning for osseointegrated implants in the maxilla. A tomographic evaluation of available alveolar bone and morphological relations in the maxilla. *International Journal of Oral and Maxillofacial Surgery* **15**, 722-6.

Ekestubbe, A. & Gröndahl, H-G. (1993). Reliability of spiral tomography with the Scanora® technique for dental implant planning. *Clinical Oral Implant Research* **4**, 195-202.

Ekestubbe, A., Gröndahl, K., Ekholm, S., Johansson, P.E. & Gröndahl, H-G. (1996). Low-dose tomographic techniques for dental implant planning. *International Journal of Oral and Maxillofacial Implants* **5**, 650-659.

Ekestubbe, A., Thilander, A., Gröndahl, K. & Gröndahl, H-G. (1993). Absorbed doses from computed tomography for dental implant surgery: comparison with conventional tomography. *Dentomaxillofacical Radiology* **22**, 13-17.

Esposito, M., Ekestubbe, A. & Gröndahl, K. (1993). Radiological evaluation of marginal bone loss at tooth surfaces facing single Brånemark implants. *Clinical Oral Implant Research* **4**, 151-157.

Fredriksen, N.L., Benson, B.W. & Solokowski, T.W. (1995). Effective dose and risk assessment from computed tomography of the maxillofacial complex. *Dentomaxillofacial Radiology* **24**, 55-58.

Gröndahl, K., Ekestubbe, A. & Gröndahl, H-G. (1996). *Radiography in oral endosseuos prosthetics*. Göteborg: Nobel Biocare.

Gröndahl, K., Ekestubbe, A., Gröndahl, H-G. & Johnsson, T. (1991). Reliability of hypocycloidal tomography for the evaluation of the distance from the alveolar crest to the mandibular canal. *Dentomaxillofacial Radiology* **19**, 200-204.

Ivanoff, C.J, Sennerby, L. & Lekholm, U. (1996). Influence of mono- and bicortical anchorage on the integration of titanium implants. A study in the rabbit tibia. *International Journal of Oral and Maxillofacial Surgery* **25**, 229-235.

Lindh, C., Petersson, A. & Klinge, B. (1992). Visualisation of the mandibular canal by different radiographic techniques. *Clinical Oral Implant Research* **3**, 90-97.

Lindh, C., Petersson, A. & Klinge, B. (1995). Measurements of distances related to the mandibular canal in radiographs. *Clinical Oral Implant Research* **6**, 96-103.

Lindh, C., Petersson, A., Klinge, B. & Nilsson, M. (1996b). Trabecular bone volume and bone mineral density in the mandible. *Dentomaxillofacial Radiology* **26**, 101-106.

Lindh, C., Petersson, A. & Rohlin, M. (1996a). Assessment of the trabecular pattern prior to endosseous implant treatment. *Dentomaxillofacial Radiology* **82**, 335-343.

Sennerby, L., Thomsen, P. & Ericson, L. (1992). A morphometrical and biomechanical comparison of titanium implants inserted in rabbit cortical and cancellous bone. *International Journal of Oral and Maxillofacial Surgery* **7**, 62-71.

Sundén, S., Gröndahl, K. & Gröndahl, H-G. (1995). Accuracy and precision in the radiographic diagnosis of clinical instability in Brånemark dental implants. *Clinical Oral Implant Research* **6**, 220-226.

Tronje, G. (1982). Image distortion in rotational panoramic radiography. *Dentomaxillofacial Radiology* Suppl 3.

van der Stelt, P. (1979). *Periapical bone lesions*. Dissertation. Amsterdam: University of Amsterdam.

Wenzel, A. & Gröndahl, H-G. (1995). Direct digital radiography in the dental office. *International Dental Journal* **45**, 27-34.

CHAPTER 37

The Surgical Site

ULF LEKHOLM

Preoperative examination
   Primary judgment
   Secondary assessment
   Treatment planning

Implant placement
   Flap design

Bone drilling
Implant position
Implant direction
Cortical stabilization
Implant selection
Healing time

PREOPERATIVE EXAMINATION

The two main prerequisites for proper implant treatment are: well-performed preoperative examination and thorough pretreatment planning. In part, the outcome is also dependent on the medical condition of the patient as well as the local health and bone morphology of the area considered for implants. Consequently, adequate preoperative assessments, adapted to individual needs, have to be performed before any implant treatment is offered. When carried out, the examinations have to be cost effective and mainly based on conventional techniques, at least in the routine situation. The below protocol, based on experience of the Brånemark implant system, may constitute one practical way of working in the partially edentulous patient. In essence, the same principles can, of course, also be valid when working with other oral implant protocols. The following preoperative examination levels are thereby recommended:

1. primary judgment (prosthetic level)
2. secondary assessment (surgical level)
3. treatment planning (combined surgical-prosthetic level)

Primary judgment

When patients are referred – seeking implant treatment – the restorative dentist/prosthodontist must first of all identify the specific oral problems that the patient is having. It is also important to discuss his or her esthetic and functional demands in case of being treated, i.e. to elucidate what the patient really is expecting of the treatment. The patient can first then be presented with alternative prosthetic solutions, implant therapy being only one option. If implants are considered, there should be clear motivations given, as implant treatment ought not to be routinely offered just because a tooth or some teeth are missing. Indications for oral implants may, for example, be present in partially edentulous situations, when removable partial dentures are not accepted and fixed prosthetic reconstructions are wanted, but where remaining teeth are either too few or are so located that they can not support conventional fixed bridgework. Implants may also be indicated in connection with single tooth losses or small gap situations, especially in younger individuals, in order to avoid unnecessary mutilation of intact neighboring teeth. Furthermore, if interdental diastemas are to be preserved, only implants seem to give an acceptable solution.

However, before suggesting any implant treatment it is important to roughly judge whether it is realistic to perform the procedure, from both medical and anatomic points of view. It is also necessary to check whether the wishes/prerequisites of the patient match the potentials of the technique offered. Any sign of unrealistic expectation, including too cosmetically-oriented demands, must be identified and discussed, as otherwise problems may later arise in the patient-doctor relationship or in the patient's appreciation of performed treatment. Regarding the medical history, the same principles as in connection with any type of oral and maxillofacial surgery can be followed. The anatomic state within the area considered for implants can roughly be checked with regard to the available bone volume via palpation and/or probing through the mucosa, together with evaluation of obtained panoramic and periapical radiographs (for X-ray techniques, see Chapter 36). If implant treatment is regarded as possible, the X-rays are also used to study the health condition of remaining teeth and edentulous areas, as the need for pretreatment must be considered. No ongoing pathology, such as denture-induced stomatitis, candidosis, hyperplasia or similar mucosal disorders, root remnants, periodontitis, periapical lesions, residual jaw infections or cysts, benign or malignant tumors, etc. can be accepted at the time of implant placement. Consequently, the entire oral situation, and not only the edentulous area aimed for implants, must be examined and evaluated, i.e. a total oral rehabilitation plan should be offered to the patient. Information on possible results and risks with the treatment, as well as on expected costs and treatment duration, must also be included, before the patient is left with the decision of whether or not to accept the offered tentative treatment plan.

Before continuing with secondary assessments, there should be signs of ongoing healing regarding all pathology treated. Depending on the nature and extent of the pretreatment, the time before advancing to the next level will vary. Mucosal lesions mostly need a few weeks of healing, whereas conditions involving bone formation may take months to heal, depending on how much bone restoration is desired. In the case of tooth extractions, various modalities have been advocated regarding how soon after the tooth removal implants can be inserted. Everything from immediate placement to delayed and/or late insertion of implants has been suggested. The advantages of immediate placement may be that the patient only has to use provisional removable or fixed constructions for a short period, and that the postextraction resorption of the alveolar bone may be limited. However, various levels of implant failures (2-7%) have been found with the immediate implant insertion technique (Krump & Barnett 1991, Gelb 1993, Watzek et al. 1995), which is why delayed (5-6 weeks of healing) or even late implant insertion (9-10 months of healing) seem to be recommended in the long term. In connection with endodontic treatment of periapical lesions, at least the beginning of bone fill within the previous defect should radiographically be detected before implants are to be inserted, to prevent residual tooth infections from migrating to and contaminating the inserted implants during healing. If periodontal treatment is needed, positive results from that must be recognizable as well, and the patient should be deemed capable of continuously maintaining good oral hygiene at remaining teeth and prosthetic constructions, before any implant surgery is started. Unfavorable plaque control and ongoing periodontitis may otherwise adversely affect the implant treatment outcome (Berglund 1993, Hardt et al. 2002).

Summary: primary judgment
The specific oral problems of the patient must first be identified by the prosthodontist/restorative dentist, after which different treatment alternatives can be presented. If implant therapy is preferred, there should be clear motivations for this, together with a rough estimation of how realistic it would be to carry it out. A total treatment plan must always be offered to the patient, not just implant therapy of edentulous areas. Unrealistic expectations of the discussed treatment have to be identified and explored in order to establish a well-functioning future patient-doctor relationship. Any necessary pretreatment must be initiated and signs of healing seen, before continuing to the second examination level. Furthermore, costs and timetables for suggested treatment should be indicated before the patient is left with the decision whether or not to accept the offered tentative treatment plan.

Secondary assessment

Following the primary judgment and suggested pretreatment, the patient will advance to secondary assessments, where the medical condition of the patient as well as the local health and bone morphology of future implant sites will be analyzed in more detail from a surgical standpoint.

Medical condition
The patients must meet the physical demands for surgery in general and have such a psychological constitution that they can cope with proposed surgical procedures, i.e. show *general operability*. The same principles as in connection with any type of oral and maxillofacial surgery may thereby be followed. So far no specific condition has been identified which would exclusively prevent implant surgery, should conventional oral surgery be possible. In connection with this, patient gender does not seem to have any influence on the outcome, though theoretically women after menopause are more prone to develop osteoporotic conditions (Lekholm et al. 1994, Friberg et al. 1997, Sennerby & Rasmusson 2001). Furthermore, age does not seem to be influential for the establishment of osseointegration, as implants become bone anchored both in young (Thilander et al. 1994) as well as in elderly individuals (Köndell et al. 1988, Jemt 1993). Still, it must be remembered that elderly patients are more susceptible to infections and/or slow healing, and therefore may constitute potential risks for problems peroperatively and postoperatively (Sennerby & Rasmusson 2001). It must also be observed that implants inserted in growing individuals may end up in infra-occlusion (Ödman 1994), as they will not follow the growth and development of the jaws, but rather react like ankylotic teeth. Consequently, it is not the chronological age but rather the dental and skeletal maturation that must be considered when osseointegrated implants are to be inserted in adolescents (Thilander et al. 1994). Individual growth curves should be studied together with radiographs of the growth zones of the hand bones, to check that the body growth has ceased or is

close to completion, before any titanium implants are inserted in adolescents in general. It is only in very specific situations, and then due to psychosocial reasons mainly, that implants may be inserted in even younger individuals (Koch et al. 1996).

For implant surgery as well as other types of oral operations, there are some absolute and relative contraindications for treatment that have to be identified. As examples of absolute contraindications, the following conditions can be mentioned:

1. Systemic diseases such as developing cancer and Aids. Even HIV-positive patients ought not to be considered, as there may be future complications due to their impaired immunology defense mechanisms, resulting in increased risks for infections and impaired healing around the implants.
2. Cardiac diseases, if not otherwise stated by a responsible medical doctor. Implant surgery should be carefully considered in patients with heart valve replacements and should not be performed on patients having suffered from recent infarcts, i.e. within the latest 6-month period.
3. Deficient hemostasis and blood dyscrasias, such as hemophilia, thrombocytopenia, acute leukemia and agranulocytosis, are situations which present risks for bleeding or may limit the healing capacity of the tissues. If these conditions are suspected, the patient should be checked via laboratory tests and the responsible physician consulted.
4. Anticoagulant medication or any medication leading to impaired hemostasia, such as ASA, may result in extended peroperative and postoperative bleeding as well as enlarged postoperative hematoma formation. If anamnestic information regarding such medication is at hand, tests of coagulation and/or primary hemostasia should be carried out and the medication be interrupted, if implants are to be inserted.
5. Psychological diseases may carry potential risks as well, as such patients often have difficulties co-operating and/or lack interest in maintaining sufficient oral hygiene. They may also be using medication which could interfere with the anesthesia needed during the surgical procedure.
6. Uncontrolled acute infections, as in the respiratory tract, may negatively influence the surgical procedure or may affect the treatment result and are thus a contraindication for surgical treatment.

There are relative contraindications for implant surgery in connection with some medical and clinical situations as well as chronic health conditions. However, as long as conventional precautions for the treatment of these situations are fully considered during the surgical interventions, it may still be possible to perform implant placement.

In the case of diabetes, when there may be an increased risk for infection and reduced healing, it is still possible to perform implant surgery if the operation is carried out under antibiotic cover, and provided that the diabetic condition can be controlled via insulin medication and/or via the diet (Adell 1992, Sennerby & Rasmusson 2001). However, if unregulated diabetes is present, implant surgery ought to be avoided.

Irradiation of the jaw may be another potential risk factor for implant treatment, specifically if the jaw has been exposed to irradiation over the level of 50 Gy (Adamo & Szal 1979, Sennerby & Rasmusson 2001), due to the risk of developing osteoradionecrosis. However, it has been suggested that with the use of hyperbaric oxygen treatment preceding implant therapy, the failure rate can be reduced from around 60% to about 5% (Granström 1992). Furthermore, reports have indicated (Franzén et al. 1995) a lower risk for failures if the preoperative irradiation has been less than 40 Gy and carried out 2 years or more prior to the implant placement. However, whenever treating irradiated patients, a specific follow-up protocol is strongly recommended postoperatively, in order to detect possible problems early.

Chemotherapy has been reported (Wolfaardt et al. 1996) to have little effect on the osseointegration of implants if these have been inserted either before or after the medication period. However, if the implants are placed during the medication, or if chemotherapy is given in combination with irradiation, higher failure rates have been indicated (Wolfaardt et al. 1996).

Smoking has been found to negatively affect the long-term prognosis of osseointegration as well as the marginal bone remodeling around implants (Bain & Moy 1993, Lindqvist et al. 1996). Furthermore, it has been reported that if the patient can stop smoking just during healing, the implant survival rate may improve (Bain 1996). Other abuse situations such as the misuse of alcohol and/or drugs must be discussed too; there are potential risks for complications in such patients due to their higher propensity for bleeding, infections and/or impaired healing. Co-operation is also often lacking in affected persons, and therefore it is recommended to refer them to a psychiatrist for analysis to see if their misuse can be related to the edentulous state, and if implant treatment can help them to recover.

The cutaneous lesion lichen planus, especially the erosive type, has in some single cases resulted in total implant losses; the reason for this is not fully understood at the present time. Changes in the capacity of the epithelium to adhere to the titanium surface may be the problem, as the losses seem to occur first after some time of clinical function. However, there are also lichen patients, mainly of the reticular type, in whom implants have been inserted without creating any late problems, which is why the condition cannot be regarded as an absolute contraindication for implant treatment. Still, potential implant patients having the disease should be informed that they might experience late implant failures if treated. It has to be mentioned, too, that conditions such as pemphigus, lupus erythematosus, erythema multiforme, aphthous stomatitis, herpes zoster and herpes labialis ought to be handled with caution due to the lack of knowledge regarding these disorders in combination with oral implant placement.

Long-standing steroid medication has often been connected with the gradual development of poor bone quality, i.e. osteoporosis (Mori et al. 1997), which is why the medication may also affect the establishment and/or maintenance of implant osseointegration. However, patients suffering from severe osteoporosis have been treated with implants without developing any negative results in the long term (Friberg et al. 2001, Sennerby & Rasmusson 2001). Therefore, steroid medication/osteoporosis may not always have a deteriorating effect on implant treatment, at least not when performed in edentulous jaws.

Local health and bone morphology

It is also important to examine the intraoral health status of the soft and hard tissues as well as of the bone morphology in future implant areas, i.e. to judge the *local operability*. This is mainly done using both clinical and radiographic parameters.

The clinical assessments include inspection and palpation of the edentulous areas considered for implants, in order first of all to decide that no persisting pathology is present. Via the palpation, a second estimation of the available bone volume is performed, and any defects should thereby be identified in order to contemplate the need for augmentation procedures. If during implant placement, minor fenestrations or marginal dehiscences would occur, resulting in some exposed threads, these can in general be left unattended, as in follow-up studies no real adverse mucosal reactions have been observed due to their presence (Lekholm et al. 1996), at least not as long as good oral hygiene is provided for in the area. Consequently, it does not seem necessary to perform bone augmentations just because a few implant threads have become exposed during implant insertion. However, if the jaws contain defects of such a magnitude that the implants cannot be placed in favorable positions without having major parts of their surfaces exposed, some kind of guided bone regeneration or local bone grafting procedure might be recommended (Buser et al. 1994, Deporter 2001).

Furthermore, the clinical examination must include a judgment of the interarch and interdental spaces to see that there is accessibility for the instruments as well as for the future prosthetic construction. First of all, the patient must be able to open up sufficiently to allow access of the hand piece together with the drills. When occluding, the minimum interarch distance must be at least 5 mm to harbor the implant-supported bridgework. The smallest interdental space that can be accepted, without damaging the periodontal support of neighboring teeth, is around 7 mm, if implants of about 4 mm in diameter are to be used. It is also important to carefully study the jaw relation, as that will have an influence on the implant direction (fur-

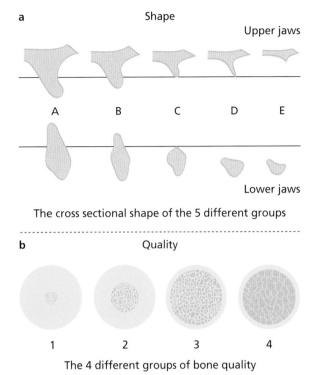

Fig. 37-1. Schematic drawings showing: (a) residual jaw shape classification, and (b) jaw bone quality classification, according to Lekholm & Zarb (1985).

ther discussed below). The final step of the clinical assessment is to take impressions for stone cast models which will later be used during the treatment planning and for the possible manufacturing of surgical position and direction stents.

Based on the radiographic assessments performed (for techniques, see Chapter 36) it is possible to also study the bone volume and the bone quality present for implants, i.e. to elucidate the *radiographic operability*. A grading into five groups depending on the resorption rate (Fig. 37-1a) has been presented for the residual jaw shape, together with a corresponding grading into four groups (Fig. 37-1b) regarding the jaw bone quality (Lekholm & Zarb 1985). Even if not specifically adapted to the partially edentulous situation, these classifications may still be roughly applied also there. The base for the radiographic examinations is mainly the panoramics and the intraoral apical images from which, besides the shape and quality parameters, important anatomic landmarks surrounding the edentulous area designated for implants can be identified. Such structures are, for example, the floor of sinusal and nasal cavities, incisive nerve, inferior alveolar nerve, roots and apices of neighboring teeth, and top of the alveolar crest. From the two-dimensional pictures it is also possible to get information about the height available for implants, but three-dimensional X-rays, tomographs mainly, are necessary to study the bone volume. Consequently, no final judgment of the operability can in critical situations be based on just intraoral radiographs and orthopantomograms, especially not if it is of crucial importance

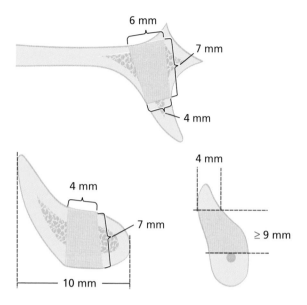

Fig. 37-2. Schematic drawings showing minimum bone volume needed for standard implants of the Bråne-mark System.

to decide the bone volume present for implants. The location of the inferior alveolar nerve must, for example, be studied via tomography in order to avoid inserting the implants in such a way that the sensation of the lower lip and neighboring soft tissues is impaired. Tomography may also be used when the clinical palpation has indicated that small bone volumes are present in other areas, e.g. in the lateral or posterior regions of the maxilla.

The minimum bone volume needed for a standard Brånemark implant (7 mm long and 3.75 mm in diameter) is where the bone height is 7-9 mm and the buccal-lingual width amounts to at least 4 mm (Fig. 37-2). When working above the inferior alveolar nerve, a minimum height of 9-10 mm is needed for a 7 mm long implant. If less height is present, no standard implant can be placed without damaging the nerve, as the drills extend about 2 mm deeper than the length of the implant. Heights of 7-9 mm may only be accepted if working in between the mental foraminae or when working in the maxillae, where it is possible to perforate the second cortex without damaging any important structures.

From the obtained radiographs, it is possible to discuss tentative locations of the implants as well as the number and type of implants needed. This can be done first after having identified where the minimum bone volume is located in a distal direction (Fig. 37-3), keeping in mind that each implant needs a gap distance of about 7 mm. However, no definite decision regarding the number and type of implants that may be used should be made preoperatively, but instead should be made during stage one surgery and after the implant sites have been finalized (see below).

Following the second assessments, the patient is again informed about the clinical procedures, possible risks, costs involved, treatment timing, etc., in order

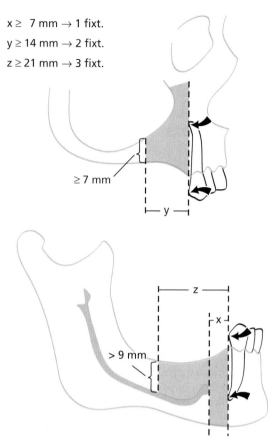

Fig. 37-3. Schematic drawings indicating location of minimum bone volume areas in distal directions, and giving distances needed for various numbers of implants. Arrows indicate prominence and apex of the nearest tooth.

to make the final decision whether or not to go on with the implant therapy suggested.

Summary: second assessment

The second level of clinical and radiographic examinations is performed in order to evaluate the operability of the patient from medical and anatomic standpoints. No specific medical condition has so far been detected that specifically excludes implant surgery. Consequently, the same absolute and relative contraindications for treatment are present when inserting implants as when performing other types of oral and maxillofacial surgery. It is recommended when treating patients at risk that trained specialists work in collaboration with the physicians responsible for the treatment of such conditions when performing the handling. The local health of edentulous areas considered for implants must be studied too, and no pathology in the soft and hard tissues of the jaws can be accepted at the time of implant placement. Radiographic evaluations are necessary in order to identify important landmarks, constituting the limits for the operation, as well as the jaw shape and bone quality in areas considered for implants. Tomography is specifically needed when working in relation to the inferior alveolar nerve, and when the clinical examination indicates small volumes of bone also in other edentulous areas of interest. The minimum bone volume required for implant surgery according to the standard protocol is about 7-9 mm of height, measured from the level where the jaw is at least 4-6 mm wide.

Treatment planning

After having collected all clinical and radiographic data, a final treatment planning is carried out by the prosthodontist/restorative dentist. As the placement of the implants is an important part of the treatment strategy, the responsible surgeon/periodontist should also take part in the detailed planning regarding implant location, i.e. participate in a team approach. It is important that the surgeon understands that the final result will never be better than what he or she establishes when placing the implants as support for the prosthetic construction. During the planning, the clinicians involved should also discuss what they want to achieve with the treatment as well as estimating whether the wishes of the patient are realistic and can be fulfilled via the proposed procedure. Unrealistic expectations must be identified and discussed with the patient, and alternative therapies suggested.

During the treatment planning, the earlier mentioned stone cast models are used to discuss what may be the best position and direction of the future implants. It is thereby the prosthodontist/restorative dentist who best knows what the prerequisites are for creating the desired prosthetic solution. The surgeon should, however, evaluate via the clinical and radiographic information obtained, whether suggested positions and directions are possible to establish in relation to the available anatomy. Possible obstacles for surgery must be identified, and alternative solutions such as local grafting and/or bone augmentation (Deporter 2001) might be suggested in case it turns out to be impossible to perform the first alternative during implant placement. The skill of the surgeon will thereby be important when having to improvise during the stage one operation.

In order to study the anticipated esthetic and functional result, a wax-up may be produced on the stone cast models, indicating the best positions and inclinations for the implants. This is specifically recommended when working in the frontal region of the maxilla, where the esthetic outcome is most obvious. The wax-up can, of course, also be used to show the patient the suggested treatment result, and it may later be used to fabricate a surgical stent too. The latter is of great help when, due to anatomic shortcomings, it is not possible to strictly follow the originally proposed guidelines for implant placement. The design of the surgical stent should be such, though, that it will not interfere with the surgical procedure. Furthermore, it should also be possible to sterilize it.

Finally, the patient is once again informed about the tentative treatment plan, possible complications, expected prognosis and protocol for annual check-ups. After obtaining the consent of the patient for suggested treatment, implant surgery can begin.

Summary: treatment planning

Based on the clinical and radiographic data collected, a final discussion regarding what is expected and possible to perform is carried out. The prosthodontist/restorative dentist conveys to the surgeon the optimal therapy for the patient, so that a team approach to the treatment planning can be established. In order to create acceptable function and esthetics, the best position and direction of the implants must be identified together with the number and type of implants that can be inserted. A wax-up may thereafter be fabricated in order to study the suggested treatment result and to show the patient the presumed outcome. Based on the waxing, a surgical stent may be fabricated, the design of which should be simple and possible to sterilize. After obtaining the consent of the patient, the implant insertion can finally be executed.

PRINCIPLE COMMENTS ON IMPLANT PLACEMENT

The main purpose of the implant surgery is to establish the anchorage for the future fixed prosthetic construction (Brånemark et al. 1985). In order to create a favorable and lasting result, it is first of all important to understand that the jawbone is a living tissue that cannot be violated during surgery. Secondly, a strict protocol for the clinical handling must be followed, based on collaboration with the general clinician/prosthodontist responsible for the restorative treatment. Consequently, all surgery must be performed according to defined and correct techniques. Those for the standard protocol of the Brånemark Implant System have been presented in detail elsewhere (Adell et al. 1985, Lekholm & Jemt 1989). In connection with the treatment of partially edentulous jaws, some factors are of specific interest as have been discussed by, for example, Palacci et al. (1995). Without giving a step-by-step presentation of how to insert the implants, the aim of the current section is to generally inform about some surgical technique aspects.

Flap design

In principle, two different flap designs can be used: vestibular or crestal incisions. At present there is no information available to indicate that one of the two techniques is more advantageous than the other. Consequently, the surgeon should select the method best suited for the individual situation. As a rule of thumb, the wider the top of the crest the more convenient it is to use a crestal incision. If the crest is high and narrow,

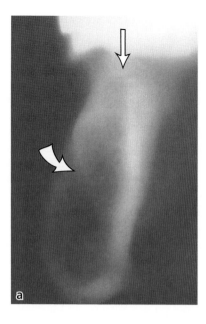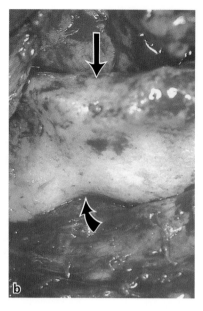

Fig. 37-4. The structure that can clearly be identified both radiographicly (a) and clinically (b) is the top of the alveolar crest, as seen in a radiograph (white thin arrow) and clinical picture (black thin arrow). In the pictures, the upper border of the mental foramina is also marked correspondingly with curved white and black arrows, respectively.

a buccal approach might be better. The decision about whether or not to place the incision within the crevicular area of close-standing teeth must be based on the space available for the implants. A general recommendation when placing implants close to teeth is to make the incision within the pocket region in order to get sufficient width of the mucosa for its nutrition and to obtain full mucosa coverage of the implant. However, whenever possible it is suggested that the gingiva of the neighboring teeth be avoided; this gives a better esthetic result for the appearance of the soft tissue margin of those teeth later on.

When elevating the mucosa, it is also necessary to properly raise the periosteum with the flap, specifically when releasing the soft tissue on the lingual side of the mandible. In this way it is possible to prevent the soft tissue from being caught by the burs or implants, should the lingual cortex be accidentally perforated during the subsequent drilling or implant installation. It is also important to detach the flap properly on the buccal side of both the maxilla and the mandible. Thereby, it will be possible to inspect any concavities and/or protrusions of the jaws, contours of tooth roots and nerve entrances, structures that may later influence the positioning of the implants. Furthermore, it will facilitate the irrigation of the bone during drilling.

In connection with the raising of the flap, a point also to consider is whether and when it is necessary to adjust the top of the alveolar crest. As a general rule of the two-stage surgical protocol, no bone should be removed from start, except when the crest is very thin. Instead, it is recommended when working in the mandible that a correction of possible sharp bone edges first takes place after the implants have been placed, i.e. at the end of stage one surgery. If possible, a few mm of bone ought to be left above the level of inserted cover screws to avoid early loading of the implants from provisional dentures. In the maxilla, the trimming should in most situations be postponed until the

second stage surgery, after checking that inserted implants have become osseointegrated. This avoids any unnecessary removal of bone which could otherwise lead to impaired prosthesis retention if, due to implant losses, the patient has to return to a conventional removable denture. In connection with an immediate implant loading technique, the bone around the implant head should be carefully adjusted so attached abutments do not have to be unnecessarily long to compensate for surrounding bone and soft tissues.

Bone drilling

It is of utmost importance to keep in mind that the bone tissue should not be exposed to adverse friction heat formation during drilling (Brånemark et al. 1985). This may easily take place, though, as the threshold level for osteocyte damage lies around 47°C, i.e. only about 10°C above the body temperature (Eriksson & Adell 1986). Consequently, all surgery must be performed at a minimum rise of temperature, which can be achieved via the use of an intermittent drilling technique, together with sharp burs, executed in a sequence of preparation steps under profuse saline irrigation (Adell et al. 1985). Whenever extremely dense bone is present, which mostly occurs in the symphysis region of the mandible, it is furthermore recommended to use an extra wide twist drill with a diameter of 3.15 mm, before pretapping and/or inserting the implants (Friberg 1994). However, when working in softer bone qualities, the drilling must be performed with the highest precision, as otherwise the entrance of the implant site may be widened too much, resulting in an unstable implant from the start. To minimize the risk of initial instability, an adjusted surgical technique using either thinner drills or wider diameter implants has been recommended (Bahat 1993, Friberg 1994, Watzek & Ulm 2001).

No implant site should be prepared in relation to

the inferior alveolar nerve without first having carried out some kind of tomographic examination, as mentioned above. The only structure that can clearly be identified both in radiographs and clinically is the top of the alveolar crest (Fig. 37-4). Consequently, that configuration has to be used as reference for all measurements, both in X-rays and when drilling. During the preparation of the site it is also of particular importance to keep an eye on the depth references of the drills in relation to the alveolar top and not only in relation to the level of the starting point for drilling. Furthermore, it must be pointed out that during the preparation of the site, the reference point for depth measurements may move in an apical direction, particularly if a narrow and drop-shaped alveolar crest is present (Fig. 37-5). When this happens, a shorter implant than originally intended must be considered, in order to ensure that it is completely bone covered on all sides and that it does not get into contact with the nerve canal.

If, during drilling in the mandible, a perforation through the lingual cortex occurs, this may be a problem, depending on where it takes place. If the perforation is located in the frontal region of the mandible, i.e. in between the canines, and provided that the periosteum has been properly released when raising the flap on the lingual side, no real adverse complications can be expected. However, if instead such a perforation occurs in the premolar or molar regions of the mandible (Fig. 37-6), an obvious risk of damaging the loop of the *vena facialis* or even *arteria submentalis* may arise, a condition which might lead to extensive and even lethal bleeding.

Implant position

If possible with regard to the anatomic situation, the implant should preferably be placed in tooth position (Fig. 37-7), both in a mesiodistal and in a buccolingual direction. To achieve this, the starting point must in most instances be located towards the buccal side of the crest in the mandible, and towards the palate in the maxilla, due to the presence of concavities that often exist in the jaws. Depending on the extent of the concavities, the starting point will be located either close to the top of the crest, as in the case of a wide alveolar process, or deeper down palatally or buccally (Fig. 37-7), if the jaw is thin in its coronal portion.

The distance between two sites should not be less than about 7 mm, measured from center to center (Fig. 37-8); otherwise there will be problems with the use of the instruments, or with the oral hygiene of the abutments later on. First the site closest to a tooth is marked, starting approximately 3.5-4 mm away from the prominence of that tooth. The following implant positions are then marked in a distal direction until reaching the area of minimum bone volume for implants, i.e. 5 versus 7(9) mm (Figs. 37-2, 37-3). The longest distance that can be accepted between two

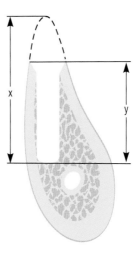

Fig. 37-5. Schematic drawing showing maximum drilling depth (x) without reaching the nerve, as measured from the top of the crest, and implant site length (y), as measured from the lowest bone level in the canal entrance.

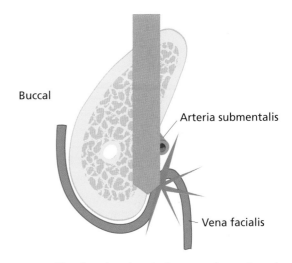

Buccal

Arteria submentalis

Vena facialis

Fig. 37-6. Sketches showing, in the premolar region of the mandible, the relation between a perforating drill tip and the loop of *vena facialis* or *arteria submentalis*.

implants has not yet been properly defined. However, the general rule is that the softer the bone, the closer the implants should be inserted. As an alternative to a reduced interimplant distance, and therefore increased number of implants, it is sometimes also possible to place wider diameter implants, as discussed below.

The second guideline regarding placement of implants in partially edentulous jaws is to insert at least three implants, instead of just two, in order to avoid overloading of the anchorage units (Rangert et al. 1989). The reason for this is that the failure rate has been reported to be higher with two than with three or more implants (Jemt & Lekholm 1993), due to the adverse biomechanics that can occur if only one rotational axis is present to distribute the loading forces. Furthermore, the implants should be placed in a tripod position (Fig. 37-8) instead of being inserted in a

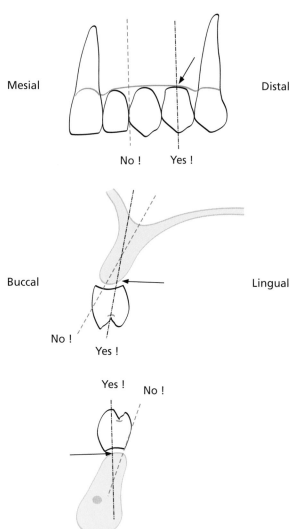

Mesial   Distal

No !   Yes !

Buccal   Lingual

No !

Yes !

Yes !   No !

Fig. 37-7. Schematic drawings showing implant positions in mesial-distal and buccal-lingual dimensions. Indicated starting points for drilling are marked with black arrows.

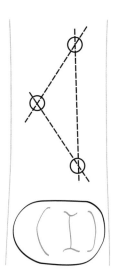

Fig. 37-8. Schematic drawing indicating a tripod placement of the implants in order to minimize individual load distribution onto each implant by creating several rotational axes.

cavities either, as no damage of surrounding tissues can be accepted just because of the wish to insert implants for prosthetic anchorage.

Implant direction

After marking the position of the implant sites it is also important, in the buccolingual and mesiodistal dimensions, to decide the direction/inclination of the implants. The general principle is still to place the implants within tooth position, which means that normally the long axis of the implant should be directed through the crown or the occlusal surface of the bridge to be. Regarding the buccolingual dimension (Fig. 37-9), the long axis of mandibular implants will mainly be directed towards the limbus part of the incisors or the palatal cusps of the teeth in the maxilla. For implants placed in the maxilla, the corresponding inclination should be towards the incisive edges of the frontal teeth or the buccal cusps of the premolars or molars of the mandible. If the starting point of the implant sites in upper jaws has been located close to the top of the crest, and if a possible concavity on the buccal side is present, the long axis of the implants may easily be leaned too far buccally to avoid fenestrations. The equivalent for the mandible may be a too lingually directed implant owing to the presence of lingual concavities. Such adverse directions can, however, impair the esthetics and function of the future bridgework (Fig. 37-7), even though angulated abutments may to some extent compensate for such a surgical error. In addition, the inclination of the implants will also be dependent on the existing jaw relation. In Applegate-Kennedy Class I, for example, the implants should be placed rather vertically in both jaws. In Class II, the implants should mainly be placed vertically in the maxilla and slightly in a buccal direc-

straight line, thereby minimizing the transmission of bending forces on to each individual implant (Rangert et al. 1989). If only one implant can be inserted, then that sole anchorage should mainly be used to support a single crown restoration. The combination of implants and teeth to support a fixed bridge construction is possible (Gunne et al. 1992, Naert et al. 1992) but ought in most cases to be avoided due to the risk of overloading the implant during function. The tooth can move via its periodontal ligament, whereas the implant is immobile due to its osseointegration. However, if a combination therapy is planned, an implant as long as possible should be inserted and the combination should be done only with a tooth that has sufficient and healthy periodontal support.

Implants should never be placed in the midline of the maxilla or the mandible, as in these positions they may either expand the suture, as between the two maxillae, and/or may compromise the esthetics. Of course, the implants should not be placed into important structures such as nerves, tooth roots and jaw

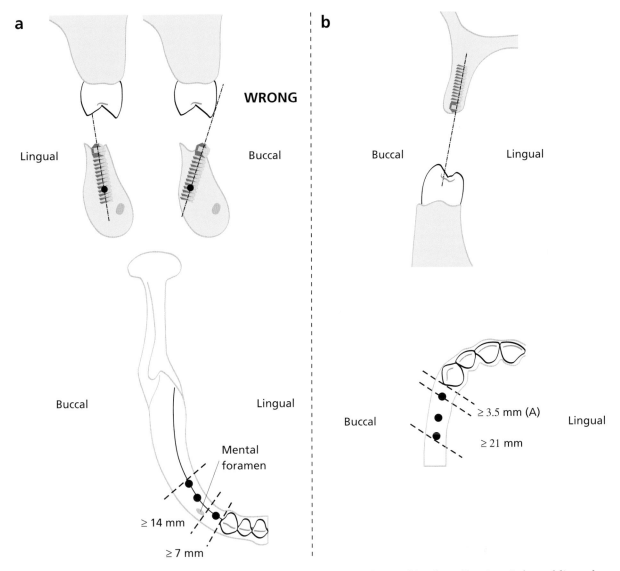

Fig. 37-9. Schematic drawings showing the most favorable starting points and implant directions in buccal-lingual dimension within (a) the mandible and (b) the maxilla. A = closest distance of a site to a tooth.

tion in the mandible, whereas in Class III, the implants should be located somewhat buccally in the maxilla and slightly lingual in the mandible. If there is too adverse a relation between the jaws, it is recommended that orthognathic surgery (Clokie 2001) be discussed with the patient prior to or in combination with the implant placement, in order to correct the abnormal jaw relation. Otherwise, too unfavorable an inclination of the implants may occur, impairing the final prosthetic function and esthetics.

For the mesiodistal dimension (Fig. 37-10), the rule is that the implant site closest to the last tooth is placed parallel to the long axis of the root of that tooth. The further distally the site is located into the molar region, on the other hand, the more violated this rule must be. In the mandible, for example, it is recommended that the most distal implants be placed in a slightly mesial direction to facilitate the connection of the abutments and the fabricated fixed bridge construction. Correspondingly, when working in the premolar regions of the maxilla, the last implant could be directed slightly distally in order to follow the mesial wall of the maxillary sinus, thereby allowing a longer implant to be placed. An alternative to this procedure would be to use some kind of sinus elevation technique (Hochwald & Davis 1992, Neukam & Kloss 2001). Finally, it has to be stressed that if the surgeon is inexperienced in directing implants, the use of a surgical stent is strongly recommended, especially when inserting implants in the front of the maxilla, where the need for an esthetic result is obvious.

Cortical stabilization

As a general recommendation, inserted implants should whenever possible be placed so they engage two cortical layers (Ivanoff et al. 1996), i.e. one at the marginal and another at the apical level of the implant. The reason for this is that studies (Sennerby et al. 1992) have shown how the cortical bone, and not the trabecular bone at least from start, provides the most

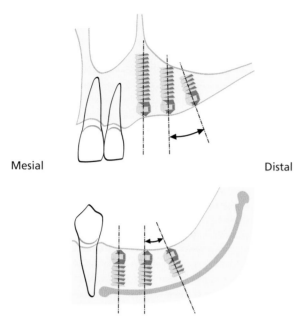

Mesial   Distal

Fig. 37-10. Drawings showing implant directions in mesial-distal dimension of posterior parts of the jaws. In the maxilla, the most distal implant is directed distally due to the orientation of the sinus wall to engage more bone. In the mandible, the implant is tilted mesially to provide better access for instruments during abutment and prosthetic procedures.

favorable anchorage of the implant. When working in the maxilla, establishing bicortical stabilization (Adell et al. 1985) is not a problem *per se* as the floor of the nasal and/or sinosal cavities can easily be perforated on purpose when drilling. However, at the same time it is necessary to point out that, after perforating the bases of the maxillae with the burs, it is important to properly measure the canal depth so that the implant does not reach above the floor of the cavities but only engages the cortical layer with its apical tip. In the frontal regions of the mandible, i.e. between the mental foraminae, it is not a problem to reach the second cortical layer either, especially when working in a slightly resorbed but low density jaw (shape group B/quality group 4; Lekholm & Zarb 1985). However, if denser bone is present as in the anterior part of the lower jaw, the implants do not have to reach all the way down to the jaw base, as long as the implants obtain good initial stability. When working above the inferior alveolar nerve, on the other hand, the requirement to engage two cortices can rarely be met for natural reasons and, therefore, implants in these regions will most often only be monocortically stabilized. It is not recommended to try to establish any contact with the cortex that surrounds the inferior alveolar nerve, as this may easily result in compression of the nerve canal. In some instances, however, the lingual cortex of the mandible can be reached and used for stabilization, especially when working with wider diameter implants. Other ways to overcome the problem with impaired monocortical stabilization are to be careful with the countersinking within the cortical layer of the entrance of the implant site, and to decide on a longer healing time before loading the implants (Sennerby et al. 1992, Friberg 1994). The nerve transpositioning technique may also be used as an alternative (Rosenquist 1994).

Implant selection

Depending on the specific condition of each site, the surgeon selects the most suitable type of implant. Whenever possible, the longest implant should as a rule be inserted, as shorter implants have a tendency to show less favorable survival rates than longer ones (Friberg et al. 1991, Lekholm et al. 1994). However, it has to be pointed out that all commercially available Brånemark System implants, including the 7 mm-long ones, have survival rates exceeding 85% after 5 years of follow-up (Lekholm 1992, Friberg et al. 2000). Consequently, it is the bone quality and not the implant length that is of importance for the outcome of the implant treatment. As a second rule, self-tapping implants are often inserted in order to minimize the time for the surgical procedure. If the bone site is very soft (quality 4; Lekholm & Zarb 1985), the longest and widest standard implant, i.e. 4 mm or 5 mm in diameter, instead ought to be placed in order to enhance the initial stability (Ivanoff et al. 1997). Conical implants and implants having a rougher surface have lately been introduced to achieve a better initial stability in soft bone situations, but so far no long-term follow-up results have been presented. If, on the other hand, the bone is of good density, shorter self-tapping implants or standard implants (after pretapping) of regular diameters (3.75 mm) will be sufficient. The latter may often be the case when working in frontal regions of the mandible. Whatever type of implant is being used, the overall aim is to reach initial stability of the implant at installation, and to create a lasting anchorage unit for the prosthetic construction via maintained osseointegration (Sennerby & Rasmusson 2001).

Healing time

The factor of most importance for how long the healing time should be, i.e. the time required before implants are loaded, is the quality of the bone of the implant site. The general and original principle has been that the softer the bone the longer the healing time. Within the mandible, the standard length of healing is 3-4 months for bone of good quality. For the maxilla the corresponding time is 5-6 months, as the bone is normally more cancellous in that jaw (Adell et al. 1985, Watzek & Ulm 2001). When soft bone is present (quality 4; Lekholm & Zarb 1985), it is recommended to extend the healing time by a month or two also in the mandible (Friberg 1994), especially if only one cortical layer is engaged by the implant. As variations may exist between different regions of the same jaw, e.g. between frontal and distal segments or even between different sites within the same region (Watzek & Ulm 2001), it is important to also individualize the healing and to allow the softest bone site to decide the timing.

By the use of resonance frequency analysis (Meredith et al. 1996) it has become possible to measure the initial implant stability of each site, i.e. the density of the bone surrounding the implant. The bone quality can thereby be repeatedly analyzed over time and the healing period individualized without using any invasive technique for the tests. An implant stability quotient (ISQ) value of above 60 has thereby been recommended (Sennerby & Meredith 2002) in order to load oral implants directly after insertion. The use of one-stage procedures for the surgical protocol is a topic of currently increasing interest (Ericsson et al. 1994, Bernard et al. 1995, Brånemark et al. 1999). Immediate loading of implants has, for example, been suggested, both in the way of using provisional constructions (Balshi & Wolfinger 1997, Schnitman et al. 1997) and/or permanent bridges for early loading (Randow et al. 1995, Ericsson et al. 2000). The latter means that the implants are unloaded only during the time it takes to fabricate the prosthesis. Favorable short-term outcome has also been presented for provisional constructions in partially edentulous jaws using temporary implants (Petrongaro 1997). However, before a general recommendation can be given for immediate protocols in partially edentulous situations, more patients representing various shape and quality groups as well as different partial jaw situations will have to be treated and followed for longer periods.

Abutment selection

Due to the great variety of abutments being available within different implant systems, it is difficult to give any detailed recommendations on what type of abutment should be selected. However, the rule of thumb should be to choose the one that gives least interference with the esthetics and function. The best choice during second-stage surgery, if uncertain about what to place, is to attach a healing abutment. This makes it possible for the prosthodontist/general practitioner to later change it to the individually best abutment, when the swelling of the soft tissue has gone down.

Summary

A well-performed surgical protocol, based on preoperative examinations and treatment planning, constitutes the prerequisite for a successful future implant treatment result. The placement of the implant within tooth position, both in mesiodistal and buccolingual dimensions, is of primary importance. Secondly, the implant should whenever possible engage two cortical layers in order to establish maximum initial stability. Thirdly, implants as long and/or as wide as possible due to anatomic conditions should also be considered, to optimize the initial stability and the subsequent osseointegration level. If surgery is performed in the correct way and using a team approach, the outcome of the surgical protocol can also be predictable and successful in partially edentulous situations, as seen in long-term follow-up studies (Naert et al. 1992, Nevins & Langer 1993, Lekholm et al. 1999). However, indications are at hand that the individual skill level of the clinician/surgeon is an important factor too for the treatment result, and consequently not only the surgical technique and/or the type of implant/implant system being utilized will influence the clinical outcome (Esposito et al. 1998).

REFERENCES

Adamo, A.R. & Szal, R.L. (1979). Timing, results and complications of mandibular reconstructive surgery. Report of 32 cases. *Journal of Oral Surgery* **37**, 755-763.

Adell, R. (1992). The surgical principles of osseointegration. In: Worthington, P. & Brånemark, P-I., eds. *Advanced Osseointegration Surgery*. Chicago: Quintessence, pp. 94-107.

Adell, R., Lekholm, U. & Brånemark, P-I. (1985). Surgical procedures. In: Brånemark, P-I., Zarb, G.A. & Albrektsson, T., eds. *Tissue-integrated Prostheses. Osseointegration in Clinical Dentistry*. Chicago: Quintessence, pp. 211-232.

Bahat, O. (1993). Treatment planning and placement of implants in the posterior maxillae: report of 732 consecutive Nobel-pharma implants. *International Journal of Oral Maxillofacial Implants* **8**, 151-161.

Bahlshi, T.J. & Wolfinger, G.J. (1997). Immediate loading of Brånemark implants in edentulous mandibles: a preliminary report. *Implant Dentistry* **6**, 83-88.

Bain, C. (1996). Smoking and implant failure – benefits of a smoking cessation protocol. *International Journal of Oral and Maxillofacial Implants* **11**, 756-759.

Bain, C.A. & Moy, P.K. (1993). The association between the failure of dental implants and cigarette smoking. *International Journal of Oral and Maxillofacial Implants* **8**, 609-616.

Berglund, T. (1993). *Studies on gingiva and peri-implant mucosa in the dog.* Thesis. Göteborg: Faculty of Odontology, University of Göteborg.

Bernard, J-P., Belser, U.C., Martinet, J-P. & Borgis, S.A. (1995). Osseointegration of Brånemark fixtures using a single step operation technique. A preliminary prospective one-year study in the edentulous mandible. *Clinical Oral Implants Research* **6**, 122-129.

Brånemark, P-I., Engstrand, P., Örnell, L-O., Gröndahl, K., Nilsson, P., Hagberg, K., Darle, C. & Lekholm, U. (1999). Brånemark Novum: A new treatment concept for rehabilitation of the edentulous mandible. Preliminary results from a prospective clinical follow-up study. *Clinical Implant Dentistry and Related Research* **1**, 2-16.

Brånemark, P-I., Zarb, G.A. & Albrektsson, T., eds. (1985). *Tissue-Integrated Prostheses. Osseointegration in Clinical Dentistry.* Chicago: Quintessence.

Buser, D., Dahlin, C. & Schenk, R.K., eds. (1994). *Guided Bone Regeneration in Implant Dentistry.* Chicago: Quintessence.

Clokie, C.M. (2001). Strategies for bone regeneration and osseointegration in completely edentulous patients. In: Zarb G., Lekholm U., Albrektsson T. & Tenenbaum H., eds. *Aging, Osteoporosis and Dental Implants.* Chicago: Quintessence, pp. 113-124.

Deporter, D. (2001). Surgical site development in the partially edentulous patient. In: Zarb G., Lekholm U., Albrektsson T. & Tenenbaum H., eds. *Aging, Osteoporosis and Dental Implants.* Chicago: Quintessence, pp. 99-112.

Ericsson, I., Randow, K., Glantz, P-O., Lindhe, J. & Nilner, K. (1994). Some clinical and radiographic features of submerged and non-submerged titanium implants. *Clinical Oral Implants Research* **5**, 185-189.

Ericsson, I., Randow, K., Nilner, K. & Peterson A. (2000). Early functional loading of Brånemark dental implants: 5-year clinical follow-up study. *Clinical Implant Dentistry and Related Research* **2**; 70-77.

Eriksson, R.A. & Adell, R. (1986). Temperatures during drilling for the placement of implants using the osseointegration technique. *Journal of Oral and Maxillofacial Surgery* **44**, 4-7.

Esposito, M., Hirsch, J-M., Lekholm, U. & Tomsen, P. (1998). Biological factors contributing to failures of osseointegrated oral implants (II). Ethiopathogenesis. *European Journal of Oral Science* **106**, 721-764.

Franzén, L., Rosenquist, J.B., Rosenquist, K.J. & Gustafsson I. (1995). Oral implant rehabilitation of patients with oral malignancies treated with radiotherapy and surgery without adjunctive hyperbaric oxygen. *International Journal of Oral and Maxillofacial Implants* **10**, 183 -187.

Friberg, B. (1994). *Bone quality evaluation during implant placement.* Odont. lic. thesis. Göteborg: Faculty of Odontology, University of Göteborg.

Friberg, B., Ekestubbe, A., Mellström, D & Sennerby, L. (2001). Brånemark implants and osteoporosis: a clinical explorative study. *Clinical Implant Dentistry and Related Research* **3**, 50-56.

Friberg, B., Gröndahl, K., Lekholm, U. & Brånemark, P-I. (2000). Long-term follow-up of severely atrophic edentulous mandibles reconstructed with short Brånemark implants. *Clinical Implant Dentistry and Related Research* **2**, 184-189.

Friberg, B., Jemt, T. & Lekholm, U. (1991). Early failures of 4641 consecutively installed Brånemark dental implants. I. A study from stage one surgery to installation of the completed prostheses. *International Journal of Oral and Maxillofacial Implants* **6**, 142-146.

Friberg, B., Nilson, H., Olsson, M. & Palmquist, C. (1997). MK II – The self-tapping Brånemark implant: 5-year results of a prospective three-center study. *Clinical Oral Implants Research* **8**, 279-285.

Gelb, D.A. (1993). Immediate implant surgery: three-year retrospective evaluation of 50 consecutive cases. *International Journal of Oral and Maxillofacial Implants* **8**, 400-408.

Granström, G. (1992). The use of hyperbaric oxygen to prevent implant loss in the irradiated patient. In: Worthington, P. & Brånemark, P-I., eds. *Advanced Osseointegration Surgery. Ap-*

plications in the Maxillofacial Region. Chicago: Quintessence, pp. 336-345.

Gunne, J., Åstrand, P., Ahlén, K., Borg, K. & Olsson, M. (1992). Implants in partially edentulous patients. A longitudinal study on bridges supported by both implants and natural teeth. *Clinical Oral Implants Research* **3**, 305-312.

Hardt, C.R.E., Gröndahl, K., Lekholm, U. & Wennström, J. (2002). Outcome of implant therapy in periodontal and non-periodontal patients. A retrospective 5-year study. *Clinical Oral Implants Research* **6**.

Hochwald, D.A. & Davis, W.H. (1992). Bone grafting in the maxillary sinus floor. In: Worthington, P. & Brånemark, P-I., eds. *Advanced Osseointegration Surgery.* Chicago: Quintessence, pp. 175-181.

Ivanoff, C.J., Sennerby, L., Johansson, C., Rangert, B. & Lekholm, U. (1997). Influence of implant diameters on the integration of screw implants. An experimental study in rabbits. *International Journal of Oral and Maxillofacial Surgery* **26**, 141-148.

Ivanoff, C.J., Sennerby, L. & Lekholm, U. (1996). Influence of mono- and bi-cortical anchorage on the integration of titanium implants. A study in the rabbit tibia. *International Journal of Oral and Maxillofacial Surgery* **25**, 229-235.

Jemt, T. (1993). Implant treatment in elderly patients. *International Journal of Prosthodontics* **6**, 456-461.

Jemt, T. & Lekholm, U. (1993). Oral implant treatment in posterior partially edentulous jaws. A 5-year follow-up report. *International Journal of Oral and Maxillofacial Implants* **8**, 635-640.

Koch, G., Bergendahl, T., Kvint, S. & Johansson, U-B., eds. (1996). *Consensus conference on oral implants in young patients.* Stockholm: Förlagshuset Gothia AB.

Köndell, P-Å., Nordenram, Å. & Landt, H. (1988). Titanium implants in the treatment of edentulousness: influence of patient's age on prognosis. *Gerodontics* **4**, 280-284.

Krump, J.L. & Barnett, B.G. (1991). The immediate implant: a treatment alternative. *International Journal of Oral and Maxillofacial Implants* **6**, 19-23.

Lekholm, U. (1992). The Brånemark Implant Technique: a standardized procedure under continuous development. In: Laney, W.R. & Tolman, D.E., eds. *Tissue Integration in Oral, Orthopedic and Maxillofacial Reconstruction.* Chicago: Quintessence, pp. 194-199.

Lekholm, U., Gunne, J., Henry, P., Higuchi, K., Lindén, U., Berström, C. & van Steenberghe, D. (1999). Survival of the Brånemark implant in partially edentulous jaws: a 10-year prospective multicenter study. *International Journal of Oral Maxillofacial Implants* **14**, 639-645.

Lekholm, U. & Jemt, T. (1989). Principles for single tooth replacement. In: Albrektsson, T. & Zarb, G.A., eds. *The Brånemark Osseointegrated Implant.* Chicago: Quintessence, pp. 117-126.

Lekholm, U., Sennerby, L., Roos, J. & Becker, W. (1996). Soft tissue and marginal bone conditions at osseointegrated implants with exposed threads. A 5-year retrospective study. *International Journal of Oral Maxillofacial Implants* **11**, 599-604.

Lekholm, U., van Steenberghe, D., Herrmann, I., Bolender, C., Folmer, T., Gunne, J., Higuchi, K., Laney, W. & Lindén, U. (1994). Osseointegrated implants in the treatment of partially edentulous jaws. A prospective 5-year multicenter study. *International Journal of Oral Maxillofacial Implants* **9**, 627-635.

Lekholm, U. & Zarb, G.A. (1985). Patient selection. In: Brånemark, P-I., Zarb, G.A. & Albrektsson, T., eds. *Tissue Integrated Prostheses. Osseointegration in Clinical Dentistry.* Chicago: Quintessence, pp. 199-209.

Lindqvist, L.W., Carlsson, G.E. & Jemt, T. (1996). The association between mandibular alveolar bone resorption around osseointegrated dental implants and cigarette smoking. *Clinical Oral Implants Research* **7**, 329-336.

Meredith, N., Alleyne, D. & Cawley, P. (1996). Quantitative determination of the stability of the implant-tissue interface using resonance frequency analysis. *Clinical Oral Implants Research* **7**, 262-267.

Mori, H., Manabe, M., Kurach, Y. & Nagumo, M. (1997). Osseointegration of dental implants in rabbit bone with low mineral density. *Journal of Oral Maxillofacial Surgery* **55**, 351-361.

Naert, J., Quirynen, M., van Steenberghe, D. & Darius, P. (1992). A six-year prosthetic study of 509 consecutively inserted implants for the treatment of partial edentulism. *Journal of Prosthetic Dentistry* **67**, 236-245.

Neukam, F.W. & Kloss, F.R. (2001). Compromised jawbone quantity and its influence on oral implant placement. In: Zarb G., Lekholm U., Albrektsson T. & Tenenbaum H., eds. *Aging, Osteoporosis and Dental Implants*. Chicago: Quintessence, pp. 85-97.

Nevins, M. & Langer, B. (1993). The successful application of osseointegrated implants to the posterior jaw. A long-term retrospective study. *International Journal of Oral and Maxillofacial Implants* **8**, 428-432.

Ödman, J. (1994). *Implants in orthodontics. An experimental and clinical study*. Thesis. Göteborg: Faculty of Odontology, University of Göteborg.

Palacci, P., Ericsson, I., Engstrand, P. & Rangert, B., eds. (1995). *Optimal Implant Positioning and Soft Tissue Management for the Brånemark System*. Chicago: Quintessence.

Petrongaro, P.S. (1997). Fixed temporization and bone-augmented ridge stabilization with transitional implants. *Practical Periodontal Aesthetic Dentistry* **9**, 1071-1078.

Randow, K., Ericsson, I., Glantz, P.-O., Lindhe, J., Nilner, K. & Pettersson, A. (1995). *Influence of early functional contacts on fixture stability, soft tissue quality and bone level integrity. A clinical pilot study*. Presented at Brånemark System 30 year Anniversary, Göteborg, Sweden.

Rangert, B., Jemt, T. & Jörneus, L. (1989). Forces and moments on Brånemark Implants. *International Journal of Oral and Maxillofacial Implants* **4**, 241-247.

Rosenquist, B. (1994). Implant placement in combination with nerve transpositioning: experience with the first 100 cases. *International Journal of Oral and Maxillofacial Implants* **9**, 522-531.

Schnitman, P.A., Wörle, P.S., Rubenstein, J.E., DaSilva, J.D. & Wang, N.H. (1997). Ten year results for Brånemark implants immediately loaded with fixed prostheses at implant placement. *International Journal of Oral Maxillofacial Implants* **12**, 495-503.

Sennerby, L. & Meredith, N. (2002). Analisi della Frequenza di Risonanza (RFA). Conoscenze attuali e implicazioni cliniche. In: Chiapasco, M. & Gatti, C., eds. *Osteointegrazione e Carico Immediato. Fondamenti biologici e applicazioni cliniche*. Milano: Masson, pp. 19-32.

Sennerby, L. & Rasmusson, L. (2001). Osseointegration surgery: Host determinants and outcome criteria. In: Zarb G., Lekholm U., Albrektsson T. & Tenenbaum H., eds. *Aging, Osteoporosis and Dental Implants*. Chicago: Quintessence, pp. 55-66.

Sennerby, L., Thomsen, P. & Ericson, L. (1992). A morphometrical and biomechanical comparison of titanium implants inserted in rabbit cortical and cancellous bone. *International Journal of Oral and Maxillofacial Implants* **7**, 62-71.

Thilander, B., Ödman, J., Gröndahl, K. & Friberg, B. (1994). Osseointegrated implants in adolescents. An alternative in replacing missing teeth? *European Journal of Orthodontics* **16**, 84-95.

Watzek, G., Haider, R., Mensdorff-Pouilly, N. & Haas, R. (1995). Immediate and delayed implantation for complete restoration of the jaw following extraction of all residual teeth: a retrospective study comparing different types of serial immediate implantation. *International Journal of Oral Maxillofacial Implants* **10**, 561-567.

Watzek, G & Ulm, C. (2001). Compromised alveolar bone quality in edentulous jaws. In: Zarb G., Lekholm U., Albrektsson T. & Tenenbaum H., eds. *Aging, Osteoporosis and Dental Implants*. Chicago: Quintessence, pp. 67-84.

Wolfaardt, J., Granström, G., Friberg, B., Narsh, J. & Tjellström, A. (1996). A retrospective study on the effect of chemotherapy on osseointegration. *Journal of Facial Somato Prosthetics* **2**, 99-107.

CHAPTER 38

Alveolar Bone Formation

NIKLAUS P. LANG, MAURÍCIO ARAÚJO AND THORKILD KARRING

During embryogenesis, in the alveolar process of the maxilla and the mandible, bone is formed within a primary connective tissue. This process is termed *intramembranous* bone formation and also occurs at the cranial vault and in the midshaft of the long bones. In contrast, bone formation in the remaining parts of the skeleton occurs via an initial deposition of a cartilage template that is subsequently replaced by bone. This process is called *endochondral* bone formation.

Alveolar bone lost as a result of disease, trauma or extensive post-extraction bone modeling may pose therapeutic problems in reconstructive and/or implant dentistry. Thus, implant placement both in the maxilla and in the mandible may be hampered by the lack of sufficient amounts of alveolar bone tissue in the recipient sites. *De novo* formation of alveolar bone in such compromised sites may be necessary and different regenerative therapies were developed to allow for bone regrowth. Various apparently successful regenerative methods may technically appear to be markedly different. They all, however, have one aspect in common: the compliance with the principles of bone biology.

BASIC BONE BIOLOGY

Bone is a specialized connective tissue that is mainly characterized by its mineralized organic matrix. The bone organic matrix is comprised of collagen, non-collagenous proteins and proteoglycans. Within this matrix, ions of calcium and phosphate are laid down in the ultimate form of hydroxyapatite. This composition allows the bone tissue (1) to resist load, (2) to protect highly sensitive organs (e.g. the central nervous system) from external forces, and (3) to participate as a reservoir of minerals that contribute to the body homeostasis.

Bone cells

Osteoblasts are the cells responsible for the formation of bone. Thus, osteoblasts synthesize the organic matrix components and control the mineralization of the matrix. Osteoblasts are located on bone surfaces exhibiting active matrix deposition and may eventually differentiate into two different types of cells: *bone lining cells* and *osteocytes*. Bone lining cells are elongated cells that cover a surface of bone tissue and exhibit no synthetic activity. Osteocytes are stellate-shaped cells that are trapped within the mineralized bone matrix but remain in contact with other bone cells by thin cellular processes. The osteocytes are organized as a syncytium that provides a very large contact area between the cells (and their processes) and the non-cellular part of the bone tissue. This arrangement allows osteocytes (1) to participate in the regulation of the blood-calcium homeostasis, and (2) to sense mechanical loading and to transmit this information to other cells within the bone.

The osteoblasts are fully differentiated cells and lack the capacity for migration and proliferation. Thus, in order to allow bone formation to occur at a given site, undifferentiated mesenchymal progenitor cells (*osteoprogenitor cells*) must migrate to the site and proliferate to become osteoblasts. Friedenstein (1973) divided osteoprogenitor cells into *determined* and *inducible osteogenic precursor cells*. The determined osteo-

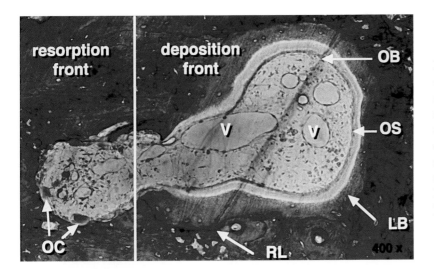

Fig. 38-1. Histological section illustrating a bone multicellular unit (BMU). Note the presence of a resorption front with osteoclast (OC) and a deposition front that contains osteoblasts (OB), and osteoid (OS). Vascular structures (V) occupy the central area of the BMU. RL = reserval line; LB = lamellar bone.

progenitor cells are present in the bone marrow, in the endosteum and in the periosteum that cover the surfaces of bone. Such cells possess an intrinsic capacity to proliferate and differentiate into osteoblasts. Inducible osteogenic precursor cells, on the other hand, represent mesenchymal cells present in other organs and tissues (e.g. muscles) that may become bone-forming cells when exposed to specific stimuli. As osteogenesis is always closely related to the ingrowth of vascular tissue, the stellate-shaped perivascular cell (the *pericyte*) is considered to be the main osteoprogenitor cell. The differentiation and development of osteoblasts from osteoprogenitor cells are dependent on the release of bone morphogenetic proteins (BMP) and other growth factors such as insulin-growth factor (IGF), platelet-derived growth factor (PDGF) and fibroblast growth factor (FGF).

The bone formation activity is consistently coupled to bone resorption that is initiated and maintained by *osteoclasts*. Osteoclasts are multinucleated cells that originate from hemopoietic precursor cells.

Modeling and remodeling

Once bone has formed, the new mineralized tissue starts to be reshaped and renewed by processes of resorption and apposition, i.e. through *modeling* and *remodeling*. Modeling represents a process that allows a change in the initial bone architecture. It has been suggested that external demands (such as load) on bone tissue may initiate modeling. Remodeling, on the other hand, represents a change that occurs within the mineralized bone without a concomitant alteration of the architecture of the tissue. The process of remodeling is important (1) during bone formation, and (2) when old bone is replaced with new bone. During bone formation remodeling enables the substitution of the primary bone (woven bone), which has low load bearing capacity, with lamellar bone which is more resistant to load.

The bone remodeling that occurs in order to allow replacement of old bone with new bone involves two processes: bone resorption and bone apposition (formation). These processes are coupled in time and are characterized by the presence of so called *bone multicellular units* (BMUs). A BMU (Fig. 38-1) is comprised of (1) a front osteoclast residing on a surface of newly resorbed bone – the resorption front, (2) a compartment containing vessels and pericytes, and (3) a layer of osteoblasts present on a newly formed organic matrix – the deposition front. Local stimuli and release of hormones, such as parathyroid hormone, growth hormone, leptin and calcitonin, are involved in the control of bone remodeling. Modeling and remodeling occur throughout life to allow bone to adapt to external and internal demands.

BONE HEALING – GENERAL ASPECTS

Healing of an injured tissue usually leads to the formation of a tissue that differs in morphology or function from the original tissue. This type of healing is called *repair*. Tissue *regeneration*, on the other hand, is a term used to describe a healing that leads to complete restoration of morphology and function.

The healing of bone tissue includes both regeneration and repair phenomena depending on the character of the injury. For example, a properly stabililized, narrow bone fracture (e.g. green stick fracture) will heal by regeneration, while a larger defect in the bone will often heal with repair. There are certain factors that may interfere with the bone tissue formation following injury, such as:

1. failure of vessels to proliferate into the wound
2. improper stabilization of the coagulum and granulation tissue in the defect
3. ingrowth of "non-osseous" tissues with a high proliferative activity
4. bacterial contamination.

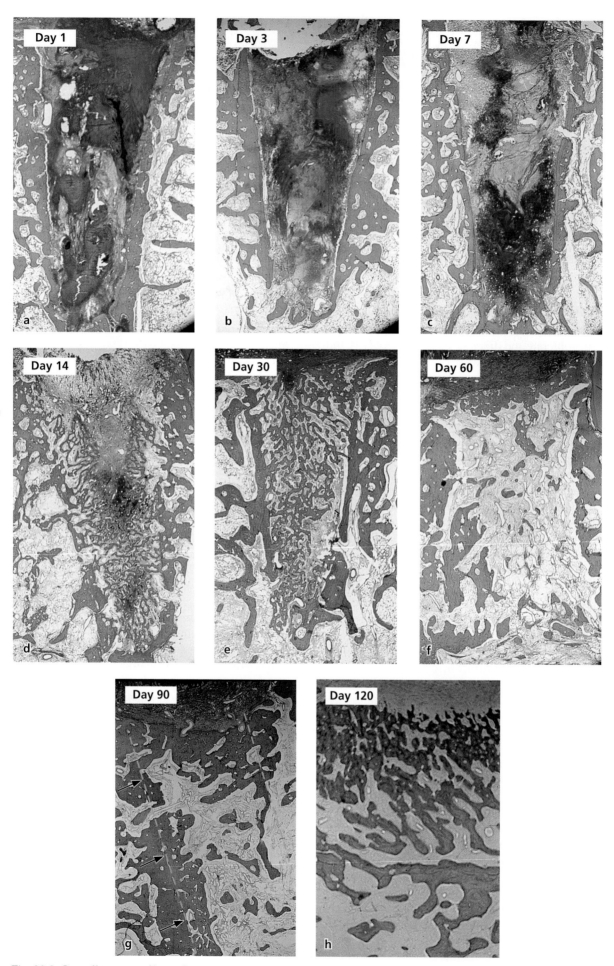

Fig. 38-2. Overall pattern of bone formation in an extraction socket. For details see text.

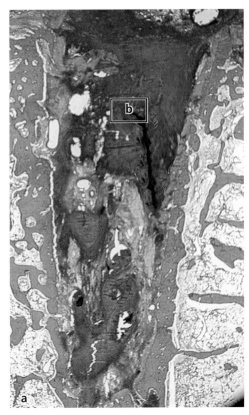

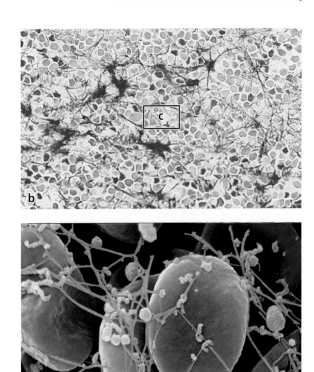

Fig. 38-3. Histologic section representing 1 day of healing (a). The socket is occupied with a blood clot that contains large numbers of erythrocytes (b) entrapped in a fibrin network, as well as platelets (blue cells in c).

The healing of a wound includes four phases:

1. blood clotting
2. wound cleansing
3. tissue formation
4. tissue modeling and remodeling.

These phases occur in an orderly sequence but, in a given site, may overlap in such a way that in some areas of the wound, tissue formation may be in progress while in other areas tissue modeling is the dominating event.

Model of bone tissue formation

The closure of an extraction socket may serve as a model to describe tissue events that lead to bone formation in a defect in the alveolar process. The healing of such an extraction socket is described in Fig. 38-2. The mandibular premolars in a group of dogs were extracted, and the healing of the extraction sites was monitored in biopsies obtained at various time intervals following tooth removal.

Overall pattern of bone formation
The empty socket was first filled with blood and a coagulum (clot) was formed (Fig. 38-2a). Inflammatory cells migrated into the coagulum and the process of wound cleansing was initiated (Fig. 38-2b). Vascular tissue and mesenchymal cells entered into the coagulum and a granulation tissue was produced (Fig. 38-2c). This granulation tissue was gradually replaced by a provisional connective tissue (Fig. 38-2d) and the formation of new bone (woven bone) started (Fig. 38-2d,e). The socket (identified by dotted lines) was gradually filled with this woven bone (Fig. 38-2e) that later on was modeled and remodeled into lamellar bone and marrow (Figs. 38-2f,g,h). Note the dotted lines and the arrows which indicate the border between the old bone and the newly formed bone

Important events in bone formation
Blood clotting: Immediately after tooth extraction, blood from the severed blood vessels will fill the cavity. Proteins derived from vessels and damaged cells initiate a series of events that lead to the formation of a fibrin network. *Platelets* form aggregates (platelet thrombi) and interact with the fibrin network to produce a *blood clot* (a coagulum) that effectively plugs the severed vessels and stops the bleeding (Fig. 38-3). The blood clot acts as a physical matrix that directs cellular movements and contains substances that are of importance for the continuation of the healing process. Thus, the clot contains substances that (1) influence mesenchymal cells (i.e. *growth factors*), and (2) affect inflammatory cells. These substances will induce and amplify the migration of various types of cells, as well as their proliferation, differentiation and synthetic activity within the coagulum.

Although the blood clot is crucial in the initial phase of wound healing, its removal is mandatory to

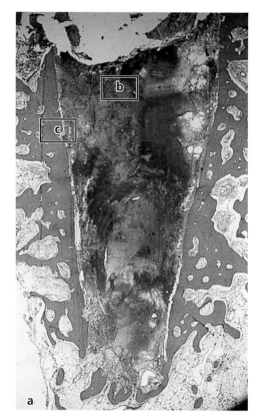

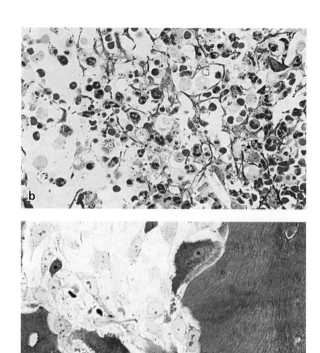

Fig. 38-4. Histologic section representing 3 days of healing (a). Note the presence of neutrophils and macrophages that engaged in wound cleansing and the breakdown of the blood clot (b). Osteoclastic activity on the surface of the walls of the old bone that lined the socket (c).

enable the formation of new tissue. Thus, within a few days after the tooth extraction, the blood clot will start to break down, i.e. "fibrinolysis" starts (Fig. 38-4).

Wound cleansing: Neutrophils and macrophages migrate into the wound, engulf bacteria and damaged tissue (Fig. 38-4) and clean the site before tissue formation starts. The neutrophils enter the wound early while macrophages come into the scene somewhat later. The macrophages are not only involved in the cleaning of the wound but they also release several growth factors and cytokines that further promote the migration, proliferation and differentiation of mesenchymal cells. Once the debris has been removed and the wound has become "sterilized", the neutrophils undergo a programmed cell death (i.e. *apoptosis*) and are removed from the site through the action of macrophages. The macrophages subsequently withdraw from the wound.

In the extraction socket, a portion of the traumatized bone facing the wound will undergo necrosis and will be removed by osteoclastic activity. Thus, osteoclasts also may participate in the wound cleansing phase of the bone healing.

Tissue formation: mesenchymal, fibroblast-like cells which migrate into the wound from, for example, the bone marrow, start to proliferate and deposit matrix components in an extracellular location (Fig. 38-5). In this manner a new tissue, i.e. *granulation tissue*, will

gradually replace the blood clot. From a didactic point of view the granulation tissue may be divided into two portions: (1) early granulation tissue, and (2) late granulation tissue. A large number of macrophages, a few mesenchymal cells, small amounts of collagen fibers and sprouts of vessels make up the early granulation tissue. The late granulation tissue contains few macrophages, but a large number of fibroblast-like cells and newly formed blood vessels present in a connective matrix. The fibroblast-like cells continue (1) to release growth factors, (2) to proliferate, and (3) to deposit a new extracellular matrix that guides the ingrowth of new cells and the further differentiation of the tissue. The newly formed vessels provide the oxygen and nutrients that are needed for the increasing number of cells in the new tissue. The intense synthesis of matrix components exhibited by these mesenchymal cells is called *fibroplasia* while the formation of new vessels is called *angiogenesis*. Through the combined fibroplasia and angiogenesis a *provisional connective tissue* is established (Fig. 38-6).

The transition of the provisional connective tissue into bone tissue occurs along the vascular structures. Thus, osteoprogenitor cells (e.g. pericytes) migrate and gather in the vicinity of the vessel. They differentiate into osteoblasts that produce a matrix of collagen fibers which takes on a woven pattern. The osteoid is hereby formed and the process of mineralization is initiated in its central portions. The osteoblasts continue to lay down osteoid and occasionally cells are

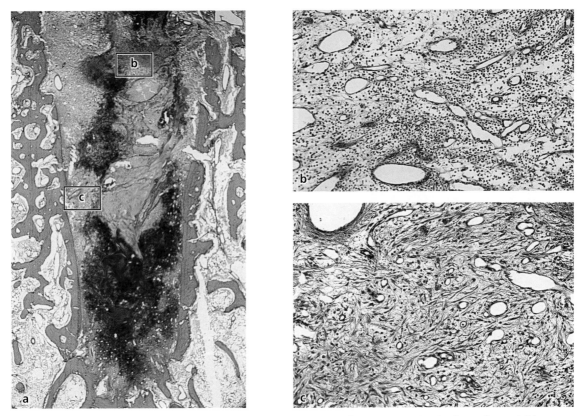

Fig. 38-5. Histologic section representing 7 days of healing (a). Note in the upper portion in the socket a richly vascularized early granulation tissue with large numbers of inflammatory cells can be seen (b), while in more apical areas a tissue including large numbers of fibroblast-like cells is present, i.e. late granulation tissue (c).

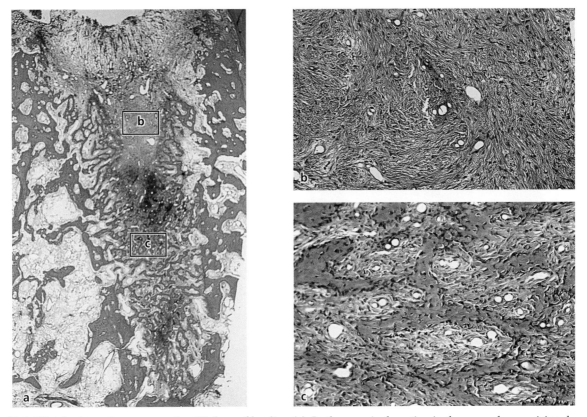

Fig. 38-6. Histologic section representing 14 days of healing (a). In the marginal portion in the wound a provisional connective tissue rich in fibroblast-like cells is formed (b). The formation of woven bone has at this time interval already begun in more apical regions of the bone defect (c).

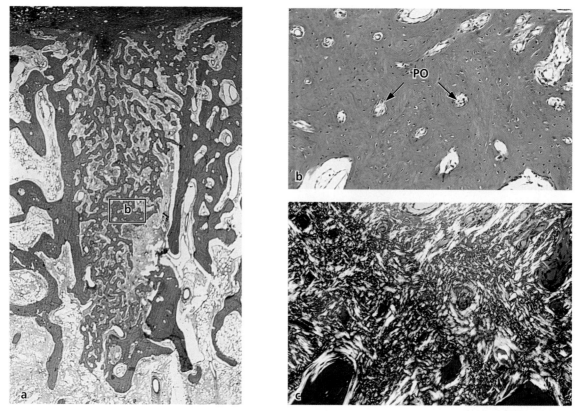

Fig. 38-7. Histologic section representing 30 days of healing (a). The socket is filled with woven bone. This woven bone contains a large number of cells and primary osteons (PO;b). The woven pattern of the collagen fibers of the woven bone is illustrated in (c) (polarized light).

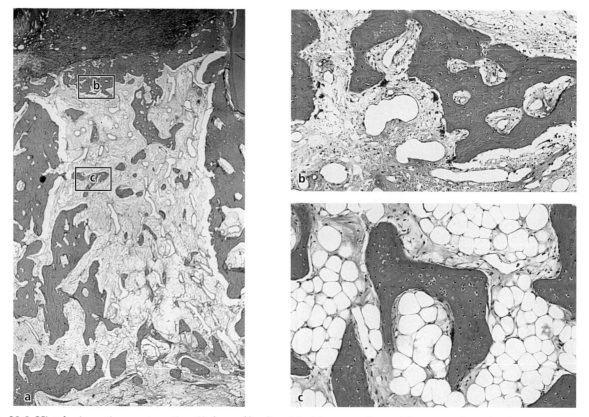

Fig. 38-8. Histologic section representing 60 days of healing (a). A large portion of the woven bone has been replaced with bone marrow through osteoclastic activity and subsequent bone marrow formation, i.e. modeling (b). Note in (c) the large number of adipocytes that reside in a tissue that still contains portions of woven bone.

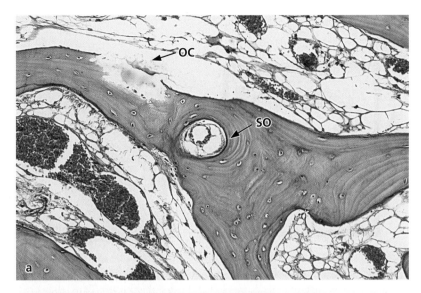

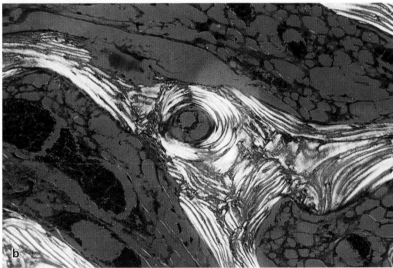

Fig. 38-9. Histologic section representing a bone tissue after 60 days of healing. Note in (a) the presence of osteoclasts (OC) on the surface of a secondary osteon (SO) within the bone trabeculae. (b) The concentric pattern of the collagen fibers of the lamellar bone within the secondary osteon (polarized light).

trapped in the matrix and become osteocytes. The newly formed bone is called *woven bone* (Fig. 38-7).

The woven bone is the first type of bone to be formed and is characterized by (1) its rapid deposition along the route of vessels, (2) the poorly organized collagen matrix, (3) the large number of osteoblasts that are trapped in its mineralized matrix, and (4) its low load-bearing capacity. The woven bone forms as finger-like projections along the newly formed vessels. Trabeculae of woven bone are shaped and encircle the vessel. The trabeculae become thicker through the deposition of further woven bone, cells (osteocyts) are entrapped and the first set of osteons, the *primary osteons* are organized. The woven bone is occasionally reinforced by the deposition of so called *parallel-fibered bone* that has its collagen fibers organized not in a woven but in a concentric pattern.

Tissue modeling and remodeling: The initial bone formation is a fast process. Within a few weeks, the entire extraction socket will be occupied with woven bone or as this tissue is also called, *primary bone spongiosa*. The woven bone offers (1) a stable scaffold, (2) a solid surface, (3) a source of osteoprogenitor cells, and (4) ample blood supply for cell function and matrix mineralization.

The woven bone with its primary osteons is gradually replaced by lamellar bone and bone marrow (Figs. 38-8, 38-9) through the processes of modeling and remodeling as described earlier (Fig. 38-10). In the remodeling process the primary osteons are replaced with secondary osteons. The woven bone is first through osteoclastic activity resorbed to a certain level. This level of the resorption front will establish the so-called reversal line, which is also the starting point for the new bone formation building up a secondary osteon. Although the modeling and remodeling may start early it will take several months until all woven bone in the extraction socket is replaced by bone marrow and lamellar bone (Fig. 38-11).

In summary: Following tooth extraction, the first 24 hours are characterized by the formation of a *blood clot* and the starting of *hemolysis* (Fig. 38-12a). Within 2-3 days the blood clot is contracting and is replaced by the *formation of a granulation tissue* with the *blood vessels* and collagen fibers (Fig. 38-12b). After 3 days, an increased density of fibroblasts is visible in the clot and the *proliferation of epithelium* from the wound mar-

Woven bone   BMU   Lamellar bone

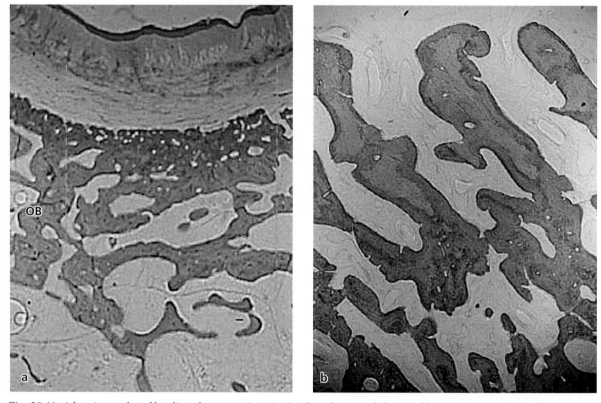

Fig. 38-10. Schematic drawing describing the transition between woven bone and lamellar bone, i.e. remodeling. Woven bone with primary osteons (PO) is transformed into lamellar bone in a process that involves the presence of BMUs. The BMU contains osteoclasts (OC), as well as vascular structures (V) and osteoblasts (OB). Thus, the osteoblasts in the BMU produce bone tissue that has a concentric orientation around the vessel, and secondary osteons (SO) within lamellar bone are hereby formed.

Fig. 38-11. After 6 months of healing the extraction site (within the area delineated by the vertical, dotted lines (a)) is more or less fully healed. The site contains lamellar bone and marrow (b) and some remaining woven bone. Through a process of modeling and remodeling the newly formed bone is now continuous with the "old bone" (OB (a)) of the neighboring areas.

gins is apparent. Remodeling of the sockets begins with the *presence of osteoclasts* inducing bone resorption (Fig. 38-12c). One week after extraction, the socket is characterized by granulation tissue consisting of a *vascular network,* young *connective tissue, osteoid* formation in the apical portion and epithelial coverage over the wound (Fig. 38-12d). One month following extraction, the socket is characterized by a *dense connective tissue* overlying the residual sockets, which are now filled with *granulation tissue.* A trabecular pattern of bone starts emerging. Wound *coverage by epithelium* is complete (Fig. 38-12e). Two months following extraction, bone formation in the socket is complete. The bony height of the original sockets has not yet been reached and the trabecular pattern is still undergoing remodeling (Fig. 38-12f).

Tooth extraction

Hemorrhagia,
Bleeding,
Blood clot

48-72 h after extraction

Blood clot,
Beginning of
granulation tissue formation

96 h after extraction

Residual blood clot,
Granulation tissue,
Epithelial proliferation

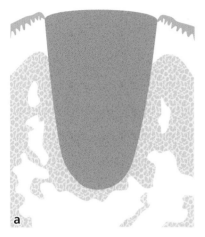

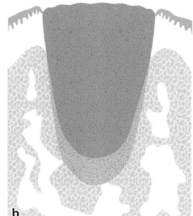

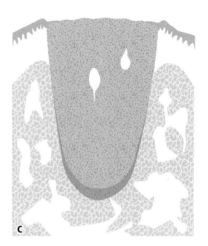

7 days after extraction

Young connective tissue,
Primary osteoid formation,
Epithelial proliferation

21 days after extraction

Connective tissue,
Osteoid start of mineralization,
Reepithelialization

6 weeks after extraction

Connective tissue,
Woven bone, trabeculae,
Reepithelialization

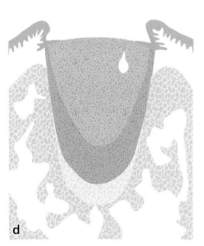

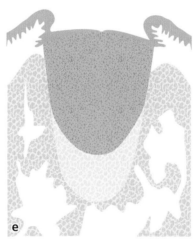

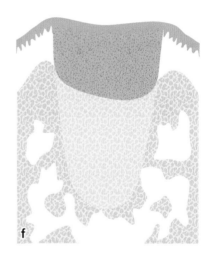

Fig. 38-12. Healing of extraction sockets (Amler 1969). (a) Bleeding and formation of a blood clot immediately after tooth extraction. Blood vessels are closed by thrombi and a fibrin network is formed. (b) Already during the first 48 hours, neutrophil granulocytes, monocytes and fibroblasts begin to migrate along the fibrin network. (c) The blood clot is slowly replaced by granulation tissue. (d) Granulation tissue forms predominantly in the apical third of the alveolus. Increased density of fibroblasts. After 4 days, contraction of the clot and beginning proliferation of the oral epithelium. Osteoclasts are visible at the margins of the alveolus. Osteoblasts and osteoids seem to appear in the bottom of the alveolus. (e) Reorganization of the granulation tissue through formation of osteoid trabeculae. Epithelial proliferation from the wound margins on top of the young connective tissue. Again, the formation of osteoid trabeculae is evident from the wall of the alveolus in a coronal direction. After 3 weeks some of the trabeculae start to mineralize. (f) Radiographically, bone formation may be visible. The soft tissue wound is closed and epithelialized after 6 weeks. However, bone fill in the alveolus takes up to 4 months and does not seem to reach the level of the neighboring teeth.

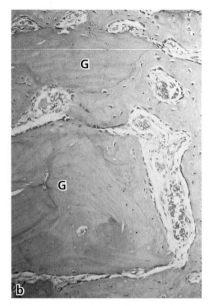

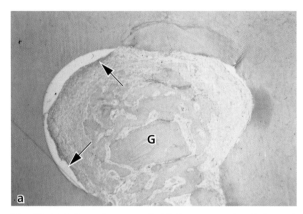

Fig. 38-13. Microphotograph (a) demonstrating bifurcation defect 3 weeks after grafting with autogenous cancellous jaw bone (G). New bone has invaded the defect, and the bone grafts have exerted an osteoconductive function. Epithelium (arrows) has migrated into one side of the defect. (b) Higher magnification of (a) showing that new bone has formed around the bone grafts (G), which have lost their vitality, indicated by the empty osteocyte lacunae.

Bone grafting

Although bone tissue exhibits a large regeneration potential and may restore its original structure and function completely, bony defects may often fail to heal with bone tissue. In order to facilitate and/or promote healing, bone grafting materials have been placed into bony defects. It is generally accepted that the biologic mechanisms forming the basis for bone grafting include three basic processes: *osteogenesis*, *osteoconduction* and *osteoinduction*.

Osteogenesis occurs when viable osteoblasts and precursor osteoblasts are transplanted with the grafting material into the defects, where they may establish centers of bone formation. Autogenous iliac bone and marrow grafts are examples of transplants with osteogenic properties (see Chapter 33).

Osteoconduction occurs when non-vital implant material serves as a scaffold for the ingrowth of precursor osteoblasts into the defect. This process is usually followed by a gradual resorption of the implant material. Autogenous cortical bone or banked bone allografts may be examples of grafting materials with osteoconductive properties (Fig. 38-13). Such grafting materials, as well as bone-derived or synthetic bone substitutes, have similar osteoconductive properties. However, degradation and substitution by viable bone is often poor. If the implanted material is not resorbable, which is the case for most porous hydroxylapatite implants, the incorporation is restricted to bone apposition to the material surface, but no substitution occurs during the remodeling phase.

Osteoinduction involves new bone formation by the differentiation of local uncommitted connective tissue cells into bone-forming cells under the influence of one or more inducing agents. *Demineralized bone matrix* (DMB) or *bone morphogenetic proteins* (BMP) are examples of such grafting materials (Bowers et al. 1989a,b, Sigurdsson et al. 1994).

It often occurs that all three basic bone-forming mechanisms are involved in bone regeneration. In fact, osteogenesis without osteoconduction and osteoinduction is unlikely to occur, since almost none of the transmitted cells of autogenous cancellous bone grafts survive the transplantation. Thus, the grafting material predominantly functions as a scaffold for invading cells of the host. In addition, the osteoblasts and osteocytes of the surrounding bone lack the ability to migrate and divide which, in turn, means that the transplant is invaded by uncommitted mesenchymal cells that later differentiate into osteoblasts.

On that basis it is appropriate to define three basic conditions as prerequisites for bone regeneration:

1. the *supply of bone-forming cells* or cells with the capacity to differentiate into bone forming cells
2. the presence of *osteoinductive stimuli* to initiate the differentiation of mesenchymal cells into osteoblasts
3. the presence of an *osteoconductive environment* forming a scaffold upon which invading tissue can proliferate and in which the stimulated osteoprogenitor cells can differentiate into osteoblasts and form bone.

The placement of bone-grafting materials to favor

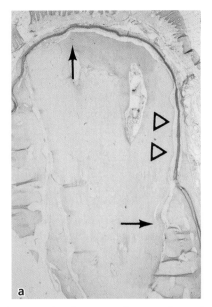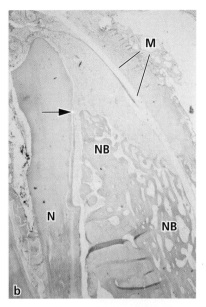

Fig. 38-14. Microphotographs showing submerged membrane-covered roots. (a) Membrane has collapsed, leaving a narrow space adjacent to the root surface (arrowheads). The formation of bone underneath the membrane is negligible, but a thin layer of new cementum covers the root surface between the arrows. (b) Root covered with a membrane (M) which has maintained considerable space adjacent to the root surface. New cementum is seen on the root surface from the notch (N) to the arrow, and considerable amounts of new bone (NB) have formed underneath the membrane. Note that in the area below the notch (N), new bone (NB) has also formed on top of the original buccal bone plate where bone has not existed before.

healing in osseous defects or to augment atrophic alveolar ridges has been evaluated in a number of experimental and clinical studies (Boyne 1970, Thompson & Casson 1970, Steinhäuser & Hardt 1977, Fazili et al. 1978, Baker et al. 1979, Mulliken & Glowacki 1980, Curtis & William 1983, Swart & Allard 1985, Block et al. 1987, Cullum et al. 1988, Hupp & McKenna 1988). However, there are several reports indicating that this type of treatment fails to predictably produce bone fill and augment alveolar ridges (Körlof et al. 1973, Curtis & Ware 1977, Steinhäuser & Hardt 1977, Taylor 1983, Davis et al. 1984, Jackson et al. 1986, Hupp & McKenna 1988). Often the bone grafts do not attach to the graft site through bony attachment and there is bone resorption and bone loss associated with grafting procedures. As a consequence, much of the intended volume is lost, and frequently the defects heal with a fibrous connective tissue instead of bone.

CONCEPT OF GUIDED TISSUE REGENERATION (GTR)

The principles of guided tissue regeneration (GTR) have been developed on the basis of a number of experimental animal studies on periodontal regeneration (see Chapter 33). In one of these studies (Gottlow et al. 1984), barrier membranes were placed over crown-resected roots in monkeys. The membrane-covered roots were then submerged. Following 3 months of healing, it was noticed that, in situations

where the membranes were collapsed, leaving a narrow space adjacent to the root surface, new cementum had formed on the root surface, but the amount of newly formed alveolar bone was negligible (Fig. 38-14a). On the other hand, in situations where the membranes had not collapsed, leaving a wider space adjacent to the root surface, considerable amounts of new bone had formed in addition to the new connective tissue attachment to the root surface, even in areas where bone had not existed before (Fig. 38-14b). This observation suggested that the GTR principle may be applied successfully in bone regeneration as well by creating a secluded space which can only be invaded by cells with bone-forming capacity from existing bone.

Animal studies

Alveolar bone defects
The application of the GTR principle for bone regeneration (guided bone regeneration (GBR)) was first investigated by Dahlin et al. (1988) in an experimental study in rats. Transmandibular defects 5 mm in diameter were surgically created bilaterally, while the test sites were covered on either side of the defect with a barrier membrane to allow the exclusive ingrowth of tissue from the mandibular bone, at the same time excluding the fibrous tissue of the area from proliferating into the defect. The control sites were left without the placement of a membrane. On the test side, almost complete bone healing was demonstrated both on defleshed mandibles and in histologic prepara-

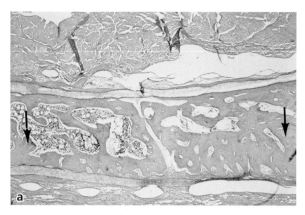

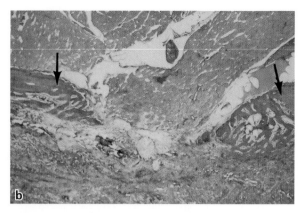

Fig. 38-15. (a) Test defects of critical size with membranes blocking the proliferation of undesired cells into the defect, resulting in complete bone regeneration after 6 weeks. (b) Control defects with residual transmandibular defects after 9 weeks due to the invasion of soft tissues into the defect space.

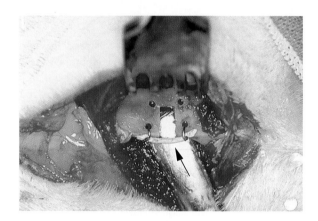

Fig. 38-16. 2 × 3 mm standardized defect produced at the inferior border of the mandible of a rat. A gutta-percha point (arrow) is placed to indicate the original level of the inferior border.

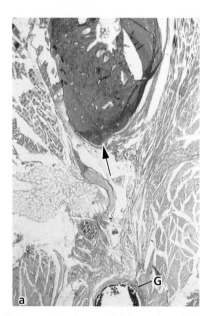

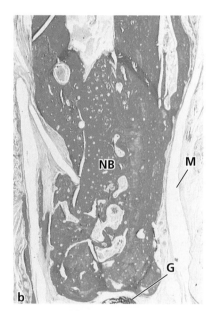

Fig. 38-17. Microphotographs of control (a) and test (b) jaw bone defects 6 months following surgery. Some new bone has formed in the bottom of the control defect (arrow) while the remaining part contains muscle and connective tissue. The gutta-percha point (G) indicates the original inferior border of the mandible. In the test defect (b), covered with a membrane (M), the newly formed bone (NB) is filling out the defect and has reached the gutta-percha point (G), indicating the original level of the inferior border of the mandible.

tions after 6 weeks (Fig. 38-15a). Control sites, on the other hand, demonstrated residual transmandibular defects, although somewhat diminished in diameter after 9 weeks due to the fact that surrounding soft tissues were invading the defects, hindering the bone-regenerating cells from occupying the wound space (Fig. 38-15b).

Similar results have been reported in an experimental model in rats where standardized mandibular defects were covered with a bio-absorbable membrane (Kostopoulos & Karring 1994a). The mandibular ramus of the rats was exposed on both sides and a 2 x 3 mm defect was created at its lower border (Fig. 38-16). A gutta-percha point was placed to indicate the original level of the border. On one side the defects were covered with a resorbable membrane, while the contralateral sides remained uncovered. The jaws were subjected to histologic analysis. In addition, defleshed specimens were prepared. These specimens revealed minimal bone fill in the control defects (Fig. 38-17a), while all test defects healed to or close to the gutta-percha point, indicating the original inferior border of the jaw (Fig. 38-17b). Likewise, the histologic analysis showed that bone regeneration in the experimental specimens occurred gradually over 7-180 days, amounting to 85% of the initial defect depth at 180 days (Fig. 38-18). In the control defects only some bone regeneration occurred within the first month following surgery. Bone regeneration in the control specimens amounted to 48% of the defect at 180 days. The rest of the control defect was filled with muscular, glandular and connective tissue (Fig. 38-17a).

Bone regeneration adjacent to implants

Titanium dental implants were inserted into the tibial bone in rabbits in such a way that three to four coronal threads were exposed on one side of each implant (Dahlin et al. 1989). At the test sites the implants were covered with a Teflon membrane, whereas at the control sites the implants remained uncovered. The overlying soft tissues were then sutured to obtain complete closure. Histologic analysis after 6 weeks revealed that, in the test sites, new bone was completely covering the exposed threads of the implants, while the threads of the implants at the control sites were covered by connective tissue. In a similar study in dogs (Becker et al. 1990), titanium implants were inserted in such a way that some of their threads remained exposed. Again, before closure of the wounds with a mucoperiosteal flap, the test sites were covered with a Teflon membrane, while the control sites remained uncovered. Following a healing period of 18 weeks, the specimens were subjected to clinical, radiographic and histologic examination. For the majority of the test implants, new bone was covering the previously exposed implant threads. The average gain in bone height was 1.37 mm for the test and 0.23 mm for the control implants. In the control sites, loosely adherent connective tissue was covering the exposed threads.

Immediate implant placement

The effect of GTR on osseointegration of titanium implants inserted into fresh extraction sockets was investigated by Warrer et al. (1991) in an experimental study in monkeys. The experimental sites were covered with a Teflon membrane, while the controls remained uncovered at the time of complete wound closure. Following 3 months of healing, histologic

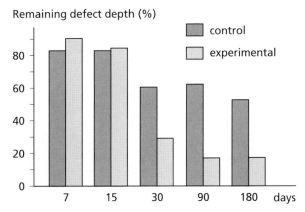

Fig. 38-18. Diagram showing the regeneration of bone in experimental and control defects. The columns indicate the remaining defect area, not filled with bone at various observation times. It can be seen that bone formation in the control defects is arrested after 1 month, while new bone continues to fill out the experimental defects.

analysis of the experimental sites revealed complete bone regeneration to the top of the implants and complete osseointegration. However, when exposure of the membrane had occurred during healing, less bone regeneration was observed and the coronal part of the fixtures was not osseointegrated. The controls also exhibited incomplete osseointegration. The authors concluded that osseointegration may be achieved predictably on dental implants placed into extraction sockets and covered with a membrane, provided the membrane is kept without communication to the oral cavity during healing. These results are in agreement with the results of other experimental studies in dogs (Becker et al. 1991, Gotfredsen et al. 1993), where titanium dental implants were placed in fresh extraction sockets or where HA-coated implants were placed in stimulated sockets before coverage with e-PTFE membranes (Caudill & Meffert 1991, Caudill & Lancaster 1993). Again, substantial amounts of new bone formed under the membranes, while minimal amounts were seen in control sites.

A comparison of e-PTFE membranes alone or in combination with platelet-derived growth factor (PDGF) and insulin-like growth factor (IGF-I) or demineralized freeze-dried bone (DFDB) in stimulating bone formation around immediate extraction socket implants was investigated in dogs by Becker et al. (1992). Following 18 weeks of healing, the histologic analysis revealed that e-PTFE membranes alone or e-PTFE membranes combined with PDGF/IGF-I were equally effective in promoting bone growth around the implants. Bone regeneration in the DFDB-treated specimens was highly variable and did not improve the efficacy of the Teflon membranes. The authors concluded that, on the basis of these results, the clinical use of DFDB must be questioned.

A study in monkeys has indicated that bony defects similar to those occurring around failed implants can

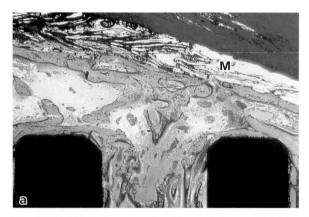
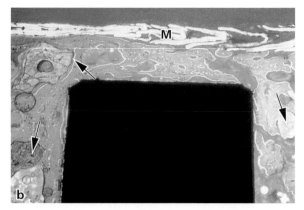

Fig. 38-19. Microphotographs of bone defects around implants covered with membranes (M). The defect seen in (b) was grafted with hydroxylapatite (arrows). Both non-grafted (a) and grafted (b) defects are filled with bone which extends coronally to the implant, to the level of the membrane (M).

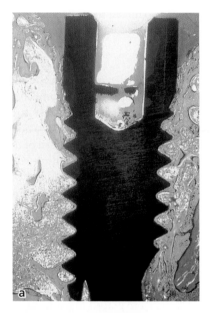
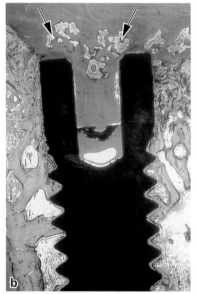

Fig. 38-20. Microphotographs of bone defects around implants treated without membranes. (b) Defect grafted with hydroxylapatite (arrows). (a) Non-grafted defect shows incomplete bone fill, while new bone has formed in the grafted defect (b) to the top of the implant. Some hydroxylapatite particles (arrows) are seen in the soft tissue coronal to the implant.

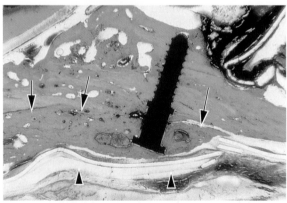

Fig. 38-21. Microphotograph showing that the space between the membrane (arrowheads) and the original border of the mandible (arrows) is filled with new bone, and the naturally existing curvature is eliminated.

also be successfully treated with membranes (Gotfredsen et al. 1991). Standardized bony defects were prepared in the alveolar ridge of edentulous areas in monkeys. A titanium dental implant was then placed

in the middle of these defects. In each monkey one defect was covered with a membrane. Another was grafted with hydroxylapatite particles before coverage with a membrane. A third defect was grafted with hydroxylapatite only and a fourth defect, serving as control, was covered only by the raised tissue flaps. Histologic analysis after 3 months of healing showed that all bony defects treated only with a membrane (Fig. 38-19a) and the majority of those grafted with hydroxylapatite and subsequently covered with a membrane were completely filled with bone (Fig. 38-19b). The defects treated with hydroxylapatite alone (Fig. 38-20b) and the control defects (Fig. 38-20a) often demonstrated incomplete bone fill in the defects. Thus, the placement of hydroxylapatite in the defects in addition to membrane coverage did not improve the healing results.

Localized ridge augmentation
The principle of GBR was applied in localized ridge augmentation in dogs (Seibert & Nyman 1990). Surgically created alveolar ridge defects in the mandibles of dogs were covered with e-PTFE membrane alone,

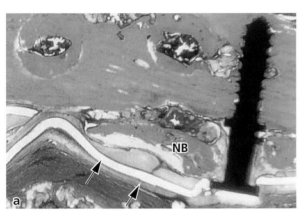
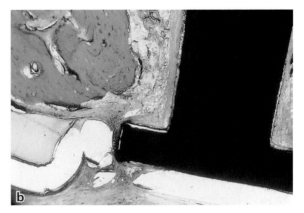

Fig. 38-22 a,b. Microphotographs showing new bone formation (NB) between the membrane (arrows) and the mandibular border. A rupture in the membrane, seen at high magnification in (b), has allowed soft connective tissue to invade the space underneath the membrane, thereby preventing osseointegration between the newly formed bone and the surface of the micro-titanium implant.

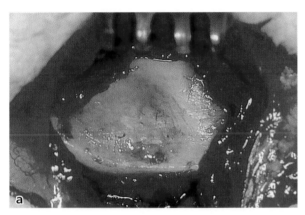
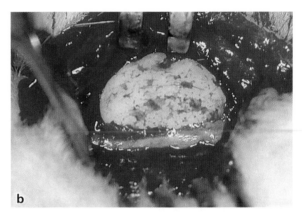

Fig. 38-23. After elevation of a musculo-periosteal flap exposing the mandibular ramus (a), a non-porous Teflon capsule is placed with its opening facing the mandibular ramus (b).

or treated with a combination of membrane placement and porous hydroxylapatite (HA) blocks, functioning as a space keeper, or with a combination of membrane and tissue growth matrix (porous PTFE). Tissue growth matrix as well as porous HA blocks were also used without membranes. In the control specimens, neither membranes nor implants were placed. Histologic analysis after 55-90 days of healing revealed that in the specimens covered only with membranes, bone had filled out the entire space underneath the membrane. At the sites where a membrane and HA were used, bone had also filled out the entire space. However, the pores of the HA adjacent to the subsurface of the membrane were only partially filled with bone. Bone deposition was mainly observed in the apical and middle part of the implant. The control specimens without membranes showed no new bone formation.

Vertical augmentation of the mandible at its inferior border using a bioresorbable membrane adapted to create a secluded space for ingrowth of bone tissue was evaluated in a study in rats (Kostopoulos & Karring 1994b). Following exposure of the mandibular ramus, a standardized titanium microimplant serving as a space maker and a fixed reference point was inserted in the naturally existing curvature at the inferior border of the mandible. The implant consisted of two parts, a threaded and a non-threaded part, separated by a stopper ring. One side of the mandible was covered with a bioabsorbable membrane, in such a way that a space was created in the curvature between the membrane and the inferior border of the mandible. The contralateral sides remained uncovered and served as controls. After 6 months of healing the specimens were defleshed and prepared for histologic analysis. The control specimens revealed minimal bone formation and the naturally existing curvature at the inferior border of the mandible had persisted. In contrast, the test specimens revealed considerable bone formation and the non-threaded part of the titanium microimplants was osseointegrated (Fig. 38-21). However, in specimens where soft tissue from the environment had escaped underneath the membrane, bone formation was reduced and osseointegration of the implants prevented (Fig. 38-22).

In order to evaluate the potential to produce bone with GTR in a space where bone has not existed before, an experimental model was developed by Kostopoulos et al. (1994). Non-porous, rigid, Teflon capsules of identical size were placed on the lateral surface of the

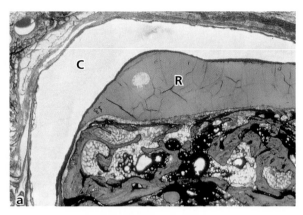
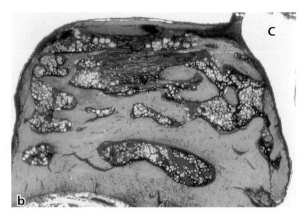

Fig. 38-24. Microphotographs of Teflon capsules 2 months (a) and 4 months (b) after placement on the mandibular ramus. After 2 months (a) the capsule (C) is about half filled with bone, while after 4 months (b) new bone is filling out the entire capsule. R: Remaining capsule space.

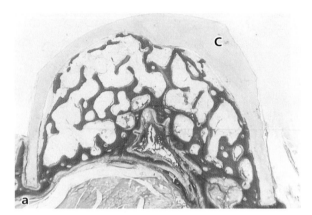
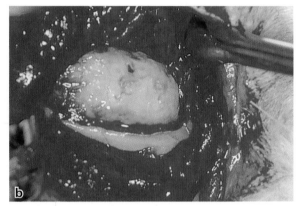

Fig. 38-25. Microphotograph of Teflon capsule (C) prior to removal after 6 months (a). The capsule is completely filled with bone. (b) Bone tuberosity present at the mandibular ramus after removal of the capsule.

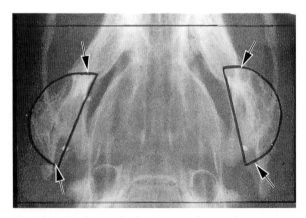

Fig. 38-26. Radiograph showing the bone tuberosities (arrows) formed on the lateral aspect of the ramus at both sides of the mandible.

mandibular ramus of rats in such a way that the open part of the capsules was adjoining the lateral surface of the mandibular ramus which was either covered with periosteum or denuded (Fig. 38-23). The histologic analysis revealed that new bone formation gradually occurred in the capsules (Fig. 38-24a). At 120 days, the capsules were filled out or almost filled out

with bone amounting to five to six times the original width of the mandibular ramus at both the periosteum-covered and the denuded sides (Fig. 38-24b). However, up to 60 days following surgery the amount of generated bone was significantly greater at the periosteum-covered sites than at the denuded sites. The authors suggested that a secluded space created adjacent to an existing bone surface, covered or not with periosteum, will inevitably be filled with newly formed bone.

The stability of such bone tuberosities produced by GTR in areas where bone has not existed before was evaluated by Lioubavina et al. (1997). Non-porous Teflon capsules were placed on the lateral surfaces of the mandibular ramus of rats. At one side the periosteum was preserved, while the other side was denuded. Histologic analysis of some of the animals after 6 months showed that the capsules were completely filled with bone (Fig. 38-25). The capsules in the remaining animals were removed by a second operation at 6 months and the structure and size of the bone tuberosities were evaluated histologically and radiographically until 1 year following removal of the capsules. The bone tuberosities diminished slightly in size immediately after capsule removal, after which

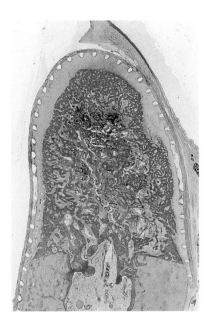

Fig. 38-27. Buccolingual section of a defect covered by a barrier membrane after 2 months. Complete bone fill in the secluded space beneath the membrane yields *primary spongiosa*. (From Schenk et al. (1994).)

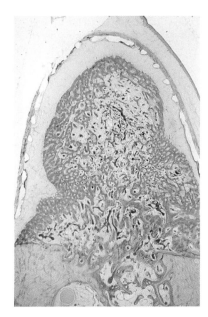

Fig. 38-28. Transformation of the primary spongework into cortical and cancellous bone. After 2 months, the peripheral spongiosa is somewhat denser than the center. (From Schenk et al. (1994).)

time no further resorption was observed (Fig. 38-26). This observation indicates that bone formed by GTR is stable over the long term.

Healing of GTR-treated bone defects
An experimental study in a canine model (Schenk et al. 1994) provided detailed information about the sequence and pattern of bone regeneration in surgically created, membrane-protected defects in the alveolar ridge. This histologic documentation confirmed that bone regeneration in membrane-protected defects followed closely the pattern of normal intramembraneous bone growth in extraction sites and a development through a similar sequence of maturation steps. Following initial organization of the blood clot, protected by the membrane, regeneration was initiated by deposition of *woven bone* along *new vascular structures* originating from the three surgically created bony walls that defined the defect margins. This *primary spongiosa* was characterized by blood vessels originating from marrow spaces (Fig. 38-27).

Secondarily, the network of woven bone was reinforced by concentrically deposited parallel-fibered *lamellar bone*, which resulted in the development of a new cortical structure at the periphery of the defects (Fig. 38-28). Finally, the onset of bone remodeling with the formation of *secondary osteons* could be observed in the newly formed bone close to the defect margins (Fig. 38-29). The duration of the maturation process obviously exceeded 4 months in the large defects created, since small remaining defects were still found in the midcrestal portion of the defect after 4 months (Fig. 38-30).

Subsequently, a similar second study was performed in dogs as well (Schenk et al. 1994) to address

questions about osseointegration of titanium implants into regenerated bone and the remodeling process of regenerated bone under functional loading conditions. In this study, complete bone fill was demonstrated in the defects after 6 months of healing, which histologically represented regular compact and cancellous bone perfectly suitable for the osseointegration of implants. Hence, all the implants inserted yielded primary stability. An intimate viable regenerated bone to implant contact was demonstrated in the histologic preparations. Secondary osteon formation and signs of ongoing remodeling were found in close proximity to the implant interface. Formation of bone trabeculae to "support" the implant was also identified in the more spongy region of the regenerated alveolar bone. The bone remodeling process, however, was not influenced by functional loading of the implants. On the other hand, regenerated control sites with no implant placement exhibited a rarefied bone structure characterized by a thin cortical layer and sparse bone trabeculae. Hence, it may be stated that the incorporation of titanium implants into newly regenerated bone may provide the necessary stimulus to activate bone maturation and remodeling.

Human experimental studies

At present, most of the information regarding the biologic events which lead to new bone formation is derived from animal studies. Results regarding bone formation collected in animal studies have to be applied with proper caution in humans. In particular, the time sequence of the various steps ultimately leading to the formation of mineralized mature bone in man

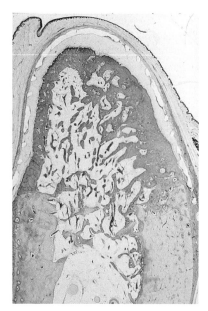

Fig. 38-29. Cortical bone formation and *secondary spongiosa* after 4 months. A compact bone layer in the periphery including haversian remodeling confines a cancellous bone in the center with well-defined trabeculae and bone marrow. (From Schenk et al. (1994).)

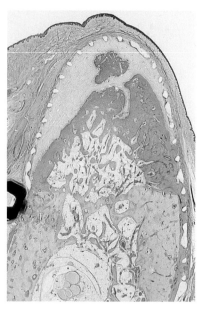

Fig. 38-30. The barrier membrane separates an outer gingival compartment from the compartment that is mainly accessible from the marrow space. In the latter, a well-vascularized connective tissue derived from bone marrow forms a periosteal envelope along the bone surface. (From Schenk et al. (1994).)

is different from that in all experimental animal systems known. A few human specimens, often harvested under poorly controlled conditions, contribute relatively little to the understanding of the biologic events of bone regeneration in humans.

A model system was designed to obtain human specimens of regenerated and also newly generated alveolar bone for the study of the biologic events under a variety of conditions (Hämmerle et al. 1996). A mucoperiosteal flap was raised in the retromolar area of the mandible of nine healthy volunteers. Following flap reflection, a standardized hole was drilled through the cortical bone into the bone marrow. Congruent test cylinders were firmly placed into the prepared bony bed, yielding primary stability; 1½-2 mm of the test device were submerged below the level of the surrounding bone, leaving 2-3 mm above the bone surface. The bone-facing end of the cylinder was left open, while the coronal soft tissue-facing end was closed by an ePTFE-membrane. The flap was sutured to obtain primary wound closure. In order to prevent infection, penicillin was prescribed systemically and oral rinses of chlorhexidine were administered. After 2, 7 and 12 weeks, one test device, including the regenerated tissue, was surgically harvested, while after 16, 24 and 36 weeks, respectively, two devices were harvested and processed for soft or hard tissue histology or histochemistry. The tissue generated after 2 and 7 weeks (Fig. 38-31) presented with a cylindrical shape, whereas the specimens harvested at 12 weeks and thereafter resembled the form of an hourglass. Specimens of 12 weeks and less regeneration time were

almost entirely composed of soft tissue, while specimens with a regeneration time of 4 months and more were composed of both soft and increasing amounts of mineralized tissue (Fig. 38-32). It was concluded that the model system is suitable for studying temporal dynamics and tissue physiology of bone regeneration in humans with minimal risk of complications or adverse effects for the volunteers.

In a retrospective re-entry study (Lang et al. 1994a), the bone volume regenerated using non-bioresorbable membrane barriers was assessed. Nineteen patients with jaw bone defects of various sizes and configurations were included. Combined split-thickness/full-thickness mucosal flaps were elevated in the area of missing bone. The size of the defects was assessed geometrically. Following the placement of Gore-Tex® augmentation material as a barrier, the maximum possible volume for bone regeneration was calculated. At the time of membrane removal (3-8 months later), the same measurements were performed and the percentages of regenerated bone in relation to the possible volume for regeneration determined. In six patients in whom the membranes had to be removed early, between 3 and 5 months, due to an increased risk of infection, bone regeneration varied between 0 and 60%. In 13 patients in whom the membranes were left for 6-8 months, regenerated bone filled 90-100% of the possible volume. It was concluded that successful bone regeneration consistently occurred with an undisturbed healing period of at least 6 months.

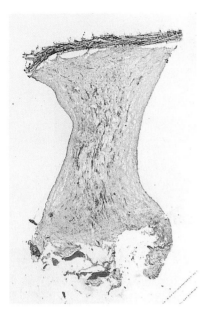

Fig. 38-31. Histologic section of a 7-week specimen, comprising non-mineralized connective tissue in the shape of an hourglass. Note the covering e-PTFE membrane.

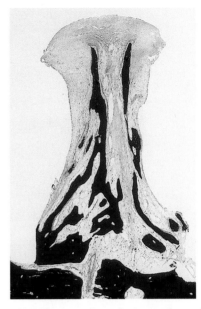

Fig. 38-32. Histologic section of a 9-month specimen. The height of the mineralized tissue has reached the top 20% of the cylinder space area.

CLINICAL APPLICATIONS

As a result of the animal studies elaborated above, several clinical applications of the principle of "guided tissue regeneration", in conjunction with the treatment of oral defects prior to or concomitantly with the placement of oral implants, have been developed to produce predictable treatment outcomes. These include:

- Alveolar bone defect closure
- Enlargement or augmentation of alveolar ridges
- Alveolar bone dehiscences or fenestrations in association with oral implants
- Immediate implant placement following tooth extraction.

Alveolar bone defect closure

A clinical example is described in Figs. 38-33a-i. The defect is self-limited and presents with well-defined bony borders.

An ankylosed retained canine (Fig. 38-33a) had to be removed (Fig. 38-33b), leaving a cavity the size of a cherry which extended into the edentulous ridge of tooth 23 (Fig. 38-33c). An e-PTFE membrane was tightly adapted to cover the palatal defect completely (Fig. 38-33d). After 6 months, the membrane was removed (Fig. 38-33e), and a bed for a one-stage transmucosal implant was prepared (Fig. 38-33f). The central bone core of the ITI hollow screw implant was processed histologically (Fig. 38-33g). Regular intramembraneous bone formation with woven bone and remodeling processes evidenced by the apposition of

lamellar bone was seen. Fig. 38-33h-i documents the clinical and radiographic appearance of a stable implant 8 years after the placement into the regenerated bone. It should be mentioned that no bone substitutes have been used as fillers or scaffold in this self-containing defect.

Enlargement or augmentation of alveolar ridges

In areas with a partially resorbed alveolar ridge, the bone volume is often insufficient to contain an implant. Therefore, enlargement of the alveolar ridge is frequently necessary prior to the placement of an implant.

As opposed to a self-contained jaw bone defect guaranteeing the maintenance of the secluded space into which exclusively osteogenic cells may proliferate, such a space will first have to be created for the enlargement of atrophic jaw bone crests.

A series of case reports and clinical studies (Nyman et al. 1990, Buser et al. 1991, 1993, 1995a,b, 1996a,b) were initiated to develop a surgical protocol resulting in predictable treatment outcomes of localized ridge augmentation and, later on, to validate the technique (Buser et al. 1994). In all these trials, ePTFE membranes were closely adapted to the bone surfaces and fixed with fixation screws or pins, while the space under the membrane was provided by means of specially designed supporting screws (Memfix®, Straumann Institute, Waldenburg, Switzerland) (Buser et al. 1994). In order to prevent membrane collapse, autogenous bone grafts were also used as support under the membranes. The clinical experience regarding optimal treatment outcomes was presented in a methodologic

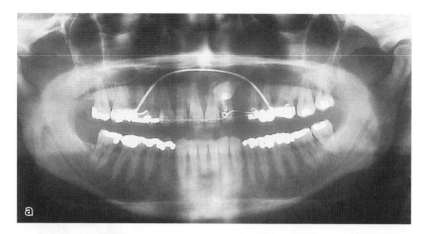

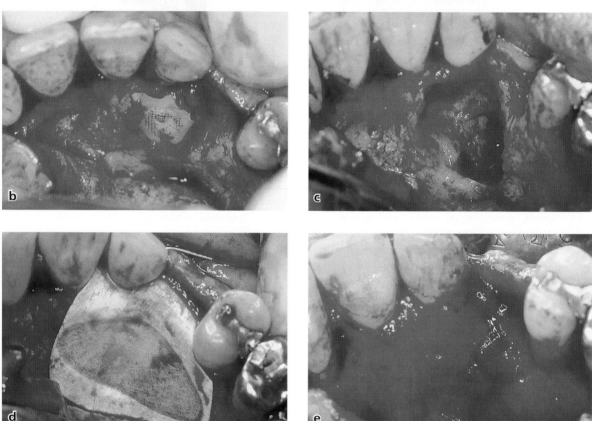

Fig. 38-33. Alveolar bone defect closure. (a) Orthopantomogram of an ankylosed retained maxillary canine. (b) Following flap elevation the crown of the ankylosed canine (23) is prepared free from its bony coverage. (c) A large defect extending into the edentulous ridge of tooth 23 is visible. (d) The self-containing defect is covered with a membrane barrier (e-PTFE). (e) At removal of the membrane after 6 months the defect has been filled with new bone. (f) Implantation of a hollow cylinder implant (ITI) is now possible. (g) Histologic preparation of the central bone core of the implant bed showed woven bone undergoing remodeling. (h) Clinical appearance of the crowned implant in position of tooth 23, 8 years after implant placement. (i) Radiographic documentation after 8 years showing implant stability.

report (Buser et al. 1995a,b). The essential criteria for success were:

1. Achievement of primary soft tissue healing to avoid membrane exposure by utilizing a lateral incision technique
2. Creation and maintenance of a secluded space under the membrane to avoid collapse of the membrane by utilizing appropriate membrane support

with or without autogenous bone grafts or osteoconductive substitutes
3. Stabilization and close adaptation of the membrane to the supporting bone to prevent the ingrowth of competing non-osteogenic cells into the defect area by utilizing fixation screws or pins
4. Allowance of an adequate healing period of at least 6-7 months to obtain complete bone regeneration and bone maturation.

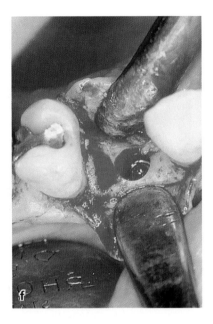

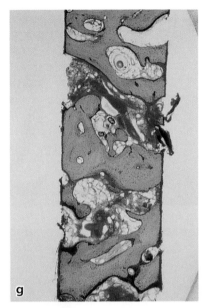

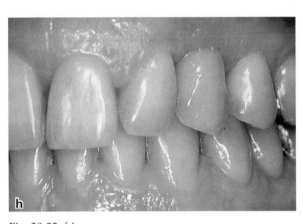

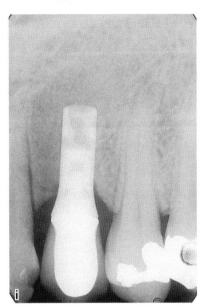

Fig. 38-33, f-i.

The technique advocated involves a combined split-thickness/full-thickness mucoperiosteal flap extending between the teeth adjacent to the defect. Care is taken to place the initial incision over intact bone remote from the bone defect. No vertical releasing incisions are placed, but the incisions extend into the gingival sulcus of the neighboring teeth.

Following flap elevation, soft tissue within the defect is carefully removed (Fig. 38-34a). A barrier membrane is adjusted and adapted to cover the bony defect and 3-4 mm of the surrounding intact bone, but avoiding contact with the adjacent teeth (Fig. 38-34c). In situations where there is a possible risk of collapse of the membrane barrier into the defect, miniscrews (Memfix®, Straumann Institute, Waldenburg, Switzerland) are placed to support the membrane for maintenance of the secluded space created (Fig. 38-34b).

Cortical bone lining the defect is perforated into the subjacent cancellous bone (Fig. 38-34b). The mucope-

riosteal flaps are subsequently repositioned and tightly sutured with mattress sutures. Postsurgical plaque control includes two daily rinsings with a chlorhexidine solution. Care is exercised not to touch or press the surgical site while using temporary reconstructions. The sutures are removed after 14 days. Postsurgical visits at monthly intervals to check the course of healing and the patient's plaque control are advocated (Fig. 39-34d). The removal of the membranes is performed 6-8 months after surgery (Fig. 38-34e).

In the case of exposure of the membrane prior to the scheduled removal, special efforts have to be made to prevent infection of the treated area by using antimicrobial therapy. At the time of membrane removal, the volume of newly formed bone corresponds to approximately 90-100% of the space created by the barrier membrane. Occasionally, a soft tissue coverage most likely originating from the bone marrow is seen

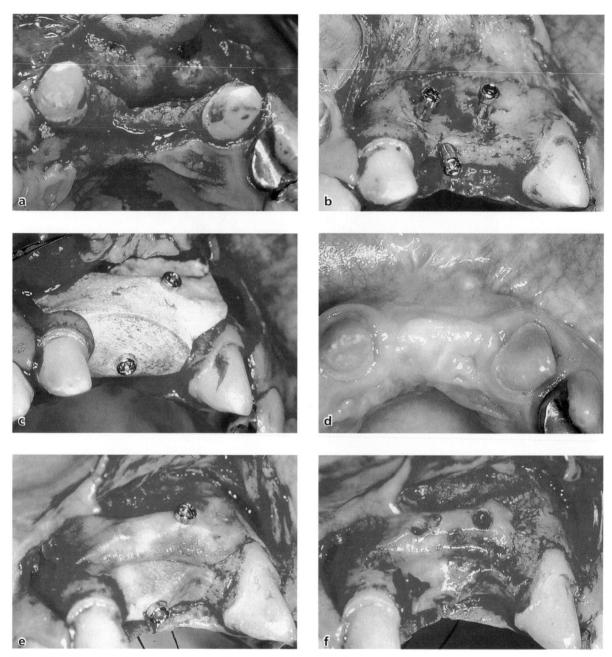

Fig. 38-34. Alveolar ridge augmentation. (a) Bony defect (156 mm³) in the maxilla of a 45-year-old woman following flap elevation. (b) Mini-supporting screws placed for the support and fixation of a membrane. (c) Placement of fixation-screws to adapt the membrane. (d) Soft tissue healing of the augmented ridge prior to membrane removal. (e) Regenerated bone under the membrane at the time of removal 8 months postsurgically. Effective new bone volume: 144 mm³, or 92% of the space volume. (f) Appearance of a thin, dense layer of nonmineralized tissue located between the regenerated bone surface and the inner surface of the membrane.

under the membrane (Fig. 38-34f). This well-vascularized connective tissue forms a periosteal envelope along the bone surface (Schenk et al. 1994). Provided an undisturbed healing of 6-8 months is observed, remarkable volumes of new alveolar bone may be generated by the GTR principle, resulting in an adequate volume for implant placement. Using this technique a clinical study of 40 partially edentulous patients was presented (Buser et al. 1996a,b). The patients who were admitted consecutively to the study had 66 augmented sites which were used for implant placement 7-13 months following the augmentation

of the alveolar crest. All but one patient showed complication-free soft tissue healing with an enlargement of the crest width ranging from 3.5 mm to 7.1 mm. The outcome of the procedure allowed the placement of a non-submerged titanium implant in all situations.

Another retrospective study (Lang et al. 1994b) utilizing the same technique also confirmed a 6-8-month period of undisturbed healing as a prerequisite for a successful treatment outcome. Between 90% and 100% of the volume created by the membrane was filled with regenerated bone after this time, while a shorter undisturbed healing period (3-5 months) yielded a

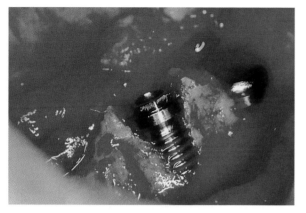

Fig. 38-35. Alveolar bone dehiscence exposing the threads of an implant.

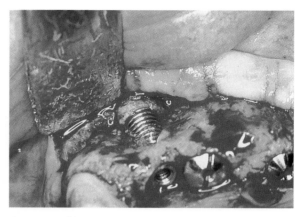

Fig. 38-36. Alveolar bone fenestration exposing an implant buccally.

regenerated volume of unpredictable magnitude (0-60%). Infection after membrane exposure was the major source of complication. A publication (Buser et al. 1996a,b), presenting 5-year results of the first group of 12 patients with alveolar ridge enlargement, has documented the long-term stability of the results.

Alveolar bone dehiscences and fenestrations in association with oral implants

An implant dehiscence is defined as exposure of the implant surface from the top of the implant head to the point where the implant is totally covered by bone (Fig. 38-35). An implant fenestration or window of exposed implant surface results from either insufficient buccolingual alveolar width or inadvertent misdirection of implant placement (Fig. 38-36).

Jovanovic et al. (1993) evaluated the potential for bone regeneration at dehisced dental implant sites in a clinical study including 11 patients. Nineteen titanium dental implants with exposed threads were studied. In order to create a secluded space for bone formation, a barrier membrane was placed over the exposed implant sites and secured with an implant cover screw. Subsequently the implants were completely covered with the surgical flaps. Clinical evaluation of the treatment was performed 4½-6 months after initial surgery. Fourteen out of 19 dehisced implant sites revealed 100% bone fill of the space created by the membrane. In addition, alveolar ridge augmentation had occurred at these sites. However, in cases where the membrane and the implant were exposed, minimal bone regeneration occurred. Six to 12 months after prosthesis connection, 12 of the 19 implants were available for radiographic analysis, and an average bone loss of 1.73 mm was measured.

In a prospective multicenter study (Dahlin et al. 1995), implant dehiscences and fenestrations were evaluated 3 years following alveolar bone augmentation therapy. Out of 54 augmented sites, six membranes were exposed and four implants were lost at the time of abutment connection, corresponding to an

implant failure rate of 7.4% after 1 year. The cumulative survival rates after 2 years were 85% and 95% for the maxilla and the mandible, respectively. At 3 years, the rates decreased to 76% and 83%, respectively. These rates are clearly lower than those regularly reported for implant placement into a bone volume of sufficient dimension. Hence, it has to be considered that augmenting bone at exposed implant threads may involve additional risk factors for the longevity of the implants placed.

Immediate implant placement following tooth extraction

Placement of implants at the time of tooth extraction is called "immediate implant placement".

Several authors have reported placement of implants into extraction sockets and augmentation of these sites with barrier membranes (Lazzara 1989, Becker & Becker 1990, Nyman et al. 1990). The rationale for this procedure is to decrease the restorative time, to promote bone-to-implant contact and to preserve alveolar bone height. Indications for extraction and immediate implant placement are: failed endodontically-treated teeth, teeth with advanced periodontal disease, root fractures and advanced caries beneath the gingival margin. However, teeth with suppuration or large periapical infections are not candidates for extraction and immediate replacement with implants. A prospective clinical multicenter study (Becker et al. 1994) evaluated implants which were placed into extraction sockets and augmented by GTR. Out of 49 implants, three were lost prior to loading. These implants had premature membrane exposure. At 3 years, 93.9% of the implants remained functional. Bone formation adjacent to the implants was related to barrier membrane retention. Sites where the barrier remained unexposed had greater amounts of bone fill in the sockets (average of 4.8 mm) when compared with sites where the membranes became prematurely exposed and were removed (average of 4.0 mm). Recently, 109 Nobel Biocare implants

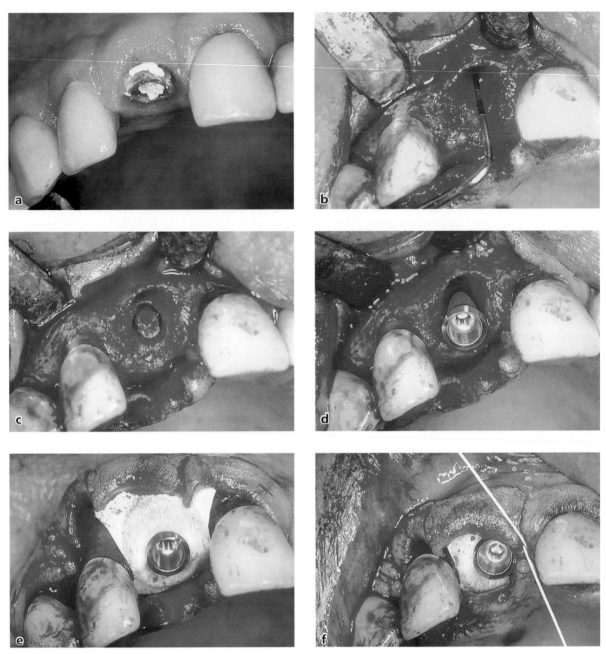

Fig. 38-37. (a) Root fracture following trauma of tooth 11. (b) Extraction socket 11 following careful removal of the tooth after raising a flap. (c) Preparation of the implant bed into the palatal socket wall. (d) Considerable lack of bone on the buccal aspect. (e) Barrier membrane shaped and adapted around the neck of the hollow cylinder implant demonstrating primary stability. (f) Single interrupted sutures mesial and distal to the implant. (g) The membrane has been *in situ* for 6 months. Infection was prevented by chemical plaque control. A flap was raised and the membrane removed from the soft and underlying hard tissue. (h) Radiographic appearance of new bone generated underneath the membrane after 10 years. The entire plasma-sprayed surface of the implant is still covered with bone. (i) Final reconstruction: porcelain fused to metal crown seated 7 months after the tooth extraction and maintained for 6 years.

immediately placed into extraction sockets were evaluated up to 5½ years (average 2½ years) following the treatment (Rosenquist & Grenthe 1996). The survival rate was 94% and the success rate 92%. Even though implants immediately placed into extraction sockets have been reported to have predictable healing in a *submerged* environment, the *non-submerged* placement of an implant into an extraction socket would offer a number of advantages. A series of

methodologic reports and clinical studies evaluated the healing of immediate one-stage transmucosal implants (Cochran & Douglas 1993, Lang et al. 1994a, Tritten et al. 1995, Brägger et al. 1996, Hämmerle et al. 1998).

One prospective study (Lang et al. 1994a) on the installation of immediate transmucosal implants in combination with GTR evaluated 21 implants in 16 patients after 2½ years. By meticulous antimicrobial

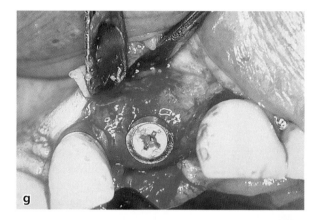

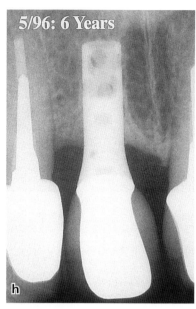

5/96: 6 Years

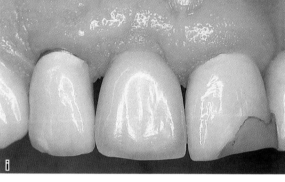

Fig. 38-37, g-i.

prophylactic procedures, including regular and prolonged topical use of antiseptics in conjunction with postsurgical administration of antibiotics, membrane removal was generally performed after 6 months. With the exception of one implant, complete fill of the extraction socket was achieved without the use of any autogenous or heterologous filler materials.

Another study on 10 patients with re-entry after 6 months following the placement of one-stage transmucosal implants into extraction sockets revealed a mean filling-up of 6.7 mm of the bone missing at the extraction sites, which corresponded to 94% of the volume estimates of bone fill at these sites (Hämmerle et al. 1997). Most of these studies were performed using non-resorbable occlusive barrier membranes to cover the self-containing defects at the extraction sites. However, bio-resorbable collagen barriers in conjunction with the application of deproteinized bone mineral as a supporting material also resulted in predictable treatment outcomes (Hämmerle & Lang 2001).

When compared to the standard placement of transmucosal implants, immediate transmucosal implants yielded very similar favorable clinical conditions in both groups of patients in a cross-sectional study after 1 year (Brägger et al. 1996). Low plaque and mucositis indices, similar amounts of recession, probing pocket depths and clinical attachment levels were registered in 41 patients.

In summary, five determining factors were identified to be prerequisites for positive treatment out-

comes in the placement of *one-stage non-submerged* implants placed *immediately* into extraction sockets:

1. Preservation of the bony margins of the alveolus during extraction to provide the necessary support for the barrier membrane.
2. Primary implant stability by precise preparation of an implant bed in the apical portion or along the walls of the socket.
3. Tight circumferential adaptation of a barrier membrane as a collar around the neck of the implant extending over the borders of the alveolus by 3-4 mm.
4. Careful management of the soft tissue flap and close flap adaptation to the neck of the implant. If the latter cannot be achieved, the extraction socket should be left to heal for 1 month to obtain a soft tissue coverage of the wound. The implant may then be placed into this recent extraction site (Wilson & Weber 1993).
5. Meticulous plaque control for the entire healing period of approximately 6 months. This is achieved by postsurgical antibiotic coverage, daily oral rinses with chlorhexidine and daily application of chlorhexidine gel under the base of the temporary restoration.

A clinical situation in which tooth 11 was lost owing to a long fracture (Fig. 38-37a) may illustrate the clinical procedure. A mucoperiosteal flap is raised on both the buccal and oral aspects ranging from tooth 13 to

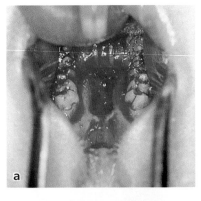
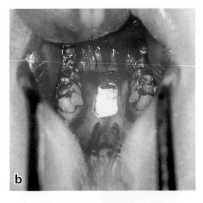
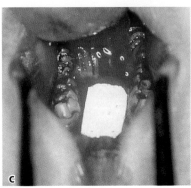
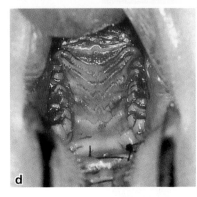

Fig. 38-38. An osseous submucous cleft palate is produced surgically (a). A membrane is placed both on the nasal (b) and palatal aspects (c) of the defect before the raised tissue flap is repositioned and sutured (d).

tooth 21. Tooth 11 is carefully extracted using fine elevators and small desmosomes to avoid the breakage of the buccal bony plate (Fig. 38-37b). If present, granulation tissue is removed. Immediately following the extraction and after rinsing the socket with sterile saline, an implant bed is prepared at the bottom or into the walls of the sockets (Fig. 38-37c) to obtain primary stability by intimate bone-to-implant contact (Fig. 38-37d).

In order to obtain bone fill of the circumferential defects adjacent to the implant and osseointegration also in the coronal part of the exposed plasma-sprayed implant surface, a barrier membrane is individually adapted to surround the neck of the implant tightly and to cover the bony defect around the implant (Fig. 38-37e). Care is taken to extend the barrier membrane 3-4 mm beyond the bony edges of the defect. Also, any contact of the membrane material with the adjacent teeth is avoided. Subsequently, the soft tissue flap is adapted snugly around the collar of the implants, allowing for transmucosal integration of these one-stage implants. Individual interrupted sutures are placed (Fig. 38-37f).

To prevent colonization with microorganisms leading to infection in the wound area, the patients should receive systemic antibiotics (amoxicillin) for 5-10 days. In addition, the patients should rinse twice daily with a chlorhexidine solution for at least 3 weeks after placement of the implants. A 1% chlorhexidine gel may be applied topically twice daily from the time of surgery and until the prosthetic appliance is incorporated. Since GTR may require longer periods of undisturbed healing for bone than for periodontal ligament regeneration (Lang et al. 1994a), the barrier membrane is intended to be left for periods of at least 6-8 months.

During this healing phase, the patients are checked once a month for plaque removal. During the healing period, the implants are functionally not loaded, i.e. the patients are provided with temporary removable partial dentures with no contact between the base of the denture and the soft tissue surrounding the immediate implants. The barrier membrane is removed under local anesthesia (Fig. 38-37g). The newly generated bone adjacent to the implant may be seen. Following resuturing, the flap adapting the soft tissues around the neck of the implant at the site is allowed to heal for 2-3 weeks. Subsequently, the final reconstruction is installed. After 6 years the radiographic documentation demonstrates stability of the bone level (Fig. 38-37h) and the peri-implant mucosal tissues are clinically healthy (Fig. 38-37i).

PERSPECTIVES IN BONE REGENERATION WITH GTR

In the studies described above, jaw bone defects in rats and monkeys healed with complete bone fill when covered with Teflon® membranes, whereas soft tissue invaded control defects treated without membranes (Dahlin et al. 1988, 1989, Kostopoulos & Karring 1994a,b). This observation suggests that GTR can be applied successfully in the field of cranio- and maxillofacial surgery. In fact, a study (Matzen et al. 1996) has demonstrated that healing of osseous submucous cleft palate defects with bone can be achieved by GTR. Osseous submucous cleft palate defects were produced surgically in rats (Fig. 38-38a). Barrier membranes were placed so that they covered both the nasal

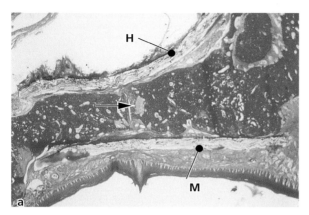
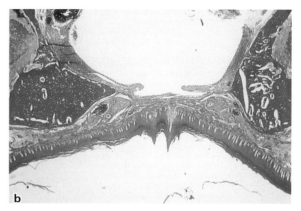

Fig. 38-39. (a) Microphotograph showing a membrane (M)-covered defect completely filled with new bone with a suture-like tissue (arrow) in the middle. (b) Control defect invaded by soft tissue.

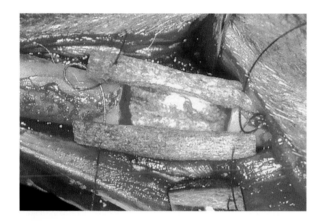

Fig. 38-40. A segmental, 1-cm osteoperiosteal defect produced in the radius of a rabbit and subsequently covered with a bioabsorbable membrane.

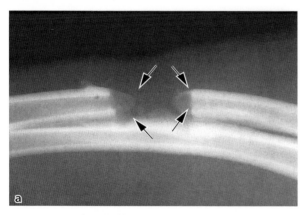
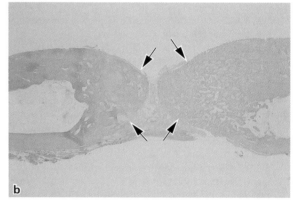

Fig. 38-41. Radiograph (a) and microphotograph (b) of a control defect treated without a membrane. The defect displays a characteristic non-union with rounded bone ends (arrows) separated by soft tissue.

(Fig. 38-38b) and the palatal (Fig. 38-38c) aspect of the defect before the raised palatal mucoperiosteal flap was repositioned and sutured (Fig. 39-38d). Histologic and macroscopic examination of defleshed specimens showed that complete healing of the defects with a suture-like tissue in the middle (Fig. 38-39a) was accomplished in all the membrane-treated defects, while soft tissue had invaded the control defects treated without a membrane (Fig. 38-39b).

There are also reasons to believe that the principle of GTR can be successfully applied in orthopedic surgery. This view is based on the results of studies in rabbits in which healing of long bone segmental de-

fects was accomplished by connecting the bone fragments with a bioabsorbable membrane tube (Nielsen 1992, Nielsen et al. 1992). Segmental 1-cm osteoperiosteal defects were produced in both radii of rabbits. One defect was covered with a bioabsorbable membrane (Fig. 38-40), while the contralateral defect without a membrane served as control. Nine out of 10 control defects displayed non-union (Fig. 38-41), whereas all membrane-treated defects healed by a callus external to the membrane, producing continuity between the bone fragments. However, loose connective tissue was predominant in the gap underneath the membrane. When, in a second experiment, demin-

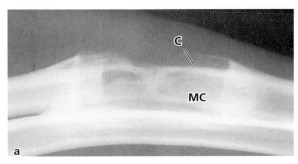
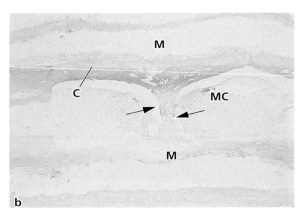

Fig. 38-42. Radiograph (a) and microphotograph (b) of a test defect treated with a membrane (M) and the placement of demineralized bone in the defect. The defect displays osseous continuity with the formation of a cortical (C) bone cylinder surrounding a marrow canal (MC). A narrow zone of woven bone with a central transverse disk of cartilagenous tissue remains in the midportion of the defect (arrows).

eralized bone matrix (DMB) was placed in the gap inside the tube, all membrane-covered defects exhibited osseous continuity with the formation of a cortical bone cylinder surrounding a marrow canal inside the tube (Fig. 38-42a).

A narrow midline zone of woven bone with a central transverse disk of cartilaginous tissue remained in some of the covered defects after 12 weeks (Fig. 38-42b). Histologic examination of this zone revealed that bone formation resembling endochondral ossification at growth plates was taking place in this area. These observations suggest that the combined use of GTR and DMB may have a clinical application in the treatment of large bony defects in long-bone fractures and in bone-lengthening procedures.

References

Amler, M.H. (1969). The time sequence of tissue regeneration in human extraction wounds. *Oral Surgery* **27**, 309-318.

Baker, R.D., Terry, B.C., Davis, W.H. & Connole, P.W. (1979). Long-term results of alveolar ridge augmentation. *Journal of Oral Surgery* **37**, 486-489.

Becker, W. & Becker, B. (1990). Guided tissue regeneration for implants placed into extraction sockets and for implant dehiscences: Surgical techniques and case reports. *International Journal of Periodontics and Restorative Dentistry* **10** (5), 377-391.

Becker, W., Becker, B.E., Handelsman, M., Celletti, R., Ochsenbein, C., Hardwick, R. & Langer, B. (1990). Bone formation at dehisced dental implant sites treated with implant augmentation material: a pilot study in dogs. *International Journal of Periodontics and Restorative Dentistry* **10**, 93-101.

Becker, W., Becker, B.E., Handelsman, M., Ochsenbein, C. & Albrektsson, T. (1991). Guided tissue regeneration for implants placed into extraction sockets. A study in dogs. *Journal of Periodontology* **62**, 703-709.

Becker, W., Dahlin, C., Becker, B.E., Lekholm, U., van Steenberghe, D., Higuchi, K. & Kultje, C. (1994). The use of ePTFE barrier membranes for bone promotion around titanium implants placed into extraction sockets: A prospective multicenter study. *International Journal of Oral Maxillofacial Implants* **9**, 31-40.

Becker, W., Lynch, S.E., Lekholm, U., Becker, B.E., Cafesse, R., Donath, K. & Sanchez, R. (1992). A comparison of e-PTFE membranes alone or in combination with platelet-derived growth factors and insulin-like growth factor-I or demineralized freeze-dried bone in promoting bone formation around immediate extraction socket implants. *Journal of Periodontology* **63**, 929-940.

Block, M.S., Kent, J.N., Ardoin, R.C. & Davenport, W. (1987). Mandibular augmentation in dogs with hydroxylapatite combined with demineralized bone. *Journal of Oral and Maxillofacial Surgery* **45**, 414-420.

Bowers, G.M., Chadroff, B., Carnevale, R., Mellonig, J., Corio, R., Emerson, J., Stevens, M. & Romberg, E. (1989a). Histologic evaluation of new attachment apparatus formation in humans. Part II. *Journal of Periodontology* **60**, 675-682.

Bowers, G.M., Chadroff, B., Carnevale, R., Mellonig, J., Corio, R., Emerson, J., Stevens, H. & Romberg, E. (1989b). Histologic evaluation of new attachment apparatus formation in humans. Part III. *Journal of Periodontology* **60**, 683-693.

Boyne, P.J. (1970). Autogenous cancellous bone and marrow transplants. *Journal of Clinical Orthopedics* **73**, 199-212.

Brägger, N., Hämmerle, C.H.F. & Lang, N.P. (1996). Immediate transmucosal implants using the principle of guided tissue regeneration (II). A cross-sectional study comparing the clinical outcome 1 year after immediate to standard implant placement. *Clinical Oral Implants Research* **7**, 268-276.

Buser, D., Brägger, U., Lang, N.P. & Nyman, S. (1991). Regeneration and enlargement of jaw bone using guided tissue regeneration. *Clinical Oral Implants Research* **1**, 22-32.

Buser, D., Dula, K., Belser, U., Hirt, H.P. & Berthold, H. (1993). Localized ridge augmentation using guided bone regeneration. I. Surgical procedure in the maxilla. *International Journal of Periodontics and Restorative Dentistry* **13**, 29-45.

Buser, D., Dula, K., Belser, H., Hirt, H.P. & Berthold, H. (1995a). Localized ridge augmentation using guided bone regeneration. II. Surgical procedures in the mandible. *International Journal of Periodontics and Restorative Dentistry* **15**, 13-29.

Buser, D., Dula, K., Hirt, H.P. & Berthold, H. (1994). Localized ridge augmentation using guided bone regeneration. In: Buser, D., Dahlin, C. & Schenk, R.K., eds. *Guided Bone Regeneration in Implant Dentistry.* Berlin: Quintessence, pp. 189-233.

Buser, D., Dula, K., Hirt, H.P. & Schenk, R.K. (1996a). Lateral ridge augmentation using autografts and barrier membranes: A clinical study with 40 partially edentulous patients. *Journal of Oral and Maxillofacial Surgery* **54**, 420-434.

Buser, D., Dula, K., Lang, N.P. & Nyman, S. (1996b). Long-term stability of osseointegrated implants in bone regenerated with the membrane technique. 5-year results of a prospective study with 12 implants. *Clinical Oral Implants Research* **7**, 175-183.

Buser, D., Hirt, H.P., Dula, K. & Berthold, H. (1992). Gleichzeitige Anwendung von Membranen bei Implantaten mit peri-implantären Knochendefekten. *Schweizer Monatsschrift für Zahnmedizin* **102**, 1490-1505.

Buser, D., Ruskin, J., Higinbottom, F., Hardwick, R., Dahlin, C. & Schenk, R.K. (1995b). Osseointegration of titanium implants in bone regenerated in membrane-protected defects. A histologic study in the canine mandible. *International Journal of Oral and Maxillofacial Implants* **10**, 666-681.

Caudill, R. & Lancaster, D. (1993). Histologic analysis of the osseointegration of endosseous implants in simulated extraction sockets with and without e-PTFE barriers. Part II. Histomorphometric findings. *Clinical Oral Implants Research* **19**, 209-215.

Caudill, R.F. & Meffert, R.M. (1991). Histologic analysis of the osseointegration of endosseous implants in simulated extraction sockets with and without e-PTFE barriers. Part I. Preliminary findings. *International Journal of Periodontics & Restorative Dentistry* **11**, 207-215.

Cochran, D.L. & Douglas, H.B. (1993). Augmentation of osseous tissue around non-submerged endosseus dental implants. *International Journal of Periodontis and Restorative Dentistry* **13**, 506-519.

Cullum, P.E., Frost, D.E., Newland, T.B., Keane, T.M. & Ehler, W.J. (1988). Evaluation of hydroxylapatite particles in repair of alveolar clefts in dogs. *Journal of Oral and Maxillofacial Surgery* **46**, 290-296.

Curtis, T.A. & Ware, D.H. (1977). Autogenous bone graft procedures for atrophic edentulous mandibles. *Journal of Prosthetic Dentistry* **38**, 366-379.

Curtis, T.A. & William, R.W. (1983). Autogenous bone grafts for atrophic edentulous mandibles: A review of twenty patients. *Journal of Prosthetic Dentistry* **49**, 212-216.

Dahlin, C., Gottlow, J., Lindhe, A. & Nyman, S. (1990). Healing of maxillary and mandibular bone defects using a membrane technique. An experimental study in monkeys. *Scandinavian Journal of Plastic Reconstructive and Hand Surgery* **24**, 13-19.

Dahlin, C., Lekholm, U., Becker, W., Becker, B., Higuchi, K., Callens, A. & van Steenberghe, D. (1995). Treatment of fenestration and dehiscence bone defects around oral implants using the guided tissue regeneration technique: A prospective multicenter study. *International Journal of Oral and Maxillofacial Implants* **3**, 312-318.

Dahlin, C., Linde, A., Gottlow, J. & Nyman, S. (1988). Healing of bone defects by guided tissue regeneration. *Plastic and Reconstructive Surgery* **81**, 672-676.

Dahlin, C., Sennerby, L., Lekholm, U., Linde, A. & Nyman, S. (1989). Generation of new bone around titanium implants using a membrane technique: An experimental study in rabbits. *International Journal of Oral Maxillofacial Implants* **4**, 19-25.

Davis, W.H., Martinoff, J.I. & Kaminishi, R.M. (1984). Long term follow-up of transoral rib grafts for mandibular atrophy. *Journal of Oral and Maxillofacial Surgery* **42**, 606-609.

Eggli, P.S., Müller, W. & Schenk, R.K. (1988). Porous hydroxylapatite and tricalcium phosphate cylinders with two different pore size ranges implanted in the cancellous bone of rabbits. A comparative histomorphometric and histologic study of bony ingrowth and implant substitution. *Clinical and Orthopedically Related Research* **232**, 127.

Fazili, M., Overvest-Eerdmans, G.R., Vernooy, A.M., Visser, W.J. & Waas, M.A.J. (1978). Follow-up investigation of reconstruction of the alveolar process in the atrophic mandible. *International Journal of Oral Surgery* **7**, 400-404.

Friedenstein, A.J. (1973). Determined and inducible osteogenic precursor cells. In: *Hand Tissue Growth Repair and Remineralisation*. Aba Foundation Symposium 11, pp. 169-181.

Gotfredsen, K., Nimb, L., Buser, D. & Hjørting-Hansen, E. (1993). Evaluation of guided bone regeneration around implants placed into fresh extraction sockets: An experimental study in dogs. *Journal of Oral and Maxillofacial Surgery* **51**, 879-884.

Gotfredsen, K., Warrer, K., Hjørting-Hansen, E. & Karring, T. (1991). Effect of membranes and porous hydroxylapatite on healing in bone defects around titanium dental implants. An experimental study in monkeys. *Clinical Oral Implants Research* **2**, 172-178.

Gottlow, J., Nyman, S. & Karring, T. (1992). Maintenance of new attachment gained through guided tissue regeneration. *Journal of Clinical Periodontology* **19**, 315-317.

Gottlow, J., Nyman, S., Karring, T. & Lindhe, J. (1984). New attachment formation as the result of controlled tissue regeneration. *Journal of Clinical Periodontology* **11**, 494-503.

Hämmerle, C.H.F., Brägger, U., Schmid, B. & Lang, N.P. (1998). Successful bone formation at immediate transmucosal implants: A clinical report. *International Journal of Oral and Maxillofacial Implants* **13**, 522-530.

Hämmerle, C.H.F., Fourmousis, I., Winkler, J.R., Weigel, C., Brägger, U. & Lang, N.P. (1995). Successful bone-fill in late peri-implant defects using guided tissue regeneration. A short communication. *Journal of Periodontology* **66**, 303-308.

Hämmerle, C.H.F. & Lang, N.P. (2001). Single stage surgery combining transmucosal implant placement with guided bone regeneration and bioresorbable materials. *Clinical Oral Implants Research* **12**, 9-18.

Hämmerle, C.H.F., Schmid, J., Olah, A.J. & Lang, N.P. (1996). A novel model system for the study of experimental guided bone formation in humans. *Clinical Oral Implants Research* **7**, 38-47.

Hjørting-Hansen, E., Warsaae, N. & Lemons, J.E. (1990). Histologic response after implantation of porous hydroxylapatite ceramic in humans. *International Journal of Oral and Maxillofacial Implants* **5**, 255-263.

Hupp, J.T. & McKenna, S.J. (1988). Use of porous hydroxylapatite blocks for augmentation of atrophic mandibles. *Journal of Oral and Maxillofacial Surgery* **46**, 538-545.

Jackson, I.T., Helden, G. & Marx, R. (1986). Skull bone grafts in maxillofacial and craniofacial surgery. *Journal of Oral and Maxillofacial Surgery* **44**, 949-960.

Jensen, S.S., Åboe, M., Pinholt, E.M., Hjørting-Hansen, E., Melsen, F. & Ruyter, I.E. (1996). Tissue reaction and material characteristics of four bone substitutes. *International Journal of Oral and Maxillofacial Implants* **11**, 55-66.

Jovanovic, S.A., Kenney, E.B., Carranza, F.A. & Donath, K. (1993). The regenerative potential of plaque-induced peri-implant bone defects treated by a submerged membrane technique: An experimental study. *International Journal of Oral and Maxillofacial Implants* **8**, 13-18.

Jovanovic, S.A., Spiekermann, H. & Richter, J.E. (1992). Bone regeneration around titanium dental implants in dehisced defect sites: A clinical study. *International Journal of Oral and Maxillofacial Implants* **7**, 233-245.

Körlof, B., Nylen, B. & Rietz, K.A. (1973). Bone grafting of skull defects: A report on 55 cases. *Journal of Plastic and Reconstructive Surgery* **52**, 378-383.

Kostopoulos, L. & Karring, T. (1994a). Guided bone regeneration in mandibular defects in rats using a bioresorbable polymer. *Clinical Oral Implants Research* **5**, 66-74.

Kostopoulos, L. & Karring, T. (1994b). Augmentation of the rat mandible using the principle of guided tissue regeneration. *Clinical Oral Implants Research* **5**, 75-82.

Kostopoulos, L., Karring, T. & Uraguchi, R. (1994). Formation of jaw bone tuberosities using "Guided Tissue Regeneration". An experimental study in the rat. *Clinical Oral Implants Research* **5**, 245-253.

Lang, N.P., Brägger, U., Hämmerle, C.H.F. & Sutter, F. (1994a). Immediate transmucosal implants using the principle of guided tissue regeneration. I. Rationale, clinical procedures and 30-month results. *Clinical Oral Implants Research* **5**, 154-163.

Lang, N.P., Hämmerle, C.H.F., Brägger, U., Lehmann, B. & Nyman, S.R. (1994b). Guided tissue regeneration in jaw bone defects prior to implant placement. *Clinical Oral Implants Research* **5**, 92-97.

Lazzara, R.J. (1989). Immediate implant placement into extraction sites: surgical and restorative advantages. *International Journal of Periodontics and Restorative Dentistry* **9**, 333-343.

Lehmann, B., Brägger, U., Hämmerle, C.H.F., Fourmousis, I. & Lang, N.P. (1992). Treatment of an early implant failure according to the principles of guided tissue regeneration (GTR). *Clinical Oral Implants Research* **3**, 42-48.

Lioubavina, N., Kostopoulos, L., Wenzel, A. & Karring, T. (1997). Long-term stability of jaw bone tuberosities formed at the lateral aspect of the rat mandibular ramus by "guided tissue regeneration". *Clinical Oral Implants Research* **8** (in press).

Matzen, M., Kostopoulos, L. & Karring, T. (1996). Healing of osseous submucous cleft palates with guided tissue regeneration. *Scandinavian Journal of Plastic and Reconstructive Hand Surgery* **30**, 161-167.

Mulliken, J.B. & Glowacki, J.B. (1980). Induced osteogenesis for repair and construction in the craniofacial region. *Journal of Plastic and Reconstructive Surgery* **65**, 553-559.

Nielsen, F.F. (1992). *Guided bone induction – a method in the treatment of diaphysial long-bone defects.* Thesis. Royal Dental College, University of Aarhus, Denmark, 128 pp..

Nielsen, F.F., Karring, T. & Gogolewski, S. (1992). Biodegradable guide for bone regeneration. Polyurethane membranes tested in rabbit radius defects. *Acta Orthopedica Scandinavica* **63**, 66-69.

Nyman, S., Lang, N.P., Buser, D. & Brägger, U. (1990). Bone regeneration adjacent to titanium dental implants using guided tissue regeneration: a report of two cases. *International Journal of Oral and Maxillofacial Implants* **5**, 9-14.

Pinholt, E.M., Ruyter, I.E., Haanaer, H.R. & Bang, G. (1992). Chemical, physical and histopathological studies on four commercial apatites intended for alveolar ridge augmentation. *Journal of Oral and Maxillofacial Surgery* **50**, 859-867.

Rosenquist, B. & Grenthe, B. (1996). Immediate placement of implants into extraction sockets: Implant survival. *International Journal of Oral and Maxillofacial Implants* **11**, 205-209.

Schenk, R.K. (1994). Bone regeneration: Biologic basis. In: Buser, D., Dahlin, C., Schenk, R.K., eds. *Guided Bone Regeneration in Implant Dentistry.* Berlin: Quintessence, pp. 49-100.

Schenk, R.K., Buser, D., Hardwick, W.R. & Dahlin, C. (1994). Healing pattern of bone regeneration in membrane-protected defects. A histologic study in the canine mandible. *International Journal of Oral and Maxillofacial Implants* **9**, 13-29.

Seibert, J. & Nyman, S. (1990). Localized ridge augmentation in dogs. A pilot study using membranes and hydroxylapatite. *Journal of Periodontology* **61**, 157-165.

Sigurdsson, T., Hardwick, R., Bogle, G. & Wikesjö, U. (1994). Periodontal repair in dogs: Space provision by reinforced ePTFE membranes enhances bone and cenentum regeneration in large supraalveolar defects. *Journal of Periodontology* **65**, 350-356.

Steinhäuser, E. & Hardt, N. (1977). Secondary reconstruction of cranial defects. *Journal of Maxillofacial Surgery* **5**, 192-198.

Swart, L.G.N. & Allard, R.H.B. (1985). Subperiosteal onlay augmentation of the mandible: A clinical and radiographic survey. *Journal of Oral and Maxillofacial Surgery* **43**, 183-187.

Taylor, G.I. (1983). The current status of free vascularized bone grafts. *Journal of Clinical Plastic Surgery* **10**, 185-196.

Thompson, N. & Casson, J. (1970). Experimental onlay bone grafts to the jaws. A preliminary study in dogs. *Journal of Plastic and Reconstructive Surgery* **46**, 341-349.

Tritten, C.B., Brägger, U., Fourmousis, I. & Lang, N.P. (1995). Guided bone regeneration around an immediate transmucosal implant for single tooth replacement: A case report. *Practical Periodontics and Aesthetic Dentistry* **7**, 29-38.

Wachtel, H.C., Langford, A., Bernimoulin, J-P. & Reichart, P. (1991). Guided bone regeneration next to osseointegrated implants in humans. *International Journal of Oral and Maxillofacial Implants* **6**, 127-134.

Warrer, K., Gotfredsen, K., Hjørting-Hansen, E. & Karring, T. (1991). Guided tissue regeneration ensures osseointegration of dental implants placed into extraction sockets. An experimental study in monkeys. *Clinical Oral Implants Research* **2**, 166-171.

Wetzel, A.C., Stich, H. & Caffesse, R.G. (1995). Bone apposition onto oral implants in the sinus area filled with different grafting materials. *Clinical Oral Implants Research* **6**, 155-163.

Wilson, T.G. & Weber, H.P. (1993). Classification of and therapy for areas of deficient bony housing prior to dental implant placement. *International Journal of Periodontics and Restorative Dentistry* **13**, 451-458.

CHAPTER 39

Procedures Used to Augment the Deficient Alveolar Ridge

MASSIMO SIMION

General considerations

Case reports

Alveolar ridge augmentation for single tooth restoration in the anterior maxilla

Alveolar ridge augmentation for implant restoration in the anterior maxilla

Alveolar ridge augmentation for implant restoration of multiple adjacent maxillary teeth

Vertical ridge augmentation in the anterior area of the mandible

Vertical ridge augmentation to allow implant placement in the posterior segments of the mandible

A variety of surgical techniques used for horizontal and vertical ridge augmentation have been described by different authors (e.g. Buser et al. 1990, 1993, 1995, 1996, Nevins & Mellonig 1992, 1994, Mellonig & Triplett 1993, Lang et al. 1994, Rominger & Triplett 1994, Simion et al. 1994, 1998, Tinti et al. 1996, Tinti & Parma-Benfenati 1998). Such procedures often include the use of autogenous bone grafts or grafts including different biomaterials as well as the placement of barrier membranes (guided bone regeneration (GBR), see Chapter 38). In the present chapter, ridge augmentation techniques will be described that can be performed either before or in combination with implant placement and that include the use of autogenous bone grafts.

GENERAL CONSIDERATIONS

All ridge augmentation procedures should be performed in a proper surgical setting and in patients with a dentition free of signs of destructive periodontitis. Before the surgical session, the perioral skin must be cleaned with the use of a disinfectant. The patient must rinse his or her mouth for 2 minutes with a 0.12-0.2% solution of chlorhexidine gluconat. The patient is subsequently covered with sterile sheets to minimize bacterial contamination from extraoral sites. The surgical procedure is in most cases performed on a lightly sedated patient and under local anesthesia.

Flap design

A full thickness crestal incision is placed within the keratinized mucosa of the edentulous ridge. In a partially dentate patient the crestal incision is extended into an intrasulcular incision – mesially and/or distally – to involve one or two adjacent teeth. Vertical releasing incisions are made at the mesial and distal ends of the crestal incision. In order to get proper access to the surgical site the releasing incisions are frequently made in buccal as well as in lingual (palatal) direction.

Initial preparation of the recipient site

A meticulous preparation of the recipient site is crucial for the successful outcome of a ridge augmentation procedure. Thus, following placement of the incisions, the buccal and palatal (lingual) flaps are reflected with the use of an elevator, to allow a proper exposure of the surgical site. During flap elevation care must be taken not to damage the palatine artery, and the mental nerve in patients with a severely reabsorbed maxilla and/or mandible. Further, the soft tissue flaps must be handled gently to minimize trauma and to avoid perforations and lacerations.

Once exposed, the cortical bone at the recipient site is curetted with a chisel to remove all remnants of granulation tissue and portions of adherent periosteum.

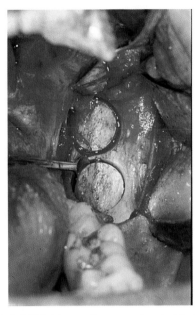

Fig. 39-1. A full thickness flap was elevated in the ramus of the mandible. The osteotomy was performed with the use of trephines.

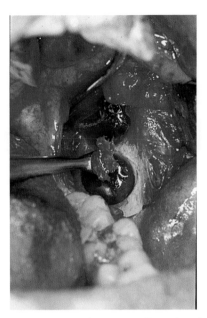

Fig. 39-2. The bone samples were collected with a Molt curette.

Positioning of the barrier membrane

The barrier membrane most frequently used in ridge augmentation procedures is made of expanded polytetrafluoroethylene (e-PTFE; Gore-Tex, W.L. Gore Ass., Flagstaff, AZ, US) and often the titanium reinforced variety of the e-PTFE membrane (TR GTAM; Gore-Tex, W.L. Gore Ass., Flagstaff, AZ, USA) is placed to obtain optimal stability of the wound in the recipient site.

Mini-screws made of stainless steel (or titanium) are often used to support the membrane in the center of the defect. The mini-screws are, thus, positioned in the recipient site and left to protrude from the bone surface at the intended height of the new bone. As an alternative to the use of mini-screws, a block of autogenous bone can be placed to stabilize the membrane. The bone block must be firmly anchored to the bone of the recipient site with fixation screws.

Before the placement of graft material, the cortical bone of the recipient site must be perforated with a round bur to expose the cancellous bone and induce a bleeding hard tissue surface (Rompen et al. 1999). When a titanium reinforced e-PTFE membrane is used, the barrier is adjusted with the use of pliers and adapted to the intended shape of the augmented ridge. The membrane is trimmed with scissors and adjusted to extend at least 4-5 mm beyond the margins of the defect.

Once positioned at the surgical site, the membrane is fixed to the *lingual/palatal* aspect of the bone crest with mini-screws. This will allow the graft to be placed in the recipient site from a buccal direction.

Preparation of the donor site

Both *extraoral* and *intraoral* sites have been proposed as possible donor sites for the harvesting of autogenous bone.

The use of *extraoral* sites, including the iliac crest, the tibia and the calvaria, allows the harvesting of large volumes of bone. The use of such donor sites, however, (1) increases the morbidity associated with the procedure, and (2) requires general anesthesia and often the hospitalization of the patient

The most frequently used *intraoral* donor sites include:

1. the ramus (the retromolar region)
2. the symphysis of the mandible.

Before bone is harvested, a comprehensive clinical and radiographic examination (a panoramic radiograph is generally, but not always, sufficient) of the intraoral donor site must be performed. In this examination the following issues must be considered:

1. the position of the alveolar nerve in relation to the bone crest
2. the position of the mental foramen in relation to an obvious landmark (e.g. a neighboring tooth)
3. the length of the roots and the position of the apices of the mandibular incisors in relation to the lower border of the mandible
4. the volume of bone that can be harvested.

Surgical procedure in the region of the ramus

Bone collection from the mandibular ramus is normally performed only when the third molar is missing and when only a limited amount of bone is required to graft the recipient site.

A crestal incision is made. The incision should start about 2-3 mm distal of the second molar and be extended in distal and lateral direction following the lateral margin of the ramus. A vertical releasing incision is made at the mesial aspect of the crestal incision. After the elevation of a full thickness flap, the osteotomy can be accomplished with the use of trephines or thin carbide burs. Bone harvesting must be carried out in a gentle and careful manner and during irrigation of the surgical site with sterile saline (Figs. 39-1, 39-2). The dimension (amount) of the bone graft that can be harvested is dependent on (1) the buccal-lingual dimension of the ramus, and (2) the position of the inferior alveolar nerve. Thus, at least 3 mm of intact bone must remain over the alveolar nerve to avoid neurological complications. It is also essential not to penetrate the lingual wall of the ramus region and thereby sever blood vessels in this region.

When a particulate bone graft is harvested, the round osteotomies – prepared with a trephine – should overlap in order to reduce the size of each individual hard tissue block, and to facilitate their collection and grinding. After the bone collection procedure is completed, the flaps are replaced and closed with interrupted sutures.

Surgical procedure in the region of the symphysis of the mandible

An incision is placed about 10 mm below the mucogingival junction and is extended between the distal aspect of the two mandibular canines. A full thickness flap is elevated with a periosteal elevator and is reflected from the incision line to the inferior border of the mandible.

When the intention is to prepare a particulate bone graft, the osteotomy can be accomplished with medium-sized trephines (8 mm diameter). During bone sampling the surgical site is irrigated with saline. The circular osteotomy cuts should overlap to facilitate the removal of the bone tissue (see above). The depth of each cut (≤ 5-6 mm) must consistently be related to the buccal-lingual dimension of the donor site (Figs. 39-3, 39-4). The apical limit of the bone harvesting is located 5 mm coronal to the inferior border of the chin. The coronal limit of the osteotomy is 5 mm apical of the apex of the anterior teeth, and the lateral limit is 5 mm mesial to the mental foramen (Hunt & Jovanovic 1999). The bone harvesting is normally made with a curette. The small hard tissue portions are subdivided into small bone chips.

When the intention is to harvest a block of bone, a bone saw can be used to prepare a rectangular shaped graft of desired dimensions (Figs. 39-5, 39-6).

Before wound closure, a collagen sponge is placed as hemostatic agent in the donor site. This sponge will reduce postoperatory swelling and hematoma forma-

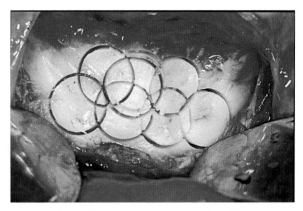

Fig. 39-3. Round osteotomies were made with the use of an 8 mm diameter trephine. The cuts overlapped and reached a depth of 5-6 mm.

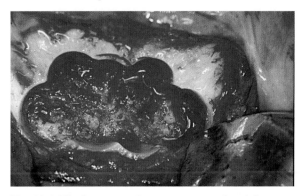

Fig. 39-4. The bone samples were removed and the cancellous bone was collected with the use of a surgical spoon.

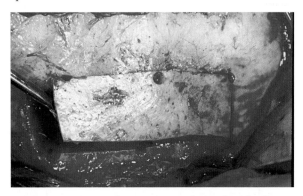

Fig. 39-5. A rectangular cut was performed with a bone saw to collect a large bone block.

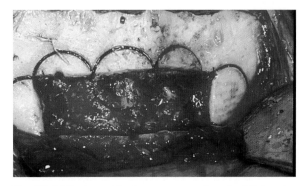

Fig. 39-6. The bone block was removed and additional round cuts were prepared with the trephine. The round bone samples will be ground with the use of a bone mill to obtain bone chips.

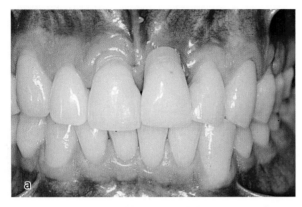 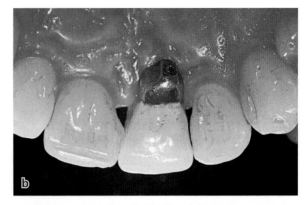

Fig. 39-7. (a) 39-year-old patient exhibiting an implant-supported restoration of tooth 21. The esthetic appearance was compromised by the "overcontoured" crown. (b) Palatal aspect of the same crown.

tion. The closure of the flaps includes a two-layer suturing technique, one internal and one external suture. For the internal suture a resorbable suture material is used. The internal suture often has the design of a horizontal mattress and is intended to close the periosteum and the severed muscles. For the external suture, that is intended for closure of the incision wounds, a non-resorbable material is used. A continuous or an interrupted suturing technique may be adopted.

During the immediate post-operative period (10 days) most patients will experience some swelling and discoloration of the chin area. Paresthesia of the lower anterior tooth region can persist for periods exceeding 6 months.

Positioning of the bone graft in the recipient site

The barrier membrane is first anchored to the lingual bone wall of the defect with mini-screws. After the harvesting of the small bone blocks and the preparation of bone chips (particulated graft), the graft particles are packed on the perforated hard tissue surface of the bone crest of the recipient site. The membrane is subsequently adjusted to cover the graft and is finally anchored to the buccal bone wall with mini-screws placed at the mesiobuccal and distobuccal rims. This will provide optimal stability of the membrane and ideal protection of the grafts.

In regions where the recipient site is located close to a natural tooth, a 2 mm wide zone of crestal bone next to the tooth must be left uncovered by the membrane so that the graft and the membrane will not interfere with the periodontal tissues of the natural tooth.

Closure of the recipient site

Releasing incision
Before the wound is closed, a releasing incision must be made in the periosteum at the base of the buccal flap (sometimes also of the lingual/palatal flap) to facilitate soft tissue management and to achieve a tension-free soft tissue adaptation. The periosteal incision must join the vertical releasing incisions at the mesial and distal margins of the flap. Particular attention must be paid when such releasing incisions are placed in the lower jaw in order to avoid damage of the inferior alveolar nerve at its exit from the mental foramen. Moreover, the incisions at the lingual aspect of the mandible must be placed so as to avoid damage of the vascular plexa at the floor of the mouth.

Suturing
Wound closure is often accomplished with horizontal mattress sutures, alternated with interrupted sutures. Horizontal mattress sutures are applied to achieve proper flap position. Interrupted sutures are placed between the mattress sutures and to close the vertical releasing incisions.

Postoperative care

After the completion of the procedure, the patient should receive an antibiotic to prevent infection and an anti-inflammatory agent to reduce edema and swelling, for a period of about 1 week.

Chemical plaque control including the use of chlorhexidine mouth rinses (0.12% solution twice a day) is instituted for 2 weeks. The sutures are removed after 12-15 days. The e-PTFE membrane is usually removed after 6 months of healing. Implants may then be placed in the augmented ridge, according to directions provided in the manual for the different implant systems used.

CASE REPORTS

Patient 1 – Alveolar ridge augmentation for single tooth restoration in the anterior maxilla

The 39-year-old man expressed concern about the esthetic outcome of an implant-supported restoration that had been placed in the maxillary left central incisor region. The patient also complained about the bulky palatal surface of the same restoration (Fig. 39-7a,b). The patient was in good general health and was a non-smoker.

Initial examination
The patient's natural dentition was in good condition and he had a comparatively good oral hygiene status. Tooth 21 presented with an implant-supported crown made of porcelain fused to metal that was overcontoured both at its buccal and lingual aspects (Fig. 39-8). The peri-implant mucosa exhibited signs of inflammation.

The reason why the restoration had been overcontoured by the prosthodontist was, most likely, the improper position of the implant in the ridge between the natural teeth. In fact, during surgery the implant had been placed too far palatally as compared to the position of the adjacent teeth. The gingiva at the buccal aspect of tooth 11 and tooth 22 exhibited modest recession (Fig. 39-7a).

Treatment planning
During treatment planning different options were considered:

1. removal of the implant and placement of a conventional three-unit bridge
2. placement of a Maryland bridge restoration
3. removal of the implant, reconstruction of the soft and hard tissues at site 21 and subsequently *de novo* implant installation and crown restoration.

The different treatment options were explained to the patient. Option 3 was selected.

Treatment

Initial therapy
The patient was instructed in proper plaque control procedures. After flap elevation, the implant in site 21 was removed with the use of a calibrated trephine. The flap was repositioned coronally and closed with interrupted sutures.

Implant placement and bone regeneration
After 2 months of healing following implant removal, buccal and lingual full thickness flaps were elevated. The flaps extended from tooth 11 to tooth 22 (Figs. 39-9, 39-10) and were released with vertical incisions

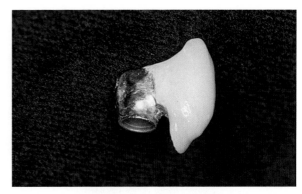

Fig. 39-8. The artificial crown was removed. It was possible to recognize the "overcontoured" surfaces on both the buccal and the palatal aspect of the crown.

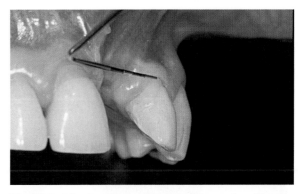

Fig. 39-9. After implant removal and 2 months of healing, the site demonstrated the presence of a deep defect in the bone. Also the soft tissue was compromised.

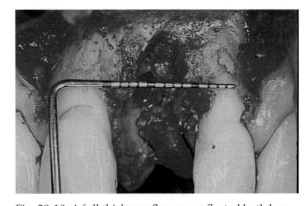

Fig. 39-10. A full thickness flap was reflected both buccally and palatally, extending from tooth 11 to tooth 22.

placed at the distal line angle of teeth 11 and 22. The bone surface was carefully curetted and all residual soft tissue was removed from the defect.

An implant (13 mm long) was placed in a proper position with the implant shoulder 3 mm apical of the free gingival margin of the adjacent teeth. This resulted in an implant exposure outside the buccal bone housing of about 8 mm (Fig. 39-11).

A reinforced e-PTFE membrane was adapted and fixed palatally with the use of titanium pins. A particulated bone graft was collected from the retromolar

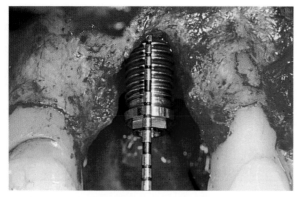

Fig. 39-11. An implant was placed with the shoulder located 3 mm apical of the free gingival margin of the adjacent teeth. This resulted in an implant exposure outside the buccal bone of about 8 mm.

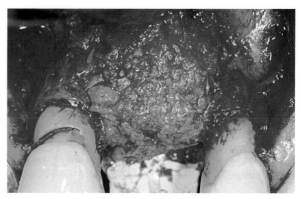

Fig. 39-12. A particulated bone graft was collected from the retromolar area in the mandible and was packed into the bone defect.

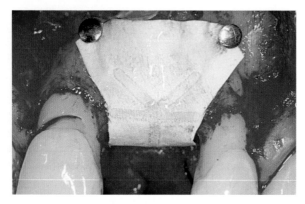

Fig. 39-13. A titanium reinforced e-PTFE membrane was placed and stabilized buccally and palatally with titanium pins.

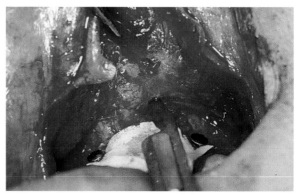

Fig. 39-14. The periosteum of the buccal flap was incised and released in order to augment the flap movability before wound closure.

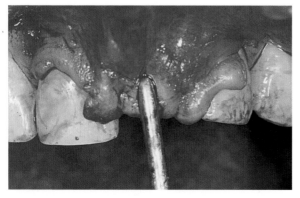

Fig. 39-15. The wound closure was performed with horizontal mattress and interrupted suture.

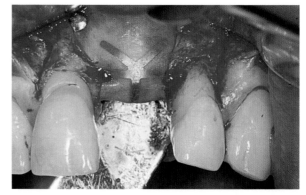

Fig. 39-16. After 6 months of uneventful healing, the e-PTFE membrane was removed.

area in the mandible and was packed into the bone defect (Fig. 39-12). The membrane was then anchored to the buccal bone wall with two titanium pins (Fig. 39-13).

The periosteum of the buccal flap was released in order to augment the movability of the flap before the wound was closed with horizontal mattress and interrupted sutures (Figs. 39-14, 39-15).

Membrane removal and abutment connection
After 6 months of healing, the e-PTFE membrane was

removed and a connective tissue graft was placed on top of the regenerated bone to increase the thickness of the mucosa (Figs. 39-16, 39-17, 39-18). After another 2 months, the cover screw was exposed and connected to a regular abutment (Fig. 39-19).

Restorative therapy
A provisional acrylic crown was prepared and inserted after one additional month of healing. The emergence profile of the crown was modified repeatedly during the next 6 months to condition the soft

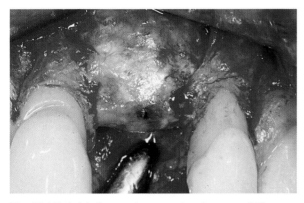

Fig. 39-17. A thin layer of connective tissue could be seen on the surface of the regenerated bone.

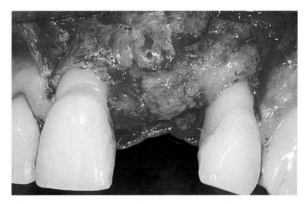

Fig. 39-18. A connective tissue graft was placed on top of the regenerated bone to increase the thickness of the mucosa.

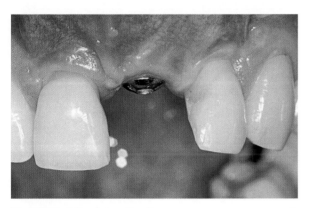

Fig. 39-19. After 2 months the cover screw was exposed and connected with a regular abutment.

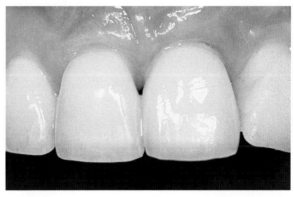

Fig. 39-20. A Procera® made full porcelain crown was inserted.

tissue, and finally a "Procera® crown" (Nobel Biocare, Gothenburg, Sweden) was fabricated and inserted (Fig. 39-20).

Concluding remarks

This case showed that GBR techniques can also be effectively used for the treatment of peri-implant bone defects in the anterior region of the maxilla. The treatment included a series of surgical and prosthetic steps but resulted in proper function and an optimal esthetic outcome.

Patient 2 – Alveolar ridge augmentation for implant restoration in the anterior maxilla

A 22-year-old man had been involved in a motorcycle accident in which the two upper central incisors, together with the associated buccal bone plate had been lost. The patient was otherwise in good general health and was a non-smoker.

Initial examination

The patient presented with his natural dentition in good condition. There were no clinical signs of periodontitis and dental caries. The clinical findings were confirmed in the radiographic examination. The oral

hygiene examination revealed the presence of modest amounts of soft and hard supragingival deposits.

The upper central incisors were missing and the edentulous ridge in this region was insufficient, both in width and height, for implant installation. The upper lateral incisors were vital, exhibiting minute crown fractures that had been restored with composite.

Treatment planning

The patient was informed about the lack of sufficient bone tissue in the upper front tooth region. The different treatment modalities that were available were described. These included bone augmentation, implant installation and crown restoration. Further, the anticipated long-term result and alternative treatment options were discussed.

After having evaluated the options, it was decided that a ridge augmentation procedure including GBR should be performed with subsequent implant placement and prosthetic reconstruction.

Treatment

Initial therapy

This treatment included patient information, oral hygiene instruction and professional tooth debridement

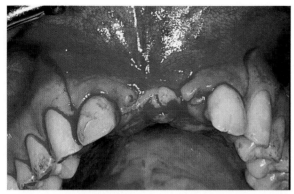

Fig. 39-21. A 22-year-old man had a motorcycle accident and the two upper central incisors and the buccal bone plate were lost. A full thickness flap was elevated both buccally and palatally from tooth 12 to tooth 22.

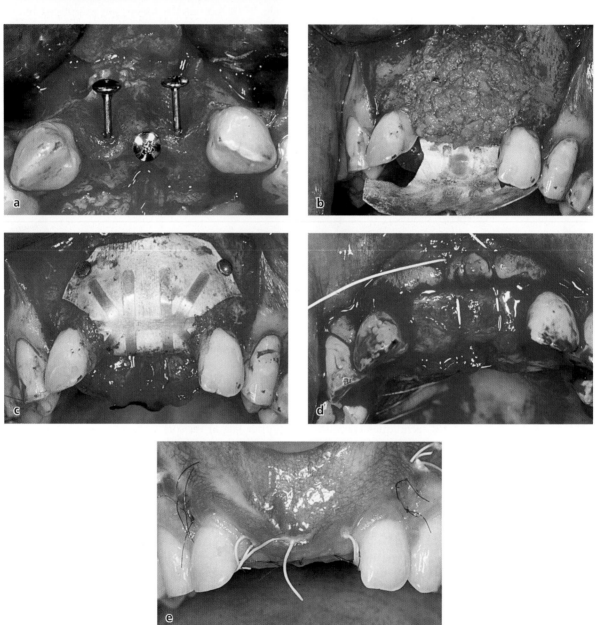

Fig. 39-22. (a) Three mini-screws were applied to the buccal defect and on top of the bone crest in order to support a membrane and to avoid its collapse into the defect. (b) A titanium reinforced e-PTFE membrane was adapted and fixed to the palatal aspect of the edentulous bone crest with titanium pins. A particulate autogenous bone graft was packed into the defect. (c) The membrane was anchored buccally with two titanium pins. (d) A connective tissue graft was harvested from the palate and positioned on top of the crest to augment the thickness of the mucosa. (e) The flaps were closed with horizontal mattress and interrupted sutures.

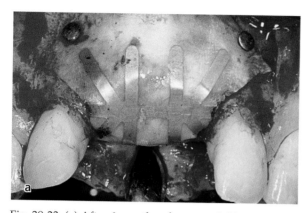
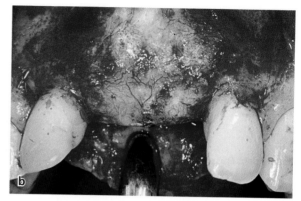

Fig. 39-23. (a) After 6 months of uneventful healing, a full thickness flap was elevated and the membrane exposed. (b) The membrane was removed. The mini-screws appear embedded in the regenerated bone.

A Maryland bridge was fabricated and inserted as a provisional restoration in the upper incisor region.

Ridge augmentation
A full thickness flap was elevated both buccally and palatally and extended from tooth 12 to tooth 22 (Fig. 39-21). A titanium reinforced e-PTFE membrane was adapted and fixed to the palatal aspect of the edentulous bone crest with titanium pins. Three mini-screws were applied to the buccal defect and on top of the bone crest in order to support the membrane and to avoid its collapse into the defect (Fig. 39-22a). A particulated bone graft was collected from the mandibular symphysis region and placed in the ridge defect (Fig. 39-22b). The membrane was then fixed buccally with two titanium pins (Fig. 39-22c). A connective tissue graft was harvested from the palate and positioned on top of the crest to augment the thickness of the soft tissue (Fig. 39-22d). Releasing incisions were placed in the periosteum and the flaps were closed with horizontal mattress and interrupted sutures (Fig. 39-22e). The sutures were removed after 2 weeks.

Membrane removal and implant placement
After 6 months of uneventful healing, a full thickness flap was elevated and the membrane, pins and screws were removed (Fig. 39-23a,b). Two 13 mm long implants were placed in region 11 and 21 (Fig. 39-24).

After 6 months, abutment connection was performed (Fig. 39-25a,b). In addition, the fornix was

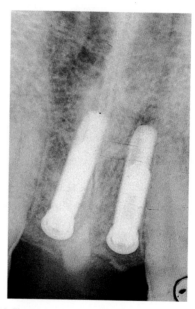

Fig. 39-24. Two 13 mm long implants were placed in region 11 and 21.

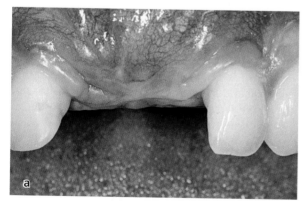
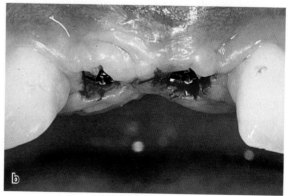

Fig. 39-25. (a)After 6 months of healing, the abutment connection was performed. (b) Two healing abutments were placed.

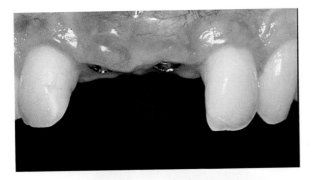

Fig. 39-26. The fornix was deepened with a partial thickness flap. After one month the mucosa had healed.

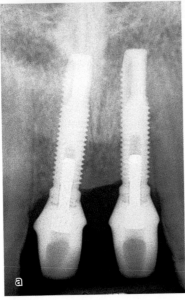

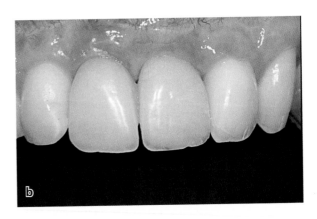

Fig. 39-27. (a) Periapical radiograph demonstrating the amount of new bone formation as well as the provisional restoration. (b) Two acrylic crowns were inserted.

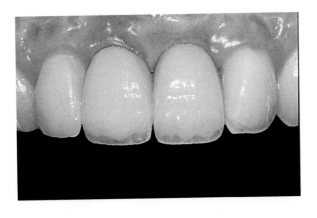

Fig. 39.28. The final prosthetic restoration including two independent (porcelain fused to metal) crowns, was placed after 4 months of soft tissue conditioning.

deepened using a partial thickness flap procedure (Fig. 39-26).

Restorative therapy

The peri-implant tissues were left to heal and mature for 1 month before two provisional crowns were fabricated and inserted (Fig. 39-27a,b). The final prosthetic restorations, including two single crowns (porcelain fused to metal), were placed after 4 months of soft tissue maturation (Fig. 39-28).

The patient was incorporated in a supportive care program that included recall appointments every 6 months.

Concluding remarks

This case describes the different phases included in the surgical and prosthetic reconstruction of a site which included two adjacent missing teeth in the upper jaw. In this particular case the esthetic outcome was of great importance. Therefore, a number of different procedures were required to reconstruct both the hard and the soft tissues.

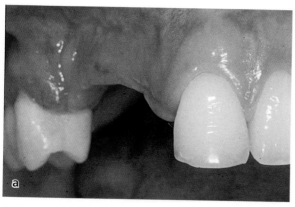

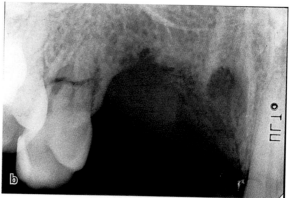

Fig. 39-29. Clinical picture of a 25-year-old woman demonstrating the presence of an edentulous ridge with advanced bone loss at sites 11, 12 and 13. (b) Periapical radiograph demonstrating the bone defect and a horizontal root fracture at the middle of the root of tooth 14.

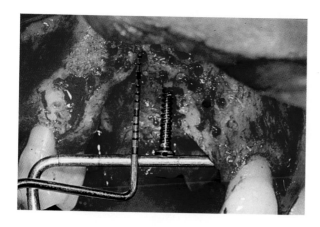

Fig. 39-30. A mucoperiosteal flap was raised both buccaly and palatally. A 20 mm long titanium screw was positioned, projecting from the bone crest.

Patient 3 – Alveolar ridge augmentation for implant restoration of multiple adjacent maxillary teeth

A 25-year-old woman had lost teeth 11, 12 and13 and fractured the root of tooth 14 in a car accident. She was a non-smoker, in good general health and required restoration of function and esthetics in the central maxillary tooth region.

Initial examination

The remaining dentition was in good condition. The patient had a good oral hygiene standard and exhibited no open carious lesions or periodontitis. The clinical examination and the radiographs demonstrated the presence of an edentulous ridge with advanced bone loss at sites 11, 12 and 13. Tooth 14 presented with a horizontal root fracture at the middle of the root (Fig. 39-29a,b).

Treatment planning

The patient was informed about the steps included in ridge augmentation and implant therapy. Particular attention was paid to explaining the risks, the failure rate and the possible outcome of a suboptimal esthetic result.

Due to the small amount of residual bone a two-stage approach for bone regeneration and implant placement was considered.

Treatment

Initial treatment
A Maryland bridge was placed as a provisional restoration.

Horizontal and vertical ridge augmentation
Following the placement of crestal and releasing incisions, buccal and palatal mucoperiosteal flaps were raised. The flaps extended one tooth mesial and two teeth distal of the defect.

The bone defect was exposed and debrided with a chisel. The cortical bone was perforated to expose the cancellous bone and to stimulate bleeding. A 20 mm long titanium screw was positioned in the recipient site, projecting from the defect (Fig. 39-30) and was intended to support the titanium reinforced e-PTFE membrane that was subsequently placed and anchored to the palatal bone. The defect was filled with autogenous bone chips harvested from the chin, and the membrane was anchored to the buccal bone wall of the defect area (Figs. 39-31a,b,c). The periosteum was released and the flaps were closed with horizontal mattress and interrupted sutures. After one month of healing the fractured tooth in site 14 was extracted.

Implant placement
After 6 months of healing, full thickness flaps were elevated and the membrane was removed. Three 13

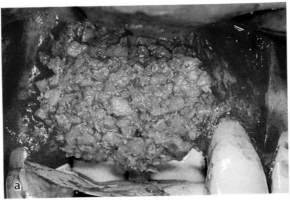

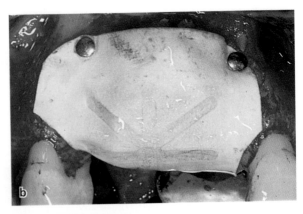

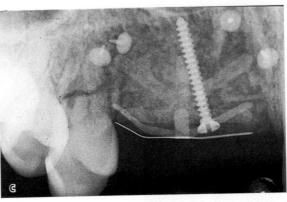

Fig. 39-31. (a) The bone defect was filled with autogenous bone chips harvested from the chin. (b) A titanium reinforced e-PTFE membrane was anchored buccally and palatally with the use of titanium pins. (c) Periapical radiograph demonstrating the bone fill immediately after the surgery.

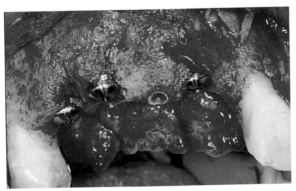

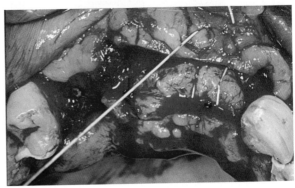

Fig. 39-32. After 6 months of healing flaps were elevated and the membrane removed. Three implants, 13 mm long, were placed in sites 11, 13 and 14.

Fig. 39-33. A connective tissue graft harvested from the palatal mucosa was positioned on top of the bone crest to augment the thickness of the soft tissue.

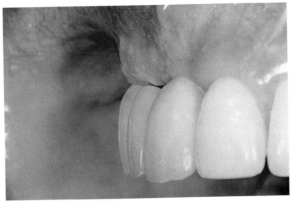

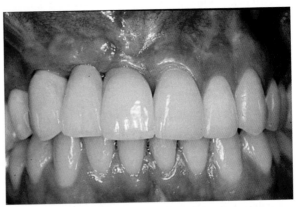

Fig. 39-34. After the abutment connection was performed, the patient used a provisional acrylic bridge for six months.

Fig. 39-35. Full ceramic abutments were inserted to support a (porcelain fused to metal) four-unit bridge.

mm long implants were placed in sites 11, 13 and 14 (Fig. 39-32). Before the wound was closed, a connective tissue graft, harvested from the palatal mucosa, was positioned on top of the bone crest to augment the thickness of the mucosa (Fig. 39-33).

Restorative therapy
Abutment connection was performed after 4 months. The patient used a provisional acrylic bridge for 6 months (Fig. 39-34). During this interval the emergence profiles of the temporary crowns were adjusted to the correct shape of the soft tissue margin. For the final restoration full ceramic abutments were used to support a four-unit bridge (Fig. 39-35).

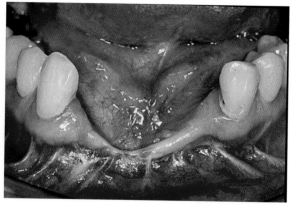

Fig. 39-36. A 36-year-old woman presenting with a fractured mandible. She had lost all the lower incisors and the buccal alveolar bone plate.

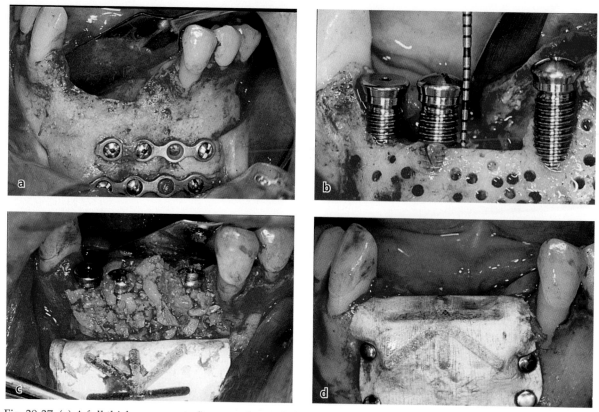

Fig. 39-37. (a) A full thickness remote flap was elevated. (b) Three 15 mm long implants, were placed in position 31, 41 and 42, 6-8 mm of the implants project outside the bone surface. (c) A titanium reinforced e-PTFE membrane was adjusted to the defect. The space under the membrane was filled with autogenous bone chips collected from the chin. (d) The membrane was anchored buccally with four titanium pins.

Patient 4 – Vertical ridge augmentation in the anterior area of the mandible

This 36-year-old woman had been involved in a car accident. She presented with a fractured mandible and, in addition, she had lost all the lower incisors together with the buccal alveolar bone plate in the mandibular front tooth region. The fracture was treated with osteosynthesis and healed uneventfully.

The patient was a non-smoker and was in good general health. She asked for a fixed restoration in the lower front tooth region.

Initial examination
The remaining dentition appeared to be in reasonably good condition. There were no signs of additional tooth fracture or soft tissue damage. The patient's oral hygiene status was below optimal standard. Thus, large amounts of supragingival plaque were observed in most segments of the dentition. The clinical and radiographic examination revealed the presence of a

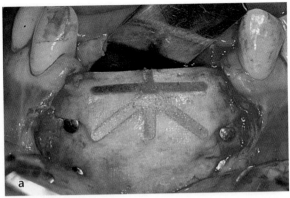

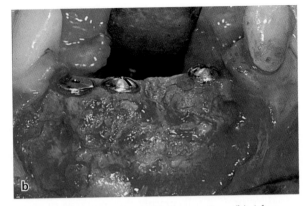

Fig. 39-38. (a) After 6 months the tissues adjacent to the membrane exhibited no signs of inflammation. (b) After membrane removal, it was possible to assess the complete coverage of the implants with newly formed bone.

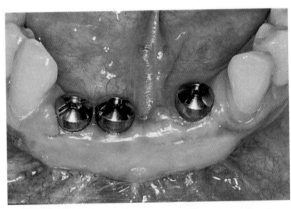

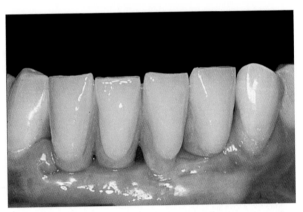

Fig. 39-39. After one further month of healing, the abutments were inserted.

Fig. 39-40. The final prosthetic rehabilitation was made with porcelain-fused-to-metal crowns.

deep and wide ridge defect in the frontal region of the mandible. The defect was covered with a non-keratinized mucosa (Fig. 39-36).

Treatment planning and treatment

An implant-supported restoration was chosen as the optimal treatment alternative. The adjacent teeth, therefore, were not to be included in the final restoration. It was further decided that a vertical ridge augmentation procedure had to be performed to improve the height of the ridge and to allow for proper implant installation and prosthetic rehabilitation.

Implant placement and vertical ridge augmentation
After the elevation of a full thickness flap (Fig. 39-37a), three 15 mm long implants were placed in the defect and in positions 31, 41 and 42. The implant shoulders were positioned 3 mm apical of the cemento-enamel junction of the adjacent teeth; 6-8 mm of the "coronal" portions of the implants were not invested in bone but projected into the defect space (Fig. 39-37b). A titanium reinforced e-PTFE membrane was adjusted and anchored to the lingual wall of the defect. The implants supported the membrane and prevented it

from collapsing into the defect. The space under the membrane was filled with autogenous bone chips collected from the chin in the same surgical site (Fig. 39-37c). The membrane was fixed buccally with four titanium pins (Fig. 39-37d). Releasing incisions were placed in the periosteum at the base of the buccal and lingual flaps,. The wound was closed with horizontal mattress and interrupted sutures.

Membrane removal and restorative therapy
The membrane was removed after six months (Fig. 39-38a,b). After one further month, healing abutments were inserted in a second-stage surgery, and a free gingival graft, collected from the palatal mucosa, was placed outside the buccal aspects of the abutments (Fig. 39-39). The final prosthetic reconstruction included porcelain-fused-to-metal crowns (Fig. 39-40).

Concluding remarks

This case showed how a large defect in the ridge can be augmented using a one-step technique that involved (1) implant placement, (2) the use of autogenous bone graft, and (3) the use of a membrane to protect the graft.

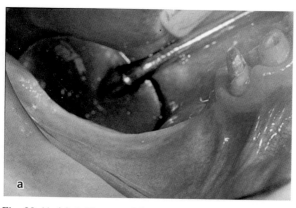 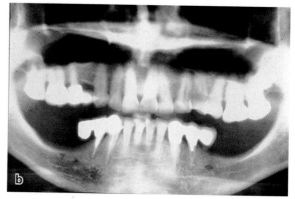

Fig. 39-41. (a) A 62-year-old woman exhibiting advanced crestal bone atrophy in the posterior regions of the mandible. (b) Orthopantomogram demonstrating the bilateral bone atrophy. The inferior alveolar nerves were located about 4 mm apical of the bone crest.

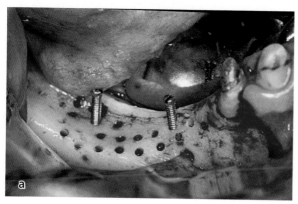 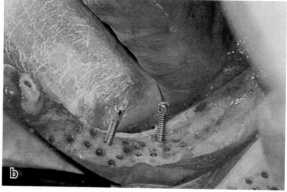

Fig. 39-42. A mucoperiosteal flap was elevated both buccally and lingually. Two 10 mm long mini-screws of titanium were placed in the bone, projecting from the bone crest by about 7 mm.

Patient 5 – Vertical ridge augmentation to allow implant placement in the posterior segments of the mandible

A 62-year-old woman had been wearing a removable partial denture in the lower jaw for about 15 years, and expressed the desire to replace this denture with a fixed bridge. She was in good general health and was a non-smoker.

Initial examination

The clinical examination revealed that the patient's oral hygiene was poor. Thus, large amounts of supragingivally located accumulations of plaque and calculus were seen in all segments of the remaining dentition. There were also signs of a generalized gingivitis, but the probing pocket depth measurements revealed that there were no pathologically deepened pockets.

The crown and bridge restorations that were present in the posterior segments of the maxilla were of acceptable quality. The following teeth were missing in the mandible: 35, 36, 37, 38 and 45, 46, 47, 48. Teeth 33, 34 and 43, 44 presented with proper root fillings, posts and cores.

In the orthopantomogram, it was observed that the edentulous areas of the mandible exhibited advanced crestal bone resorption (Fig. 39-41a,b). Further, the inferior alveolar nerve was located about 4 mm apical of the bone crest.

Treatment planning

The natural dentition and the crown and bridge restorations in the maxilla were maintainable. A cause-related periodontal therapy was required. This should include oral hygiene instruction as well as scaling and root planing. Implant-supported fixed bridge reconstruction in the posterior mandible would require vertical ridge augmentation prior to implant installation.

The patient was informed about the risks involved in this treatment and alternative treatment options.

Treatment

Initial therapy
The cause-related periodontal therapy was performed in order to achieve periodontal health before the initiation of the ridge augmentation procedure.

Vertical ridge augmentation
In both sides of the posterior mandible a crestal incision was made in the keratinized mucosa of the ridge. The crestal incision was extended along the natural teeth. Two vertical releasing incisions were made at

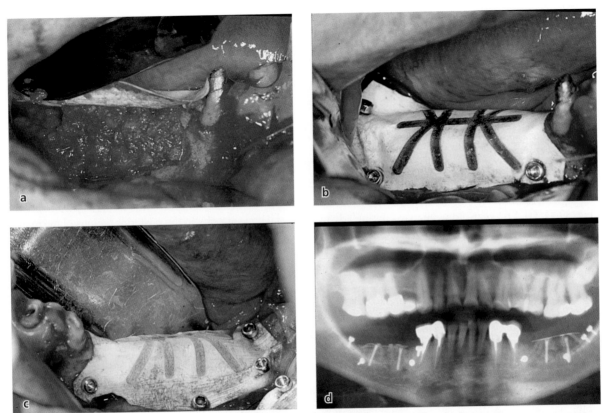

Fig. 39-43. (a) A particulate autogenous bone graft, collected from the chin, was placed on top of the crest. (b,c) The membrane was stabilized buccally and lingually with the use of mini-screws. (d) Ortopanthomogram demonstrating the bilateral vertical ridge augmentation immediately after the surgery.

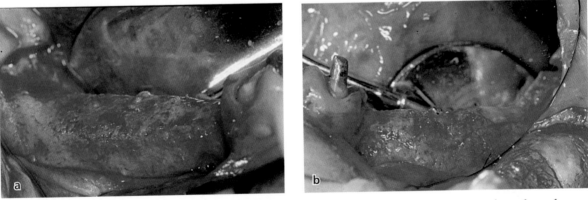

Fig. 39-44. After 6 months of uneventful healing the membrane was removed. Note the amount of new bone formation.

the mesial and distal ends of the crestal incision. Buccal and lingual mucoperiosteal flaps were elevated. The lingual flap was gently reflected beyond the mylohyoid insertion of the omohyoid muscle. This was done in order to enhance the movability of the flap and to manage a subsequent coronal advancement of the lingual flap.

Two mini-screws made of titanium and 10 mm long were placed in the remaining bone. The screws projected from the bone crest by about 7 mm (Fig. 39-42). A titanium reinforced e-PTFE membrane was retained to the lingual bone wall with fixation screws. A particulated autogenous bone graft, collected from the chin, was placed on top of the crest and the membrane

was stabilized to the buccal bone wall pins (Fig. 39-43a,b,c). Care was taken not to sever the alveolar nerve in particular at the region of the mental foramen. A releasing incision was placed in the buccal periosteum. The buccal and lingual flaps were closed with horizontal mattress and interrupted sutures.

Membrane removal and implant placement
After 6 months of healing, incisions were made, flaps were elevated, the membranes, pins and mini-screws were removed, and the amount of new bone that had formed was assessed (Fig. 39-44). Four implants (10 mm long) were placed in sites 35, 36 and 45, 46 (Fig. 39-45). The sites were left to heal for 6 months.

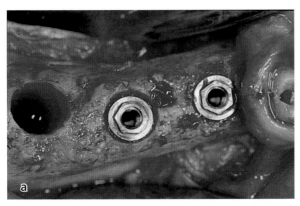
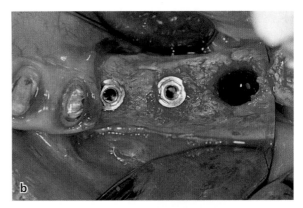

Fig. 39-45. Four implants, 10 mm long, were placed in sites 35, 36 and 45, 46 according to the standard surgical technique.

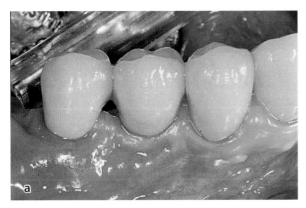
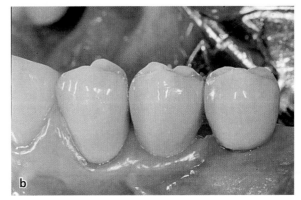

Fig. 39-46. Porcelain-fused-to-metal crowns were inserted. The implant-supported crowns were left without fixed contact with the natural teeth.

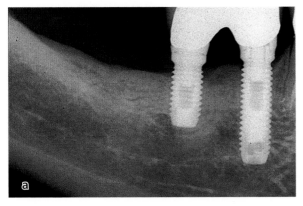
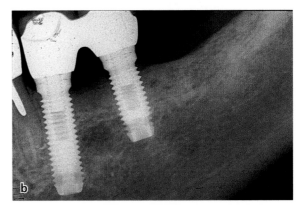

Fig. 39-47. Periapical radiographs demonstrating the implants in the regenerated bone after 3 years of function.

Restorative therapy

After abutment connection, provisional crowns were placed and left in function for a period of 3 months. Finally, porcelain-fused-to-metal crowns were inserted. The implant supported crowns were not connected to the natural teeth (Fig. 39-46, 39-47).

Concluding remarks

This case illustrates how vertical ridge augmentation including a GBR technique can be used to restore a partially edentulous ridge and how implant installation and crown restoration can be performed subsequently in the augmented region.

REFERENCES

Buser D., Bragger U., Lang N.P. & Nyman S. (1990). Regeneration and enlargement of jaw bone using guided tissue regeneration. *Clinical Oral Implants Research* **1**, 22-32.

Buser, D., Dula, K., Belser, U., Hirt, H.P. & Berthold, H. (1993). Localized ridge augmentation using guided bone regeneration. I. Surgical procedure in the maxilla. *International Journal of Periodontics and Restorative Dentistry* **13**, 29-45.

Buser, D., Dula, K., Belser, U., Hirt, H.P. & Berthold, H. (1995). Localized ridge augmentation using guided bone regeneration. II. Surgical procedure in the mandible. *International Journal of Periodontics and Restorative Dentistry* **15**, 11-29.

Buser, D., Dula, K., Hirt, H.P. & Schenk, R.K. (1996). Lateral ridge augmentation using autografts and barrier membranes: A clinical study with 40 partially edentulous patients. *Journal of Oral and Maxillofacial Surgery* **54**, 420-432.

Hunt, D.R. & Jovanovic, S.A. (1999). Autogenous bone harvesting: a chin graft technique for particulate and monocortical bone blocks. *International Journal of Periodontics and Restorative Dentistry* **19**, 165-173.

Lang, N.P., Hammerle, C.H.F., Bragger, U., Lehmann, B. & Nyman, S.R. (1994). Guided tissue regeneration in jawbone defects prior to implant placement. *Clinical Oral Implant Research* **5**, 92-97.

Mellonig, J.T. & Triplett, J. (1993). Guided tissue regeneration and endosseous dental implants. *International Journal of Periodontics and Restorative Dentistry* **13**, 109-119.

Nevins, M. & Mellonig, J.T. (1992). Enhancement of the damaged edentulous ridge to receive dental implants: A combination of allograft and the Gore-Tex membrane. *International Journal of Periodontics and Restorative Dentistry* **12**, 12-17.

Nevins, R. & Mellonig, J.T. (1994). The advantage of localized ridge augmentation prior to implant placement: A two stage event. *International Journal of Periodontics and Restorative Dentistry* **14**, 97-111.

Rominger, J.W. & Triplett, R.G. (1994). The use of guided tissue regeneration to improve implant osseointegration. *Journal of Oral and Maxillofacial Surgery* **52**, 106-112.

Rompen, E. H., Biewer, R., Vanheusden, Zahedi, S. & Nusgens, B. (1999). The influence of cortical perforations and of space filling with peripheral blood on the kinetics of guided bone regeneration. A comparative histometric study. *Clinical Oral Implant Research* **10**, 85-94.

Simion, M., Trisi, P. & Piattelli, A. (1994). Vertical ridge augmentation using a membrane technique associated with osseointegrated implants. *International Journal of Periodontics and Restorative Dentistry* **14**, 497-511.

Simion, M., Jovanovic, S.A., Trisi, P., Scarano, A. & Piattelli, A. (1998). Vertical ridge augmentation around dental implants using a membrane technique and autogenous bone or allografts in humans. *International Journal of Periodontics and Restorative Dentistry* **18**, 9-23.

Tinti, C. & Parma-Benfenati, S. (1998). Vertical ridge augmentation: Surgical protocol and retrospective evaluation of 48 consecutively inserted implants. *International Journal of Periodontics and Restorative Dentistry* **18**, 445-443.

Tinti, C., Parma-Benfenati, S. & Polizzi, G. (1996). Vertical ridge augmentation: What is the limit? *International Journal of Periodontics and Restorative Dentistry* **16**, 221-229.

CHAPTER 40

Implant Placement in the Esthetic Zone

URS BELSER, JEAN-PIERRE BERNARD AND DANIEL BUSER

BASIC CONCEPTS

The clinical replacement of lost natural teeth by osseointegrated implants has represented one of the most significant advances in restorative dentistry. Numerous studies on various clinical indications have documented high implant survival and success rates with respect to specific application criteria (Ekfeldt et al. 1994, Laney et al. 1994, Andersson et al. 1995, Brånemark et al. 1995, Lewis 1995, Jemt et al. 1996, Lindqvist et al. 1996, Buser et al. 1997, Ellegaard et al. 1997a,b, Levine et al. 1997, Andersson et al. 1998, Bryant & Zarb 1998, Eckert & Wollan 1998, Ellen 1998, Lindh et al. 1998, Mericske-Stern 1998, ten Bruggenkate et al. 1998, Wyatt & Zarb 1998, Gunne et al. 1999, Lekholm et al. 1999, Van Steenberghe et al. 1999, Wismeijer et al. 1999, Behneke et al. 2000, Hosny et al. 2000, Hultin et al. 2000, Weber et al. 2000, Boioli et al. 2001, Gomez-Roman et al. 2001, Kiener et al. 2001, Mengel et al. 2001, Oetterli et al. 2001, Zitzmann et al. 2001, Bernard & Belser 2002, Buser et al. 2002, Haas et al. 2002, Leonhardt et al. 2002, Romeo et al. 2002). Several recently published studies have focused on treatment outcome of implant therapy in partially edentulous patients in general, and related to maxillary anterior implant restorations in particular. Belser (1999) reviewed selected publications which appear to have impact when it comes to the discussion of es-

thetic aspects which will be addressed in this chapter. In a prospective longitudinal study involving a total of 94 implants (50 in the anterior maxilla) restored with fixed partial dentures (FPDs), Zarb and Schmitt (1993) published an average success rate of 91.5% for an observation period up to 8 years. The respective data concerning the maxillary implants demonstrated a success rate of 94% (100% for the prosthesis success). It was concluded that implant therapy in anterior partial edentulism can replicate the data established in the literature for fully edentulous patients. The same authors (Schmitt & Zarb 1993) published an 8-year implant survival rate of 97.9% for single-tooth replacement in partially edentulous patients. These results were confirmed by Avivi-Arber and Zarb in 1996.

Andersson et al. (1998) published similarly favorable prospective 5-year data on single-tooth restorations, performed either in a specialist clinic or in general practices, while Eckert and Wollan (1998) presented a retrospective evaluation up to 11 years on a total of 1170 implants inserted in partially edentulous patients, and found no differences in survival rates with respect to the anatomical location of the implants. A meta-analysis concerning implants placed for the treatment of partial edentulism was carried out by Lindh et al. (1998). The 6–7-year survival rate for single implant crowns corresponded to 97.5%, while the survival rate of implant-supported fixed partial

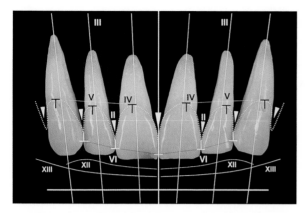

Fig. 40-1. The esthetic checklist, describing a number of respective fundamental objective criteria as they relate to the maxillary anterior segment (detailed description presented in Table 40.1). (Reprinted from Magne & Belser 2002, with permission.)

Table 40.1. Fundamental objective esthetic criteria (Magne & Belser 2002)

1. Gingival health
2. Interdental closure
3. Tooth axis
4. Zenith of the gingival contour
5. Balance of the gingival levels
6. Level of the interdental contact
7. Relative tooth dimensions
8. Basic features of tooth form
9. Tooth characterization
10. Surface texture
11. Color
12. Incisal edge configuration
13. Lower lip line
14. Smile symmetry

Subjective criteria (esthetic integration)

Variations in tooth form
Tooth arrangement and positioning
Relative crown length
Negative space

dentures (FPDs) was 93.6%. The influence of implant design and surface texture was investigated by Norton (1998) by means of a radiographic follow-up of 33 implants loaded for up to 4 years. A most favorable maintenance of marginal bone around the conical collar was revealed, with a mean marginal bone loss of 0.32 mm mesially and 0.34 mm distally for the whole group.

Soft tissue stability around implant restorations and adjacent teeth is of paramount importance within the appearance zone (Bengazi et al. 1996, Chang et al. 1999, Ericsson et al. 2000, Grunder 2000, Choquet et al. 2001, Cooper et al. 2001, Mericske-Stern et al. 2001, Bernard & Belser 2002, Engquist et al. 2002, Haas et al.

2002, Krenmair et al. 2002). Scheller et al. (1998) specifically addressed this parameter in their 5-year prospective multicenter study on 99 implant-supported single-crown restorations. The authors reported overall cumulative success rates of 95.9% for implants and 91.1% for implant crowns. Soft tissue levels around implant restorations and adjacent teeth remained stable over the entire evaluation period. Wyatt and Zarb (1998) published a longitudinal study on 77 partially edentulous patients, involving a total of 230 implants and 97 fixed partial dentures, with an observation period of up to 12 years (mean 5.41 years) after loading. The average implant success rate was 94%, while the continuous stability of the prostheses (fixed partial dentures) corresponded to 97%. This study comprised 70 anterior and 31 posterior maxillary implants. No significant differences with respect to longevity could be detected either between anterior and posterior locations or between maxillary and mandibular implant restorations.

Along with osseointegration and restoration of function, the patient's subjective satisfaction is a key element of the success of implant therapy. Especially when the implant is located in the anterior part of the oral cavity, an essential part of the therapy aims at creating appropriate conditions, so that finally the implant prosthesis cannot be distinguished from the adjacent natural teeth. In this context, a variety of specific procedures have been developed, including novel bone augmentation protocols, connective tissue grafting and reconstruction of lost papillary tissue (Bahat et al. 1993, Salama & Salama 1993, Bahat & Daftary 1995, Salama et al. 1995, Price & Price 1999, Choquet et al. 2001).

Being part of a comprehensive textbook about clinical periodontology, this chapter will focus primarily on fixed implant restorations located in the esthetic zone.

General esthetic principles and related guidelines

The basic parameters related to dental and gingival esthetics in general and to the maxillary anterior segment in particular are well established in the dental literature (Goldstein 1976, Belser 1982, Schärer et al. 1982, Seibert & Lindhe 1989, Goodacre 1990, Rüfenacht 1990, Nathanson 1991, Magne et al. 1993a,b, Chiche & Pinault 1994, Magne et al. 1994, Kois 1996, Kokich 1996, Magne et al. 1996, Kokich & Spear 1997, Jensen et al. 1999) and have been recently summarized in the form of an updated integral check-list by Magne & Belser (2002). When it comes to the characteristics of the natural maxillary anterior dentition, a number of fundamental objective criteria, including gingival health and its normal morphology as well as dimension, form, specific structural composition, color, opalescence, translucency, transparency and surface texture of incisors and canines, have been identified (Ta-

Table 40.2. Patient expectations related to maxillary anterior edentulous segments

- Long-lasting esthetic and functional result with a high degree of predictability

- Minimal invasiveness (preservation of tooth structure)

- Maximum subjective comfort

- Minimum risk for complications associated with surgery and healing phase

- Avoidance of removable prostheses

- Optimum cost effectiveness

Table 40.3. Therapeutic modalities for tooth replacement in the esthetic zone

- Conventional fixed partial dentures (FPDs), comprising cantilever units

- Resin-bonded ("adhesive") bridges

- Conventional removable partial dentures (RPDs)

- Tooth-supported overdentures

- Orthodontic therapy (closure of edentulous spaces)

- Implant-supported prostheses (fixed, retrievable or removable suprastructures)

- Combinations of the above

Table 40.4. Criteria favoring implant-borne restorations

- Normal wound healing capacity

- Intact neighboring teeth

- Unfavorable ("compromised") potential abutment teeth

- Extended edentulous segments

- Missing strategic abutment teeth

- Presence of diastemas

ble 40-1, Fig. 40-1). This list is completed by an addition of subjective criteria associated with esthetic integration, such as variations in the arrangement and positioning of front teeth, relative crown length and negative space.

Depending on the type of a given initial clinical situation requiring the replacement of one or several teeth, the patient's expectations may vary from the achievement of an almost perfect illusion, i.e. that the untrained eye cannot easily distinguish the restoration from the surrounding natural dentition, to the acceptance of various degrees of compromise from a purely esthetic point of view. The latter case is not infrequent after multiple anterior tooth loss in combination with significant hard and soft tissue deficiencies. In relation to maxillary anterior edentulous segments, patients expect in general a long-lasting functional and esthetic result with a high level of predictability (Table 40-2). To this primary objective are normally added a number of secondary goals which include parameters such as minimal invasiveness, low risk associated to eventual surgery, overall simplicity and cost effectiveness.

Prior to selecting an implant-based solution, one should comprehensively review all of the possible treatment modalities available (Table 40-3) which have the potential to solve a given clinical problem, and carefully ponder their respective advantages and eventual shortcomings, and only then take the decision together with the adequately informed patient. Currently, the restorative spectrum in the case of missing maxillary anterior teeth comprises conventional FPDs, resin-bonded bridges, removable partial dentures (RPDs), tooth-supported overdentures and implant-supported fixed or removable prostheses. Furthermore, one should not forget that occasionally orthodontic therapy, e.g. closure of limited edentulous spaces, can represent an effective and elegant alternative or adjunction to a prosthetic treatment. However, the availability of scientific evidence – when possible at its highest level – for the planned treatment modality, should be the key parameter for the final choice.

In this clinical decision-making process certain criteria, as for example the compromised structural, periodontal and/or endodontic status of potential natural

abutments, or the extended dimension of the edentulous segment, are among the factors favoring an implant-borne restoration rather than a tooth-supported fixed prosthesis (Table 40-4).

Esthetic considerations related to maxillary anterior implant restorations

In the context of the natural dentition, long clinical crowns, the irregular contour of the gingival margin, i.e. any abrupt change in vertical tissue height between neighboring teeth, and the loss of papillary tissue often have an adverse influence on dental-facial esthetics (Seibert & Lindhe 1989). Furthermore, the same authors have underlined that in the case of a *high scalloped gingival morphotype* (in contrast to a rather *low scalloped gingival morphotype*) there is mostly an unpredictable relationship between the underlying bone and the gingival contour, often leading to so called "black hole cases" and presenting a high risk for losing soft tissue (e.g. gingival or mucosal recession at the labial aspect of teeth or implants), particularly in relation to restorative procedures, as for example insertion of retraction cords and impression taking.

Another esthetically relevant concern lies in the fact that under normal conditions a maxillary front tooth extraction leads on average to approximately 2 mm loss in vertical tissue height. The mean length of the clinical crown of a maxillary central incisor is 10.2 mm, the one of a lateral incisor 8.2 mm and that of a canine

Table 40.5. Evaluation of anterior tooth-bound edentulous sites prior to implant therapy

- Mesio-distal dimension of the edentulous segment, including its comparison with existing contralateral control teeth
- Three-dimensional analysis of the edentulous segment regarding soft tissue configuration and underlying alveolar bone crest (ref. "bone-mapping")
- Neighboring teeth:
  - volume (relative tooth dimensions), basic features of tooth form and three-dimensional position and orientation of the clinical crowns
  - structural integrity and condition
  - surrounding gingival tissues (course/scalloping of the gingival line)
  - periodontal and endodontic status/conditions
  - crown-to-root ratio
  - length of roots and respective inclinations in the frontal plane
  - eventual presence of diastemata
- Interarch relationships:
  - vertical dimension of occlusion
  - anterior guidance
  - interocclusal space
- Esthetic parameters:
  - height of upper smile line ("high lip" versus "low lip")
  - lower lip line
  - course of the gingival-mucosa line
  - orientation of the occlusal plane
  - dental versus facial symmetry
  - lip support

Table 40.6. Optimal three-dimensional implant positioning ("restoration-driven implant placement") in anterior maxillary sites. *Implant = apical extension of the ideal future restoration*

- Correct vertical position of implant shoulder (sink depth) using the cemento-enamel junction of adjacent teeth as reference:
  - no visible metal
  - gradually developed, flat axial profile
- Correct oro-facial position of point of emergence for future suprastructure from the mucosa:
  - similar to adjacent teeth
  - flat emergence profile
- Implant axis compatible with available prosthetic treatment options (ideally: implant axis identical with "prosthetic axis")

Price & Price 1999, Belser et al. 2000, Tarnow et al. 2000).

In view of maxillary anterior implant restorations, the systematic and comprehensive evaluation of edentulous sites, including the surrounding natural dentition, is of paramount importance (Table 40-5). Key parameters comprise the mesio-distal dimension of the edentulous segment, the three-dimensional analysis of the underlying alveolar bone crest, the status of the neighboring teeth, and interarch relationships as well as specific esthetic parameters.

As one should consider the implant as the apical extension of the ideal future restoration and not the opposite, a respective optimal three-dimensional ("restoration-driven") implant position is mandatory (Table 40-6). Consequently, parameters addressing vertical (sink-depth) and oro-facial implant shoulder location, have been defined, as well as guidelines related to the long axis of the implant, as the latter has a significant impact on the subsequent technical procedures during suprastructure conception and fabrication.

Recently, the ITI Consensus Conference has approved the distinctly submucosal implant shoulder location in the maxillary anterior segment in order to respond to natural esthetic demands (Buser & von Arx 2000). As the current implant design – in contrast to the scalloped cemento-enamel junction – features a straight horizontal, "rotation-symmetrical" restorative interface, interproximal implant crown margins are often located several millimeters submucosally, and thus difficult to reach by the patient's routine oral hygiene efforts (Belser et al. 1998). Mainly for this reason a screw-retained implant suprastructure (Sutter et al. 1993, Hebel & Gajjar 1997, Keller et al. 1998) is preferred to a cemented one, as it benefits from the surface quality and marginal fidelity of prefabricated, machined components, and avoids potential problems associated with cement excess that may be difficult to reach and thoroughly eliminate.

10.4 mm. Consequently, any kind of maxillary anterior restoration should aim at staying within reasonable limits of these average morphological dimensions, if a harmonious and esthetically pleasing result is to be achieved. Ultimately, an anterior implant restoration should correspond closely to an ovate pontic of a conventional FPD with respect to the relevant soft tissue parameters (Kois 1996).

Numerous publications, mostly in the form of textbooks, book chapters, reviews, case reports and descriptions of clinical and laboratory procedures and techniques, have addressed various aspects specifically related to esthetics and osseointegration (Parel & Sullivan 1989, Gelb & Lazzara 1993, Jaggers et al. 1993, Vlassis et al. 1993, Bichacho & Landsberg 1994, Ghalili 1994, Landsberg & Bichacho 1994, Neale & Chee 1994, Studer et al. 1994, Carrick 1995, Corrente et al. 1995, De Lange 1995, Garber 1995, Garber & Belser 1995, Jansen & Weisgold 1995, Khayat et al. 1995, Touati 1995, Brugnolo et al. 1996, Davidoff 1996, Grunder et al. 1996, Hess et al. 1996, Marchack 1996, Mecall & Rosenfeld 1996, Bain & Weisgold 1997, Bichacho & Landsberg 1997, Chee et al. 1997, Garg et al. 1997, Spear et al. 1997, Salinas & Sadan 1998, Jemt 1999,

ANTERIOR SINGLE-TOOTH REPLACEMENT

Favorable 5-year multicenter results for 71 single-tooth replacements in the anterior maxilla (implant success rate of 96.6%) were reported by Henry et al. (1996); however, this group mentioned an associated 10% esthetic failure rate. In a retrospective study on 236 patients treated with single-tooth implant restorations in the anterior maxilla (Walther et al. 1996), a Kaplan-Meier survival rate of 89% was found for an observation period of 10 years. The failure rate for lateral incisor replacement was lower than the one for central incisors. Furthermore, 5% of the related prosthetic suprastructures had to be replaced during the 10 years of observation. Kemppainen et al. (1997) prospectively documented 102 implants (ASTRA/ ITI) for single-tooth replacement in the anterior maxilla of 82 patients and found survival rates of 97.8% and 100%, respectively, after 1 year. Still related to single-tooth maxillary anterior implants, a prospective study on 15 patients revealed a 100% implant survival rate after two years of function (Palmer et al. 1997). At crown insertion (6 months after implant placement) the mean bone level was located 0.47 mm apically to the top of the implants. No significant additional changes in crestal bone level occurred during the remainder of the study.

Today, it is generally accepted that the final implant shoulder sink depth for esthetic fixed single-tooth restorations can be determined primarily by the location of the cemento-enamel junction (CEJ) of the neighboring teeth and by the level of the free gingival margin at the vestibular aspect of these same teeth. This means that the implant shoulder is positioned 1-2 mm more apically to the labial CEJ of the adjacent teeth (Belser et al. 1998, 2000). However, the noticeable esthetic progress made in this kind of implant restoration is the result of recent developments in the absence of extensive long-term documentation. Because the exclusive use of clinical signs for establishing peri-implant health or disease may not be sufficient, the evaluation of additional objective parameters is needed. A number of diagnostic tests have been utilized by clinicians to supplement clinical signs with objective methods. These tests include microbiologic monitoring, proteolytic bacterial enzyme markers, markers of tissue destruction, and finally, markers of tissue repair and regeneration. In this context peri-implant crevicular fluid (PICF) analysis has become the focus of intense investigation. It has been observed that the volume of crevicular fluid did not differ between implant sites and natural teeth and that the features of inflammation seem to be the same around teeth and implants. In addition, the histologic arrangement of peri-implant soft tissues resembles basically that observed around natural teeth, although featuring also some aspects of scar tissue (Abraham-

Table 40.7 Basic considerations related to anterior single-tooth replacement

Achievements	Predictable and reproducible results regarding both esthetic parameters and longevity in sites without significant vertical tissue deficienies Well defined and well established surgical protocols: • *restoration-driven* implant placement Adequate and versatile restorative protocols and prosthetic components: • occclusal/transverse screw-retention • angulated abutments • high-strength ceramic components
Sites with buccal bone deficienies	Lateral bone augmentation using *autografts* and *barrier membranes*: • technique offers efficacy and predictability • *simultaneous* or *staged approach* depending on defect extension and defect morphology Lateral bone augmentation by means of *alveolar bone crest splitting* and/or various *osteotome techniques*: • limited clinical long-term documentation
Limitations	Combined vertical bone and soft tissue deficienies: • following removal of ankylosed teeth or failing implants • advanced loss of periodontal tissues, including gingival recession, on neighboring teeth • limited scientific documentation related to *vertical bone augmentation* and *distraction osteogenesis*

son et al. 1996, Berglundh & Lindhe 1996, Abrahamson et al. 1997, Lindhe & Berglundh 1998).

Giannopoulou et al. (2002) investigated the effect of intracrevicular restoration margins on peri-implant health of 61 maxillary anterior implants – mainly single-tooth replacements – in 45 patients up to 9 years. Results revealed that the only statistically significant differences between baseline and follow-up examination concerned pocket probing depth (PPD) and the distance between the implant shoulder and the mucosal margin (DIM measurements), which slightly increased over time. The remainder of the clinical measurements and almost all of the microbiologic and biochemical parameters analysed did not significantly change. Probably the most critical parameter from a purely esthetic point of view is the DIM value, particularly on the labial aspect of the maxillary anterior implants investigated in this study. A mean value of –1.5 ± 1.1 mm was found at baseline examination, and a slight increase (–1.7 ± 1.1 mm) at the follow-up. This indicates that the risk for exposure of the implant-to-crown interface or margin can be considered low. These findings corroborate recently pub-

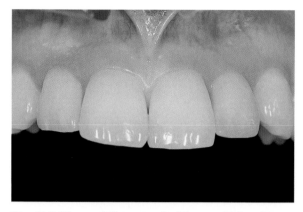

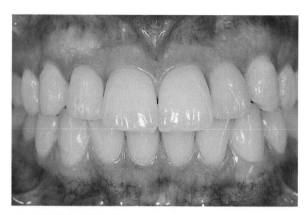

Fig. 40-2. 10-year follow-up of a 28-year-old female patient. Both congenitally missing lateral incisors were replaced by implants, restored with screw-retained porcelain-fused-to-metal crowns.

Fig. 40-3. The frontal view in centric occlusal position documents the harmonious integration of the two implant restorations after 10 years of clinical service.

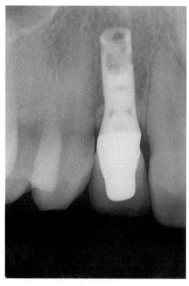

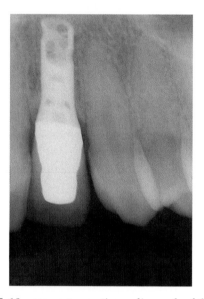

Fig. 40-4. 10-year postoperative radiograph of the maxillary right lateral single-tooth implant restoration.

Fig. 40-5. 10-year postoperative radiograph of the maxillary left lateral single-tooth implant restoration.

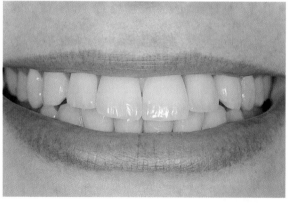

Fig. 40-6. During unforced smiling an adequate balance between implant-crowns and natural dentition can be noticed.

lished data addressing similar parameters (Grunder 2000). The consistently negative Periotest scores confirmed the stability and osseointegrated status of the implants examined. Furthermore, no associations were observed between the above results and the number of years that the implants had been in function. Based on these clinical, microbiologic and biochemical data, and on an observation period of 4-9

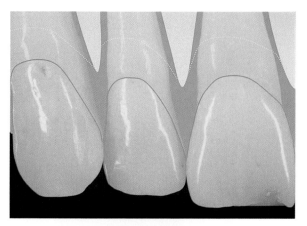

Fig. 40-7. Schematic representation of an intact maxillary right anterior segment. The alveolar bone follows the scalloped course of the cemento-enamel junction for a distance of approximately 2 mm (white dotted line), whereas, accordingly, the gingival tissue occupies completely the interdental area.

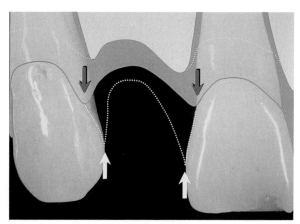

Fig. 40-8. Schematic representation of the same segment after loss of the lateral incisor. While the interproximal bone height has basically been maintained, the corresponding gingival tissue is flattened due to a lack of support originally provided by the now missing tooth.

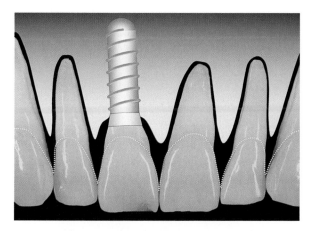

Fig. 40-9. The treatment objective in the case of an anterior single-tooth replacement is an implant restoration with a gradually developed, flat emergence profile from the implant shoulder to the peri-implant mucosal surface. Ideally, the clinical crown of the implant restoration should aim at replicating the clinical crown of the corresponding contralateral tooth.

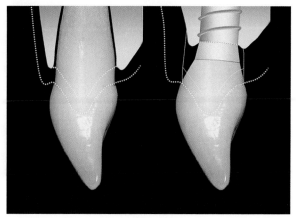

Fig. 40-10. Schematic comparison in the sagital plane between a natural maxillary incisor and a respective implant borne single-tooth restoration. The decrease of alveolar bone height on the labial and palatal aspect following tooth loss leads to a more palatal implant position when compared to the original root position, which in turn influences the axial profile of the restoration.

years (mean: 6.8 years), it was concluded that in patients with appropriate oral hygiene, implant-supported maxillary anterior crowns with distinctly intracrevicular margins did not predispose to unfavorable peri-implant host and microbial responses. In particular, overall healthy and stable peri-implant tissue conditions – a paramount criterion when it comes to esthetic implant crowns – were consistently encountered and maintained longitudinally. One of the patients participating in this study and who recently passed the 10-year clinical and radiographic follow-up control, is presented in Figs. 40-2 to 40-6. An adequate esthetic integration of the two single-tooth restorations, replacing the congenitally missing lateral incisors, could be achieved and maintained over time.

In a simplistic way, the morphologic and esthetic consequences in the frontal plane of the loss of a single maxillary incisor, when compared to the original intact situation, can be summarized as follows: maintenance of the tooth-sided interproximal bone height at the neighboring teeth, and vertical loss ("flattening") of the corresponding gingival tissue due to a lack of support originally provided by the now missing tooth (Figs. 40-7 and 40-8). In case of an anterior single-tooth replacement, the related implant restoration should aim at replicating the clinical crown of the contralateral control tooth from the line of soft tissue emergence to the incisal border. Additionally, a gradually developed, flat emergence profile from the implant shoulder to the peri-implant mucosal margin is mandatory (Figs. 40-9 and 40-10).

The basic considerations related to maxillary ante-

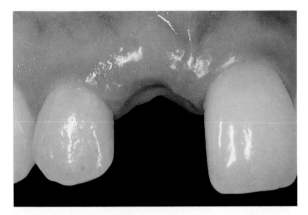

Fig. 40-11. Preoperative close-up view of the upper right anterior region of a 22-year-old female patient with a missing right central incisor. The scalloped course of the gingiva is maintained, featuring interproximal soft tissue at the level of the cemento-enamel junction.

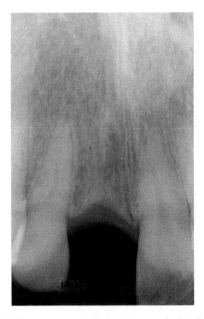

Fig. 40-12. The corresponding radiograph displays favorable bony conditions in view of implant therapy. Note in particular the interproximal bone height, following the cemento-enamel junction for a distance of less than 2 mm.

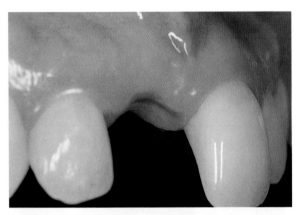

Fig. 40-13. The oblique close-up view confirms optimal conditions for the insertion of an implant, namely interproximal soft tissue height and no significant loss of the buccal bone plate.

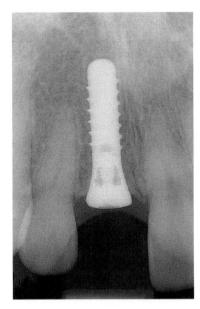

Fig. 40-15. The corresponding radiograph displays a continuous close contact between bone and implant and confirms that the vertical interproximal bone level has been maintained.

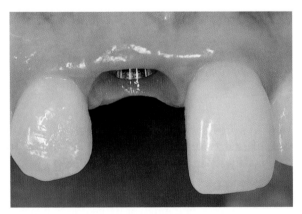

Fig. 40-14. Clinical view of the maxillary anterior implant site 8 weeks after insertion of a solid screw implant according to a one-stage transmucosal surgical protocol. A harmonious peri-implant soft tissue profile has been established by means of a titanium healing cap featuring a respective emergence profile and thus offering adequate interproximal soft tissue support.

rior single-tooth replacement, including the respective general achievements and limitations, and ad-

dressing edentulous segments with different types of labial bone deficiencies, are presented in Table 40-7.

Sites without significant tissue deficiencies

An increasing body of evidence indicates that the most determinant parameter for achieving an esthetic single-tooth restoration is the interproximal bone height at the level of the teeth confining the edentulous gap. The related bone should be within a physiologic dis-

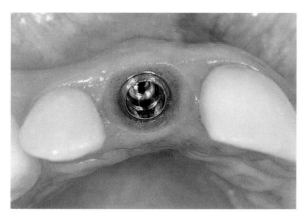

Fig. 40-16. The occlusal view reveals an implant position in the orofacial plane that is in accordance with the adjacent natural roots and thus permits development of a flat emergence profile.

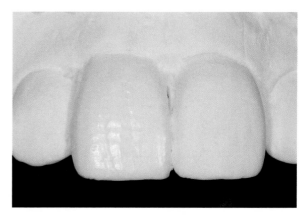

Fig. 40-17. On a stone model derived from the clinical situation, the laboratory technician defines the treatment objective in wax. At this stage priority is given to esthetic principles and maintenance of symmetry rather than to the actual position of the underlying implant.

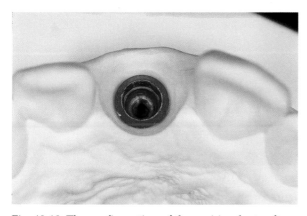

Fig. 40-18. The configuration of the peri-implant soft tissue is subsequently adapted on the stone model according to the diagnostic wax-up. Ultimately, it will be the restoration itself that completes the last phase of soft tissue conditioning by subtle respective physical displacement.

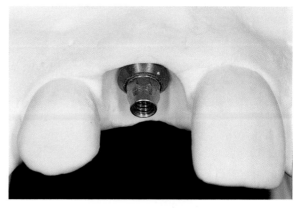

Fig. 40-19. An appropriate secondary titanium component (abutment) is selected as support for the planned screw-retained implant restoration.

tance, i.e. approximately 2 mm, of the cemento-enamel junction (CEJ) and thus be providing the essential support for the overlaying soft tissue compartments. Consequently, preoperative diagnosis will include interproximal radiographic bone height assessment and periodontal probing of the soft tissue attachment level.

If the comprehensive presurgical analysis of a given maxillary anterior single-tooth gap has confirmed on the one hand a favorable vertical level of both soft tissue and underlying alveolar bone at the interproximal aspect of the two adjacent teeth (Figs. 40-11, 40-12, 40-13), and no major vestibular bone deficiencies on the other hand, the site can be considered compatible with a straightforward implant surgical protocol. In order to ensure the best probability of a successful and long-lasting esthetic treatment outcome, the actual implant placement has to be carried out meticulously according to the surgical guidelines defined in Table 40-6. These guidelines include key-parameters such as

low-trauma surgical principles in general and precise three-dimensional ("restoration-driven") implant positioning in particular. In the case of standard single-tooth sites, most surgeons do not advocate the use of a surgical guide or stent, as the adjacent teeth and associated anatomical structures normally offer sufficient morphologic landmarks to safely reach the therapeutic objective. As far as the detailed surgical protocol is concerned, readers are referred to Chapter 37, "The surgical site". Buser and von Arx (2000) have published the surgical step-by-step procedure related to maxillary anterior single-tooth implants, and insisted on a slightly palatal incision technique to preserve a maximum of keratinized mucosa on the labial aspect of the future implant restoration. Another crucial parameter is the maintenance of at least 1 mm of bone plate on the vestibular aspect of the implant in order to minimize the risk for peri-implant soft tissue recessions, a factor parameter when it comes to esthetics. Under such conditions one may consistently

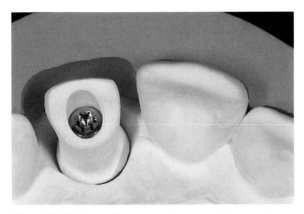

Fig. 40-20. Using a silicon template as guide, a prefabricated ceramic blank is inserted and subsequently reduced to provide adequate space for the external layers of cosmetic porcelain.

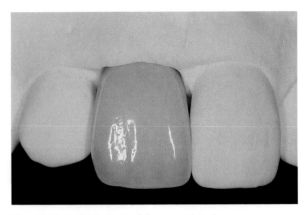

Fig. 40-21. Labial view of the completed ceramo-ceramic restoration on the master cast.

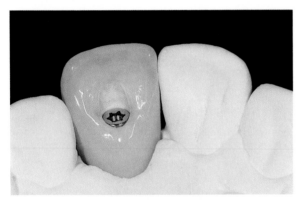

Fig. 40-22. In particular, the completed screw-retained all-ceramic restoration displays a high degree of translucency on its incisal third.

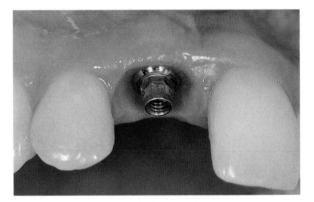

Fig. 40-23. A titanium abutment will serve as infrastructure for the transocclusally screw-retained high-strength all-ceramic restoration.

achieve postsurgical treatment outcomes featuring unaltered vertical soft tissue and underlying bone levels at the interproximal aspect of the adjacent natural teeth (Figs. 40-14, 40-15, 40-16).

Once osseointegration is confirmed radiologically and clinically, the clinical situation is transferred to the master model by means of an impression, normally assisted by auxiliary components in the form of prefabricated impression copings. On the master model, which in turn contains a replica (analogue) of the implant, the laboratory technician defines the final configuration of the single-tooth implant restoration by means of a diagnostic wax-up (Fig. 40-17). Under normal circumstances, i.e. when the natural contralateral control tooth corresponds mostly to the esthetic and functional requirements of an appropriate "target model", the technician basically copies the clinical crown of this control tooth in wax, regardless of the actual underlying implant position. At this stage a close-to-ideal restoration is planned, while its connection to the underlying implant will be addressed later. This approach comprises the minute shaping of the peri-implant soft tissue configuration (on the master model in the form of stone), in view of an identical emergence from the labial and interproximal soft tissue margin, like the one observed on the natural tooth

site (Fig. 40-18). Only after having completed this preparatory step, will the ceramist select the most adequate secondary component (i.e. abutment), depending on the three following cardinal criteria (Fig. 40-19):

1. implant shoulder depth in relation to the labial mucosal margin
2. oro-facial implant shoulder position with respect to the future line of emergence of the suprastructure
3. long axis of the implant.

In most instances, preference will be given to a screw-retained implant suprastructure, unless a combination of mesiostructure and cemented restoration is chosen. Screw-retention is primarily preferred due to a marked submucosally located implant shoulder, in particular at the interproximal aspect, which may render the removal of excess cement difficult, and which is mostly not within reach of the patient's routine oral hygiene measures. In addition, screw-retained suprastructures benefit from the close-to-perfect surface quality characteristics and the marginal precision of machined, prefabricated components. Nowadays several of the leading implant systems also offer high-strength ceramic tertiary components which may

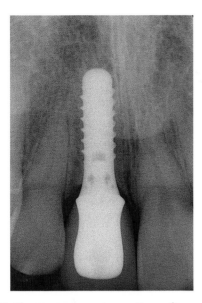

Fig. 40-24. The one-year postoperative radiograph confirms favorable conditions at the bone-to-implant interface. Note a high degree of radio-opacity of the all-ceramic substrate, permitting the evaluation of the fidelity of the marginal adaptation.

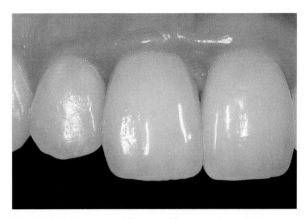

Fig. 40-25. An acceptable overall integration of the metal-free implant-borne restoration on site 11 can be noted.

positively contribute to the esthetic treatment outcome, particularly in the case of a rather thin labial peri-implant mucosa (Fig. 40-20). Another parameter which is of primary importance when it comes to esthetic considerations relates to maxillary anterior implant restorations and is associated with the suprastructure design itself at the interproximal aspect. In order to provide optimal conditions for the related soft tissue, a long interdental contact line is established, located slightly more towards the palatal aspect of the restoration (Figs. 40-21, 40-22). This design offers optimal support for the interproximal soft tissue and thereby reduces the potential hazard of a so-called "black triangle" (Figs. 40-23, 40-24, 40-25). In this context some studies have indicated that there exists a predictable relationship between the location of the interdental contact point and the associated alveolar bone crest when it comes to presence or absence of interdental papillae fully occupying the interdental space of maxillary anterior teeth (Tarnow et al. 1992, Tarnow & Eskow 1995).

Sites with localized horizontal deficiencies

In a case of a localized (minor) horizontal deficiency, i.e. a confined vestibular alveolar bone crest defect at the vestibular aspect of a maxillary anterior single-tooth gap, one prefers to place the implant and simultaneously undertake a lateral bone augmentation procedure, on condition that several well-defined prerequisites are fulfilled. These include an implant placement in accordance with the guidelines presented in Table 40-6 ("restoration-driven" implant placement), the achievement of an adequate primary stability and a resulting cervical dehiscence-type bony defect

which is compatible with a predictable bone augmentation procedure. More specifically, the dehiscence should have the form of a two-wall bony defect, whereas the labial aspect of the inserted implant should not exceed the surrounding bone contours. Under such conditions, the treatment of choice consists of the application of autogenous bone chips, harvested at the site of the implant surgical intervention. The bone chips which can be combined with one of the numerous available bone substitutes (e.g. BioOss®) if necessary, will provide adequate support for a subsequently adapted barrier membrane. The described grafting material is finally complemented with "bone slurry", constantly collected during the entire procedure. Subsequently, a bioabsorbable membrane is applied prior to repositioning and tension-free suturing of the mucoperiosteal flap. This implicates a rather extended flap design, comprising vertical releasing incisions.

In conclusion, a simultaneous lateral augmentation procedure is recommended if the three following conditions are present:

1. ideal three-dimensional ("restoration-driven") implant position
2. adequate primary implant stability
3. localized two-wall bony defect, exceeding the labial contour of the implant and hereby assuring an appropriate bone regeneration potential and providing the necessary stability to the applied bone graft.

Under these specific conditions, the implant can be functionally loaded after 2-4 months, depending on size and configuration of the respective bone defect.

It is not infrequent in the anterior maxilla, due to its specific alveolar bone crest morphology, that "restoration-driven" rather than "bone-driven" implant positioning leads to a fenestration-type defect in the apical area of the implant. If adequate primary implant stability can be obtained, a similar simultaneous lateral bone augmentation procedure, as described for localized dehiscence-type defects, appears feasible. Under

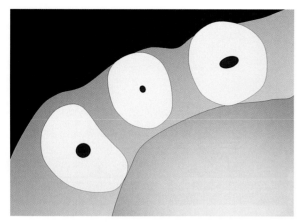

Fig. 40-26. Schematic representation of a horizontal section at the cemento-enamel junction level of the maxillary right anterior segment.

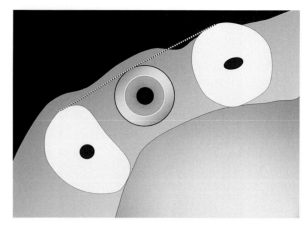

Fig. 40-27. "Restoration-driven" implant placement in the horizontal plane at the site of the maxillary right lateral incisor. In order to maintain at least 1 mm of alveolar bone also on the labial aspect, the implant has to be inserted approximately 1-2 mm more to the palate when compared to the adjacent roots.

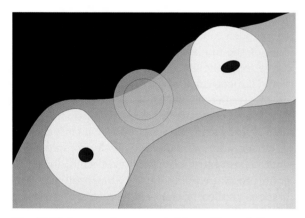

Fig. 40-28. In case of an extended lateral bone deficiency, where an adequately placed implant would largely exceed the vestibular border of the alveolar bone crest, a lateral bone augmentation procedure (staged approach) is indicated

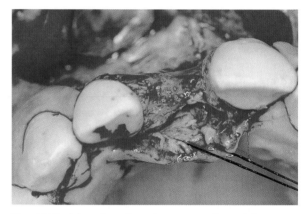

Fig. 40-29. After elevation of a mucoperiosteal flap a severe extended resorption – namely on the vestibular aspect – of the edentulous alveolar ridge becomes apparent. Such a morphology is hardly compatible with "restoration-driven" implant placement.

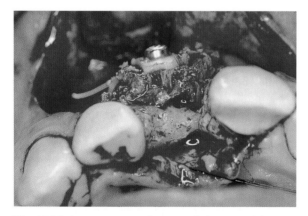

Fig. 40-30. An autogenous bone graft, harvested from the patient's chin region, has been secured with a fixation screw and its periphery filled in with additional bone chips prior to membrane placement.

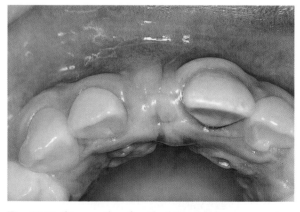

Fig. 40-31. Six months after the lateral ridge augmentation procedure the clinical occlusal view documents that uneventful healing has occurred and that the orofacial ridge profile has been improved.

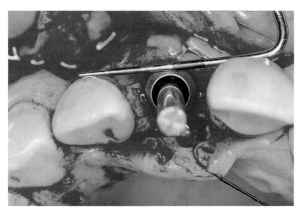

Fig. 40-32. During implant surgery one can note that all key parameters characterizing an optimal implant position (shoulder sink depth, orofacial point of emergence, implant axis) could be satisfied.

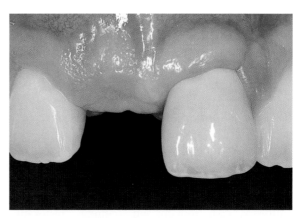

Fig. 40-33. After three months of healing the labial view documents a slight excess of keratinised peri-implant mucosa in a coronal direction, which is a prerequisite for the development of the final esthetic soft tissue contours. The first step of the subsequent procedure will consist of the insertion of a longer titanium healing cap, following a minor mucosaplasty.

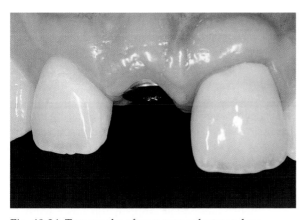

Fig. 40-34. Two weeks after mucosaplasty and exchange of healing caps the initiation of a harmoniously scalloped labial soft tissue course is apparent. Furthermore, the access from the surface to the underlying implant shoulder has been established.

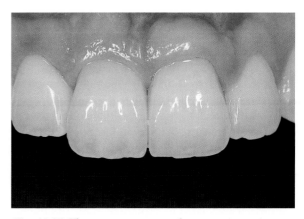

Fig. 40-35. The two ceramo-metal crown restorations – one tooth borne (site 21) and one implant borne (site 11) – display little difference in appearance since symmetry has been respected from the line of mucosal emergence to the incisal edge.

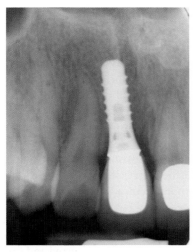

Fig. 40-36. The 1-year follow-up radiograph confirms the stability of the osseointegrated 10-mm titanium screw implant.

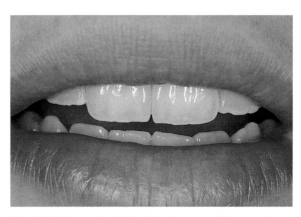

Fig. 40-37. An esthetically pleasing overall integration of the two maxillary anterior restorations is underlined by a close-up view of the patient's unforced smile.

such circumstances the healing time prior to functional implant loading remains the same as advocated for standard implant protocols (i.e. two months for SLA-coated screw-type titanium implants).

Sites with extended horizontal deficiencies

In a case of more extended horizontal alveolar bone crest deficiencies, a simultaneous implant placement and lateral bone augmentation procedure becomes technically more difficult and less predictable, as the ultimate goal remains an optimal "restoration-driven" implant positioning (Figs. 40-26, 40-27). The described extended horizontal bone deficiency may often, on the one hand, not permit an acceptable primary implant stability to be achieved, and on the other hand may lead to a vestibular bone dehiscence that does not have a distinct two-wall morphology. Furthermore, the labial implant contour would be more prominent than the respective surrounding bone (Fig. 40-28). Under these specific circumstances the principal prerequisites for a simultaneous approach are clearly not present, thus leading to the recommendation to proceed according to a staged surgical protocol, which will address the lateral bone augmentation first and the actual implant placement in a second stage.

This may represent a major problem for some patients, as two surgical interventions, normally separated by approximately six months, are necessary, leading to a total treatment time of eight months or more. It is therefore indispensable to thoroughly inform the patient about both the reasons for the staged approach associated to implant therapy, and the possible conventional prosthodontic alternatives (e.g. a traditional tooth-borne FPD, eventually in combination with a connective tissue grafting procedure to optimize the deficient edentulous ridge in view of an optimal and esthetic pontic). The patient will then be in a position to give his or her informed consent to either of the two therapeutic modalities, according to individual preference.

In a case of implant therapy, the first step consists of the elevation of a rather extended mucoperiosteal flap featuring vertical releasing incisions, as the added site volume (due to the block graft and barrier membrane) will require subsequent splitting of the periosteum prior to flap repositioning and suturing (Fig. 40-29). Numerous studies reporting results of various bone augmentation techniques and related materials have been published (Hürzeler et al. 1994, Buser et al. 1996, Ellegaard et al. 1997b, Chiapasco et al. 1999, 2001, von Arx et al. 2001a,b, Zitzmann et al. 2001). To date, autogenous bone block grafts, mostly harvested from the chin or the retromolar area, in combination with e-PTFE barrier membranes, still have the best clinical long-term documentation (Buser et al. 2002). These authors presented prospectively documented 5-year data of 40 consecutively treated patients, according to a staged protocol. On all laterally augmented sites

implants could be subsequently inserted. It was concluded that the clinical results of implants placed in regenerated bone were comparable to those reported for implants in non-regenerated bone. A clinical example of the described approach is presented in Figs. 40-29 to 40-37.

Sites with major vertical tissue loss

When it comes to maxillary anterior single-tooth gaps with significant vertical tissue loss, the predictable achievement of an esthetically pleasing treatment outcome, ideally providing a so-called perfect illusion with respect to its integration in the surrounding natural dentition, gets difficult. As pointed out earlier in this chapter, there exists a close relationship between the interproximal bone height and the associated soft tissue level (Figs. 40-7, 40-8). If the coronal border of the alveolar bone is no longer within the physiological distance of approximately 2 mm from the interproximal CEJ of the teeth confining the edentulous space, there is an increased risk for an altered respective soft tissue course (due to a lack of underlying bony support) and its adverse impact on the appearance. Such situations can be encountered following the removal of ankylosed teeth or failing implants, or in case of advanced periodontal tissue loss – including gingival recession – on neighboring teeth. Under these specific circumstances, the final decision whether or not to use implants will ultimately depend on the one hand on the careful and comprehensive evaluation of all of the therapeutic modalities available for anterior tooth replacement (Table 40-3), and on the other hand the patient's individual smile line and expectations. This process includes an objective analysis of the advantages and eventual shortcomings associated with each modality.

To illustrate these clinically relevant aspects, the initial situation and the subsequent implant treatment of a 35-year-old female patient consulting with an ankylosed maxillary deciduous left canine, are presented in Figs. 40-38 to 40-46. The preoperative analysis had led to the conclusion that the fabrication of a conventional tooth-borne three-unit FPD, using the intact lateral incisor and first premolar as abutments and featuring a canine pontic, was not opportune from several points of view. Among these should be particularly mentioned aspects related to the questionable mechanical resistance of the resulting conventional prosthesis, specific occlusal considerations (e.g. canine guidance in a pontic area), lack of esthetic superiority when compared to a virtual implant-borne fixed restoration, and last but not least the conflict with the general principle of minimal invasiveness (maximum preservation of intact tooth structure).

Once the decision was made, both the implant surgical and the restorative strategies focused on improving or at least optimally exploiting the pre-existing

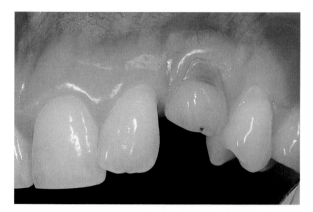

Fig. 40-38. Preoperative view of a 35-year-old female patient consulting with a persisting primary tooth in the position of the maxillary left canine. Note the irregular course of the adjacent gingiva in general and the loss in vertical tissue height in particular.

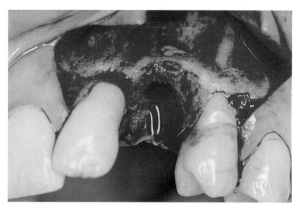

Fig. 40-39. One month after removal of the deciduous canine, the root of which was severely resorbed, a mucoperiosteal flap with vertical releasing incisions is elevated and the preparation of a calibrated implant bed performed. One can note an increased distance between the cemento-enamel junction and the coronal border of the alveolar bone and the left lateral incisor.

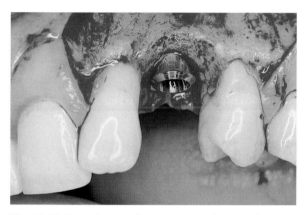

Fig. 40-40. Buccal view after insertion of the implant.

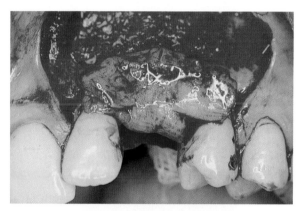

Fig. 40-41. In a case of rather thin mucosa, the utilization of a connective tissue graft, harvested from the palate, may be indicated to create a sufficient thickness of soft tissue at the implant site.

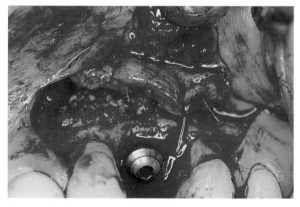

Fig. 40-42. Prior to flap closure, the connective tissue graft is secured to the flap with bioabsorbable sutures.

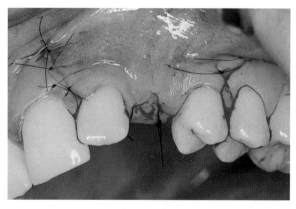

Fig. 40-43. Coverage of most of the healing cap during suturing is recommended, leading to a submerged or at least to a "semi-submerged" healing mode.

limited esthetic potential of the site. From the surgical side, this comprised a deeper than normal implant shoulder sink depth (Fig. 40-40), the use of a connective tissue graft on the vestibular aspect (Fig. 40-41), a localized lateral bone augmentation (simultaneous approach) procedure (Fig. 40-42) and a coronally repositioned flap (Fig. 40-43). The metal-ceramic implant restoration featured a transverse screw-reten-

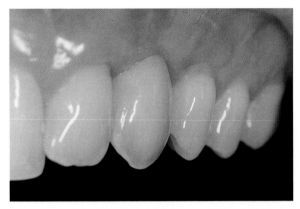

Fig. 40-44. The clinical aspect after insertion of the cera-mometal implant crown reveals stable and esthetic peri-implant soft tissue contours.

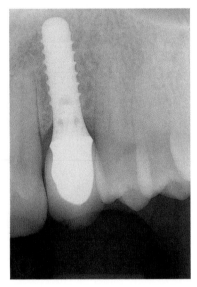

Fig. 40-45. The 2-year follow-up radiograph confirms the stability of the osseointegrated 10 mm solid screw titanium implant.

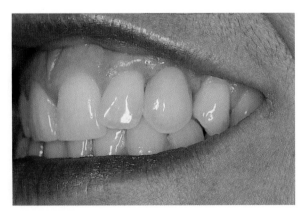

Fig. 40-46. On a left-lateral view, during the patient's forced smiling, one can note that the lack of vertical soft tissue in the interproximal area has been compensated for with an apically extended interdental contact line.

tion to provide maximum space for esthetic porcelain stratification and a long contact line on the mesial

aspect to compensate for the missing interdental soft tissue height (Figs. 40-44 to 40-46).

A more severe preoperative situation of vertical tissue deficiency, combined with a marked horizontal bone defect, is presented in Figs. 40-47 and 40-49. This 19-year-old female patient lost her maxillary right lateral incisor due to a localized periodontal problem. Again, the comprehensive site analysis concluded that a single-tooth implant restoration was the best compromise in view of major disadvantages associated with all of the conventional prosthodontic options. From a purely esthetic point of view, none of the therapeutic modalities had the potential to predictably lead to a perfect re-establishment of a symmetrical, harmoniously scalloped soft tissue course at its original physiological level. However, a rather low lip-line during the patient's normal communication and unforced smiling permitted the least invasive approach to be chosen. Following a lateral connective tissue and bone augmentation procedure (Fig. 40-50), an implant could be inserted in an acceptable position and subsequently restored with a screw-retained crown. The final frontal view, allowing a direct comparison between the intact (Fig. 40-51) and the restored side, clearly demonstrates the current esthetic limitations associated with implant therapy in sites with a marked vertical tissue deficiency (Fig. 40-52).

MULTIPLE-UNIT ANTERIOR FIXED IMPLANT RESTORATIONS

The normal consequence following loss of two or more adjacent upper anterior teeth comprises a flattening of the edentulous segment. In particular one can observe the disappearance, in an apical direction, of the crestal bone originally located between the incisor teeth. This phenomenon is not, or only minimally, present at the interproximal aspect of the remaining anterior teeth and thus explains the fundamental difference between a maxillary anterior single-tooth gap and a multi-unit edentulous segment.

If two standard screw-type titanium implants are inserted to replace two missing maxillary central incisors (Figs. 40-53, 40-54), an additional peri-implant bone remodeling process will take place. In the frontal plane, two different characteristic processes, one between the natural tooth and the implant and the other between the two implants, can be distinguished. At the site between tooth and implant, the tooth-sided interproximal bone height should theoretically remain at its original location, i.e. within 2 mm from the CEJ, from where the implant-sided interproximal bone height drops in an oblique manner towards the first implant-to-bone contact, normally located approximately 2 mm apically of the junction ("microgap") between the implant shoulder and the abutment or suprastructure. This phenomenon has been referred to in the literature as "saucerization" or establ-

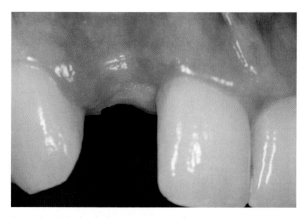

Fig. 40-47. Labial close-up view of the maxillary right anterior region of a 19-year-old female patient. The interdental soft tissue height distal to the central incisor and the corresponding underlying alveolar bone height are markedly reduced, leading to exposure of the cemento-enamel junction.

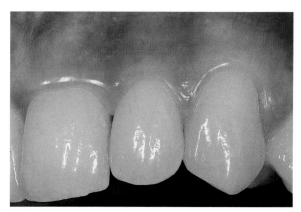

Fig. 40-48. The contralateral side of the dental arch shows perfectly intact and harmonious conditions with respect to the course of the gingiva.

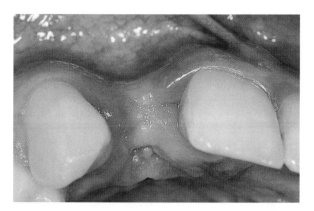

Fig. 40-49. On the occlusal view of the edentulous site a significant lateral crest deficiency becomes apparent, which calls for both a bone and soft tissue augmentation procedure, particularly if an implant solution is planned.

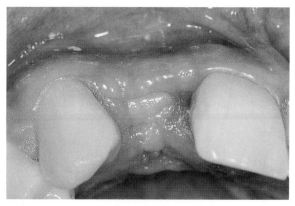

Fig. 40-50. Six months after combined lateral bone and soft tissue augmentation, the site appears to be compatible with "restoration-driven" implant placement.

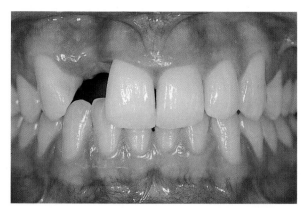

Fig. 40-51. The buccal view in centric occlusion position before therapy summarizes the problems associated with localized vertical tissue deficiencies: lack of a harmoniously scalloped soft tissue course in general and missing interdental papillae in particular.

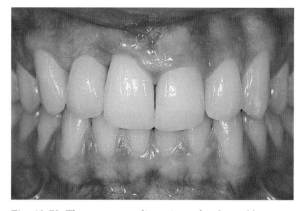

Fig. 40-52. The corresponding view after lateral bone and soft tissue augmentation on the one hand and insertion of an implant borne single-tooth restoration on the site of the right lateral incisor on the other hand, underlines the resulting shortcomings with respect to esthetic parameters. Vertical tissue deficiencies – which at present cannot be predictably compensated for – clearly compromise the overall integration of an otherwise successful treatment.

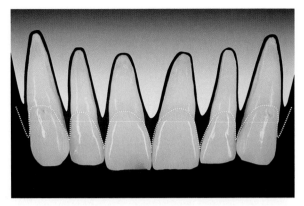

Fig. 40-53. Schematic representation of the six maxillary anterior teeth, including their bony support and the course of the marginal soft tissue, corresponding ideally approximately to the cemento-enamel junction (dotted line).

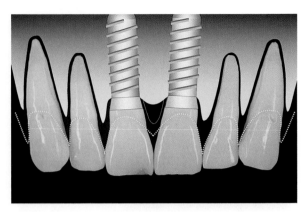

Fig. 40-54. Loss of the two central incisors and their subsequent replacement by implant restorations normally leads to well-defined bone loss ("micro-gap", establishment of a "biologic width") around the implant sites. The main consequence from an esthetic point of view consists of vertical soft tissue deficiencies, namely between adjacent implants (dotted lines).

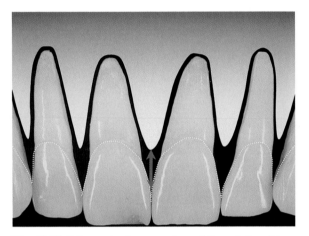

Fig. 40-55. Schematic close-up view of the relationship between cemento-enamel junction, alveolar bone and course of the gingiva in the maxillary incisor area.

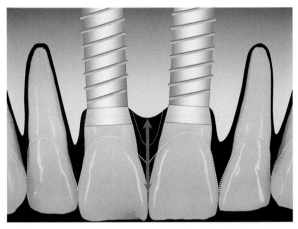

Fig. 40-56. Same area after implant therapy. The red arrow represents the distance between the interimplant bone crest and the interdental contact point. The lack of bony support for the interdental soft tissue often causes the appearance of black triangles, compromising the esthetic treatment outcome.

Table 40.8. Basic considerations related to anterior fixed multiple-unit implant restorations in sites with horizontal and/or vertical soft and hard tissue deficiencies

Achievements	Predictable and reproducible results regarding lateral bone augmentation using barrier membranes supported by autografts: • allows implant placement in patients with a low lip line
Limitations	Vertical bone augmentation is difficult to achieve and related surgical techniques lack prospective clinical long-term documentation Interimplant papillae cannot predictably be re-established as of yet

ishment of a "biologic width" (Hermann et al. 1997, 2000, 2001a,b). In contrast, the interimplant bone height normally decreases further in an apical direction, once the respective abutments or suprastructures are connected to the implant shoulder. This process is mostly accompanied by a loss of interimplant soft tissue height and hence may lead to unsightly, so-called "black interdental triangles". The schematic close-up views comparing the original dentate situation with the status after integration of two adjacent implant restorations, clearly demonstrate the negative consequences on the course of the marginal soft tissue line in a case of multiple adjacent maxillary anterior implants (Figs. 40-55 and 40-56).

The basic considerations related to the current state of achievements and limitations of maxillary anterior fixed multiple-unit implant restorations in sites with and without horizontal and/or vertical soft and hard tissue deficiencies are summarized in Table 40-8.

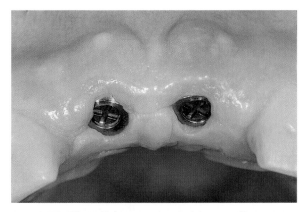

Fig. 40-57. Clinical close-up view of the maxillary anterior segment of a 32-year-old female patient following placement of two 12 mm solid screw implants according to a one-stage transmucosal surgical protocol.

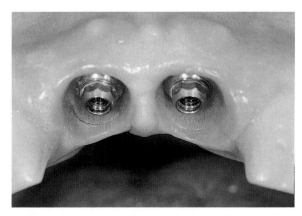

Fig. 40-58. The conditioning of the peri-implant mucosa in view of the future restorations has been performed by means of auxiliary plastic components featuring the possibility of individualizing the emergence profile.

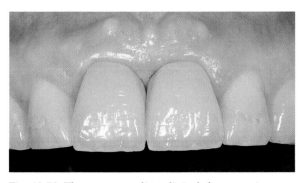

Fig. 40-59. The corresponding clinical close-up view, taken shortly after insertion of the two screw-retained ceramometal restorations, documents the effect of a long interdental contact line, the presence of pronounced mesial ridges and a slight increase of color saturation in the cervico-interdental area. Such technical measures contribute to the compensation of a flat and more apically located labial mucosa line.

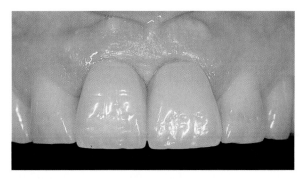

Fig. 40-60. Clinically, a slight fill-in of interimplant mucosa and an overall stable soft tissue situation can be noted after 6 years of clinical service.

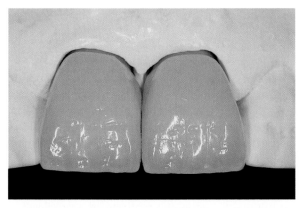

Fig. 40-61. In order to compensate for the reduced height of the interimplant soft tissue, the ceramist has used an apically prolonged interdental contact line in the form of so-called "mini-wings". These interdental ceramic extensions are made of a more saturated root-like porcelain and are slightly displaced to the palatal aspects of the crowns. This approach results in restorations that integrate successfully, although being physically larger than the original anatomical crowns.

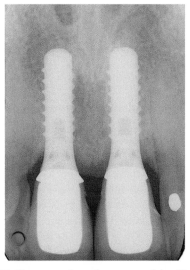

Fig. 40-62. Six years after placement of the 12 mm solid screw titanium implants, the respective radiographs reveal stable conditions at the osseointegrated interface and adequate marginal adaptation.

Sites without significant tissue deficiencies

Due to the previously described shortcomings inherent in multiple adjacent implant restorations, the clinical decision-making process will thus address both the height of the patient's smile-line (low, medium, high) and the individual gingival phenotype ("thick and low scalloped or thin and high scalloped"). In the presence of a favorable gingival morphotype, some restorative "tricks", including peri-implant soft tissue conditioning and particular interproximal crown design, need to be implemented to predictably achieve an acceptable esthetic compromise (Figs. 40-57 to 40-62). Peri-implant soft tissue conditioning is primarily achieved by using either healing caps featuring an appropriately shaped, continuously increasing (in a coronal direction) axial emergence profile, or by means of plastic components permitting the customization of the best suited axial contour in the region from the implant shoulder or abutment to the mucosal margin (Fig. 40-58). The particular suprastructure design concerns the interimplant aspect, where instead of an interdental contact point a long and slightly palatal contact line is developed in the form of two adjacent "wings", which are more color-saturated in order to create a discrete shade transition ("blending-in") at the mucosal margin. If the mesial oblique triangular ridges of the two adjacent implant restorations are located at their normal location, the ceramic crowns will not – despite their increased vestibular diameter – optically appear larger (Fig. 40-61). This design reduced the interimplant cervical triangle to a minimum at the moment of the crown insertion (Fig. 40-59), and favoured a coronal soft tissue increase, clearly visible at the 6-year clinical follow-up (Fig. 40-60).

Sites with extended horizontal deficiencies

If the absence of multiple adjacent teeth in the anterior maxilla is accompanied by a marked, but primarily horizontal, resorption of the edentulous alveolar bone crest towards the palate, one can adopt two different strategies. One consists of a so-called "bone-driven" implant placement which will lead to a distinct palatal implant position. In most instances this strategy calls for an implant assisted overdenture-type prosthesis which can more easily compensate for the discrepancy between the required position of the teeth to be replaced and the actual implant location, when compared to a fixed implant prosthesis. Furthermore, the denture flange can solve quite efficiently shortcomings related to esthetics, phonetics and/or insufficient labial and facial tissue support. Normally, denture stability and subjective comfort are excellent and – owing to its removable nature – access for oral hygiene is easy (Mericske-Stern 1998, Kiener et al. 2001). One should be aware, however, that this approach also has its inherent limits and has to take into account crucial parameters such as phonetics and minimal room required for the tongue. As this chapter focuses primarily on fixed maxillary anterior implant restorations, we refer to the relevant respective literature.

Another approach consists of one of the various lateral bone augmentation procedures reported in the literature (Buser et al. 1996, 1999, Chiapasco et al. 1999, von Arx et al. 2001a,b, Zitzmann et al. 2001, Buser et al. 2002), which ultimately should lead to a more "restoration-driven" implant placement, ideally compatible with a straightforward fixed implant prosthesis featuring a continuous, flat axial emergence profile. To date a scalloped course of the peri-implant mucosa cannot be predictably achieved around multiple adjacent maxillary anterior fixed implant restorations, and as an increased clinical crown length is normally inherent in this approach as well, the preoperative assessment of the patient's lip line or smile line (Jensen et al. 1999) is of primary importance during the related decision-making process.

Sites with major vertical tissue loss

The replacement of multiple missing adjacent maxillary anterior teeth with a fixed implant prosthesis still represents a major therapeutic challenge in the presence of combined major horizontal and vertical alveolar ridge deficiencies. Vertical bone augmentation techniques, as for example the distraction osteogenesis procedure (Chiapasco et al. 2001), hold promise for the future but at present are lacking clinical long-term documentation.

As a consequence, the treatment of choice consists in most instances of an implant assisted (e.g. spherical attachments, bar devices) removable overdenture.

CONCLUSIONS AND PERSPECTIVES

When it comes to implants to be inserted within the esthetic zone in view of a fixed restoration, a deep placement – close to or at the alveolar bone crest level – of the shoulder of implants often specifically designed for this indication, permits the suprastructure margin below the mucosa to be hidden, and the development of a gradual harmonious emergence profile from the implant shoulder to the surface, so that the resulting clinical crown replicates the profile of the natural control tooth despite a slightly more palatal implant position. This in turn leads to a secondary peri-implant bone loss or bone remodeling – particularly in a case of multiple adjacent implants – due to the reorganization of a biologic width (Hermann et al. 1997, 2000, 2001a,b). Under these particular circumstances, screw-retained restorations, based on prefabricated, machined components, will assure a maximum marginal adaptation, favoring the maintenance

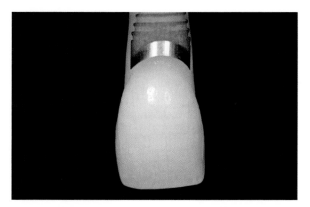

Fig. 40-63. Instead of the traditional implant design, featuring a flat rotation symmetrical coronal aspect, a scalloped connection, inspired by the natural cemento-enamel junction, may lead to a more superficial implant insertion and by this to the preservation of more bone in the interproximal area.

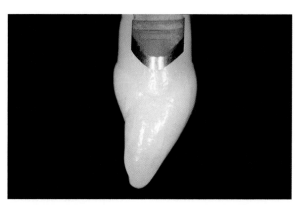

Fig. 40-64. Comparison in the sagital plane of a natural maxillary central incisor and a titanium implant featuring a scalloped design at its coronal end. The radius corresponds to the amount of bone which might theoretically be preserved.

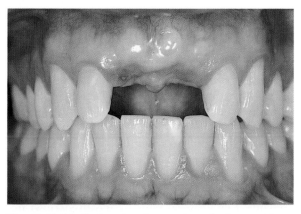

Fig. 40-65. Vestibular view in centric occlusion position of a 24-year-old male patient. The two maxillary central incisors have been lost due to a traumatic injury.

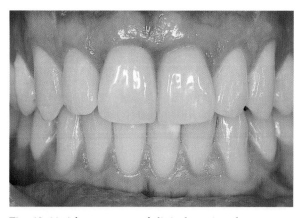

Fig. 40-66. After one year of clinical service, the presence of a harmoniously scalloped marginal soft tissue course, including the most critical interimplant area, can be noted.

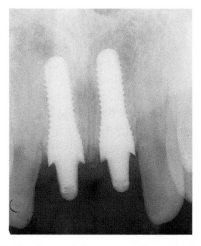

Fig. 40-67. The 1-year follow-up radiograph shows prototype of titanium implants featuring a scalloped design at their coronal end. This design permits a more superficial implant insertion, aiming at a better preservation of interimplant alveolar bone.

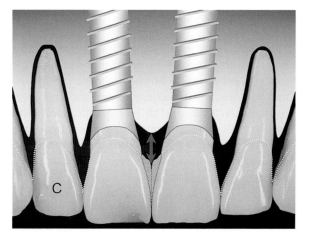

Fig. 40-68. Schematic representation of the theoretical advantages of a scalloped implant design: more superficial implant placement, increased bone and soft tissue preservation particularly in the interimplant area, and improved esthetics (in combination with interdental "mini-wings").

of the long-term stability of the esthetic result (Belser 1999, Belser et al. 1998, 2000). The currently flat, "rotation-symmetrical" design of standard screw-type titanium implants, leading to a marked submucosal implant shoulder position at the interproximal aspect, may not represent, however, the optimal design, in particular in the context of multiple adjacent implants.

Scalloped implant design

As pointed out earlier in this chapter, the traditional implant design may lead to esthetic shortcomings in a case of multiple adjacent maxillary anterior fixed implant restorations. One could hypothesize in this context whether a modified design at the coronal end of the implant, in the sense of a scalloped, more "CEJ-like" configuration, might lead to an improved preservation of peri-implant bone at the interproximal aspect in general, and between adjacent implants in particular. One of the possible design solutions and its anticipated theoretical impact on bone and esthetic parameters are presented in Figs. 40-63, 40-64 and 40-68. More specifically, this approach ultimately aims at creating an interimplant bone height and resulting soft tissue level situation compatible with generally accepted esthetic criteria. Among these one should primarily mention the establishment and/or maintenance of a harmoniously scalloped course of the marginal peri-implant mucosa. At present, the combination of the following three elements appears important:

1. screw-type titanium implant body, featuring optimal surface characteristics
2. tooth-colored transmucosal portion with adequate axial emergence profile and scalloped coronal end
3. mechanically sound suprastructure-connection, permitting both screw-retention and cementation.

The clinical potential of such a novel, scalloped implant design is anecdotally documented in Figs. 40-65 to 40-67, presenting a 24-year-old male patient who had lost his two maxillary central incisors in the course of an accident. The 1-year clinical and radiographic follow-up appears to support – at least short-term – the hypothesis that such an approach may preserve to a certain extent interimplant crestal bone and overlaying soft tissue.

Segmented fixed implant restorations in the edentulous maxilla

Another particular challenge from both a surgical and a prosthodontic point of view represents the implant-supported fixed prosthetic rehabilitation of the edentulous maxilla. Undoubtedly esthetic considerations and certain aspects associated with the patient's subjective comfort – both during the actual treatment phase and once the prosthesis is completed – also play a major role in this context. We will limit our reflections to (1) specific aspects of pre-implant diagnosis, (2) the importance of implant number, alignment and spatial distribution, and (3) conception of the suprastructure.

These elements are addressed in the form of a respective clinical case presentation, involving a 67-year-old female patient, edentulous in the maxilla (Figs. 40-69 to 40-89). Besides the traditional clinical and radiologic investigation, an in-mouth try-in of the envisioned treatment objective in the form of a set-up of teeth without vestibular denture-type flange is of primary importance (Fig. 40-73). Among other aspects, this approach will allow the visualization of the length of the clinical crowns of the future fixed implant prosthesis, and the evaluation of whether a fixed prosthesis will provide sufficient lip and facial support (Fig. 40-74). A surgical guide, derived from the described tooth set-up, will guarantee that the future implant positions are in accordance with the determined tooth positions. Whenever possible, parallelism of implants is recommended, as it permits an eventual early or immediate loading approach (Szmukler-Moncler et al. 2000, Cooper et al. 2001, Andersen et al. 2002, Cochran et al. 2002), and facilitates the subsequent clinical and laboratory procedures. Although little scientific evidence exists to indicate how many implants of which dimension and in what position are required for a predictable and long-lasting fixed implant rehabilitation of an edentulous maxilla, some clinical trends – mostly derived from traditional prosthodontic experience – do exist. If one plans to extend the prosthesis to the first molar area, and if the anatomical conditions allow the use of standard-size (length and diameter) implants, between six and eight implants seems reasonable. However, in order to increase the overall prosthetic versatility and to be able to apply the principle of segmenting, which includes the ease of eventual reinterventions in a case of localized complications (Priest 1996, Goodacre et al. 1999, Lang et al. 2000, Johnson & Persson 2001), eight implants may be considered adequate. The recommended respective positions are on both sides of the jaw – the sites of the central incisors, the canines, the first premolars and the first molars (Fig. 40-76). This approach will ultimately allow the fabrication of four independent three-unit FPDs, with all the related technical and clinical advantages (Figs. 40-78 to 40-89). Some of the scientific data available to date and supporting the concept of smaller segments rather than full-arch splinting will be presented and discussed in Chapter 41.

In conclusion, the concepts and therapeutic modalities do exist nowadays to solve – by means of implants – elegantly as well as predictably a majority of clinical situations requiring the replacement of missing teeth in the esthetic zone, and the most promising novel approaches and perspectives can already be identified on a not too distant horizon.

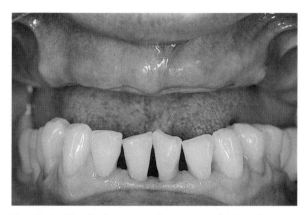

Fig. 40-69. Vestibular view of a 67-year-old female patient, edentulous in the maxilla since 18 months. Date when the pre-existing fixed prosthetic rehabilitation had to be removed due to periodontal disease and was replaced by an immediate complete upper denture to which she never adapted. In the mandible a natural dentition until the premolar area is present.

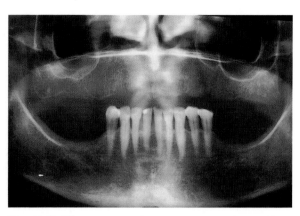

Fig. 40-70. The corresponding panoramic radiograph reveals – at least as far as the vertical bone volume is concerned – favourable conditions in view of implant therapy in both the upper and the lower posterior jaw.

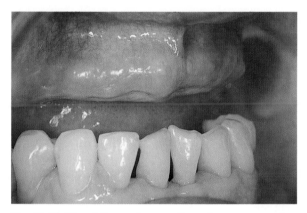

Fig. 40-71. The oblique view confirms the presence of an appropriate intermaxillary relationship which is essential for a fixed implant supported prosthesis.

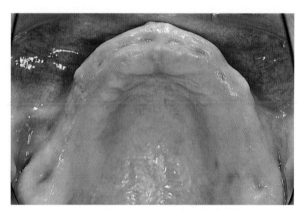

Fig. 40-72. On the occlusal view of the edentulous maxilla, one can note on the one hand overall favorable conditions for implant therapy and on the other hand the clinical signs of the recently performed tooth extractions.

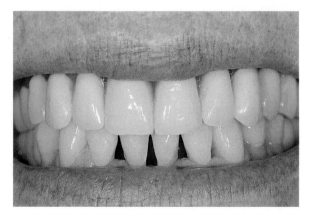

Fig. 40-73. During an unforced smile, the height of the smile line and the eventual need for additional lip support, are evaluated. Both parameters are decisive for the selection between a fixed implant prosthesis or an implant overdenture.

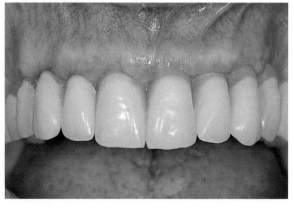

Fig. 40-74. In order to evaluate the feasibility of a fixed implant prosthesis, the clinical try-in of a diagnostic tooth set-up is of paramount importance. One should perform this tooth set-up without vestibular denture flange, so that the patient can realize how long the clinical crowns will be.

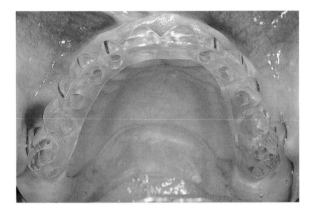

Fig. 40-75. A duplicate of the diagnostic tooth set-up in transparent acrylic will serve as a surgical guide. For optimal stability during surgery, the guide is extended to the posterior palate, an area which will not be concerned by the flap elevation.

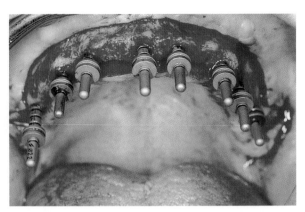

Fig. 40-76. Intrasurgical view of the edentulous maxilla, prepared for the insertion of eight implants to support a fixed prosthesis. Particular attention has been paid to achieving optimal parallelism of the implants by means of a respective surgical guide.

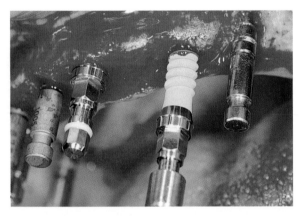

Fig. 40-77. Insertion of a titanium solid screw implant, featuring an SLA surface, in the area of the maxillary left canine.

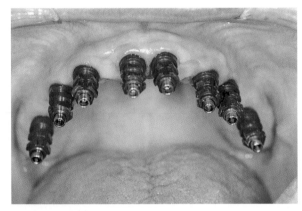

Fig. 40-78. Eight weeks after implant surgery osseointegration is confirmed radiologically and clinically. Screw-retained impression copings are inserted to perform an implant-level impression.

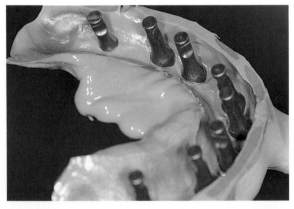

Fig. 40-79. Prior to the master cast fabrication, color-coded implant replicas (analogues) are secured to the respective impression copings.

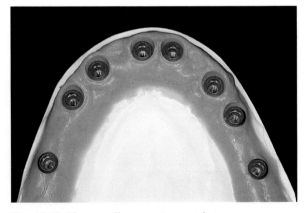

Fig. 40-80. The maxillary master cast features a removable silicon representation of the peri-implant soft tissues.

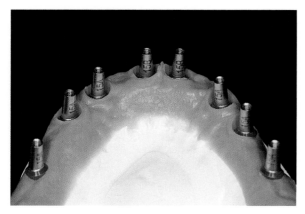

Fig. 40-81. After mounting the master cast in a second-generation, semi-adjustable articulator, the most suitable secondary components (abutments) in view of a cementable fixed implant prosthesis are selected.

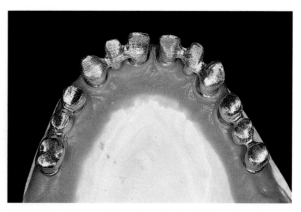

Fig. 40-82. Using a silicon key, derived from the diagnostic wax-up, as a guide, the laboratory technician has fabricated the cast metal framework in the form of four independent three-unit segments. Each segment will be supported by two implants.

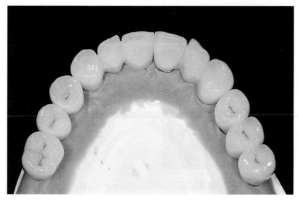

Fig. 40-83. The completed ceramometal implant prosthesis on the master cast, ready to be inserted in the patient's mouth.

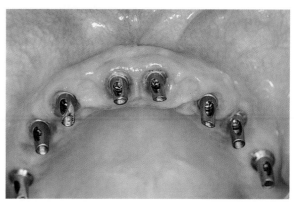

Fig. 40-84. Prior to cementation of the described ceramometal suprastructure, the secondary implant components (abutments) are tightened to 35 Ncm with a calibrated torque wrench.

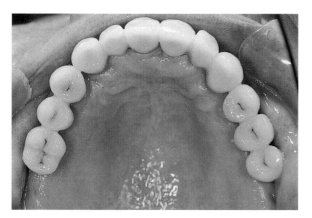

Fig. 40-85. The corresponding clinical view documents that a design similar to that applied in the natural dentition has been used.

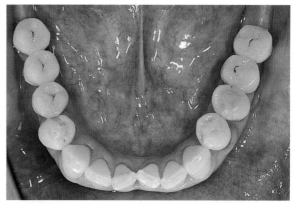

Fig. 40-86. In the mandible the bilaterally shortened arch has been prolonged to the first molar area by means of two fixed cemented ceramometal implant prostheses.

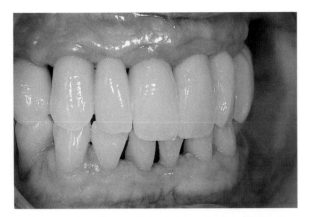

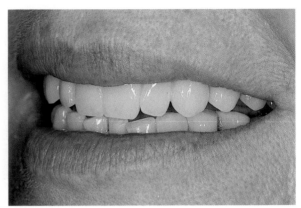

Fig. 40-87. The oblique clinical close-up view of the final implant restoration reveals an acceptable integration both from a functional and an esthetic point of view.

Fig. 40-88. Finally, an esthetically pleasing result could be achieved by means of a fixed implant-supported prosthesis.

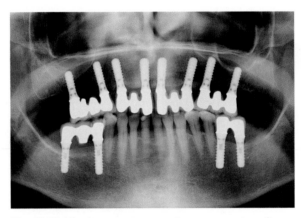

Fig. 40-89. The 1-year postoperative panoramic radiograph confirms osseointegration and documents that the maxillary prosthesis has been completed in four independent segments.

REFERENCES

Abrahamson, I., Berglundh, T. & Lindhe, J. (1997). The mucosal barrier following abutment dis/reconnection. An experimental study in dogs. *Journal of Clinical Periodontology* 24, 568-572.

Abrahamson, I., Berglundh, T., Wennström, J. & Lindhe, J. (1996). The peri-implant hard and soft tissues at different implant systems. *Clinical Oral Implants Research* 7, 212-219.

Andersen, E., Haanæs, H.R. & Knutsen, B.M. (2002). Immediate loading of single-tooth ITI implants in the anterior maxilla: a prospective 5-year pilot study. *Clinical Oral Implants Research* 13, 281-287.

Andersson, B., Ödman, P., Lindvall, A.M. & Brånemark, P.I. (1998). Five-year prospective study of prosthodontic and surgical single-tooth implant treatment in general practices and at a specialist clinic. *International Journal of Prosthodontics* 11, 351-365.

Andersson, B., Ödman, P., Lindvall, A.M. & Lithner, B. (1995). Single-tooth restorations supported by osseointegrated implants: results and experiences from a prospective study after 2 to 3 years. *International Journal of Oral and Maxillofacial Implants* 10, 702-711.

Avivi-Arber, L. & Zarb, G.A. (1996). Clinical effectiveness of implant-supported single-tooth replacement: the Toronto study. *International Journal of Oral and Maxillofacial Implants* 11, 311-321.

Bahat, O. & Daftary, F. (1995). Surgical reconstruction – a prerequisite for long-term implant success: a philosophic approach. *Practical Periodontics and Aesthetic Dentistry* 7, 21-31.

Bahat, O., Fontanesi, R.V. & Preston, J. (1993). Reconstruction of the hard and soft tissues for optimal placement of osseointegrated implants. *International Journal of Periodontics and Restorative Dentistry* 13, 255-275.

Bain, C.A. & Weisgold, A.S. (1997). Customized emergence profile in the implant crown – a new technique. *Compendium for Continuing Education in Dentistry* 18, 41-46.

Behneke, A., Behneke, N. & d'Hoedt, B. (2000). The longitudinal clinical effectiveness of ITI solid screw implants in partially edentulous patients: A 5-year follow-up report. *International Journal of Oral and Maxillofacial Implants* 15, 633-645.

Belser, U.C. (1982). Esthetics checklist for the fixed prosthesis. Part II: Biscuit-bake try-in. In: Schärer, P., Rinn, L.A., Kopp, F.R., eds. *Esthetic Guidelines for Restorative Dentistry*. Carol Stream, Ill: Quintessence Publishing Co., pp. 188-192.

Belser, U.C. (1999). Esthetic implant restorations. In: Lang, N.P., Karring, T. & Lindhe, J., eds. *Proceedings of the 3rd European Workshop on periodontology*. Berlin: Quintessence, pp. 304-332.

Belser, U.C., Buser, D., Hess, D., Schmid, B., Bernard, J.P. & Lang, N.P. (1998). Aesthetic implant restorations in partially edentulous patients – a critical appraisal. *Periodontology 2000* **17**, 132-150.

Belser, U.C., Mericske-Stern, R., Bernard, J.P. & Taylor, T.D. (2000). Prosthetic management of the partially dentate patient with fixed implant restorations. *Clinical Oral Implants Research* **11** (suppl. I), 126-145.

Bengazi, F., Wennström, J.L. & Lekholm, U. (1996). Recession of the soft tissue margin at oral implants. A 2-year longitudinal prospective study. *Clinical Oral Implants Research* **7**, 303-310.

Berglundh, T. & Lindhe, J. (1996). Dimension of the periimplant mucosa. Biological width revisited. *Journal of Clinical Periodontology* **23**, 971-983.

Bernard, J.P. & Belser, U. (2002). Twelve years of clinical experience with the ITI Dental Implant System at the University of Geneva. *Journal de Parodontologie et d'Implantologie orale* **21**, 1-27.

Bichacho, N. & Landsberg, C.J. (1994). A modified surgical/prosthetic approach for an optimal single implant-supported crown. Part II. The cervical contouring concept. *Practical Periodontics and Aesthetic Dentistry* **6**, 35-41.

Bichacho, N. & Landsberg, C.J. (1997). Single implant restorations: prosthetically induced soft tissue topography. *Practical Periodontics and Aesthetic Dentistry* **9**, 745-754.

Boioli, L.T., Penaud, J. & Miller N. (2001). A meta-analytic, quantitative assessment of osseointegration establishment and evolution of submerged and non-submerged endosseous titanium oral implants. *Clinical Oral Implants Research* **12**, 579-588.

Brånemark, P.I, Svensson, B. & van Steenberghe, D. (1995). Ten-year survival rates of fixed prostheses on four or six implants ad modum Brånemark in full edentulism. *Clinical Oral Implants Research* **6**, 227-231.

Brugnolo, E., Mazzocco, C., Cordioll, G. & Majzoub, Z. (1996). Clinical and radiographic findings following placement of single-tooth implants in young patients – case reports. *International Journal of Periodontics and Restorative Dentistry* **16**, 421-433.

Bryant, R.S. & Zarb, G.A. (1998). Osseointegration of oral implants in older and younger adults. *International Journal of Oral and Maxillofacial Implants* **13**, 492-499.

Buser, D., Dula, K., Hess, D., Hirt, H.P. & Belser U.C. (1999). Localized ridge augmentation with autografts and barrier membranes. *Periodontology 2000* **19**, 151-163.

Buser, D., Dula, K., Hirt, H.P. & Schenk, R.K. (1996). Lateral ridge augmentation using autografts and barrier membranes: a clinical study with 40 partially edentulous patients. *Journal of Oral and Maxillofacial Surgery* **54**, 420-432.

Buser, D., Ingimarsson, S., Dula, K., Lussi, A., Hirt, H.P. & Belser, U.C. (2002). Long-term stability of osseointegrated implants in augmented bone: A 5-year prospective study in partially edentulous patients. *International Journal of Periodontics and Restorative Dentistry* **22**, 108-117.

Buser, D., Mericske-Stern, R., Bernard, J.P., Behneke, A., Behneke, N., Hirt, H.P., Belser, U.C. & Lang, N.P. (1997). Long-term evaluation of non-submerged ITI implants. Part I: 8-year life table analysis of a prospective multi-center study with 2359 implants. *Clinical Oral Implants Research* **8**, 161-172.

Buser, D. & von Arx, T. (2000). Surgical procedures in partially edentulous patients with ITI implants. *Clinical Oral Implants Research* **11** (suppl. I), 83-100.

Carrick, J.L. (1995). Post-trauma replacement of maxillary central incisors utilizing implants: a case report. *Practical Periodontics and Aesthetic Dentistry* **7**, 79-85.

Chang, M., Wennström, J.L., Oedman, P. & Andersson, B. (1999). Implant supported single-tooth replacements compared to contralateral natural teeth. Crown and soft tissue dimensions. *Clinical Oral Implants Research* **10**, 185-194.

Chee, W.W., Cho, G.C. & Ha, S. (1997). Replicating soft tissue contours on working casts for implant restorations. *Journal of Prosthodontics* **6**, 218-220.

Chiapasco, M., Abati, S., Romeo, E. & Vogel, G. (1999). Clinical outcome of autogenous bone blocks or guided regeneration with e-PTFE membranes for reconstruction of narrow edentulous ridges. *Clinical Oral Implants Research* **10**, 278-288.

Chiapasco, M., Romeo, E. & Vogel, G. (2001). Vertical distraction osteogenesis of edentulous ridges for improvement of oral implant positioning: A clinical report of preliminary results. *International Journal of Oral and Maxillofacial Implants* **16**, 43-51.

Chiche, G. & Pinault, A. (1994). *Esthetics of Anterior Fixed Prosthodontics*. Carol Stream, Ill: Quintessence Publishing Co.

Choquet, V., Hermans, M., Adrienssens P., Daelemans, P., Tarnow, D.P. & Malevez, C. (2001). Clinical and radiographic evaluation of the papilla level adjacent to single-tooth dental implants. A retrospective study in the maxillary anterior region. *Journal of Periodontology* **72**, 1364-1371.

Cochran, D.L., Buser, D., ten Bruggenkate, C.M., Weingart, D., Taylor, T. M., Bernard, J.P., Peters, F. & Simpson, J.P. (2002). The use of shortened healing times on ITI implants with a sandblasted and acid-etched (SLA) surface. Early results from clinical trials on ITI SLA implants. *Clinical Oral Implants Research* **13**, 144-153.

Cooper, L., Felton, D.A., Kugelberg, C.F., Ellner, S., Chaffee, N., Molina, A.L., Moriarty, J.D., Paquette, D. & Palmqvist, U. (2001). A multicenter 12-months evaluation of single-tooth implants restored 3 weeks after 1-stage surgery. *International Journal of Oral and Maxillofacial Implants* **16,** 182-192.

Corrente, G., Vergnano, L., Pascetta, R. & Ramadori, G. (1995). A new custom-made abutment for dental implants: a technical note. *International Journal of Oral and Maxillofacial Implants* **10,** 604-608.

Davidoff, S.R. (1996). Late stage soft tissue modification for anatomically correct implant-supported restorations. *Journal of Prosthetic Dentistry* **76**, 334-338.

De Lange, G.L. (1995). Aesthetic and prosthetic principles for single tooth implant procedures: an overview. *Practical Periodontics and Aesthetic Dentistry* **7**, 51-62.

Eckert, S.E. & Wollan, P.C. (1998). Retrospective review of 1170 endosseous implants placed in partially edentulous jaws. *Journal of Prosthetic Dentistry* **79**, 415-421.

Ekfeldt, A., Carlsson, G.E. & Börjesson, G. (1994). Clinical evaluation of single-tooth restorations supported by osseointegrated implants: a retrospective study. *International Journal of Oral and Maxillofacial Implants* **9**, 179-183.

Ellegaard, B., Baelum, V. & Karring, T. (1997a). Implant therapy in periodontally compromised patients. *Clinical Oral Implants Research* **8**, 180-188.

Ellegaard, B., Kølsen-Petersen, J. & Baelum, V. (1997b). Implant therapy involving maxillary sinus lift in periodontally compromised patients. *Clinical Oral Implants Research* **8**, 305-315.

Ellen, R.P. (1998). Microbial colonization of the peri-implant environment and its relevance to long-term success of osseointegrated implants. *International Journal of Prosthodontics* **11**, 433-441.

Engquist, B, Åstrand, P., Dahlgren, S., Engquist, E., Feldman, H. & Gröndahl, K. (2002). Marginal bone reaction to oral implants: a prospective comparative study of Astra Tech and Brånemark System implants. *Clinical Oral Implants Research* **13**, 30-37.

Ericsson, I., Nilson, H., Nilner, K. & Randow, K. (2000). Immediate functional loading of Brånemark single tooth implants. An 18 months' clinical pilot follow-up study. *Clinical Oral Implants Research* **11**, 26-33.

Garber, D.A. (1995). The esthetic implant: letting restoration be the guide. *Journal of the American Dental Association* **126**, 319-325.

Garber, D.A. & Belser, U.C. (1995). Restoration-driven implant placement with restoration-generated site development. *Compendium of Continuing Education in Dentistry* **16**, 796-804.

Garg, A.K., Finley, J. & Dorado, L.S. (1997). Single-tooth implant-supported restorations in the anterior maxilla. *Practical Periodontics and Aesthetic Dentistry* **9**, 903-912.

Gelb, D.A. & Lazzara, R.J. (1993). Hierarchy of objectives in implant placement to maximize esthetics: use of pre-angulated abutments. *International Journal of Periodontics & Restorative Dentistry* **13**, 277-287.

Ghalili, K.M. (1994). A new approach to restoring single-tooth implants: report of a case. *International Journal of Oral and Maxillofacial Implants* **9**, 85-89.

Giannopoulou, C., Bernard, J.P., Buser, D., Carrel, A. & Belser, U.C. (2002). Effect of intracrevicular restoration margins on peri-implant health: Clinical, biochemical and microbiological findings around esthetic implants up to 9 years. Submitted to *International Journal of Oral & Maxillofacial Implants*.

Goldstein, R. (1976). *Esthetics in Dentistry*. Philadelphia, PA: Lippincott Publ.

Gomez-Roman, G., Kruppenbacher, M., Weber, H. & Schulte, W. (2001). Immediate postextraction implant placement with root-analog stepped implants: Surgical procedure and statistical outcome after 6 years. *International Journal of Oral and Maxillofacial Implants* **16**, 503-513.

Goodacre, C.A. (1990). Gingival esthetics. *Journal of Prosthetic Dentistry* **64**, 1-12.

Goodacre, C.J., Kan, J.I.K. & Rungcharassaeng, K. (1999). Clinical complications of osseointegrated implants. *Journal of Prosthetic Dentistry* **81**, 537-552.

Grunder, U. (2000). Stability of the mucosal topography around single-tooth implants and adjacent teeth: 1-year results. *International Journal of Periodontics and Restorative Dentistry* **20**, 11-17.

Grunder, U., Spielmann H.P. & Gaberthuel, T. (1996). Implant-supported single tooth replacement in the aesthetic region: a complex challenge. *Practical Periodontics and Aesthetic Dentistry* **8**, 835-842.

Gunne, J., Åstrand, P. Lindh, T., Borg, K. & Olsson, M. (1999). Tooth-implant and implant supported fixed partial dentures: A 10-year report. *International Journal of Prosthodontics* **12**, 216-221.

Haas, R., Polak C., Fürhauser, R., Mailath-Pokorny, G., Dörtbudak, O. & Watzek, G. (2002). A long-term follow-up of 76 Brånemark single-tooth implants. *Clinical Oral Implants Research* **13**, 38-43.

Hebel, K.S. & Gajjar, R.C. (1997). Cement-retained versus screw-retained implant restorations: achieving optimal occlusion and esthetics in implant dentistry. *Journal of Prosthetic Dentistry* **77**, 28-35.

Henry, P.J., Laney, W.R., Jemt, T., Harris, D., Krogh, P.H.J., Polizzi, G., Zarb, G.A. & Herrmann, I. (1996). Osseointegrated implants for single-tooth replacement: a prospective 5-year multicenter study. *International Journal of Oral and Maxillofacial Implants* **11**, 450-455.

Hermann, J.S., Buser, D., Schenk, R.K., Higginbottom, F.L. & Cochran, D.L. (2000). Biologic width around titanium implants. A physiologically formed and stable dimension over time. *Clinical Oral Implants Research* **11**, 1-11.

Hermann, J.S., Buser, D., Schenk, R.K., Schoolfield, J.D. & Cochran, D.L. (2001a). Biologic width around one- and two-piece titanium implants. A histometric evaluation of unloaded nonsubmerged and submerged implants in the canine mandible. *Clinical Oral Implants Research* **12**, 559-571.

Hermann, J.S., Cochran, D.L., Nummikoski, P.V. & Buser, D. (1997). Crestal bone changes around titanium implants. A radiographic evaluation of unloaded nonsubmerged and submerged implants in the canine mandible. *Journal of Periodontology* **68**, 1117-1130.

Hermann, J.S., Schoolfield, J.D., Nummikoski, P.V., Buser, D., Schenk, R.K & Cochran, D.L. (2001b). Crestal bone changes around titanium implants: A methodological study comparing linear radiographic with histometric measurements. *International Journal of Oral and Maxillofacial Implants* **16**, 475-485.

Hess, D., Buser, D., Dietschi, D., Grossen, G., Schönenberger, A. & Belser, U.C. (1996). Aesthetischer Einzelzahnersatz mit Implantaten – ein "Team-Approach". *Implantologie* **3**, 245-256.

Hosny, M., Duyck, J., van Steenberghe, D. & Naert, I. (2000). Within-subject comparison between connected and nonconnected tooth-to-implant fixed partial prostheses: Up to 14-year follow-up study. *International Journal of Prosthodontics* **13**, 340-346.

Hultin, M., Gustafsson, A. & Klinge, B. (2000). Long-term evaluation of osseointegrated dental implants in the treatment of partially edentulous patients. *Journal of Clinical Periodontology* **27**, 128-133.

Hürzeler, M.B., Quinones, C.R. & Strub, J.R. (1994). Advanced surgical and prosthetic management of the anterior single tooth osseointegrated implant: a case presentation. *Practical Periodontics and Aesthetic Dentistry* **6**, 13-21.

Jaggers, A., Simons, A.M. & Badr, S.E. (1993). Abutment selection for anterior single tooth replacement. A clinical report. *Journal of Prosthetic Dentistry* **69**, 133-135.

Jansen, C.E. & Weisgold, A. (1995). Presurgical treatment planning for the anterior single-tooth implant restoration. *Compendium of Continuing Education in Dentistry* **16**, 746-764.

Jemt, T. (1999). Restoring the gingival contour by means of provisional resin crowns after single-implant treatment. *International Journal of Periodontics and Restorative Dentistry* **19**, 21-29.

Jemt, T., Heath, M.R., Johns, R.B., McNamara, D.C., van Steenberghe, D. & Watson, R.M. (1996). A 5-year prospective multicenter follow-up report on overdentures supported by osseointegrated implants. *International Journal of Oral and Maxillofacial Implants* **11**, 291-298.

Jensen, J., Joss, A. & Lang, N.P. (1999). The smile line of different ethnic groups depending on age and gender. *Acta Medicinae Dentium Helvetica* **4**, 38-46.

Johnson, R.H. & Persson, G.R. (2001). A 3-year prospective study of a single-tooth implant – prosthodontic complications. *International Journal of Prosthodontics* **14**, 183-189.

Keller, W., Brägger, U. & Mombelli, A. (1998). Peri-implant microflora of implants with cemented and screw retained suprastructures. *Clinical Oral Implants Research* **9**, 209-217.

Kemppainen, P., Eskola, S. & Ylipaavalniemi, P. (1997). A comparative prospective clinical study of two single-tooth implants: a preliminary report of 102 implants. *Journal of Prosthetic Dentistry* **77**, 382-387.

Khayat, P., Nader, N. & Exbrayat, P. (1995). Single tooth replacement using a one-piece screw-retained restoration. *Practical Periodontics and Aesthetic Dentistry* **7**, 61-69.

Kiener, P., Oetterli, M., Mericske, E. & Mericske-Stern, R. (2001). Effectiveness of maxillary overdentures supported by implants: maintenance and prosthetic complications. *International Journal of Prosthodontics* **14**, 133-140.

Kois, J.C. (1996). The restorative-periodontal interface: biological parameters. *Periodontology 2000* **11**, 29-38.

Kokich, V.G. (1996). Esthetics: the orthodontic-periodontic restorative connection. *Seminars in Orthodontics* **2**, 21-30.

Kokich, V.G. & Spear, F.M. (1997). Guidelines for managing the orthodontic-restorative patient. *Seminars in Orthodontics* **3**, 3-20.

Krenmair, G., Schmidinger, S. & Waldenberger, O. (2002). Single-tooth replacement with the Frialit-2 System: A retrospective clinical analysis of 146 implants. *International Journal of Oral and Maxillofacial Implants* **17**, 78-85.

Landsberg, C.J. & Bichacho, N. (1994). A modified surgical/prosthetic approach for an optimal single implant supported crown. Part I: The socket seal surgery. *Practical Periodontics and Aesthetic Dentistry* **6**, 11-17.

Laney, W.R., Jemt, T., Harris, D., Henry, P.J., Krogh, P.H.J., Polizzi, G., Zarb, G.A. & Herrmann, I. (1994). Osseointegrated implants for single-tooth replacement: progress report from a multicenter prospective study after 3 years. *International Journal of Oral and Maxillofacial Implants* **9**, 49-54.

Lang, N.P., Wilson, T. & Corbet, E.F. (2000). Biological complications with dental implants: their prevention, diagnosis and treatment. *Clinical Oral Implants Research* **11** (suppl. I), 146-155.

Lekholm, U., Gunne, J., Henry, P., Higuchi, K., Linden, U., Bergstrom, C. & van Steenberghe, D. (1999). Survival of the Brånemark implant in partially edentulous jaws: a 10-year prospective multicenter study. *International Journal of Oral and Maxillofacial Implants* **14**, 639-645.

Leonhardt, Å., Gröndahl, K., Bergström, C. & Lekholm, U. (2002). Long-term follow-up of osseointegrated titanium implants using clinical, radiographic and microbiological parameters. *Clinical Oral Implants Research* **13**, 127-132.

Levine, R.A., Clem, D.S., Wilson, T.G., Higginbottom, F. & Saunders, S.L. (1997). A multicenter retrospective analysis of the ITI implant system used for single-tooth replacements: preliminary results at 6 or more months of loading. *International Journal of Oral and Maxillofacial Implants* **12**, 237-242.

Lewis, S. (1995). Anterior single-tooth implant restorations. *International Journal of Periodontics and Restorative Dentistry* **15**, 30-41.

Lindh, T., Gunne, J., Tillberg, A. & Molin, M. (1998). A meta-analysis of implants in partial edentulism. *Clinical Oral Implants Research* **9**, 80-90.

Lindhe, J. & Berglundh, T. (1998). The interface between the mucosa and the implant. *Periodontology 2000* **17**, 47-53.

Lindqvist, L.W., Carlsson, G.E. & Jemt, T. (1996). A prospective 15-year follow-up study of mandibular fixed prostheses supported by osseointegrated implants. Clinical results and marginal bone loss. *Clinical Oral Implants Research* **7**, 329-336.

Magne, P. & Belser, U.C. (2002). *Bonded Porcelain Restorations in the Anterior Dentition. A Biomimetic Approach.* Chicago/Berlin: Quintessence Books.

Magne, P., Magne, M. & Belser, U.C. (1993a). Natural and restorative oral esthetics. Part I: Rationale and basic strategies for successful esthetic rehabilitations. *Journal of Esthetic Dentistry* **5**, 161-173.

Magne, P., Magne, M. & Belser, U.C. (1993b). Natural and restorative oral esthetics. Part II: Esthetic treatment modalities. *Journal of Esthetic Dentistry* **5**, 239-246.

Magne, P., Magne, M. & Belser, U.C. (1994). Natural and restorative oral esthetics. Part III: Fixed partial dentures. *Journal of Esthetic Dentistry* **6**, 15-22.

Magne, P., Magne, M. & Belser, U.C. (1996). The diagnostic template: a key element to the comprehensive esthetic treatment concept. *International Journal of Periodontics and Restorative Dentistry* **16**, 561-569.

Marchack, C.B. (1996). A custom titanium abutment for the anterior single-tooth implant. *Journal of Prosthetic Dentistry* **76**, 288-291.

Mecall, R.A. & Rosenfeld, A.L. (1996). Influence of residual ridge resorption pattern on fixture placement and tooth position. Part III: Presurgical assessment of ridge augmentation requirements. *International Journal of Periodontics and Restorative Dentistry* **16**, 322-337.

Mengel, R., Schröder, T. & Flores-de-Jacoby, L. (2001). Osseointegrated implants in patients treated for generalized chronic periodontitis and generalized aggressive periodontitis: 3- and 5-year results of a prospective long-term study. *Journal of Periodontology* **72**, 977-989.

Mericske-Stern, R. (1998). Treatment outcomes with implant-supported overdentures: clinical considerations. *Journal of Prosthetic Dentistry* **79**, 66-73.

Mericske-Stern, R., Grütter, L., Rösch, R. & Mericske, E. (2001). Clinical evaluation and prosthetic complications of single tooth replacement by non submerged implants. *Clinical Oral Implants Research* **12**, 309-318.

Nathanson, D. (1991). Current developments in esthetic dentistry. *Current Opinions in Dentistry* **1**, 206-211.

Neale, D. & Chee, W.W. (1994). Development of implant soft tissue emergence profile: a technique. *Journal of Prosthetic Dentistry* **71**, 364-368.

Norton, M.R. (1998). Marginal bone levels at single tooth implants with a conical fixture design. The influence of surface macro- and microstructure. *Clinical Oral Implants Research* **9**, 91-99.

Oetterli, M., Kiener, P. & Mericske-Stern, R. (2001). A longitudinal study on mandibular implants supporting an overdenture: The influence of retention mechanism and anatomic-

prosthetic variables on periimplant parameters. *International Journal of Prosthodontics* **14**, 536-542.

Palmer, R.M., Smith, B.J., Palmer, P.J. & Floyd, P.D. (1997). A prospective study of Astra single tooth implants. *Clinical Oral Implants Research* **8**, 173-179.

Parel, S.M. & Sullivan, D.Y. (1989). *Esthetics and Osseointegration*. Dallas, TX: Taylor Publishing.

Price, R.B.T. & Price, D.E. (1999). Esthetic restoration of a single-tooth dental implant using a subepithelial connective tissue graft: a case report with 3-year follow-up. *International Journal of Periodontics and Restorative Dentistry* **19**, 93-101.

Priest, G.F. (1996). Failure rates of restorations for single-tooth replacement. *International Journal of Prosthodontics* **9**, 38-45.

Romeo, E., Chiapasco, M., Ghisolfi, M. & Vogel, G. (2002). Long-term clinical effectiveness of oral implants in the treatment of partial edentulism. Seven-year life table analysis of a prospective study with ITI® Dental Implant System used for single-tooth restorations. *Clinical Oral Implants Research* **13**, 133-143.

Rüfenacht, C.R. (1990). *Fundamentals of Esthetics*. Carol Stream, Ill: Quintessence Publishing Co.

Salama, H. & Salama, M. (1993). The role of orthodontic extrusive modeling in the enhancement of soft and hard tissue profiles prior to implant placement: a systematic approach to the management of extraction site defects. *International Journal of Periodontics and Restorative Dentistry* **13**, 312-334.

Salama, H., Salama, M. & Garber, D.A. (1995). Techniques for developing optimal peri-implant papillae within the esthetic zone. Part I, guided soft tissue augmentation: the three-stage approach. *Journal of Esthetic Dentistry* **7**, 3-9.

Salinas, T.J. & Sadan, A. (1998). Establishing soft tissue integration with natural tooth-shaped abutments. *Practical Periodontics and Aesthetic Dentistry* **10**, 35-42.

Schärer, P., Rinn, L.A. & Kopp, F.R. (eds). (1982). Esthetic guidelines for restorative dentistry. Carol Stream, Ill: Quintessence Publishing Co., Inc.

Scheller, H., Urgell, J.P., Kultje, C., Klineberg, I., Goldberg, P.V., Stevenson-Moore, P., Alonso, J.M., Schaller, M., Corria, R.M., Engquist, B., Toreskog, S., Kastenbaum, F. & Smith, C.R. (1998). A 5-year multicenter study on implant-supported single crown restorations. *International Journal of Oral and Maxillofacial Implants* **13**, 212-218.

Schmitt, A. & Zarb, G.A. (1993). The longitudinal clinical effectiveness of osseointegrated implants for single-tooth replacement. *International Journal of Prosthodontics* **6**, 197-202.

Seibert, J. & Lindhe, J. (1989). Esthetics and periodontal therapy. In: Lindhe, J., ed. *Textbook of Clinical Periodontology*, 2nd edn. Copenhagen: Munksgaard, pp. 477-514.

Spear, F.M., Mathews, D.M. & Kokich, V.G. (1997). Interdisciplinary management of single-tooth implants. *Seminars in Orthodontics* **3**, 45-72.

Studer, S., Pietrobon, N. & Wohlwend, A. (1994). Maxillary anterior single-tooth replacement: comparison of three treatment modalities. *Practical Periodontics and Aesthetic Dentistry* **6**, 51-62.

Sutter, F., Weber, H.P., Sorensen, J. & Belser, U.C. (1993). The new restorative concept of the ITI Dental Implant System: Design and engineering. *International Journal of Periodontics and Restorative Dentistry* **13**, 409-431.

Szmukler-Moncler, S., Piatelli, J.A., Favero, J.H. & Dubruille, J.H. (2000). Considerations preliminary to the application of early and immediate loading protocols in dental implantology. *Clinical Oral Implants Research* **11**, 12-25.

Tarnow, D.P., Cho, S.C. & Wallace, S.S. (2000). The effect of inter-implant distance on the height of inter-implant bone crest. *Journal of Periodontology* **71**, 546-549.

Tarnow, D.P. & Eskow, R.N. (1995). Considerations for single-unit esthetic implant restorations. *Compendium of Continuing Education in Dentistry* **16**, 778-788.

Tarnow, D.P., Magner, A.W. & Fletcher, P. (1992). The effect of the distance from the contact point to the crest of bone on the presence or absence of the interproximal dental papilla. *Journal of Periodontology* **63**, 995-996.

ten Bruggenkate, C.M., Asikainen, P., Foitzik, C., Krekeler, G. & Sutter, F. (1998). Short (6 mm) non-submerged dental implants: results of a multicenter clinical trial of 1-7 years. *International Journal of Oral and Maxillofacial Implants* **13**, 791-798.

Touati, B. (1995). Improving aesthetics of implant-supported restorations. *Practical Periodontics and Aesthetic Dentistry* **7**, 81-92.

Van Steenberghe, D., Quirynen, M. & Wallace, S.S. (1999). Survival and success rates with oral endosseous implants. In: Lang, N.P., Karring, T. & Lindhe, J., eds. *Proceedings of the 3rd European Workshop on Periodontology*. Berlin: Quintessence, pp. 242-254.

Vlassis, J.M., Lyzak, W.A. & Senn, C. (1993). Anterior aesthetic considerations for the placement and restoration of nonsubmerged endosseous implants. *Practical Periodontics and Aesthetic Dentistry* **5**, 19-27.

von Arx, T., Cochran, D.L., Hermann, J.S., Schenk, R.K. & Buser, D. (2001b). Lateral ridge augmentation using different bone fillers and barrier membrane application. A histologic and histomorphometric pilot study in the canine mandible. *Clinical Oral Implants Research* **12**, 260-269.

von Arx, T., Cochran, D.L., Hermann, J., Schenk, R.K., Higginbottom, F. & Buser, D. (2001a). Lateral ridge augmentation and implant placement: An experimental study evaluating implant osseointegration in different augmentation materials in the canine mandible. *International Journal of Oral and Maxillofacial Implants* **16**, 343-354.

Walther, W., Klemke, J., Wörle, M. & Heners, M. (1996). Implant-supported single-tooth replacements: risk of implant and prosthesis failure. *Journal of Oral Implantology* **22**, 236-239.

Weber, H.P., Crohin, C.C. & Fiorellini, J.P. (2000). A 5-year prospective clinical and radiographic study of non-submerged dental implants. *Clinical Oral Implants Research* **11**, 144-153.

Wismeijer, D., van Waas, M.A.J., Mulder, J., Vermeeren, I.J.F. & Kalk, W. (1999). Clinical and radiological results of patients treated with three treatment modalities for overdentures on implants of the ITI dental implant system. A randomised controlled clinical trial. *Clinical Oral Implants Research* **10**, 297-306.

Wyatt, C.L. & Zarb, G.A. (1998). Treatment outcomes of patients with implant-supported fixed partial prostheses. *International Journal of Oral and Maxillofacial Implants* **13**, 204-211.

Zarb, G.A. & Schmitt, A. (1993). The longitudinal clinical effectiveness of osseointegrated dental implants in anterior partially edentulous patients. *International Journal of Prosthodontics* **6**, 180-188.

Zitzmann, N.U., Schärer, P. & Marinello, C.P. (2001). Long-term results of implants treated with guided bone regeneration: A 5-year prospective study. *International Journal of Oral and Maxillofacial Implants* **16**, 355-366.

Acknowledgements

The authors wish to acknowledge and thank Drs Jean-Paul Martinet, Nicholas Roehrich and Dimitri Thiébaud (all of them clinicians at School of Dental Medicine, University of Geneva, and involved in the treatment of some of the patients presented in this chapter) for their contributions. We would also like to thank the laboratory technicians and ceramists Michel Bertossa, Michel Magne and Alwin Schönenberger, for their expertise and meticulous execution of the implant suprastructures presented in this chapter. Furthermore, our gratitude is extended to Dr Pascal Magne (Senior Lecturer, University of Geneva) for his competent assistance in development of the schematic illustrations.

CHAPTER 41

Implants in the Load Carrying Part of the Dentition

URS BELSER, DANIEL BUSER AND JEAN-PIERRE BERNARD

BASIC CONCEPTS

General considerations

The overall favorable long-term survival and success rates reported in the recent literature for osseointegrated implants in the treatment of various types of edentulism (Brånemark et al. 1995, Jemt et al. 1996, Lindqvist et al. 1996, Buser et al. 1997, Andersson et al. 1998, Buser et al. 1998b, Eckert & Wollan 1998, Lindh et al. 1998, Mericske-Stern 1998, ten Bruggenkate et al. 1998, Wyatt & Zarb 1998, Gunne et al. 1999, Lekholm et al. 1999, Van Steenberghe et al. 1999, Wismeijer et al. 1999, Behneke et al. 2000, Hosny et al. 2000, Hultin et al. 2000, Weber et al. 2000, Boioli et al. 2001, Gomez-Roman et al. 2001, Kiener et al. 2001, Mengel et al. 2001, Oetterli et al. 2001, Zitzmann et al. 2001, Bernard & Belser 2002, Buser et al. 2002, Haas et al. 2002, Leonhardt et al. 2002, Romeo et al. 2002) nowadays permit consideration of dental implants as one of the reliable therapeutic modalities during the establishment of any prosthetic treatment plan. In numerous clinical situations implants can clearly contribute to a notable simplification of therapy, frequently enabling removable prostheses to be avoided, keeping it less invasive with respect to remaining tooth structure or rendering the treatment both more elegant and versatile as well as more predictable (Belser et al. 2000).

As part of a textbook focusing essentially on clinical periodontics, this chapter will address primarily implant therapy performed in the posterior segments of partially edentulous patients. In this context, the use of implants may often significantly reduce the inherent risk of a "borderline" conventional tooth-borne fixed prosthesis (e.g. compromised or missing "strategic" abutment teeth, long-span fixed partial dentures, cantilevers) by implementing the principle of segmentation. It is currently widely accepted that – in comparison with extended splinted prosthetic segments – small ones are preferable as they are easier to

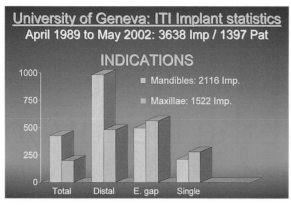

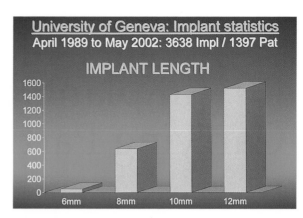

Fig. 41-1. University of Geneva implant statistics, 1989-2002.

Fig. 41-2. Implant length distribution.

fabricate, generally provide improved "passive fit" and marginal fidelity, offer better access for the patient's oral hygiene, and ultimately are less complicated to handle in case of need for reintervention. When it comes to treatment planning in general, and to the choice *implant versus tooth-borne fixed partial denture (FPD) versus tooth* in particular, the related decision-making criteria should be essentially derived from scientific evidence and objective prosthetically-oriented risk assessment in the broad sense, including additional parameters such as simplicity, cost-effectiveness and quality of life. Beyond any doubt, the advent of osseointegration has had a fundamental impact on the therapeutic approach and strategies implemented today in the field of prosthetic rehabilitation of the compromised posterior dentition. The implant statistics of the University of Geneva School of Dental Medicine, for example, reveal that from April 1989 until May 2002 more than 3600 implants of 6-12 mm length have been inserted in about 1400 patients presenting with different types of edentulism (Figs. 41-1, 41-2). This treatment predicament is increasingly applied worldwide and has had a tremendous influence on traditional prosthodontic attitudes (Beumer et al. 1993, Zarb & Schmitt 1995, Tarnow et al. 1997, Zitzmann & Marinello 1999, Belser et al. 2000, Schwarz-Arad & Dolev 2000, Brägger et al. 2001, Deporter et al. 2001, Zitzmann & Marinello 2002). Since nowadays most of the established dental implant systems comprise a wide range of mostly screw-type implants with different diameters and dimensions to replace missing premolars and molars (Fig. 41-3), the versatility of implant therapy in the load carrying part of the dentition of partially edentulous patients has been significantly enhanced.

Numerous other indications have been added to the so-called classical indications for the use of implants, i.e. the severely atrophied edentulous jaws, missing teeth in otherwise intact dentitions (congenitally missing teeth; tooth loss due to trauma or due to a localized endodontic/restorative/periodontal complication or failure) and the distally shortened dental arch (particularly when premolars are missing). Among these other indications one should mention all

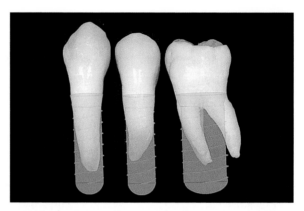

Fig. 41-3. Different implant diameters are available for the replacement of posterior teeth.

the strategies aiming at either reducing the prosthodontic risk in general or rendering the treatment simpler and more cost-effective. Virtually no limits for the placement of implants seem to exist any more owing, for example, to advanced bone augmentation techniques, comprising anterior sinus floor elevation and distraction osteogenesis (Buser et al. 1993, 1995, 1996, 1998a, Chiapasco et al. 1999, Buser & von Arx 2000, Chiapasco et al. 2001a, Simion et al. 2001, von Arx et al. 2001a,b, Buser et al. 2002).

When it comes to the technique of placing implants in the posterior segments of the jaws, a one-step non-submerged surgical protocol can be associated with notable advantages. On the one hand, healing of the peri-implant soft tissues occurs simultaneously with osseointegration, and on the other hand the location of the junction between the implant shoulder and the secondary components is normally positioned close to the mucosal surface. It is ultimately the position of this junction which determines the apical migration of the peri-implant epithelium and the crestal bone level, once the so-called biologic width has been established (Abrahamson et al. 1997, Hermann et al. 1997, Lindhe & Berglundh 1998, Hermann et al. 2000, 2001a,b, Engquist et al. 2002, Wyatt & Zarb 2002). Positioning of the transition between implant shoulder and secondary components at the level of the mucosa rather than at the crestal bone also represents a biomechani-

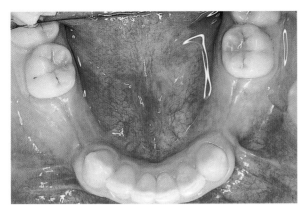

Fig. 41-4. Occlusal view of the mandible of a 22-year-old male patient. All premolars are congenitally missing, the remainder of the dentition is intact.

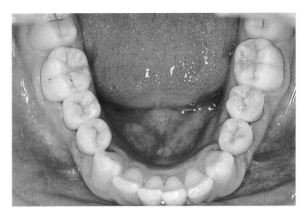

Fig. 41-5. Final view after insertion of four implants, restored with cemented metal-ceramic suprastructures.

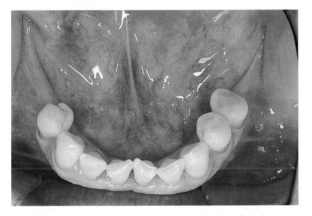

Fig. 41-6. Bilaterally distally shortened dental arch in the mandible of a 66-year-old female patient.

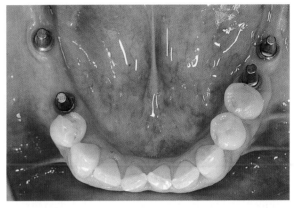

Fig. 41-7. Four implants have been inserted to lengthen the arch bilaterally to the region of the first molars.

cal advantage, as it contributes to the reduction of the lever effect and resulting bending moments acting on the junction between implant and suprastructure. This is clinically relevant, as one should be aware of the existence of an increasing body of evidence reporting technical complications, such as loosening/fracture of screws or fracture of components/veneers, related to implant-supported prosthetic suprastructures (Lundgren & Laurell 1994, Wie 1995, Hebel & Gajjar 1997, Rangert et al. 1997, Bosse & Taylor 1998, Glantz & Nilner 1998, Taylor 1998, Brägger 1999, Goodacre et al. 1999, Isidor 1999, Keith 1999, Schwarz 2000, Johnson & Persson 2001). Besides mechanical type of complications, a number of other conditions that are rather biological in nature, like for example peri-implantitis, are reported in the recent literature (Ellegaard et al. 1997a,b, Ellen 1998, Lang et al. 2000, Brägger et al. 2001, Quirynen et al. 2001, 2002). As these are addressed in detail in another chapter, we will only focus on aspects related to fixed posterior implant restoration design and maintenance.

It is the aim of this chapter to present clinically oriented guidelines and procedures for implant therapy of various types of edentulism located in the load carrying part of the dentition, addressing primarily the partially dentate patient and mainly focusing on fixed implant-supported prostheses.

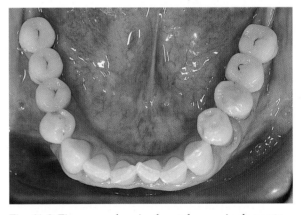

Fig. 41-8. Five premolar-sized metal-ceramic elements were used to restore the four implants.

Indications for implant restorations in the load carrying part of the dentition

When it comes to partial edentulism in the posterior segments of the jaws, implants are increasingly used to either preserve sound mineralized tooth structure or to avoid removable partial dentures (RPDs) and high-risk conventional fixed partial dentures (FPDs). This includes situations with missing teeth in otherwise intact dentitions (Figs. 41-4, 41-5), the distally shortened dental arch (Figs. 41-6 to 41-8), extended

Table 41-1. Indications for posterior implants

- Replacement of missing teeth in intact dentitions (e.g. congenitally missing premolars), i.e. preservation of tooth structure
- Avoidance of removable partial dentures (RPDs)
- Increase of the number of abutments:
  - reduction of the prosthetic risk
  - application of the principle of segmenting
  - ease of eventual reinterventions
- Maintenance of pre-existing crowns and FPDs
- Following prosthetic complications and failures

Table 41.2. Impact of dental implants related to the treatment of posterior partial edentulism

- Favorable overall long-term results
- Preservation of mineralized tooth structure
- "Mechanical" advantages:
  - commercially pure (c.p.) titanium (biocompatibility, mechanical properties, no risk for caries)
  - reproducible, prefabricated ("machined") primary, secondary and tertiary components and auxiliary parts
- Simplified clinical and laboratory protocols

Table 41.3. "High risk" conventional fixed partial dentures (FPDs)

- Long-span fixed partial bridges
- Cantilever units (mainly distal extensions)
- Missing "strategic" tooth abutments
- Structurally/periodontally/endodontically compromised tooth abutments
- Reduced inter-arch distance
- Presence of occlusal parafunctions/bruxism

edentulous segments, missing "strategic" tooth abutments and structurally, endodontically or periodontally compromised potential abutment teeth (Table 41-1).

The rapid advance in terms of the broad utilization of dental implants is not exclusively based on the associated favorable long-term reports for this treatment modality. Other parameters such as purely "mechanical" advantages and the availability of prefabricated components and auxiliary parts, which in turn contribute notably to the simplification of the treatment, had a significant impact on current concepts and strategies as well (Table 41-2). Furthermore, clinical decision making based on prosthetically oriented risk assessment (Table 41-3), frequently leads to the need for an increased number of abutments. The objective is to reduce the overall risk associated with a given prosthetic solution on the one hand, and to implement the principle of segmenting on the other.

A representative clinical example is given in Figs. 41-9 and 41-10. Instead of a conventional five-unit FPD, replacing the missing maxillary left first and second premolars as well as the absent first molar, three implants have been inserted. This approach allowed the avoidance of a long span bridge, a full coverage preparation of the second molar and an associated surgical crown lengthening procedure. The additional cost related to the three implants was justified by an overall reduced prosthodontic risk. The question about adequate number, size and distribution of implants will be addressed later in this chapter. Prosthetically oriented risk assessment comprises the comprehensive evaluation of potential natural abutment teeth, including their structural, restorative, periodontal and endodontic status. As often several well-documented treatment modalities are possible to replace missing posterior teeth, this objective evaluation is of primary importance and represents an ever increasing challenge to the clinician. This is illustrated by a maxillary posterior segment where both the first premolar and the first molar were missing (Figs 41-11 to 41-14). The insertion of a five-unit tooth-borne FPD was discarded because of its too invasive nature related to the intact canine, and owing to a slightly questionable status of the endodontically treated second premolar in view of its eventual use as so-called "peer-abutment". Finally, an implant has been placed at the site of the missing first premolar and subsequently restored with a single-unit restoration. As the proximity of the maxillary sinus at the location of the missing first molar would have required a grafting procedure to make an implant installation possible, a three-unit tooth supported FPD was – after having duly discussed the respective advantages and shortcomings with the patient – ultimately chosen. Having attributed to the moderately compromised second premolar a "strategic value" by using it as abutment of a short span bridge, there was still a difficulty in consistently establishing clinical treatment plans that were fully based on scientific evidence.

Still under the influence of the high level of predictability and longevity reported for implant therapy, the clinician is currently not only pondering implant-borne restorations versus conventional FPDs, but increasingly implant versus maintaining a compromised tooth (Figs. 41-15, 41-16). In this particular clinical case, the evaluation focused on whether or not it was objectively opportune to restore the structurally compromised root of a maxillary second premolar. This would have required – after elimination of the decayed dentin – a surgical crown lengthening procedure to create access to the margin, which in turn would have included the risk for an adverse effect (furcation proximity of the adjacent first molar) on the neighboring teeth. Furthermore, a three-unit FPD was out of the question for obvious reasons. Based on this rationale and in the context of a more comprehensive analysis of the situation, it was finally decided to extract a *per se* treatable root and to replace it by an

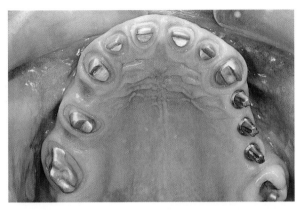

Fig. 41-9. Maxillary occlusal view displaying natural and implant abutments prior to the insertion of an extended porcelain-fused-to-metal restoration. In order to avoid a high-risk long-span FPD, three implants have been added in the left posterior segment.

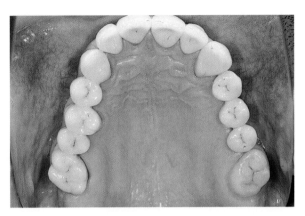

Fig. 41-10. A similar restorative design has been chosen for both natural and implant-supported metal-ceramic suprastructures.

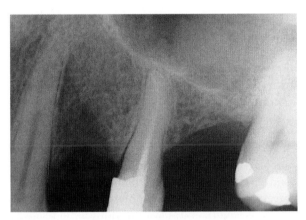

Fig. 41-11. Preoperative radiograph of the left maxilla, revealing two missing dental elements. One should note in particular an intact canine, a structurally reduced second premolar and an extended recessus of the sinus in the area of the missing first molar.

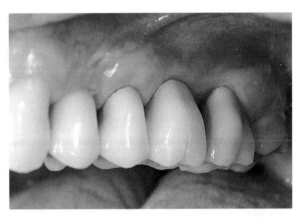

Fig. 41-12. Vestibular view of the prosthetic rehabilitation of the maxillary left quadrant: an implant-supported single-tooth restoration on the site of the first premolar, and a three-unit tooth-borne FPD to replace the missing first molar.

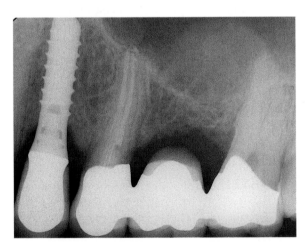

Fig. 41-13. The postoperative radiograph documents that an endodontic revision has been performed on the second premolar prior to its restoration with an adhesive carbon-fibre-post based build-up and a metal-ceramic crown (bridge retainer).

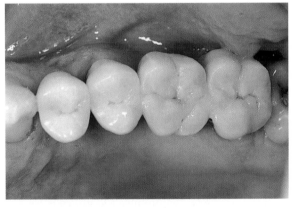

Fig. 41-14. An identical prosthetic design has been applied for both the implant-supported and the tooth-supported restoration.

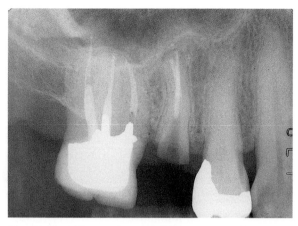

Fig. 41-15. Ad hoc radiograph of the upper right posterior sextant. One notes the presence of a structurally compromised second premolar. The treatment of that particular root would require build-up and crown-lengthening (margin exposure, creation of an adequate ferrule) which in turn would negatively affect the adjacent teeth.

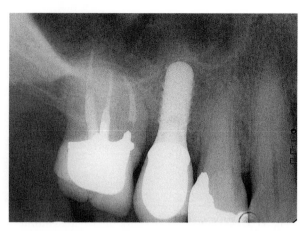

Fig. 41-16. The postoperative radiograph documents that the root of the second premolar has been replaced by a single-tooth implant restoration. In particular, the pre-existing metal-ceramic crown on the first molar could be maintained by this approach.

Table 41.4. Controversial issues related to posterior implant restorations

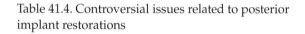

- Adequate number, size (length/diameter), configuration and distribution of implants
- Cemented versus screw-retained (transocclusal/transverse screw-retention)
- Single units versus splinted adjacent implant restorations
- Longest possible versus shorter implants
- Impact of implant axis
- Optimal implant shoulder sink depth
- Minimal ratio between implant length and suprastructure height
- Combination of natural teeth and implants in the same restoration
- Design of the optimal abutment-to-implant connection
- Implant-specific occlusal concepts, including occluding restorative materials, non-axial loading, type of guidance during mandibular excursions
- Healing times prior to functional loading (immediate/early/delayed)
- Significance of offset/staggered implant positioning

tulous patient is an overall highly predictable treatment modality, several conceptional issues remain controversial to date (Table 41-4). These controversial issues include open questions addressing adequate number, size and distribution of implants for optimal therapy of a given type and configuration of partial edentulism, as well as parameters related to occlusion and occlusal materials, to implant axis, to the minimal acceptable ratio between suprastructure height and implant length, and – last but not least – related to questions focusing more specifically on the mechanical aspects and requirements of posterior implant prosthodontics. Among these, the kind of connection between implant and abutment have to be mentioned in particular. Most of these questions will be discussed in the remainder of this chapter, at length where possible and appropriate, or more superficially when solid information is missing or when the topic is more adequately covered by other authors in this book.

RESTORATION OF THE DISTALLY SHORTENED ARCH WITH FIXED IMPLANT-SUPPORTED PROSTHESES

As pointed out earlier in this chapter, from 1989 to 2002 the distally shortened arch represented the most frequent indication for the use of implants at the University of Geneva School of Dental Medicine. In fact, out of a total of 3638 implants, almost 1500 were placed in distally shortened arches, with close to 1000 implants inserted in the mandible and about 500 in the posterior maxilla (Fig. 41-1). Implants were primarily used when premolars were also missing. Whenever possible, the adopted treatment strategy consisted of

implant. One should never forget, however, that this trend to consider, under certain circumstances, an implant as a better solution than treating "acrobatically" a severely compromised tooth, calls for well defined evidence-based respective criteria and represents a non-negligible ethical responsibility for the clinician.

Controversial issues

Despite the ever-growing body of scientific evidence indicating that implant therapy in the partially eden-

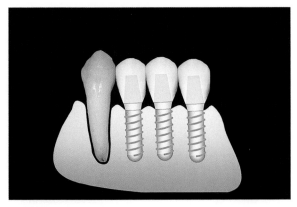

Fig. 41-17. Schematic representation of the distally shortened dental arch. One therapeutic option consists of replacing each missing occlusal unit up to the first molar area with an implant.

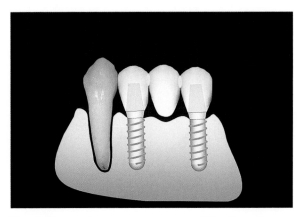

Fig. 41-18. An alternative option would be the replacement of the three missing occlusal units by two implants to support a three-unit suprastructure with a central pontic.

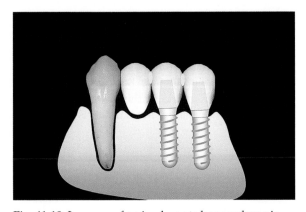

Fig. 41-19. In a case of an inadequate bone volume in the area of the missing first premolar, the placement of two distal implants may be considered, leading to a three-unit suprastructure with a mesial cantilever.

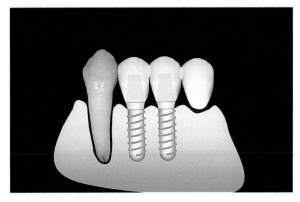

Fig. 41-20. In a case of an inadequate bone volume in the area of the missing first molar, the placement of two mesial implants may be considered, leading to a three-unit suprastructure with a distal cantilever.

restoring the shortened dental arch to the region of the first molars. Occasionally, implant therapy was restricted to the premolar area, according to the principles of the well-established premolar occlusion concept, or extended to the second molar area if an antagonistic contact had to be established for an opposing natural second molar.

Number, size and distribution of implants

Although it is still unclear to date how many implants of which dimension at which localization are required to optimally rehabilitate a given edentulous segment in the load carrying part of the dentition, a number of different respective recommendations and related strategies are currently in use, mostly derived from traditional prosthodontic experience and attitudes, and based on so-called clinical experience and common sense rather than on solid scientific evidence. In defense of the situation one should be aware, however, that it is often difficult to design and carry out randomized clinical trials evaluating exclusively and

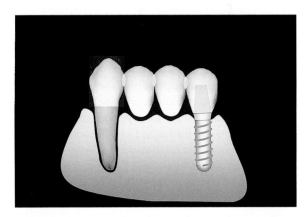

Fig. 41-21. In a case of inadequate bone volume in the area of the two missing premolars, the placement of a distal implant may be considered, leading to a four-unit suprastructure with a mixed (tooth and implant) support.

without interference one specific parameter of conceptual relevance.

In a situation where the canine is the most distal remaining tooth of a dental arch, at least five different options can be taken into consideration if one plans to

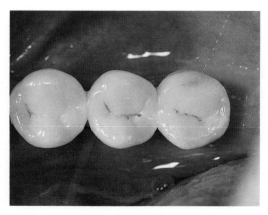
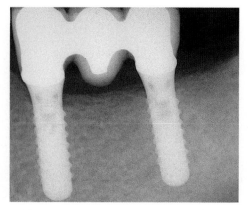

Fig. 41-22. (a) Occlusal view of a cemented three-unit metal-ceramic FPD, supported by a mesial and a distal implant. (b) The corresponding 3-year follow-up radiograph confirms stable conditions at the implant to bone interface of the two 12 mm solid screw implants.

replace the missing teeth up to the first molar area (Figs. 41-17 to 41-21). These include the replacement of each missing occlusal unit by one implant (Fig. 41-17), a mesial and a distal implant to support a three-unit FPD with a central pontic (Fig. 41-18), two distal implants to permit the insertion of a three-unit FPD with a mesial cantilever (Fig. 41-19), two mesial implants to sustain a three-unit FPD with a distal cantilever (Fig. 41-20) and, finally, only one distally inserted implant in view of a four-unit FPD combining implant and natural tooth support (Fig. 41-21).

As far as the recommendation to use premolar-sized units for implant-borne posterior FPDs is concerned, it has proven its practical validity in more than ten years of clinical experience (Buser et al. 1997, Bernard & Belser 2002). In fact, a crown featuring a mesio-distal diameter of 7-8 mm at its occlusal surface allows the optimal generation of a harmonious axial profile, gradually emerging from the standard implant shoulder (Ø 4-5 mm on average) to the maximum circumference. In addition, the width of the occlusal table is confined, limiting thereby the risk for unfavorable bending moments to the implant-abutment-suprastructure complex (Belser et al. 2000).

Based on an increasing body of scientific evidence, most clinicians' first choice represents the mesial and distal implant and the respective FPD with the central pontic (Figs. 41-22a,b). Prospective long-term multicenter data (Buser et al. 1997, Bernard & Belser 2002) have confirmed the efficacy and predictability of this specific modality. In fact, it permits the defined treatment objective with a minimal number of implants and associated costs. Although presently still lacking formal evidence at the level of prospectively documented, randomized clinical trials, it appears from clinical experience that the use of two implants to support a four-unit FPD with two central pontics (Figs. 41-23, 41-24) may be adequate in certain clinical situations. Clinicians tend to use this approach in the presence of favorable bone conditions, permitting standard-size or wide-diameter implants with appropriate length (i.e. 8 mm or more).

If the alveolar bone crest dimension is also suffi-cient in an oro-facial direction, the utilization of wide-diameter/wide-platform implants is preferred. Due to their increased dimensions a more adapted suprastructure volume and improved axial emergence profile of the implant restoration – when compared to a so-called premolar unit – can be achieved in the molar area (Figs. 41-25, 41-28). By this token the intercuspation with an opposing natural molar is facilitated as well.

Implant restorations with cantilever units

There is strong evidence in the relevant dental literature that cantilever units – in particular distal extensions – of conventional tooth-borne FPDs are associated with a significantly higher complication rate when compared to FPDs featuring a mesial and a distal abutment and a central pontic. Respective failure rates could be attributed to decisive factors such as non-vital abutment teeth as well as specific occlusal conditions such as a reduced interarch distance and/or occlusal parafunctions (Glantz & Nilner 1998). These authors concluded in their review of the current relevant literature that risks were lower for mechanical failures with cantilevered implant-borne reconstructions than with comparable conventional fixed situations. The risks, however, do exist. As loss of retention, which was one of the frequent complications encountered on conventional cantilevered prostheses, can easily be prevented when it comes to implant-supported restorations of this type, the latter seem to be a viable alternative in cases where the local alveolar bone crest conditions do not allow the insertion of an implant at the most favorable location. In such situations the clinician has to ponder whether a bone augmentation procedure can be objectively justified or if the risk for complications of a more simple, straightforward approach can be considered low.

The 6-year clinical and radiographic follow-up of a three-unit FPD featuring a mesial cantilever is presented in Figs. 41-29 and 41-30.

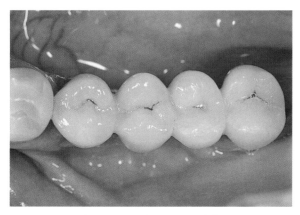

Fig. 41-23. Occlusal view of a cemented four-unit metal-ceramic FPD supported by a mesial and a distal implant.

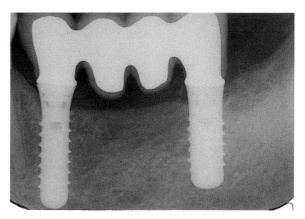

Fig. 41-24. The related 2-year follow-up radiograph documents that at the distal site a 10 mm solid screw implant with an increased diameter ("wide body implant") has been used.

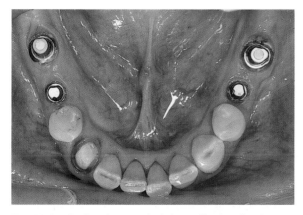

Fig. 41-25. Occlusal view of a bilaterally distally shortened mandibular arch. Two implants have been placed on either side to restore the arch to the area of the first molars. The two distal implants feature an increased diameter, better suited for the replacement of a missing molar.

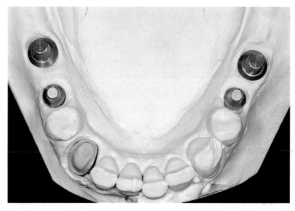

Fig. 41-26. The master model comprises color-coded aluminum laboratory analogues at the implant sites, facilitating the technician's work in view of the suprastructure fabrication. This is in contrast to the site of the prepared natural abutment.

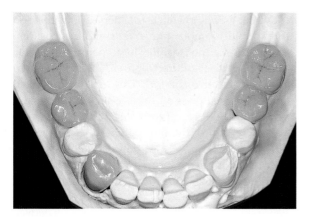

Fig. 41-27. Once the metal-ceramic restorations are completed, no noticeable design difference between implant-supported and tooth-supported suprastructures is apparent.

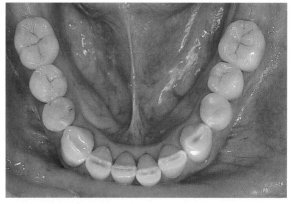

Fig. 41-28. The respective clinical view confirms an acceptable integration of the four implant restorations in the existing natural dentition.

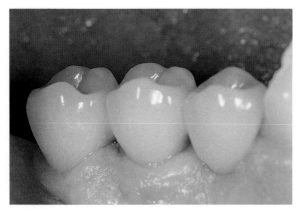

Fig. 41-29. Six-year clinical follow-up view of a mandibular three-unit FPD supported by two distal implants.

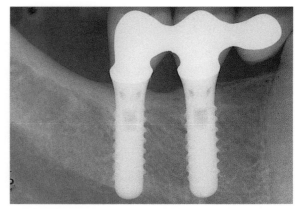

Fig. 41-30. The 6-year radiograph displays stable bony conditions around the two implants supporting a cemented suprastructure with a premolar-sized mesial cantilever unit.

Combination of implant and natural tooth support

There is general agreement that, from a purely scientific point of view, the combination of implants and natural teeth to support a common FPD is feasible. Clinical studies reporting prospectively documented long-term data did not show adverse effects of splinting teeth to implants (Olsson et al. 1995, Gunne et al. 1997, 1999, Hosny et al. 2000, Lindh et al. 2001, Naert et al. 2001a,b, Tangerud et al. 2002). The issue of connecting implants and teeth by means of rigid or nonrigid connectors, however, remains controversial to date, but intrusion of natural roots has been reported in the literature as a potential hazard of non-rigid connection (Sheets & Earthman 1993). Most of the recently published respective literature reviews conclude with the general clinical recommendation that one should avoid, whenever possible, the direct combination of implants and teeth as it may frequently lead to a more complicated type of prosthesis. If there is no viable alternative available, a rigid type of connection is preferred to prevent an eventual intrusion of the involved abutment teeth (Lundgren & Laurell 1994, Gross & Laufer 1997).

Furthermore, it has been demonstrated that despite the fundamental difference between an osseointegrated implant and a tooth surrounded by a periodontal ligament, the assumption that when these two structures are combined, the entire occlusal load will ultimately go to the implant and hence create an unfavorable "cantilever-type" situation, is not valid from a scientific point of view (Richter, Isidor, Brägger). In fact, under normal function, such as during mastication, the tooth abutment is similarly load-bearing. This may change, however, during severe occlusal parafunctions, like nocturnal bruxism.

Sites with extended horizontal bone volume deficiencies and/or anterior sinus floor proximity

It is not infrequent that distally shortened dental arches do not feature an adequate local bone volume at the prospective implant sites. This may refer to bone height, bone width, alveolar bone crest axis or to the vicinity of noble structures such as the mandibular alveolar nerve canal or the anterior part of the maxillary sinus. Often a combination of several of the mentioned limitations is encountered. As implant insertion is clearly a three-dimensional surgical and restorative procedure on the one hand, and as "restoration-driven" rather than "bone-driven" implant placement is widely recommended on the other hand, a meticulous presurgical site analysis – based on the envisioned treatment objective – is of primary importance. In order to keep the treatment as easy and finally also as cost-effective as possible, one should comprehensively evaluate whether a minor deviation from the ideal implant position could be considered acceptable, i.e. not leading to a compromise which might adversely affect predictability, longevity and/or subjective comfort. This approach may still permit in some cases a professionally defendable result, but without a complexity of treatment that would be difficult to bear by some patients.

Advanced invasive procedures like lateral bone augmentation, anterior sinus floor elevation, alveolar ridge splitting or distraction osteogenesis, require a high level of skills and respective experience and hence should only be deployed if the relation between benefit and risk/cost is soundly balanced (Buser et al. 1993, 1995, 1996, 1999, 2002, Chiapasco et al. 1999, 2001a, Simion et al. 2001, von Arx et al. 2001a,b, Zitzmann et al. 2001).

In this specific context, a complex implant treatment of a 67-year-old male patient whose most distal remaining tooth in the left maxilla was an endodontically treated canine, is shown in Figs. 41-31 to 41-44. Preoperative diagnosis revealed the necessity to perform – according to a staged approach – first a combined lateral bone augmentation procedure and anterior sinus floor elevation and, after a six months' healing period, the insertion of implants. For the sinus floor elevation the so-called "trap-door" technique was used and the created space grafted with autogenous bone chips and BioOss®. The lateral bone augmentation comprised the fixation of a large block graft in the area of the first premolar. After application of an ePTFE barrier membrane, primary wound closure was achieved by sectioning of the periosteum of the respective muco-periosteal flap. This often leads to a lack of attached keratinized mucosa on the vestibular aspect of the surgical site, which has to be subsequently corrected, most conveniently at the moment of implant placement. When it comes to sites that have been previously grafted, the majority of surgeons advocate inserting one implant per missing occlusal unit. This attitude appears to be based more on the reflection that the overall heaviness of the approach would largely justify this additional security and/or on the hypothesis that augmented bone may not have exactly the same "load-bearing" capacity as the pre-existing bone, than on irrefutable scientific evidence. Accordingly, three adjacent screw-type implants – the most distal one an increased-diameter titanium screw – had been placed and subsequently restored by a three-unit splinted metal-ceramic FPD (Figs. 41-38 to 41-44).

Results from a recently published longitudinal clinical study (Buser et al. 2002) on 40 consecutively

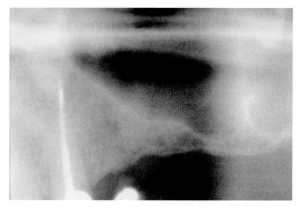

Fig. 41-31. Initial radiograph of the maxillary left posterior segment of a 67-year-old male patient. The canine represents the most distal remaining tooth element. Note the marked extension of the anterior recessus of the sinus.

enrolled patients, who were first treated with a lateral bone augmentation procedure and subsequently, in a second stage, received implants inserted in the previously augmented area. In the totality of treated sites implants could finally be placed as planned, and at the 5-year clinical and radiographic follow-up examination a 97% success rate was revealed. It was thus concluded that lateral bone augmentation is indeed a predictable procedure and that implants subsequently inserted in augmented sites do have similar success rates to implants placed in comparable non-augmented sites.

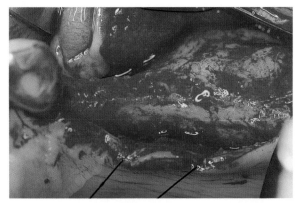

Fig. 41-32. After elevation of a mucoperiosteal flap, an insufficient horizontal bone volume in the region of the premolars becomes apparent.

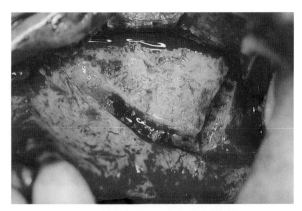

Fig. 41-33. In view of an anterior sinus floor elevation procedure, the first step for a respective osteotomy is performed. Attention is given not to perforate the Schneiderian membrane.

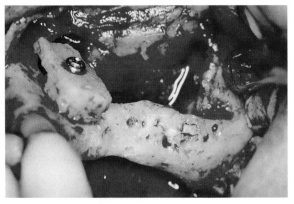

Fig. 41-34. After the so-called "hinge-door" procedure in the region of the maxillary sinus, an autogenous bone block graft, harvested from the patient's retromolar area, is positioned and then immobilized by a fixation screw at the location of the missing first premolar.

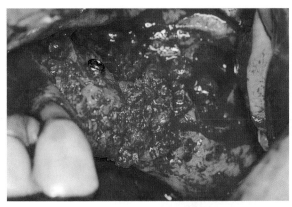

Fig. 41-35. The lateral bone augmentation procedure is completed by adding a combination of autogenous bone chips, bone slurry and BioOss®.

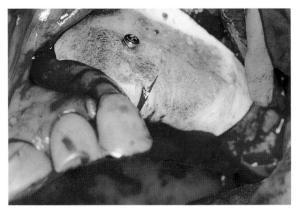

Fig. 41-36. Prior to flap repositioning and suturing, a barrier membrane is applied.

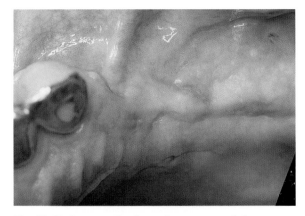

Fig. 41-37. One month after primary wound closure and uneventful healing, the involved soft tissues have recovered their normal appearance.

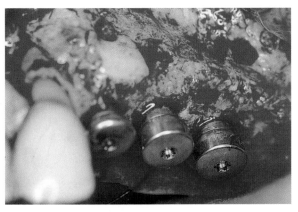

Fig. 41-38. Eight months following the combined anterior sinus floor elevation and lateral bone augmentation procedure, the site is reopened and three implants are inserted.

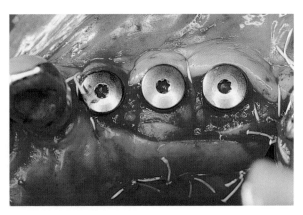

Fig. 41-39. In order to increase the amount of keratinized mucosa on the vestibular aspect of the implants, the flap is repositioned accordingly. The resulting deficiency on the palatal aspect is compensated for by means of a connective tissue being part of the partial thickness flap.

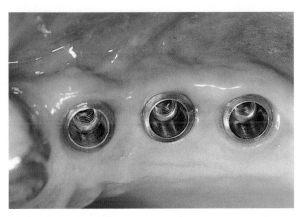

Fig. 41-40. Three months after implant placement, favorable peri-implant soft tissue conditions have been re-established.

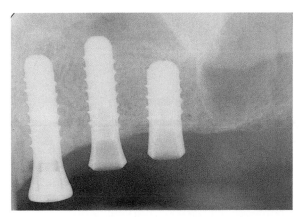

Fig. 41-41. The corresponding radiograph confirms successful osseointegration of the three implants that are mostly located in augmented bone.

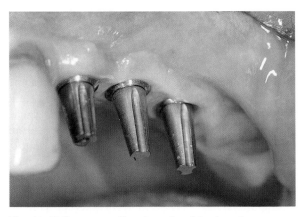

Fig. 41-42. In a case of implant shoulder location compatible with cementation, respective solid abutments are selected and tightened to 35 Ncm with a calibrated torque wrench.

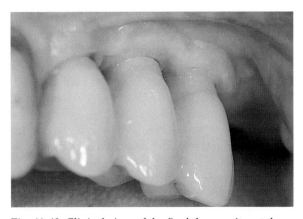

Fig. 41-43. Clinical view of the final three-unit metal-ceramic implant suprastructure, featuring a flat and continuous emergence profile and adequate access for interimplant oral hygiene.

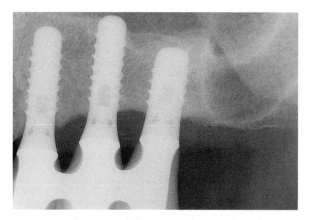

Fig. 41-44. The 4-year follow-up radiograph confirms stable conditions at the osseointegrated interface.

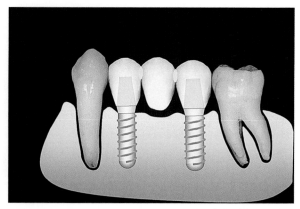

Fig. 41-45. Schematic representation of a tooth-bound posterior edentulous segment, restored by two implants and a three-unit FPD with a central pontic.

MULTIPLE-UNIT TOOTH-BOUND POSTERIOR IMPLANT RESTORATIONS

Number, size and distribution of implants

When it comes to implant therapy in extended posterior edentulous segments confined mesially and distally by remaining teeth, the question about optimal number, size and distribution of implants has to be raised again. Among the key parameters to be addressed during the decision-making process are the mesio-distal dimension of the edentulous segment, the precise alveolar bone crest volume (including bone height and crest width in an oro-facial direction), the opposing dentition (premolars or molars), interarch distance and specific occlusal parameters, as well as the periodontal, endodontic and structural conditions of the neighboring teeth.

One feasible approach consists of segmenting the edentulous space in premolar-size units of approximately 7 mm of mesio-distal diameter at the level of the occlusal plane, and of approximately 5 mm at the prospective implant shoulder. As on posterior locations clinicians increasingly prefer a rather superficial implant shoulder location or in many instances even a supramucosal one, the respective measurements can be carried out at the crest level of study casts. It is important during this process to anticipate a minimal distance between implant shoulders of approximately 2 mm, and between a natural tooth and an implant of about 1.5 mm (to be measured at the interproximal soft tissue level). Again, the treatment objective, i.e. a long-lasting implant-supported FPD, should be predictably reached on the one hand with optimal efficacy and on the other hand with a minimum of invasiveness and cost. The still existing controversy of whether each missing occlusal unit should be replaced by one implant or whether a minimal number of implants should be used, has already been addressed earlier in this chapter.

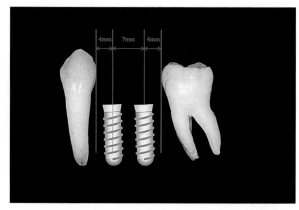

Fig. 41-46. If a given tooth-bound edentulous space only permits the insertion of two adjacent implants, a minimal interimplant distance of 2 mm and a minimal implant-to-tooth distance of 1.5 mm (at the interproximal soft tissue level) should be respected.

In the case of three missing occlusal units and in the absence of other particular restrictive conditions such as limited local bone volume, the authors recommend the insertion of a mesial and a distal implant to support a three-unit FPD with a central pontic (Fig. 41-45). This approach permits the fabrication of three metal-ceramic elements featuring a mesio-distal diameter of about 7 mm each. Based on an average implant shoulder dimension of approximately 5 mm, one can anticipate a gradually increasing, harmonious emergence profile from the implant shoulder to the occlusal surface. In order to satisfy the remaining important dimensional conditions, i.e. respecting the minimal distance between adjacent implants and in between teeth and implants, one needs to dispose of a minimal total mesio-distal gap distance of 21-22 mm (Fig. 41-47).

In the case of two missing occlusal units, one should try as a general rule to select the largest possible implant diameters with respect to the total mesio-distal distance of the given tooth-bound edentulous segment. Decisive parameters are again interimplant distance and space between implants and adjacent teeth, as well as oro-facial crest width at the two prospective implant sites. For a total gap diameter of about 14-15

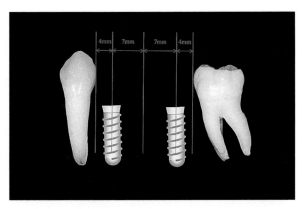

Fig. 41-47. In the case of three missing occlusal units, an implant-supported FPD with a central pontic (approximately 7 mm in width) may be considered as a viable solution.

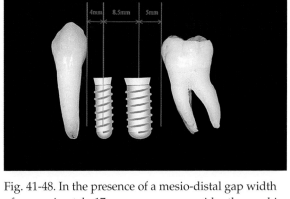

Fig. 41-48. In the presence of a mesio-distal gap width of approximately 17 mm, one may consider the combination of a standard and an increased-diameter ("wide neck") implant. The same minimal interimplant and implant-to-tooth distances have to be respected.

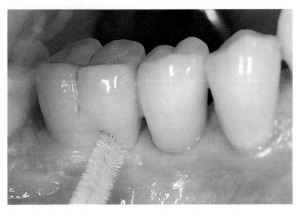

Fig. 41-49. Vestibular aspect of a metal-ceramic restoration supported by two screw-type implants. Due to an excess of mesio-distal space, the implants have been separated by approximately 4 mm. Instead of a traditional pontic, a root imitation has been performed close to the distal implant, providing an adequate guide for an interdental brush in view of an efficient plaque control at the marginal area of the implant restoration.

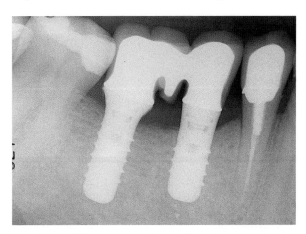

Fig. 41-50. With respect to cleansibility, the respective prosthesis design is clearly visible on the postoperative radiograph.

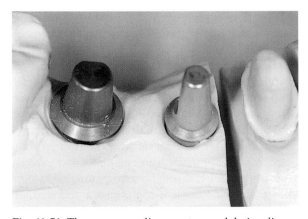

Fig. 41-51. The corresponding master model visualizes the different dimensions and distances involved in this individual case.

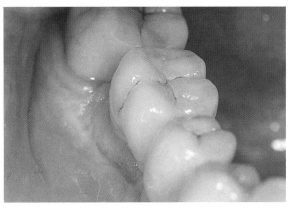

Fig. 41-52. On an oblique view the vestibular axial profile of the implant restoration becomes visible. Soft tissue (cheek and tongue) support and harmony with adjacent teeth are of paramount importance.

mm, two standard-size implants are most suitable (Fig. 41-46), while for one of 17 to 18 mm the combi- nation of one standard and one wide-diameter/wide-platform implant is considered adequate (Fig. 41-48).

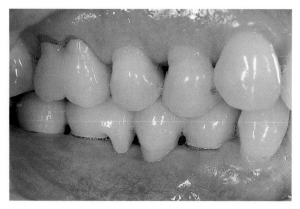

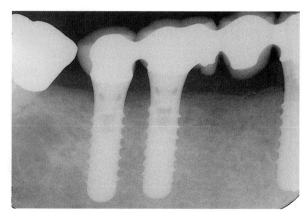

Fig. 41-53. Buccal view of an extended edentulous right mandibular tooth-bound gap treated with an implant restoration. In the pontic area a design favoring the efficacy of an interdental brush close to the implant margins has been applied.

Fig. 41-54. The related radiograph illustrates the chosen design in the pontic area in terms of access to and efficacy of interproximal plaque control.

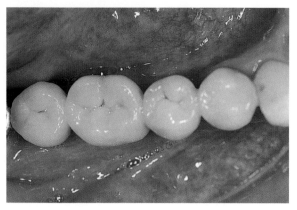

Fig. 41-55. Occlusal view of the completed 4-unit implant-borne fixed porcelain-fused-to-metal prosthesis.

Table 41.5. Splinting of multiple adjacent posterior implants

Parameters to consider:

- access for oral hygiene
- marginal adaptation/"passive fit"
- technical simplicity/ease of eventual reinterventions
- "overload" of the osseointegrated interface
- "rotational forces" on implant components
- screw-loosening/fatigue fractures

It goes without saying that the latter choice requires also the respective oro-facial bone volume.

These are just frequently encountered clinical examples, but in the function of other morphology and dimensions of edentulous tooth-bound segments, additional approaches and implant combinations may be envisioned. Two such particular clinical situations are presented in Figs. 41-49 to 41-52 and Figs. 41-53 to 41-55. In the first case, the gap diameter required the two adjacent implants to be spaced wider than the

normally advocated interproximal 2 mm. The laboratory technician compensated for this excess of space with a root-imitation pontic which in turn provided an excellent guide facilitating the use of an interdental brush (Fig. 41-49). In the second case, only the placement of three standard-size implants was possible due to a restricted bone volume in oro-facial direction. Again, the technician could optimally distribute the different restoration volumes but still comply with basic prerequisites such as a flat axial emergence profile and optimal access for the patient's oral hygiene (Figs. 41-53, 41-54).

Splinted versus single-unit restorations of multiple adjacent posterior implants

Another persisting controversial issue relates to the question whether multiple adjacent implants in the load carrying part of the dentition should support splinted or segmented single-unit restorations (Table 41-5). There still appears to be a confrontation between rather "biological" considerations versus more "mechanical" thinking.

Generally speaking, the biologically oriented considerations, insisting on easy access for oral hygiene and optimal marginal adaptation, represent probably the more scientifically-based point of view. Clinicians advocating splinting of multiple adjacent implants do so primarily for mechanical reasons. They hypothesize that this approach decreases forces and force moments at the level of the suprastructures and the various underlying implant components, and that relatively frequent mechanical complications such as screw-loosening and fractures may be significantly reduced or prevented by this measure. The related literature does not at present provide a clear answer, as randomized long-term clinical trials addressing this particular parameter are still scarce. Some more general reports do exist, however, addressing mainly

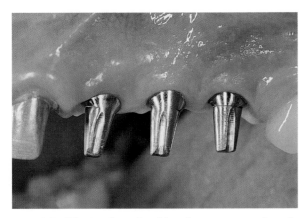

Fig. 41-56. The implant shoulder-abutment complex of the three left maxillary posterior implants has been prepared with fine-grain diamond burrs under abundant water cooling in order to facilitate the configuration of the related suprastructure. Particular emphasis was given to margins following closely the scalloped course of the soft tissue.

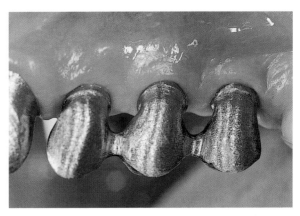

Fig. 41-57. In a case of reduced-diameter implants, splinting of adjacent units may reduce the risk for technical complications. A metal framework try-in prior to the application of the ceramic veneering may help to detect and eliminate an eventual non-passive fit at an early stage.

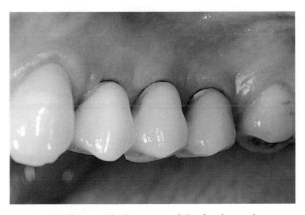

Fig. 41-58. The vestibular view of the final metal-ceramic restoration illustrates the impact on esthetics of a metal margin. This aspect should be discussed with the patient before treatment. In case of a high smile line, one may consider an increased sink depth during implant surgery.

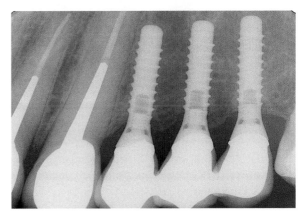

Fig. 41-59. On the 1-year follow-up radiograph an acceptable marginal fidelity can be assessed.

type and frequency of mechanical complications (Goodacre et al. 1999).

Among the frequently forwarded arguments to plead the case of splinting are reduced-diameter (Figs. 41-56 to 41-59) or short (i.e. less than 8 mm) implants, implants inserted in low-density bone, implants placed in augmented or grafted (e.g. after anterior sinus floor elevation) bone, or implant restorations in the posterior segments of patients with verified notable occlusal parafunctions or bruxism. One should be aware, however, that the majority of these arguments are primarily based on clinical opinions and eventually common sense, and that to date they are lacking formal scientific evidence. In fact, there is increased indication, derived from prospective multicenter studies (although not addressing this parameter in particular), that splinting does not appear to be a prerequisite for preventing excessive crestal bone resorption or even loss of osseointegration. Nowadays,

the authors would seriously reconsider their respective choice related to the suprastructure design presented in Figs. 41-60 and 41-61. Definitely, in the presence of standard-size (i.e. addressing both diameter and length) implants, which are placed in normal density original (non-augmented or grafted) bone, single-unit restorations are recommended as they comply better with the various parameters that are important from a more biological point of view, as demonstrated by the clinical example presented in Figs. 41-62 and 41-63.

POSTERIOR SINGLE-TOOTH REPLACEMENT

At the time when most implant systems had basically only one "standard" dimension at disposition, this

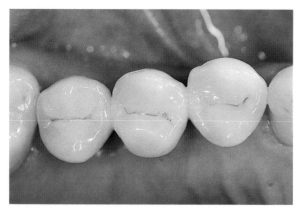

Fig. 41-60. Occlusal view of a right maxillary posterior three-unit implant restoration featuring premolar-sized segments.

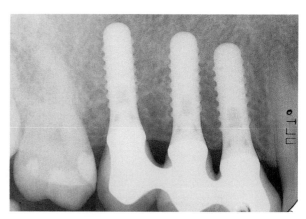

Fig. 41-61. The corresponding follow-up radiograph confirms acceptable peri-implant conditions.

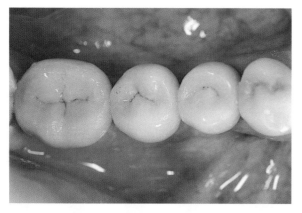

Fig. 41-62. Occlusal view of three independent, implant-supported fixed metal-ceramic restorations in the right posterior mandible.

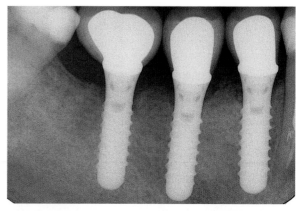

Fig. 41-63. As confirmed by the follow-up radiograph, an increased (more molar-like) dimension has been given to the most distal restoration, despite the fact that a standard-sized implant had to be used for restricted bone volume reasons.

corresponded to approximately 4–5 mm at the implant shoulder and thus was optimally suited for premolar-size restorations, featuring a continuously increasing (towards coronally) flat axial emergence profile and a mesio-distal diameter of about 7–8 mm at the occlusal surface. Clinicians were not infrequently faced with posterior single-tooth sites, however, that did not comply with these dimensions, for example in the case of missing first molars or after the loss of persisting deciduous (primary) second molars. As a consequence, the resulting implant restorations featured either unfavorable excessive interproximal overcontour or wide open embrasures. The first situation was difficult to clean, while the second led to undesired food retention (impaction). Nowadays most of the leading implant manufacturers offer wide-body/wide-platform implants designed for the replacement of multirooted teeth (Fig. 41-3).

Premolar-size single-tooth restorations

When it comes to posterior single-tooth gaps that dimensionally correspond to an average premolar,

standard-size screw-form implants are well suited. The respective implant dimensions which include both the intrabony part and the implant shoulder, offer the additional advantage of being mostly compatible with a limited bone volume in oro-facial direction. Whenever feasible, a straightforward low-maintenance restorative design is advocated, which normally consists of a cementable porcelain-fused-to-metal crown with vestibular and oral axial contours that are in harmony with the adjacent teeth and thus provide adequate guidance for cheek and tongue (Figs. 41-64 to 41-66).

Molar-size single-tooth restorations

If a given posterior single-tooth gap corresponds rather to the mesio-distal dimension of a molar, it is recommended, for the reasons quoted in the previous paragraph, that the insertion of a wide-neck implant is planned (Bahat & Handelsman 1996). This approach, however, also requires the respective bone volume in an oro-facial direction. If this is not the case, the presurgical site analysis, eventually in the form of

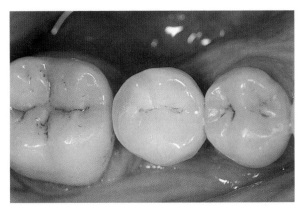

Fig. 41-64. Occlusal view of a single-tooth implant restoration replacing a missing mandibular right second premolar.

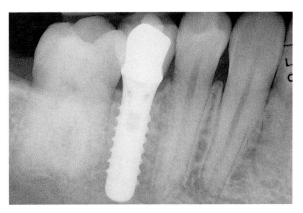

Fig. 41-65. The 5-year radiographic follow-up displays favorable bony conditions around this 12 mm solid screw implant.

a bone-mapping, should identify whether it is possible to have an implant placement in combination with a lateral bone augmentation procedure according to a simultaneous approach. If the local bone anatomy requires a bone augmentation according to a staged protocol, one has to carefully ponder and discuss with the patient if this additional effort, risk and ultimately also cost can be justified by an anticipated implant restoration featuring close-to-ideal axial contours and embrasures.

A clinical example demonstrating the potential of increased-diameter implants for the optimal replacement of a single missing mandibular molar is given in Figs. 41-67 and 41-68.

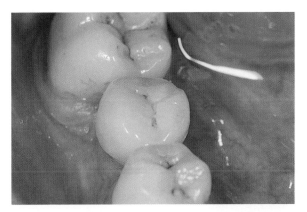

Fig. 41-66. On the oblique view one can notice that an axial contour similar to that present on the adjacent natural teeth has been applied to facilitate oral hygiene and to assure adequate soft tissue (cheek and tongue) guidance and support.

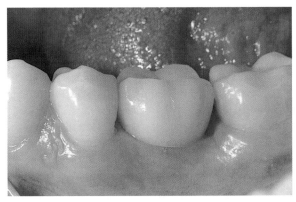

Fig. 41-67. In a case of the replacement of a single missing molar, ideally the use of an implant with corresponding dimensions is recommended to permit a restoration featuring optimal subjective comfort and cleansibility.

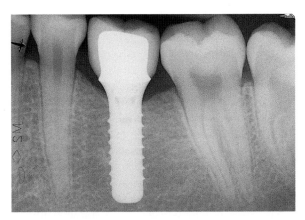

Fig. 41-68. On the 1-year radiographic follow-up a diameter-increased ("wide neck") implant can be noted which is essential for a suprastructure design without extremely open interdental embrasures, which would be prone to food retention and oral parafunctions.

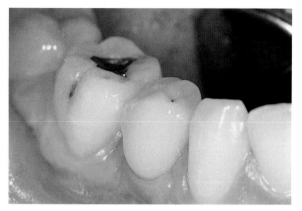

Fig. 41-69. Clinical aspect of a single-tooth implant restoration in the mandibular right premolar area.

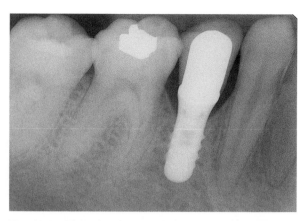

Fig. 41-70. The related 2-year follow-up radiograph shows a so-called unfavorable relationship between the height of the suprastructure and the length of the supporting implant. The placement of a longer implant was not possible due to the limited local bone conditions.

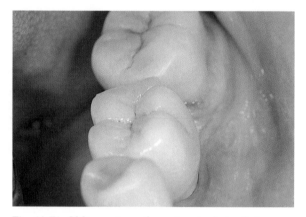

Fig. 41-71. Oblique view of a molar single-tooth implant restoration in the left mandible.

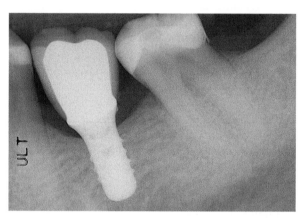

Fig. 41-72. A short diameter-increased screw implant supporting a long molar-sized suprastructure is displayed on the 1-year follow-up radiograph. Note that a normal level of the first bone-to-implant contact has been maintained.

Sites with limited vertical bone volume

Quite frequently the clinician is confronted with posterior single-tooth gaps that present all of the major prerequisites for successful implant therapy listed earlier in this chapter, with the exception of sufficient vertical bone height for the insertion of an implant featuring what is broadly accepted as an adequate length of the implant itself and in relation to the prospective length of the suprastructure. The question that arises is whether there is a minimal implant length required in the context of posterior single-tooth restorations and whether the ratio between implant length and suprastructure length has an influence on crestal bone resorption and ultimately on the longevity of the entire implant-suprastructure complex. The

analysis of the respective implant data collected at the University of Geneva School of Dental Medicine in the frame of a prospective multicenter study from 1989 to 2002, permitted the conclusion that shorter implants (6-8 mm) did not show more average crestal bone resorption than longer implants (10-12 mm), and that a so-called unfavorable ratio between implant length and suprastructure height did not lead to more pronounced crestal bone resorption (Bernard et al. 1995a, Bernard & Belser 2002). This data is corroborated by other recently published reports (ten Bruggenkate et al. 1998, Bischof et al. 2001, Deporter et al. 2001).

Two examples of respective clinical anecdotal-type evidence, one premolar-size and one molar-size single-tooth restoration, are presented in Figs. 41-69 and 41-70 and Figs. 41-71 and 41-72.

Table 41.6. Indications for screw-retained posterior fixed implant restorations

Parameters to consider:

- implant shoulder location incompatible with a cemented suprastructure, i.e. inaccessible for meticulous excess cement removal (> 2 mm submucosally)
- reduced intermaxillary distance (< 5 mm)
- foreseeable need for reintervention at the respective implant site
- extended implant-supported rehabilitations, involving numerous implants
- high overall level of complexity (e.g. non-parallel implants)

CLINICAL APPLICATIONS

Screw-retained implant restorations

For many years there was a strong tendency to design most of the fixed implant restorations as screw-retained suprastructures. Retrievability, and by this maintaining the possibility for modification, extension or eventually repair of the prosthesis, was the main rationale for this strategy. One should be aware, however, that this approach also encompasses notable specific inconveniences: colonization of the inner compartments of the implant-abutment-suprastructure complex with mostly anaerobic microorganisms, risk for loosening or fracture of screws, increased technical complexity and related costs, possible interference with structural parameters (weakening of the metal-ceramic design) and esthetics, as well as a "higher maintenance profile" (Sutter et al. 1993, Wie 1995, Hebel & Gajjar 1997, Keller et al. 1998). As far as the microbial colonization is concerned, it remains unknown to date whether and under which conditions this may have an adverse effect on the longevity of osseointegrated implants.

For these reasons there exists currently a distinct trend towards cementable fixed implant restorations in the load carrying part of the dentition.

The main indications for screw-retention are listed in Table 41-6.

Transocclusal screw-retention
If for one of the aforementioned reasons a transocclusally screw-retained suprastructure is adopted, several parameters should be taken into consideration. First, the screw-access channel should be centred on the occlusal surface in order not to interfere too much with the area to be occupied by the cuspids.

A typical clinical example documenting an indication for a screw-retained posterior single-tooth restoration is given in Figs. 41-73 to 41-75. A reduced interarch distance has led to a deeper than usual implant shoulder location which in turn is neither accessible for well-controlled excess cement removal nor in reach

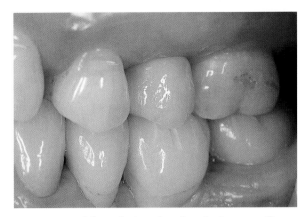

Fig. 41-73. Left lateral view showing the intermaxillary relationship of a young patient in centric occlusion. The missing maxillary second premolar has been replaced by a single-tooth, screw-retained implant restoration. Screw-retention was chosen for two reasons: limited interocclusal distance and implant shoulder location incompatible with cementation.

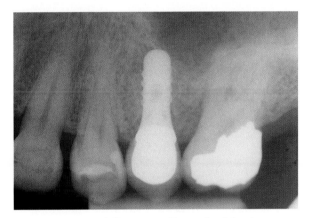

Fig. 41-74. 1-year follow-up radiograph of the described 8 mm solid screw implant.

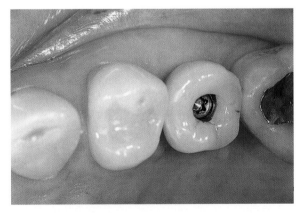

Fig. 41-75. Ideally, the screw-access channel should be located in the center of the occlusal surface. This reduces both the risk for interference with an appropriate metal-ceramic design in general, and the risk for porcelain fractures in particular.

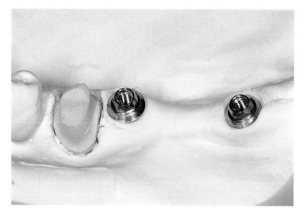

Fig. 41-76. Occlusal view of a mandibular master model comprising two posterior implant analogues and a prepared natural second premolar abutment. Note the proximity of the mesial implant and the second premolar on the one hand, and the distinct lingual position of the two implants on the other.

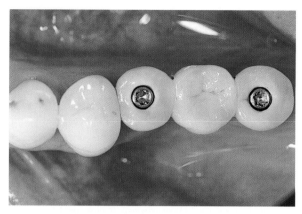

Fig. 41-77. The clinical view of the completed transocclusally screw-retained three-unit implant-supported FPD demonstrates that the lingual implant position did not allow for a suprastructure that is in line with the adjacent teeth. Furthermore, the screws are reaching the occlusal surface, leaving no space for an esthetic coverage with composite resin.

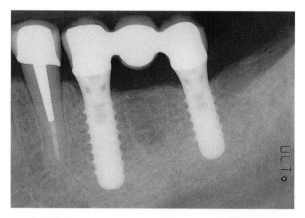

Fig. 41-78. The related 3-year follow-up radiograph documents an only minimal distance between implant shoulder and occlusal surface. Under such conditions, a slight reduction of the alveolar ridge prior to implant placement would have provided more vertical leeway for compensating the lingual implant position and ultimately for covering the occlusal screw.

for the patient's routine oral hygiene. In order to benefit from their superior surface quality characteristics and marginal precision, prefabricated machined cast-on components have been used for the respective suprastructure fabrication. Ideally, the screw-access channel occupies a restricted area in the centre of the occlusal table, and the distance from the head of the screw to the occlusal surface should be sufficient for a subsequent composite cover-restoration (Fig. 41-75).

Furthermore, the principles of the metal-ceramic technology require a well-defined space for developing an adequate metal support for a uniform thickness of the overlaying stratification of porcelain. Even in a case of a well-centred occlusal perforation, the latter occupies close to half of the mesio-distal and oro-facial diameter of the occlusal table, and thereby significantly weakens the overall mechanical resistance of

the structure. If the screw-access channel is not centered, however, additional problems are created in the sense of both weakening the restoration and interfering with esthetical criteria. Under such circumstances one should consider, for example, the use of angled abutments as currently offered by most of the leading implant systems.

Another key parameter represents the interarch distance, or more specifically, the distance between the implant shoulder and the plane of occlusion. According to our experience this distance should be at least equal to 5 mm. This is minimal and does not permit – for esthetic reasons – the occlusal screw to be subsequently covered with a composite resin restoration. In this context 6-7 mm are clearly more adequate.

A combination of several well-known problems, which are frequently encountered after implant placement in the posterior mandible, are shown in Figs. 41-76 to 41-78. Two implants have been inserted to restore a distally shortened arch with a three-unit FPD. Owing to the local bone anatomy, the implants were placed in a more lingual position than the original teeth (Fig. 41-76). The – for these particular circumstances – too superficial implant shoulder location did not provide sufficient distance to gradually correct the discrepancy between the actual implant shoulder position and the ideal occlusal location. Furthermore, the necessity to keep the screw-access in the center of the occlusal table, and the insufficient room for composite screw-head coverage, ultimately led to a considerable compromise (Fig. 41-77). The final radiograph (Fig. 41-78) clearly shows that the presurgical bone volume would have permitted a vertical reduction of the edentulous bone crest to be performed prior to implant insertion. By this token the suboptimal implant position could have been partially corrected by the implant restoration, and the occlusal screw covered by composite resin, or a screw-retained restoration even-

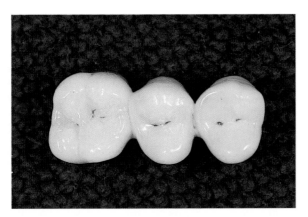

Fig. 41-79. Occlusal configuration of a three-unit metal-ceramic implant restoration designed for transversal screw-retention. Note the absence of any interference due to screws on the occlusal aspect of the restoration.

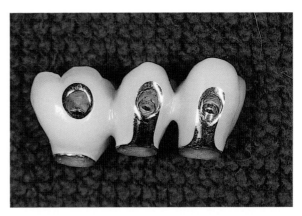

Fig. 41-80. The oral aspect of that same prosthesis features the decisive elements related to the transverse screw-retention: improved esthetics, no weakening of the ceramo-metal design. The screw-access channels are completely protected by the metal framework.

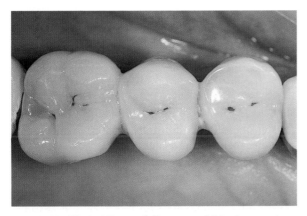

Fig. 41-81. Clinical 5-year follow-up of this three-unit implant restoration. No significant changes can be noticed on the occlusal surface.

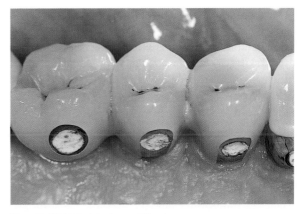

Fig. 41-82. Palatal view of the transverse screw-retained implant prosthesis after 5 years of clinical service. The screw-access channels are blocked out by a temporary material.

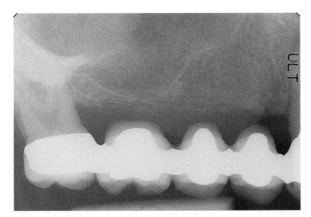

Fig. 41-83. Preoperative radiograph of the patient's maxillary right posterior segment, revealing a tooth-borne long-span FPD which had failed after four years of function due to loss of retention and subsequent damage on the mesial abutment.

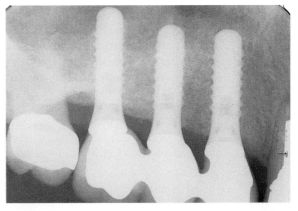

Fig. 41-84. Five-year follow-up radiograph of the same quadrant, now restored with a three-unit transverse screw-retained metal-ceramic implant suprastructure. Note that the distal retainer of the original tooth-borne FPD could be maintained.

tually avoided due to now adequate conditions for a cemented suprastructure.

Transverse screw-retention

When it comes to screw-retained posterior implant restorations one should not forget the option of transverse screw-retention (Figs. 41-79 to 41-84). This specific technical approach leaves the occlusal surface of the restoration free from any screw and permits the design of a screw-access channel on the oral aspect, featuring a metal protection on the entire circumference of the perforation (Fig. 41-80). These two factors improve significantly both the overall mechanical resistance and the esthetic appearance. Furthermore, the metal protects the surrounding porcelain during removal and tightening of the transverse screw and thereby prevents the induction of fissures prone to subsequent propagation and ultimately leading to ceramic fractures. One has to be aware, however, that from a purely technical and economic point of view, transverse screw-retained restorations require additional, more complex components and advanced technical skills, and are more expensive. On the other hand the distinct advantages should in the long-term clearly outweigh these inconveniences in numerous clinical situations.

Abutment-level impression versus implant shoulder-level impression

Most of the leading implant systems currently offer the possibility of taking impressions either at the level of a previously inserted abutment or at the level of the implant shoulder itself (Figs. 41-85 and 41-86). The former approach is mostly indicated if the patient does not wear a removable temporary prosthesis and in the case of optimally – "restoration-driven" – placed implants, comprising accessibility of the implant shoulder, point of emergence from the soft tissue, implant axis, interarch distance and overall easy access for use of simple "pop-on" plastic transfer cop-

ings. As shown later, a clear preference is given to cemented suprastructures under such simple, straightforward conditions. In fact, the clinician is only required to keep a limited stock of components, i.e. cementable titanium abutments of various heights and injection-molded impression copings, in his office. Whenever the clinical situation deviates notably from the previously described conditions, one may consider taking an impression directly at the level of the implant shoulder. For that approach, only transfer copings have to be available in the dental practice. In fact, the patient is leaving the office after the impression session exactly as he came in, i.e. with the same cover screw and with the same unaltered temporary prosthesis. The technician will then – after master model fabrication and articulator mounting – select in the laboratory the most appropriate secondary components and ultimately deliver the finished restoration together with the respective supporting abutments.

Cemented multiple-unit posterior implant prostheses

In recent years, an increasing trend towards cemented posterior implant restorations, using either temporary or permanent luting agents, could be observed. The associated original paradigm, indicating that maintaining "retrievability" was one of the fundamental advantages of implant-borne suprastructures, permitting reintervention, modification and/or extension at any time, has been lately challenged by parameters such as increased clinical and technical simplicity, low-maintenance design of the restorations and superior cost effectiveness. The more implants are utilized in clinical situations where conventional FPDs would also be easily possible, but where the latter have become second choice, the more the sites are favorable for this type of therapy and the more these implants come close to the characteristics currently termed as "restoration-driven". Parallel to this improved mas-

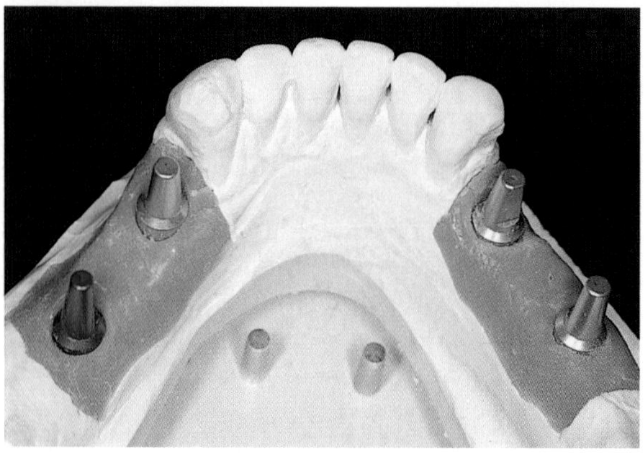

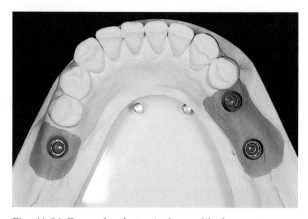

Fig. 41-85. Example of a typical mandibular master model, derived from an impression at the abutment level, comprising four colour-coded implant-abutment analogues.

Fig. 41-86. Example of a typical mandibular master model, derived from an impression at the implant shoulder level, comprizing three colour-coded implant analogues.

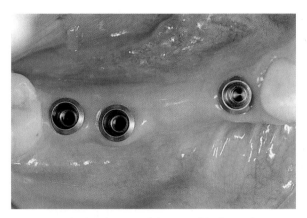

Fig. 41-87. Occlusal view of the mandibular right posterior quadrant with three implants that had been placed according to a single-step transmucosal surgical protocol.

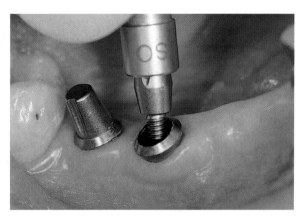

Fig. 41-88. In accordance with the available interocclusal space, adequately dimensioned solid abutments are selected, inserted and subsequently tightened to 35 Ncm in view of a cemented suprastructure.

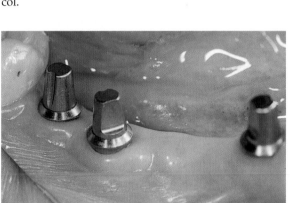

Fig. 41-89. With the solid abutments in place, the interimplant parallelism is confirmed. Note the easily accessible implant shoulders which will facilitate the following impression and restorative procedures.

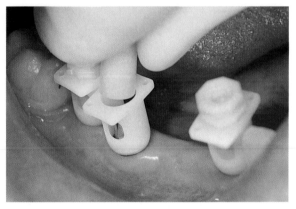

Fig. 41-90. Prefabricated injection-molded, self-centering impression copings and related color-coded positioning cylinders are inserted prior to impression taking with a stock tray.

tering of the three-dimensional implant positioning, secondary components such as abutments that are optimally designed for subsequent cemented restorations have been developed, in combination with auxiliary parts such as simplified impression copings, laboratory analogues and burn-out patterns. A typical clinical example of the treatment of an extended toothbound posterior segment by means of implants and a subsequently cemented suprastructure is presented in Figs. 41-87 to 41-94. Three screw-type implants have been inserted according to a single-step transmucosal (non-submerged) surgical protocol, leading 8 weeks after implant installation to a clinical situation which is well suited for a restorative procedure similar to the one traditionally used in the context of natural tooth abutments. More particularly, all of the involved implant shoulders are easily accessible (Figs. 41-87 to 41-90) for restorative procedures and later for maintenance, and the surrounding peri-implant mucosa healing and tissue maturation has occurred simultaneously with implant osseointegration, both being key factors in facilitating prosthetic procedures. Furthermore, the superficially located interface between implant shoulder and suprastructure or abutment will

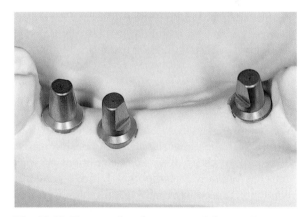

Fig. 41-91. The completed master model comprises color-coded aluminum implant analogues.

reduce the length of suprastructure leverage and by this the resulting bending moments. Under the assumption that presurgical site analysis and, derived from that, prosthetic treatment planning has predictably led to an optimal implant positioning, the resulting implant prosthesis should almost by definition feature a gradually increasing, flat axial emergence

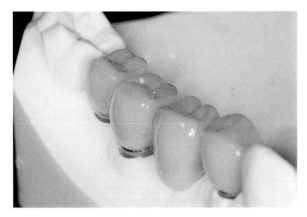

Fig. 41-92. Based on prefabricated burn-out patterns, the final metal-ceramic restoration has been completed. Note the continuous flat axial emergence profile of the individual elements.

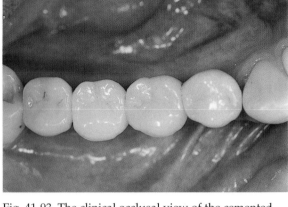

Fig. 41-93. The clinical occlusal view of the cemented four-unit implant prosthesis composed by premolar-sized segments.

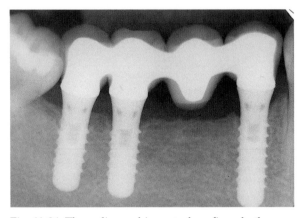

Fig. 41-94. The radiographic control confirms both successful osseointegration of the involved implants and accurate marginal adaptation of the suprastructure.

profile, adequate embrasures and overall design and occlusal characteristics similar to those advocated for tooth-borne FPDs (Figs. 41-92 to 41-94).

Angulated abutments

It is not infrequent that all of the parameters defining an optimal three-dimensional implant position cannot be readily reached. Under such conditions the clinician has basically three options. Either a bone augmentation procedure is undertaken, or a conventional tooth-borne prosthesis is chosen, or one evaluates carefully whether a minor positional compromise can be considered acceptable. The related parameters have to be objectively pondered prior to taking the respective decision together with the duly informed patient. The heaviness of a so-called "site-development" procedure (e.g. lateral or vertical bone augmentation or anterior sinus floor elevation) should definitely be put in direct relation with the expected benefit. This approach in some instances allows significantly invasive procedures to be avoided. Particularly in situations where only the implant axis interferes

with an otherwise optimal implant positioning, the subsequent use of angled abutments may still lead to a largely acceptable treatment outcome (Figs. 41-95 to 41-98). In other terms, there appears to exist some limited room for sometimes considering a slightly "bone-driven" instead of a purely "restoration-driven" implant placement in order to render implant therapy bearable for a given individual patient.

Angled abutments, encompassing various inclinations and dimensions, are currently part of the armamentarium of most of the leading implant systems. They are frequently used and compatible with both a cementable or a screw-retained suprastructure design.

High-strength all-ceramic implant restorations

Additional options, such as milled titanium frameworks as infrastructures for metal-ceramic prostheses or high-strength all-ceramic restorations, have also become recently available in the context of posterior implant restorations. Some of these approaches are based on computer-assisted design and computer-assisted machining (CAD/CAM) technology. As implants and their secondary components are mostly industrially produced or machined, and as their related dimensions and tolerances are well defined, they appear particularly well-suited to this kind of technology. In this context, and in order to explain the particular interest associated with this type of technology, it has to be underlined that using either the same metal (i.e. c.p. titanium) or no metal at all for the suprastructure fabrication, would be highly preferable. The still widely spread high-gold containing porcelain-fused-to-metal alloys is primarily utilized due to its superior casting ability.

It would go beyond the scope of this textbook to describe in detail the current evolution in the field of CAD/CAM systems in general and to their impact on implant dentistry in particular. A representative clinical example, however, is given in Figs. 41-99 to 41-105.

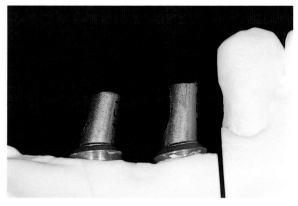

Fig. 41-95. Lateral view of a master model comprising implant level analogues in the right mandibular posterior sextant. Angulated abutments have been selected to correct a too distal implant axis.

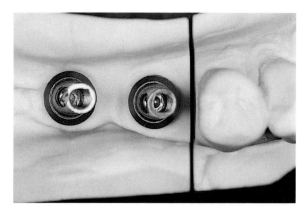

Fig. 41-96. The corresponding occlusal aspect visualizes the amount of axis correction achieved.

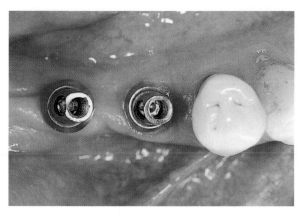

Fig. 41-97. Using an appropriate index, the two angulated abutments are transferred intraorally and subsequently tightened to 35 Ncm with a torque wrench.

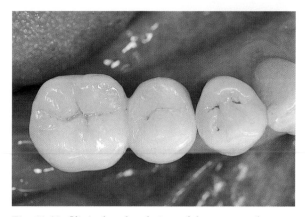

Fig. 41-98. Clinical occlusal view of the cemented two-unit metal-ceramic implant restoration.

All-ceramic implant suprastructures are still preferred as single-unit restorations, primarily for purely technical reasons.

Orthodontic and occlusal considerations related to posterior implant therapy

As one increasingly strives for the best possible biological, functional and esthetic integration of a given implant restoration in the pre-existing dentition, three-dimensional preoperative site analysis is of paramount importance. It is not infrequent that this subsequently calls for a pluridisciplinary approach termed "site development", which may also include presurgical orthodontic therapy (Figs. 41-106 to 41-119). The objective is clearly to create local conditions that are best suited for the type of therapy chosen. If implants are to be involved, the local bone and soft tissue anatomy as well as the mesio-distal and oro-facial distances of a given edentulous segment have to comply optimally with the respective most appropriate implant dimensions. Quite often mesio-distal gap dimensions have to be optimized orthodontically and neighboring roots aligned, so that they will not inter-

fere with "restoration-driven" implant positioning. Site development in the broad sense of the term comprises also parameters associated with intermaxillary relationships such as occlusal plane, interarch space and occlusal guidance during mandibular excursions. As osseointegrated implants do provide excellent anchorage for orthodontic appliances (Melsen & Lang 2001), and thus can significantly contribute to the efficacy and simplicity of such a treatment, one may also consider implant insertion prior to orthodontic therapy. This, however, requires a meticulous preoperative analysis and precise three-dimensional implant positioning, anticipating perfectly the ideal location with respect to the final treatment objective.

When it comes to occlusal considerations related to posterior implant restorations, one should note that most of the relevant literature available to date is addressing eventual effects of occlusal loading on the various components of the implant-abutment-suprastructure complex (Brägger 1999, 2001, Bassit et al. 2002, Wiskott et al. 2002). In fact, a variety of recommendations are derived from such studies, including various occlusal restorative materials, type and mechanical characteristics of different abutment to im-

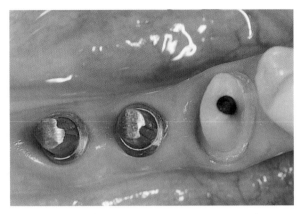

Fig. 41-99. Mandibular right posterior segment, featuring a full-coverage preparation on the non-vital second premolar and two implants equipped with solid abutments in the area of the missing first molar.

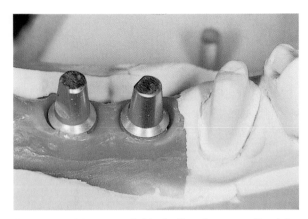

Fig. 41-100. Master model including the stone die of the prepared premolar and the two implant analogues.

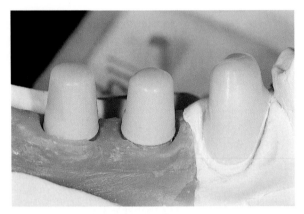

Fig. 41-101. Three respective aluminous oxyde copings have been fabricated according to the PROCERA® technique.

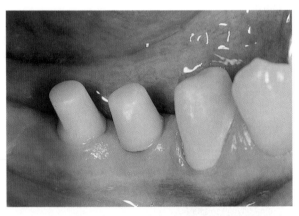

Fig. 41-102. Clinical try-in of the high-strength porcelain infrastructures.

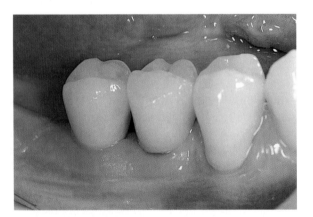

Fig. 41-103. Vestibular view of the cemented final all-ceramic restorations.

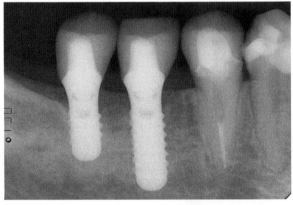

Fig. 41-104. The 1-year radiographic follow-up displays sufficient radio-opacity of the all-ceramic substrate to evaluate the marginal adaptation of the three single-unit restorations.

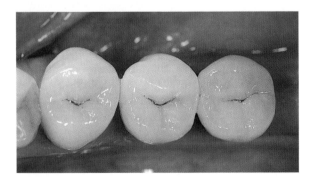

Fig. 41-105. Occlusal view of the two posterior implant-borne premolar-sized suprastructures and the tooth-supported ceramic restoration on the second premolar.

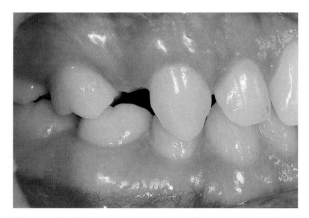

Fig. 41-106. Right lateral view of a 19-year-old female patient, congenitally missing all four permanent maxillary premolars. One can note both an inadequate mesio-distal gap width and a reduced interarch distance.

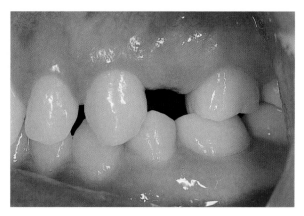

Fig. 41-107. A similar situation regarding interarch distance is present on the patient's left side.

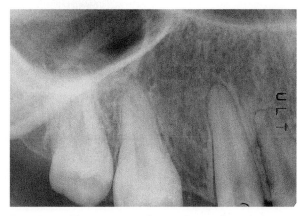

Fig. 41-108. The corresponding radiograph underlines the need for additional orthodontic therapy prior to the insertion of an implant in order to optimize the gap width and the interradicular distance.

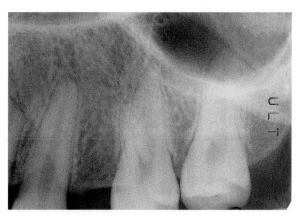

Fig. 41-109. Although to a lesser degree, presurgical orthodontic therapy is also indicated on the maxillary left posterior segment.

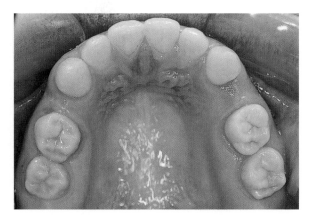

Fig. 41-110. The clinical occlusal view displays the bilateral edentulous spaces in the premolar area. Despite a previously performed orthodontic therapy, aiming at reducing the edentulous spaces to the size of one premolar, the mesio-distal gap width on the right side is insufficient for the insertion of an implant.

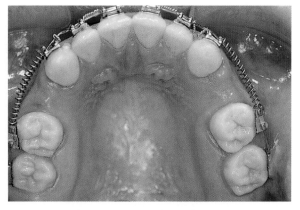

Fig. 41-111. After six months of additional orthodontic treatment using an upper fixed full-arch appliance, the dimensions of the two prospective implant sites appear compatible with this kind of therapy.

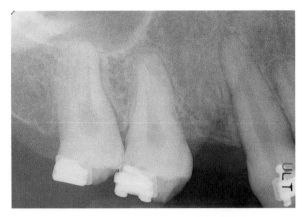

Fig. 41-112. The respective radiograph confirms adequate space in the upper right premolar region for the placement of a standard single-tooth implant.

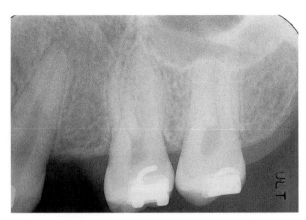

Fig. 41-113. A similar presurgical situation is radiographically confirmed for the upper left premolar site.

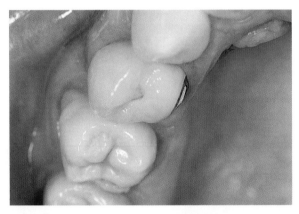

Fig. 41-114. The right oblique occlusal view of the implant restoration clearly demonstrates the advantage of the transverse screw-retention design: no occlusal screw access channel interfering with the functional occclusal morphology and esthetics or with structural requirements inherent to the metal-ceramic technology.

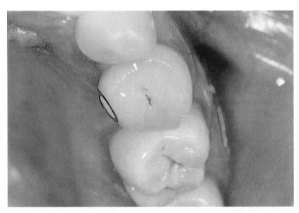

Fig. 41-115. As described for the patient's right side, the left maxillary fixed single-tooth implant restoration integrates appropriately the existing natural dentition.

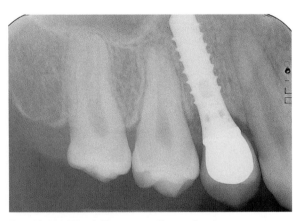

Fig. 41-116. The follow-up radiograph taken one year after the insertion of the 12 mm solid screw implant, shows adequate marginal fidelity and stable conditions at the bone-to-implant interface.

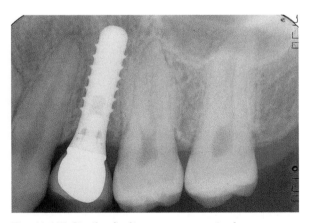

Fig. 41-117. Similar findings are present in the corresponding left-sided follow-up radiograph.

plant connections, as well as general guidelines for optimal suprastructure design.

Regarding an eventual direct relationship between occlusal loading and maintenance of osseointegration in general and occurrence of peri-implant crestal bone resorption in particular, little information is presently available (Wiskott & Belser 1999, Duyck et al. 2001, Engel et al. 2001, Gotfredsen et al. 2001a-c, O'Mahony

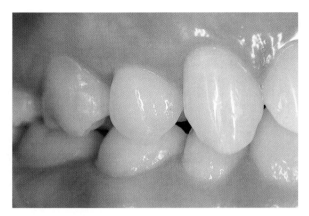

Fig. 41-118. The final right lateral view in centric occlusion features acceptable general interarch conditions and related intercuspation.

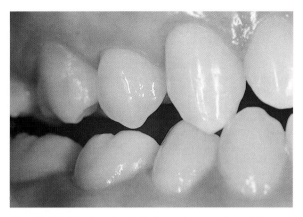

Fig. 41-119. During the right lateral excursion of the mandible (working-side movement), a canine guidance could be established.

et al. 2001, Engquist et al. 2002, Wright et al. 2002). Attempts have been made to take into account the fundamental differences between a tooth surrounded by a periodontal ligament and an "ankylosed" osseointegrated implant, the latter disposing neither of local mechanoreceptors nor of a so-called "damping" capacity. This led to a hypothetical implant-specific occlusal concept (Table 41-7), featuring parameters such as lighter contacts in centric occlusion when compared with the surrounding natural dentition, and no or only minimal contacts on implant restorations during mandibular excursions. One should clearly note, however, that these guidelines are primarily derived from clinical experience, subjective opinions and eventually common sense, and that there is little or no solid scientific evidence available to date which would support such a concept (Taylor et al. 2000).

CONCLUDING REMARKS AND PERSPECTIVES

Early and immediate fixed implant restorations

Currently, one can observe a strong tendency towards shortened healing delays and ultimately towards immediate loading or at least "immediate restoration" protocols in association with dental implants (Tarnow et al. 1997, Ericsson et al. 2000, Gatti et al. 2000, Szmukler-Moncler et al. 2000, Bernard et al. 2001, Chiapasco et al. 2001b, Ganeles et al. 2001, Gomez-Roman et al. 2001, Roccuzzo et al. 2001, Romanos et al. 2002). Improved implant surface characteristics have contributed to this evolution (Buser et al. 1998a, Deporter et al. 2001, Gotfredsen et al. 2001b, Roccuzzo et al. 2001, Cochran et al. 2002). Numerous studies have reported that such an approach can be considered predictable under certain well-defined conditions. Under these

Table 41.7. Hypothetical implant-specific occlusal concept

- "Light infraocclusion" in centric occlusion position (CO) on posterior implant restorations
- "Narrow" occlusal table
- Only "axial" loading on implant restorations
- No or only "minimal contacts" on implant restorations during "mandibular excursions"
  - no canine guidance on implants
  - eventually "minimal" group function on the working side

conditions fall four to six implants inserted in the interforaminal part of the edentulous mandible and which are subsequently splinted with a bar device (Gatti et al. 2000), as well as multiple implants evenly distributed around an edentulous arch and then immediately restored – according to the principle of "cross-arch stabilization" – with a splinted full-arch FPD (Tarnow et al. 1997). Achieving adequate primary stability at the moment of implant installation, and confining, during the crucial first healing period, an eventual mobility below the threshold of approximately 50 microns, appear to be among the decisive parameters for predictably achieving osseointegration (Szmukler et al. 2000). With regard to the routine application of immediate loading protocols for posterior single-tooth restorations, it appears advisable to wait for scientific confirmation of its respective potential in the form of randomized controlled clinical trials.

In conclusion, the possibility of performing highly predictable treatments which are more simple, require less time and which can be conducted in a standard dental practice set-up, as well as the associated quality of treatment outcomes, have nowadays made implant therapy in the load carrying part of the dentition an integral part of the restorative spectrum for any kind of edentulism. This evolution is most dynamic and holds promise for further significant developments.

REFERENCES

Abrahamson, I., Berglundh, T. & Lindhe, J. (1997). The mucosal barrier following abutment dis/reconnection. An experimental study in dogs. *Journal of Clinical Periodontology* **24**, 568-572.

Andersson, B., Ödman, P., Lindvall, A.M. & Brånemark, P.I. (1998). Five-year prospective study of prosthodontic and surgical single-tooth implant treatment in general practices and at a specialist clinic. *International Journal of Prosthodontics* **11**, 351-365.

Bahat, O. & Handelsman, M. (1996). Use of wide implants and double implants in the posterior jaw: a clinical report. *International Journal of Oral and Maxillofacial Implants* **11**, 379-386.

Bassit, R., Lindström, H. & Rangert, B. (2002). In vivo registration of force development with ceramic and acrylic resin occlusal materials on implant-supported prostheses. *International Journal of Oral and Maxillofacial Implants* **17**, 17-23.

Behneke, A., Behneke, N. & d'Hoedt, B. (2000). The longitudinal clinical effectiveness of ITI solid screw implants in partially edentulous patients: A 5-year follow-up report. *International Journal of Oral and Maxillofacial Implants* **15**, 633-645.

Belser, U.C., Mericske-Stern, R., Bernard, J.P. & Taylor, T.D. (2000). Prosthetic management of the partially dentate patient with fixed implant restorations. *Clinical Oral Implants Research* **11** (suppl. I), 126-145.

Bernard, J.P. & Belser, U. (2002). Twelve years of clinical experience with the ITI Dental Implant System at the University of Geneva. *Journal de Parodontologie et d'Implantologie orale* **21**, 1-27.

Bernard, J.P., Belser, U.C., Smukler-Moncler, S., Martinet, J.P., Attieh, A. & Schaad, P.J. (1995a). Intérêt de l'utilisation d'implants ITI de faible longueur dans les secteurs postérieurs: resultats d'une etude clinique à trois ans. *Médecine Buccale & Chirurgie Buccale* **1**, 11-18.

Bernard, J.P., Szmukler-Moncler, S. & Samson, J. (2001). A 10-year life-table-analysis on TPS coated implants inserted in type IV bone. *Clinical Oral Implants Research* **12**, 395 (abstract no. 10).

Beumer III, J., Hamada, M.O. & Lewis, S. (1993). A prosthodontic overview. *The International Journal of Prosthodontics* **6**, 126-130.

Bischof, M., Nedir, R., Smukler-Moncler, S. & Bernard, J.P. (2001). A 5-year life-table-analysis of ITI implants. Results from a private practice with emphasis on the use of short implants. *Clinical Oral Implants Research* **12**, 396 (abstract no. 13).

Boioli, L.T., Penaud, J. & Miller, N. (2001). A meta-analytic, quantitative assessment of osseointegration establishment and evolution of submerged and non-submerged endosseous titanium oral implants. *Clinical Oral Implants Research* **12**, 579-588.

Bosse, L.P. & Taylor, T.D. (1998). Problems associated with implant rehabilitation of the edentulous maxilla. *Dental Clinics of North America* **42**, 117-127.

Brägger, U. (1999). Technical failures and complications related to prosthetic components of implant systems and different types of suprastructures. In: Lang, N.P., Karring, T. & Lindhe, J., eds. *Proceedings of the 3rd European Workshop on Periodontology*. Berlin: Quintessence, pp. 304-332.

Brägger, U., Aeschlimann, S., Bürgin, W., Hämmerle, C.H.F. & Lang, N.P. (2001). Biological and technical complications and failures with fixed partial dentures (FPD) on implants and teeth after 4-5 years of function. *Clinical Oral Implants Research* **12**, 26-34.

Brägger, U., Bürgin, W.B., Hämmerle, C.H.F. & Lang, N.P. (1997). Associations between clinical parameters assessed around implants and teeth. *Clinical Oral Implants Research* **8**, 412-421.

Brånemark, P.I, Svensson, B. & van Steenberghe, D. (1995). Ten-year survival rates of fixed prostheses on four or six implants ad modum Brånemark in full edentulism. *Clinical Oral Implants Research* **6**, 227–231.

Buser, D., Belser, U.C. & Lang, N.P. (1998b). The original one-stage dental implant system and its clinical applications. *Periodontology 2000* **17**, 106-118.

Buser, D., Dula, K., Belser, U.C., Hirt, H.P. & Berthold, H. (1993). Localized ridge augmentation using guided bone regeneration. I. Surgical procedure in the maxilla. *International Journal of Periodontics and Restorative Dentistry* **13**, 29-45.

Buser, D., Dula, K., Belser, U.C., Hirt, H.P. & Berthold, H. (1995). Localized ridge augmentation using guided bone regeneration. II. Surgical procedure in the mandible. *International Journal of Periodontics and Restorative Dentistry* **15**, 13-29.

Buser, D., Dula, K., Hess, D., Hirt, H.P. & Belser U.C. (1999). Localized ridge augmentation with autografts and barrier membranes. *Periodontology 2000* **19**, 151-163.

Buser, D., Dula, K., Hirt, H.P. & Schenk, R.K. (1996). Lateral ridge augmentation using autografts and barrier membranes: a clinical study with 40 partially edentulous patients. *Journal of Oral and Maxillofacial Surgery* **54**, 420-432.

Buser, D., Ingimarsson, S., Dula, K., Lussi, A., Hirt, H.P. & Belser, U.C. (2002). Long-term stability of osseointegrated implants in augmented bone: A 5-year prospective study in partially edentulous patients. *International Journal of Periodontics and Restorative Dentistry* **22**, 108-117.

Buser, D., Mericske-Stern, R., Bernard, J.P., Behneke, A., Behneke, N., Hirt, H.P., Belser, U.C. & Lang, N.P. (1997). Long-term evaluation of non-submerged ITI implants. Part I: 8-year life table analysis of a prospective multi-center study with 2359 implants. *Clinical Oral Implants Research* **8**, 161-172.

Buser, D., Nydegger, T., Oxland, T., Schenk, R.K., Hirt, H.P., Cochran, D.L., Snétivy, D. & Nolte, L.P. (1998a). Influence of surface characteristics on the interface shear strength between titanium implants and bone. A biomechanical study in the maxilla of miniature pigs. *Journal of Biomedical Materials Research* **45**, 75-83.

Buser, D. & von Arx, T. (2000). Surgical procedures in partially edentulous patients with ITI implants. *Clinical Oral Implants Research* **11** (suppl. I), 83-100.

Chiapasco, M., Abati, S., Romeo, E. & Vogel, G. (1999). Clinical outcome of autogenous bone blocks or guided regeneration with e-PTFE membranes for reconstruction of narrow edentulous ridges. *Clinical Oral Implants Research* **10**, 278-288.

Chiapasco, M., Abati, S., Romeo, E. & Vogel, G. (2001b). Implant-retained mandibular overdentures with Brånemark System MKII implants: A prospective study between delayed and immediate loading. *International Journal of Oral and Maxillofacial Implants* **16**, 537-546.

Chiapasco, M., Romeo, E. & Vogel, G. (2001a). Vertical distraction osteogenesis of edentulous ridges for improvement of oral implant positioning: A clinical report of preliminary results. *International Journal of Oral and Maxillofacial Implants* **16**, 43-51.

Cochran, D.L., Buser, D., ten Bruggenkate, C.M., Weingart, D., Taylor, T. M., Bernard, J.P., Peters, F. & Simpson, J.P. (2002). The use of shortened healing times on ITI implants with a sandblasted and acid-etched (SLA) surface. Early results from clinical trials on ITI SLA implants. *Clinical Oral Implants Research* **13**, 144-153.

Deporter, D., Pilliar, R.M., Todescan, R., Watson, P. & Pharoah, M. (2001). Managing the posterior mandible of partially edentulous patients with short, porous-surfaced dental implants: Early data from a clinical trial. *International Journal of Oral and Maxillofacial Implants* **16**, 653-658.

Duyck, J., Rønold, H.J., Van Oosterwyck, H., Naert, I., Vander Sloten, J. & Ellingsen, J.E. (2001). The influence of static and dynamic loading on marginal bone reactions around osseointegrated implants: an animal experimental study. *Clinical Oral Implants Research* **12**, 207-218.

Eckert, S.E. & Wollan, P.C. (1998). Retrospective review of 1170 endosseous implants placed in partially edentulous jaws. *Journal of Prosthetic Dentistry* **79**, 415-421.

Ellegaard, B., Baelum, V. & Karring, T. (1997a). Implant therapy in periodontally compromised patients. *Clinical Oral Implants Research* **8**, 180-188.

Ellegaard, B., Kolsen-Petersen, J. & Baelum, V. (1997b). Implant therapy involving maxillary sinus lift in periodontally compromised patients. *Clinical Oral Implants Research* **8**, 305-315.

Ellen, R.P. (1998). Microbial colonization of the peri-implant environment and its relevance to long-term success of osseointegrated implants. *International Journal of Prosthodontics* **11**, 433-441.

Engel, E., Gomez-Roman, G. & Axmann-Krcmar, D. (2001). Effect of occlusal wear on bone loss and periotest values of dental implants. *International Journal of Prosthodontics* **14**, 444-450.

Engquist, B, Åstrand, P., Dahlgren, S., Engquist, E., Feldman, H. & Gröndahl, K. (2002). Marginal bone reaction to oral implants: a prospective comparative study of Astra Tech and Brånemark System implants. *Clinical Oral Implants Research* **13**, 30-37.

Ericsson, I., Nilson, H., Nilner, K. & Randow, K. (2000). Immediate functional loading of Brånemark single tooth implants. An 18 months' clinical pilot follow-up study. *Clinical Oral Implants Research* **11**, 26-33.

Ganeles, J., Rosenberg, M.M., Holt, R.L. & Reichman, L.H. (2001). Immediate loading of implants with fixed restorations in the completely edentulous mandible: Report of 27 patients from a private practice. *International Journal of Oral and Maxillofacial Implants* **16**, 418-426.

Gatti, C., Haefliger, W. & Chiapasco, M. (2000). Implant-retained mandibular overdentures with immediate loading: a prospective study of ITI implants. *International Journal of Oral and Maxillofacial Implants* **15**, 383-388.

Glantz, P.O. & Nilner, K. (1998). Biomechanical aspects of prosthetic implant-borne reconstructions. *Periodontology 2000* **17**, 119-124.

Gomez-Roman, G., Kruppenbacher, M., Weber, H. & Schulte, W. (2001). Immediate postextraction implant placement with root-analog stepped implants: Surgical procedure and statistical outcome after 6 years. *International Journal of Oral and Maxillofacial Implants* **16**, 503-513.

Goodacre, C.J., Kan, J.I.K. & Rungcharassaeng, K. (1999). Clinical complications of osseointegrated implants. *Journal of Prosthetic Dentistry* **81**, 537-552.

Gotfredsen, K., Berglundh, T. & Lindhe, J. (2001a). Bone reactions adjacent to titanium implants subjected to static load. A study in the dog (I). *Clinical Oral Implants Research* **12**, 1-8.

Gotfredsen, K., Berglundh, T. & Lindhe, J. (2001b). Bone reactions adjacent to titanium implants with different surface characteristics subjected to static load. A study in the dog (II). *Clinical Oral Implants Research* **12**, 196-201.

Gotfredsen, K., Berglundh, T. & Lindhe, J. (2001c). Bone reactions adjacent to titanium implants subjected to static load of different duration. A study in the dog (III). *Clinical Oral Implants Research* **12**, 552-558.

Gross, M. & Laufer, B.Z. (1997). Splinting osseointegrated implants and natural teeth in rehabilitation of partially edentulous patients. Part I: Laboratory and clinical studies. *Journal of Oral Rehabilitation* **24**, 863-870.

Gunne, J., Åstrand, P., Lindh, T., Borg, K. & Olsson, M. (1999). Tooth-implant and implant supported fixed partial dentures: A 10-year report. *International Journal of Prosthodontics* **12**, 216-221.

Gunne, J., Rangert, B., Glantz, P-O. & Svensson, A. (1997). Functional load on freestanding and connected implants in three-unit mandibular prostheses opposing complete dentures: An in vivo study. *International Journal of Oral and Maxillofacial Implants* **12**, 335-341.

Haas, R., Polak, C., Fürhauser, R., Mailath-Pokorny, G., Dörtbudak, O. & Watzek, G. (2002). A long-term follow-up of 76 Brånemark single-tooth implants. *Clinical Oral Implants Research* **13**, 38-43.

Hebel, K.S. & Gajjar, R.C. (1997). Cement-retained versus screw-retained implant restorations: achieving optimal occlusion and esthetics in implant dentistry. *Journal of Prosthetic Dentistry* **77**, 28-35.

Hermann, J.S., Buser, D., Schenk, R.K., Higginbottom, F.L. & Cochran, D.L. (2000). Biologic width around titanium implants. A physiologically formed and stable dimension over time. *Clinical Oral Implants Research* **11**, 1-11.

Hermann, J.S., Buser, D., Schenk, R.K., Schoolfield, J.D. & Cochran, D.L. (2001a). Biologic width around one- and two-piece titanium implants. A histometric evaluation of unloaded nonsubmerged and submerged implants in the canine mandible. *Clinical Oral Implants Research* **12**, 559-571.

Hermann, J.S., Cochran, D.L., Nummikoski, P.V. & Buser, D. (1997). Crestal bone changes around titanium implants. A radiographic evaluation of unloaded nonsubmerged and submerged implants in the canine mandible. *Journal of Periodontology* **68**, 1117-1130.

Hermann, J.S., Schoolfield, J.D., Nummikoski, P.V., Buser, D., Schenk, R.K & Cochran, D.L. (2001b). Crestal bone changes around titanium implants: A methodological study comparing linear radiographic with histometric measurements. *International Journal of Oral and Maxillofacial Implants* **16**, 475-485.

Hosny, M., Duyck, J., van Steenberghe, D. & Naert, I. (2000). Within-subject comparison between connected and nonconnected tooth-to-implant fixed partial prostheses: Up to 14-year follow-up study. *International Journal of Prosthodontics* **13**, 340-346.

Hultin, M., Gustafsson, A. & Klinge, B. (2000). Long-term evaluation of osseointegrated dental implants in the treatment of partially edentulous patients. *Journal of Clinical Periodontology* **27**, 128-133.

Isidor, F. (1999). Occlusal loading in implant dentistry. In: Lang, N.P., Karring, T. & Lindhe, J., eds. *Proceedings of the 3rd European Workshop on Periodontology.* Berlin: Quintessence, pp. 358-375.

Jemt, T., Heath, M.R., Johns, R.B., McNamara, D.C., van Steenberghe, D. & Watson, R.M. (1996). A 5-year prospective multicenter follow-up report on overdentures supported by osseointegrated implants. *International Journal of Oral and Maxillofacial Implants* **11**, 291-298.

Johnson, R.H. & Persson, G.R. (2001). A 3-year prospective study of a single-tooth implant – Prosthodontic complications. *International Journal of Prosthodontics* **14**, 183-189.

Keith, S.E., Miller, B.H., Woody, R.D. & Higginbottom, F.L. (1999). Marginal discrepancy of screw-retained and cemented metal-ceramic crowns on implant abutments. *International Journal of Oral and Maxillofacial Implants* **14**, 369-378.

Keller, W., Brägger, U. & Mombelli, A. (1998). Peri-implant microflora of implants with cemented and screw retained suprastructures. *Clinical Oral Implants Research* **9**, 209-217.

Kiener, P., Oetterli, M., Mericske, E. & Mericske-Stern, R. (2001). Effectiveness of maxillary overdentures supported by implants: maintenance and prosthetic complications. *International Journal of Prosthodontics* **14**, 133-140.

Lang, N.P., Wilson, T. & Corbet, E.F. (2000). Biological complications with dental implants: their prevention, diagnosis and treatment. *Clinical Oral Implants Research* **11** (suppl. I), 146-155.

Lekholm, U., Gunne, J., Henry, P., Higuchi, K., Linden, U., Bergstrøm, C. & van Steenberghe, D. (1999). Survival of the Brånemark implant in partially edentulous jaws: a 10-year prospective multicenter study. *International Journal of Oral and Maxillofacial Implants* **14**, 639-645.

Leonhardt, Å., Gröndahl, K., Bergström, C. & Lekholm, U. (2002). Long-term follow-up of osseointegrated titanium implants using clinical, radiographic and microbiological parameters. *Clinical Oral Implants Research* **13**, 127-132.

Lindh, T., Bäck, T., Nyström, E. & Gunne, J. (2001). Implant versus tooth-implant supported prostheses in the posterior maxilla: a 2-year report. *Clinical Oral Implants Research* **12**, 441-449.

Lindh, T., Gunne, J., Tillberg, A. & Molin, M. (1998). A meta-analysis of implants in partial edentulism. *Clinical Oral Implants Research* **9**, 80-90.

Lindhe, J. & Berglundh, T. (1998). The interface between the mucosa and the implant. *Periodontology 2000* **17**, 47-53.

Lindqvist, L.W., Carlsson, G.E. & Jemt, T. (1996). A prospective 15-year follow-up study of mandibular fixed prostheses supported by osseointegrated implants. Clinical results and marginal bone loss. *Clinical Oral Implants Research* **7**, 329-336.

Lundgren, D. & Laurell, L. (1994). Biomechanical aspects of fixed bridgework supported by natural teeth and endosseous implants. *Periodontology 2000* **4**, 23-40.

Melsen, B. & Lang, N.P. (2001). Biological reactions of alveolar bone to orthodontic loading of oral implants. *Clinical Oral Implants Research* **12**, 144-152.

Mengel, R., Schröder, T. & Flores-de-Jacoby, L. (2001). Osseointegrated implants in patients treated for generalized chronic periodontitis and generalized aggressive periodontitis: 3- and 5-year results of a prospective long-term study. *Journal of Periodontology* **72**, 977-989.

Mericske-Stern, R. (1998). Treatment outcomes with implant-supported overdentures: clinical considerations. *Journal of Prosthetic Dentistry* **79**, 66-73.

Merz, B.R., Hunenbart, S. & Belser, U.C. (2000). Mechanics of the connection between implant and abutment – an 8γ morse taper compared to a butt joint connection. *International Journal of Oral and Maxillofacial Implants* **15**, 519-526.

Morneburg, T.R. & Pröschel, P.A. (2002). Measurement of masticatory forces and implant loads: A methodological clinical study. *International Journal of Prosthodontics* **15**, 20-27.

Naert, I.E., Duyck, J.A.J., Hosny, M.M.F., Quirynen, M. & van Steenberghe, D. (2001b). Freestanding and tooth-implant connected prostheses in the treatment of partially edentulous patients. Part II: An up to 15-years radiographic evaluation. *Clinical Oral Implants Research* **12**, 245-251.

Naert, I.E., Duyck, J.A.J., Hosny, M.M.F. & van Steenberghe, D. (2001a). Freestanding and tooth-implant connected prostheses in the treatment of partially edentulous patients. Part I: An up to 15-years clinical evaluation. *Clinical Oral Implants Research* **12**, 237-244.

Oetterli, M., Kiener, P. & Mericske-Stern, R. (2001). A longitudinal study on mandibular implants supporting an overdenture: The influence of retention mechanism and anatomic-prosthetic variables on periimplant parameters. *International Journal of Prosthodontics* **14**, 536-542.

Olsson, M., Gunne, J., Åstrand, P. & Borg, K. (1995). Bridges supported by free standing implants vs. bridges supported by tooth and implants. A five-year prospective study. *Clinical Oral Implants Research* **6**, 114-121.

O'Mahony, A.M., Williams, J.L. & Spencer, P. (2001). Anisotropic elasticity of cortical and cancellous bone in the posterior mandible increases peri-implant stress and strain under oblique loading. *Clinical Oral Implants Research* **12**, 648-657.

Quirynen, M., De Soete, M. & van Steenberghe, D. (2002). Infectious risks for oral implants: a review of the literature. *Clinical Oral Implants Research* **13**, 1-19.

Quirynen, M., Peeters, W., Naert, I., Coucke, W. & van Steenberghe, D. (2001). Peri-implant health around screw-shaped c.p. titanium machined implants in partially edentulous patients with or without ongoing periodontitis. *Clinical Oral Implants Research* **12**, 589-594.

Rangert, B., Sullivan, R.M. & Jemt, T.M. (1997). Load factor control for implants in the posterior partially edentulous segment. *International Journal of Oral and Maxillofacial Implants* **12**, 360-370.

Roccuzzo, M., Bunino, M., Prioglio, F. & Bianchi, S.D. (2001). Early loading of sandblasted and acid-etched (SLA) implants: a prospective split-mouth comparative study. *Clinical Oral Implants Research* **12**, 572-578.

Romanos, G.E., Toh, C.G., Siar, C.H., Swaminathan, D. & Ong, A.H. (2002). Histologic and histomorphometric evaluation of peri-implant bone subjected to immediate loading: An experimental study with *macaca fascicularis*. *International Journal of Oral and Maxillofacial Implants* **17**, 44-51.

Romeo, E., Chiapasco, M., Ghisolfi, M. & Vogel, G. (2002). Long-term clinical effectiveness of oral implants in the treatment of partial edentulism. Seven-year life table analysis of a prospective study with ITI® Dental Implant System used for single-tooth restorations. *Clinical Oral Implants Research* **13**, 133-143.

Schwarz, M.S. (2000). Mechanical complications of dental implants. *Clinical Oral Implants Research* **11 (suppl. I)**, 261-264.

Schwartz-Arad, D. & Dolev, E. (2000). The challenge of endosseous implants placed in the posterior partially edentulous maxilla: a clinical report. *International Journal of Oral and Maxillofacial Implants* **15**, 261-264.

Sheets, C.G. & Earthman, J.C. (1993). Natural tooth intrusion and reversal in implant-assisted prosthesis: evidence of and a hypothesis for the occurrence. *Journal of Prosthetic Dentistry* **70**, 513-522.

Simion, M., Jovanovic, S.A., Tinti, C. & Parma Benfenati, S. (2001). Long-term evaluation of osseointegrated implants inserted at the time of or after vertical ridge augmentation. A retrospective study on 123 implants with 1-5 year follow-up. *Clinical Oral Implants Research* **12**, 35-45.

Sutter, F., Weber, H.P., Sørensen, J. & Belser, U.C. (1993). The new restorative concept of the ITI Dental Implant System: Design and engineering. *International Journal of Periodontics and Restorative Dentistry* **13**, 409-431.

Szmukler-Moncler, S., Piatelli, J.A., Favero, J.H. & Dubruille, J.H. (2000). Considerations preliminary to the application of early and immediate loading protocols in dental implantology. *Clinical Oral Implants Research* **11**, 12-25.

Tangerud, T., Grønningsæter, A.G. & Taylor, Å. (2002). Fixed partial dentures supported by natural teeth and Brånemark System implants: A 3-year report. *International Journal of Oral and Maxillofacial Implants* **17**, 212-219.

Tarnow, D.P., Emtiaz, S. & Classi, A. (1997). Immediate loading of threaded implants at stage 1 surgery in edentulous arches: ten consecutive case reports with 1- to 5-year data. *International Journal of Oral and Maxillofacial Implants* **12**, 319-324.

Taylor, T.D. (1998). Prosthodontic problems and limitations associated with osseointegration. *Journal of Prosthetic Dentistry* **79**, 74-78.

Taylor, T.D., Belser, U.C. & Mericske-Stern, R. (2000). Prosthodontic considerations. *Clinical Oral Implants Research* **11** (suppl. I), 101-107.

ten Bruggenkate, C.M., Asikainen, P., Foitzik, C., Krekeler, G. & Sutter F. (1998). Short (6 mm) non-submerged dental implants: results of a multicenter clinical trial of 1-7 years. *International Journal of Oral and Maxillofacial Implants* **13**, 791-798.

Van Steenberghe, D., Quirynen, M. & Wallace, S.S. (1999). Survival and success rates with oral endosseous implants. In: Lang, N.P., Karring, T. & Lindhe, J., eds. *Proceedings of the 3rd European Workshop on Periodontology*. Berlin: Quintessence, pp. 242-254.

von Arx, T., Cochran, D.L., Hermann, J., Schenk, R.K., Higginbottom, F. & Buser, D. (2001a). Lateral ridge augmentation and implant placement: An experimental study evaluating implant osseointegration in different augmentation materials in the canine mandible. *International Journal of Oral and Maxillofacial Implants* **16**, 343-354.

von Arx, T., Cochran, D.L., Hermann, J.S., Schenk, R.K. & Buser, D. (2001b). Lateral ridge augmentation using different bone fillers and barrier membrane application. A histologic and histomorphometric pilot study in the canine mandible. *Clinical Oral Implants Research* **12**, 260-269.

Weber, H.P., Crohin, C.C. & Fiorellini, J.P. (2000). A 5-year prospective clinical and radiographic study of non-submerged dental implants. *Clinical Oral Implants Research* **11**, 144-153.

Wie, H. (1995). Registration of localization, occlusion and occluding materials for failing screw joints in the Brånemark implant system. *Clinical Oral Implants Research* **6**, 47-63.

Wiskott, A.H.W. & Belser, U.C. (1999). Lack of integration of smooth titanium surfaces: a working hypothesis based on strains generated in the surrounding bone. *Clinical Oral Implants Research* **10**, 429-444.

Wiskott, A.H.W., Perriard, J, Scherrer, S.S., Dieth, S. & Belser, U.C. (2002). In vivo wear of three types of veneering materials using implant-supported restorations. A method evaluation. *European Journal of Oral Sciences* **110**, 61-67.

Wismeijer, D., van Waas, M.A.J., Mulder J., Vermeeren I.J.F. & Kalk, W. (1999). Clinical and radiological results of patients treated with three treatment modalities for overdentures on implants of the ITI dental implant system. A randomised controlled clinical trial. *Clinical Oral Implants Research* **10**, 297-306.

Wright, P.S., Glantz, P-O., Randow, K. & Watson, R.M. (2002). The effects of fixed and removable implant-stabilised prostheses on posterior mandibular residual ridge resorption. *Clinical Oral Implants Research* **13**, 1169-1174.

Wyatt, C.L. & Zarb, G.A. (1998). Treatment outcomes of patients with implant-supported fixed partial prostheses. *International Journal of Oral and Maxillofacial Implants* **13**, 204-211.

Wyatt, C.L. & Zarb, G.A. (2002). Bone level changes proximal to oral implants supporting fixed partial prostheses. *Clinical Oral Implants Research* **13**, 162-168.

Zarb, G.A. & Schmitt, A. (1995). Implant prosthodontic treatment options for the edentulous patient. *Journal of Oral Rehabilitation* **22**, 661-671.

Zitzmann, N.U. & Marinello, C.P. (1999). Treatment plan for restoring the edentulous maxilla with implant supported restorations: removable overdenture versus fixed partial denture design. *Journal of Prosthetic Dentistry* **82**, 188-196.

Zitzmann, N.U. & Marinello, C.P. (2002). A review of clinical and technical considerations for fixed and removable implant prostheses in the edentulous mandible. *International Journal of Prosthodontics* **15**, 65-67.

Zitzmann, N.U., Schärer, P. & Marinello, C.P. (2001). Long-term results of implants treated with guided bone regeneration: A 5-year prospective study. *International Journal of Oral and Maxillofacial Implants* **16**, 355-366.

ACKNOWLEDGEMENTS

The authors wish to acknowledge and thank Drs Viviana Coto-Hunziker, Stephan Dieth, Thierry Doumas, German Gallucci, Robin Jaquet, Nikolaos Perakis and Valérie Wouters (all of them clinicians at School of Dental Medicine, University of Geneva, and involved in the treatment of some of the patients presented in this chapter) for their contributions. We would also like to thank the laboratory technicians and ceramists Michel Bertossa, Cédric Bertsch, Pierre Martini, Roger Renevey, Alwin Schönenberger and Gérard Verdel, for their expertise and meticulous execution of the implant suprastructures presented in this chapter. Furthermore, our gratitude is extended to Dr Pascal Magne (Senior Lecturer, University of Geneva) for his competent assistance in development of the schematic illustrations.

CHAPTER 42

Rehabilitation by Means of Implants: Case Reports

CHRISTOPH H. F. HÄMMERLE, TORD BERGLUNDH, JAN LINDHE AND INGVAR ERICSSON

Patient 1
Implants used to restore function in the mandible

Patient 2
Fixed restorations on implants and teeth

Patient 3
Implants used to restore function in the maxilla

Patient 4
Implants used in a cross-arch bridge restoration

Patient 5
Implants used to solve restorative problems occurring during maintenance therapy

Patient 6
Implants used to solve problems associated with accidental root fractures of important abutment teeth

---

PATIENT 1
IMPLANTS USED TO RESTORE FUNCTION IN THE MANDIBLE

The 56-year-old woman sought help to solve her periodontal and esthetic problems. She was systemically healthy and in good physical condition. She had been a smoker since age 18.

Initial examination

The patient presented with a full denture in the maxilla and a cross-arch fixed porcelain-fused-to-metal restoration in the mandible (Fig. 42-1a-d). The initial examination included inspection of the oral mucosa and the periodontal tissues (pocket depths, furcation involvements, radiographs), vitality testing, caries diagnosis and evaluation of the restoration (Table 42-1). This examination revealed the presence of hard and soft supragingival and subgingival deposits throughout the dentition (plaque score 75%), severe inflammation (Bleeding on probing – BoP – 84%) and advanced destruction of the periodontal tissues at several teeth.

At various locations the restoration showed subgingivally located, overcontoured and ill-fitting margins.

Initial prognosis
Teeth 33, 43, 44 and 45 could be maintained; teeth 41, 42, 46 and 47 were questionable due to periodontal and endodontic problems; number 37 could not be maintained.

Treatment planning

In order to achieve a situation that allowed for proper self-performed plaque removal by the patient, it seemed reasonable to remove the plaque retention factors brought about by the ill-fitting cross-arch bridge. The loss of tooth 37 called for the placement of dental implants to make possible the placement of a new cross-arch bridge. Evaluation of the remaining teeth or roots as abutments for the new bridge was postponed until the existing bridge had been removed.

The patient was informed regarding her status, problems specific to her situation, and the etiology of oral and especially periodontal diseases, as is commonly done for patients with periodontitis. The treatment plan as well as possible treatment alternatives

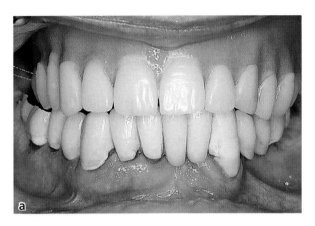

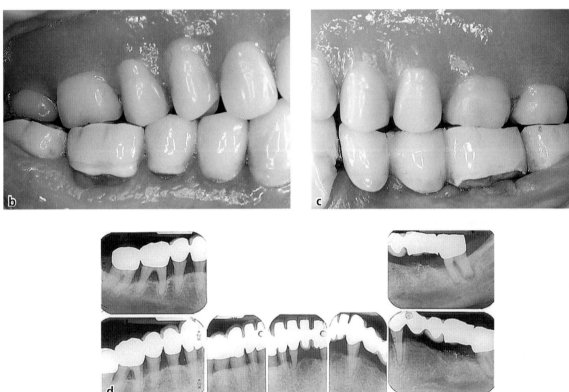

Fig. 42-1. (a-c) Clinical pictures of patient 1 at initial examination. (d) Radiographs of patient 1 at initial examination.

were also thoroughly discussed with the patient. In particular, the requirements for a successful long-term result of the therapy were emphasized: excellent personal plaque removal, proper healing of the periodontal tissues and optimal tissue integration of the implants. Finally, the importance of continuous supportive care to prevent the recurrence of periodontal and peri-implant disease was explicitly addressed.

Treatment

No precautions due to systemic conditions were necessary.

Initial therapy (cause related)
A program training the patient in proper oral hygiene measures was initiated. The cross-arch fixed bridge was removed and replaced by an acrylic temporary restoration. Tooth 37 was extracted. All remaining roots were carefully scaled and planed under local anesthesia. After completion of this treatment phase, the patient was enrolled in a maintenance care program with appointments scheduled every 3 months.

Corrective therapy and implantation
A re-examination after 4 months revealed that only minor reductions in pocket depth had occurred and that BoP was only slightly reduced (68%) (Table 42-2). Hence, flap surgery was performed to allow for improved removal of plaque and calculus from all root surfaces. During this surgical intervention, teeth 41, 42 and 47 were removed due to advanced periodontal destruction. The furcation of tooth 46 was eliminated by hemisection, and the mesial root was extracted. In order to replace the strategically important abutments in the third quadrant, two implants of the ITI® Dental

Table 42-1. Initial examination, periodontal diagnosis and prognosis

		Clinical periodontal examination				Diagnosis				Prognosis		
						Gingivitis	Parodontitis levis	Parodontitis gravis	Parodontitis compl.	extraction	questionable	maintain
Tooth	m	b	d	l	Furcation involvement							
47	8	6	5	8	b,l					x	x	
46	6	4	6	7	b,l					x	x	
45	7	3	6	7				x				x
44	6	3	6	6			x					x
43	6	3	8	6				x				x
42	5	4	6	3			x				x	
41	5	3	4	5			x				x	
33	5	3	5	5			x					x
37	8	6	4	8	b,l				x	x		

Table 42-2. Re-evaluation after 4 months

		Clinical periodontal examination			
		Pocket depth			Furcation involvement
Tooth	m	b	d	l	
47	8	6	5	8	b,l
46	4	3	3	6	b,l
45	4	2	4	5	
44	4	2	5	4	
43	4	2	3	6	
42	4	3	5	3	
41	3	2	4	4	
·33	5	2	5	5	

Table 33-3. Periodontal findings and prognosis at completion of active therapy

		Clinical periodontal examination				Prognosis	
		Pocket depth				questionable	maintain
Tooth	m	b	d	l			
46	4	4	4	3			x
45	5	2	3	2			x
44	3	2	3	4			x
43	3	2	3	3			x
33	3	2	2	2			x
I34	3	2	3	4			x
I36	3	1	2	3			x

Implant System were placed in regions 34 (hollow cylinder 8 mm long) and 36 (hollow screw 8 mm long).

Restorative therapy
After the periodontal and peri-implant tissues were given sufficient time to heal properly (Fig. 42-2), three porcelain-fused-to-metal fixed bridges were made and inserted. One bridge was purely implant borne (I34-x-I36), and two bridges were purely tooth borne (33-xxxx-43, 44-45-x-46). Concomitantly, a new maxillary full denture was manufactured.

Maintenance therapy
During the 5 documented years of maintenance care, supportive therapy consisted of recall appointments

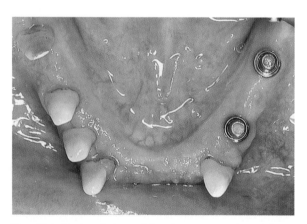

Fig. 42-2. Occlusal view of the abutment teeth and the two implants in patient 1 prior to insertion of the fixed bridges.

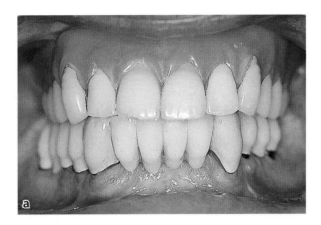

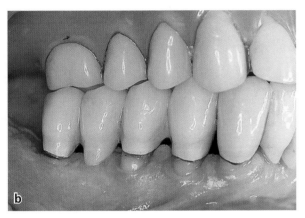

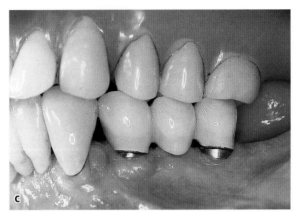

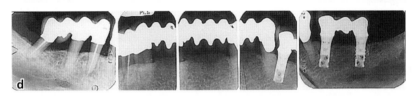

Fig. 42-3. (a-c) Clinical pictures of patient 1, 5 years following completion of active therapy. (d) Radiographs of patient 1, 5 years following completion of active therapy.

with the dental hygienist every 3-4 months, including standard procedures for periodontal patients with implants and fixed reconstructions. In addition, tooth 44 lost its vitality and was given root canal therapy. The alignment of the front teeth of the maxillary full denture was readjusted for esthetic reasons. No additional incidents arose calling for therapeutic interventions. The situation 5 years after completion of active therapy is shown in Fig. 42-3a-d and Table 42-3 (plaque score 7%, BoP 15%). Based on the clinical and radiographic findings as well as on the excellent plaque control performed by the patient, all teeth and implants were given a good prognosis.

Concluding remarks

This case illustrates how the loss of strategically important abutments can be compensated by the placement of dental implants, thus allowing treatment with fixed bridgework. In addition, proper attention to personal and professional plaque removal will maintain a successful treatment outcome of combined periodontal, prosthetic and implant therapy for prolonged periods of time also in patients who are susceptible to diseases caused by plaque infections.

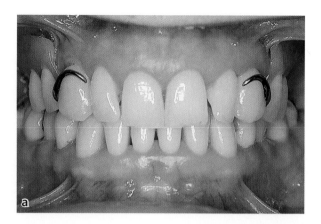

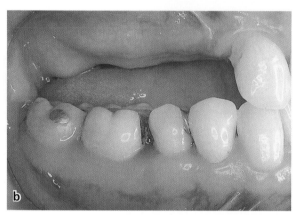

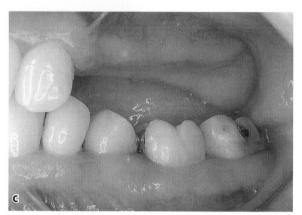

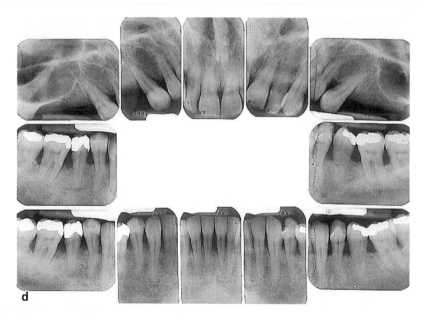

Fig. 42-4. (a-c) Clinical pictures of patient 2 at initial examination. (d) Radiographs of patient 2 at initial examination.

PATIENT 2
FIXED RESTORATIONS ON IMPLANTS AND TEETH

The 35-year-old woman complained about the esthetics and function of the removable partial denture (RPD) in the maxilla. She had been wearing this prosthesis for 4 years but had been unable to adapt to it.

The posterior teeth in the maxilla had been lost due to periodontal disease. The patient was suffering from hypertension but was otherwise in good physical condition.

Initial examination

The patient presented with a removable partial denture in the maxilla (Fig. 42-4a-d). The cast denture

Table 42-4. Initial examination, periodontal diagnosis and prognosis

	Clinical periodontal examination					Diagnosis				Prognosis		
	Pocket depth				Furcation involvement	Gingivitis	Parodontitis levis	Parodontitis gravis	Parodontitis compl.	extraction	questionable	maintain
Tooth	m	b	d	l								
13	4	3	3	4			x					x
12	3	2	2	3		x						x
11	3	2	2	3		x						x
21	3	2	3	2		x						x
22	3	2	3	3		x						x
23	4	2	2	4			x					x
47	3	3	3	3	b	x						x
46	7	2	6	2	l			x			x	
45	3	2	5	2			x					x
44	3	2	4	2			x					x
43	4	2	4	2			x					x
42	3	2	5	2			x					x
41	4	2	3	3			x					x
31	5	4	3	2			x					x
32	4	2	3	2			x					x
33	2	2	4	2			x					x
34	4	2	5	3			x					x
35	6	3	5	3				x				x
36	6	2	6	4	b,l			x			x	
37	5	3	5	4	b,l			x			x	

replaced teeth 17, 16, 15, 14 and 24, 25, 26, 27 and was anchored to the canines by clasps. The initial examination included inspection of the oral mucosa and the periodontal tissues (pocket depths, furcation involvements, radiographs), vitality testing and caries diagnosis (Table 42-4). This examination revealed the presence of hard and soft deposits both supragingivally and subgingivally throughout the dentition (plaque score 48%). Gingival inflammation was moderate exept where the RPD was in contact with the marginal periodontium (BoP 532); there it was severe. Destruction of the periodontal tissues was mild to moderate throughout the dentition.

Initial prognosis
All teeth in the maxilla and mandible except for teeth 36, 37 and 47 could be maintained; 36, 37 and 47 were questionable due to deep pockets with angular bone defects and furcation involvements.

Treatment planning

Before any form of prosthetic treatment could be considered, the periodontal disease had to be treated and further disease development prevented. Based on the premise of successful periodontal therapy, the treatment plan foresaw placement of dental implants in regions 14 and 24, allowing the restoration of two premolar units bilaterally, i.e. pursuing the concept of a shortened dental arch.

The patient was informed regarding her status, problems specific to her situation, and the etiology of oral and especially periodontal diseases, as is commonly done for patients with periodontitis. The treatment plan as well as possible treatment options involving removable partial dentures or elevation of the sinus floors for the placement of additional implants were also thoroughly discussed with the patient. In particular the conditions for a successful long-term result of the therapy were explained, including: excellent personal plaque removal, proper healing of the periodontal tissues and optimal tissue integration of the implants. Finally, the importance of continuous

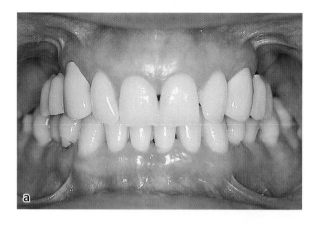
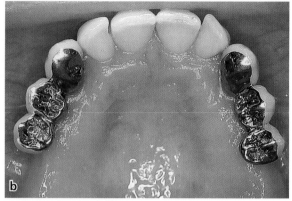
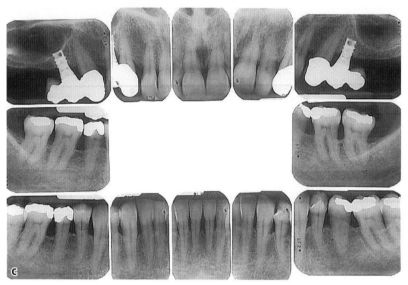

Fig. 42-5. (a-b) Clinical pictures of patient 2, 4½ years following completion of active therapy. (c) Radiographs of patient 2, 4½ years following completion of active therapy.

supportive care to prevent periodontal and peri-implant diseases was explicitly addressed.

Treatment

No precautions for standard dental and oral surgical interventions were necessary due to the systemic condition of the patient.

Initial therapy (cause related)

The patient was enrolled in a program training her to perform proper oral hygiene procedures. In order to test the functional and esthetic feasibility of a shortened dental arch, the existing removable partial denture was altered, i.e. the molars were removed from the denture. Hard and soft deposits were removed from all tooth surfaces and the exposed root surfaces were carefully scaled and planed under local anesthesia. After completion of this treatment, the patient was enrolled in a maintenance care program with appointments scheduled every 3 months.

Corrective therapy and implantation

A re-examination performed after 3 months revealed that the inflammatory processes were resolved (plaque 9%, BoP 12%). Marked recession of the marginal gingiva had occurred and the probing depths were reduced. No periodontal surgical intervention was necessary. Two implants of the ITI® Dental Implant System were placed in regions 14 (hollow screw 6 mm long) and 24 (hollow screw 6 mm long).

Restorative therapy

After 4 months, two porcelain-fused-to-metal fixed bridges were inserted. Both bridges (13-I14-×× and 23-I24-×) were seated on mixed support, i.e. one natural tooth abutment, one implant abutment.

Maintenance therapy

During the 4½ documented years after completion of active therapy, supportive care consisted of recall appointments with the dental hygienist every 3-4 months. No therapeutic interventions apart from regular recall activities were necessary. The situation 4½ years after completion of active therapy is shown in Fig. 42-5a-c and Table 42-5 (plaque 14%, BoP 19%). Based on the clinical and radiographic findings as well as on the plaque control performed by the patient, all teeth and implants were given a good prognosis.

Table 42-5. Periodontal findings and prognosis at completion of active therapy

| | Clinical periodontal examination | | | | | Prognosis | |
| | Pocket depth | | | | Furcation involvement | questionable | maintain |
Tooth	m	b	d	l			
l14	3	2	2	3			x
13	3	2	2	2			x
12	2	1	2	2			x
11	2	2	2	1			x
21	2	1	2	1			x
22	2	1	2	1			x
23	2	2	2	2			x
l24	3	2	3	2			x
47	4	3	4	2	b		x
46	4	2	3	2	l		x
45	3	2	4	2			x
44	3	2	3	1			x
43	3	2	2	1			x
42	2	1	3	1			x
41	2	2	2	1			x
31	2	1	3	1			x
32	2	2	3	1			x
33	3	2	3	1			x
34	3	1	3	2			x
35	3	2	4	3			x
36	4	2	3	2	l		x
37	3	3	3	3	l		x

Concluding remarks

This case demonstrates the sequence of therapy when dental implants are to be placed in patients with periodontal disease. Successful completion of cause-related therapy including professional as well as personal plaque removal represents a *conditio sine qua non* for implantation with predictable success. Furthermore, in situations where minimal amounts of bone are available for implant placement, the concept of shortened dental arches will limit therapy to standard dental procedures. Finally, proper attention to personal and professional plaque removal will allow the maintenance of a successful treatment outcome.

PATIENT 3
IMPLANTS USED TO RESTORE FUNCTION IN THE MAXILLA

Initial examination

The condition of the dentition of this 49-year-old woman is illustrated in the radiographs of Fig. 42-6 and the periodontal status (pocket depth, furcation

involvement, tooth mobility and diagnoses) from the clinical examination in Fig. 42-7. The analysis of the data discloses a case of moderately advanced periodontal disease. The overall plaque score was 35% and the corresponding bleeding on probing (BoP) score was 60%.

Treatment planning

The combined periodontal, endodontal and caries lesions in both tooth 16 and the root fractures in teeth 15 and 14 called for extraction of these three teeth. In the maxilla the following teeth were judged as maintainable: teeth 13, 12, 11, 21, 22, 23. Tooth 26, which displayed both periodontal and endodontal lesions, was regarded as questionable.

In the mandibular dentition both first molars (36 and 46) were furcation involved and displayed signs of periapical pathology. In the mandible the following teeth could be maintained: 47, 45... 35 and 37. From a rehabilitation point of view, the mandible offered no marked problem. The maxillary restoration, however, was more difficult. Different alternatives were considered.

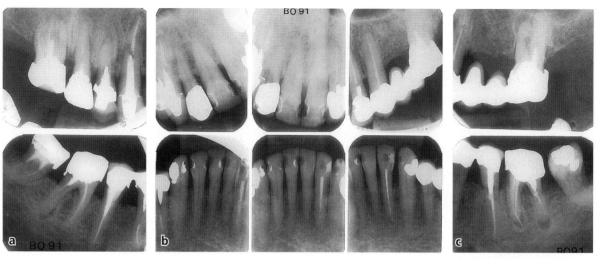

Fig. 42-6a-c.

Case: B.O. female, 49 years   PLI: 35%   BoP: 60%

Tooth	Pocket depth M B D L				Furcation involvement	Tooth mobility
18						
17						
16	6	7	6	11	m,b,d: III	3
15	6		6			1
14	5		5	8		2
13	6	4	6	4		1
12	5	4	6	4		1
11	4		5	4		1
21	5		5	5		1
22	6		5	5		
23	6		5	5		
24						
25						
26	6	4	8	5	m: II, b: I	
27						
28						

Periodontal charting

Tooth	Pocket depth M B D L				Furcation involvement	Tooth mobility
48						
47	6	4	6	4		
46	4	5	4	4	b, l: II	
45	6		6			
44	5		6	4		
43	4		4			
42	5		5			1
41	5	4	5			1
31	5		4			1
32	4	4	6	4		1
33	4		4			
34	5		6	4		
35	6		6	4		
36	4		4		III	
37						
38	5		5	4		

Diagnosis

	16	15	14	13	12	11	21	22	23		26	
Gingivitis												
Parodontitis levis				×	×	×	×	×	×		×	
Parodontitis gravis	×	×	×									
... et complicata	×	×	×								×	

	47	46	45	44	43	42	41	31	32	33	34	35	36		38
Gingivitis															
Parodontitis levis	×	×	×	×	×	×				×	×	×	×		×
Parodontitis gravis							×	×	×						
... et complicata		×											×		×

Fig. 42-7.

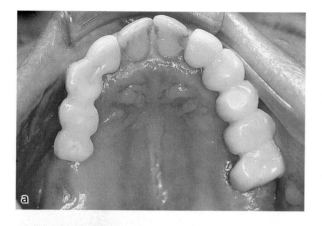

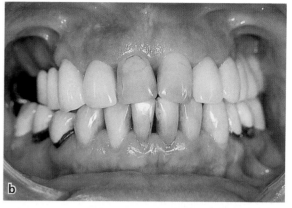

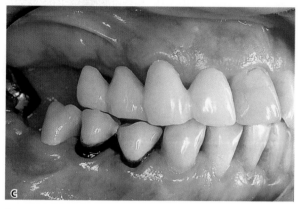

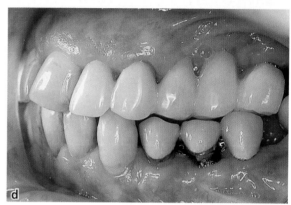

Fig. 42-8a-d.

Alternative 1

A removable partial denture anchored with attachments or clasps to the canines/incisiors. This solution was not readily acceptable to the patient.

Alternative 2

A fixed, cross-arch bridge extending from tooth 13 (with cantilever in position 14) to tooth 26 (palatal root).

Alternative 3

One implant-supported bridge distal of tooth 13, and one tooth-supported fixed bridge extending from 23 to 26 (provided that at least one root in the molar tooth could be maintained following furcation therapy and root resection).

Treatment

Initial therapy

The cause-related therapy included oral hygiene instruction and meticulous scaling and root planing. Teeth 16, 15 and 14 were extracted and a temporary restoration placed on 13 and 12 with cantilevers on positions 15 and 14 (Fig. 42-8). The cantilever in position 15 was in infraocclusion. The existing restoration 22...26 was removed and replaced with a temporary reconstruction in acrylic. Teeth 26, 36 and 46 were exposed to endodontic therapy.

Corrective therapy

A re-examinmation performed 3 months after the end of the initial therapy phase disclosed that the patient's self-performed plaque control was excellent. Several deep pockets with positive BoP still existed. Flap surgery was performed in both the maxilla and mandible to get access for proper scaling and root planing. During surgery tooth 26 was subjected to root resection and the remaining roots were subsequently fitted with a post.

Implant therapy

The edentulous region of the right maxilla was anesthetized. An incision, extending from region 13 to region 16, was made at the top of the crest and full thickness flaps were raised. Three fixture sites were prepared in positions 14, 15 and 16. Fixtures of the Astra Tech Implants® Dental System were installed; diameter = 3.5 mm; length = 13 mm (position 14), 11 mm (position 15), and 11 mm (position 15). Abutment connection was 6 months later in a second stage procedure.

Restorative therapy

Two bridges – porcelain fused to gold – were fabricated; one for the implant section (position 14... 16) (Fig. 42-9) and one for the tooth section (22... 26) (Fig. 42-10). In addition, single crowns were produced for teeth 13 and 12 (Fig. 42-11).

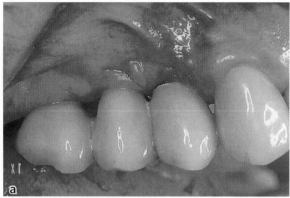

Fig. 42-9a,b.

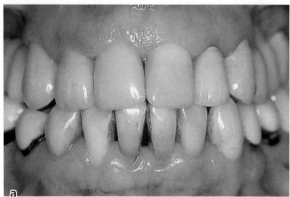

Fig. 42-10a,b.

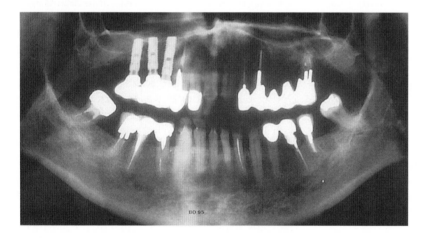

Fig. 42-11.

Maintenance therapy

The supportive care included recall appointments with the dental hygienist every 3 months for plaque control evaluation and, if indicated, professional debridement at tooth sites exhibiting positive BoP values.

Concluding remarks

This case illustrates how implants can be used to restore function in a periodontally compromised patient, and how the design of the restoration – both in the implant and the tooth segments – will allow the patient to exercise proper plaque control (Fig. 42-12).

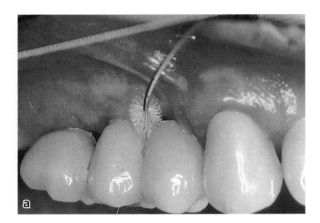
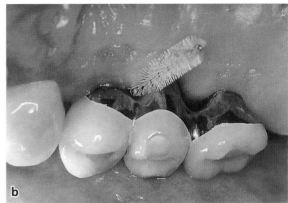
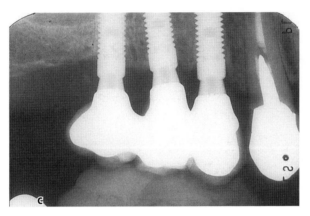

Fig. 42-12a-c.

PATIENT 4
IMPLANTS USED IN A CROSS-ARCH BRIDGE RESTORATION

Initial examination

The clinical and radiographic characteristics of this 58-year-old man are illustrated in Figs. 42-13 and 42-14 and the periodontal conditions (pocket depth, furcation involvement, tooth mobility and diagnoses) from the initial examination in Fig. 42-15. The analysis of the data disclosed a case of severely advanced periodontal disease. At several teeth the destruction of the periodontal tissues had reached a level close to their apices. Tooth 15 exhibited a wide apico-marginal communication, all remaining molars exhibited furcation involvement of degree III. The overall plaque score was 92% and the corresponding bleeding on probing – BoP – score was 86%.

Treatment planning

Tooth 15 required immediate endodontic therapy, although the prognosis was very questionable. The root canal was debrided, widened and a calcium hydrox-

ide filling was placed. A clinical and radiographic examination 8 weeks later disclosed that no proper healing had occurred, the apico-marginal communication persisted and tooth 15 was extracted (Fig. 42-16). The severely involved mandibular molars (47, 46 and 37) as well as teeth 31 and 41 could not be maintained and were scheduled for extraction. Teeth 13, 26 and 27 were regarded as questionable from a treatment point of view. The remaining teeth in the maxilla and mandible could be maintained following periodontal therapy.

The prosthetic rehabilitation of the case was considered difficult but different options could be examined.

Alternative 1
A fixed, cross-arch bridge extending from tooth 13 (with cantilever in position 14) to tooth 26 (27) could have been considered, had the prognosis for tooth 13 been good. This particular tooth, however, was root filled, exhibited advanced marginal bone loss and was not regarded as a proper final abutment for a cross arch splint.

Alternative 2
A removable partial denture anchored with attachments to a fixed bridge extending from tooth 11 to 25. This would allow the extraction of the two questionable maxillary molars (26, 27).

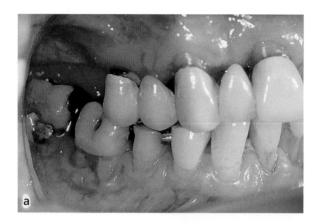
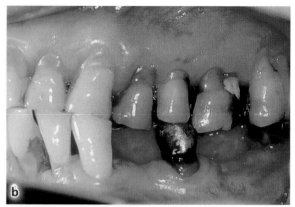
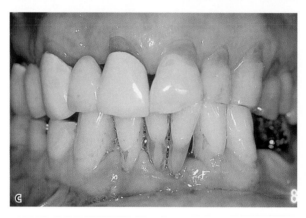

Fig. 42-13a-c.

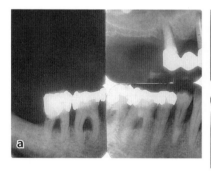
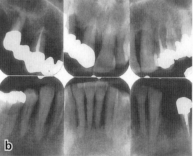
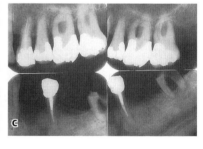

Fig. 42-14a-c.

Alternative 3

One implant-supported bridge distal of tooth 11, and one tooth-supported fixed bridge extending from 11 to 25 (alternatively to 26/27, provided that at least one root in this region could be maintained following furcation therapy and root resection).

Treatment

Initial therapy

The cause-related therapy included oral hygiene instruction and meticulous scaling and root planing. Teeth 15, 13, 47, 46, 31, 41 and 37 were extracted. A temporary fixed bridge extending from 11 to 27 was inserted (Fig. 42-17) and a removable partial denture was produced to restore function in the right maxilla. A temporary fixed bridge for the mandible extending

from 35 to 45 was also inserted. Teeth 26 and 27 were exposed to endodontic therapy.

Corrective therapy

A re-examination performed 3 months after the end of the initial therapy phase disclosed that the patient's self-performed plaque control was excellent. Although a marked pocket depth reduction had occurred, several deep pockets still existed. Flap surgery was performed in both the maxilla and mandible to get access for proper scaling and root planing. During surgery it was observed that all roots of 26 had to be removed, while the palatal root of 27 could be maintained. This root was subsequently fitted with a post.

Implant therapy

The edentulous region of the right maxilla was anesthetized. An incision, extending from region 11 to 16,

Case: L.F. male, 58 years   PLI: 92%   BoP: 86%

Periodontal charting

Tooth	Pocket depth M B D L	Furcation involvement	Tooth mobility
~~18~~			
~~17~~			
~~16~~			
15	6 _ 8 6		1
~~14~~			
13	8 _ 7 7		1
12			
11	8 _ 8 7		1
21	6 _ 6 6		
22	6 _ 8 6		
23	10 _ 8 8		
24	7 _ 5 8		
25	6 _ 7 6		
26	8 8 8 8	m,b,d: III	
~~27~~	9 8 10 4	m,b,d: III	
~~28~~			

Tooth	Pocket depth M B D L	Furcation involvement	Tooth mobility
~~48~~			
47	6 _ 6 6	III	
46	5 6 8 8	III	
45	6 _ 6 5		
44	8 _ 6 5		
43	8 _ 6 6		
42	6 _ 8 4		1
41	6 _ 6 4		3
31	6 _ 6 6		3
32	6 4 6 5		1
33	5 _ 4		
~~34~~			
35	4 _ 4		
~~36~~			
37	not probed		
~~38~~			

Diagnosis

	15	13	11	21	22	23	24	25	26	27
Gingivitis										
Parodontitis levis										
Parodontitis gravis	×	×	×	×	×	×	×	×	×	×
... et complicata	×	×				×			×	×

	47	46	45	44	43	42	41	31	32	33	35	37
Gingivitis												
Parodontitis levis			×							×	×	
Parodontitis gravis	×	×		×	×	×	×	×	×			×
... et complicata	×	×										×

Fig. 42-15.

was made at the top of the crest and full thickness flaps were raised. Three fixture sites were prepared in position 12, 13 and 15. Fixtures of the Astra Tech Implants® Dental System were installed; diameter = 3.5 mm; length = 13 mm (position 12), 15 mm (position 13), and 9 mm (position 15). Abutment connection was made 6 months later in a second stage procedure (Fig. 42-18).

Restorative therapy

A cross-arch bridge made of porcelain fused to gold was fabricated for the mandible. This bridge extended from 35 to 45 and had one cantilever unit distal to both 35 and 45.

In the maxilla, two bridges – porcelain fused to gold – were fabricated; one for the implant section and one for the tooth section (Fig. 42-19). The two bridges were connected with an attachment that allowed movement in apicocoronal direction but prevented horizontal deflection (Fig. 42-20). The restoration at the try-in appointment is illustrated in Fig. 42-21. The outcome

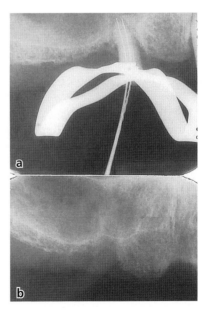

Fig. 42-16a,b.

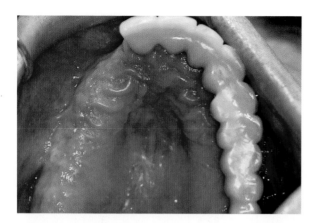

Fig. 42-17.

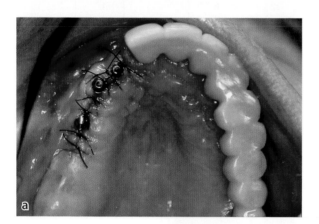

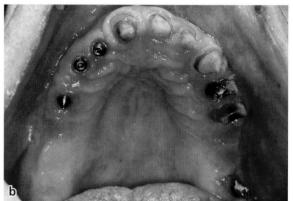

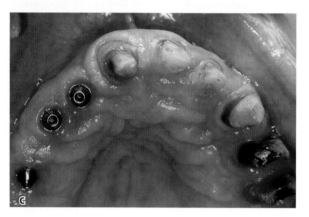

Fig. 42-18a-c.

of treatment is illustrated in clinical photographs and radiographs in Figs. 42-22 and 42-23.

Maintenance therapy

The supportive care included recall appointment with the dental hygienist every 3 months for plaque control evaluation and, if indicated, professional debridement at tooth sites exhibiting positive BoP values.

Concluding remarks

This case illustrates how implants can be (1) used to restore function in a periodontally compromised patient, (2) combined with a conventional bridge with an attachment that allows apicocoronal movement of the tooth-carrying segment but prevents horizontal deflection.

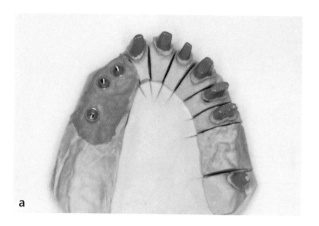
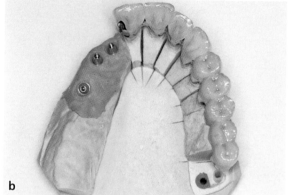
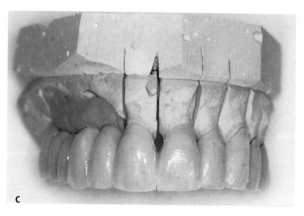

Fig. 42-19a-c.

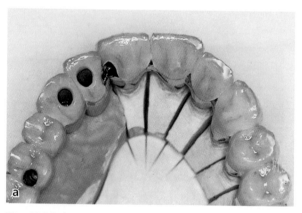
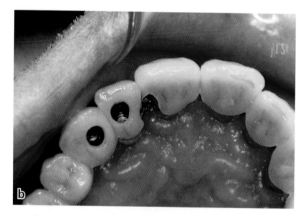

Fig. 42-20a,b.

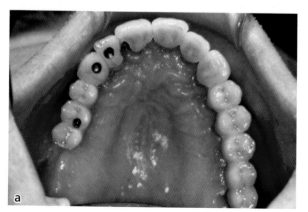
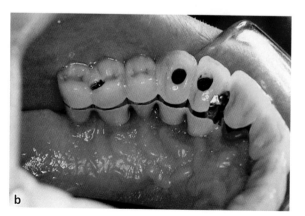

Fig. 42-21a,b.

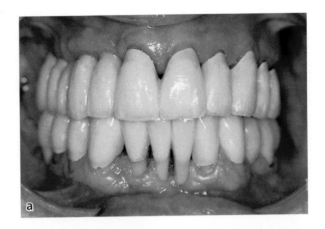

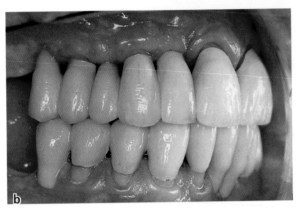

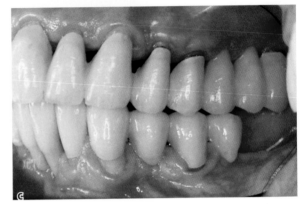

Fig. 42-22a-c.

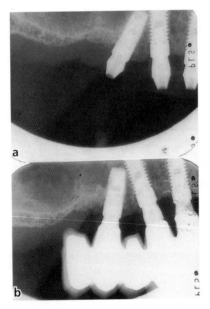

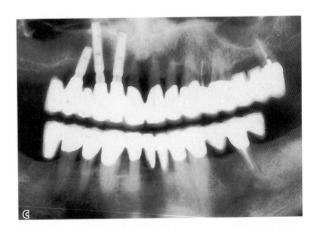

Fig. 42-23a-c.

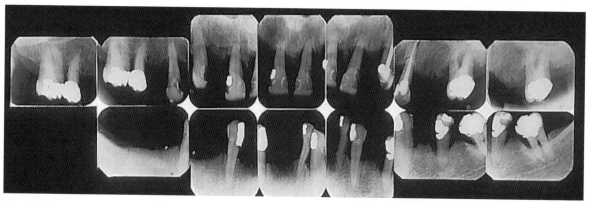

Fig. 42-24.

Case: L.T

Initial Examination: 751009

PLI: 100%   BoP: 100%

Periodontal charting

Tooth	Pocket depth M B D L	Furcation involvement	Tooth mobility
18			
17			
16	8 5 6	b1	
15	5 6 6		
14			
13	10 8 10		
12			
11	8 6 7		1
21	8 8 10		2
22			
23	6 6 9		
24			
25			
26			
27	10 8 8	m II, d II	2
28			

Tooth	Pocket depth M B D L	Furcation involvement	Tooth mobility
48			
47			
46			
45			
44			
43	4 6		1
42			
41			
31			
32	4		2
33	6 6 6		
34			
35	10 6 8		
36			
37	10 10 4 7	III	
38			

Fig. 42-25.

PATIENT 5
IMPLANTS USED TO SOLVE RESTORATIVE PROBLEMS OCCURRING DURING MAINTENANCE THERAPY

The periodontal condition of this 48-year-old man in 1975 is illustrated by the radiographs (Fig. 42-24), the measurements included in the periodontal chart (Fig. 42-25), and the clinical photograph (Fig. 42-26) from the examination of October 10. An analysis of the data from this examination disclosed a patient with advanced periodontal disease which at most teeth had progressed to a level where only the apical third, or less, of the roots had remaining periodontal tissue support.

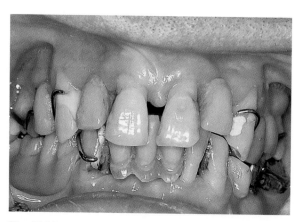

Fig. 42-26.

Treatment planning

Following careful planning of the treatment it was decided that (1) initially no teeth had to be removed; (2) several teeth were questionable, i.e. 13, 11, 21, 23, 27 as well as 35 and 37; (3) teeth 16, 15 as well as 33,

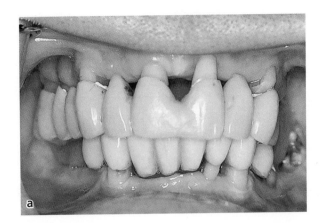

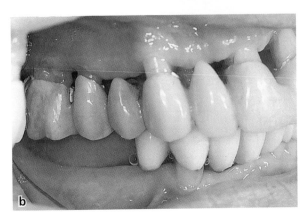

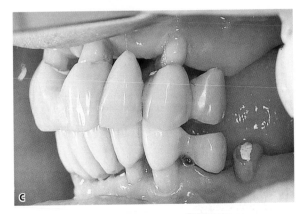

Fig. 42-27a-c.

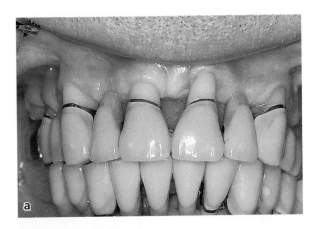

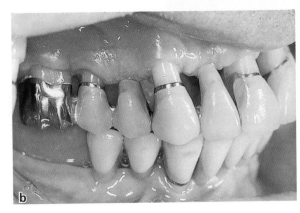

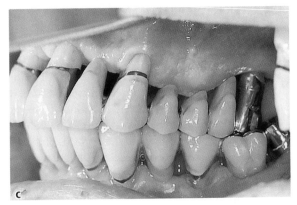

Fig. 42-28a-c.

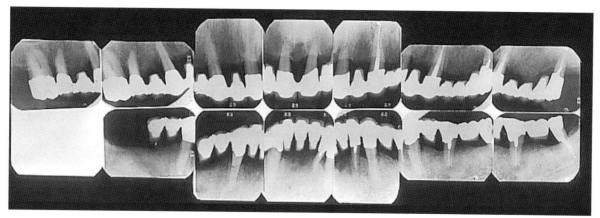

Fig. 42-29.

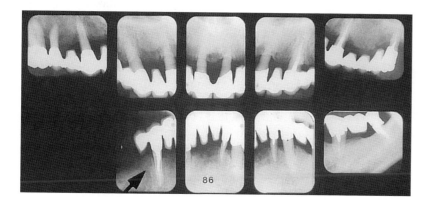

Fig. 42-30.

32, 43 could be maintained; (4) the patient should after the completion of periodontal therapy be restored with fixed cross-arch splints in the maxilla and mandible.

Treatment (1)

Following case presentation and oral hygiene instruction, temporary bridges were prepared for both the maxilla and mandible. The maxillary bridge extended from 16 to 24, and the mandibular bridge from 44 to 34 (Figs. 42-27a-c). Teeth 27, 35 and 37 were subjected to endodontic therapy.

Mucoperiosteal flaps were elevated, the root surfaces were carefully debrided and planed. Root separation and hemisection was performed at 27 and 37. After 6 months of healing, permanent restorations were inserted (Figs. 42-28a-c and 42-29). Note that the mandibular bridge was designed with two cantilever units in the 4th quadrant (for details regarding the design of the occlusion and the cantilever extension see Chapter 41).

The patient was enrolled in a maintenance care program which included recall visits (1) once every 3 months to the dental hygienist and (2) once a year to the dentist.

During a 9-year interval no sign of recurrent periodontal disease was observed.

In 1984, an acute marginal abscess originating from a periapical lesion occurred at tooth 43. Endodontic

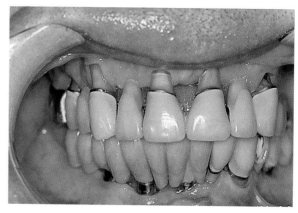

Fig. 42-31.

therapy was performed, the lesion was resolved, a post was placed in 43, and the most distal cantilever unit (45) was removed. Two years later, in 1986, the root of tooth 43 exhibited a long fracture and was extracted (Fig. 42-30). The bridge in the mandible had to be separated mesial of tooth 32. The abutments available in the mandible were 32, 33, 35 and the distal root of 37.

Two treatment alternatives were possible at this interval:

1. Removable partial denture
2. Implant-supported fixed bridge in quadrant 4.

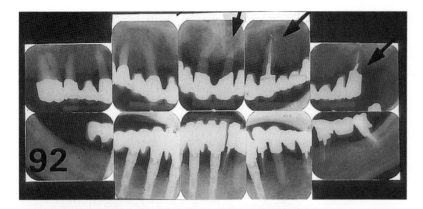

Fig. 42-32.

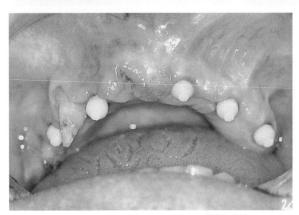

Fig. 42-33.

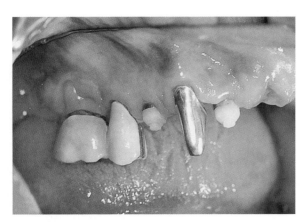

Fig. 42-34.

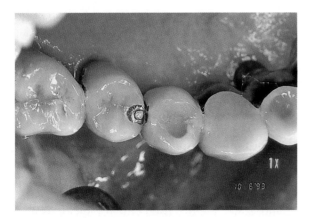

Fig. 42-35.

Treatment (2)

Three fixtures a.m. Brånemark (Brånemark System® Nobel Biocare) were placed in the area between the foramen mentale in quadrant 4 and the lateral incisor (32) in quadrant 3. Four months later a fixed bridge was connected to the implants (Fig. 42-31). This restoration extended from 45 to 31.

The installation of the implant-retained bridge apparently resulted in an altered occlusion and a force distribution (and magnitude) which – despite repeated occlusal adjustment – caused an increasing mobility (arrows) of the left segment of the maxillary splint. This condition is illustrated in a radiograph in Fig. 42-32, which was obtained in 1992.

Treatment (3)

At this time interval teeth 11, 21 and the palatal root of 27 could no longer be maintained and were extracted. Only teeth 16, 15 and 13 could be maintained in the maxilla.

Implants were placed in positions 14, 12, 21 23 and 25 (Fig. 42-33). Following 6 months of healing, abutment connection was performed. A two-unit bridge was placed on 16 and 15. This bridge was designed with a mesial sliding attachment (Fig. 42-34). Tooth 13 was fitted with an inner crown (Fig. 42-34). An implant-supported bridge extending from position 14 to 26 (including 13 as a telescoping unit) was inserted and connected to the bridge on 16/15 via the attachment (Figs. 42-35 and 42-36). Figs. 42-37 and 42-38a-c illustrate the clinical and radiographical appearance 3 years after treatment (3).

Concluding remarks

This case demonstrates that during the course of a "successful" maintenance care program unexpected and unanticipated problems may occur. This particular patient honored all recall visits, and the dentist and dental hygienist consistently carried out proper supportive care measures. The vitality of the pulp of tooth 43 was lost – reason unknown – the tooth was root filled through the restoration and a post placed. This

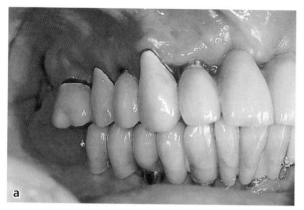

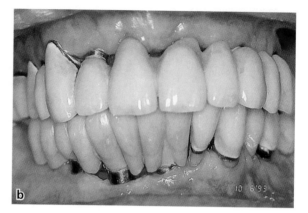

Fig. 42-36.

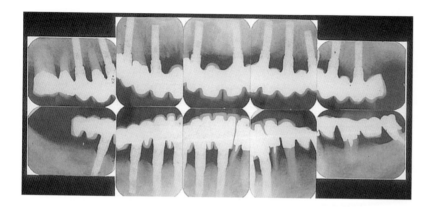

Fig. 42-37.

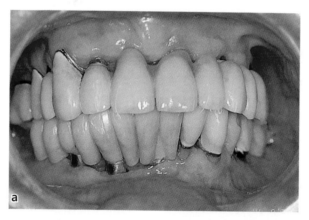

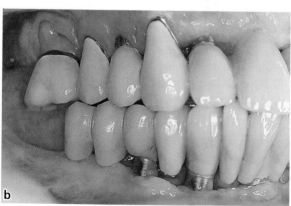

Fig. 42-38a-c.

obviously compromised the support and retention for the bridge in the mandible and a situation developed which eventually resulted in a long fracture of this distal endabutment (43). Implant treatment was used as an alternative to a removable partial denture. An implant-supported bridge – ankylotic – now occluded

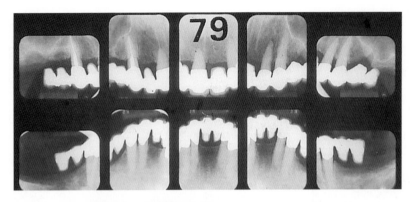

Fig. 42-39.

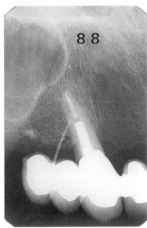

Fig. 42-40.

against a tooth-supported maxillary splint with compromised abutments. The forces elicited during occlusion were difficult to control and eventually jeopardized the stability of the maxillary splint.

PATIENT 6
IMPLANTS USED TO SOLVE PROBLEMS ASSOCIATED WITH ACCIDENTAL ROOT FRACTURES OF IMPORTANT ABUTMENT TEETH

Initial examination

Following proper periodontal treatment of this 57-year-old woman in 1976, only four teeth could be maintained in the maxilla, i.e. 13, 11, 22 and 23. These two teeth were used as abutments for a fixed cross-arch bridge extending from 15 to 25. In the mandible the teeth 43, 42, 32 and 33 were maintained and used as abutments for a fixed bridge extending from 45 to 35. In both the maxillary and mandibular restorations, two cantilever units were placed on each side of the

midline. The condition, 3 years following initial therapy (i.e. in 1979), is illustrated by the radiographs shown in Fig. 42-39.

Following this treatment the patient was placed in a maintenance care program which called for appointments with the dental hygienist once every 3 months and with the dentist once a year.

After 10 years of supportive dental care, the retention of the bridge at tooth 13 was lost due to a compromised cement lock. The bridge was removed. A new post was placed in 13 and a new bridge inserted. This bridge had an extension identical to that of the original one.

After another 2 years (i.e. 1988) a marginal abscess occurred at the distal/palatal aspect of 13. Note in Fig. 42-40 the gutta-percha point that was inserted in the lesion. After flap elevation, a fracture could be identified in the root of 13; the tooth was subsequently removed.

Treatment planning and treatment

At this stage, 11, 22 and 23 were available as abutments. The bridge was separated distal of tooth 11 and four fixtures (Brånemark® System, Nobel Biocare) were inserted in positions 16, 15, 13 and 12. After 6 months of healing, abutment connection was performed, and a six-unit implant-supported bridge, extending from position 17 to position 12, was fabricated and attached to the implant pillars (Figs. 42-41 and 42-42).

Following this treatment the patient was again placed in the maintenance care program.

Figs. 42-43 and 42-44a,b demonstrate the clinical and radiographic appearance of the resonstruction 20 years following initial therapy.

Concluding remarks

This case illustrates how implants can be used to solve difficult problems in patients who during a maintenance care program experience unexpected tooth loss.

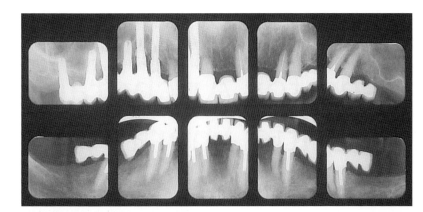

Fig. 42-41.

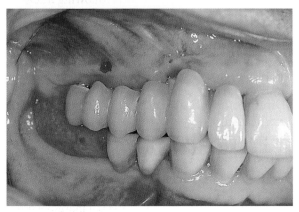

Fig. 42-42.

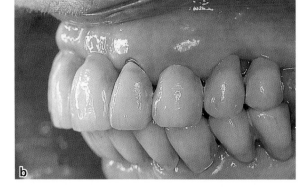

Fig. 42-43.

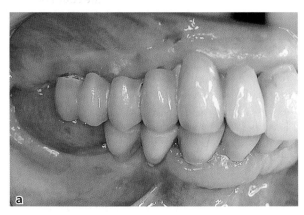

Fig. 42-44a,b.

CHAPTER 43

Implants Used for Anchorage in Orthodontic Therapy

HEINER WEHRBEIN

Implants for orthodontic anchorage

Orthodontic-prosthetic implant anchorage (OPIA)

Orthodontic implant anchorage (OIA)

Direct and indirect orthodontic implant anchorage

Palatal orthodontic implant anchors

Anchorage is a fundamental problem in the treatment of dental and skeletal dysgnathia. The loading of the anchorage unit is based on conditions of static equilibrium (action = reaction) as defined by Newton as long ago as 1687 (cf. Diedrich 1993).

If teeth are used for anchorage purposes, their reactive load with respect to quantity, direction, type and duration is yielded by the forces and moments applied through the orthodontic biomechanics for the active tooth movements. This problem has to be taken into account in any anchorage planning. If the periodontal anchorage potential is inadequate with respect to the treatment goal, additional intraoral and/or extraoral anchorage aids may be needed if negative side effects are to be avoided (Diedrich 1993).

Additional anchorage aids such as headgear and intermaxillary elastics are, however, characterized by potential disadvantages: visibility, compliance dependence, and the risk of undesirable side effects. Intraoral anchorage aids such as Class II elastics are not visible but are also compliance-dependent and may be accompanied by certain side effects: tipping of the occlusal plane, protrusion of mandibular incisors, and extrusion of teeth.

The aim of this chapter is to demonstrate and discuss how implants as positionally stable, intraoral (invisible) and compliance-independent anchorage units may be integrated into orthodontic treatment tasks, with some of the disadvantages listed above being avoided.

IMPLANTS FOR ORTHODONTIC ANCHORAGE

Case reports and prospective clinical studies as well as experiments on animals have shown that osseointegrated implants remain positionally stable under orthodontic and even orthopedic loading conditions (e.g. Linkow 1970, Turley et al. 1980, 1988, Roberts et al. 1984, 1990a,b, Ödman et al. 1988, 1994, Shapiro & Kokich 1988, Van Roeckel 1989, Haanaes et al. 1991, Wehrbein & Diedrich 1993, Wehrbein 1994, De Pauw et al. 1999, Majzoub et al. 1999, Wehrbein et al. 1999a,b). They can thus be used as orthodontic anchorage elements as well as anchors for orthopedic treatment tasks in the maxillofacial complex.

From the clinical standpoint it is of some relevance whether implants are used only temporarily as orthodontic anchorage elements for the correction of a malocclusion, and subsequently as abutments to support a fixed prosthetic appliance (orthodontic-prosthetic implant anchorage (OPIA)), or whether they are to function exclusively as orthodontic anchorage elements (orthodontic implant anchorage (OIA)). These aspects determine factors such as insertion site and implant type and dimension, as well as the type of orthodontic implant anchorage.

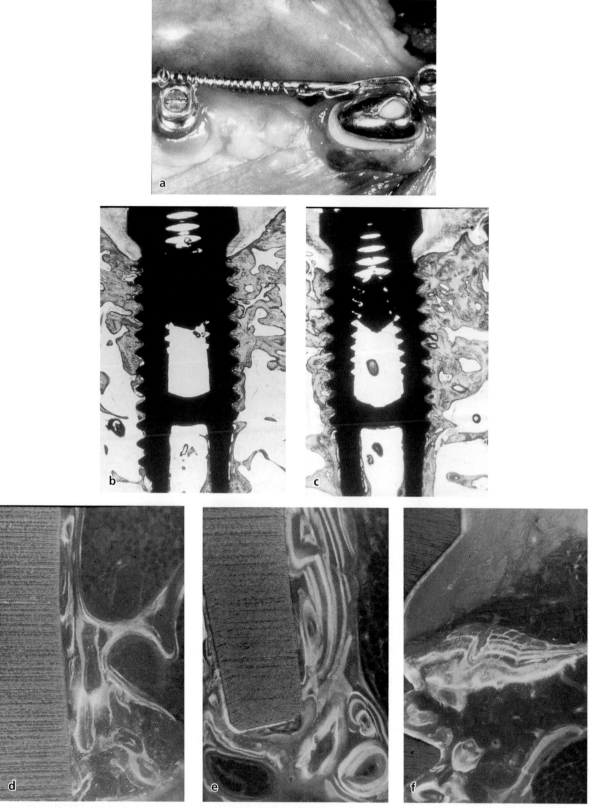

Fig. 43-1. (a) Osseointegrated prosthetic implant (Brånemark, length 10 mm) used as orthodontic anchor to distalize premolars in an experimental study in dogs. Horizontal loading of 2 N for 26 weeks. (b,c) Histologic sections (staining: toluidine blue, original magnification × 2, orientation: sagittal plane) of a non-loaded control (b) and loaded test implant (c). The test implant reveals a broader peri-implant hard tissue casing. (d,e) Fluorescent micrographs (× 25) from the apical part of the control (d) and the test implant (e). Note the higher remodeling activity and the multiple bony apposition lines at the test implant. (f) Fluorescent micrograph (× 25) from the marginal bone (pressure side) of a test implant. Note the multiple bony apposition lines adjacent to the implant. Such an amount of apposition was not detected in any of the controls (material from the study by Wehrbein & Diedrich 1993).

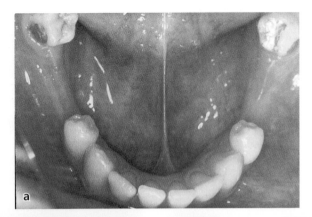

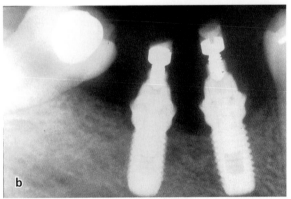
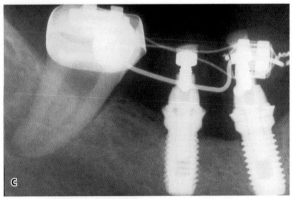

Fig. 43-2. Orthodontic-prosthetic implant anchorage. (a) Bilaterally missing P2, M1 and M2. Both M3 are tipped to mesial. Radiograph (b) before and (c) after uprighting. Uprighting was done by moving the molar root mesially through the bone. This type of uprighting needs high-capacity anchorage units. The advantage of using implants as anchors is that the anterior dentition is not loaded for anchorage purposes, therefore side effects such as protrusion of the anterior teeth are avoided.

ORTHODONTIC-PROSTHETIC IMPLANT ANCHORAGE (OPIA)

In the OPIA technique, the insertion site is determined fundamentally by the subsequent use of the implant as a prosthetic abutment. For this reason conventional prosthetic implants are inserted into the alveolar part of the mandible or the maxilla. However, the number of implants and their position within the alveolar process have to be selected with reference to prospective aspects, i.e. the position of the teeth after orthodontic treatment is dictated by the number of implants and their position. It may be helpful in this context to prepare a preimplantologic set-up.

For OPIA, an orthodontic attachment such as a bracket or band is fixed at the provisional crown or prefabricated bonding bases. The orthodontic force system acts at the superstructure of the implant. The reactive moments and forces applied in moving teeth are thus transmitted directly to the implant and its surrounding bone. Biomechanically speaking, this is a direct implant anchorage type.

Potential peri-implant reactions/orthodontic load

As occlusal loading conditions are not comparable to orthodontic loading conditions, it is important to know what effects long-term orthodontic loading conditions (e.g. magnitude of loading: up to 5 N; type of loading: continuous; duration of loading: more than 6 months; loading directions: intrusive/extrusive horizontally as well as rotational) may have on the peri-implant bone. This question is of special interest because the orthodontic load should not have a negative impact on the peri-implant bone and as such impair the long-term prognosis of the implant as a prosthetic abutment. In an experimental study, Wehrbein & Diedrich (1993) investigated the positional stability and the effect of long-term orthodontic loading on the peri-implant bone of osseointegrated prosthetic implants (titanium screws, length: 10 mm). The orthodontically loaded test implants were compared with non-loaded controls after a 26-week implant loading period with horizontally acting continuous forces of 2 N. The findings were positional stability and maintenance of osseointegration of loaded implants. In comparison with the control implants, some test implants revealed a broader peri-implant hard tissue fraction and marginal bone apposition (Fig. 43-1). Analysis of bone labeling fluorochromes documented that bone apposition took place in the orthodontic loading period, as bone markers were administered exclusively in that period. These results suggest that long-term orthodontic loading may induce endosseous and even marginal hard tissue apposition. The latter was also observed by Majzoub et al. (1999) at the pressure surfaces of orthodontically loaded osseointegrated short implants in a short-term trial (8 weeks of continuous horizontal loading with around 1.5 N). So far, no negative effects of orthodontic loading on the peri-implant bone of osseointegrated prosthetic implants are known.

Indications for orthodontic-prosthetic implant anchorage

Orthodontic-prosthetic implant anchorage may be indicated in the partially edentulous patient with, for example:

- malpositioned anterior teeth and either unilateral or bilateral free-end situations, or
- malpositioned anterior or posterior teeth in association with edentulous spaces (gaps of two or more missing teeth), most frequently in the posterior mandible or maxilla.

Fig. 43-2 gives an example of how prosthetic implants may be used for orthodontic anchorage purposes before serving as abutments for a fixed oral rehabilitation.

Age and orthodontic-prosthetic implant anchorage

Implants should not be inserted into the alveolar bone before the completion of growth, because they impair the development of the surrounding bone and even that of adjacent teeth (Ödman et al. 1991, Thilander et al. 1994). In clinical terms, early implant placement will lead to infraocclusion of the implant and adjacent teeth with development of an open bite.

ORTHODONTIC IMPLANT ANCHORAGE (OIA)

With respect to the insertion site, implant dimension, biomechanical type of implant anchorage and duration of use, there are fundamental differences between OPIA and exclusively OIA.

Insertion sites

Since regular orthodontic patients have a full dentition or extraction sites to be closed, no edentulous alveolar bone section is available for insertion of a prosthetic implant. Therefore, orthodontic implant anchors have to be inserted into other topographical regions.

The following insertion sites have been described:

- the interradicular septum (e.g. Bousquet et al. 1996, Kanomi 1997)
- the supra-apical and infra-zygomatical area (e.g. Kanomi 1997, Costa et al. 1998)
- the retromolar area in the mandible (Roberts et al. 1990b, Higuchi & Slack 1991)
- the median or paramedian anterior palate (Triaca et al. 1992, Block & Hoffman 1995, Hoffman 1995, Glatzmaier et al. 1996, Wehrbein et al. 1996, 1999b).

Fig. 43-3 presents some insertion sites of orthodontic implant anchors in patients and a histologic section of the median and paramedian region of the anterior part of the palate.

Implant designs and dimensions

As the insertion sites listed above have significantly less vertical or horizontal supporting bone than the alveolar bone, orthodontic implant anchors differ from prosthetic implants in their design and dimension. Depending on the insertion site, length-reduced and/or diameter-reduced implants (e.g. length < 6 mm; diameter < 2 mm) are essential if adjacent anatomical structures are not to be violated.

As diameter-reduced orthodontic implant anchors, titanium pins (Bousquet et al. 1996) and titanium mini-screws (Kanomi 1997, Costa et al. 1998) have been described. Various types of length-reduced orthodontic implant anchors have been used:

- titanium flat screw (Triaca et al. 1992)
- resorbable orthodontic implant anchor (Glatzmaier et al. 1996)
- T-shaped orthodontic implant (Wehrbein et al. 1996, 1999b).

The onplant described by Block and Hoffman (1995) and by Hoffman (1995) has a special status. In view of its design principle, this fixture is not an endosseous implant but a subperiosteal orthodontic anchorage element.

Aspects relating to the use of orthodontic implant anchors

In addition to their diameter-reduced and length-reduced characteristics, orthodontic anchorage implants should still fulfill the following requirements: positional stability despite their small dimensions, minimum strain on the patient, reliable fixation of orthodontic wires, and anchorage facilities for many types of tooth movement with one implant.

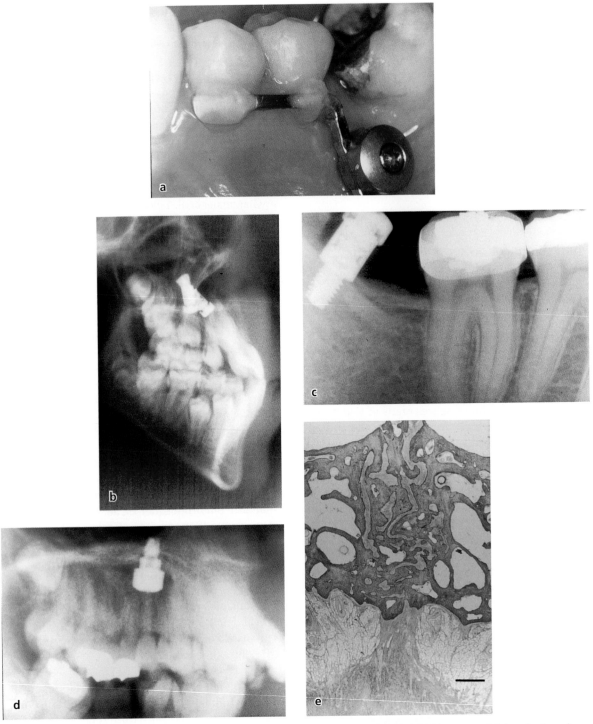

Fig. 43-3. Potential insertion sites for orthodontic/orthopedic implant anchorage. (a) Transseptal (alveolar bone) area to reinforce the premolars for molar uprighting. (b) Intrazygomatical area to protract the maxilla (radiograph). (c) Retromolar area to distalize molars (radiograph). (d) Palate to retract and intrude incisors and canines (radiograph). (e) Transversal histologic section of the median palate from a 40-year-old male. At the center of the figure, the suture is seen to be penetrating through the bone from the nasal to the oral surface. In the broad median suture zone, the bone is relatively dense as compared to the more paramedian regions. Therefore, this is the area of choice for palatal orthodontic implant placement in adults. Staining: toluidine blue, bar 1000 μ.

Positional stability/small dimension

Despite their small dimensions, orthodontic implant anchors must maintain positional stability under orthodontic loading. As connective tissue encapsulation would initiate implant dislocation, osseointegration is vital. Histologic examination of explanted human orthodontic implant bone specimens with Orthosystem® implants (length 4 or 6 mm) inserted palatally, in the retromolar area of the mandible or the infrazygomatic region, revealed that osseointegration was maintained during long-term orthodontic and orthopedic loading under clinical conditions. The percentage of implant-to-bone contact at the removed implants in patients was between 34% and 93% with an average of 75% (Wehrbein et al. 1998, 1999b).

Minimizing strain on patients
Strain on patients can be *minimized* during *implantation and/or explantation* by applying an atraumatic surgical technique (Fig. 43-4). Using a mucosal punch during insertion or a standardized system-compatible trephine during explantation permits surgical interventions involving both hard and soft tissues to be minimized (Feifel et al. 1998, Bernhard et al. 2000) (Fig. 43-4c). As no findings on "sleeping orthodontic implants" have been published to date, orthodontic anchorage implants should be retrieved after use. In a prospective clinical-radiological study, palatal implant anchorage reinforcement was investigated in nine adult patients (Wehrbein et al. 1999a), with the surgeon applying the atraumatic implantation and explantation procedure specified above. Following insertion, five of the nine patients reported no postoperative pain, while four required 1-2 paracetamol tablets to achieve total postoperative painlessness. All implants were successfully osseointegrated and had to be retrieved after orthodontic treatment. Primary wound healing after retrieval was observed in eight patients. No postoperative bleeding or other complications were recorded in these patients. In one of the nine patients secondary wound healing was observed. Two weeks after local treatment the bone defect had healed.

Attachment of orthodontic wires
Reliable three-dimensional attachment of orthodontic wires at the orthodontic implant is of major clinical relevance when the indirect implant anchorage system is to be applied (e.g. Wehrbein et al. 1996a, Wehrbein & Merz 1998a). The underlying principle is that the orthodontic force systems are applied at anchorage teeth which are not to be moved and which are kept in position through a rigid connection with the implant (e.g. transpalatal arch or lingual arch). Three-dimensional attachment of the orthodontic wires to the implant may be guaranteed by using a clamping cap or a welding and soldering cap (Figs. 43-4d,g).

In the case of indirect implant anchorage, the connecting element between implant and anchorage teeth is of crucial significance. Besides offering reliable fixing of the connecting element to the implant abutment, the connecting element itself must be sufficiently rigid to prevent deflection. With .032 × .032" stainless steel TPAs, a mean anchorage loss of about 1 mm was registered in the retraction or in the torquing of incisors to the buccal teeth (Wehrbein et al. 1999). Although this anchorage loss was clinically irrelevant, the use of thicker wires (.051 × .051" = 1.2 × 1.2 mm; Figs. 43-4d,g) is recommended. Other TPA configurations may further reduce the deformation of the connecting element.

DIRECT AND INDIRECT ORTHODONTIC IMPLANT ANCHORAGE

Comprehensive anchorage facilities using one single orthodontic implant anchor for many different types and directions of active orthodontic tooth movement during the same treatment can be achieved only by the indirect implant anchorage method. This is due to the anchorage teeth being supported by the implant, so that conventional intra-arch appliance designs allowing many different types and directions of orthodontic tooth movement may be used. However, a connecting element (e.g. transpalatal arch) is mandatory if any benefit is to be derived from these practical advantages.

As the force systems act between the teeth to be moved and the implant(s) in direct orthodontic implant anchorage, the types and directions of active tooth movement are somewhat limited with one implant. As the implant position determines the direction of potential tooth movements, the implants have sometimes to be positioned in topographical areas such as the infrazygomatic or infranasal bone (e.g. Costa et al. 1998). In this context the risk of discomfort and infection in relation to different topographical areas and their specific soft tissue covering conditions have to be considered. Furthermore, the orthodontic force systems (e.g. coil springs) may run unfavorably and cause some discomfort. The restricted facilities of direct implant anchorage may, however, be extended by using lever arms.

Treatment schedule and anchorage facilities with palatal orthodontic implant anchors

Interdisciplinary treatment with palatal implant anchors using the indirect implant anchorage method most frequently runs as follows: evaluation of the vertical bone quantity in the lateral cephalogram (Wehrbein et al. 1999a), atraumatic implant insertion, 2-3 months of unloaded implant healing, impression taking for transpalatal arch construction, integration of the transpalatal arch, and start of orthodontic treatment. Depending on the treatment goal and schedule, different transpalatal arches may be necessary during one course of treatment in one and the same patient. Implant removal may be carried out during the orthodontic retention period. An overview of the possibilities of preoperative diagnosis and surgical procedures with three different implant systems used in the palate was presented by Bernard et al. (2000).

The treatment facilities involved in one single palatal implant anchor using the indirect anchorage method are relatively comprehensive: preparation of a stationary posterior anchorage unit to retract canines and incisors or to torque incisors. Using this method,

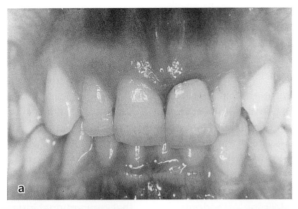

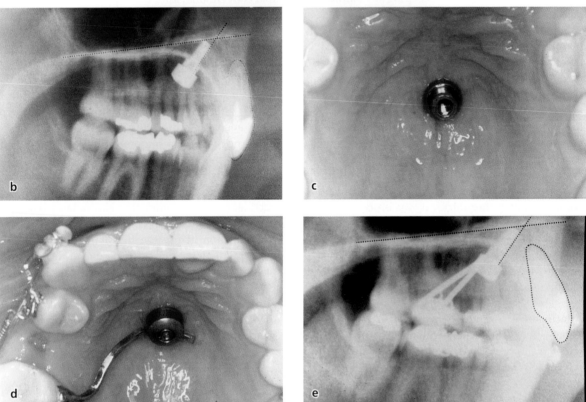

Fig. 43-4. Young woman with "impaired smile" and too much tooth display. Clinical findings: Class II of ¾ premolar width on the right side, nearly Class I on the left side; deep bite, retroinclined upper and lower incisors with upper and lower crowding and midline deviation (a). Treatment goal: extraction of tooth 15, midline correction in the maxilla (to the right), leveling, space closure and deep bite correction through pure incisor intrusion. Situation directly after atraumatic implant insertion using a punch for soft tissue removal (b,c). Three-month implant healing period, insertion of a unilateral palatal bar, and at start of orthodontic treatment (d). The TPA is three-dimensionally fixed with a clamping cap to the implant abutment; reduced orthodontic appliance in this treatment phase due to a stable osseous-periodontal anchorage unit (implant supported 16). Conventional orthodontics would require bonding of a large part of the dentition for anchorage purposes and wearing of Class II elastics or headgear to prevent mesial migration of 16. Cephalogram (e) after midline correction, deep bite treatment and superimposed tracings (f) from before orthodontic treatment, and after midline correction as well as deep bite treatment: significant incisor root torque and intrusion without extrusion of posterior teeth, normal overbite. Modified TPA now for preparation of an anterior implant-supported anchorage unit for residual space closure from distal (g). The TPA is welded to the abutment cap and bonded at the premolars. Occlusal view (h) and cephalogram (i) three months after implant removal: healed palatal mucosa in former insertion area; radiologically, the former osseous explantation cavity seems to be filled with bone (i). Frontal view after implant anchored orthodontic treatment (j): compare to initial finding (a). Differential (alternated) anchorage support of different teeth or tooth groups during different treatment phases by only one implant through TPA modification offers maximum treatment control and predictability without compliance.

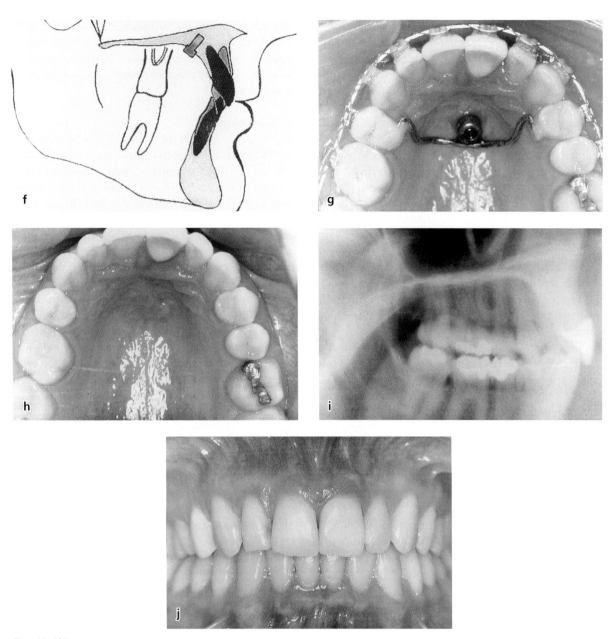

Fig. 43-4f-j.

deep bite can be corrected with incisor intrusion alone, with no posterior tooth extrusion. Furthermore, preparation of a stationary anterior anchorage unit can be used to mesialize, distalize or intrude posterior teeth (Fig. 43-4).

Periodontal considerations for orthodontic implant anchorage
It is clear that implant supported teeth receive continuous osseous reinforcement, with unfavorable jiggling forces on anchor teeth – as might be found with headgear or temporarily worn Class II elastics – being reduced or even avoided. This may play a more decisive role in cases where the periodontal anchorage potential is compromised (e.g. reduced attachment level due to periodontitis or other problems impairing the anchorage capacity of the remaining teeth). When direct orthodontic implant anchorage is used, no teeth are integrated into the anchorage unit.

Palatal implants in adolescents
The use of palatal implants in adult patients has been reported by various authors (e.g. Triaca et al. 1992, Wehrbein et al. 1996, 1999b, Bernard et al. 2000). When this technology is to be applied in adolescents, interactions with residual growth changes have to be reduced to a clinically irrelevant level. That may well be the case when the fully erupted teeth include the second molars. Furthermore, the implant should not be placed in the median but in the paramedian (parasutural) area of the anterior palate to prevent interactions with potential residual intermaxillary suture growth changes (transversal plane).

The most important maxillary growth changes, however, occur in the vertical plane through displacement and cortical drift. In specific areas, different mean amounts of growth from the age of four to adulthood were measured (Björk 1977): sutural lowering of the maxilla (displacement) by 11.2 mm, apposition at the orbit floor (drift) 6.4 mm, apposition at the infrazygomatic crest (displacement) 2.5 mm, resorptive lowering of the nasal floor (drift) 4.6 mm, and appositional increase of alveolar bone height 14.6 mm. If it is speculated that one third of these growth changes has still to be realized from the age of 12 to adulthood, then that implies a residual vertical growth of about 1.5 mm in the palate and of about 5 mm in the alveolar bone (both by drift). As an osseointegrated implant is not involved in the growth of its site because it behaves like an ankylosed tooth, a palatal implant would remain 1.5 mm behind its surrounding bone whereas an alveolar bone implant would produce an infraocclusion of 5 mm in the same time unit. Furthermore the time factor has to be considered. In comparison with an alveolar bone prosthetic implant, a palatal orthodontic implant remains *in situ* for only 1-2 years. Thus, potential growth impairment is likely to be limited to values of less than 1 mm.

First experiences with palatal implants in growing individuals aged 12 years or more, using the paramedian orthodontic implant placement technique, produced the following clinical and radiologic observations: implant stability, no clinically detectable growth impairment in the implant-surrounding bone of the palate and no tendency to implant submersion, but migration of the palatal complex with its implant to a more forward and downward position, probably due to the growth of more cranially located bony structures leading to displacement and drift.

At present, however, the use of palatal orthodontic implants in clinical practice should be confined to patients whose growth is completed or approaching completion, since no long-term results are available, e.g. effects on residual growth after implant removal.

Advantages

In addition to dispensing with compliance dependent intraoral and extraoral anchorage aids, some other advantages have to be discussed. If an anchorage unit is stable, its behavior can be controlled by the clinician and is no longer left to chance, so that the orthodontic treatment outcome is more predictable. Furthermore, a positionally stable anchorage unit allows en masse retraction to be performed without the risk of clinically significant anchorage loss. This may reduce the treatment time as compared with fractional retraction of canines and incisors. In some situations the orthodontic appliances can be reduced temporarily or for the whole treatment, enhancing the comfort of the orthodontic appliance as well as its esthetic appearance. Finally, a combination of palatal implant and lingual appliance conceals both the anchorage and the appliance.

Disadvantages

If they are to benefit from the above advantages, patients have to undergo two minor surgical procedures. The main risks of any orthodontic implant anchorage treatment are loss of the implant and peri-implant infection. The success rate of palatal orthodontic anchorage implants was investigated in a clinical-radiological study (Wehrbein et al. 2001). Each of the 22 adult patients enrolled in the study received one Orthosystem® implant (length 4 or 6 mm) in the median palate. Insertion was done by two experienced surgeons. In all patients primary stability was recorded. In 2 of the 22 patients mobility and subdued percussion sound were found at the 1-month control session. In the remaining 20 patients the fixtures underwent osseointegration and were used as orthodontic anchors. In the orthodontic loading period no loosening or positional changes of the implants were recorded. The success rate after the first insertion was thus 91%. In the two patients with implant loss, reinsertion was performed after a 2-month healing period, after which the implants osseointegrated and were positionally stable during the orthodontic treatment period.

Conclusions

Osseointegrated implants are a tool providing absolutely stable osseous orthodontic anchorage and are thus superior to any kind of tooth-borne anchorage facilities. Indications for orthodontic-prosthetic or purely orthodontic implant anchorage include: inadequate periodontal anchorage facilities, non-acceptance of extraoral anchorage aids, prevention of potential side effects of conventional intraoral anchorage aids, and esthetic aspects. Preconditions for a high acceptance of this promising, relatively new technology are: simplicity in use, minimum strain on patients, high success rate and reliability of the respective method under clinical conditions. This may be realized by a close interdisciplinary co-operation, and profound know-how in the fields of both implantology and orthodontics.

REFERENCES

Bernhard, T., Dörtbudak, O., Wehrbein, H., Baier, C., Bantleon, H-P. & Kucher, G. (2000). Das Gaumenimplantat. Informationen aus Orthodontie & Kieferorthopädie **32**, 209-229.

Björk, A. (1977). Growth of the maxilla in three dimensions as revealed radiographically by the implant method. *British Journal of Orthodontics* **4**, 53-64.

Block, M.S. & Hoffman, D.R. (1995). A new device for absolute anchorage for orthodontics. *American Journal of Orthodontics and Dentofacial Orthopedics* **3**, 251-258.

Bousquet, F., Bousquet, P., Mauran, G. & Parquel, P. (1996). Use of an impacted post for anchorage. *Journal of Clinical Orthodontics* **5**, 261-265.

Buser, D., Nydegger, T., Hirt, H.P., Cochran, D.L. & Nolte, L.P. (1998). Removal of torque values of titanium implants in the maxilla of miniature pigs. A direct comparison of sandblasted and acid-etched with machined and acid-etched screw implants. *International Journal of Oral and Maxillofacial Implants* **13**, 611-619.

Costa, A., Raffini, M. & Melsen, B. (1998). Miniscrews as orthodontic anchorage. A preliminary report. *International Journal of Adult Orthodontics and Orthognathic Surgery* **13**, 201-209.

De Pauw, G.A.M., Dermaut, L., De Bruin, H. & Johansson, C. (1999). Stability of implants as anchorage for orthopedic traction. *The Angle Orthodontist* **69**, 401- 407.

Diedrich, P. (1993). Verschiedene orthodontische Verankerungssysteme – eine kritische Betrachtung. *Fortschritte der Kieferorthopädie* **54**, 156-171.

Feifel, H., Wehrbein, H., Jänicke, S. & Riediger, R. (1998). Surgical experience with the Orthosystem, a new palatal implant for orthodontic anchorage. (Abstract) *Journal of Craniomaxillofacial Surgery* **26** (Suppl. 1), 90-91.

Glatzmaier, J., Wehrbein, H. & Diedrich, P. (1996). Biodegradable implants for orthodontic anchorage. A preliminary biomechanical study. *European Journal of Orthodontics* **18**, 465-469.

Haanaes, H.R., Stenvik, A., Beyer-Olson, E.S., Tryti, S. & Raehn, O. (1991). The efficacy of two-stage titanium implants as orthodontic anchorage in the preprosthodontic correction of third molars in adults – a report of three cases. *European Journal of Orthodontics* **13**, 287-296.

Higuchi, K.W. & Slack, J.M. (1991). The use of titanium fixtures for intraoral anchorage to facilitate orthodontic tooth movement. *International Journal of Maxillofacial Implants* **6**, 338-344.

Hoffman, D. (1995). Implants and Orthodontics. In: Block, M.S. & Kent, J.K., eds. *Endosseous implants for maxillofacial reconstruction.* Philadelphia, London, Toronto, Sydney, Tokyo: W.B. Saunders, pp. 382-399.

Kanomi, R. (1997). Mini-implants for orthodontic anchorage. *Journal of Clinical Orthodontics* **11**, 763-767.

Linkow, L.I. (1970). Implanto-orthodontics. *Journal of Clinical Orthodontics* **4**, 685-705.

Majzoub, Z., Finotti, M., Miotti, F., Giardino, R., Aldini, N.N. & Cordolini, G. (1999). Bone response to orthodontic loading of endosseous implants in the rabbit calvaria: early continuous distalizing forces. *European Journal of Orthodontics* **21**, 223-230.

Ödman, J., Gröndahl, K., Lekholm, U. & Thilander, B. (1991). The effect of osseointegrated implants on the dento-alveolar development. A clinical and radiological study in growing pigs. *European Journal of Orthodontics* **13**, 279-286.

Ödman, J., Lekholm, U., Jemt, T., Brånemark. P-I. & Thilander. B. (1988). Osseointegrated titanium implants – A new approach in orthodontic treatment. *European Journal of Orthodontics* **10**, 98-105.

Ödman, J., Lekholm, U., Jemt, T. & Thilander, B. (1994). Osseointegrated implants as orthodontic anchorage in treatment of partially edentulous adult patients. *European Journal of Orthodontics* **3**, 187-201.

Roberts, W.E., Helm, F.R., Marshal, K.J. & Gongloff, R.K. (1990a). Rigid endosseous implants for orthodontic and orthopedic anchorage. *The Angle Orthodontist* **59**, 247-256.

Roberts, W.E., Marshall, K.J. & Mozsary, P.G. (1990b). Rigid endosseous implant utilized as anchorage to protract molars and close an atrophic extraction site. *The Angle Orthodontist* **60**, 135-152.

Roberts, W.E., Smith, R.K., Silberman, Y., Mozsary, P-G. & Smith, R.S. (1984). Osseous adaptation to continuous loading of rigid endosseous implants. *American Journal of Orthodontics* **86**, 95-111.

Shapiro, P.A. & Kokich, V.G. (1988). Uses of implants in Orthodontics. *Dental Clinics of North America* **32**, 539-550.

Smalley, W., Shapiro, P.A., Hohl, T. & Kockich, V.G. (1988). Osseointegrated titanium implants for maxillofacial protraction. *American Journal of Orthodontics* **94**, 285-295.

Thilander, B., Ödman, J., Gröndahl, K. & Lekholm, U. (1994). Osseointegrated implants in adolescents. An alternative in replacing missing teeth? *European Journal of Orthodontics* **16**, 84-95.

Triaca, A., Antonini, M. & Wintermantel, E. (1992). Ein neues Titan-Flachschraubenimplantat zur Verankerung am anterioren Gaumen. *Informationen aus Orthodontie und Kieferorthopädie* **24**, 251-257.

Turley, P.K., Kean, C., Schnur, J., Stefanac, J., Gray, J., Hermes, J. & Poon, C. (1988). Orthodontic force application to titanium endosseous implants. *Angle Orthodontist* **58**, 151-162.

Turley, P.K., Shapiro, P.A. & Moffett, B.C. (1980). The loading of bioglass coated aluminium oxide implants to produce sutural expansion of the maxillary complex in pigtail (Macaca nemestrina). *Archives of Oral Biology* **25**, 459-469.

Van Roeckel, N.B. (1989). The use of Brånemark system implants for orthodontic anchorage. Report of a case. *International Journal of Oral and Maxillofacial Implants* **4**, 341-344.

Wehrbein, H. (1994). Enossale Titanimplantate als orthodontische Verankerungselemente. Experimentelle Untersuchungen und klinische Anwendung. *Fortschritte der Kieferorthopädie* **5**, 236-250.

Wehrbein, H. & Diedrich P. (1993). Endosseous titanium implants during and after orthodontic load – an experimental study in dog. *Clinical Oral Implants Research* **4**, 76-82.

Wehrbein, H., Feifel, H. & Diedrich, P. (1999b). Palatal implant anchorage reinforcement of posterior teeth. A prospective study. *American Journal of Orthodontics & Dentofacial Orthopedics* **116**, 678-686.

Wehrbein, H., Glatzmaier, J., Mundwiller, U. & Diedrich, P. (1996). The Orthosystem – a new implant system for orthodontic anchorage in the palate. *Journal of Orofacial Orthopedics* **57**, 142-153.

Wehrbein, H., Glatzmaier, J. & Yildirim, M. (1997). Anchorage capacity of short titanium screw implants in the maxilla. An experimental study in the dog. *Clinical Oral Implants Research* **8**, 131-141.

Wehrbein, H. & Merz, B.R. (1998). Aspects of the use of endosseous palatal implants in orthodontic therapy. *Journal of Esthetic Dentistry* **6**, 315-324.

Wehrbein, H., Merz, B.R. & Diedrich, P. (1999a). Palatal bone support for orthodontic implant anchorage reinforcement. A clinical and radiological study. *European Journal of Orthodontics* **27**, 65-70.

Wehrbein, H., Merz, B.R., Hämmerle, C.H.F. & Lang, P.N. (1998). Bone-to-implant contact of orthodontic implants in humans subjected to horizontal loading. *Clinical Oral Implants Research* **9**, 348-353.

Wehrbein, H., Moradi Sabzevar, M. & Diedrich, P. (2001). Success rate of palatal orthodontic implant anchors (Abstract). *European Journal of Orthodontics* **23**, 468.

Wilke, H.J., Claes, L. & Steinemann, S. (1990). The influence of various implant surfaces on the interface shear strength between implant and bone. In: Heinke, G., Soltesz, U. & Lee, A.J.C., eds. *Advances in Biomaterials.* Amsterdam: Elsevier Science Publishers.

CHAPTER 44

Mucositis and Peri-implantitis

TORD BERGLUNDH, JAN LINDHE, NIKLAUS P. LANG AND LISA MAYFIELD

Excessive load

Infection

Peri-implant mucositis

Peri-implantitis

Treatment of peri-implant tissue inflammation
　Resolution of the inflammatory lesion
　Re-osseointegration

Microbial aspects associated with implants in humans
　Microbial colonization

Failure sometimes happens in implant therapy. Such failures occur due to complications that take place either early following the installation of the implant device or later when the implant supported reconstruction has been in function for various periods of time.

Early implant failures are the result of events that may jeopardize or prevent osseointegration from occurring and include among others:

1. Improper preparation of the recipient site which results in undue hard tissue damage such as necrosis of the bone
2. Bacterial contamination and extensive inflammation of the wound that may delay healing of the soft and hard tissues
3. Improper mechanical stability of the implant following its insertion
4. Premature loading of the implant.

Late failures occur in situations during which osseointegration of a previously stable and properly functioning implant is lost. It was suggested (Proceedings of the 3rd European Workshop on Periodontology; Flemmig & Renvert (1999)) that such late failures are often the result of excessive load and/or infection.

EXCESSIVE LOAD

Forces applied to the restoration placed on implants are, at least in part, transferred to the bone (Skalak 1985). It is realized that although "excessive load" may be difficult to define and may vary from one subject

and site to the next, factors such as occlusal force (trauma from occlusion) in relation to (1) size of implant, (2) surface features of implant, and (3) quality of the host bone, must obviously be considered. Clinical studies have indicated that peri-implant bone loss may be associated with load (e.g. Lindquist et al. 1988, Sanz et al. 1991, Quirynen et al. 1992, Rangert et al. 1995). A few experimental studies have indicated that a relationship may exist between load and bone loss (e.g. Hoshaw et al. 1994, Isidor 1997, Miyata et al. 2000). But other investigators have been unable to confirm this association (e.g. Asikainen et al. 1997, Wehrbein et al. 1997, Hürzeler at al. 1998, Gotfredsen et al. 2001, 2002).

The peri-implant tissue response to excessive load released during function is thus not fully understood but may involve the bone tissue around the entire implant. The tissue in the zone of osseointegration is, due to the load, broken down and *implant mobility* becomes the cardinal feature.

INFECTION

The host response to biofilm formation on the implant includes a series of inflammatory reactions which initially occur in the soft tissue but which may subsequently progress and lead to loss of supporting bone. The tissue destruction in the bone compartment starts in the "marginal", i.e. neck region, of the implant and crater-like bone defects develop and become visible in the radiograph. Implant stability may be maintained for long periods of time.

Peri-implant mucositis is a term used to describe

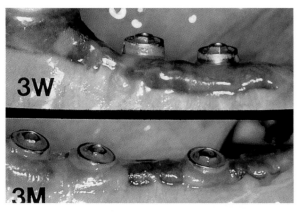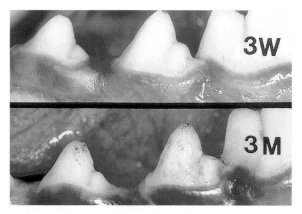

Fig. 44-1. A clinical view illustrating 3 weeks (3 W) and 3 months (3 M) of undisturbed plaque formation on the implants and the teeth of a beagle dog.

reversible inflammatory reactions in the mucosa adjacent to an implant. *Peri-implantitis* is defined as an inflammatory process that (1) affects the tissues around an osseointegrated implant in function, and (2) results in loss of supporting bone (Albrektsson & Isidor 1994).

The prevalence of *peri-implantitis* in man is difficult to estimate but may vary between 2% and 10% of all implants inserted (Esposito et al. 1998, Mombelli & Lang 1998). Clinical studies have documented that *peri-implantitis* may lead to implant failure and loss. Thus findings from, for example, a multicenter study by van Steenberge et al. (1993) including 159 patients and 558 implants (Brånemark system®) revealed that during the second and third year (1) as many as 2% of the remaining implants failed, and (2) failure occurred more frequently in subjects with a high degree of plaque accumulation. Weyant & Burt (1993) and Weyant (1994) reported data from 598 subjects and 2098 implants that were monitored during a 5-year period. The authors found that close to 4% of the implants failed and that risk factors for implant loss included plaque, smoking and local factors. Brägger et al. (2001) described biological and technical complications that may occur with fixed partial dentures placed on tooth abutments or implant abutments or on a combination of teeth and implants. This study included 85 patients and measurements were made on 142 teeth and 103 implants that supported a total of 116 fixed partial dentures. During the course of a follow-up period of about 5 years, ten (about 9%) implant sites (peri-implantitis) and six (about 4%) tooth sites (periodontitis) exhibited signs of advanced inflammation and tissue breakdown, i.e. bleeding on probing, suppuration and increased probing depth. Findings made in a 5-year retrospective study (Hardt et al. 2002) further demonstrated that implants placed in "periodontitis-susceptible" patients exhibited a higher failure rate (8%) than similar type implants that were placed in periodontally healthy subjects (3.3%). In this study it was also pointed out that the amount of bone loss that occurred around implants during the 5 years correlated well with the amount of bone loss that had occurred at the remaining teeth at the time of implant installation. The observations by Hardt et al. (2002) are important because they do indicate that similar mechanisms may be involved in periodontal and peri-implant tissue breakdown.

PERI-IMPLANT MUCOSITIS

The response of the gingiva and the peri-implant mucosa to early and more long-standing periods of plaque formation was analyzed both in experiments in animals and in studies in man.

In experiments in the dog, Berglundh et al. (1992) and Ericsson et al. (1992) compared the reaction of the gingiva and the peri-implant mucosa to 3 weeks and 3 months of *de novo* plaque formation. The mandibular premolars in one side of the mandible were extracted, leaving the premolars on the contralateral side as controls. After 3 months of healing, fixtures (Brånemark® system) were inserted and, another 3 months later, abutment connection was performed in a second-stage procedure. The animals were placed in a careful plaque control program to allow for ideal healing of the mucosa at the implants and to prevent gingivitis from occurring in the tooth segments of the dentition. Four months after abutment connection, the dogs were examined clinically and samples from the minute plaques that were present on the marginal portion of the implant and tooth surfaces were harvested. The plaque control program was terminated and the animals given a soft diet, which allowed gross plaque formation. Re-examinations, including clinical assessment (Fig. 44-1) and sampling of plaque bacteria from teeth and implants as well as biopsy, were performed after 3 weeks and 3 months.

During the course of the study, it was observed that similar amounts of plaque formed on the tooth and implant segments of the dog dentition. The composition of the two developing plaques was also similar. It was therefore concluded that early microbial coloni-

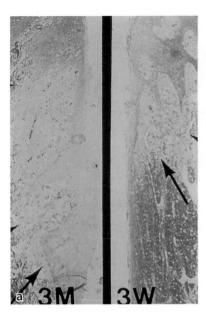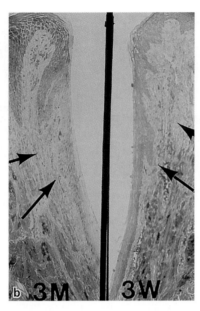

Fig. 44-2. Microphotographs illustrating the establishment of inflammatory cell infiltrates (ICT) in the peri-implant mucosa (a) and the gingiva (b) (3W = 3 weeks; 3M = 3 months). Note, in the microphotographs representing 3 months, the infiltrate in the peri-implant mucosa extends much deeper into the tissue than is the case in the gingiva.

zation on titanium implants followed the same patterns as that on teeth (Leonhardt et al. 1992).

Both the gingiva and the peri-implant mucosa responded to this microbial colonization with the establishment of overt inflammatory lesions, i.e. infiltrates of leukocytes in the connective tissue. The lesions in the gingiva and in the peri-implant mucosa were in this early phase (up to 3 weeks) matched both with respect to size and location. Hence, both lesions were consistently found in the "knee" between the keratinized oral epithelium and the junctional or barrier epithelium (Fig. 44-2a,b).

Similar observations were made by Pontoriero et al. (1994) in a clinical study in human volunteers. Twenty partially edentulous subjects who had been restored with implants in one or several segments of the dentition were asked to participate. After a baseline examination they refrained from all oral hygiene measures for 3 weeks. It was observed that plaque formation (amount and composition) and the soft tissue response to plaque, i.e. inflammation, developed in a similar manner in the tooth and implant segments.

Zitzmann et al. (2001) examined the tissue reaction to *de novo* plaque formation at implants and teeth in humans using immunohistochemical techniques. Twelve subjects with healthy periodontal and peri-implant conditions were asked to refrain from tooth/implant cleaning for a period of 3 weeks. Soft tissue biopsies were sampled at baseline and on day 21. It was demonstrated that plaque formation was associated with clinical signs of soft tissue inflammation. The lesions in the gingival and in the peri-implant mucosa increased in size in a similar manner during the 3 weeks of experiment. *In other words, in a given individual, the early soft tissue response to plaque seems to be similar in the mucosa at implants and in the gingiva of the teeth.*

With increasing duration of plaque build-up (3 months) in the dog model, the lesions in the peri-implant mucosa expanded more and progressed further

"apically" than was the case in the gingiva (Fig. 44-2a,b). The *composition* of the lesions in the two tissues, the gingiva and the peri-implant mucosa, differed mainly with respect to their content of fibroblasts. Thus, the lesion in the peri-implant mucosa was found to have a much smaller number of fibroblasts than the corresponding compartment in the gingiva.

It may be anticipated that in an inflammatory tissue lesion of long standing, periods of breakdown and periods of repair interchange. The gingival lesion in the dog model retained its size unchanged between 3 weeks and 3 months of plaque exposure. It is suggested, therefore, that in the gingival lesion, the amount of tissue destruction that occurred during a breakdown phase was more or less fully compensated by tissue build-up occurring during a subsequent phase of repair. In the lesion within the peri-implant mucosa, the tissue breakdown that occurred during the 3 months of plaque exposure was not fully recovered by reparative events. The small number of fibroblasts present in this particular lesion may simply have been unable to produce enough collagen and matrix during the reparative phase. This reduced build-up resulted in an additional propagation and spread of the inflammatory cell infiltrate in the peri-implant mucosa.

Conclusion

The peri-implant mucosa seems less effective than the gingiva in encapsulating plaque-associated lesions.

Peri-implantitis

In order to study the ability of the peri-implant mucosa to respond to more longstanding plaque exposure and to manage the associated inflammatory lesions, an experimental periodontitis/peri-implantitis model was developed in the dog (Lindhe et al. 1992)

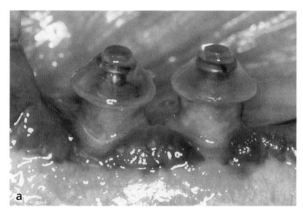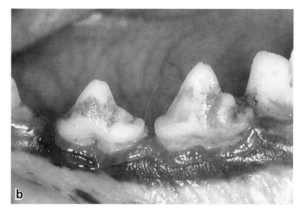

Fig. 44-3. (a) A clinical view describing features of experimental peri-implantitis in the beagle dog. (b) A clinical view describing features of experimental periodontitis in the beagle dog.

and in the monkey (Lang et al. 1993, Schou et al. 1993). Although the experiments had somewhat varying design, the outcome of the studies was almost identical and, hence, only the result from the dog model will be reported.

In the *dog model*, the premolars were extracted in one side of the mandible, fixtures (Brånemark system®) were inserted and abutment connection performed 3 months later as described above (Berglundh et al. 1991). During the healing phase a strict plaque control regimen was maintained and healthy tissue conditions were hereby established in all tooth and implant sites to be monitored.

On a given day, the periodontitis and peri-implantitis lesions were induced. This was accomplished by (1) terminating the plaque control regimen, and (2) placing cotton floss ligatures around the neck of both the premolar teeth and the implants. The ligatures were forced into a position apical of the soft tissue margins. A "pocket" between the tooth/gingiva and implant/mucosa was thereby created, a submarginal microbiota rapidly formed and inflammatory lesions developed in the neighboring tissues. Radiographs obtained after 6 weeks of experiment revealed that a substantial amount of bone tissue had been lost at both teeth and implant sites. The ligatures were removed. After another 4 weeks, the animals were re-examined (Fig. 44-3a,b), radiographs obtained, bacteria sampled and biopsies of tooth and implant sites harvested.

It was observed that the plaque that had formed in the deep "pockets" was similar at tooth and implant sites and was dominated by Gram-negative and anaerobic species (Leonhardt et al. 1992). This observation is consistent with findings indicating that in humans, the microbiota at teeth and implants has many features in common but also that the microbiota at healthy and diseased sites – tooth sites as well as implant sites – is very different. Thus, implants and teeth that are surrounded by healthy soft tissues are associated with biofilms including small amounts of Gram-positive coccoid cells and rods. Sites with extensive periodontal and peri-implant inflammation harbor biofilms with large numbers of Gram-negative anaerobic bacteria (for review see Mombelli 1999).

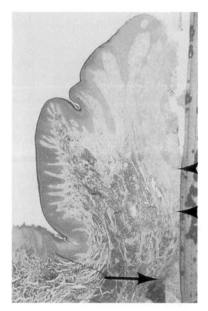

Fig. 44-4. Microphotograph (buccal/lingual section) illustrating the periodontitis lesion. Note the apical extension of the infiltrate (arrow) but also the presence of a zone of normal connective tissue between the infiltrate and the bone crest (arrow).

bor biofilms with large numbers of Gram-negative anaerobic bacteria (for review see Mombelli 1999).

The histopathologic examination of the biopsy samples from the dog study (Lindhe et al. 1992) revealed that there were marked differences in the size and location of the inflammatory lesions of the two sites. Thus, while the lesions in the periodontal sites (Fig. 44-4) were consistently separated from the alveolar bone by a zone, about 1 mm high, of non-inflamed connective tissue, the lesion in the peri-implant tissue in most situations extended into and involved the marrow spaces of the alveolar bone.

It was concluded that the pattern of spread of inflammation was different in periodontal and peri-implant tissues. The lesions in plaque-associated periodontitis were limited to the connective tissue, while in the peri-implant tissues the lesions involved, in addi-

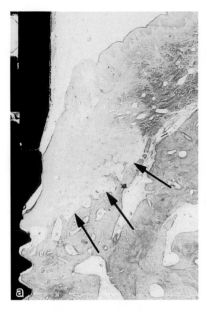
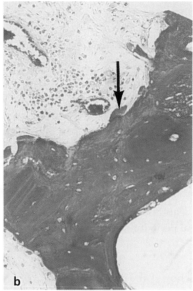

Fig. 44-5. (a) Ground section illustrating a peri-implantitis lesion. The implant is positioned to the left and the apical portions of the infiltrate (arrows) extend into contact with the bone. (b) Close up of (a) illustrating the presence of inflammatory cells and osteoclasts (arrow) on the bone surface.

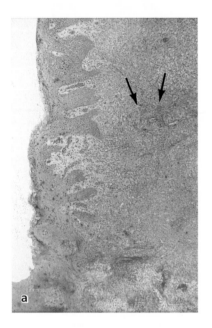
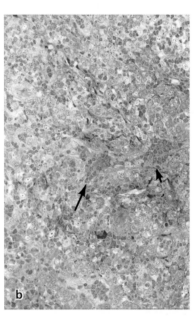

Fig. 44-6. Microphotograph illustrating a human peri-implantitis lesion. Note the large inflammatory infiltrate lateral to the pocket epithelium (a). The implant was positioned to the left. Arrows indicate vascular units illustrated in a larger magnification in (b).

tion, the alveolar bone (Fig. 44-5a,b). It was suggested that the peri-implant tissues, in variance with the periodontal tissues, are poorly organized to resolve progressive, plaque-associated lesions. In subsequent studies (Marinello et al. 1995, Ericsson et al 1996, Persson et al. 1996, Gotfredsen et al. 2002), using similar models but allowing for different periods of tissue breakdown, the validity of this conclusion was substantiated.

Histopathologic analyses of tissues sampled from peri-implantitis sites in humans revealed the presence of large inflammatory cell infiltrates in the mucosa. Sanz et al. (1991) analyzed soft tissue biopsies from six patients with peri-implantitis and reported that 65% of the connective tissue portion was occupied by an inflammatory cell infiltrate. Piattelli et al. (1998) described histopathologic characteristics of tissues from 230 retrieved implants. It was reported that at sites where implants were removed due to peri-implantitis, "an inflammatory infiltrate, composed of macro-

phages, lymphocytes and plasma-cells, was found in the connective tissue around the implants". In a study on human peri-implantitis lesions, Berglundh et al. (2003) found that the mucosa contained large lesions with numerous plasma cells, lymphocytes and macrophages (Fig. 44-6a,b). It was further demonstrated that the inflammatory cell infiltrate consistently extended to an area apical of the pocket epithelium and that the apical part of the soft lesion frequently reached the bone tissue. Berglundh et al. (2003) also observed that numerous PMN cells were present in the human peri-implantitis lesion. Such cells occurred not only in the pocket epithelium and associated areas of the lesions, but also in peri-vascular compartments distant from the implant surface. Further, in the apical part of the lesion the inflamed connective tissue appeared to be in direct contact with the biofilm on the implant surface. Gualini & Berglundh (2003) used immunohistochemical techniques to analyze the composition of lesions occurring in the peri-implant mucosa sampled

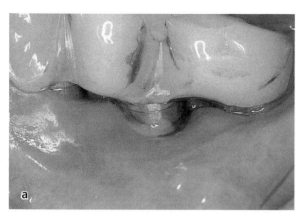
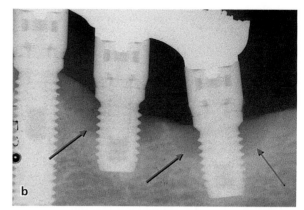

Fig. 44-7. Clinical (a) and radiographic (b) characteristics of two implant sites with peri-implantitis in the left side of the mandible. Note the presence of swelling and suppuration in the peri-implant mucosa (a) and the crater-formed bone destruction around the implants in the radiograph (arrows) (b).

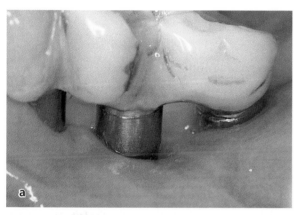
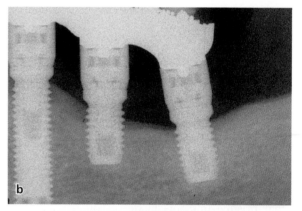

Fig. 44-8. Clinical and radiographic characteristics of the two implant sites illustrated in Fig. 42-7 at 6 months after treatment. Note the recession of the peri-implant mucosa (a) and the altered outline of the peri-implant bone (b).

from sites with peri-implantitis in six volunteers. The elastase marker, indicating PMN cells, was found in a large number of cells in the central portions of the infiltrate. This finding indicates a high PMN cell activity at sites with peri-implantitis and is in agreement with observations made by Hultin et al. (2002). They analyzed crevicular fluid that was sampled from implant sites in 17 patients with peri-implantitis and in 19 patients with "stable marginal tissue conditions". The authors found that sites with peri-implantitis had higher elastase activity and concentration of lactoferrin than control sites.

The findings described above – large numbers of neutrophils in the peri-implantitis lesion and the absence of an epithelial lining between the lesion and the biofilm – indicate that the peri-implantitis lesions have features that are different from those of periodontitis lesions.

Conclusion
Peri-implantitis lesions are poorly encapsulated, extend into the marginal bone tissue and may, if they are allowed to progress, lead to the loss of the implant. Symptoms of peri-implantitis relate to the infectious/inflammatory nature of the lesion. Thus, there

is radiographic evidence of bone loss and the bone loss consistently takes the shape of a crater. Swelling and redness of the mucosa as well as bleeding on gentle probing and suppuration frequently occur. The implant may remain stable over long periods.

TREATMENT OF PERI-IMPLANT TISSUE INFLAMMATION

Resolution of the inflammatory lesion

In dog experiments by Ericsson et al (1996) and Persson et al. (1996, 1999), peri-implantitis lesions were first produced according to the technique previously described (Lindhe et al. 1992). The peri-implantitis lesions were subsequently exposed to therapy. Thus, antibiotics (amoxicillin and metronidazole) were administered via the systemic route to the animals but local treatment was provided to only some of the diseased implant sites. Following several months of healing, it was observed that in implant sites also given local therapy, i.e. submarginal debridment, the inflammatory lesions were resolved. In implant sites not exposed to local debridement, however, the inflammatory infiltrate in the mucosa as well as in the bone tissue persisted.

These observations clearly demonstrate that a treatment regimen that is restricted to systemic administration of antibiotics is not effective in the management of peri-implantitis, but must always be combined with meticulous removal of the biofilm from the contaminated implant surface.

In this context it must be remembered that in the treatment of chronic periodontitis administration of systemic antibiotics but no local therapy (i.e. scaling and root planning) is an improper regimen. It will fail to resolve the inflammatory lesion in the gingiva and fail to arrest the further progression of tissue breakdown (Lindhe et al. 1983a,b, Berglundh et al. 1998).

Re-osseointegration

In the animal experiments it was noted that even though a combined systemic and local antimicrobial therapy successfully resolved the inflammatory lesion, this regimen failed to promote "re-osseointegration", i.e. the formation of new bone in contact with the previously contaminated titanium surface. It is likely that the biofilm that formed on the implant during the tissue breakdown phase altered the surface characteristics of the titanium body. It is well known that pristine implants made of commercially pure titanium are covered with a thin layer of titanium dioxide. This dioxide layer gives the implant a high surface energy that facilitates the interaction between the implant and the cells of the host tissues (Bair & Meyer 1988). Contamination of a titanium surface, however, markedly alters its characteristics. An implant with a low surface energy results. Such a surface may not allow tissue integration to occur but rather provokes a foreign body reaction (Bair & Meyer 1988, Sennerby & Lekholm 1993).

Different techniques have been proposed for a local therapy aimed at "re-juvenating" a once contaminated implant surface. Such techniques have included mechanical brushing of the surface, the use of air-powder abrasives, the application of chemicals such as citric acid, chlorhexidine and delmopinol (Persson et al. 1999, Wetzel et al. 1999). These local therapies were effective in cleaning the titanium surface and to allow soft tissue healing and bone fill in the defects, but only limited amounts of re-osseointegration occurred.

The techniques described above regarding treatment of peri-implantitis lesions including systemic antibiotics and local therapy (debridement and removal of granulation tissue) are apparently effective and have been utilized also in humans. Fig. 44-7a,b shows two implant sites with peri-implantitis in the left side of the mandible. The clinical and radiographic characteristics of the two implant sites at 6 months

after treatment (antibiotics and local therapy) are presented in Fig. 44-8a,b. The recession of the peri-implant mucosa is evident and probing at the two sites did not result in bleeding (a). Note the altered outline of the peri-implant bone in (b).

Conclusion

Current knowledge has documented that the use of antibacterial treatment procedures will effectively resolve the inflammatory component of the peri-implantitis lesions. Re-osseointegration to a once contaminated implant surface is difficult and the outcome of such regenerative procedures is difficult to predict.

MICROBIAL ASPECTS ASSOCIATED WITH IMPLANTS IN HUMANS

Microbial colonization

Successful implants

Biofilms consist of highly organized microcolonies of bacteria within a glycocalyx matrix. They form on all hard, non-shedding surfaces situated within an aqueous environment. Thus, a biofilm will readily form on the portion of an implant exposed to the oral cavity. The microbial colonization of titanium implants has been studied in humans using microscopy, culture techniques and DNA analysis.

Mombelli et al. (1988) investigated the early colonization of titanium implants placed in edentulous mandibles. The composition of the biofilm associated with healthy peri-implant tissues was established within 7 days of implantation. It consisted of mainly Gram-positive facultatively anaerobic rods and cocci, and showed no shifts in composition over time. Gram–negative anaerobic rods accounted for only a small proportion of the microflora. This microbiological profile associated with successful implants is similar to that found at periodontally healthy teeth and has been confirmed by others (Apse et al. 1989, Bower et al. 1989, Mombelli & Mericske-Stern 1990, Sordyl et al. 1995).

Peri-implant infections

The composition of the microflora associated with peri-implant infection is markedly different to that associated with successful implants. In overview, there is a transition from small quantities of plaque, predominantly Gram-positive cocci, with low proportions of Gram-negative species, to a larger amount of plaque with increased proportions of Gram-negative anaerobic and facultative anaerobic species (Rams & Link 1983, Rams et al. 1984, Mombelli et al. 1987, Alcoforado et al. 1991, George et al. 1994, Augthun & Conrads 1997, Salcetti et al. 1997). The microflora associated with peri-implantitis is similar to that associated with periodontal disease. Opportunistic periodontal pathogens such as *Actinobacillus actinomycetemcomitans*, *Porphyromonas gingivalis*, *Bacteroides forsythus*, *Prevotella intermedia*, *Peptostreptcoccus micros* and *Fusobacterium nucleatum* have been identified in association with peri-implantitis in partially edentulous patients (van Winkelhoff & Wolf 2000, van Winkelhoff et al. 2000).

In addition, microorganisms primarily not associated with periodontitis, such as *Staphylococcus* spp., enterics and *Candida* spp., have also been suggested to play a role in peri-implantitis (Rams et al. 1990, Alcoforado et al. 1991, Rosenberg et al. 1991, Leonhardt et al. 1999, Kronström et al. 2001).

There is evidence that potential pathogens identified around remaining teeth may colonize implants within 6 months of placement of implants (Apse et al. 1989, Quirynen & Listgarten 1990, Koka et al. 1993, Leonhardt et al. 1993, Kohavi et al. 1994, Mombelli et al. 1995, van Winkelhoff et al. 2000). Proliferation of these opportunistic pathogens results in an inflammatory response and may lead to peri-implant infection. This emphasizes the importance of the establishment of healthy periodontal conditions prior to placement of implants in partially edentulous patients, and the importance of a regular maintenance program thereafter.

Treatment of peri-implant infection
The goal of therapy is the suppression of the opportunistic pathogens associated with the infection, and the establishment of a local environment and microflora compatible with health. Treatment should begin with an infection control program including oral hygiene instruction, mechanical debridement and removal of the biofilm within the peri-implant pocket, and the regular application of an antimicrobial agent such as chlorhexidine gel or mouthrinse. In most cases of peri-implant mucositis this infection control regimen will be sufficient to reduce the quantity of plaque and to establish a microflora associated with healthy peri-implant tissues.

Additional treatment for peri-implantitis may include the use of adjunctive antibiotic therapy, either systemically or locally administered (see CIST protocol, Chapter 45). As is the case in periodontal therapy, antibiotics used alone are ineffective. The nature of a biofilm affords protection to its co-inhabitants, and they may develop resistance to antimicrobial agents via a number of mechanisms. Therefore, antibiotics

should always be prescribed in conjunction with disruption of the biofilm by mechanical debridement. Furthermore, a microbiological diagnosis may be of value for guidance in the choice of antimicrobial treatment for patients with peri-implant infection.

There are only two studies monitoring the changes in the microflora following treatment of peri-implantitis in humans. Mombelli & Lang (1992) observed a reduction in the quantity and proportions of anaerobic bacteria following systemic administration of ornidazole, an antibiotic that specifically targets Gram-negative anaerobic organisms. The alteration in the microbial composition was accompanied by a sustained clinical improvement over a 1-year period.

In the second study, peri-implantitis treatment using local delivery of tetracycline demonstrated a positive effect on clinical and microbiological parameters (Mombelli et al. 2001). The local delivery device Actisite® (fibers containing polymeric tetracycline HCl) resulted in significantly lower total anaerobic bacterial counts than at baseline. A significant decrease in frequency of detection was observed for *Prevotella intermedia/nigrescens*, *Fusobacterium* sp., *Bacteroides forsythus*, and *Campylobacter rectus*.

In order for a local delivery device to be effective against the microorganisms within a biofilm, the active agent must reach the peri-implant pocket in sufficient concentration for a long enough time. Thus the kinetics of the local delivery device are critical. A number of local antibiotic therapies are currently available; however, the tetracycline fibers are, to date, the only local delivery device evaluated for the treatment of peri-implantitis (see Chapter 45).

Conclusion

Bacteria play a major role in the etiology of peri-implant mucositis and peri-implantitis. There are distinct differences in the microflora associated with successful implants and implants with peri-implantitis. Remaining teeth with periodontal disease may provide a reservoir for colonization of implants by opportunistic periodontal pathogens. Periodontal health should therefore be achieved prior to implant placement. Treatment of peri-implant infection aims at suppression of the Gram-negative anaerobic bacteria and the establishment of a local environment and microflora conducive to peri-implant health.

REFERENCES

Albrektsson, T. & Isidor, F. (1994). Consensus report: Implant therapy. In: Lang, N.P. & Karring, T., eds. *Proceedings of the 1st European Workshop on Periodontology*. Berlin: Quintessence, pp. 365-369.

Alcoforado, G.A., Rams, T.E., Feik, D. & Slots, J. (1991). Microbial

aspects of failing osseointegrated dental implants in humans. *Journal de Parodontologie* 10, 11-18.

Apse, P., Ellen, R.P., Overall, C.M. & Zarb, G.A. (1989). Microbiota and crevicular fluid collagenase activity in the osseointegrated dental implant sulcus: a comparison of sites in edentulous and partially edentulous patients. *Journal of Periodontal Research* **24**, 96-105.

Asikainen, P., Klemetti, E., Vuillemin, T., Sutter, F., Rainio, V. & Kotilainen, R. (1997). Titanium implants and lateral forces. An experimental study with sheep. *Clinical Oral Implants Research* **8**, 465-468.

Augthun, M. & Conrads, G. (1997). Microbial findings of deep peri-implant bone defects. *International Journal of Oral and Maxillofacial Implants* **12**, 106-112.

Bair, R. E. & Meyer, A. E. (1988). Implant surface preparation. *The International Journal of Oral and Maxillofacial Implants* **3**, 9-20.

Berglundh, T., Gislason, Ö., Lekholm, U., Sennerby, L. & Lindhe, J. (2003). Some histopathological characteristics of human periimplantitis lesions. *Clinical Oral Implants Research* (in press).

Berglundh, T., Krok, L., Liljenberg, B., Westfelt, E., Serino, G. & Lindhe, J. (1998). The use of metronidazole and amoxicillin in the treatment of advanced periodontal disease. A prospective, controlled clinical trial. *Journal of Clinical Periodontology* **25**, 354-362.

Berglundh, T., Lindhe, J., Ericsson, I, Marinello, C.P., Liljenberg, B. & Thomsen, P. (1991). The soft tissue barrier at implants and teeth. *Clinical Oral Implants Research* **2**, 81-90.

Berglundh, T., Lindhe, J., Ericsson, I, Marinello, C.P. & Liljenberg, B. (1992). Soft tissue reactions to de novo plaque formation at implants and teeth. An experimental study in the dog. *Clinical Oral Implants Research* **3**, 1-8.

Bower, R.C., Radny, N.R., Wall, C.D. & Henry, P.J. (1989). Clinical and microscopic findings in edentulous patients 3 years after incorporation of osseointegrated implant-supported bridgework. *Journal of Clinical Periodontology* **16**, 580-587.

Brägger, U., Aeschlimann, S., Bürgin, W., Hämmerle, C. & Lang, N.P. (2001). Biological and technical complications and failures with fixed partial dentures (FPD) on implants and teeth after four to five years of function. *Clinical Oral Implants Research* **12**, 26-34.

Ericsson, I, Berglundh, T., Marinello, C.P., Liljenberg, B. & Lindhe, J. (1992). Long-standing plaque and gingivitis at implants and teeth in the dog. *Clinical Oral Implants Research* **3**, 99-103.

Ericsson, I, Persson, L.G., Berglundh, T., Edlund, T. & Lindhe, J. (1996). The effect of antimicrobial therapy on peri-implantitis lesions. An experimental study in the dog. *Clinical Oral Implants Research* **7**, 320-328.

Esposito, M., Hirsch, J.M., Lekholm, U. & Thomsen, P. (1998). Biological factors contributing to failures of osseointegrated oral implants. (I) Success criteria and epidemiology. *European Journal of Oral Sciences* **106**, 527-551.

Flemmig, T. & Renvert, S. (1999). Consensus report: Maintenance and complications. In: Lang, N.P., Karring, T. & Lindhe, J., eds. *Proceedings of the 3rd European Workshop on Periodontology.* Berlin: Quintessence, pp. 347-351.

George, K., Zafiropoulos, G.G., Murat, Y., Hubertus, S. & Nisengard, R.J. (1994). Clinical and microbiological status of osseointegrated implants. *Journal of Periodontology* **65**, 766-770.

Gotfredsen, K., Berglundh, T. & Lindhe, J. (2001). Bone reactions adjacent to titanium implants subjected to static load of different duration. An experimental study in the dog. III. *Clinical Oral Implants Research* **12**, 552-558.

Gotfredsen, K., Berglundh, T. & Lindhe, J. (2002). Bone reactions at implants subjected to experimental peri-implantitis and static load. An experimental study in the dog. IV. *Journal of Clinical Periodontology* **29**, 144-151.

Gualini, F. & Berglundh, T. (2003). Immunohistochemical characteristics of inflammatory lesions at implants. *Journal of Clinical Periodontology* (in press).

Hardt, C., Gröndahl, K., Lekholm, U. & Wennström, J. (2002). Outcome of implant therapy in relation to experienced loss of periodontal bone support. A retrospective 5-year study. *Clinical Oral Implants Research* (in press).

Hoshaw, S.J., Brunski, J.B. & Cochran G.V.B. (1994). Mechanical

loading of Brånemark implants affects interfacial bone modeling and remodeling. *International Journal of Oral and Maxillofacial Implants* **9**, 345-60.

Hultin, M., Gustafsson, A., Hallström, H., Johansson, L-Å, Ekfeldt, A. & Klinge, B. (2002). Microbiological findings and host response around failing implants. *Clinical Oral Implants Research* (in press).

Hürzeler, M.B., Quinones, C.R., Kohal, R.J., Rohde, M., Strub, J.R., Teuscher, U. & Caffesse, R.G. (1998). Changes in peri-implant tissues subjected to orthodontic forces and ligature breakdown in monkeys. *Journal of Periodontology* **69**, 396-404.

Isidor, F. (1997). Histological evaluation of peri-implant bone at implants subjected to occlusal overload or plaque accumulation. *Clinical Oral Implants Research* **8**, 1-9.

Kohavi, D., Greenberg, R., Raviv, E. & Sela, M.N. (1994). Subgingival and supragingival microbial flora around healthy osseointegrated implants in partially edentulous patients. *International Journal of Oral and Maxillofacial Implants* **9**, 673-678.

Koka, S., Razzoog, M.E., Bloem, T.J. & Syed, S. (1993). Microbial colonization of dental implants in partially edentulous subjects. *Journal of Prosthetic Dentistry* **70**, 141-144.

Kronström, M., Svensson, B., Hellman, M. & Persson, G.R. (2001). Early implant failures in patients treated with Brånemark System titanium dental implants: a retrospective study. *International Journal of Oral and Maxillofacial Implants* **16**, 201-207.

Lang, N.P., Brägger, U, Walther, D., Beamer, B. & Kornman, K. (1993). Ligature-induced peri-implant infection in cynomolgus monkeys. *Clinical Oral Implants Research* **4**, 2-11.

Lang, N.P., Wetzel, A.C., Stich, H. & Caffesse, R.G. (1994). Histologic probe penetration in healthy and inflamed peri-implant tissues. *Clinical Oral Implants Research* **5**, 191-201.

Leonhardt, A., Adolfsson, B., Lekholm, U., Wikstrom, M. & Dahlen, G. (1993). A longitudinal microbiological study on osseointegrated titanium implants in partially edentulous patients. *Clinical Oral Implants Research* **4**, 113-120.

Leonhardt, Å., Berglundh, T., Ericsson, I. & Dahlén, G. (1992). Putative periodontal pathogens on titanium implants and teeth in experimental gingivitis and periodontitis in beagle dogs. *Clinical Oral Implants Research* **3**, 112-119.

Leonhardt, A., Renvert, S. & Dahlen, G. (1999). Microbial findings at failing implants *Clinical Oral Implants Research* **10**, 339-345.

Lindhe, J., Berglundh, T., Ericsson, I., Liljenberg, B. & Marinello, C.P. (1992). Experimental breakdown of periimplant and periodontal tissues. A study in the beagle dog. *Clinical Oral Implants Research* **3**, 9-16.

Lindhe, J., Liljenberg, B. & Adielsson, B. (1983b). Effect of longterm tetracycline therapy of human periodontal disease. *Journal of Clinical Periodontology* **10**, 590-601.

Lindhe, J., Liljenberg, B., Adielsson, B. & Börjesson, I. (1983a). Use of metronidazole as a probe in the study of human periodontal disease. *Journal of Clinical Periodontology* **10**, 100-112.

Lindqvist, L., Rockler, B. & Carlsson, G. (1988). Bone resorption around fixtures in edentulous patients treated with mandibular fixed tissue-integrated prosthesis. *Journal of Prosthetic Dentistry* **59**, 59-63.

Marinello, C.P., Berglundh, T., Ericsson, I., Klinge, B., Glantz, P.O. & Lindhe, J. (1995). Resolution of ligature-induced peri-implantitis lesions in the dog. *Journal of Clinical Periodontology* **22**, 475-480.

Miyata, T., Kobayashi, Y., Araki, H., Ohto, T. & Shin, K. (2000). The influence of controlled occlusal overload on peri-implant tissue. Part 3. A histologic study in monkeys. *International Journal of Oral and Maxillofacial Implants* **15**, 425-431.

Mombelli, A. (1999). Prevention and therapy of peri-implant infections. In: Lang, N.P., Karring, T. & Lindhe, J., eds. *Proceedings of the 3rd European Workshop on Periodontology.* Berlin: Quintessence, pp. 281-303.

Mombelli, A., Buser, D. & Lang, N.P. (1988). Colonisation of osseointegrated titanium implants in edentulous patients. Early results. *Oral Microbiology and Immunology* 3, 113-120.

Mombelli, A., Feloutzis, A., Brägger, U. & Lang, N.P. (2001). Treatment of peri-implantitis by local delivery of tetracycline. Clinical, microbiological and radiological results. *Clinical Oral Implants Research* 12, 287-294.

Mombelli, A. & Lang, N.P. (1992). Antimicrobial treatment of peri-implant infections. *Clinical Oral Implants Research* 3, 162-168.

Mombelli, A. & Lang, N.P. (1998). The diagnosis and treatment of periimplantitis. *Periodontology* 17, 63-76.

Mombelli, A., Marxer, M., Gaberthuel, T., Grunder, U. & Lang, N.P. (1995) The microbiota of osseointegrated implants in patients with a history of periodontal disease. *Journal of Clinical Periodontology* 22, 124-130.

Mombelli, A. & Meriscke-Stern, R. (1990). Microbiological features of stable osseointegrated implants used as abutments for overdentures. *Clinical Oral Implants Research* 1, 1-7.

Mombelli, A., van Oosten, M.A., Schurch, E. Jr & Lang, N.P. (1987). The microbiota associated with successful or failing osseointegrated titanium implants. *Oral Microbiology and Immunology* 2, 145-151.

Persson, L.G., Araújo, M., Berglundh, T., Gröhndal, K. & Lindhe, J. (1999). Resolution of periimplantitis following treatment. An experimental study in the dog. *Clinical Oral Implants Research* 10, 195-203.

Persson, L.G., Ericsson, I., Berglundh, T. & Lindhe, J. (1996). Guided bone generation in the treatment of periimplantitis, *Clinical Oral Implants Research* 7, 366-372.

Piattelli, A., Scarano, A. & Piattelli, M. (1998). Histologic observations on 230 retrieved dental implants: 8 years' experience (1989-1996). *Journal of Periodontology* 69, 178-184.

Pontoriero, R., Tonelli, M.P., Carnevale, G., Mombelli, A., Nyman, S. & Lang, N.P. (1994) Experimentally induced peri-implant mucositis. A clinical study in humans. *Clinical Oral Implants Research* 5, 254-259.

Quirynen, M. & Listgarten, M.A. (1990). Distribution of bacterial morphotypes around natural teeth and titanium implants ad modum Brånemark. *Clinical Oral Implants Research* 1, 8-12.

Quirynen, M., Naert, I. & van Steenberge, D. (1992). Fixture design and overload influence marginal bone loss and fixture success in the Brånemark system. *Clinical Oral Implants Research* 3, 104-111.

Rams, T.E., Feik, D. & Slots, J. (1990). Staphylococci in human periodontal diseases. *Oral Microbiology and Immunology* 5, 29-32.

Rams, T.E. & Link, C.C. Jr. (1983). Microbiology of failing dental implants in humans: electron microscopic observations. *Journal of Oral Implantology* 11, 93-100.

Rams, T.E., Roberts, T.W., Tatum, H. Jr. & Keyes, P.H. (1984). The subgingival microbial flora associated with human dental implants. *Journal of Prosthetic Dentistry* 51, 529-534.

Rangert, B., Krogh, P.H., Langer, B. & van Roekel, N. (1995). Bending overload and implant fracture: a retrospective clinical analysis. *International Journal of Oral and Maxillofacial Implants* 10, 326-334.

Rosenberg, E.S., Torosian, J.P. & Slots, J. (1991). Microbial differences in two clinically distinct types of failures of osseointegrated implants. *Clinical Oral Implants Research* 2, 135-144.

Salcetti, J.M., Moroarty, J.D., Cooper, L.F., Smith, F.W., Collins, J.G., Socransky, S.S. & Offenbacher, S. (1997). The clinical, microbial, and host response characteristics of the failing implant. *International Journal of Oral and Maxillofacial Implants* 12, 32-42.

Sanz, M., Aladez, J., Lazaro, P., Calvo, J.L., Quirynen, M. & van Steenberghe, D. (1991). Histopathologic characteristics of peri-implant soft tissues in Brånemark implants with two distinct clinical and radiological patterns. *Clinical Oral Implants Research* 2, 128-134.

Schou, S., Holmstrup, P., Stoltze, K., Hjørting-Hansen, E. & Kornman, K. S. (1993). Ligature-induced marginal inflammation around osseointegrated implants and anckylosed teeth. Clinical and radiographic observations in Cynomolgus monkeys. *Clinical Oral Implants Research* 4, 12-22.

Sennerby, L. & Lekholm, U. (1993). The soft tissue response to titanium abutments retrieved from humans and reimplanted in rats. A light microscopic pilot study. *Clinical Implants Research* 4, 23-27.

Skalak, R. (1985). Aspect of biomechanical considerations. In: Brånemark, P.I., Zarb, G. & Albrektsson, T., eds. *Tissue-integrated Prosthesis. Osseointegration in Clinical Dentistry*. Chicago: Quintessence, pp. 117-128.

Sordyl, C.M., Simons, A.M. & Molinari, J.A. (1995). The microflora associated with stable endosseous implants. *Journal of Oral Implantology* 21, 19-22.

van Steenberge, D, Klinge, B, Lindén, U., Quirynen, M., Herrmann, I. & Garpland, C. (1993). Periodontal indices around natural titanium abutments: A longitudinal multicenter study. *Journal of Periodontology* 64, 538-541.

van Winkelhoff, A.J., Goene, R.J., Benschop, C. & Folmer, T. (2000). *Clinical Oral Implants Research* 11, 511-520.

van Winkelhoff, A.J. & Wolf, J.W. (2000). *Actinobacillus actinomycetemcomitans*-associated peri-implantitis in an edentulous patient. A case report. *Journal of Clinical Periodontology* 27, 531-535.

Wehrbein, H., Glatzmaier, J. & Yildirim (1997). Orthodontic anchorage capacity of short titanium titanium screw implants in the maxilla. An experimental study in the dog. *Clinical Oral Implants Research* 8, 131-141.

Wetzel, A.C., Vlassis, J., Caffesse, R.G., Hämmerle, C.H.F. & Lang, N.P. (1999). Attempts to obtain re-osseointegration following experimental periimplantitis in dogs. *Clinical Oral Implants Research* 10, 111-119.

Weyant, R.J. (1994). Characteristics associated with the loss and peri-implant tissue health of endosseous dental implants. *International Journal of Oral and Maxillofacial Implants* 9, 95-102.

Weyant, R.J. & Burt, B.A. (1993). An assessment of survival rates and within-patient clustering of failures for endosseous oral implants. *Journal of Dental Research* 72, 2-8.

Zitzmann, N.U., Berglundh, T., Marinello, C.P. & Lindhe, J. (2001). Experimental periimplant mucositis in man. *Journal of Clinical Periodontology* 28, 517-523.

CHAPTER 45

Maintenance of the Implant Patient

Niklaus P. Lang and Jan Lindhe

Since their introduction in the 1970s, endosseous oral implants have become an integral part of reconstructive dentistry. Initially, implant therapy was predominantly intended for the fully edentulous patient. In recent years, however, the partially dentate patient has also become a candidate for implant placement. In such a patient, both dental and implant abutments are used to reconstruct the compromised dentition. This blend of teeth and implants is, in particular, critical in the periodontally susceptible patient in whom the submarginal biofilms may harbor putative periodontal pathogens which may also be involved in the processes associated with the resorption of the bony support for the implant.

The objective of this chapter is to describe the prevention and therapy of problems around implants that arise from microbial colonization on teeth and implants in the periodontally susceptible patient.

GOALS

Inflammatory lesions occurring in the peri-implant tissues were described in Chapter 44. Such processes are the result of opportunistic infections and may, if left untreated, progress deep into the supporting bone and lead to implant loss. It is, therefore, imperative that the tissues around implants be monitored at regular intervals to discover arising biological complications and to interfere with the disease process at an early stage. The appropriate therapy instituted following the diagnosis must be aimed towards the reduction of the submucosal biofilm and the alteration of the ecological conditions for the bacterial habitat.

THE DIAGNOSTIC PROCESS

The examination of the tissues around implants has many features in common with the periodontal examination (Chapter 18) and must include parameters relevant to the pathogenic process of the peri-implant infection. It should be understood that, while advanced peri-implant lesions are easily recognized on radiographs, early alterations in the mucosa are often site specific and discrete. Hence, they require for their detection a systematic examination that should include assessments of:

- Bleeding on probing (BoP)
- Suppuration
- Probing depth (PPD)
- Radiographic bone loss
- Implant mobility.

Assessments of BoP, suppuration and PPD must be made at four surfaces (mesial, buccal, distal and lingual) of each implant, while radiographic interpretation is limited to the evaluation of the mesial and distal aspects.

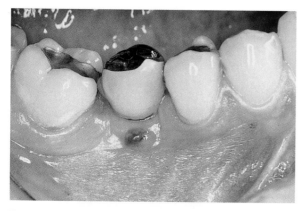

Fig. 45-1. Suppuration in combination with the development of a fistula indicates clinical signs of active peri-implant infection.

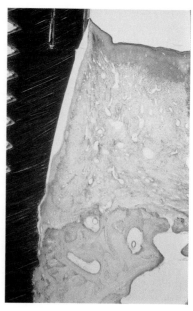

Fig. 45-2. Clinical probing of the peri-implant sulcus results in complete epithelial attachment after 5-7 days, thus not damaging the transmucosal soft tissue seal. From Etter et al. 2002.

Bleeding on probing (BoP)

Bleeding on probing (BoP+) occurring following the application of the probe with a light pressure (0.25 N) reveals the presence of an inflammatory lesion in the gingiva around teeth (Lang et al. 1991). Although this symptom (BoP+) may have a limited predictive value for periodontal disease progression (Lang et al. 1986), its absence (BoP–) indicates periodontal stability (Lang et al. 1990). With regard to the mucosa around implants, the diagnostic accuracy of BoP appears to be even better than that of BoP in a periodontal examination (Luterbacher et al. 2000). Hence, a peri-implant site that following probing is BoP negative is considered healthy and stable.

Suppuration

As indicated in Chapter 44, peri-implant infections are characterized by inflammatory processes that contain a variety of leukocytes. In the inflammatory lesions collagen is destroyed and tissue necrosis results. This process leads to pus formation, suppuration and the development of a fistula (Fig. 45-1). Hence, suppuration must be associated with episodes of active tissue destruction and indicates a need for anti-infective therapy.

Probing depth

As stated in Chapter 35, probing in the peri-implant sulcus must be made with a light probing force (about 0.2-0.3 N) to avoid undue tissue damage and overextension into the healthy tissues (Mombelli et al. 1997).

If a light probing pressure is applied during probing, the epithelial attachment of the transmucosal tissue seal will be disrupted but will heal within 5-7 days (Etter et al. 2002). This means that – as is the case in probing around teeth (Taylor & Campbell 1972) – probing the peri-implant tissue can be performed

without causing permanent damage to the integrity of the transmucosal attachment.

Clinical probing must thus be regarded as an important and reliable diagnostic parameter in the continuous monitoring of both periodontal and peri-implant tissues (Fig. 45-2).

The diagnostic value of probing the mucosa around implants was also described in Chapter 35. Thus, at sites with healthy mucosa or mucositis, the tip of the probe may identify the location of the apical level of the barrier epithelium (Ericsson & Lindhe 1993, Lang et al. 1994). Since the barrier epithelium is about 2-3 mm long, the probing depth at such sites should be ≤ 3 mm. At sites with peri-implantitis, however, the probe will penetrate apical to the epithelium and reach the base of the inflammatory lesion at the alveolar bone crest (Lang et al. 1994). Consequently, an increased probing depth will result.

Radiographic interpretation

The preservation of marginal bone height is crucial for implant maintenance and is often used as a primary success criterion for different implant systems. A mean marginal bone loss amounting to less than 0.2 mm annually following the first year of service was originally proposed as one of the major success criteria (Albrektsson et al. 1986, Lekholm et al. 1986). This success criterion has been questioned, since recent longitudinal studies have demonstrated that loss of alveolar bone may be almost absent or minimal in well-maintained patients.

In this context, it is important to realize that in the individual patient, a mean alveolar bone loss/year may be a misleading parameter, since peri-implant

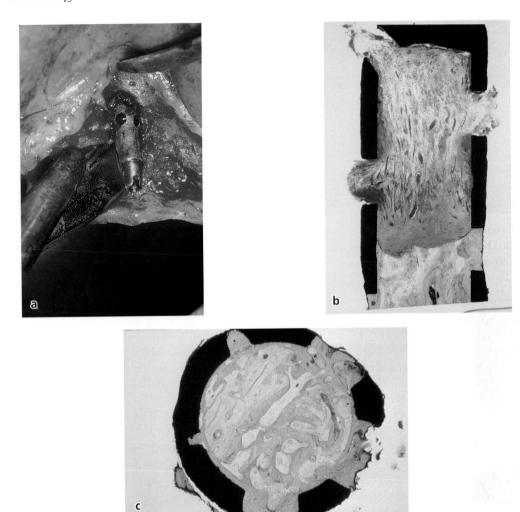

Fig. 45-3. Peri-implantitis resulting in the loss of an old titanium implant after 8 years of function. (a) Loss of alveolar bone and peri-implant lesion progressing into the implant concavity. Clinical signs of advanced peri-implant infection. (b) Explanted implant of (a) affected by peri-implantitis. Active infective lesion in the coronal part of the implant (granulation tissue: red, bacterial colonization: brown) and perfect osseointegration in the apical part (alveolar bone: green). (c) Cross-sectional ground section through the apical portion of the explanted implant from (a) indicating perfect osseointegration. As a consequence, the implant remains clinically stable. Hence, mobility represents a diagnostic test with poor sensitivity.

infections are implant specific. Hence, in a given patient the mean bone loss may be small, but one of multiple implant sites may be severely affected and in need of anti-infective therapy. Radiographic interpretation should not be the only parameter to estimate the performance of implants. In the absence of clinical signs of infection, it is recommended to take radiographs 1 year after implant installation and no more than every other year thereafter (Chapter 36). Additional radiographs may be obtained to determine the extent of marginal bone loss if clinical parameters (e.g. BoP+, suppuration, and increased probing depth) indicate peri-implant infection.

Mobility

Implant mobility indicates lack of osseointegration. Even if peri-implantitis has progressed relatively far, implants may still appear clinically stable due to some remaining direct bone to implant contact (Fig. 45-3a,b,c). Mobility, therefore, is a specific diagnostic test for loss of osseointegration and is decisive in the decision to remove the affected implant.

CUMULATIVE INTERCEPTIVE SUPPORTIVE THERAPY (CIST)

Preventive and therapeutic strategies

Depending on the clinical, and eventually the radiographic diagnosis, protocols for preventive and therapeutic measures were designed to intercept the development of peri-implant lesions. This system of supportive therapy is cumulative in nature and includes four steps which should not be used as single procedures, but rather as a sequence of therapeutic proce-

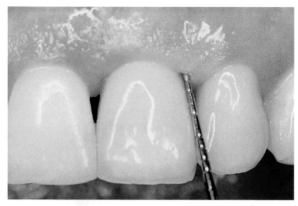

Fig. 45-4. Clinically stable implant with VMK crown (region 21) characterized by absence of bleeding on probing, suppuration, and a peri-implant probing depth not exceeding 3 mm.

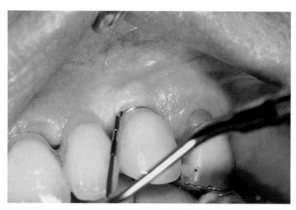

Fig. 45-5. Peri-implant mucositis characterized by presence of bleeding on probing, absence of suppuration and a peri-implant probing depth of 4 mm.

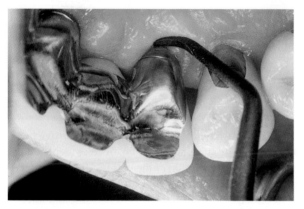

Fig. 45-6. Calculus deposits may be chipped off using carbon fiber curettes with the aim of not scratching the implant surface.

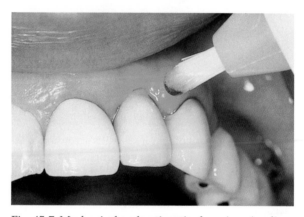

Fig. 45-7. Mechanical and antiseptic cleansing. Application of chlorhexidine gel (Plakout®, 0.2%) to a site with peri-implant mucositis.

dures with increasing anti-infective potential depending on the severity and extent of the lesion. Diagnosis, therefore, represents a key feature of this supportive therapy program.

The major clinical parameters to be used have been discussed above and include:

1. Presence of a biofilm
2. Presence or absence of BoP
3. Presence or absence of suppuration
4. Increased peri-implant probing depth
5. Evidence and extent of radiographic alveolar bone loss.

Oral implants without plaque and calculus and surrounded by healthy peri-implant tissues, as evidenced by (1) absence of BoP, (2) absence of suppuration, and (3) probing depth usually not exceeding 3 mm, should be considered clinically stable. Such sites should not be exposed to therapeutic measures (Fig. 45-4).

Mechanical debridement; CIST protocol A
Implants with plaque and calculus deposits and surrounded by a mucosa that is BoP positive but suppu-

ration negative and with a PPD ≤ 4 mm are to be subjected to mechanical debridement (Fig. 45-5). While calculus may be chipped off using carbon fiber (Fig. 45-6) or plastic curettes, plaque is removed by polishing the implant surface with rubber cups and a polishing paste. Carbon fiber curettes do not sever the implant surface. They may be sharpened and are strong enough to remove most accumulations of calculus. Conventional steel curettes or ultrasonic instruments with metal tips should not be used because they may cause severe damage to the implant surface (Matarasso et al. 1996).

Antiseptic therapy; CIST protocol A+B
At implant sites, which are BoP positive, exhibit an increased probing depth (4-5 mm) and may or may not demonstrate suppuration, antiseptic therapy is delivered in addition to mechanical debridement. Thus, a 0.2% solution of chlorhexidine digluconate is prescribed for daily rinsing, or a 0.2% gel of the same antiseptic is recommended for application in the affected site (Fig. 45-7).

Generally, 3-4 weeks of antiseptic therapy are necessary to achieve positive treatment results.

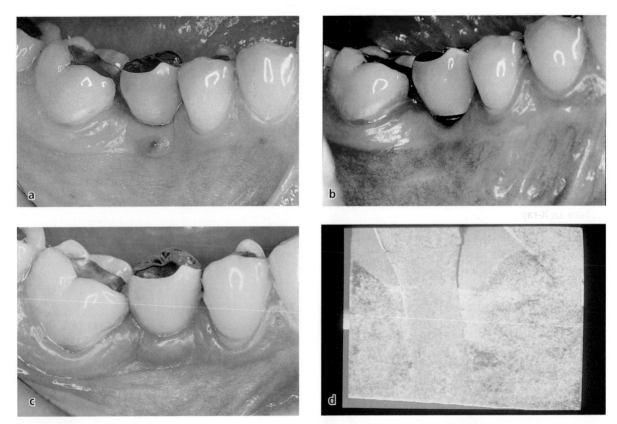

Fig. 45-8. Treatment of peri-implantitis according to the protocol of CIST (cumulative interceptive supportive therapy): (a) Clinical diagnosis of peri-implantitis: presence of bleeding on probing, suppuration, development of a fistula, loss of alveolar bone. Peri-implant probing depth 7 mm. (b) Clinical resolution of the peri-implant infection one year following the mechanical and antiseptic cleansing and followed by the systemic application of antibiotics (500 mg Tiberal® b.i.d for 10 days). Some recession is visible. (c) Documentation of the healed peri-implant infection by contrast–enhanced subtraction radiography. The intrabony crater has been completely filled 1 year after therapy. (d) Absence of mucositis, reduced peri-implant probing depth to 3 mm and bone-fill of the lesion.

Antibiotic therapy; CIST protocol A+B+C

At BoP positive implant sites with deep pockets (PPD ≥ 6 mm) (suppuration may or may not be present), there are frequently also signs of radiographic bone loss. Such pockets represent an ecological habitat, which is conducive for the colonization of Gram-negative and anaerobic putative periodontal pathogens (Mombelli et al. 1987). The anti-infective treatment must include the use of antibiotics to eliminate or reduce the pathogens in this habitat. This, in turn, will allow soft tissue healing as demonstrated in a clinical study by Mombelli & Lang (1992). Prior to administering antibiotics the mechanical (CIST A) and the antiseptic (CIST B) protocols have to be applied.

During the last 10 days of the antiseptic treatment regimen, an antibiotic directed against the anaerobic bacteria (e.g. metronidazole or ornidazole) is used. Thus for instance, 350 mg t.i.d. of Flagyl® (Rhone-Poulenc) or 500 mg b.i.d. of Tiberal® (Roche) is administered via the systemic route. A site treated according to the above protocol is depicted in Figs. 45-8a-d. A fistula can be seen in the buccal aspect of implant site 45 (Fig. 45-8a). The site exhibited BoP+ and had a probing depth of 7 mm. After therapy the inflammation is resolved (Fig. 45-8b) and some recession of the

mucosal margin has occurred. In Fig. 45-8c the bone fill that took place in the angular defect is illustrated in a subtraction radiography image using contrast enhancing. Fig. 45-8d presents the site 8 years after active therapy.

An alternative to the systemic administration is the controlled, local delivery of antibiotics. It must be realized, however, that only devices with proper release kinetics must be used to assure successful clinical results. The antibiotic must thus remain at the site of action for at least 7-10 days and in a concentration high enough to penetrate the submucosal biofilm (Mombelli et al. 2001). An example of such a controlled-release device is the tetracycline-containing periodontal fiber (Actisite®; Alza). The therapeutic effect of this controlled-release device appears to be identical to the effect obtained by the systemic use of antibiotics (Mombelli et al. 2001).

Regenerative or resective therapy; CIST protocol A+B+C+D

It is imperative to understand that regenerative or resective therapy is not instituted until the peri-implant infection is under control. Thus, before surgical intervention is planned, the previously diseased site

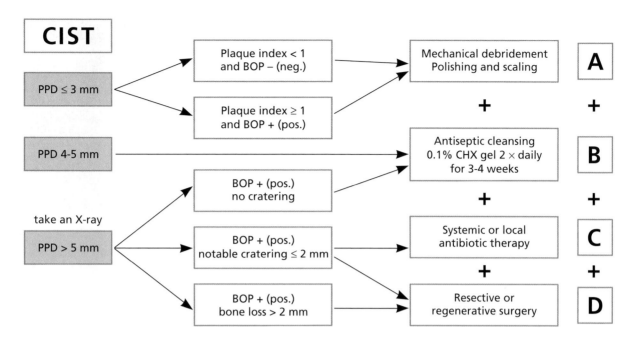

Fig. 45-9. Decision tree for Cumulative Interceptive Supportive Therapy (CIST). Depending on the mucosal condition and probing depth, either regime A or regime A+B, regime A+B+C or regime A+B+C+D are performed. A: Mechanical debridement; B: Antiseptic cleansing; C: Antibiotic therapy; D: Resective or regenerative surgery.

should have become BoP negative, exhibit no suppuration and disclose a reduced probing depth. Depending on the extent and severity of the local bone loss, a decision is made whether regenerative or resective measures are to be applied.

In this context it must be realized that the goal of regenerative therapy, including the use of barrier membranes is new bone formation in the crater-like defect around the implant, although *de novo* osseointegration may occur to a limited extend (Persson et al. 1999, Wetzel et al. 1999).

Conclusions

An implant patient must always be enrolled in a supportive therapy program that involves recall visits at regular intervals. Each recall visit must start with an examination to assess whether the implant sites are healthy or exhibit signs of inflammation.

Cumulative Interceptive Supportive Therapy (CIST) includes a series of four protocols to be used when the examination and the diagnostic process are completed.

Fig. 45-9 outlines (1) the decision process to be used for the peri-implant tissue diagnosis and (2) the different therapeutic measures that are available to treat and/or prevent peri-implant infections.

REFERENCES

Albrekstsson, T., Zarb, G., Worthington, P. & Eriksson, A.R. (1986). The long term efficacy of currently used dental implants; a review and proposed criteria of success. *International Journal of Oral and Maxillofacial Implants* 1, 11-25.

Ericsson, I. & Lindhe, J. (1993). Probing depth at implants and teeth. An experimental study in the dog. *Journal of Clinical Periodontology* 20, 623-627.

Etter, T.H., Håkanson, I., Lang, N.P., Trejo, P.M. & Caffesse, R.J. (2002). Healing after standardized clinical probing of the periimplant soft tissue seal – a histomorphometric study in dogs. *Clinical Oral Implants Research* 13, 573-582.

Lang, N.P., Adler, R., Joss, R.A. & Nyman, S. (1990). Absence of bleeding on probing. An indicator of periodontal stability. *Journal of Clinical Periodontology* 1, 714-721.

Lang, N.P., Joss, A., Orsanic, T., Gusberti, F.A. & Siegrist, B.E. (1986). Bleeding on probing. A predictor for the progression of periodontal disease? *Journal of Clinical Periodontology* 13, 590-596.

Lang, N.P., Nyman, S., Senn, C. & Joss, A. (1991). Bleeding on probing as it relates to probing pressure and gingival health. *Journal of Clinical Periodontology* 18, 257-261.

Lang, N.P., Wetzel, A.C., Stich, H. & Caffesse, R.J. (1994). Histologic probe penetration in healthy and inflamed periimplant tissues. *Clinical Oral Implants Research* 5, 191-201.

Lekholm, U., Adell, R., Lindhe, J., Brånemark, P.I., Eriksson, B., Rockler, B., Lindwall, A-M & Yoneyama, T. (1986). Marginal tissue reactions at osseointegrated titanium fixtures. *International Journal of Oral and Maxillofacial Surgery* 15, 53-61.

Luterbacher, S., Mayfield, L., Brägger, U. & Lang, N.P.(2000). Diagnostic characteristics of clinical and microbiological tests for monitoring periodontal and periimplant mucosal tissue conditions during supportive periodontal therapy (SPT). *Clinical Oral Implants Research* 11, 521-529.

Matarasso, S., Quaremba, G., Coraggio, F., Vaia, E., Cafiero, C. & Lang, N.P. (1996). Maintenance of implants: an in vitro study of titanium implant surface modifications, subsequent to the application of different prophylaxis procedures. *Clinical Oral Implants Research* **7**, 64-72.

Mombelli, A., Feloutzis, A., Brägger, U. & Lang, N.P. (2001). Treatment of peri-implantitis by local delivery of tetracycline. Clinical, microbiological and radiological results. *Clinical Oral Implants Research* **12**, 287-294.

Mombelli, A. & Lang, N.P. (1992). Anti-microbial treatment of peri-implant infections. *Clinical Oral Implants Research* **3**, 162-168.

Mombelli, A., Mühle, T., Brägger, U., Lang, N.P. & Bürgin, W.B. (1997). Comparison of periodontal and peri-implant probing by depth-force pattern analysis. *Clinical Oral Implants Research* **8**, 448-455.

Mombelli, A., van Oosten, M.A.C., Schürch, E. & Lang, N.P. (1987). The microbiota associated with successful or failing ossoeintegrated titanium implants. *Oral Microbiology and Immunology* **2**, 145- 151.

Persson, L.G., Araújo, M., Berglundh, T., Gröndahl, K. & Lindhe, J. (1999). Resolution of peri-impatitis following treatment. An experimental study in the dog. *Clinical Oral Implants Research* **10**, 195-203.

Taylor, A.C. & Campbell, M.M. (1972). Reattachment of gingival epitheölium to the tooth. *Journal of Periodontology* **43**, 281-293.

Wetzel, A.C., Vlassis, .J., Caffesse, R.J., Hämmerle, C.H.F. & Lang, N.P. (1999). Attempts to obtain re-osseointegration following experimental peri-implantitis in dogs. *Clinical Oral Implants Research* **10**, 111-119.

Index